VOLUME 3

CLINICAL NURSING SKILLS

A Concept-Based Approach to Learning

SECOND EDITION

Barbara Callahan, MEd, RN, NCC, CHSE
Lenoir Community College
Kinston, North Carolina

PEARSON

Boston Columbus Indianapolis New York San Francisco Hoboken
Amsterdam Cape Town Dubai London Madrid Milan Munich Paris Montreal Toronto
Delhi Mexico City Sao Paulo Sydney Hong Kong Seoul Singapore Taipei Tokyo

Publisher: Julie Alexander
Executive Editor: Kelly Trakalo
Development Editor: Rachel Bedard
Program Manager: Melissa Bashe
Editorial Assistant: Kevin Wilson
Director of Marketing: David Gesell
Senior Marketing Manager: Phoenix Harvey
Marketing Specialist: Michael Sirinides
Director, Product Management Services: Etain O'Dea
Project Management Team Lead: Cynthia Zonneveld
Project Manager: Maria Reyes
Manufacturing Manager: Maura Zaldivar-Garcia
Art Director/Cover and Interior Design: Mary Siener
Cover Art: Aaron Craven/Vetta/Getty Images
Lead Digital Project Manager: Karen Bretz
Full-Service Project Management: Kelly Ricci
Composition: iEnergizer Aptara®, Inc.
Printer/Binder: LSC Communications/Kendallville
Cover Printer: LSC Communications/Kendallville

Library of Congress Cataloging-in-Publication Data
Clinical nursing skills (2015)
    Clinical nursing skills : a concept-based approach to learning.
        p.; cm.
    Includes bibliographical references.
    ISBN 978-0-13-517203-2—ISBN 0-13-517203-9
    I. Pearson Education, Inc., publisher.   II. Title.
    [DNLM: 1. Nursing Process. WY 100.1]
    RT40
    610.73—dc23
                            2014013118

1   18

PEARSON

ISBN 13: 978-0-13-517203-2
ISBN 10:   0-13-517203-9

PREFACE

As you flip through the pages of this book, you will readily see that this is not just another "how-to" book filled only with skills and checklists. This book has additional features throughout, including cultural and developmental considerations and setting of care, to support the process of individualizing nursing care to obtain the best client outcomes. Safety, nursing, legal, and clinical alerts are integrated into the skills. Client teaching sections are included to help organize teaching plans for clients. Practice guidelines and evidence-based nursing practice boxes provide suggestions for best practice from available evidence. Features are color-coded for easy recognition. In addition, skills include tables, boxes, and figures for better understanding and visual reinforcement of information.

The Table of Contents is unique in its categorization of the skills listed. Chapter titles support concepts and are in alphabetical order. Associated skills have been organized into subgroups within chapters. Subgroups are listed to reflect sequence of thinking, such as assessment skills being listed before intervention skills in the chapters. As an example, here is the path for finding the skill about using a nasal cannula for supplemental oxygen therapy:

- Concept—Oxygenation, Chapter 13
- Subgroup—Supplemental Oxygen Therapy
- Skill—Administering Oxygen by Nasal Cannula, Face Mask, or Face Tent, Skill 13.9
- VARIATION—Using a Nasal Cannula

Chapters are color-coded and organized with the same series of headings, beginning with Related Concepts and Exemplars, Skills-at-a-Glance, and Expected Outcomes. As appropriate, skills then progress through Delegation, Equipment, Preparation, and Procedure. Chapters end with a table of Critical Thinking Options for Unexpected Outcomes. This feature provides selected expected outcomes, some problems that might occur instead, and possible nursing actions to resolve them. As such, it is a good tool for review and practice in clinical decision making.

It has been a pleasure to be on the team that revised, reorganized, improved, enhanced, and refreshed this second edition of *Clinical Nursing Skills: A Concept-Based Approach to Learning*. This updated skills book provides readers with quality content, not only about the "how" of doing nursing skills but also about the all-important "who, what, when, and why" indications of the skills. Elements of nursing reasoning, problem solving, and critical thinking are integrated to support nursing thinking processes. And now, the safe and effective application of these skills is up to you, the nurse, in your quest to achieve the best client outcomes.

ACKNOWLEDGMENTS

Thanks to Barbara Callahan for her strong organization of the second edition and for her willingness to take on the role of Editor. She was a continually positive force for improvement. Thanks to Rachel Bedard and her team at Editorial Consultants, and to Pearson Project Manager Maria Reyes, Program Manager Melissa Bashe, and Editorial Assistant Kevin Wilson for doing everything needed to make this book happen.

CONTENTS

1 Assessment

RELATED CONCEPTS

The Biophysical Concepts

The Psychological Concepts

The Social Functioning Concepts

The Developmental Concepts

The Spiritual Concepts

The Health, Wellness, and Illness Concepts

Exemplars

All concepts found in the Individual Domain are related to the Assessment Concept. Throughout all these concepts, assessment data is gathered from a variety of sources. Cognitive functions of analyzing, interpreting, and making clinical judgments are done to determine appropriate interventions for best individual client outcomes.

Skills-at-a-Glance

(continued on next page)

Skills-at-a-Glance *(continued)*

Health assessment, the collection and interpretation of data regarding the client's previous and current health status, is one of the most important professional responsibilities of the registered nurse. Vigilance in performing relevant assessment techniques, determining the meaning of the findings, and taking appropriate action based on the evaluation of the data are central aspects of effective nursing care and cannot be delegated to those without the requisite skills and knowledge.

In order for the process of assessment to be more client focused than nurse focused, we must guide our intentions. Rather than viewing this process as simply gathering information and data, the nurse should view it as a process of discovery in which the nurse and client identify patterns, accessing what is already known to the client. The nurse uses listening skills to hear clients' stories and beliefs about what is going on inside their bodies and to seek clarification and verification. The nurse may also use intuitive skills to enhance the pattern recognition process.

It is essential for the nurse to access information about the client's spiritual health and well-being along with information about physical health. Accrediting organizations specify that a spiritual assessment be conducted on all clients. The assessment need not take much time, and many resources are available to assist nurses in spiritual assessment and care (Dossey & Keegan, 2008).

The nurse is able to perform a comprehensive assessment of each individual body system. In practice, however, the generalist nurse performs a brief screening assessment of all systems (sometimes referred to as a head-to-toe assessment) when first encountering the client and then more detailed focused assessments of particular systems as indicated by the client's condition. Independent clinical judgment drives the selection of those components for which an assessment is indicated. **Box 1–1** ● presents the order generally followed in performing a head-to-toe assessment. Advance practice nurses such as nurse practitioners may perform much more in-depth assessments of selected systems.

The traditional vital signs are body temperature, pulse, respirations, and blood pressure. Many agencies such as the

---

BOX 1–1 Head-to-Toe Framework

GENERAL SURVEY INCLUDING VITAL SIGNS

Areas below are assessed and include a determination of current complaints and inspection. Palpation, percussion, and auscultation are used if indicated.

- Head
  - Hair and face
  - Eyes and vision
  - Ears and hearing
  - Nose
  - Mouth and oropharynx
- Neck
  - Muscles
  - Lymph nodes
  - Trachea
  - Thyroid gland
  - Carotid arteries
  - Neck veins
- Upper extremities
  - Skin and nails
  - Muscle strength and tone
  - Joint range of motion
  - Brachial and radial pulses
  - Sensation
- Chest and back
  - Skin
  - Thorax shape and size
  - Lungs
  - Heart
  - Spinal column
  - Breasts and axillae
- Abdomen
  - Skin
  - Abdominal sounds
  - Femoral pulses
- External genitals
- Anus
- Lower extremities
  - Skin and toenails
  - Gait and balance
  - Joint range of motion
  - Popliteal, posterior tibial, and dorsalis pedis pulses

Veterans Administration, American Pain Society, and the Joint Commission have designated pain as a fifth vital sign. In addition, the effectiveness of respirations and circulation is commonly measured noninvasively through pulse oximetry (see Skill 1.11 and Chapter 13 on oxygenation) at the same time as other vital signs. These signs, which should be looked at both individually and collectively, enable nurses to monitor the functions of the body. Vital signs reflect changes that otherwise might not be observed. Monitoring a client's vital signs should not be an automatic or routine procedure; it should be a thoughtful, scientific assessment. Vital signs should be evaluated with reference to the client's present and prior health status and compared to accepted standards

- On admission to a healthcare agency to obtain baseline data
- When a client has a change in health status or reports symptoms such as chest pain or feeling hot or faint
- Before and after surgery or an invasive procedure
- Before and/or after the administration of a medication that could affect the respiratory or cardiovascular systems; for example, before giving a digitalis preparation
- Before and after any nursing intervention that could affect the vital signs (e.g., ambulating a client who has been on bed rest)

(**Box 1–2** ●). If findings appear inconsistent with those anticipated, they should immediately be rechecked. Some of the vital signs that are confirmed to vary from expected values will require a nursing care plan, and a few represent medical emergencies.

▶ CULTURAL NORMS IN NONVERBAL COMMUNICATION

Here are a few examples of different cultural norms in nonverbal communication. Cultural norms will vary within a culture, and from generation to generation. Therefore, it is extremely important to observe carefully, ask your client about preferences, and not make assumptions. Your assessment and care will benefit greatly from this awareness of differences.

Eye Contact

Keep in Mind   Eye contact and the handshake have different meanings for different cultures. For example, some communities consider direct eye contact an invasion of privacy and a firm handshake aggressive. Other cultures avoid eye contact as a sign of respect for the other individual. Some nurses might misinterpret that a client who avoids direct eye contact is somewhat suspicious, or that a weak handshake signifies disinterest. In some countries, direct eye contact is common and accepted.

Nursing Implications   Be careful not to assume things about your client based on the norms for your own cultural group. For example, if you value eye contact as a sign of interest, you may incorrectly assume your client is disinterested if he or she does not maintain eye contact. In fact, the client may be trying to show respect for you. Observing your client with family and other individuals is a helpful way to learn about his or her usual pattern of eye contact.

Touch and Personal Space

Keep in Mind   Many Americans tend to keep a certain amount of space between themselves and others, typically 3 feet, and they use touch sparingly. Others feel comfortable standing very close to others and are comfortable touching. Some cultural groups may consider excessive touching offensive, especially from the opposite sex.

Nursing Implications   Note patterns of touch between family members, or individuals of the same culture. Just as with eye contact, it may be difficult for you to change your habits of touch and personal space. However, if you sense unease in your clients, reevaluate your actions to be more sensitive to their comfort level. When in doubt, ask your client if he or she feels comfortable in the situation.

Use of Body Language

Keep in Mind   Body language can easily be misinterpreted during the assessment, so pay careful attention to the assumptions you are making based on your own cultural norms. For example, many individuals that live in the United States typically nod to indicate agreement or approval. Others may nod to be polite, but this may not actually indicate agreement.

Nursing Implications   Make sure that you are not relying solely on nonverbal clues to determine if your client understands or agrees with you. Instead of asking "Did you understand how we will test your blood?" and relying on a nod for affirmation, you might ask "Can you explain how we will test your blood?" Also try to follow up on your questions so that you actually hear a verbal "yes" or "no" response.

▶ GENERAL ASSESSMENT

Expected Outcomes

1. Assessment data of the client's appearance reveal expected normal findings.
2. Height and weight are obtained and recorded.
3. Client's weight shows expected losses, gains, or stabilization.

SKILL 1.1 Assessing Appearance and Mental Status

Procedure

1. Prior to performing the procedure, introduce self and verify the client's identity using agency protocol. Explain to the client what you are going to do, why it is necessary, and how he or she can participate. Discuss how the results will be used in planning further care or treatments.
2. Perform hand hygiene and observe appropriate infection control procedures.
3. Provide for client privacy.

ASSESSMENT	NORMAL FINDINGS	DEVIATIONS FROM NORMAL
4. Observe body build, height, and weight in relation to the client's age, lifestyle, and health.	Proportionate, varies with lifestyle	Excessively thin or obese
5. Observe client's posture and gait, standing, sitting, and walking.	Relaxed, erect posture; coordinated movement	Tense, slouched, bent posture; uncoordinated movement; tremors, unbalanced gait
6. Observe client's overall hygiene and grooming.	Clean, neat	Dirty, unkempt
7. Note body and breath odor in relation to activity level.	No body odor or minor body odor relative to work or exercise; no breath odor	Foul body odor; ammonia odor; acetone breath odor; foul breath
8. Observe for signs of distress in posture or facial expression.	No apparent distress	Bending over because of abdominal pain, wincing, frowning, or labored breathing
9. Note obvious signs of health or illness (e.g., in skin color or breathing).	Well developed, well nourished, intact skin, easy breathing	**Pallor** (paleness), weakness, lesions, cough
10. Assess the client's attitude (frame of mind).	Cooperative, able to follow instructions	Negative, hostile, withdrawn, anxious
11. Note the client's affect/mood; assess the appropriateness of the client's responses.	Appropriate to situation	Inappropriate to situation, sudden mood changes, paranoia
12. Listen for speech quantity (amount and pace) and quality (loudness, clarity, inflection).	Understandable, moderate pace; clear tone and inflection	Rapid or slow pace; overly loud or soft
13. Listen for relevance and organization of thoughts.	Logical sequence, relevant answers, has sense of reality	Illogical sequence, flight of ideas, confusion, generalizations, vague
14. Document findings in the client record using handwritten or electronic forms and checklists supplemented by narrative notes when appropriate ❶.		

Developmental Considerations

INFANTS

- Observation of children's behavior can provide important data for the general survey, including physical development, neuromuscular function, and social and interactional skills.
- It may be helpful to have parents hold older infants and very young children for part of the assessment.
- Measure height of children under age 2 in the supine position with knees fully extended.
- Weigh without clothing.
- Include measurement of head circumference until age 2. Standardized growth charts include head circumference up to age 3.

CHILDREN

- Anxiety in preschool-age children can be decreased by letting them handle and become familiar with examination equipment.

- School-age children may be very modest and shy about exposing parts of the body.
- Adolescents should be examined without parents present unless the adolescent requests their presence.
- Weigh children without shoes and with as little clothing as possible.

OLDER ADULTS (OVER AGE 65)

- Allow extra time for clients to answer questions.
- Adapt questioning techniques as appropriate for clients with hearing or visual limitations.
- Older adults with osteoporosis can lose several inches in height. Be sure to document height and ask if they are aware of becoming shorter.
- When asking about weight loss, be specific about amount and time frame, for example, "Have you lost more than five pounds in the last two months?"

SKILL 1.1 Assessing Appearance and Mental Status (continued)

ADMISSION DATA

Date 4-16-11 Time 3:15 p.m. Primary Language English

Arrived Via: ☐ Wheelchair ☐ Stretcher ☑ Ambulatory

From: ☐ Admitting ☐ ER ☑ Home ☐ Nursing Home ☐ Other

Admitting M.D. R. Katz Time Notified 5 p.m.

ORIENTATION TO UNIT

	YES	NO		YES	NO
Arm Band Correct	☑	☐	Visiting Hours	☑	☐
Allergy Band	☑	☐	Smoking Policy	☑	☐
Telephone	☑	☐	TV, Lights, Bed Controls,		
Electrical Policy	☑	☐	Call Lights, Side Rails	☑	☐
Educational Mat'l	☑	☐	Nurses Station	☑	☐
(TV Brochure)	☑	☐			

Family M.D. R. Katz

Weight 125 lb. Height 5 ft. 2 in. BP:R — L 122/80

Temp. 103F Pulse 92, weak Resp 28, shallow

Source Providing Information ☑ Patient ☐ Other

Unable to Obtain History ☐

Reason for Admission (Onset, Duration, Pt.'s Perception) "Chest cold" X2 weeks S.O.B on exertion. "Lung pain, fever," "Dr. says I have pneumonia."

ALLERGIES & REACTIONS

Drugs Penicillin

Food/Other

Signs & Symptoms rash, nausea

Blood Reaction ☐ Yes ☑ No Dyes/Shellfish ☐ Yes ☑ No

MEDICATIONS

Current Meds	Dose/Freq.	Last Dose
Synthroid	0.1 mg. daily	4-16, 8 a.m.

Disposition of Meds: ☑ Home ☐ Pharmacy ☐ Safe *At Bedside

MEDICAL HISTORY

☑ No Major Problems   ☐ Gastro
☐ Cardiac   ☐ Arthritis
☐ Hyper/Hypotension   ☐ Stroke
☐ Diabetes   ☐ Seizures
☐ Cancer   ☐ Glaucoma
☐ Respiratory   ☑ Other Childbirth-2003

Surgery/Procedures	Date
Appendectomy	1999
Partial thyroidectomy	2005

SPECIAL ASSISTIVE DEVICES

☐ Wheelchair ☐ Contacts ☐ Venous ☐ Dentures
☐ Braces ☐ Hearing Aid Access ☐ Partial
☐ Cane/Crutches ☐ Prosthesis Device ☐ Upper
☐ Walker ☐ Glasses ☐ Epidural Catheter ☐ Lower
☐ Other None

VALUABLES

Patient informed Hospital not responsible for personal belongings.

Valuables Disposition: ☐ Patient ☐ Safe ☐ Given to

Patient/SO Signature None

PSYCHOSOCIAL HISTORY

Recent Stress None

Coping Mechanism Not assessed because of fatigue

Support System Husband, coworkers, friends

Calm: ☑ Yes ☐ No

Anxious: ☐ Yes ☐ No Facial muscles tense; trembling

Religion Catholic. Would want Last Rites

Tobacco Use: ☐ Yes ☑ No

Alcohol Use: ☐ Yes ☑ No

Drug Use: ☐ Yes ☑ No

NEUROLOGICAL

Oriented: ☑ Person ☑ Place ☑ Time ☐ Confused ☐ Sedated
☐ Alert ☐ Restless ☑ Lethargic ☐ Comatose

Pupils: ☑ Equal ☐ Unequal ☑ Reactive ☐ Sluggish
☐ Other 3mm.

Extremity Strength: ☑ Equal ☐ Unequal

Speech: ☑ Clear ☐ Slurred ☐ Other

MUSCULO-SKELETAL

Normal ROM of Extremities ☑ Yes ☐ No

☑ Weakness ☐ Paralysis ☐ Contractures ☐ Joint Swelling ☑ Pain
☐ Other ↓ related to fatigue when coughing

RESPIRATORY

Pattern: ☐ Even ☐ Uneven ☑ Shallow ☑ Dyspnea
☑ Other diminished breath sounds

Breathing Sounds: ☐ Clear ☑ Other inspiratory crackles

Secretions: ☐ None ☑ Other pink, thick sputum

Cough: ☐ None ☑ Productive ☐ Nonproductive

CARDIOVASCULAR

Pulses: Apical Rate 92-W ☑ Reg. ☐ Irregular ☐ Pacemaker
S = Strong W = Weak A = Absent D = Doppler

Radial R 92 L — Pedal R — L —

Edema: ☑ Absent ☐ Present Site

Perfusion: ☐ Warm ☐ Dry ☑ Diaphoretic ☐ Cool (Hot)

GASTROINTESTINAL

Oral Mucosa ☐ Normal ☑ Other pale and dry

Bowel Sounds: ☑ Normal ☐ Other Abd. soft

Wt. Change: ☐ ☑ N/V Stool Frequency/Character 1/day; soft

Last B/M 4-15-11 ☐ Ostomy (type)

Equip.

GENITOURINARY

Urine: Last Voided This morning

☐ Normal ☐ Anuria ☐ Hematuria ☐ Dysuria ☐ Incontinent
☑ Other ↓ amount & frequency since ill
☐ Catheter (type) Other

LMP 4-1-11 ☐ Vaginal/Penile Discharge

Other

SELF CARE

Need Assist with: ☐ Ambulating ☐ Elimination
☐ Meals ☑ Hygiene ☐ Dressing
While fatigued

Amanda Aquilini [F. age 28]
#4637651 DOB 11-02-82

☆ **NORTH BROWARD HOSPITAL DISTRICT**
NURSING ADMINISTRATION ASSESSMENT

❶ Nursing assessment form.

(continued on next page)

SKILL 1.1   Assessing Appearance and Mental Status (continued)

NUTRITION

General Appearance: ☑ Well Nourished   ☐ Emaciated
☐ Other _____
Appetite: ☐ Good   ☐ Fair   ☑ Poor -x2 days
Diet _Liquid_____   Meal Pattern _3/day_
☐ Feeds Self   ☐ Assist   ☐ Total Feed

SKIN ASSESSMENT

Color: ☐ Normal ☐ Flushed ☑ Pale ☐ Dusky ☐ Cyanotic
☐ Jaundiced ☑ Other _Cheeks flushed, hot_
General Description _Surgical scars:_
RLQ abdomen; anterior neck
_____
_____
_____
Note Cultures Obtained _____
_____
_____

PRESSURE SORE ™AT RISK SCREENING CRITERIA

OVERALL SKIN CONDITION

Grade
0	Turgor (elasticity adequate, skin warm and moist)
✓ 1	Poor turgor, skin cold & dry
2	Areas mottled, red or denuded
3	Existing skin ulcer/lesions

BOWEL AND BLADDER CONTROL

Grade
✓ 0	Always able to ask for bedpan
1	Incontinence of urine
2	Incontinence of feces
3	Totally incontinent Confined to bed

REHABILITATIVE STATE

Grade
0	Fully ambulatory
✓ 1	Ambulated with assistance
2	Chair to bed ambulation only
3	Confined to bed
4	Immobile in bed

NUTRITIONAL STATE

Grade
0	Eats all
✓ 1	Eats very little
2	Refuses food often
3	Tube feeding
4	Intravenous feeding

MENTAL STATE

Grade
✓ 0	Alert and clear
1	Confused
2	Disoriented/senile
3	Stuporous
4	Unconcious

CHRONIC DISEASE STATUS (i.e. COPD, ASCVD. Peripheral Vascular Disease, Diabetes, or Renal Disease, Cancer, Motor or Sensory Deficits, Elderly, Other)

Grade
✓ 0	Absent
1	One Present
2	Two Present
3	Three or more Present

TOTAL ___3___   Refer to Skin Care Protocol

FALLS SCREENING

If one or more of the following are checked institute fall precautions/plan of care
☐ History of Falls ☐ Unsteady Gait ☐ Confusion/Disorientation ☐ Dizziness

If two or more of the following are checked institute fall precautions/plan of care
☐ Age over 80
☐ Impaired vision
☐ Multiple Diagnoses
☐ Inability to understand or follow directions
☐ Utilizes cane, walker, w/c
☐ Impaired hearing
☐ Sleeplessness
☐ Urgency/frequency in elimination
☐ Medication/Sedative /Diuretic etc.

NURSE SIGNATURE/TITLE	DATE	TIME
Mary Medina, RN	4-16-11	3:30pm
NURSE SIGNATURE/TITLE	DATE	TIME

EDUCATION/DISCHARGE PLANNING

1. What do you know about your present illness? "Dr. says I have pneumonia." "I will have an I.V."
2. What information do you want or need about your illness? _____
3. Would you like family/SO involved in your care? Husband, Michael
4. How long do you expect to be in the hospital? "1-2 days"
5. What concerns do you have about leaving the hospital? _____

CHECK APPROPRIATE BOX

Will patient need post discharge assistance with ADLs/physical functioning? ☐ Yes ☑ No ☐ Unknown
Does patient have family capable of and willing to provide assistance post discharge?
☑ Yes ☐ No ☐ Unknown ☐ No family
Is assistance needed beyond that which family can provide?
☐ Yes ☑ No ☐ Unknown
Previous admission in the last six months?
☐ Yes ☑ No ☐ Unknown
Patient lives with _Husband and 1 child_
Planned discharge to _Home_
Comments: _Fatigue and anxiety may have interfered with learning. Re-teach anything covered at admission, later._

Social Services Notified   ☐ Yes ☑ No

NARRATIVE NOTES

S--c/o sharp chest pain when coughing and dyspnea on exertion. States unable to carry out regular daily exercise for past week. Coughing relieved "if I sit up and sit still." Nausea associated with coughing. Having occasional "chills." Occasionally becomes frightened, stating, "I can't breathe." Well groomed but "too tired to put on make-up." Assesses own supports as "good" (eg, relationship c̄ husband). Is "worried" about daughter. States husband will be out of town until tomorrow. Left 8-year-old daughter with neighbor. Concerned too about her work (is attorney). "I'll never get caught up." Had water at noon—no food today.
O--Chest expansion < 3cm, no nasal flaring or use of accessory muscles. Breath sounds and insp. crackles in ® upper and lower chest. Capillary refill 5 seconds.

✿ **NORTH BROWARD HOSPITAL DISTRICT**
NURSING ADMINISTRATION ASSESSMENT

❶ Nursing assessment form (continued).

SKILL 1.2   Measuring Height for Infant, Child, and Adult

Equipment

- Stadiometer or platform scale with stature-measuring device.

Preparation

- Have the child remove shoes and hat.

Procedure

1. Have the child stand straight with the back to the wall. The head should be held erect and in the midline position.
2. The shoulders, buttocks, and heels should touch the wall. The outer canthus of the eyes should be on the same horizontal plane as the external auditory canals. **Rationale:** *Positioning the head properly helps ensure consistency in placement of the headpiece on the crown of the head.*
3. Move the headpiece down to touch the crown.
4. Make the height reading to the nearest 0.5 cm or ¼ inch.
5. Plot the measurement for the child's age on the standardized growth curve.

Note: In the older child and adolescent, as well as in adults, height is often measured using a platform scale ❶ with an attached stature-measuring device. Have the child stand erect, facing forward. Move the stature-measuring device to the top of the head. Have the child step off the scale, and read the height in centimeters or inches.

VARIATION: MEASURING LENGTH OF AN INFANT OR SMALL CHILD

Equipment

- Measuring board or other length-measuring device

Preparation

- Have the parent remove any hat or shoes the infant or small child is wearing.

Procedure

1. When using a measuring board, place the head against the top of the board.
2. After positioning the head, gently push down on the knees until the legs are straight ❷. **Rationale:** *Because of their normally flexed posture, an infant's body must be extended to obtain an accurate measurement.*
3. Position the heels of the feet on the footboard, and record the length to the nearest 0.5 cm or ¼ inch.
4. Repeat the measurement for accuracy. If a difference between the two readings is found, take the average reading for documentation.
5. Plot the measurement for the child's age on the standardized growth curve.

Note: If such a measuring device is not available, place the infant or child on a paper sheet, stabilizing in the same manner as when using the board. Carefully holding the pen that touches the child's head and feet at a right angle to the surface, make one mark at the vertex of the head and another at the heel. Then measure the distance between the two marks. Record the length in centimeters or inches.

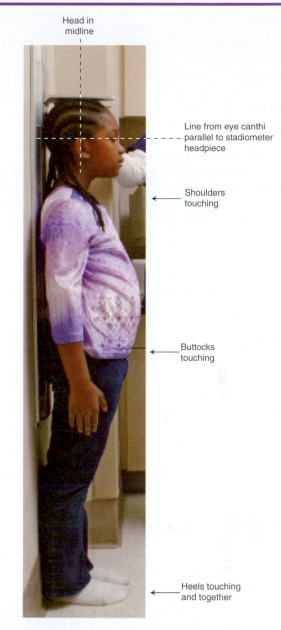

Head in midline

Line from eye canthi parallel to stadiometer headpiece

Shoulders touching

Buttocks touching

Heels touching and together

❶ Measuring a child's height. Position the head in an erect and midline position while the shoulders, buttocks, and heels touch the wall. Move the headpiece down to touch the crown.

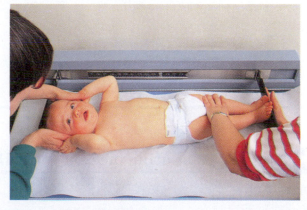

❷ Measuring an infant's length.

SKILL 1.3 **Measuring Weight for Infant, Child, and Adult**

Equipment

- Infant scale for infants
- Paper
- Standing scale for older children and adults

Preparation

FOR INFANTS

- Check the balance of the scale before using it.
- Have the parent or assistant remove all of the infant's clothing and diaper. Weigh toddlers in their underclothes. Weigh older children and adults in their street clothes with heavy clothing and shoes removed. Infants with acute diarrheal disease or a chronic health problem may need to be weighed nude for accuracy. **Rationale:** *It is important to try to minimize the amount of clothing worn by children when weighing them to improve comparisons with previous weights taken.*
- Clean the infant scale tray between uses. Place a paper cover over the scale tray.

Procedure

1. Place the infant on the scale and keep a hand close ❶. **Rationale:** *Infants move quickly and it is essential to protect them from falling.*
2. Distract the infant, and take the reading when the infant stops moving. **Rationale:** *It takes a few seconds of inactivity for the scale to settle on the infant's actual weight.*
3. Record the weight in the nearest 10 g or ½ oz.

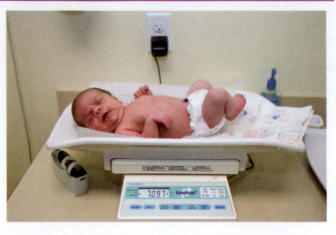

❶ A platform scale is used to weigh an infant. © Daniel Dempster Photography/Alamy.

4. Plot the measurement for the child's age in months on the standardized growth curve.

FOR OLDER CHILDREN AND ADULTS

The older child can be weighed on a standing scale.

1. Provide privacy.
2. Have the child or adult stand still on the scale.
3. View the digital reading or move the weights until the scale is balanced.
4. Record the weight to the nearest 0.1 kg or ¼ lb.

SKILL 1.4 **Measuring Body Mass Index**

The body mass index (BMI) uses a formula of kilograms per square meter (kg/m²) to assess nutritional status and total body weight relative to height. Beginning at age 2 years, the BMI can be easily determined after plotting the length and weight, or height and weight, on the standardized growth curves. **Rationale:** *Tracking the change in BMI can often provide clues to nutritional problems, including obesity, health promotion issues, or illness.*

> **CLINICAL ALERT**
> To calculate body mass index (BMI) manually, follow these steps:
>
> 1. Be sure that weight is in kilograms. If it is in pounds, divide that number by 2.2 to get kilograms.
> 2. Change height measurement to meters. Since 1 meter = 39.37 inches (or 0.0254 meter = 1 inch), you need to multiply the height in inches by 0.0254 to obtain height in meters.
> 3. Now square the number of meters.
> 4. You are ready to calculate BMI. Divide kilograms of weight by height in meters squared. If, for example, a child weighs 26.5 pounds, convert to kg (26.5 pounds = 12 kg). The child's height is 34.5 inches (0.8763 meter). Then meters² = 0.7679. Divide 12 by 0.7679; the BMI = 15.63.

SKILL 1.5   **Measuring the Newborn's Head, Chest, and Abdomen**

Preparation

- For head measurement, remove any hat, braids, or barrettes the infant is wearing.
- For chest, measurement, remove all clothing from the child's chest.
- For abdominal measurement, remove all clothing from the abdomen.

SKILL 1.5   Measuring the Newborn's Head, Chest, and Abdomen (*continued*)

Equipment

- Disposable, nonstretching measuring tape with centimeter and millimeter markings

Procedure

HEAD CIRCUMFERENCE

1. Wrap the tape around the head at the supraorbital prominence above the eyebrows, above the ears, and around the occipital prominence ❶. Be sure to prevent the tape from slipping or causing a paper cut. **Rationale:** *This is usually the point of largest circumference of the head.*

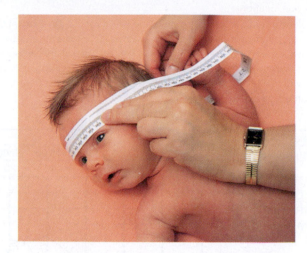

❶ Measuring head circumference.

2. Record the circumference to the nearest 0.5 cm or 1/8 inch. Repeat the measurement to confirm the reading.
3. Plot the measurement for the child's exact age in months on the standardized growth curve.

CHEST CIRCUMFERENCE

1. Wrap the tape measure around the chest, placed just under the axilla and at the nipple line ❷.

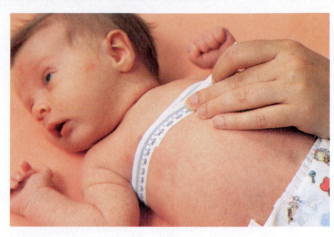

❷ Measuring chest circumference.

2. Record the circumference measurement to the nearest 0.5 cm or ⅛ inch.
3. Compare the chest circumference to the head circumference measurement. **Rationale:** *The head is approximately 2 cm greater than the chest circumference at birth. The head and chest circumference are approximately equal until after 2 years of age, when the chest circumference begins to surpass head circumference* (Barness, Gilbert-Barness, & Fauber, 2009, p. 20).

ABDOMEN CIRCUMFERENCE

1. Wrap the tape around the abdomen at the level of the umbilicus, taking care to prevent a paper cut.
2. If the measurement is taken at another location on the abdomen, place ink marks at the location of the measurement. **Rationale:** *This action will enable you or another nurse to take a future measurement at the same location.*
3. Record the measurement to the nearest 0.5 cm or ¼ inch. Compare the reading to those taken previously to determine a change in size.

▶ VITAL SIGNS

Expected Outcomes

1. Temperature is within normal range.
2. Appropriate method of temperature taking is determined for each client.
3. Pulse is palpated without difficulty.
4. Pulse rate is within normal range and rhythm is regular.
5. Respiratory rate, rhythm, and depth are within normal limits.
6. Labored, difficult, or noisy respirations are assessed.
7. Accurate readings are taken by using the correct cuff size and procedure.
8. The presence of factors that can alter blood pressure readings is identified.

SKILL 1.6   Assessing Body Temperature

Delegation

Routine measurement of the client's temperature can be delegated to unlicensed assistive personnel (UAP) or to family members/caregivers in nonhospital settings. The nurse must explain the appropriate type of thermometer and site to be used and ensure that the person knows when to report an abnormal temperature and how to record the finding. The interpretation of an abnormal temperature and determination of appropriate responses are done by the nurse.

(*continued on next page*)

SKILL 1.6 Assessing Body Temperature (*continued*)

Equipment

- Thermometer
- Thermometer sheath or cover
- Water-soluble lubricant for a rectal temperature
- Clean gloves for a rectal temperature
- Towel for axillary temperature
- Tissues/wipes

Preparation

- Check that all equipment is functioning normally.

Procedure

1. Prior to performing the procedure, introduce self and verify the client's identity using agency protocol. Explain to the client what you are going to do, why it is necessary, and how he or she can participate. Discuss how the results will be used in planning further care or treatments.
2. Perform hand hygiene and observe other appropriate infection control procedures. Apply gloves if performing a rectal temperature.
3. Provide for client privacy.
4. Place the client in the appropriate position (e.g., lateral or Sims' position for inserting a rectal thermometer).
5. Place the thermometer.
   - Apply a protective sheath or probe cover if appropriate.
   - Lubricate a rectal thermometer.
6. Wait the appropriate amount of time. Electronic and tympanic thermometers will indicate that the reading is complete by means of a light or tone. Check package instructions for length of time to wait prior to reading chemical dot or tape thermometers.
7. Remove the thermometer and discard the cover or wipe with a tissue if necessary. If gloves were applied, remove and discard gloves. Perform hand hygiene.

8. Read the temperature and record it on your worksheet. If the temperature is obviously too high, too low, or inconsistent with the client's condition, recheck it with a thermometer known to be functioning properly.

9. Wash the thermometer if necessary and return it to the storage location.
10. Document the temperature in the client record ❶. A rectal temperature may be recorded with an "R" next to the value or with the mark on a graphic sheet circled. An axillary temperature may be recorded with "A" or marked on a graphic sheet with an X. Tympanic route is recorded as "T" and scanner method as "S."

❶ Vital signs graphic record.

SKILL 1.6   Assessing Body Temperature (continued)

VARIATION: MEASURING AN INFANT OR CHILD'S TEMPERATURE

Equipment

- Digital or electronic thermometer with disposable probe cover or scanner temperature ❷
- Water-soluble lubricant
- Gloves, if necessary

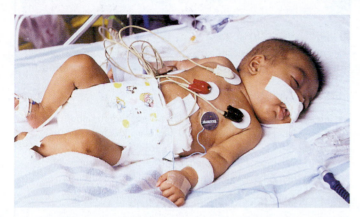

❷ The new scanner method is often used for children who are unconscious, have seizures, or have a structural abnormality.

Procedure

1. Determine appropriate thermometer and route for client (**Box 1–3** ● and **Table 1–1** ●). **Rationale:** *Oral route is appropriate for child over 3 years of age and electronic, nonbreakable thermometer is preferred.*
2. Perform hand hygiene and identify client with two forms of ID.
3. Explain procedure at client's level of understanding.
4. Remove probe from cover or attach probe tip to electronic thermometer ❸.

FOR ORAL ROUTE (ONLY FOR CLIENT AGE 3 OR OLDER)

a. Place probe under client's tongue, one side or the other.
b. Have client close mouth and either hold thermometer in place or monitor while taking temperature.
c. Leave digital thermometer in place 45 to 90 seconds or remove electronic thermometer when audible signal occurs.

> **CLINICAL ALERT**
> The temperature of an unconscious client is never taken by mouth. The rectal, tympanic, or scanner method is preferred.

FOR RECTAL ROUTE

a. Place infant or child in prone or side-lying position.
b. Lubricate probe.
c. Insert thermometer ¼ to ½ inch into rectum for infant or ½ to 1 inch for child, and hold in place.
d. Turn on scanner and follow directions.
e. Remove probe when tone or beep is heard.

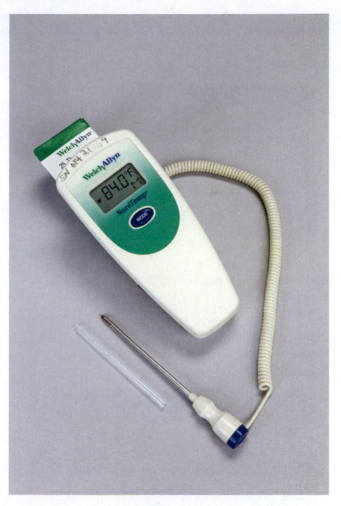

❸ An electronic thermometer. Note the probe and probe cover.

> **CLINICAL ALERT**
> Only use client's own dedicated electronic thermometer (including rectal and oral) if diagnosis includes *Clostridium difficile*–associated diarrhea because of the potential for spreading the bacteria and increasing the risk of transmitting an HAI (nosocomial infection) to others.

FOR AXILLARY ROUTE

a. Assist client to a comfortable position and expose axilla.
b. Dry axilla if necessary. **Rationale:** *A moist axillary area can produce a false low reading.*
c. Place thermometer in center of axilla. Lower client's arm down and across the chest. **Rationale:** *This position ensures that thermometer remains in contact with large vessels of the axilla.*
d. Leave in place 1 to 2 minutes or until tone is heard. **Rationale:** *Axillary temperature readings take longer to register than oral or rectal.*

5. Read and record temperature, indicate method.
6. Discard probe cover into trash by pushing ejection button, or return digital thermometer to its case.

(continued on next page)

SKILL 1.6 Assessing Body Temperature (*continued*)

BOX 1–3 Thermometer Placement

ORAL

- Place the bulb on either side of the frenulum Ⓐ.

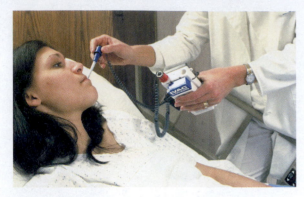

Ⓐ Oral thermometer placement.

RECTAL

- Apply clean gloves.
- Instruct the client to take a slow deep breath during insertion Ⓑ.
- Never force the thermometer if resistance is felt.
- Insert 3.5 cm (1.5 in.) in adults.

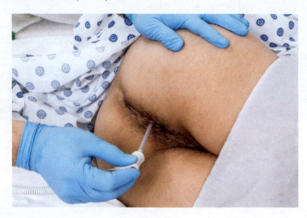

Ⓑ Inserting a rectal thermometer.

AXILLARY

- Pat the axilla dry if very moist.
- Place the bulb in the center of the axilla Ⓒ.

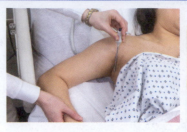

Ⓒ Placing the bulb of the thermometer in the center of the axilla.

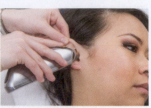

Ⓓ Pull the pinna of the ear up and back while inserting the tympanic thermometer.

TYMPANIC MEMBRANE

- Pull the pinna slightly down and back for children under 3 years, and slightly upward and backward for client over 3 years Ⓓ.
- Point the probe slightly anteriorly, toward the eardrum.
- Insert the probe slowly using a circular motion until snug.

TEMPORAL ARTERY

Brush hair aside if covering the temporal artery area. With the probe flush on the center of the forehead, depress the red button; keep depressed. Slowly slide the probe midline across the forehead to the hairline, not down the side of the face. Lift the probe from the forehead and touch on the neck just behind the earlobe. Release the button Ⓔ.

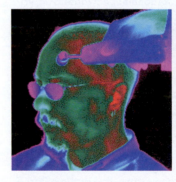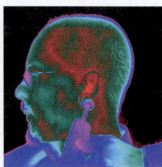

Ⓔ Positioning a temporal artery thermometer. Copyright © Courtesy of Illinois State Library digital archives.

TABLE 1–1 Potential Disadvantages of Sites for Body Temperature Measurement

SITE	DISADVANTAGES
Oral	Inaccurate if client has just ingested hot or cold food or fluid or smoked. Could injure the mouth following oral surgery.
Rectal	Inconvenient and more unpleasant for clients; difficult for client who cannot turn to the side. Could injure the rectum following rectal surgery. Presence of stool may interfere with thermometer placement and accuracy of reading.
Axillary	The thermometer must be left in place 3 to 5 minutes to obtain an accurate measurement.
Tympanic membrane	Can be uncomfortable and involves risk of injuring the membrane if the probe is inserted too far. Right and left measurements can differ. Presence of cerumen can affect the reading.
Temporal scanner	Requires electronic equipment that may be expensive or unavailable; variation in technique needed if the client has perspiration on the forehead.

SKILL 1.6   Assessing Body Temperature *(continued)*

VARIATION: USING AN INFRARED THERMOMETER FOR TYMPANIC TEMPERATURE

Note: A tympanic thermometer measures the infrared energy that naturally radiates from the tympanic membrane and surrounding tissues.

- Perform hand hygiene and identify client with two forms of ID.
- Attach disposable cover centering probe on film and press firmly until backing frame of probe cover engages base of probe. **Rationale:** *Cover protects client from transmission of microorganisms.*
- Turn the client's head to one side and stabilize the client's head.
- Pull pinna upward and backward for an adult ❹ or down and backward for a child. **Rationale:** *This procedure provides better access to the ear canal and tympanic membrane.*

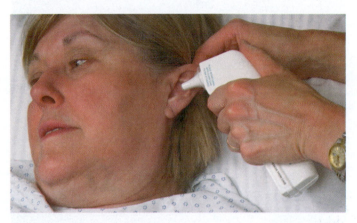

❹ Position adult client so ear canal is easily seen and pull pinna back and up.

- Center probe and gently advance into ear canal to make a firm seal, directing probe toward tympanic membrane ❺. **Rationale:** *Pressure close to the tympanic membrane seals ear canal and allows for accurate reading.*

CLINICAL ALERT

Correct Technique for Taking a Tympanic Temperature
The ear tug (pulling the pinna upward and backward for an adult and down and backward for a child) is essential for an accurate reading. Eliminating this step will not allow the thermometer to be aimed directly at the tympanic membrane.

Do not use ear thermometer in infected or draining ear or if adjacent lesion or incision exists.

- Press and hold temperature switch until green light flashes and temperature reading displays (approximately 3 seconds). **Rationale:** *Method records core body temperature.*
- Remove thermometer. Discard probe cover.
- Return thermometer to home base or storage unit for recharge.
- Keep lens clean using lint-free wipe or alcohol swab, then wipe dry. Do not use povidone-iodine (Betadine).

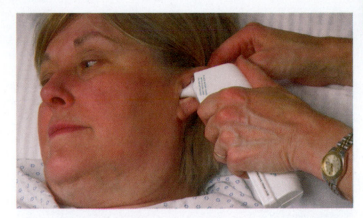

❺ Place probe in client's ear and advance into ear canal to make a firm seal.

- Perform hand hygiene.
- May be used for clients over 3 months of age.

Evidence-Based Practice

Taking a Tympanic Temperature

Temperature readings obtained by tympanic thermometer have many potential benefits. The tympanic membrane, which receives its blood supply from the carotid artery, is protected from radiant heat loss and therefore may correlate closely with core body temperature. It is a fast and easy process that is less likely to cause cross-infection than the rectal route and is less influenced by environmental factors (oral, axillary, cutaneous methods). The one barrier to having a tympanic thermometer be regarded as standard for body temperature measurement is that some studies have reported inaccuracies, mainly in children under 3 years of age.

The size and shape of the child's skull develop rapidly during the first few years of life. The direction of the ear canal and therefore the angle for visualization of the tympanic membrane are different for a small child than for an adult. Errors in tympanic temperature measurement can occur if the probe is not directed toward the tympanic membrane.

If this problem is addressed—for example, if a sensor is developed to indicate when the probe is correctly positioned facing the tympanic membrane—the tympanic method could very well become the gold standard for obtaining temperature.

(Data from El-Radhi & Barry, 2006).

VARIATION: USING AN INFRARED SCANNER THERMOMETER

- Check orders for scanner device (may be used with children to check temperature without waking) ❻.
- Press power button to turn device on. Check to see thermometer is in person mode (see symbol in window).
- Press and hold scan button; "00" will be displayed.
- Aim infrared lens at client's forehead, holding thermometer 2 to 3 inches away.
- Release scan button and note reading that is displayed ❼.
- Clean device with antiseptic wipe.

(continued on next page)

SKILL 1.6 Assessing Body Temperature (continued)

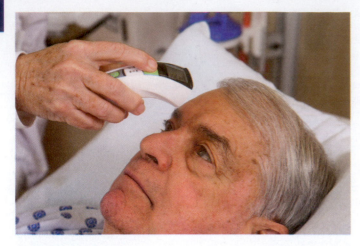

6 Follow manufacturer's directions for scanner device.

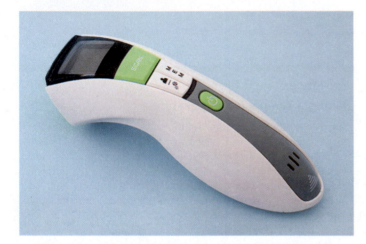

7 After releasing scan button, note reading in window.

- Place strip on forehead or deep in client's axilla—may stay in place for 2 days **8**.
- Read correct temperature by checking color changes or dots that turn from green to black **9**.
- Record temperature on appropriate form or record.

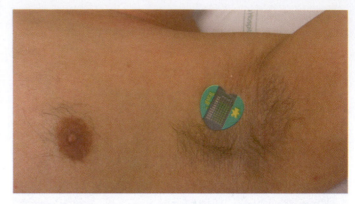

8 Place Traxit®, a continuous-reading wearable thermometer, deep in the client's axilla.

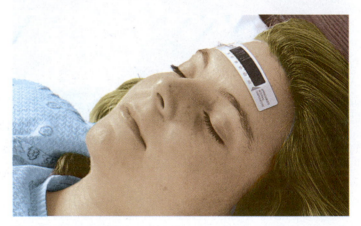

9 Liquid crystal thermometer is placed against lower forehead for 15 seconds. The temperature is read by noting color changes on the device.

Evidence-Based Practice

Cutaneous Infrared Scanners

A prospective study of more than 2,000 clients in an emergency department was done to determine the diagnostic accuracy of infrared thermal imaging using a cutaneous scanner. In the study, tympanic measurements in the left and the right ear were taken as reference points, and temporal scanning measurements of the forehead region were performed.

Results showed that the infrared thermometer underestimated body temperature at low values and overestimated it at high values. The cutaneous scanner gave a high proportion of false-positive results. Furthermore, both the person's age and environmental temperature affected the accuracy of measurements.

The study concluded that infrared thermometry does not reliably detect febrile clients, and that nurses using that method should anticipate a high number of false-positive readings.

(Data from Hausfater et al., 2008).

VARIATION: USING A HEAT-SENSITIVE WEARABLE THERMOMETER

- Check orders for continuous-reading thermometer and identify client with two forms of identification.
- Dry forehead or axilla area, if necessary.

Documentation for Temperature

- Site designated: "O" (oral), "R" (rectal), "A" (axillary), "T" (tympanic), or "S" (scanner)
- Temperature recorded on temp sheet and graph
- Nursing interventions used for alterations in temperature
- Condition of skin related to alterations from normothermia (e.g., diaphoresis)
- Signs and symptoms associated with alterations in temperature (e.g., shivering, dehydration)

CLINICAL ALERT

The temperature of an unconscious client is never taken by mouth. The rectal, tympanic, or scanner method is preferred.

Only use client's own dedicated electronic thermometer (including rectal and oral) if diagnosis includes *Clostridium difficile*–associated diarrhea because of the potential for spreading the bacteria and increasing the risk of transmitting an HAI (nosocomial infection) to others.

SKILL 1.6 Assessing Body Temperature *(continued)*

LEGAL ALERT
Nurse's Negligence

The client had a transthoracic vagotomy after which the physician ordered vital signs every 15 minutes x 1 hour and every hour for 10 hours. Vital signs were recorded 4 times for 1 day. The next day the client's temperature was 102°F and it remained there until the third day when it was 105°F. The nurse administered aspirin when it rose to 106°F. The nurse then contacted the physician who found signs of serious wound infection. The client suffered organic brain syndrome as a direct result of the continued high temperature. The court found that the nurses breached standard of care then they failed to notify the physician of the client's high temperature.

Client Teaching

- Teach the client accurate use and reading of the type of thermometer to be used. Examine the thermometer used by the client in the home for safety and proper functioning. Facilitate the replacement of mercury thermometers with nonmercury ones.
- Observe the client/caregiver taking and reading a temperature. Reinforce the importance of reporting the site and type of thermometer used and the value of using the same thermometer consistently.
- Discuss means of keeping the thermometer clean, such as warm water and soap, and avoiding cross-contamination.
- Instruct the client or family member to notify the healthcare provider if the temperature is higher than a specified level, for example, 38.5°C (101.3°F).
- Check that the client knows how to record the temperature. Provide a recording chart/table if indicated.
- Discuss environmental control modifications that should be taken during illness or extreme climate conditions (e.g., heating, air conditioning, appropriate clothing and bedding).

Developmental Considerations

INFANTS

- The body temperature of newborns is extremely labile (changeable), and newborns must be kept warm and dry to prevent hypothermia.
- Using the axillary site, you need to hold the infant's arm against the chest to keep the thermometer in place.
- The axillary route may not be as accurate as other routes for detecting fevers in children.
- The tympanic route is fast and convenient. Place the infant supine and stabilize the head. Pull the pinna straight back and slightly downward. Remember that the pinna is pulled upward for children over 3 years of age and adults but downward for children younger than 3. Direct the probe tip anteriorly and insert far enough to seal the canal. The tip will not touch the tympanic membrane.
- Avoid the tympanic route in a child with active ear infections or tympanic membrane drainage tubes.
- The tympanic membrane route may be more accurate in determining temperature in febrile infants.
- When using a temporal artery thermometer, touching only the forehead or behind the ear is needed.
- The rectal route is least desirable in infants.

CHILDREN

- Tympanic or temporal artery sites are preferred.
- For the tympanic route, have an adult hold the child in his or her lap with the child's head held gently against the adult for support. Pull the pinna straight back and upward for children over age 3.
- Avoid the tympanic route in a child with active ear infections or tympanic membrane drainage tubes.
- The oral route may be used for children over age 3, but nonbreakable, electronic thermometers are recommended.

- For a rectal temperature, place the child prone across your lap or in a side-lying position with the knees flexed. Insert the thermometer 1 inch into the rectum.

OLDER ADULTS

- Temperatures tend to be lower than those of middle-aged adults.
- Temperatures are strongly influenced by both environmental and internal temperature changes. Their thermoregulation control processes are not as efficient as when they were younger, and they are at higher risk for both hypothermia and hyperthermia.
- Significant buildup of ear cerumen can develop and interfere with tympanic thermometer readings.
- Older adults are more likely to have hemorrhoids. Inspect the anus before taking a rectal temperature.
- Temperatures may not be a valid indication of the seriousness of the pathology of a disease. Older adults may have pneumonia or a urinary tract infection and have only a slight temperature elevation. Other symptoms, such as confusion and restlessness, may be displayed and need follow-up to determine if there is an underlying process.

Setting of Care

- Ensure that the client has water-soluble lubricant if using a rectal thermometer.
- When making a home visit, take a thermometer with you in case the client does not own a functional thermometer.
- Consider whether environmental conditions such as lack of heat or air conditioning are affecting the client's temperature or temperature measurement.
- Pacifier thermometers are being used more in the home setting for children under 2 years old. The manufacturer's instructions must be followed carefully since many require adding 0.5°F in order to estimate rectal temperature.

SKILL 1.7   Assessing an Apical Pulse

Delegation

Due to the degree of skill and knowledge required, UAP are generally not responsible for assessing apical pulses.

Equipment

- Watch with a second hand or indicator
- Stethoscope
- Antiseptic wipes
- If a DUS, the transducer probe, the stethoscope headset, transmission gel, and tissues/wipes

Preparation

- If using the DUS, check that the equipment is functioning normally.

Procedure

1. Prior to performing the procedure, introduce self and verify the client's identity using agency protocol. Explain to the client what you are going to do, why it is necessary, and how he or she can participate. Discuss how the results will be used in planning further care or treatments.
2. Perform hand hygiene and observe other appropriate infection control procedures.
3. Provide for client privacy.
4. Position the client appropriately in a comfortable supine position or in a sitting position. Expose the area of the chest over the apex of the heart.
5. Locate the apical impulse ❶. This is the point over the apex of the heart where the apical pulse can be most clearly heard.
   - Palpate the angle of Louis (the angle between the manubrium, the top of the sternum, and the body of the sternum). It is palpated just below the suprasternal notch and is felt as a prominence.
   - Slide your index finger just to the left of the sternum, and palpate the second intercostal space ❷.

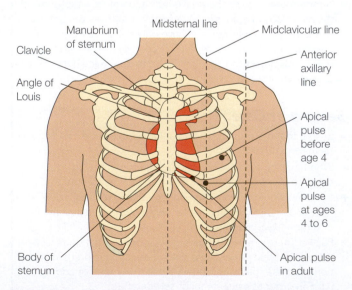

❶ Location of apical pulse for a child under 4 years, a child 4 to 6 years, and an adult.

Labels: Manubrium of sternum · Midsternal line · Midclavicular line · Clavicle · Angle of Louis · Anterior axillary line · Apical pulse before age 4 · Apical pulse at ages 4 to 6 · Body of sternum · Apical pulse in adult

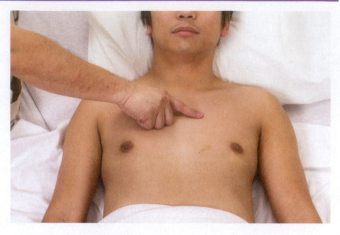

❷ Palpating the point of maximal impulse or PMI: second intercostal space.

- Place your middle or next finger in the third intercostal space ❸, and continue palpating downward until you locate the fifth intercostal space.

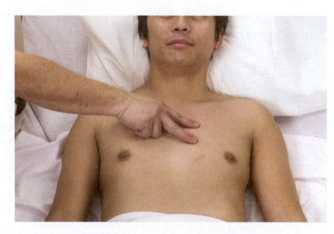

❸ Third intercostal space.

- Move your index finger laterally along the fifth intercostal space toward the midclavicular line (MCL) ❹. Normally, the apical impulse is palpable at or just medial to the MCL.

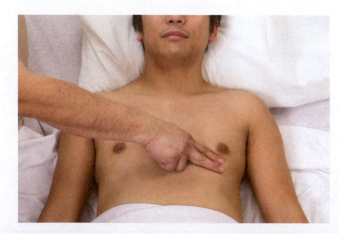

❹ Fifth intercostal space: MCL.

SKILL 1.7   Assessing an Apical Pulse *(continued)*

TABLE 1–2	Normal Heart Rates by Age	
AGE	HEART RATE RANGE (BPM)	AVERAGE HEART RATE (BPM)
Newborns	100–170	120
Infants to 2 years	80–130	110
2–6 years	70–120	100
6–10 years	70–110	90
10–16 years	60–100	85
17 years to adult	60–100	80
Older adult	60–100	70

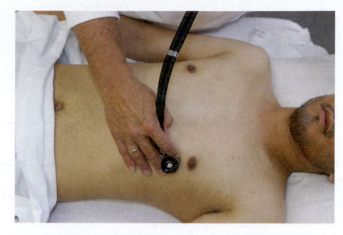

 Taking an apical pulse using the diaphragm of the stethoscope. Note how the diaphragm is held against the chest.

6. Auscultate and count heartbeats (**Table 1–2** ⬤).
   - Use antiseptic wipes to clean the earpieces and diaphragm of the stethoscope if their cleanliness is in doubt. **Rationale:** *The diaphragm needs to be cleaned and disinfected if soiled with body substances. Both earpieces and diaphragm have been shown to harbor pathogenic bacteria* (Whittington et al., 2009).
   - Warm the diaphragm of the stethoscope by holding it in the palm of the hand for a moment. **Rationale:** *The metal of the diaphragm is usually cold and can startle the client when placed immediately on the chest.*
   - Insert the earpieces of the stethoscope into your ears in the direction of the ear canals, or slightly forward, *to facilitate hearing.*
   - Tap your finger lightly on the diaphragm. **Rationale:** *This is to be sure it is the active side of the stethoscope head.* If necessary, rotate the head to select the diaphragm side ⑤.
   - Place the diaphragm of the stethoscope over the apical impulse and listen for the normal S₁ and S₂ heart sounds, which are heard as "lub-dub" ⑥ **Rationale:** *The heartbeat is normally loudest over the apex of the heart. Each lub-dub is counted as one heartbeat.* **Rationale:** *The two heart sounds are produced by*

closure of the heart valves. The S₁ heart sound (lub) occurs when the atrioventricular valves close after the ventricles have been sufficiently filled. The S₂ heart sound (dub) occurs when the semilunar valves close after the ventricles empty.
   - If you have difficulty hearing the apical pulse, ask the supine client to roll onto the left side or the sitting client to lean slightly forward. **Rationale:** *This positioning moves the apex of the heart closer to the chest wall.*
   - If the rhythm is regular, count the heartbeats for 30 seconds and multiply by 2. If the rhythm is irregular or for giving certain medications such as digoxin, count the beats for 60 seconds. **Rationale:** *A 60-second count provides a more accurate assessment of an irregular pulse than a 30-second count.*

7. Assess the rhythm and the strength of the heartbeat.
   - Assess the rhythm of the heartbeat by noting the pattern of intervals between the beats. A normal pulse has equal time periods between beats.

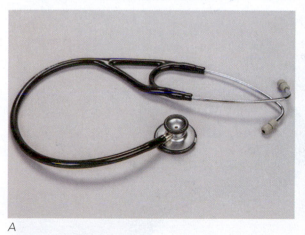

A

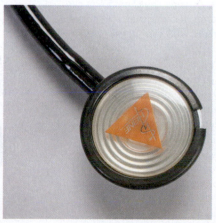

B

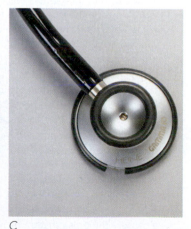

C

⑤ *A,* Stethoscope with both a bell and diaphragm; *B,* close-up of a diaphragm; *C,* close-up of a bell.

(continued on next page)

SKILL 1.7   Assessing an Apical Pulse *(continued)*

- Assess the strength (volume) of the heartbeat. Normally, the heartbeats are equal in strength and can be described as strong or weak.
8. Document the apical pulse rate and rhythm and nursing actions in the client record. Also record pertinent related data such as variation in pulse rate compared to normal for the client and abnormal skin color and skin temperature.

Sample Documentation

2/24/15 1000 Radial pulse 116 & irregular. Had been 82 & regular at 0600. T, R, & BP within client's usual range. C/o slight dizziness. Skin warm & dry. Apical pulse 120, irregular, with slight pause after q 3rd beat. MD notified & ECG ordered.

——————————————————— G. Chapman, RN

SKILL 1.8   Assessing Peripheral Pulses

Delegation

Measurement of the client's radial or brachial pulse can be delegated to UAP or be performed by the client/family members/caregivers in nonhospital settings. Reports of abnormal pulse rates or rhythms require reassessment by the nurse, who also determines appropriate action if the abnormality is confirmed. UAP are generally not delegated these assessment techniques due to the skill required in locating and interpreting peripheral pulses other than the radial or brachial artery and in using Doppler ultrasound devices.

Equipment

- Watch with a second hand or indicator
- If using a Doppler ultrasound stethoscope (DUS), the transducer probe, the stethoscope headset, transmission gel, and tissues/wipes

Procedure

1. Prior to performing the procedure, introduce self and verify the client's identity using agency protocol. Explain to the client what you are going to do, why it is necessary, and how he or she can participate. Discuss how the results will be used in planning further care or treatments.
2. Perform hand hygiene and observe other appropriate infection control procedures.
3. Provide for client privacy.
4. Select the pulse point. Normally, the radial pulse is taken, unless it cannot be exposed or circulation to another body area is to be assessed.
5. Assist the client to a resting position. When the radial pulse is assessed, with the palm facing downward, the client's arm can rest alongside the body or the forearm can rest at a 90-degree angle across the chest. For the client who can sit, the forearm can rest across the thigh, with the palm of the hand facing downward or inward.
6. Palpate and count the pulse. Place two or three middle fingertips lightly and squarely over the pulse point ❶. **Rationale:** *Use of the thumb is contraindicated because the nurse's thumb has a pulse that could be mistaken for the client's pulse.*
   - Count for 15 seconds and multiply by 4. Record the pulse in beats per minute on your worksheet. If taking a client's pulse for the first time, when obtaining baseline data, or if the pulse is irregular, count for a full minute. If an irregular pulse is found, also take the apical pulse.
7. Assess the pulse rhythm and volume.
   - Assess the pulse rhythm by noting the pattern of the intervals between the beats. A normal pulse has equal time periods between beats. If this is an initial assessment, assess for 1 minute.

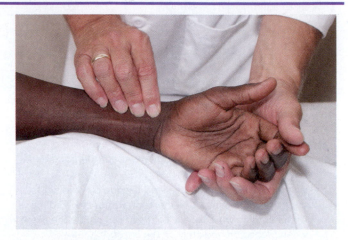

❶ *A, radial*

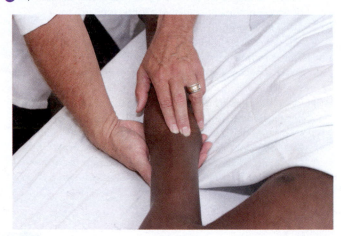

❶ *B, brachial*

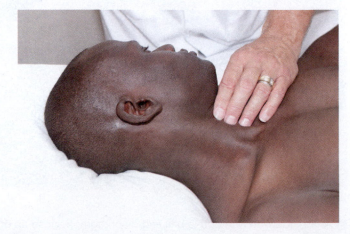

❶ *C, carotid*

SKILL 1.8 Assessing Peripheral Pulses (continued)

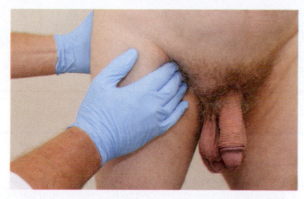

❶ D, femoral

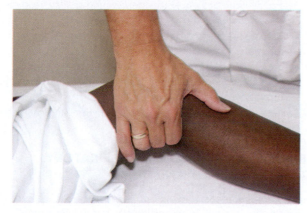

❶ E, popliteal

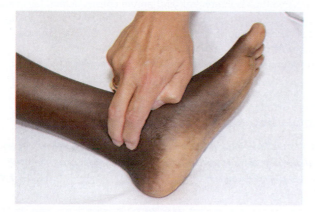

❶ F, posterior tibial

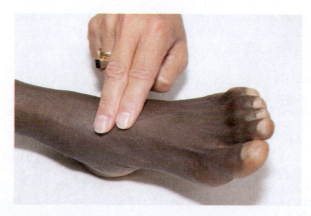

❶ G, pedal (dorsalis pedis)

- Assess the pulse volume. A normal pulse can be felt with moderate pressure, and the pressure is equal with each beat. A forceful pulse volume is full; an easily obliterated pulse is weak. Record the rhythm and volume on your worksheet.

8. Document the pulse rate, rhythm, and volume and your actions in the client record. Also record in the nurse's notes pertinent related data such as variation in pulse rate compared to normal for the client and abnormal skin color and skin temperature.

VARIATION: USING A DOPPLER ULTRASOUND DEVICE (DUS)

- If used, plug the stethoscope headset into one of the two output jacks located next to the volume control ❷.

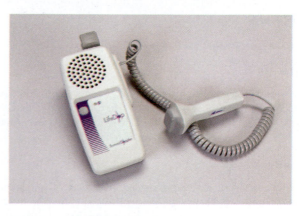

❷ A Doppler ultrasound (DUS) stethoscope

- Apply transmission gel either to the probe at the narrow end of the plastic case housing the transducer, or to the client's skin. **Rationale:** *Ultrasound beams do not travel well through air. The gel makes an airtight seal, which then promotes optimal ultrasound wave transmission.*
- Press the "on" button.
- Hold the probe against the skin over the pulse site. Use a light pressure, and keep the probe in contact with the skin ❸. **Rationale:** *Too much pressure can stop the blood flow and obliterate the signal.*

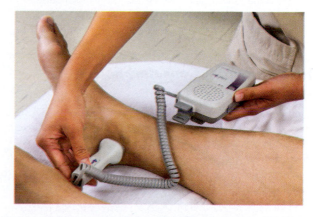

❸ Using a DUS to assess the posterior tibial pulse.

- Adjust the volume if necessary. Distinguish artery sounds from vein sounds. The artery sound (signal) is distinctively pulsating and has a pumping quality. The venous sound is

(continued on next page)

SKILL 1.8   Assessing Peripheral Pulses (*continued*)

intermittent and varies with respirations. Both artery and vein sounds are heard simultaneously through the DUS because major arteries and veins are situated close together throughout the body. If arterial sounds cannot be easily heard, reposition the probe.

- After assessing the pulse, remove all gel from the probe to prevent damage to the surface. Clean the transducer with water-based solution. **Rationale:** *Alcohol or other disinfectants may damage the face of the transducer. Remove all gel from the client.*

SKILL 1.9   Assessing Respirations

Delegation

Counting and observing respirations may be delegated to UAP. The follow-up assessment, interpretation of abnormal respirations, and determination of appropriate responses are done by the nurse.

Equipment

- Watch with a second hand or indicator

Preparation

- For a routine assessment of respirations, determine the client's activity schedule and choose a suitable time to monitor the respirations. A client who has been exercising will need to rest for a few minutes to permit the accelerated respiratory rate to return to normal.

Procedure

1. Prior to performing the procedure, introduce self and verify the client's identity using agency protocol. Explain to the client what you are going to do, why it is necessary, and how he or she can participate. Discuss how the results will be used in planning further care or treatments.
2. Perform hand hygiene and observe other appropriate infection control procedures.
3. Provide for client privacy.
4. Observe or palpate and count the respiratory rate.
   - The client's awareness that the nurse is counting the respiratory rate could cause the client to purposefully alter the respiratory pattern. If you anticipate this, place a hand against the client's chest to feel the chest movements with breathing, or place the client's arm across the chest and observe the chest movements while supposedly taking the radial pulse.
   - Count the respiratory rate for 30 seconds if the respirations are regular. Count for 60 seconds if they are irregu-

lar. An inhalation and an exhalation count as one respiration.

5. Observe the depth, rhythm, and character of respirations.
   - Observe the respirations for depth by watching the movement of the chest. **Rationale:** *During deep respirations, a large volume of air is exchanged; during shallow respirations, a small volume is exchanged.*
   - Observe the respirations for regular or irregular rhythm. **Rationale:** *Normally, respirations are evenly spaced.*
   - Observe the character of respirations—the sound they produce and the effort they require. **Rationale:** *Normally, respirations are silent and effortless.*
6. Document the respiratory rate, depth, rhythm, and character on the appropriate record.

VARIATION: ASSESSING THE RESPIRATORY RATE OF AN INFANT AND CHILD

The procedure for measuring a child's respiratory rate is essentially the same as for an adult. However, keep in mind these points:

- Observe the abdomen, rather than the chest, rise and fall in an infant and young child. **Rationale:** *Since an infant's and young child's respirations are diaphragmatic, the abdomen moves more than the chest with breathing.*
- Abdominal movement in a child will be irregular.
- Count breaths for 1 full minute, or count for 30 seconds and multiply by 2.

Sample Documentation

5/17/15 1320 Respirations irregular, varying from 18–34/min in past hour. Shallower resp. during tachypnea. Slight wheezing noted. Resp. therapist called to provide treatment. _____ D. Katano, RN

Developmental Considerations

INFANTS

- An infant or child who is crying will have an abnormal respiratory rate and rhythm and needs to be quieted before respirations can be accurately assessed.
- Infants use their diaphragms for inhalation and exhalation. If necessary, place your hand gently on the infant's abdomen to feel the rapid rise and fall during respirations.
- Most newborns are complete nose breathers, and nasal obstruction can be life threatening.
- Some newborns display "periodic breathing" in which they pause for a few seconds between respirations. This condition can be normal, but parents should be alert to prolonged or frequent pauses (apnea) that require medical attention.

- Compared to adults, infants have fewer alveoli and their airways have a smaller diameter. As a result, infants' respiratory rate and effort of breathing will increase with respiratory infections.

CHILDREN

- Because young children are diaphragmatic breathers, observe the rise and fall of the abdomen. If necessary, place your hand gently on the abdomen to feel the rapid rise and fall during respirations.
  - Abdominal movement in a child will be irregular.
  - Count breaths for 1 full minute, or count for 30 seconds and multiply by 2.

The range of normal respiratory rates based on age is listed in **Table 1–3** ●. Abnormal patterns and sounds are provided in **Table 1–4** ●.

SKILL 1.9 Assessing Respirations (continued)

TABLE 1–3	Normal Respiratory Rate Changes for Each Age Group
AGE	**RESPIRATORY RATE PER MINUTE**
Newborn	30–80
1 year	20–40
3 years	20–30
6 years	16–22
10 years	16–20
17 years and older	12–20

- Count respirations prior to other uncomfortable procedures so that the respiratory rate is not artificially elevated by the discomfort.

OLDER ADULTS

- Ask the client to remain quiet, or count respirations after taking the pulse.
- Older adults experience anatomical and physiological changes that cause the respiratory system to be less efficient. Any changes in rate or type of breathing should be reported immediately.

TABLE 1–4	Altered Breathing Patterns and Sounds	
BREATHING PATTERNS		**BREATH SOUNDS**

BREATHING PATTERNS	BREATH SOUNDS
Rate - Tachypnea—quick, shallow breaths - Bradypnea—abnormally slow breathing - Apnea—cessation of breathing **Volume** - Hyperventilation—overexpansion of the lungs characterized by rapid and deep breaths - Hypoventilation—underexpansion of the lungs, characterized by shallow respirations **Rhythm** - Cheyne-Stokes breathing—rhythmic waxing and waning of respirations, from very deep to very shallow breathing and temporary apnea **Ease or Effort** - Dyspnea—difficult and labored breathing during which the individual has a persistent, unsatisfied need for air and feels distressed - Orthopnea—ability to breathe only in upright sitting or standing positions	**Audible without Amplification** - Stridor—a shrill, harsh sound heard during inspiration with laryngeal obstruction - Stertor—snoring or sonorous respiration, usually due to a partial obstruction of the upper airway - Wheeze—continuous, high-pitched musical squeak or whistling sound occurring on expiration and sometimes on inspiration when air moves through a narrowed or partially obstructed airway - Bubbling—gurgling sounds heard as air passes through moist secretions in the respiratory tract **Chest Movements** - Intercostal retraction—indrawing between the ribs - Substernal retraction—indrawing beneath the breastbone - Suprasternal retraction—indrawing above the clavicles **Secretions and Coughing** - Hemoptysis—the presence of blood in the sputum - Productive cough—a cough accompanied by expectorated secretions - Nonproductive cough—a dry, harsh cough without secretions

Setting of Care

- Monitor respiratory rate following the administration of respiratory depressants such as morphine.
- Assess the home setting for factors that could interfere with breathing such as exhaust, gas, or paint fumes or individuals who smoke.

- If the client has just come in from another room, allow the client to rest a minute or two before counting respirations.
- Have an adult hold a child gently to reduce movement while counting respirations.

SKILL 1.10 Assessing Blood Pressure

Delegation

Blood pressure measurement may be delegated to UAP. The interpretation of abnormal blood pressure readings and determination of appropriate responses are done by the nurse.

Equipment

- Stethoscope or DUS
- Blood pressure cuff

The blood pressure cuff consists of a rubber bag, called a bladder, that can be inflated with air ①. It is covered with cloth and has two tubes attached to it. One tube connects to a rubber bulb that inflates the bladder. A small valve on the side of this bulb traps and releases the air in the bladder. The other tube is attached to a sphygmomanometer.

Blood pressure cuffs come in various sizes (newborn, infant, child, small adult, adult, large adult, thigh) because the bladder

(continued on next page)

SKILL 1.10 Assessing Blood Pressure (continued)

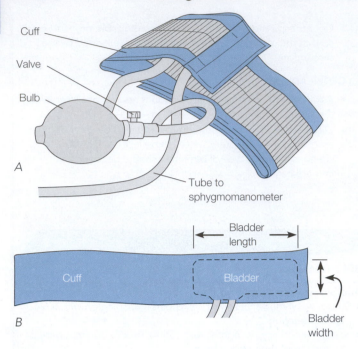

A

Cuff
Valve
Bulb

Tube to sphygmomanometer

Bladder length

Cuff   Bladder

B

Bladder width

1 *A*, Blood pressure cuff and bulb; *B*, The bladder inside the cuff.

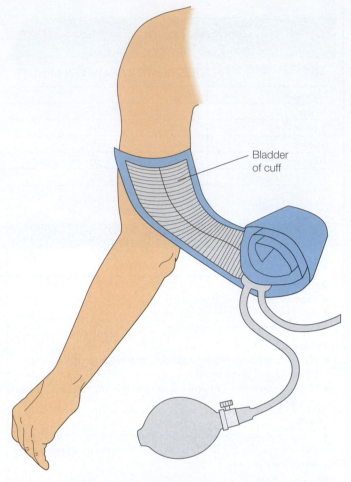

Bladder of cuff

2 Determining that the bladder of a blood pressure cuff is 40% of the arm circumference or 20% wider than the diameter of the midpoint of the limb.

must be the correct width and length for the client's arm. The width should be 40% of the circumference, or 20% wider than the diameter of the midpoint, of the limb on which it is used. The arm circumference, not the age of the client, should always be used to determine bladder size. Lay the cuff lengthwise at the midpoint of the upper arm, and hold the outermost side of the bladder edge laterally on the arm. With the other hand, wrap the width of the cuff around the arm, and ensure that the width is 40% of the arm circumference **2**.

The length of the bladder also affects the accuracy of measurement. The bladder should be sufficiently long to cover at least two thirds of the limb's circumference.

Blood pressure cuffs are made of nondistensible material so that an even pressure is exerted around the limb. Most cuffs are held in place by hooks, snaps, or Velcro. Others have a cloth bandage that is long enough to encircle the limb several times; this type is closed by tucking the end of the bandage into one of the bandage folds.

- Sphygmomanometer

The sphygmomanometer indicates the pressure of the air within the bladder. The aneroid sphygmomanometer is a calibrated dial with a needle that points to the calibrations **3**.

The pumping action to inflate the blood pressure cuff can be used as a prompt for self-care. As the nurse inflates a manual cuff, taking a few slow and complete breaths will help the nurse remain calm and focused, and to really tune into the whole person as vital signs are accessed.

Many agencies use digital (electronic) sphygmomanometers **4**, which eliminate the need to listen for the sounds of the client's systolic and diastolic blood pressures through a stethoscope. Electronic blood pressure devices should be calibrated periodically to check accuracy. All healthcare facilities should have manual blood pressure equipment available as backup.

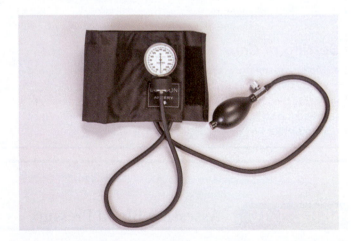

3 Blood pressure equipment: an aneroid sphygmomanometer and cuff.

Preparation

- Ensure that the equipment is intact and functioning properly. Check for leaks in the tubing of the sphygmomanometer.

SKILL 1.10 Assessing Blood Pressure *(continued)*

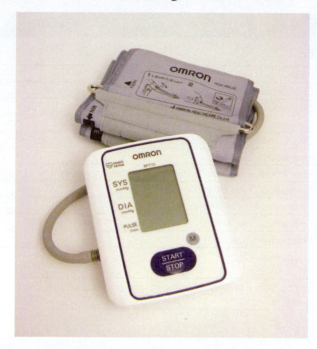

④ Electronic blood pressure monitors register blood pressures.

■ Make sure that the client has not smoked or ingested caffeine within 30 minutes prior to measurement. **Rationale:** *Smoking constricts blood vessels, and caffeine increases the pulse rate. Both of these cause a temporary increase in blood pressure.*

Procedure

1. Prior to performing the procedure, introduce self and verify the client's identity using agency protocol. Explain to the client what you are going to do, why it is necessary, and how he or she can participate. Discuss how the results will be used in planning further care or treatments.
2. Perform hand hygiene and observe other appropriate infection control procedures.
3. Provide for client privacy.
4. Position the client appropriately.
   • The adult client should be sitting unless otherwise specified. Both feet should be flat on the floor. **Rationale:** *Sitting with legs crossed at the knee results in elevated systolic and diastolic blood pressures* (Pinar, Ataalkin, & Watson, 2010).
   • The elbow should be slightly flexed with the palm of the hand facing up and the forearm supported at heart level. Readings in any other position should be specified. The blood pressure is normally similar in sitting, standing, and lying positions, but it can vary significantly by position in certain individuals (Adiyaman et al., 2007).
   • Expose the upper arm.
5. Wrap the deflated cuff evenly around the upper arm. Locate the brachial artery. Apply the center of the bladder directly over the artery. **Rationale:** *The bladder inside the cuff must be directly over the artery to be compressed if the reading is to be accurate.*

   • For an adult, place the lower border of the cuff approximately 2.5 cm (1 in.) above the antecubital space.
6. If this is the client's initial examination, perform a preliminary palpatory determination of systolic pressure. **Rationale:** *The initial estimate tells the nurse the maximal pressure to which the sphygmomanometer needs to be elevated in subsequent determinations. It also prevents underestimation of the systolic pressure or overestimation of the diastolic pressure should an auscultatory gap occur.*
   • Palpate the brachial artery with the fingertips.
   • Close the valve on the bulb.
   • Pump up the cuff until you no longer feel the brachial pulse. At that pressure the blood cannot flow through the artery. Note the pressure on the sphygmomanometer at which the pulse is no longer felt. **Rationale:** *This gives an estimate of the systolic pressure.*
   • Release the pressure completely in the cuff, and wait 1 to 2 minutes before making further measurements. **Rationale:** *A waiting period gives the blood trapped in the veins time to be released. Otherwise, falsely high systolic readings will occur.*
7. Position the stethoscope appropriately.
   • Cleanse the earpieces with antiseptic wipe.
   • Insert the ear attachments of the stethoscope in your ears so that they tilt slightly forward. **Rationale:** *Sounds are heard more clearly when the ear attachments follow the direction of the ear canal.*
   • Ensure that the stethoscope hangs freely from the ears to the diaphragm. **Rationale:** *If the stethoscope tubing rubs against an object, the noise can block the sounds of the blood within the artery.*
   • Place the bell side of the amplifier of the stethoscope over the brachial pulse site. **Rationale:** *Because the blood pressure is a low-frequency sound, it is best heard with the bell-shaped diaphragm.*
   • Place the stethoscope directly on the skin, not on clothing over the site. **Rationale:** *This is to avoid noise made from rubbing the amplifier against cloth.*
   • Hold the diaphragm with the thumb and index finger.
8. Auscultate the client's blood pressure.
   • Pump up the cuff until the sphygmomanometer reads 30 mmHg above the point where the brachial pulse disappeared.
   • Release the valve on the cuff carefully so that the pressure decreases at the rate of 2 to 3 mmHg per second. **Rationale:** *If the rate is faster or slower, an error in measurement may occur.*
   • As the pressure falls, identify the manometer reading at Korotkoff phases 1, 4, and 5. **Rationale:** *There is no clinical significance to phases 2 and 3.*

> ### CLINICAL ALERT
> The American Heart Association recommends routine use of the *bell* of the stethoscope for blood pressure (Korotkoff sounds) auscultation.

(continued on next page)

SKILL 1.10   Assessing Blood Pressure (continued)

TABLE 1–5   Selected Sources of Error in Blood Pressure Assessment

ERROR	EFFECT
Bladder cuff too narrow	Erroneously high
Bladder cuff too wide	Erroneously low
Arm unsupported	Erroneously high
Insufficient rest before the assessment	Erroneously high
Repeating assessment too quickly	Erroneously high systolic or low diastolic readings
Cuff wrapped too loosely or unevenly	Erroneously high
Deflating cuff too quickly	Erroneously low systolic and high diastolic readings
Deflating cuff too slowly	Erroneously high diastolic reading
Failure to use the same arm consistently	Inconsistent measurements
Arm above level of the heart	Erroneously low
Arm below heart level	Erroneously high
Assessing immediately after a meal or while client smokes or has pain	Erroneously high
Failure to identify auscultatory gap	Erroneously low systolic pressure and erroneously low diastolic pressure

- Deflate the cuff rapidly and completely. Document results.
- Wait 1 to 2 minutes before making further determinations. **Rationale:** *This permits blood trapped in the veins to be released.*
- Repeat the above steps to confirm the accuracy of the reading—especially if it falls outside the normal range (although this may not be routine procedure for hospitalized or well clients). If the difference between the two readings is greater than 5 mmHg, additional measurements may be taken and the results averaged. Selected sources of error are listed in **Table 1–5** ●.

9. If this is the client's initial examination, repeat the procedure on the client's other arm. There should be a difference of no more than 10 mmHg between the arms. The arm found to have the higher pressure should be used for subsequent examinations.

VARIATION: OBTAINING A BLOOD PRESSURE BY THE PALPATION METHOD

- If it is not possible to use a stethoscope to obtain the blood pressure or if Korotkoff's sounds cannot be heard, palpate the radial or brachial pulse site as the cuff pressure is released. The manometer reading at the point where the pulse reappears is an estimate of the systolic blood pressure.

VARIATION: TAKING A THIGH BLOOD PRESSURE

- Help the client to assume a prone position. If the client cannot assume this position, measure the blood pressure while the client is in a supine position with the knee slightly flexed. Slight flexing of the knee will facilitate placing the stethoscope on the popliteal space.
- Expose the thigh, taking care not to expose the client unduly.
- Locate the popliteal artery.
- Wrap the cuff evenly around the midthigh with the compression bladder over the posterior aspect of the thigh and the bottom edge above the knee. **Rationale:** *The bladder must be directly over the posterior popliteal artery if the reading is to be accurate.*

- If this is the client's initial examination, perform a preliminary palpatory determination of systolic pressure while palpating the popliteal artery.
- In adults, the systolic pressure in the popliteal artery is often 20 to 30 mmHg higher than that in the brachial artery; the diastolic pressure is usually the same.

VARIATION: USING AN ELECTRONIC BLOOD PRESSURE MONITORING DEVICE

- Place the blood pressure cuff on the extremity according to the manufacturer's guidelines.
- Turn on the blood pressure switch.
- If appropriate, set the device for the desired number of minutes between blood pressure determinations.
- When the device has determined the blood pressure reading, note the digital results.
- Electronic/automatic blood pressure cuffs can be left in place for many hours. Remove the cuff and check skin condition periodically.

10. Remove the cuff from the client's arm.
11. Wipe the cuff with an approved disinfectant. **Rationale:** *Cuffs can become significantly contaminated.* Many institutions use disposable blood pressure cuffs. The client uses a disposable cuff for the length of stay and then it is discarded. **Rationale:** *This decreases the risk of spreading infection by sharing cuffs.*
12. Document and report pertinent assessment data according to agency policy. Record two pressures in the form "130/80" where "130" is the systolic (phase 1) and "80" is the diastolic (phase 5) pressure. Record three pressures in the form "130/90/0," where "130" is the systolic, "90" is the first diastolic (phase 4), and sounds are audible even after the cuff is completely deflated. Use the abbreviations RA or RL for right arm or right leg, respectively, and LA or LL for left arm or left leg, respectively. Record a difference of greater than 10 mmHg between the two arms or legs.

SKILL 1.10 Assessing Blood Pressure *(continued)*

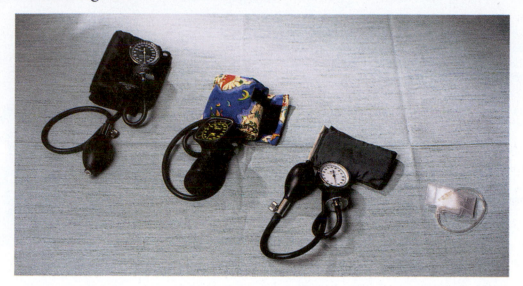

5 Blood pressure cuffs are available in various types and sizes for pediatric clients.

VARIATION: ASSESSING BLOOD PRESSURE OF INFANT AND CHILD

Preparation

- To select the proper cuff size, compare the cuff to the size of the child's upper arm or thigh.
- The bladder of the cuff should encircle 80%–100% of the extremity used and have a width that covers two thirds of the length of the extremity used (Kavey, Daniels, & Flynn, 2010). **Rationale:** *If the bladder is too small, the blood pressure reading will be falsely high; if it is too large, the pressure will be falsely low.*

EQUIPMENT

- Various sizes blood pressure cuffs with air squeezed out of the bladder **5**
- Electronic blood pressure monitor
- Sphygmomanometer and stethoscope
- Blood pressure values by age, sex, and height percentiles

Oscillometry

Procedure

Electronic equipment is often used to obtain the systolic blood pressure for infants and young children. With this technique, a transducer uses pressure oscillations received and transmitted by the blood pressure cuff to identify the mean arterial pressure and estimate the systolic and diastolic blood pressure (Ogedegbe & Pickering, 2010) **6**.

1. Wrap the cuff around the right arm or upper leg directly against the skin with the center of the bladder over the artery of the extremity. The lower edge of the cuff should be 2 to 3 cm above the antecubital or popliteal fossa. **Rationale:** *The right arm is preferred, as this is the extremity used for standardizing the blood pressure tables. The upper leg is not a preferred site to obtain the blood pressure. It is used to measure the blood pressure and contrast with the arm blood pressure to detect coarctation of the aorta.*

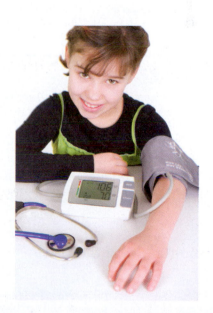

6 Measuring blood pressure using oscillometric technique.
© st-fotograf/Fotolia

(continued on next page)

SKILL 1.10   Assessing Blood Pressure (continued)

2. Place the arm with the antecubital fossa at heart level with muscles relaxed. Stabilize the arm, because movement interferes with the reading.
3. Ensure that the tubing is free of kinks, and activate the equipment according to the manufacturer's recommendations.
4. Pressure is recorded as the number over "D."
5. Document the blood pressure reading and compare values for age, sex, and height percentile. A blood pressure reading over the 90th percentile for age, sex, and height percentiles should be verified by auscultation using a manual sphygmomanometer (Howlin, 2010).

Manual Sphygmomanometer

Procedure

1. Wrap the cuff snugly around the desired extremity directly against the skin with the bladder centered over the extremity's artery.
2. Hold the arm with the antecubital fossa at heart 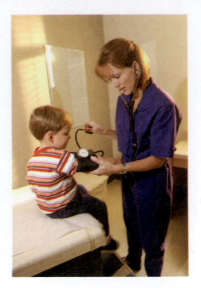. If taking the blood pressure in the thigh, the child should be lying down flat.
3. Palpate for the pulse and inflate the cuff until the pulse is occluded and no longer felt. Note the reading. Release the cuff pressure. This is the palpated systolic blood pressure, and it can be recorded as blood pressure over "P."
4. Wait a minute and place the stethoscope over the pulse area. Avoid using too much pressure against the pulse area to improve the quality of sounds heard.
5. Close the air escape valve. Pump the cuff with the bulb until the gauge rises 30 mmHg above the level of the palpated systolic blood pressure. Slowly release the air through the valve at 2 to 3 mm/sec while watching the falling gauge. **Rationale:** *The palpated reading helps improve accuracy in the recognition of the first Korotkoff sound.*
6. Continue slowly releasing the air. The fifth Korotkoff sound (the disappearance of all sound) is the diastolic pressure. It

❼ Measuring blood pressure with a manual cuff. Note the arm is at the same level as the heart.

may be 0 in children under age 12 years. For these children the fourth Korotkoff sound is considered the diastolic pressure.
7. Document the blood pressure reading and compare to values for age, sex, and height percentile.

Client Teaching

- Explain to the client and family what the equipment actually does and the information it provides.
- Instruct clients with automatic blood pressure devices such as the type often used in emergency departments to keep the elbow extended when the cuff inflates.

Forearm Blood Pressure

Statistical analysis has shown that blood pressure taken in the upper arm vs. the forearm varies by 14 to 20 mmHg. The two pressures are therefore not interchangeable. If the appropriate cuff size is not available and the forearm has to be used, document the site used.

Source: Schell, K., Bradley, E., Bucher, L., Seckel, M., Lyons, D., Wakai, S., . . . Simpson, K. (2005). Clinical comparison of automatic, noninvasive blood pressure in the forearm and upper arm. *Am. J. Crit. Care, 14*(3), 232–241.

Developmental Considerations

INFANTS

- Use a pediatric stethoscope with a small diaphragm.
- The lower edge of the blood pressure cuff can be closer to the antecubital space of an infant.
- Use the palpation method if auscultation with a stethoscope or DUS is unsuccessful.

- Arm and thigh pressures are equivalent in children under 1 year of age.
- The systolic blood pressure of a newborn ranges between 50 and 80 mmHg; the diastolic between 25 and 55 mmHg (D'Amico & Barbarito, 2011).
- Use only the first and fifth Korotkoff sounds for children ages 1 to 6 months (Knecht, Seller, & Alpert, 2009).

CHILDREN

- Blood pressure should be measured in all children over 3 years of age and in children less than 3 years of age with certain medical conditions (e.g., congenital heart disease, renal malformation, medications that affect blood pressure).
- Explain each step of the process and what it will feel like. Demonstrate on a doll.
- Use the palpation technique for children under 3 years old.
- Cuff bladder width should be 40% and length should be 80%–100% of the arm circumference.

SKILL 1.10 Assessing Blood Pressure (continued)

- Take the blood pressure prior to other uncomfortable procedures so that the blood pressure is not artificially elevated by the discomfort.
- In children, the diastolic pressure is considered to be the onset of phase 4, where the sounds become muffled.
- In children, the thigh pressure is about 10 mmHg higher than the arm.

OLDER ADULTS

- Skin may be very fragile. Do not allow cuff pressure to remain high any longer than necessary.
- Determine if the client is taking antihypertensives and, if so, when the last dose was taken.
- Medications that cause vasodilation (antihypertensive medications) along with the loss of baroreceptor efficiency in older adults place them at increased risk for having orthostatic hypotension (significant fall in blood pressure when changing from supine to sitting or standing). Measuring blood pressure while the client is in the lying, sitting, and standing positions—and noting any changes—can determine this.

- If the client has arm contractures, assess the blood pressure by palpation, with the arm in a relaxed position. If this is not possible, take a thigh blood pressure.

Setting of Care

- If the client takes blood pressure readings at home, the nurse should use the same equipment or calibrate it against a system known to be accurate.
- Observe the client or family member taking the blood pressure and provide feedback if further instruction is needed.
- Home blood pressure measurement done by the client or family can be more accurate than blood pressure measured in a clinic or office setting. This is because so-called "white coat" hypertension can occur, which is an elevation in blood pressure due to mild anxiety associated with the healthcare provider's presence—who historically wore a white laboratory coat.
- If the client is in a chair or low bed, position yourself so that you maintain the client's arm at heart level and you can read the sphygmomanometer at eye level.

SKILL 1.11 Using a Pulse Oximeter

Delegation

Application of the pulse oximeter sensor and recording of the SpO_2 value may be delegated to UAP. The interpretation of the oxygen saturation value and determination of appropriate responses are done by the nurse.

Equipment

- Nail polish remover as needed
- Alcohol wipe
- Sheet or towel
- Pulse oximeter

Pulse oximeters with various types of sensors are available from several manufacturers ❶. The *oximeter unit* consists of an inlet connection for the sensor cable, a faceplate that indicates (a) the oxygen saturation measurement (expressed as a percentage) and (b) the pulse rate. Cordless units are also available. A preset alarm system signals high and low SpO_2 measurements and a high and low pulse rate. The high and low SpO_2 levels are generally preset at 100% and 85%, respectively, for adults. The high and low pulse rate alarms are usually preset at 140 and 50 bpm for adults. These alarm limits can, however, be changed according to the manufacturer's directions.

Preparation

- Check that the oximeter equipment is functioning normally.

Procedure

1. Prior to performing the procedure, introduce self and verify the client's identity using agency protocol. Explain to the

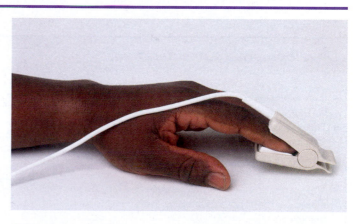

❶ Fingertip oximeter sensor. (Andy Crawford © Dorling Kindersley).

client what you are going to do, why it is necessary, and how he or she can participate. Discuss how the results will be used in planning further care or treatments.

2. Perform hand hygiene and observe other appropriate infection control procedures.
3. Provide for client privacy.
4. Choose a sensor appropriate for the client's weight, size, and desired location. Because weight limits of sensors overlap, a pediatric sensor could be used for a small adult.
   - If the client is allergic to adhesive, use a clip or sensor without adhesive. If using an extremity, assess the proximal pulse and capillary refill at the point closest to the site.

(continued on next page)

SKILL 1.11   Using a Pulse Oximeter (continued)

- If the client has low tissue perfusion due to peripheral vascular disease or therapy using vasoconstrictive medications, use a nasal sensor or a reflectance sensor on the forehead. Avoid using lower extremities that have compromised circulation and extremities that are used for infusions or other invasive monitoring.

5. Prepare the site.
   - Clean the site with an alcohol wipe before applying the sensor.
   - It may be necessary to remove a female client's dark nail polish (Valdez-Lowe, Ghareeb, & Artinian, 2009). **Rationale:** *It can interfere with accurate measurements.*
   - Alternatively, position the sensor on the side of the finger rather than perpendicular to the nail bed.

6. Apply the sensor, and connect it to the pulse oximeter.
   - Make sure the LED and photodetector are accurately aligned, that is, opposite each other on either side of the finger, toe, nose, or earlobe. Many sensors have markings to facilitate correct alignment of the LEDs and photodetector.
   - Attach the sensor cable to the connection outlet on the oximeter. Turn on the machine according to the manufacturer's directions. Appropriate connection will be confirmed by an audible beep indicating each arterial pulsation. Some devices have a wheel that can be turned clockwise to increase the pulse volume and counterclockwise to decrease it.
   - Ensure that the bar of light or waveform on the face of the oximeter fluctuates with each pulsation.

7. Set and turn on the alarm when using continuous monitoring.
   - Check the preset alarm limits for high and low oxygen saturation and high and low pulse rates. Change these alarm limits according to the manufacturer's directions as indicated. Ensure that the audio and visual alarms are on before you leave the client. A tone will be heard and a number will blink on the faceplate.

8. Ensure client safety.
   - Inspect and/or move or change the location of an adhesive toe or finger sensor every 4 hours and a spring-tension sensor every 2 hours.
   - Inspect the sensor site tissues for irritation from adhesive sensors.

9. Ensure the accuracy of measurement.
   - Minimize motion artifacts by using an adhesive sensor, or immobilize the client's monitoring site. **Rationale:** *Movement of the client's finger or toe may be misinterpreted by the oximeter as arterial pulsations.*
   - If indicated, cover the sensor with a sheet or towel to block large amounts of light from external sources (e.g., sunlight, procedure lamps, or bilirubin lights in the nursery). **Rationale:** *Bright room light may be sensed by the photodetector and alter the SpO_2 value.*
   - Compare the pulse rate indicated by the oximeter to the radial pulse periodically. **Rationale:** *A large discrepancy between the two values may indicate oximeter malfunction.*

10. Document the oxygen saturation on the appropriate record at designated intervals.

Developmental Considerations

INFANTS

- If an appropriate-sized finger or toe sensor is not available, consider using an earlobe or forehead sensor.
- The high and low SpO_2 alarm levels are generally preset at 95% and 80% for neonates.
- The high and low pulse rate alarms are usually preset at 200 and 100 for neonates.
- The oximeter may need to be taped, wrapped with an elastic bandage, or covered by a stocking to keep it in place.

CHILDREN

- Instruct the child that the sensor does not hurt. Disconnect the probe whenever possible to allow for movement.

OLDER ADULTS

- Use of vasoconstrictive medications, poor circulation, or thickened nails may make finger or toe sensors inaccurate.

Setting of Care

- Pulse oximetry is a quick, inexpensive, noninvasive method of assessing oxygenation. Like an automatic blood pressure cuff, it also provides a pulse rate reading. Use in the ambulatory or home setting whenever indicated.
- If the client requires frequent or continuous home monitoring, teach the client and family how to apply and maintain the equipment. Remind them to rotate the site periodically and assess for skin trauma.

▶ COMPLETE ASSESSMENT

Expected Outcomes

1. Assessment data include nursing history and behavioral and physical data.
2. Physical assessment data are collected through inspection, palpation, percussion, and auscultation.
3. All systems of the body are included in the complete assessment.
4. Normal and abnormal assessment data are documented.
5. Complete assessment data documentation is available to other disciplines taking care of the client.
6. Developmental considerations are made for the pediatric client.

SKILL 1.12   Assessing the Skin

Delegation

Due to the substantial knowledge and skill required, assessment of the skin is not delegated to UAP. However, the skin is observed during usual care and UAP should record their findings. Abnormal findings must be validated and interpreted by the nurse.

Equipment

- Millimeter ruler
- Clean gloves
- Magnifying glass

Procedure

1. Prior to performing the procedure, introduce self and verify the client's identity using agency protocol. Explain to the client what you are going to do, why it is necessary, and how he or she can participate. Discuss how the results will be used in planning further care or treatments.

2. Perform hand hygiene and observe other appropriate infection control procedures.

3. Provide for client privacy.

4. Inquire if the client has any history of the following: pain or itching; presence and spread of lesions, bruises, abrasions, pigmented spots; previous experience with skin problems; associated clinical signs; family history; presence of problems in other family members; related systemic conditions; use of medications, lotions, home remedies; excessively dry or moist feel to the skin; tendency to bruise easily; association of the problem with season of year, stress, occupation, medications, recent travel, housing, and so on; recent contact with allergens (e.g., metal paint).

ASSESSMENT	NORMAL FINDINGS	DEVIATIONS FROM NORMAL
5. Inspect skin color (best assessed under natural light and on areas not exposed to the sun).	Varies from light to deep brown or black; from light pink to ruddy pink; from yellow overtones to olive	Pallor, cyanosis, jaundice, erythema
6. Inspect uniformity of skin color.	Generally uniform except in areas exposed to the sun; areas of lighter pigmentation (palms, lips, nail beds) in dark-skinned people	Areas of either hyperpigmentation or hypopigmentation
7. Assess edema, if present (i.e., location, color, temperature, shape, and the degree to which the skin remains indented or pitted when pressed by a finger) ❶. Measuring the circumference of the extremity with a millimeter tape may be useful for future comparison.	No edema	See the scale for describing edema.
8. Inspect, palpate, and describe skin lesions ❷. Apply gloves if lesions are open or draining. Palpate lesions to determine shape and texture ❸. Describe lesions according to location, distribution, color, configuration, size, shape (**Table 1–6** ●; see **Box 1–4** ●). Use the millimeter ruler to measure lesions. If gloves were applied, remove and discard gloves. Perform hand hygiene.	Freckles, pigmented birthmarks that have not changed since childhood, and some long-standing vascular birthmarks such as strawberry or port-wine hemangiomas, some flat and raised nevi (moles); no abrasions or other lesions	Various interruptions in skin integrity; irregular, multicolored, or raised nevi, some pigmented birthmarks such as melanocystic nevi, and some vascular birthmarks such as cavernous hemangiomas. Even these deviations from normal may not be dangerous or require treatment. Assessment by an advanced-level practitioner is required.

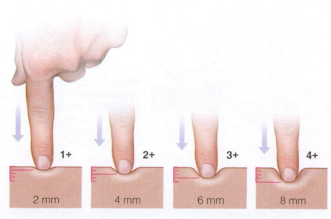

❶ Scale for grading edema.

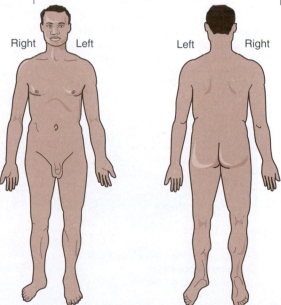

Right   Left   Left   Right

❷ Diagram for charting skin lesions.

(continued on next page)

SKILL 1.12 Assessing the Skin (*continued*)

Macule, Patch Flat, unelevated change in color. Macules are 1 mm to 1 cm (0.04 to 0.4 in.) in size and circumscribed. Examples: freckles, measles, petechiae, flat moles.
Patches are larger than 1 cm (0.4 in.) and may have an irregular shape. Examples: port-wine birthmark, vitiligo (white patches), rubella. **Ⓐ**

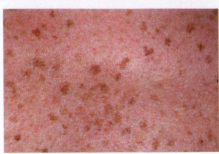

Ⓐ Multiple café-au-lait macules
(Michael P. Gadomski / Science Source)

Nodule, Tumor Elevated, solid, hard mass that extends deeper into the dermis than a papule.
Nodules have a circumscribed border and are 0.5 to 2 cm (0.2 to 0.8 in.). Examples: squamous cell carcinoma, fibroma.
Tumors are larger than 2 cm (0.8 in.) and may have an irregular border. Examples: malignant melanoma, hemangioma. **Ⓓ**

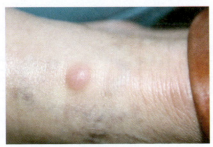

Ⓓ Peripheral neurofibromas
(DermPics / Science Source)

Cyst A 1-cm (0.4 in.) or larger, elevated, encapsulated, fluid-filled or semisolid mass arising from the subcutaneous tissue or dermis. Examples: sebaceousand epidermoid cysts, chalazion of the eyelid. **Ⓖ**

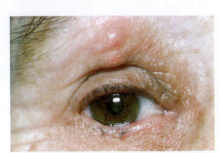

Ⓖ Digital mucous cyst
(Medical-on-Line / Alamy)

Papule Circumscribed, solid elevation of skin. Papules are less than 1 cm (0.4 in.). Examples: warts, acne, pimples, elevated moles. **Ⓑ**

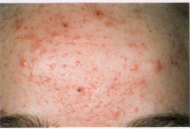

Ⓑ Papular drug eruption
(Copyright Hercules Robinson / Alamy)

Pustule Vesicle or bulla filled with pus. Examples: acne vulgaris, impetigo.

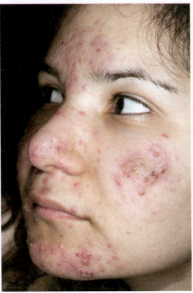

Ⓔ Chronic pustular psoriasis
(Dr. Harout Tanielian / Science Source)

Plaque Plaques are larger than 1 cm (0.4 in.). Examples: psoriasis, rubeola. **Ⓒ**

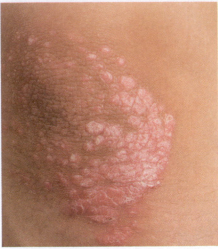

Ⓒ Psoriasis vulgaris
(Copyright olavs silis / Alamy)

Vesicle, Bulla A circumscribed, round or oval, thin translucent mass filled with serous fluid or blood.
Vesicles are less than 0.5 cm (0.2 in.). Examples: herpes simplex, early chicken-pox, small burn blister.
Bullae are larger than 0.5 cm (0.2 in.). Examples: large blister, second-degree burn, herpes simplex. **Ⓕ**

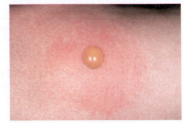

Ⓕ Bullous pemphigoid
(Scott Camazine / Science Source)

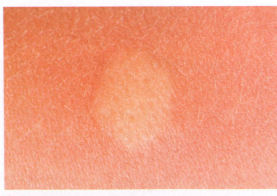

Ⓗ Allergic wheals, urticaria
(Ted Kinsman / Science Source)

Wheal A reddened, localized collection of edema fluid; irregular in shape. Size varies. Examples: hives, mosquito bites. **Ⓗ**

❸ Primary skin lesions: *A*, macule, patch; *B*, papule; *C*, plaque; *D*, nodule, tumor; *E*, pustule; *F*, vesicle, bulla; *G*, cyst; *H*, wheal.

SKILL 1.12 Assessing the Skin (continued)

ASSESSMENT	NORMAL FINDINGS	DEVIATIONS FROM NORMAL
9. Observe and palpate skin moisture.	Moisture in skinfolds and the axillae (varies with environmental temperature and humidity, body temperature, and activity)	Excessive moisture (e.g., in hyperthermia); excessive dryness (e.g., in dehydration)
10. Palpate skin temperature. Compare the two feet and the two hands, using the backs of your fingers.	Uniform; within normal range	Generalized hyperthermia (e.g., in fever); generalized hypothermia (e.g., in shock); localized hyperthermia (e.g., in infection); localized hypothermia (e.g., in arteriosclerosis)
11. Note skin turgor (fullness or elasticity) by lifting and pinching the skin on an extremity.	When pinched, skin springs back to previous state; may be slower in older adults.	Skin stays pinched or tented or moves back slowly (e.g., in dehydration). Count in seconds how long the skin remains tented.
12. Document findings in the client record using forms or checklists supplemented by narrative notes when appropriate. Draw location of skin lesions on body surface diagrams.		

CLINICAL ALERT

If possible and the client agrees, take a digital or instant photograph of significant skin lesions for the client record. Include a measuring guide (ruler or tape) in the picture to indicate lesion size.

BOX 1–4 Describing Skin Lesions

- **Type or structure.** Skin lesions are classified as primary (those that appear initially in response to some change in the external or internal environment of the skin) and secondary (those that do not appear initially but result from modifications such as chronicity, trauma, or infection of the primary lesion). For example, a vesicle (primary lesion) may rupture and cause an erosion (secondary lesion).
- **Size, shape, and texture.** Note size in millimeters and whether the lesion is circumscribed or irregular; round or oval shaped; flat, elevated, or depressed; solid, soft, or hard; rough or thickened; fluid filled or has flakes.
- **Color.** There may be no discoloration, one color (e.g., red, brown, or black), or several colors, as with ecchymosis (a bruise),

in which an initial dark red or blue color fades to a yellow color. When color changes are limited to the edges of a lesion, they are described as circumscribed; when spread over a large area, they are described as diffuse.
- **Distribution.** Distribution is described according to the location of the lesions on the body and symmetry or asymmetry of findings in comparable body areas.
- **Configuration.** Configuration refers to the arrangement of lesions in relation to each other. Configurations of lesions may be annular (arranged in a circle), clustered together or grouped, linear (arranged in a line), arc or bow shaped, or merged together or indiscrete. They may follow the course of cutaneous nerves, or be meshed in the form of a network.

TABLE 1–6 Secondary Skin Lesions

Atrophy		Ulcer	
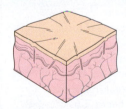	A translucent, dry, paper-like, sometimes wrinkled skin surface resulting from thinning or wasting of the skin due to loss of collagen and elastin. **Examples:** Striae, aged skin	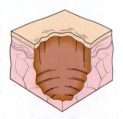	Deep, irregularly shaped area of skin loss extending into the dermis or subcutaneous tissue. May bleed. May leave scar. **Examples:** Pressure ulcers, stasis ulcers, chancres
Erosion		Fissure	
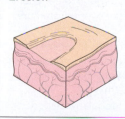	Wearing away of the superficial epidermis causing a moist, shallow depression. Because erosions do not extend into the dermis, they heal without scarring. **Examples:** Scratch marks, ruptured vesicles	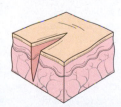	Linear crack with sharp edges, extending into the dermis. **Examples:** Cracks at the corners of the mouth or in the hands, athlete's foot

(continued on next page)

SKILL 1.12 Assessing the Skin *(continued)*

TABLE 1–6 Secondary Skin Lesions *(continued)*

Lichenification 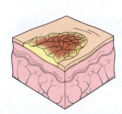	Rough, thickened, hardened area of epidermis resulting from chronic irritation such as scratching or rubbing. **Examples:** Chronic dermatitis	**Scar** 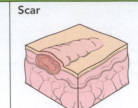	Flat, irregular area of connective tissue left after a lesion or wound has healed. New scars may be red or purple; older scars may be silvery or white. **Examples:** Healed surgical wound or injury, healed acne
Scales 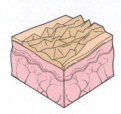	Shedding flakes of greasy, keratinized skin tissue. Color may be white, gray, or silver. Texture may vary from fine to thick. **Examples:** Dry skin, dandruff, psoriasis, and eczema	**Keloid** 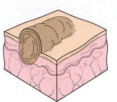	Elevated, irregular, darkened area of excess scar tissue caused by excessive collagen formation during healing. Extends beyond the site of the original injury. Higher incidence in people of African descent. **Examples:** Keloid from ear piercing or surgery
Crust 	Dry blood, serum, or pus left on the skin surface when vesicles or pustules burst. Can be red-brown, orange, or yellow. Large crusts that adhere to the skin surface are called scabs. **Examples:** Eczema, impetigo, herpes, or scabs following abrasion	**Excoriation** 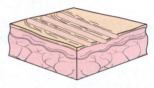	Linear erosion. **Examples:** Scratches, some chemical burns

Developmental Considerations

INFANTS

- *Physiological* jaundice may appear in newborns 2 to 3 days after birth and usually lasts about 1 week. Pathological jaundice, or that which indicates a disease, appears within 24 hours of birth and may last more than 8 days.
- Newborns may have milia (whiteheads), tiny white nodules over the nose and face, and vernix caseosa (white cheesy, greasy material on the skin).
- Premature infants may have lanugo, a fine downy hair covering their shoulders and back.
- In dark-skinned infants, areas of hyperpigmentation may be found especially on the back, in the sacral area.
- Diaper dermatitis (a rash in the groin area) may be seen in infants.
- If a rash is present, inquire in detail about immunization history.
- Assess skin turgor by pinching the skin on the abdomen.

CHILDREN

- Children normally have minor skin lesions (e.g., bruising or abrasions) on arms and legs due to their high activity level. Lesions on other parts of the body may be signs of disease or abuse, and a thorough history should be taken.
- Secondary skin lesions may occur frequently as children scratch or expose a primary lesion to microbes.
- With puberty, oil glands become more productive, and children may develop acne. Most individuals ages 12 to 24 have some acne.

- In dark-skinned children, areas of hyperpigmentation may be found on the back, especially in the sacral area.
- If a rash is present, inquire in detail about immunization history.

OLDER ADULTS

- Changes in White skin occur at an earlier age than in Black skin.
- The skin loses its elasticity and develops wrinkles. Wrinkles first appear on the skin of the face and neck, which are abundant in collagen and elastic fibers.
- The skin appears thin and translucent because of loss of dermis and subcutaneous fat.
- The skin is dry and flaky because sebaceous and sweat glands are less active. Dry skin is more prominent over the extremities.
- The skin takes longer to return to its natural shape after being pinched between the thumb and finger. This is called tenting.
- Due to the normal loss of peripheral skin turgor in older adults, assess for hydration by checking skin turgor over the sternum or clavicle.
- Flat tan to brown-colored macules, referred to as senile lentigines or melanotic freckles, are normally apparent on the back of the hand and other skin areas that are exposed to the sun. These macules may be as large as 1 to 2 cm.
- Warty lesions (seborrheic keratosis) with irregularly shaped borders and a scaly surface often occur on the face, shoulders,

SKILL 1.12   Assessing the Skin (continued)

and trunk. These benign lesions begin as yellowish to tan and progress to a dark brown or black.

- Vitiligo tends to increase with age and is thought to result from an autoimmune response.
- Cutaneous tags (acrochordons) are most commonly seen in the neck and axillary regions. These skin lesions vary in size and are soft, often flesh colored, and pedicled.
- Visible, bright red, fine dilated blood vessels commonly occur as a result of the thinning of the dermis and the loss of support for the blood vessel walls.
- Pink to slightly red lesions with indistinct borders (actinic keratoses) may appear at about age 50, often on the face, ears, backs of the hands, and arms. They may become malignant if untreated.

Setting of Care

- When making a home visit, take a penlight or examination lamp with you in case the home has inadequate lighting.
- If skin lesions are suggestive of physical abuse, follow state regulations for follow-up and reporting. Signs of abuse may include a pattern of bruises, unusual location of burns, or lesions that are not easily explainable. If lesions are present in adults or verbal-age children, conduct the interview and assessment in private.
- Document lesions by taking a photo (if client consents). Another method that can be used is to lay clean double-thick clear plastic (such as a grocery bag) over the lesion or wound and trace the shape with a permanent marker. Cut away and dispose of the bottom layer that came in contact with the client and place the top layer in the client record. Use this method only if contact with the plastic does not contaminate the wound.

Cultural Considerations

Many cultures believe that certain substances protect one's health. For example, some individuals may believe that garlic or onions eaten raw or worn on the body will prevent illness such as high blood pressure. If a client wishes to include these items in his or her diet or wear them, the nursing staff should respect this practice, since it is an important cultural tradition for many groups.

SKILL 1.13   Assessing the Hair

Delegation

Assessment of the hair is not delegated to UAP. However, many aspects are observed during usual care and may be recorded by individuals other than the nurse. Abnormal findings must be validated and interpreted by the nurse.

Equipment

- Clean gloves

Procedure

1. Prior to performing the procedure, introduce self and verify the client's identity using agency protocol. Explain to the client what you are going to do, why it is necessary, and how he or she can participate. Discuss how the results will be used in planning further care or treatments.
2. Perform hand hygiene, apply gloves, and observe other appropriate infection control procedures.
3. Provide for client privacy.
4. Inquire if the client has any history of the following: recent use of hair dyes, rinses, or curling or straightening preparations; chemotherapy; and the presence of acute or chronic conditions.

ASSESSMENT	NORMAL FINDINGS	DEVIATIONS FROM NORMAL
5. Inspect the evenness of growth over the scalp.	Evenly distributed hair	Patches of hair loss (i.e., alopecia)
6. Inspect hair thickness or thinness.	Thick hair	Very thin hair
7. Inspect hair texture and oiliness.	Silky, resilient hair	Brittle hair, excessively oily or dry hair
8. Note presence of infections or infestations by parting the hair in several areas, checking behind the ears and along the hairline at the neck.	No infection or infestation	Flaking, sores, lice, nits (louse eggs), and ringworm
9. Inspect amount of body hair.	Variable	Hirsutism (abnormal hairiness) Absent or sparse leg hair
10. Remove and discard gloves. Perform hand hygiene.		
11. Document findings in the client record using forms or checklists supplemented by narrative notes when appropriate.		

(continued on next page)

SKILL 1.13 Assessing the Hair *(continued)*

Developmental Considerations

INFANTS

- Infants exhibit a wide variation of normal hair distribution that can range from very little or none to a great deal of body and scalp hair.

CHILDREN

- As puberty approaches, axillary and pubic hair will appear.

OLDER ADULTS

- Older adults may experience a loss of scalp, pubic, and axillary hair.
- Hairs of the eyebrows, ears, and nostrils become bristle-like and coarse.

Setting of Care

- When making a home visit, ask to see the products the client usually uses on the hair. Assist the client to determine if the products are appropriate for the client's type of hair and scalp (e.g., for dry or oily hair). Provide education regarding hygiene of the hair and scalp.
- When making a home visit, examine the equipment that the client uses on the hair. Provide client teaching regarding appropriate combs and brushes and regarding safety in using electric hair-styling appliances such as hair dryers.

SKILL 1.14 Assessing the Nails

Delegation

Due to the substantial knowledge required, assessment of the nails is not delegated to UAP. However, many nail characteristics are observed during usual care and may be recorded by individuals other than the nurse. Abnormal findings must be validated and interpreted by the nurse.

Procedure

1. Prior to performing the procedure, introduce self and verify the client's identity using agency protocol. Explain to the client what you are going to do, why it is necessary, and how he or she can participate. Discuss how the results will be used in planning further care or treatments. In most situations, clients with artificial nails or polish on fingernails or toenails are not required to remove these for assessment. If the assessment cannot be conducted due to the presence of polish or artificial nails, document this in the record.

2. Perform hand hygiene and observe other appropriate infection control procedures.

3. Provide for client privacy.

4. Inquire if the client has any history of the following: presence of diabetes mellitus, peripheral circulatory disease, previous injury, or severe illness.

ASSESSMENT	NORMAL FINDINGS	DEVIATIONS FROM NORMAL
5. Inspect fingernail plate shape to determine its curvature and angle.	Convex curvature; angle of nail plate about 160° ❶ (see A)	Spoon nail (see 1B); clubbing (180° or greater) (see 1C and D)
6. Inspect fingernail and toenail texture.	Smooth texture	Excessive thickness or thinness or presence of grooves or furrows; Beau's lines (see 1E); discolored or detached nail— often due to fungus or injury
7. Inspect fingernail and toenail bed color.	Highly vascular and pink in light-skinned clients; dark-skinned clients may have brown or black pigmentation in longitudinal streaks	Bluish or purplish tint (may reflect cyanosis); pallor (may reflect poor arterial circulation)
8. Inspect tissues surrounding nails.	Intact epidermis	Hangnails; paronychia (inflammation)

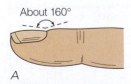 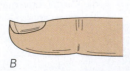 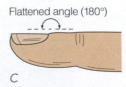 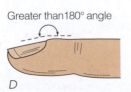 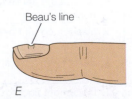

About 160°   Flattened angle (180°)   Greater than 180° angle   Beau's line

A   *B*   *C*   *D*   *E*

❶ *A*, A normal nail, showing the convex shape and the nail plate angle of about 160 degrees; *B*, a spoon-shaped nail, which may be seen in clients with iron deficiency anemia; *C*, early clubbing; *D*, late clubbing (may be caused by long-term lack of oxygen); *E*, Beau's line on nail (may result from severe injury or illness).

SKILL 1.14 Assessing the Nails *(continued)*

ASSESSMENT	NORMAL FINDINGS	DEVIATIONS FROM NORMAL
9. Perform blanch test of capillary refill. Press two or more nails between your thumb and index finger; look for blanching and return of pink color to nail bed. Count in seconds the time for the color to return completely.	Prompt return of pink or usual color (generally less than 2 seconds)	Delayed return of pink or usual color (may indicate circulatory impairment)
10. Document findings in the client record using forms or checklists supplemented by narrative notes when appropriate.		

Developmental Considerations

INFANTS

- Newborns' nails grow very quickly, are extremely thin, and tear easily.

CHILDREN

- Bent, bruised, or ingrown toenails may indicate that shoes are too tight.
- Nail biting should be discussed with an adult family member because it may be a symptom of stress.

OLDER ADULTS

- The nails grow more slowly and thicken.
- Longitudinal bands commonly develop, and the nails tend to split.

- Bands across the nails may indicate protein deficiency; white spots, zinc deficiency; and spoon-shaped nails, iron deficiency.
- Toenail fungus is more common and difficult to eliminate (although not dangerous to health).

Setting of Care

- If indicated, teach the client or family member about proper nail care including how to trim and shape the nails to avoid paronychia.
- If eyesight, fine motor control, or cognition prevents the client from safely trimming the nails, refer the client to a podiatrist or manicurist.

SKILL 1.15 Assessing the Musculoskeletal System

Delegation

Assessment of the musculoskeletal system is not delegated to UAP. However, many aspects of its functioning are observed during usual care and may be recorded by individuals other than the nurse. Abnormal findings must be validated and interpreted by the nurse.

Equipment

- Goniometer
- Tape measure

Procedure

1. Prior to performing the procedure, introduce self and verify the client's identity using agency protocol. Explain to the cli-

ent what you are going to do, why it is necessary, and how he or she can participate. Discuss how the results will be used in planning further care or treatments.
2. Perform hand hygiene and observe other appropriate infection control procedures.
3. Provide for client privacy.
4. Inquire if the client has any history of the following: presence of muscle or joint pain: onset, location, character, associated phenomena (e.g., redness and swelling of joints), and aggravating and alleviating factors; limitations to movement or inability to perform activities of daily living; previous sports injuries; loss of function without pain.

ASSESSMENT MUSCLES	NORMAL FINDINGS	DEVIATIONS FROM NORMAL
Muscles		
5. Inspect the muscles for size. Compare the muscles on one side of the body (e.g., of the arm, thigh, and calf) to the same muscle on the other side. For any discrepancies, measure the muscles with a tape.	Equal size on both sides of body	Atrophy (a decrease in size) or hypertrophy (an increase in size), Asymmetry
6. Inspect the muscles and tendons for contractures (shortening).	No contractures	Malposition of body part, (e.g., foot drop, in which the foot is flexed downward)

(continued on next page)

SKILL 1.15 Assessing the Musculoskeletal System *(continued)*

ASSESSMENT MUSCLES	NORMAL FINDINGS	DEVIATIONS FROM NORMAL
7. Inspect the muscles for tremors, for example, by having the client hold the arms out in front of the body.	No tremors	Presence of tremor
8. Test muscle strength. Compare the right side with the left side.	Equal strength on each body side	Muscle grading 25% or less of normal strength
Sternocleidomastoid: Client turns the head to one side against the resistance of your hand. Repeat with the other side.		**Grading Muscle Strength Scale**
Trapezius: Client shrugs the shoulders against the resistance of your hands.		**0:** 0% of normal strength; complete paralysis
Deltoid: Client holds arm up and resists while you try to push it down.		**1:** 10% of normal strength; no movement, contraction of muscle is palpable or visible
Biceps: Client fully extends each arm and tries to flex it while you attempt to hold arm in extension.		**2:** 25% of normal strength; full muscle movement against gravity, with support
Triceps: Client flexes each arm and then tries to extend it against your attempt to keep arm in flexion.		**3:** 50% of normal strength; normal movement against gravity
Wrist and finger muscles: Client spreads the fingers and resists as you attempt to push the fingers together.		**4:** 75% of normal strength; normal full movement against gravity and against minimal resistance
Grip strength: Client grasps your index and middle fingers while you try to pull the fingers out.		**5:** 100% of normal strength; normal full movement against gravity and against full resistance
Hip muscles: Client is supine, both legs extended; client raises one leg at a time while you attempt to hold it down.		
Hip abduction: Client is supine, both legs extended. Place your hands on the lateral surface of each knee; client spreads the legs apart against your resistance.		
Hip adduction: Client is in same position as for hip abduction. Place your hands between the knees; client brings the legs together against your resistance.		
Hamstrings: Client is supine, both knees bent. Client resists while you attempt to straighten the legs.		
Quadriceps: Client is supine, knee partially extended; client resists while you attempt to flex the knee.		
Muscles of the ankles and feet: Client resists while you attempt to dorsiflex the foot and again resists while you attempt to flex the foot.		
Bones		
9. Inspect the skeleton for structure.	No deformities	Bones misaligned
10. Palpate the bones to locate any areas of edema or tenderness.	No tenderness or swelling	Presence of tenderness or swelling (may indicate fracture, neoplasms, or osteoporosis)
Joints		
11. Inspect the joint for swelling. Palpate each joint for tenderness, smoothness of movement, swelling, crepitation, and presence of nodules.	No swelling No tenderness, swelling, crepitation or nodules Joints move smoothly	One or more swollen joints Presence of tenderness, swelling, crepitation, or nodules

SKILL 1.15 **Assessing the Musculoskeletal System** (*continued*)

ASSESSMENT MUSCLES	NORMAL FINDINGS	DEVIATIONS FROM NORMAL
12. Assess joint range of motion. Ask the client to move selected body parts. The amount of joint movement can be measured by a **goniometer**, a device that measures the angle of the joint in degrees. **❶**	Varies to some degree in accordance with person's genetic makeup and degree of physical activity ❶ A goniometer used to measure joint angle.	Limited range of motion in one or more joints
13. Document findings in the client record using forms or checklists supplemented by narrative notes when appropriate.		

Developmental Considerations

INFANTS

- Palpate the clavicles of newborns. A mass and crepitus may indicate a fracture experienced during vaginal delivery. The newborn may also have limited movement of the arm and shoulder on the affected side.
- When the arms and legs of newborns are pulled to extension and released, newborns naturally return to the flexed fetal position.
- Check muscle strength by holding the infant lightly under the arms with feet placed lightly on a table. Infants should not fall through the hands and should be able to bear body weight on their legs if normal muscle strength is present.
- Check infants for developmental dysplasia of the hip (congenital dislocation) by examining for asymmetric gluteal folds, asymmetric abduction of the legs (Ortolani and Barlow tests), or apparent shortening of the femur.
- Infants should be able to sit without support by 8 months of age, crawl by 7 to 10 months, and walk by 12 to 15 months.
- Observe for symmetry of muscle mass, strength, and function.

CHILDREN

- Pronation and "toeing in" of the feet are common in children between 12 and 30 months of age.
- Genu varum (bowleg) is normal in children for about 1 year after beginning to walk.
- Genu valgus (knock-knee) is normal in preschool and early school-age children.
- Lordosis (swayback) is common in children before age 5.
- Observe the child in normal activities to determine motor function.
- During the rapid growth spurts of adolescence, spinal curvature and rotation (scoliosis) may appear. Children should be assessed for scoliosis by age 12 and annually until their growth slows. Curvature greater than 10% should be referred for further medical evaluation.
- Muscle mass increases in adolescence, especially as children engage in strenuous physical activity, and requires increased nutritional intake.
- Children are at risk for injury related to physical activity and should be assessed for nutritional status, physical conditioning, and safety precautions in order to prevent injury.
- Adolescent girls who participate in strenuous athletic activities are at risk for delayed menses, osteoporosis, and eating disorders; assessment should include a history of these factors.

OLDER ADULTS

- Muscle mass decreases progressively with age, but there are wide variations among individuals.
- The decrease in speed, strength, resistance to fatigue, reaction time, and coordination in the older person is due to a decrease in nerve conduction and muscle tone.
- The bones become more fragile and osteoporosis leads to a loss of total bone mass. As a result, older adults are predisposed to fractures and compressed vertebrae.
- In most older adults, osteoarthritic changes in the joints can be observed.
- Note any surgical scars from joint replacement surgeries.

Setting of Care

- When making a home visit, observe the client in natural movement around the living area. To assess children, have them remove their clothes down to the underwear.
- A complete examination of joints, bone, and muscles may not be necessary. Focus the assessment on areas indicated by the history and current complaint.

SKILL 1.16   Assessing the Neurological System

Delegation

Due to the substantial knowledge and skill required, assessment of the neurological system is not delegated to UAP. However, many aspects of neurological behavior are observed during usual care and may be recorded by individuals other than the nurse. Abnormal findings must be validated and interpreted by the nurse.

Equipment (Depending on Components of Examination)

- Percussion hammer
- Wisps of cotton to assess light-touch sensation
- Sterile safety pin for tactile discrimination

Procedure

1. Prior to performing the procedure, introduce self and verify the client's identity using agency protocol. Explain to the client what you are going to do, why it is necessary, and how he or she can participate. Discuss how the results will be used in planning further care or treatments.
2. Perform hand hygiene and observe other appropriate infection control procedures.
3. Provide for client privacy.
4. Inquire if the client has any history of the following: presence of pain in the head, back, or extremities, as well as onset and aggravating and alleviating factors; disorientation to time, place, or person; speech disorder; history of loss of consciousness, fainting, convulsions, trauma, tingling or numbness, tremors or tics, limping, paralysis, uncontrolled muscle movements, loss of memory, mood swings, or problems with smell, vision, taste, touch, or hearing.

CLINICAL ALERT

All questions and tests used in a neurological examination must be age, language, education level, and culturally appropriate. Individualize questions and tests before using them.

LANGUAGE

5. If the client displays difficulty speaking:
   - Point to common objects and ask the client to name them.
   - Ask the client to read some words and to match the printed and written words with pictures.
   - Ask the client to respond to simple verbal and written commands, for example, "point to your toes" or "raise your left arm."

ORIENTATION

6. Determine the client's orientation to *time*, *place*, and *person* by tactful questioning. Ask the client the time of day, date, day of the week, city and state of residence, duration of illness, and names of family members. Ask the client why he or she is seeing a healthcare provider. Orientation is lost gradually, and early disorientation may be very subtle. "Why" questions may elicit a more accurate clinical picture of the client's orientation status than questions directed to time, place, and person. To evaluate the response, you must know the correct answer.

More direct questioning may be necessary for some people, for example, "Where are you now?" "What day is it today?" Most people readily accept these questions if initially the nurse asks, "Do you get confused at times?" If the client cannot answer these questions regarding place and time accurately, also include assessment of the *self* by asking the client to state his or her full name.

MEMORY

7. Listen for lapses in memory. Ask the client about difficulty with memory. If problems are apparent, three categories of memory are tested: immediate recall, recent memory, and remote memory.

To assess immediate recall:

- Ask the client to repeat a series of three digits (e.g., 7–4–3), spoken slowly.
- Gradually increase the number of digits (e.g., 7–4–3–5, 7–4–3–5–6, and 7–4–3–5–6–7), until the client fails to repeat the series correctly.
- Start again with a series of three digits, but this time ask the client to repeat them backward. The average person can repeat a series of five to eight digits in sequence and four to six digits in reverse order.

To assess recent memory:

- Ask the client to recall the recent events of the day, such as how the client got to the clinic. This information must be validated, however.
- Ask the client to recall information given early in the interview (e.g., the name of a physician).
- Provide the client with three facts to recall (e.g., a color, an object, and an address), and ask the client to repeat all three. Later in the interview, ask the client to recall all three items.

   To assess remote memory, ask the client to describe a previous illness or surgery (e.g., 5 years ago) or a birthday or anniversary. Generally remote memory will be intact until late in neurological pathology. It is least useful to assess for acute neurological problems.

ATTENTION SPAN AND CALCULATION

8. Test the ability to concentrate or maintain *attention span* by asking the client to recite the alphabet or to count backward from 100. Test the ability to calculate by asking the client to subtract 7 or 3 progressively from 100, that is, 100, 93, 86, 79, or 100, 97, 94, 91 (referred to as *serial sevens* or *serial threes*). Normally, an adult can complete the serial sevens test in about 90 seconds with three or fewer errors. Because educational level, language, or cultural differences affect calculating ability, this test may be inappropriate for some people.

LEVEL OF CONSCIOUSNESS

9. Apply the Glasgow Coma Scale (see Chapter 9): eye response, motor response, and verbal response. An assessment totaling 15 points indicates the client is alert and completely oriented. A comatose client scores 7 or less.

CRANIAL NERVES

10. For the specific functions and assessment methods of each cranial nerve, see **Table 1–7 ●**. Test each nerve not already evaluated in another component of the health assessment. A quick way to test cranial nerve I is shown in ❶.

SKILL 1.16 Assessing the Neurological System (continued)

TABLE 1–7 Cranial Nerve Functions and Assessment Methods

CRANIAL NERVE	NAME	TYPE	FUNCTION	ASSESSMENT METHOD
I	Olfactory	Sensory	Smell	Ask client to close eyes and identify different mild aromas, such as coffee, vanilla, peanut butter, orange/lemon, chocolate.
II	Optic	Sensory	Vision and visual fields	Ask client to read Snellen-type chart; check visual fields by confrontation; and conduct an ophthalmoscopic examination (see Skill 1.18).
III	Oculomotor	Motor	Extraocular eye movement (EOM); movement of sphincter of pupil; movement of ciliary muscles of lens	Assess six ocular movements and pupil reaction (see Skill 1.18).
IV	Trochlear	Motor	EOM; specifically, moves eyeball downward and laterally	Assess six ocular movements (see Skill 1.18).
V	Trigeminal Ophthalmic branch	Sensory	Sensation of cornea, skin of face, and nasal mucosa	While client looks upward, lightly touch the lateral sclera of the eye with sterile gauze to elicit blink reflex. To test light sensation, have client close eyes, wipe a wisp of cotton over client's forehead and paranasal sinuses.
	Maxillary branch	Sensory	Sensation of skin of face and anterior oral cavity (tongue and teeth)	Assess skin sensation as for ophthalmic branch above.
	Mandibular branch	Motor and sensory	Muscles of mastication; sensation of skin of face	Ask client to clench teeth.
VI	Abducens	Motor	EOM; moves eyeball laterally	Assess directions of gaze.
VII	Facial	Motor and sensory	Facial expression; taste (anterior two thirds of tongue)	Ask client to smile, raise the eyebrows, frown, puff out cheeks, close eyes tightly. Ask client to identify various tastes placed on tip and sides of tongue: sugar (sweet), salt, lemon juice (sour), and quinine (bitter); identify areas of taste.
VIII	Cochlear branch Sensory hearing Assess client's ability to hear spoken word and vibrations of tuning fork.	Auditory		
	Vestibular branch	Sensory	Equilibrium	Romberg test
	Cochlear branch	Sensory	Hearing	Assess client's ability to hear spoken word and vibrations of tuning fork.
IX	Glossopharyngeal	Motor and sensory	Swallowing ability, tongue movement, taste (posterior tongue)	Apply tastes on posterior tongue for identification. Ask client to move tongue from side to side and up and down.
X	Vagus	Motor and sensory	Sensation of pharynx and larynx; swallowing; vocal cord movement	Assessed with cranial nerve IX; assess client's speech for hoarseness.
XI	Accessory	Motor	Head movement; shrugging of shoulders	Ask client to shrug shoulders against resistance from your hands and turn head to side against resistance from your hand (repeat for other side).
XII	Hypoglossal	Motor	Protrusion of tongue; moves tongue up and down and side to side	Ask client to protrude tongue at midline, then move it side to side.

(continued on next page)

SKILL 1.16   Assessing the Neurological System *(continued)*

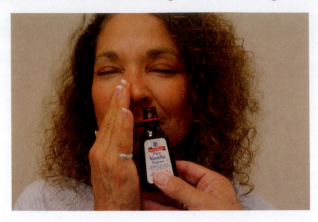

❶ Cranial nerves are tested for normal or abnormal response. For example, cranial nerve I (smell) can be tested by having the client close his or her eyes and identify different mild, familiar scents.

REFLEXES

11. Generalist nurses do not commonly assess each of the deep tendon reflexes except for the plantar (Babinski) reflex, indicative of possible spinal cord injury. Reflexes are reported using the scale below, comparing one side of the body with the other to evaluate the symmetry of response.

0 No reflex response

+1 Minimal activity (hypoactive)

+2 Normal response

+3 More active than normal

+4 Maximal activity (hyperactive)

BABINSKI REFLEX

- Use a moderately sharp object, such as the handle of the percussion hammer, a key, or an applicator stick.
- Stroke the lateral border of the sole of the client's foot, starting at the heel, continuing to the ball of the foot, and then proceeding across the ball of the foot toward the big toe ❷.

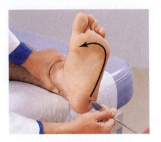

❷ Testing plantar (Babinski) reflexes.

- Observe the response. Normally, all five toes bend downward; this reaction is called a negative Babinski. In an abnormal (positive) Babinski response, the toes spread outward and the big toe moves upward.

MOTOR FUNCTION

ASSESSMENT	NORMAL FINDINGS	DEVIATIONS FROM NORMAL
12. *Gross Motor and Balance Tests:* Generally, the Romberg test and one other gross motor function and balance tests are used.		
Walking Gait		
Ask the client to walk across the room and back, and assess the client's gait.	Has upright posture and steady gait with opposing arm swing; walks unaided, maintaining balance	Has poor posture and unsteady, irregular, staggering gait with wide stance; bends legs only from hips; has rigid or no arm movements
Romberg Test		
Ask the client to stand with feet together and arms resting at the sides, first with eyes open, then closed. Stand close during this test. **Rationale:** *This prevents the client from falling.*	*Negative Romberg:* may sway slightly but is able to maintain upright posture and foot stance	*Positive Romberg:* cannot maintain foot stance; moves the feet apart to maintain stance If client cannot maintain balance with the eyes shut, client may have sensory ataxia (lack of coordination of the voluntary muscles) If balance cannot be maintained whether the eyes are open or shut, client may have cerebellar ataxia

SKILL 1.16   Assessing the Neurological System (continued)

ASSESSMENT	NORMAL FINDINGS	DEVIATIONS FROM NORMAL
Standing on One Foot with Eyes Closed		
Ask the client to close the eyes and stand on one foot. Repeat on the other foot. Stand close to the client during this test.	Maintains stance for at least 5 seconds	Cannot maintain stance for 5 seconds
Heel–Toe Walking		
Ask the client to walk a straight line, placing the heel of one foot directly in front of the toes of the other foot ❸.	Maintains heel–toe walking along a straight line ❸ Heel–toe walking test.	Assumes a wider foot gait to stay upright
Toe or Heel Walking		
Ask the client to walk several steps on the toes and then on the heels.	Able to walk several steps on toes or heels	Cannot maintain balance on toes and heels
13. *Fine Motor Tests for the Upper Extremities:*		
Finger-to-Nose Test		
Ask the client to abduct and extend the arms at shoulder height and then rapidly touch the nose alternately with one index finger and then the other. The client repeats the test with the eyes closed if the test is performed easily ❹.	Repeatedly and rhythmically touches the nose ❹ Finger-to-nose test.	Misses the nose or gives slow response
Alternating Supination and Pronation of Hands on Knees		
Ask the client to pat both knees with the palms of both hands and then with the backs of the hands alternately at an ever-increasing rate ❺.	Can alternately supinate and pronate hands at rapid pace	Performs with slow, clumsy movements and irregular timing; has difficulty alternating from supination to pronation

(continued on next page)

SKILL 1.16   Assessing the Neurological System (*continued*)

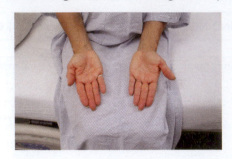
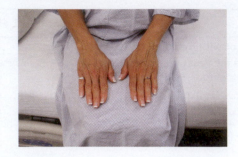

⑤ Alternating supination and pronation of hands on knees test.

ASSESSMENT	NORMAL FINDINGS	DEVIATIONS FROM NORMAL
Finger to Nose and to the Nurse's Finger		
Ask the client to touch the nose and then your index finger, held at a distance of about 45 cm (18 in.), at a rapid and increasing rate ⑥.	Performs with coordination and rapidity	Misses the finger and moves slowly
	⑥ Finger-to-nose and to the nurse's finger test.	
Fingers to Fingers		
Ask the client to spread the arms broadly at shoulder height and then bring the fingers together at the midline, first with the eyes open and then closed, first slowly and then rapidly.	Performs with accuracy and rapidity	Moves slowly and is unable to touch fingers consistently
Fingers to Thumb (Same Hand)		
Ask the client to touch each finger of one hand to the thumb of the same hand as rapidly as possible ⑦. ⑦ Fingers-to-thumb (same hand) test.	Rapidly touches each finger to thumb with each hand	Cannot coordinate this fine discrete movement with either one or both hands
14. *Fine Motor Tests for the Lower Extremities:* Ask the client to lie supine to perform these tests.		

SKILL 1.16   Assessing the Neurological System (continued)

ASSESSMENT	NORMAL FINDINGS	DEVIATIONS FROM NORMAL
Heel Down Opposite Shin		
Ask the client to place the heel of one foot just below the opposite knee and run the heel down the shin to the foot. Repeat with the other foot. The client may also use a sitting position for this test ❽.	Demonstrates bilateral equal coordination ❽ Heel down opposite shin.	Has tremors or is awkward; heel moves off shin
15. *Light-Touch Sensation:* Compare the light-touch sensation of symmetric areas of the body. **Rationale:** *Sensitivity to touch varies among different skin areas.* • Ask the client to close the eyes and to respond by saying "yes" or "now" whenever the client feels the cotton wisp touching the skin. • With a wisp of cotton, lightly touch one specific spot and then the same spot on the other side of the body ❾. • Test areas on the forehead, cheek, hand, lower arm, abdomen, foot, and lower leg. Check a distal area of the limb first (i.e., the hand before the arm and the foot before the leg). **Rationale:** *The sensory nerve may be assumed to be intact if sensation is felt at its most distal part.* • If areas of sensory dysfunction are found, determine the boundaries of sensation by testing responses about every 2.5 cm (1 in.) in the area. Make a sketch of the sensory loss area for recording purposes.	Light tickling or touch sensation ❾ Assessing light-touch sensation.	Loss of sensation (**anesthesia**); more than normal sensation (**hyperesthesia**); less than normal sensation (**hypoesthesia**); or an abnormal sensation such as burning, pain, or an electric shock (**paresthesia**)
16. *Pain Sensation* Assess pain sensation as follows: • Ask the client to close the eyes and to say "sharp," "dull," or "don't know" when the sharp or dull end of a safety pin is felt. • Alternately, use the sharp and dull end to lightly prick designated anatomical areas at random (e.g., hand, forearm, foot, lower leg, abdomen). The face is not tested in this manner. • Allow at least 2 seconds between each test to prevent summation effects of stimuli (i.e., several successive stimuli perceived as one stimulus).	Able to discriminate "sharp" and "dull" sensations	Areas of reduced, heightened, or absent sensation (map them out for recording purposes)

(continued on next page)

SKILL 1.16   Assessing the Neurological System *(continued)*

ASSESSMENT	NORMAL FINDINGS	DEVIATIONS FROM NORMAL
17. *Position or Kinesthetic Sensation:* Commonly, the middle fingers and the large toes are tested for the kinesthetic sensation (sense of position). • To test the fingers, support the client's arm and hand with one hand. To test the toes, place the client's heels on the examining table. • Ask the client to close the eyes. • Grasp a middle finger or a big toe firmly between your thumb and index finger, and exert the same pressure on both sides of the finger or toe while moving it ❿. • Move the finger or toe until it is up, down, or straight out, and ask the client to identify the position. • Use a series of brisk up-and-down movements before bringing the finger or toe suddenly to rest in one of the three positions.	Can readily determine the position of fingers and toes ❿ Position or kinesthetic sensation.	Unable to determine the position of one or more fingers or toes
18. Document findings in the client record using forms or checklists supplemented by narrative notes when appropriate. Describe any abnormal findings in objective terms, for example, "When asked to count backwards by threes, client made seven errors and completed the task in 4 minutes."		

Developmental Considerations

INFANTS

- Reflexes commonly tested in newborns include the following:
  - Rooting: Stroke the side of the face near mouth; infant opens mouth and turns to the side that is stroked.
  - Sucking: Place nipple or finger 3 to 4 cm into mouth; infant sucks vigorously.
  - Tonic neck: Place infant supine, turn head to one side; arm on side to which head is turned extends; on opposite side, arm curls up (fencer's pose).
  - Palmar grasp: Place finger in infant's palm and press; infant curls fingers around.
  - Stepping: Hold infant as if weight bearing on surface; infant steps along, one foot at a time.
  - Moro: Present loud noise or unexpected movement; infant spreads arms and legs, extends fingers, then flexes and brings hands together; may cry.
- Most of these reflexes disappear between 4 and 6 months of age.

CHILDREN

- Present the procedures as games whenever possible.
- Positive Babinski reflex is abnormal after the child ambulates or at age 2.
- For children under age 5, the Denver Developmental Screening Test II provides a comprehensive neurological evaluation—particularly for motor function.
- Note the child's ability to understand and follow directions.
- Assess immediate recall or recent memory by using names of cartoon characters. Normal recall in children is one less than age in years.

- Assess for signs of hyperactivity or abnormally short attention span.
- Children should be able to walk backward by age 2, balance on one foot for 5 seconds by age 4, heel–toe walk by age 5, and heel–toe walk backward by age 6.
- The Romberg test is appropriate over age 3.

OLDER ADULTS

- A full neurological assessment can be lengthy. Conduct in several sessions if indicated, and cease the tests if the client is noticeably fatigued.
- A decline in mental status is not a normal result of aging. Changes are more the result of physical or psychological disorders (e.g., fever, fluid and electrolyte imbalances, medications). Acute, abrupt-onset mental status changes are usually caused by delirium. These changes are often reversible with treatment. Chronic subtle insidious mental health changes are usually caused by dementia and are usually irreversible.
- Intelligence and learning ability are unaltered with age. Many factors, however, inhibit learning (e.g., anxiety, illness, pain, cultural barrier).
- Short-term memory is often less efficient. Long-term memory is usually unaltered.
- Because old age is often associated with loss of support individuals, depression is a common disorder. Mood changes, weight loss, anorexia, constipation, and early morning awakening may be symptoms of depression.
- The stress of being in unfamiliar situations can cause confusion in older adults.
- As an individual ages, reflex responses may become less intense.

SKILL 1.16 Assessing the Neurological System (continued)

- Because older adults tire more easily than younger clients, a total neurological assessment is often done at a different time from the other parts of the physical assessment.
- Although there is a progressive decrease in the number of functioning neurons in the central nervous system and in the sense organs, older adults usually function well because of the abundant reserves in the number of brain cells.
- Impulse transmission and reaction to stimuli are slower.
- Many older adults have some impairment of hearing, vision, smell, temperature and pain sensation, memory, and mental endurance.

- Coordination changes, including a reduced speed of fine finger movements. Standing balance remains intact, and Romberg's test remains negative.
- Reflex responses may slightly increase or decrease. Many show loss of Achilles reflex, and the plantar reflex may be difficult to elicit.
- When testing sensory function, the nurse needs to give older adults time to respond. Normally, older adults have unaltered perception of light touch and superficial pain, decreased perception of deep pain, and decreased perception of temperature stimuli. Many also reveal a decrease or absence of position sense in the large toes.

SKILL 1.17 Assessing the Skull and Face

Delegation

Due to the substantial knowledge and skill required, assessment of the skull and face is not delegated to UAP. However, many aspects of the skull and face are observed during usual care and may be recorded by individuals other than the nurse. Abnormal findings must be validated and interpreted by the nurse.

Procedure

1. Prior to performing the procedure, introduce self and verify the client's identity using agency protocol. Explain to the client what you are going to do, why it is necessary, and how he or she can participate. Discuss how the results will be used in planning further care or treatments.
2. Perform hand hygiene and observe other appropriate infection control procedures.
3. Provide for client privacy.
4. Inquire if the client has any history of the following: past problems with lumps or bumps, itching, scaling, or dandruff; history of loss of consciousness, dizziness, seizures, headache, facial pain, or injury; when and how any lumps occurred; length of time any other problem existed; any known cause of problem; associated symptoms, treatment, and recurrences.

ASSESSMENT	NORMAL FINDINGS	DEVIATIONS FROM NORMAL
5. Inspect the skull for size, shape, and symmetry.	Rounded (normocephalic and symmetric, with frontal, parietal, and occipital prominences); smooth skull contour	Lack of symmetry; increased skull size with more prominent nose and forehead; longer mandible (may indicate excessive growth hormone or increased bone thickness)
6. Inspect the facial features (e.g., symmetry of structures and of the distribution of hair).	Symmetric or slightly asymmetric facial features, palpebral fissures equal in size, symmetric nasolabial folds	Increased facial hair, low hair line, thinning of eyebrows, asymmetric features, exophthalmos, myxedema facies, moon face
7. Inspect the eyes for edema and hollowness.	No edema	Periorbital edema; sunken eyes
8. Note symmetry of facial movements. Ask the client to elevate the eyebrows, frown, or lower the eyebrows, close the eyes tightly, puff the cheeks, and smile and show the teeth.	Symmetric facial movements	Asymmetric facial movements (e.g., eye on affected side cannot close completely); drooping of lower eyelid and mouth; involuntary facial movements (i.e., tics or tremors)
9. Document findings in the client record using forms or checklists supplemented by narrative notes when appropriate.		

Developmental Considerations

INFANTS

- Newborns delivered vaginally can have elongated, molded heads, which take on more rounded shapes after a week or two. Infants born by cesarean section tend to have smooth, rounded heads.

- The posterior fontanel (soft spot) is about 1 cm in size and usually closes by 8 weeks. The anterior fontanel is larger, about 2 to 3 cm in size. It closes by 18 months.
- Newborns can lift their heads slightly and turn them from side to side. Voluntary head control is well established by 4 to 6 months.

SKILL 1.18 Assessing the Eyes and Vision

Delegation

Due to the substantial knowledge and skill required, assessment of the eyes and vision is not delegated to UAP. However, many aspects of eye function are observed during usual care and may be recorded by individuals other than the nurse. Abnormal findings must be validated and interpreted by the nurse.

Equipment

- Millimeter ruler
- Penlight
- Snellen or E chart
- Opaque card

Procedure

1. Prior to performing the procedure, introduce self and verify the client's identity using agency protocol. Explain to the client what you are going to do, why it is necessary, and how he or she can participate. Discuss how the results will be used in planning further care or treatments.
2. Perform hand hygiene and observe other appropriate infection control procedures.
3. Provide for client privacy.
4. Inquire if the client has any history of the following: family history of diabetes, hypertension, blood dyscrasia, or eye disease, injury, or surgery; client's last visit to an ophthalmologist; current use of eye medications; use of contact lenses or eyeglasses; hygienic practices for corrective lenses; current symptoms of eye problems (e.g., changes in visual acuity, blurring of vision, tearing, spots, photophobia, itching, or pain).

ASSESSMENT	NORMAL FINDINGS	DEVIATIONS FROM NORMAL
External Eye Structures		
5. Inspect the eyebrows for hair distribution, alignment, skin quality, and movement (ask client to raise and lower the eyebrows).	Hair evenly distributed; skin intact Eyebrows symmetrically aligned; equal movement	Loss of hair; scaling and flakiness of skin Unequal alignment and movement of eyebrows
6. Inspect the eyelashes for evenness of distribution and direction of curl.	Equally distributed; curled slightly outward	Turned inward
7. Inspect the eyelids for surface characteristics (e.g., skin quality and texture), position in relation to the cornea, ability to blink, and frequency of blinking. Inspect the lower eyelids while the client's eyes are closed.	Skin intact; no discharge; no discoloration Lids close symmetrically Approximately 15 to 20 involuntary blinks per minute; bilateral blinking When lids open, no visible sclera above corneas, and upper and lower borders of cornea are slightly covered	Redness, swelling, flaking, crusting, plaques, discharge, nodules, lesions Lids close asymmetrically, incompletely, or painfully Rapid, monocular, absent, or infrequent blinking Ptosis, ectropion, or entropion; rim of sclera visible between lid and iris
8. Inspect the bulbar conjunctiva (that lying over the sclera) for color, texture, and the presence of lesions.	Transparent; capillaries sometimes evident; sclera appears white (darker or yellowish and with small brown macules in dark-skinned clients)	Jaundiced sclera (e.g., in liver disease); excessively pale sclera (e.g., in anemia); reddened sclera (e.g., marijuana use, rheumatoid disease); lesions or nodules (may indicate damage by mechanical, chemical, allergenic, or bacterial agents)
9. Inspect the cornea for clarity and texture. Ask the client to look straight ahead. Hold a penlight at an oblique angle to the eye, and move the light slowly across the corneal surface.	Transparent, shiny, and smooth; details of the iris are visible In older people, a thin, grayish white ring around the margin, called arcus senilis, may be evident	Opaque; surface not smooth (may be the result of trauma or abrasion) Arcus senilis in clients under age 40
10. Inspect the pupils for color, shape, and symmetry of size. Pupil charts are available in some agencies. See ❶ for variations in pupil diameters.	Black in color; equal in size; normally 3 to 7 mm in diameter; round, smooth border, iris flat and round	Cloudiness, mydriasis, miosis, anisocoria; bulging of iris toward cornea; pupils less than 3 or greater than 7 mm in normal light conditions; unequal pupil size

❶ Variations in pupil diameters in millimeters.

SKILL 1.18   Assessing the Eyes and Vision (continued)

ASSESSMENT	NORMAL FINDINGS	DEVIATIONS FROM NORMAL
11. Assess each pupil's direct and consensual reaction to light to determine the function of the third (oculomotor) cranial nerve. • Partially darken the room. • Ask the client to look straight ahead. • Using a penlight and approaching from the side, shine a light on the pupil. • Observe the response of the illuminated pupil. It should constrict (direct response). • Shine the light on the pupil again, and observe the response of the other pupil. It should also constrict (consensual response).	Illuminated pupil constricts (direct response) Nonilluminated pupil constricts (consensual response)	Neither pupil constricts Unequal responses Absent responses
12. Assess each pupil's reaction to accommodation. • Hold an object (a penlight or pencil) about 10 cm (4 in.) from the bridge of the client's nose. • Ask the client to look first at the top of the object and then at a distant object (e.g., the far wall) behind the penlight. Alternate the gaze from the near to the far object. • Observe the pupil response. The pupils should constrict when looking at the near object and dilate when looking at the far object. • Next, move the penlight or pencil toward the client's nose. The pupils should converge. To record normal assessment of the pupils, use the abbreviation **PERRLA** (pupils equally round and react to light and accommodation).	Pupils constrict when looking at near object; pupils dilate when looking at far object; pupils converge when near object is moved toward nose	One or both pupils fail to constrict, dilate, or converge
Visual Fields		

13. Assess peripheral visual fields to determine function of the retina and neuronal visual pathways to the brain and second (optic) cranial nerve.
• Have the client sit directly facing you at a distance of 60 to 90 cm (2 to 3 ft).
• Ask the client to cover the right eye with a card and look directly at your nose.
• Cover or close your eye directly opposite the client's covered eye (i.e., your left eye), and look directly at the client's nose.
• Hold an object (e.g., a penlight or pencil) in your fingers, extend your arm, and move the object into the visual field from various points in the periphery. The object should be at an equal distance from the client and yourself. Ask the client to tell you when the moving object is first spotted.
  a. To test the temporal field of the left eye, extend and move your right arm in from the client's right periphery.
  b. To test the upward field of the left eye, extend and move the right arm down from the upward periphery.
  c. To test the downward field of the left eye, extend and move the right arm up from the lower periphery.
  d. To test the nasal field of the left eye, extend and move your left arm in from the periphery ❷.
• Repeat the above steps for the right eye, reversing the process.
	When looking straight ahead, client can see objects in the periphery
	Temporally, peripheral objects can be seen at right angles (90 degrees) to the central point of vision
	The upward field of vision is normally 50 degrees because the orbital ridge is in the way
	The downward field of vision is normally 70 degrees because the cheekbone is in the way
	The nasal field of vision is normally 50 degrees away from the central point of vision because the nose is in the way
	
	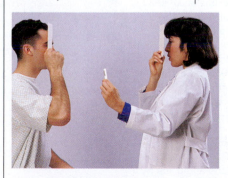
	❷ Assessing the client's left peripheral vision field.
		Visual field smaller than normal (possible glaucoma); one half vision in one of both eyes (possible nerve damage)

(continued on next page)

SKILL 1.18   Assessing the Eyes and Vision (continued)

ASSESSMENT	NORMAL FINDINGS	DEVIATIONS FROM NORMAL
Extraocular Muscle Tests		
14. Assess six ocular movements to determine eye alignment and coordination ❸. These can be performed on clients over 6 months of age. • Stand directly in front of the client and hold the penlight at a comfortable distance, such as 30 cm (1 ft) in front of the client's eyes. • Ask the client to hold the head in a fixed position facing you and to follow the movements of the penlight with the eyes only. • Move the penlight in a slow, orderly manner through the six cardinal fields of gaze, that is, from the center of the eye along the lines of the arrows in and back to the center. • Stop the movement of the penlight periodically so that nystagmus can be detected.	Both eyes coordinated, move in unison, with parallel alignment	Eye movements not coordinated or parallel; one or both eyes fail to follow a penlight in specific directions (e.g., **strabismus** [cross-eye]) **Nystagmus** (rapid involuntary rhythmic eye movement) other than at end point may indicate neurological impairment

❸ The six muscles that govern eye movement.

ASSESSMENT	NORMAL FINDINGS	DEVIATIONS FROM NORMAL
15. Assess for location of light reflex by shining penlight on pupil in corneal surface (Hirschberg test).	Light falls symmetrically on both pupils (e.g., at "6 o'clock" on both pupils)	Light falls off center on one eye (indicates misalignment)
16. Have client fixate on a near or far object. Cover one eye and observe for movement in the uncovered eye (cover test).	Uncovered eye does not move	If misalignment is present, when dominant eye is covered, the uncovered eye will move to focus on object
Visual Acuity		
17. Assess near vision by providing adequate lighting and asking the client to read from a magazine or newspaper held at a distance of 36 cm (14 in.). If the client normally wears corrective lenses, the glasses or lenses should be worn during the test.	Able to read newsprint	Difficulty reading newsprint unless due to aging process
18. Assess distance vision by asking the client to wear corrective lenses, unless they are used for reading only, that is, for distances of only 36 cm (12 to 14 in.). • Ask the client to stand or sit 6 m (20 ft) from a Snellen or character chart ❹, cover the eye not being tested, and identify the letters or characters on the chart. • Take three readings: right eye, left eye, both eyes. • Record the readings of each eye and both eyes (i.e., the smallest line from which the person is able to read one half or more of the letters). At the end of each line of the chart are standardized numbers (fractions). The top line is 20/200. The numerator (top number) is always 20, the distance the person stands from the chart. The denominator (bottom number) is the distance from which the normal eye can read the chart. Therefore, an individual who has 20/40 vision can see at 20 feet from the chart what a normal-sighted person can see at 40 feet from the chart. Visual acuity is recorded as "s̄–c" (without correction), or "c̄–c" (with correction). You can also indicate how many letters were misread in the line, for example, "visual acuity 20/40-2 c̄–c" indicates that two letters were misread in the 20/40 line by a client wearing corrective lenses.	20/20 vision on Snellen-type chart	Denominator of 40 or more on Snellen-type chart with corrective lenses
19. If the client is unable to see even the top line (20/200) of the Snellen-type chart, perform one or more of the following functional vision tests.		Functional vision only (e.g., light perception, hand movements, counting fingers at 30 cm [1 ft])

❹ Testing distance vision.

SKILL 1.18 Assessing the Eyes and Vision (continued)

ASSESSMENT	NORMAL FINDINGS	DEVIATIONS FROM NORMAL
Light Perception		
20. Shine a penlight into the client's eye from a lateral position, and then turn the light off. Ask the client to tell you when the light is on or off.		
Hand Movements		
21. Hold your hand 30 cm (1 ft) from the client's face and move it slowly back and forth, stopping it periodically. Ask the client to tell you when your hand stops moving.		
Counting Fingers		
22. Hold up some of your fingers 30 cm (1 ft) from the client's face, and ask the client to count your fingers.		
23. Document findings in the client record using forms or checklists supplemented by narrative notes when appropriate.		

Developmental Considerations

INFANTS

- Infants 4 weeks of age should gaze at and follow objects.
- Ability to focus with both eyes should be present by 6 months of age.
- Infants do not have tears until about 3 months of age.
- Visual acuity is about 20/300 at 4 months and progressively improves.

CHILDREN

- Epicanthal folds, common in people of Asian heredity, may cover the medial canthus and cause eyes to appear misaligned. Epicanthal folds may also be seen in young children of any race before the bridge of the nose begins to elevate.
- Preschool children's acuity can be checked with picture cards or the E chart. Acuity should approach 20/20 by 6 years of age.
- Always perform the acuity test with glasses on if a child has a prescription to wear lenses.
- Children should be tested for color vision deficit. From 8% to 10% of Caucasian males and from 0.5% to 1% of Caucasian females have this deficit; it is much less common in non-Caucasian children. The Ishihara or Hardy-Rand-Rittler test can be used.

OLDER ADULTS

Visual Acuity

- Visual acuity decreases as the lens of the eye ages and becomes more opaque and loses elasticity.
- The ability of the iris to accommodate to darkness and dim light diminishes.
- Peripheral vision diminishes.
- The adaptation to light (glare) and dark decreases.
- Accommodation to far objects often improves, but accommodation to near objects decreases.
- Color vision declines; older people are less able to perceive purple colors and to discriminate pastel colors.

- Many older adults wear corrective lenses; they are most likely to have hyperopia. Visual changes are due to loss of elasticity (presbyopia) and diminishing transparency of the lens.

External Eye Structures

- The skin around the orbit of the eye may darken.
- The eyeball may appear sunken because of the decrease in orbital fat.
- Skinfolds of the upper lids may seem more prominent, and the lower lids may sag.
- The eyes may appear dry and dull because of the decrease in tear production from the lacrimal glands.
- A thin, grayish white arc or ring (arcus senilis) appears around part or all of the cornea. It results from an accumulation of a lipid substance on the cornea. The cornea tends to cloud with age.
- The iris may appear pale with brown discolorations as a result of pigment degeneration.
- The conjunctiva of the eye may appear paler than that of younger adults and may take on a slightly yellow appearance because of the deposition of fat.
- Pupil reaction to light and accommodation is normally symmetrically equal but may be less brisk.
- The pupils can appear smaller in size, unequal, and irregular in shape because of sclerotic changes in the iris.

Setting of Care

- When making a home visit, take your equipment and charts with you. Also include a tape measure to lay out the 20 feet for distance vision testing.
- Use the assessment as an opportunity to reinforce proper eye care and the need for regular vision testing.

SKILL 1.19 **Assessing Visual Acuity**

Vision acuity screening should begin at about 3 years of age, when the child can cooperate with the procedure. Several procedures may be used to screen visual acuity in children.

Most states have laws regulating the ages or grades at which children must have vision screening performed, and what passing standards are accepted. Check your state laws or codes for guidelines.

VARIATION: SNELLEN LETTER CHART

The Snellen letter (alphabet) chart is the most commonly used assessment tool for visual acuity. It consists of lines of letters in decreasing size ❶.

- Most charts are designed for reading from a distance of 20 feet. When the child reads the line designated "20 feet" while standing 20 feet away, vision is 20/20. If, however, the child can only read the line labeled "40 feet" while standing 20 feet away, vision is 20/40.
- Charts are also available that can be used at a distance of 10 feet. A child who stands 10 feet from this chart and reads the 10-foot line (10/10) has vision equivalent to that of 20/20 when using the 20-foot chart.

VARIATION: HOTV, SNELLENE, OR PICTURE CHART

For toddlers and children who have not yet mastered the alphabet, the HOTV, Snellen E, or picture chart may be used, positioned either 10 or 20 feet away, matching the guidelines on the chart.

- The HOTV test uses a chart with the letters H, O, T, and V used in random order on lines in decreasing size. The child either names the letters or points to them on a card held close by. The procedure followed is the same as with the Snellen test, but because children can point to the letters on the chart in front of

them, they do not need to know the alphabet. The HOTV test can also be used, after a practice session, with children who do not speak English.

- In the Snellen E chart, the capital letter E is shown facing in different directions. The child is asked to point in the direction of the "legs" of the E. Another option is to give the child a paper with an E on it and have the child turn it in the direction the E is pointing on the chart.
- The Lea Symbols are commonly identified simple pictures (e.g., heart, square, circle, house). The child is asked to identify the pictures or point to the picture on a card held close by.

Preparation

- The procedure is explained to the child and parent. With a young child, make a game of identifying the letter, direction of the E, or the picture. Practice with the child before starting, providing positive feedback for correct responses. **Rationale:** *This ensures that the child understands the directions for the test to improve the chances of an accurate screening test result.*
- Place the chart at the child's eye level and ensure that it is well lit.

Equipment

- Screening chart
- Card or other item to cover one eye
- Card with HOTV letters, E, or Lea Symbols

Procedure

1. Place the heels of the child at the 20-foot mark (or 10-foot mark if using that chart).

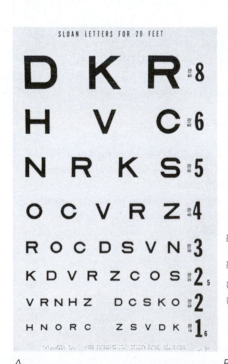

A

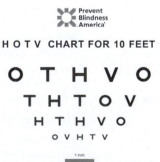

B

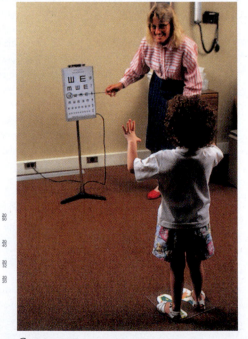

C

❶ Visual acuity charts. *A*, Snellen letter chart; *B*, HOTV chart; *C*, Snellen E chart. (*A* and *B* courtesy of the National Society to Prevent Blindness.)

SKILL 1.19   Assessing Visual Acuity (continued)

2. Assess each eye separately and then both together. If the child wears glasses, check the vision both with and without glasses. If the child is wearing contacts, leave them in and note that the results were taken with contacts in place. **Rationale:** *It is important to detect significant differences in visual acuity of the eyes of children under 5 years of age. When one eye has poorer vision than the other, the brain may decide to stop using the eye with poor vision, leading to further vision deterioration. Corrective lenses are required to enable the child to use both eyes and to preserve vision.*

3. While one eye is being tested, use the child's hand, a patch, or a piece of cardboard to cover the other eye. Tell the child to keep the covered eye open during the testing. Use a different eye cover for each child to minimize the spread of infection among children.

4. Observe for squinting, moving the head forward (to be closer to the chart), excessive blinking, or tearing during the exami-

nation. **Rationale:** *These may be signs that the child has a vision problem.*

5. Document the last line the child can read correctly (i.e., the smallest line on which the child reads at least three of five symbols). Refer the child to the pediatrician or other health-care provider (e.g., ophthalmologist or optometrist) if the following findings are noted (American Academy of Ophthalmology, 2012):
   - Age 3 to 4 years—20/50 or less in either eye
   - Age 4 to 5 years—20/40 or less in either eye
   - After age 5 years—20/30 or less in each eye
   - A difference in vision between the eyes of two lines or more on the eye chart, for example, 20/20 in one eye and 20/40 in the other eye, even when one eye is within the expected range.

SKILL 1.20   Assessing the Ears and Hearing

Delegation

Assessment of the ears and hearing is not delegated to UAP. However, many aspects of ear function are observed during usual care and may be recorded by individuals other than the nurse. Abnormal findings must be validated and interpreted by the nurse.

Equipment

- Otoscope with several sizes of ear specula

Procedure

1. Prior to performing the procedure, introduce self and verify the client's identity using agency protocol. Explain to the

client what you are going to do, why it is necessary, and how he or she can participate. Discuss how the results will be used in planning further care or treatments.

2. Perform hand hygiene and observe other appropriate infection control procedures.

3. Provide for client privacy.

4. Inquire if the client has any history of the following: family history of hearing problems or loss; presence of ear problems or pain; medication history, especially if there are complaints of ringing in ears (tinnitus); hearing difficulty (its onset, factors contributing to it, and how it interferes with activities of daily living); use of a corrective hearing device (when and from whom it was obtained).

5. Position the client comfortably, seated if possible.

ASSESSMENT	NORMAL FINDINGS	DEVIATIONS FROM NORMAL
Auricles		
6. Inspect the auricles for color, symmetry of size, and position. To inspect position, note the level at which the superior aspect of the auricle attaches to the head in relation to the eye.	Color same as facial skin Symmetrical Auricle aligned with outer canthus of eye, about 10° from vertical ❶.	Bluish color of earlobes (e.g., cyanosis); pallor (e.g., frostbite); excessive redness (inflammation or fever) Asymmetry Low-set ears (associated with a congenital abnormality, such as Down syndrome)

Normal alignment

Low-set ears and deviation in alignment

❶ Alignment of ears.

(continued on next page)

SKILL 1.20 Assessing the Ears and Hearing (continued)

ASSESSMENT	NORMAL FINDINGS	DEVIATIONS FROM NORMAL
7. Palpate the auricles for texture, elasticity, and areas of tenderness. • Gently pull the auricle upward, down-ward, and backward. • Fold the pinna forward (it should recoil). • Push in on the tragus. • Apply pressure to the mastoid process.	Mobile, firm, and not tender; pinna recoils after it is folded	Lesions (e.g., cysts); flaky, scaly skin (e.g., seborrhea); tenderness when moved or pressed (may indicate inflammation or infection of external ear)

External Ear Canal and Tympanic Membrane

ASSESSMENT	NORMAL FINDINGS	DEVIATIONS FROM NORMAL
8. Inspect the external ear canal for cerumen, skin lesions, pus, and blood.	Distal third contains hair follicles and glands Dry cerumen, grayish-tan color; or sticky, wet cerumen in various shades of brown	Redness and discharge Scaling Excessive cerumen obstructing canal
9. Visualize the tympanic membrane using an otoscope. • Attach a speculum to the otoscope. Use the largest diameter that will fit the ear canal without causing discomfort. **Rationale:** *This achieves maximum vision of the entire ear canal and tympanic membrane.* • Tip the client's head away from you, and straighten the ear canal. For an adult, straighten the ear canal by pulling the pinna up and back. **Rationale:** *Straightening the ear canal facilitates vision of the ear canal and the tympanic membrane.* • Hold the otoscope either (a) right side up, with your fingers between the otoscope handle and the client's head, or (b) upside down, with your fingers and the ulnar surface of your hand against the client's head ❷. **Rationale:** *These positions stabilize the head and protect the eardrum and canal from injury if a quick head movement occurs.* • Gently insert the tip of the otoscope into the ear canal, avoiding pressure by the speculum against either side of the ear canal. **Rationale:** *The inner two thirds of the ear canal is bony; if the speculum is pressed against either side, the client will experience discomfort.*	❷ Inserting an otoscope.	
Inspect the tympanic membrane for color and gloss.	Pearly gray color, semitransparent ❸ 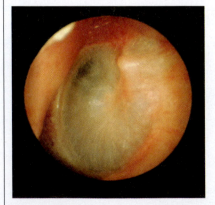 ❸ Normal tympanic membrane. (CRNI/Science Source)	Pink to red, some opacity Yellow-amber White Blue or deep red Dull surface

SKILL 1.20   Assessing the Ears and Hearing (*continued*)

ASSESSMENT	NORMAL FINDINGS	DEVIATIONS FROM NORMAL
Gross Hearing Acuity Tests		
10. Assess client's response to normal voice tones. If client has difficulty hearing the normal voice, proceed with the following tests.	Normal voice tones audible	Normal voice tones not audible (e.g., requests nurse to repeat words or statements, leans toward the speaker, turns the head, cups the ears, or speaks in loud tone of voice)
10A. *Watch tick test.* Perform the watch tick test. The ticking of a watch has a higher pitch than the human voice. • Have the client occlude one ear. Out of the client's sight, place a ticking watch 2 to 3 cm (1 to 2 in.) from the unoccluded ear. • Ask what the client can hear. • Repeat with the other ear.	Able to hear ticking in both ears	Unable to hear ticking in one or both ears
10B. *Tuning fork tests.* Perform Weber's test to assess bone conduction by examining the lateralization (sideward transmission) of sounds. • Hold the tuning fork at its base. Activate it by tapping the fork gently against the back of your hand near the knuckles or by stroking the fork between your thumb and index fingers. It should be made to ring softly. • Place the base of the vibrating fork on top of the client's head ❹ and ask where the client hears the noise. • Hold the handle of the activated tuning fork on the mastoid process of one ear ❺ A until the client states that the vibration can no longer be heard. • Immediately hold the still vibrating fork prongs in front of the client's ear canal. Push aside the client's hair if necessary. Ask whether the client now hears the sound. Sound conducted by air is heard more readily than sound conducted by bone. The tuning fork vibrations conducted by air are normally heard longer.	Sound is heard in both ears or is localized at the center of the head (Weber negative) Air-conducted (AC) hearing is greater than bone-conducted (BC) hearing, that is, AC > BC (positive Rinne)	Sound is heard better in impaired ear, indicating a bone-conductive hearing loss; or sound is heard better in ear without a problem, indicating a sensorineural disturbance (Weber positive) Bone conduction time is equal to or longer than the air conduction time, that is, BC > AC or BC = AC (negative Rinne; indicates a conductive hearing loss) *A* *B*
11. Document findings in the client record using forms or checklists supplemented by narrative notes when appropriate.	❹ Placing the base of the tuning fork on the client's skull (Weber's test).	❺ Rinne test tuning fork placement: A, Base of the tuning fork on the mastoid process; B, tuning fork prongs placed in front of the client's ear.

VARIATION: POSITIONING A CHILD FOR AN OTOSCOPIC EXAMINATION

■ If the parent is present, discuss the parent's role (e.g., holding the child or providing distraction or comfort during the procedure).

■ Make sure the person positioning and holding the child (parent or other assistant) clearly understands what body parts must be held still and how to do this safely.

For Supine Position

1. Place the child in a supine position on a bed or stretcher. Have the parent, a nurse, or an assistant lean over the child to position and hold the child's arms and body. The assistant may also assist with stabilizing the child's head.

(*continued on next page*)

SKILL 1.20 Assessing the Ears and Hearing (continued)

2. Hold the otoscope in the hand closest to the child's face. When the child is cooperative, rest the back of your hand against the child's head. **Rationale:** *This action provides additional stabilization of the child's head to prevent pain and injury when the otoscope earpiece is inserted into the auditory canal.*

3. Use your other hand to pull the pinna toward the back of the head and either up or down.

For Sitting Position

1. Have the child sit on the parent's or assistant's lap with his or her legs held firmly between the assistant's legs. The child's arms can be wrapped around the parent's or assistant's waist.

2. Have the parent or assistant hold the child's head firmly against the chest with one arm while the other arm holds the arms and upper chest. **Rationale:** *This position provides comfort to the child while securing the head.*

VARIATION: ASSESSING HEARING ACUITY IN CHILDREN

Performance of a hearing acuity screening is important to ensure that the child is able to hear so that speech and language development can occur. Newborn and infant hearing screening is performed using evoked otoacoustic emission and auditory brainstem response. Several procedures may be used to screen hearing acuity in children. Various conditions during childhood, such as frequent ear infections, could result in a hearing loss.

Pure Tone Audiometry

Equipment

- Calibrated audiometer
- Scoring sheet
- Alcohol swabs

Preparation

- When screening a large group of children, such as in a school, the machine may be taken to the classroom for demonstration and practice.
- Check the transmission of sound to be sure both earphones work properly.
- Explain the procedure in terms the child can understand. Show the earphones. Turn the sound loud enough for the child to hear and practice raising a hand or putting a block in a basket in response to the sound, which will improve test accuracy.
- If a soundproof room is not available, the audiometer should be set up in a quiet environment. **Rationale:** *It is important to reduce exposure to other sources of sound that could interfere with the child's response to the audiometer's sounds.*
- Clean the earphones with alcohol swabs between children. **Rationale:** *This practice removes most microorganisms for infection control between children.*

Procedure

1. Position the child so that his or her back is toward the machine and faced away from the tester. **Rationale:** *This position ensures that the child cannot see the examiner press the lever to present the sound, and cannot receive visual cues from the examiner's face when the sound is presented.*

2. Place the headset on the child's head and adjust for a proper fit. Note the right and left indicators on the earphones.

3. Follow directions for using the audiometer. Deliver sounds and watch for the child to raise a hand or put a block in a basket when heard. The sound cue is given to the child using a random order when testing the ears. **Rationale:** *A random order ensures that the child cannot anticipate the sound and potentially cause an inaccurate interpretation of the screening test.*

4. Test each ear at the following pitches: 500, 1,000, 2,000, and 4,000 Hz at increasing levels of loudness (decibels).

CLINICAL ALERT

The sounds of the audiometer are delivered at hertz levels, or the frequency of sound in cycles per second. Lower numbers indicate lower sounds, such as speech tones. Higher numbers indicate higher sounds, such as those heard in music. The decibels (loudness of the sounds) can also be controlled by the audiometer.

6. If the child does not pass the screening with both ears (**Table 1–8** ●), retest the child in 2 weeks. If the child still does not pass, refer for further evaluation. **Rationale:** *The child with an upper respiratory infection may not hear well and needs time for the infection to improve.* Continued failure of the screening may indicate a hearing problem.

7. Document the results of the hearing test.

Tympanometry

Tympanometry provides an estimate of middle ear pressure and an indirect measure of tympanic membrane compliance (movement). Older infants and children can be tested. Abnormal findings often indicate fluid accumulation in the middle ear that prevents the efficient transmission of sound to the inner ear. This can result in hearing loss over time.

Equipment

- Calibrated tympanometer
- Disposable earpiece
- Graph paper

Procedure

- Encourage the child to hold still during the test. The infant and young child may need assistance in holding still. **Rationale:** *Lack of movement reduces the chance of pain or injury from the earpiece in the auditory canal.*
- Gently insert the earpiece with the tympanometer probe into the auditory canal until the canal is sealed and airtight. **Rationale:** *The canal must be sealed tight to get an accurate measurement of the pressure it takes to move the tympanic membrane.*

TABLE 1–8 Passing Standards for Hearing Acuity with Pure Tone Audiometer

HERTZ	DECIBELS
500	20–25
1,000	20–25
2,000	20–25
4,000	25

SKILL 1.20   Assessing the Ears and Hearing (continued)

- Turn on the tympanometer according to manufacturer instructions and emit the tone. The pressure is measured by the probe and plots it on a graph ❻.

- Repeat the procedure in the other ear.
- Place the printout in the child's medical record and document the results of the test.

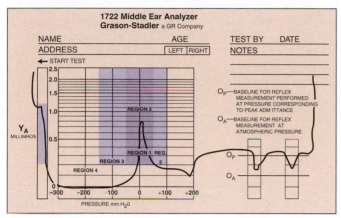

A

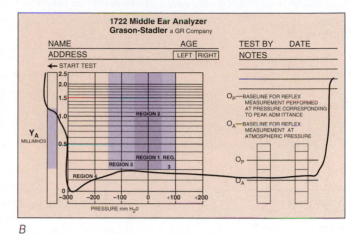

B

❻ A, This tympanogram demonstrates normal hearing as evidenced by the curve showing the tympanic membrane's movement when a sound wave is emitted into the ear canal. Mobility is between 0.2 and 1 mL, the normal range. B, In contrast, note the flat pattern in the second tympanogram, which shows very restricted mobility of the tympanic membrane in response to sound.

Developmental Considerations

INFANTS

- To assess gross hearing, ring a bell from behind the infant or have the parent call the child's name to check for a response. Newborns will quiet to the sound and may open their eyes wider. By 3 to 4 months of age, the child will turn head and eyes toward the sound.
- All newborns should have their hearing assessed using auditory brain response testing prior to discharge from the hospital.

CHILDREN

- To inspect the external canal and tympanic membrane in children less than 3 years old, pull the pinna down and back. Insert the otoscopic speculum only ¼ to ½ inch.
- Perform routine hearing checks and follow up on abnormal results. In addition to congenital or infection-related causes of hearing loss, noise-induced hearing loss is becoming more common in adolescents and young adults as a result of exposure to loud music and prolonged use of headsets at loud volumes (Daniel, 2007). Teach that music loud enough to prevent hearing a normal conversation can damage hearing.
- With pure tone audiometry, if the young child does not seem to understand what to do once screening begins, remove the headphones and practice more. Have blocks ready and instruct the child to place a block in a basket when hearing the sound. Turn up the decibel level slightly and practice until the child understands. Then turn the decibel level back to the appropriate screening level.

OLDER ADULTS

- The skin of the ear may appear dry and be less resilient because of the loss of connective tissue.
- Increased coarse and wire-like hair growth occurs along the helix, antihelix, and tragus.
- The pinna increases in both width and length, and the earlobe elongates.
- Earwax is drier.
- The tympanic membrane is more translucent and less flexible. The intensity of the light reflex may diminish slightly.
- Sensorineural hearing loss occurs.
- Generalized hearing loss (presbycusis) occurs in all frequencies, although the first symptom is the loss of high-frequency sounds: the *f*, *s*, *sh*, and *ph* sounds. To such individuals, conversation can be distorted and result in what appears to be inappropriate or confused behavior.

Setting of Care

- Ensure that the examination is conducted in a quiet place. In particular, older adults will have difficulty accurately reporting results of hearing tests if there is excessive outside noise.
- If necessary, ask the adult present with an infant or child to assist in holding the child still during the examination.
- Each state has specific laws mandating when children attending school should be screened for hearing acuity, and the hertz and decibel levels to be included. Consult your state school code for guidance about local requirements.

SKILL 1.21   Assessing the Nose and Sinuses

Delegation

Assessment of the nose and sinuses is not delegated to UAP. However, many aspects of nasal function are observed during usual care and may be recorded by individuals other than the nurse. Abnormal findings must be validated and interpreted by the nurse.

Equipment

- Nasal speculum
- Flashlight/penlight

Procedure

1. Prior to performing the procedure, introduce self and verify the client's identity using agency protocol. Explain to the client what you are going to do, why it is necessary, and how he or she can participate. Discuss how the results will be used in planning further care or treatments.
2. Perform hand hygiene and observe other appropriate infection control procedures.
3. Provide for client privacy.
4. Inquire if the client has any history of the following: allergies, difficulty breathing through the nose, sinus infections, injuries to nose or face, nosebleeds; medications taken; changes in sense of smell.
5. Position the client comfortably, seated if possible.

ASSESSMENT	NORMAL FINDINGS	DEVIATIONS FROM NORMAL
Nose		
6. Inspect the external nose for any deviations in shape, size, or color and flaring or discharge from the nares.	Symmetric and straight No discharge or flaring Uniform color	Asymmetric Discharge from nares Localized areas of redness or presence of skin lesions
7. Lightly palpate the external nose to determine any areas of tenderness, masses, and displacements of bone and cartilage.	Not tender; no lesions	Tenderness on palpation; presence of lesions
8. Determine patency of both nasal cavities. Ask the client to close the mouth, exert pressure on one naris, and breathe through the opposite naris. Repeat the procedure to assess patency of the opposite naris.	Air moves freely as the client breathes through the nares	Air movement is restricted in one or both nares
9. Inspect the nasal cavities using a flashlight or a nasal speculum. • Hold the speculum in your right hand to inspect the client's left nostril and in your left hand to inspect the client's right nostril. • Tip the client's head back. • Facing the client, insert the tip of the closed speculum (blades together) about 1 cm or up to the point at which the blade widens. Care must be taken to avoid pressure on the sensitive nasal septum ❶. • Stabilize the speculum with your index finger against the side of the nose. Use the other hand to position the head and then to hold the light. • Open the speculum as much as possible and inspect the floor of the nose (vestibule), the anterior portion of the septum, the middle meatus, and the middle turbinates. The posterior turbinate is rarely visualized because of its position ❷. • Inspect the lining of the nares and the integrity and the position of the nasal septum.	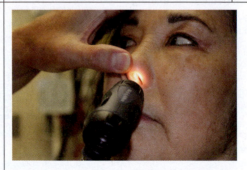 ❶ Using a nasal speculum to inspect the nasal passages. 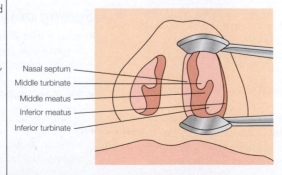 Nasal septum Middle turbinate Middle meatus Inferior meatus Inferior turbinate ❷ The inferior and middle turbinates of the nasal passage.	

SKILL 1.21 Assessing the Nose and Sinuses (continued)

ASSESSMENT	NORMAL FINDINGS	DEVIATIONS FROM NORMAL
10. Observe for the presence of redness, swelling, growths, and discharge.	Mucosa pink Clear, watery discharge No lesions	Mucosa red, edematous Abnormal discharge (e.g., pus) Presence of lesions (e.g., polys)
11. Inspect the nasal septum between the nasal chambers.	Nasal septum intact and in midline	Septum deviated to the right or to the left or septum eroded
Facial Sinuses		
12. Palpate the maxillary and frontal sinuses for tenderness.	Not tender	Tenderness in one or more sinuses
13. Document findings in the client record using forms or checklists supplemented by narrative notes when appropriate.		

Developmental Considerations

INFANTS

- A speculum is usually not necessary to examine the septum, turbinates, and vestibule. Instead, push the tip of the nose upward with the thumb and shine a light into the nares.
- Ethmoid and maxillary sinuses are present at birth; frontal sinuses begin to develop by 1 to 2 years of age; and sphenoid sinuses develop later in childhood. Infants and young children have fewer sinus problems than older children and adolescents.

CHILDREN

- A speculum is usually not necessary to examine the septum, turbinates, and vestibule, and it might cause the child to be apprehensive. Instead, push the tip of the nose upward with the thumb and shine a light into the nares.

- Ethmoid sinuses continue to develop until age 12. Sinus problems in children under this age are rare.
- Cough and runny nose are the most common signs of sinusitis in preadolescent children.
- Adolescents may have headaches, facial tenderness, and swelling, similar to the signs seen in adults.

OLDER ADULTS

- The sense of smell markedly diminishes because of a decrease in the number of olfactory nerve fibers and atrophy of the remaining fibers. Older adults are less able to identify and discriminate odors.
- Nosebleeds may result from hypertensive disease or other arterial vessel changes.

SKILL 1.22 Assessing the Mouth and Oropharynx

Delegation

Assessment of the mouth and oropharynx is not delegated to UAP. However, many aspects of mouth function are observed during usual care and may be recorded by individuals other than the nurse. Abnormal findings must be validated and interpreted by the nurse.

Equipment

- Clean gloves
- Tongue depressor
- 2 × 2 gauze pads
- Penlight

Procedure

1. Prior to performing the procedure, introduce self and verify the client's identity using agency protocol. Explain to the client what you are going to do, why it is necessary, and how he or she can participate. Discuss how the results will be used in planning further care or treatments.
2. Perform hand hygiene and observe other appropriate infection control procedures.
3. Provide for client privacy.
4. Inquire if the client has any history of the following: routine pattern of dental care, last visit to dentist; length of time ulcers or other lesions have been present; denture discomfort; medications client is receiving.
5. Position the client comfortably, seated if possible.

ASSESSMENT	NORMAL FINDINGS	DEVIATIONS FROM NORMAL
Lips and Buccal Mucosa		
6. Inspect the outer lips for symmetry of contour, color, and texture. Ask the client to purse the lips as if to whistle.	Uniform pink color (darker, e.g., bluish hue, in Mediterranean groups and dark-skinned clients) Soft, moist, smooth texture Symmetry of contour Ability to purse lips	Pallor; cyanosis Blisters; generalized or localized swelling; fissures, crusts, or scales (may result from excessive moisture, nutritional deficiency, or fluid deficit) Inability to purse lips (may indicate facial nerve damage)

(continued on next page)

SKILL 1.22 **Assessing the Mouth and Oropharynx** (*continued*)

ASSESSMENT	NORMAL FINDINGS	DEVIATIONS FROM NORMAL
7. Inspect the inner lips and buccal mucosa for color, moisture, texture, and the presence of lesions. • Apply clean gloves. • Ask the client to relax the mouth, and, for better visualization, pull the lip outward and away from the teeth. • Grasp the lip on each side between the thumb and index finger ❶. 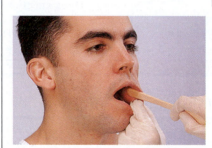 ❶ Inspecting the mucosa of the lower lip.	Uniform pink color (freckled brown pigmentation in dark-skinned clients) Moist, smooth, soft, glistening, and elastic texture (drier oral mucosa in older adults due to decreased salivation)	Pallor; leukoplakia (white patches), red, bleeding Excessive dryness Mucosal cysts; irritations from dentures; abrasions, ulcerations; nodules
Teeth and Gums		
8. Inspect the teeth and gums while examining the inner lips and buccal mucosa. • Ask the client to open the mouth. Using a tongue depressor, retract the cheek ❷. View the surface buccal mucosa from top to bottom and back to front. A flashlight or penlight will help illuminate the surface. Repeat the procedure for the other side. • Examine the back teeth. For proper vision of the molars, use the index fingers of both hands to retract the cheek ❸. Ask the client to relax the lips and first close, then open, the jaw. **Rationale:** *Closing the jaw assists in observation of tooth alignment and loss of teeth; opening the jaw assists in observation of dental fillings and caries.* Observe the number of teeth, tooth color, the state of fillings, dental caries, and tartar along the base of the teeth. Note the presence and fit of partial or complete dentures. • Inspect the gums around the molars. Observe for bleeding, color, retraction (pulling away from the teeth), edema, and lesions.	Thirty-two adult teeth Smooth, white, shiny tooth enamel Pink gums (bluish or brown patches in dark-skinned clients) Moist, firm texture to gums No retraction of gums (pulling away from the teeth) 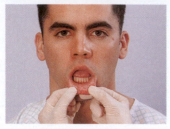 ❷ Inspecting the buccal mucosa using a tongue depressor.	Missing teeth; ill-fitting dentures Brown or black discoloration of the enamel (may indicate staining or the presence of caries) Excessively red gums Spongy texture; bleeding; tenderness (may indicate periodontal disease) Receding, atrophied gums; swelling that partially covers the teeth 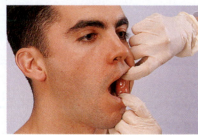 ❸ Inspecting the back teeth.
9. Inspect the dentures. Ask the client to remove complete or partial dentures. Inspect their condition, noting in particular broken or worn areas.	Smooth, intact dentures	Ill-fitting dentures; irritated and excoriated area under dentures
Tongue/Floor of the Mouth		
10. Inspect the surface of the tongue for position, color, and texture. Ask the client to protrude the tongue.	Central position Pink color (some brown pigmentation on tongue borders in dark-skinned clients); moist; slightly rough; thin whitish coating Smooth, lateral margins; no lesions Raised papillae (taste buds)	Deviated from center (may indicate damage to hypoglossal [12th cranial] nerve); excessive trembling Smooth red tongue (may indicate iron, vitamin B_{12}, or vitamin B_3 deficiency) Dry, furry tongue (associated with fluid deficit), white coating (may be oral yeast infection) Nodes, ulcerations, discolorations (white or red areas); areas of tenderness

SKILL 1.22   Assessing the Mouth and Oropharynx *(continued)*

ASSESSMENT	NORMAL FINDINGS	DEVIATIONS FROM NORMAL
11. Inspect tongue movement. Ask the client to roll the tongue upward and move it from side to side.	Moves freely; no tenderness	Restricted mobility
12. Inspect the base of the tongue, the mouth floor, and the frenulum. Ask the client to place the tip of the tongue against the roof of the mouth.	Smooth tongue base with prominent veins	Swelling, ulceration
Palates and Uvula		
13. Inspect the hard and soft palate for color, shape, texture, and the presence of bony prominences. Ask the client to open the mouth wide and tilt the head backward. Then, depress tongue with a tongue depressor as necessary, and use a penlight for appropriate visualization.	Light pink, smooth, soft palate Lighter pink hard palate, more irregular texture	Discoloration (e.g., jaundice or pallor) Palates the same color Irritations Exostoses (bony growths) growing from the hard palate
14. Inspect the uvula for position and mobility while examining the palates. To observe the uvula, ask the client to say "ah" so that the soft palate rises.	Positioned in midline of soft palate	Deviation to one side from tumor or trauma; immobility (may indicate damage to trigeminal [5th cranial] nerve or vagus [10th cranial] nerve)
Oropharynx and Tonsils		
15. Inspect the oropharynx for color and texture. Inspect one side at a time to avoid eliciting the gag reflex. To expose one side of the oropharynx, press a tongue depressor against the tongue on the same side about halfway back while the client tilts the head back and opens the mouth wide. Use a penlight for illumination, if needed.	Pink and smooth posterior wall	Reddened or edematous; presence of lesions, plaques, or drainage
16. Inspect the tonsils (behind the fauces [throat]) for color, discharge, and size.	Pink and smooth No discharge	Inflamed Presence of discharge
17. Remove and discard gloves. Perform hand hygiene.	Of normal size or not visible	Swollen
18. Document findings in the client record using forms or checklists supplemented by narrative notes when appropriate.	• *Grade 1 (normal):* The tonsils are behind the tonsillar pillars (the soft structures supporting the soft palate).	• *Grade 2:* The tonsils are between the pillars and the uvula. • *Grade 3:* The tonsils touch the uvula. • *Grade 4:* One or both tonsils extend to the midline of the oropharynx.

Client Teaching

■ Although clients may be sensitive to discussion of their personal hygiene practices, use the assessment as an opportunity to provide teaching regarding appropriate oral and dental care for the entire family. Refer clients to a dentist if indicated.

Developmental Considerations

INFANTS

■ Inspect the palate and uvula for a cleft. A bifid (forked) uvula may indicate an undetected cleft palate (i.e., a cleft in the cartilage that is covered by skin).

■ Newborns may have a pearly white nodule on their gums, which resolves without treatment.

■ The first teeth erupt at about 6 to 7 months of age. Assess for dental hygiene; parents should cleanse the infant's teeth daily with a soft cloth or soft toothbrush.

■ Fluoride supplements should be given by 6 months if the child's drinking water contains less than 0.3 part per million (ppm) fluoride.

■ Children should see a dentist by 1 year of age.

(continued on next page)

SKILL 1.22   Assessing the Mouth and Oropharynx *(continued)*

CHILDREN

- Tooth development should be appropriate for age.
- White spots on the teeth may indicate excessive fluoride ingestion.
- Drooling is common up to 2 years of age.
- The tonsils are normally larger in children than in adults and commonly extend beyond the palatine arch until the age of 11 or 12 years.

OLDER ADULTS

- The oral mucosa may be drier than that of younger individuals because of decreased salivary gland activity. Decreased salivation occurs in older adults taking prescribed medications such as antidepressants, antihistamines, decongestants, diuretics, antihypertensives, tranquilizers, antispasmodics, and antineoplastics. Extreme dryness is associated with dehydration.
- Some receding of the gums occurs, giving an appearance of increased toothiness.

- Taste sensations diminish. Sweet and salty tastes are lost first. Older adults may add more salt and sugar to food than they did when they were younger. Diminished taste sensation is due to atrophy of the taste buds and a decreased sense of smell. It indicates diminished function of the fifth and seventh cranial nerves.
- Tiny purple or bluish black swollen areas (varicosities) under the tongue, known as caviar spots, are not uncommon.
- The teeth may show signs of staining, erosion, chipping, and abrasions due to loss of dentin.
- Tooth loss occurs as a result of dental disease but is preventable with good dental hygiene.
- The gag reflex may be slightly sluggish.
- Older adults who are homebound or are in long-term care facilities often have teeth or dentures in need of repair, due to the difficulty of obtaining dental care in these situations. Do a thorough assessment of missing teeth and those in need of repair, whether they are natural teeth or dentures.

SKILL 1.23   Assessing the Neck

Delegation

Assessment of the neck is not delegated to UAP. However, many aspects of the neck are observed during usual care and may be recorded by individuals other than the nurse. Abnormal findings must be validated and interpreted by the nurse.

Procedure

1. Prior to performing the procedure, introduce self and verify the client's identity using agency protocol. Explain to the client what you are going to do, why it is necessary, and how he or she can participate. Discuss how the results will be used in planning further care or treatments.
2. Perform hand hygiene and observe other appropriate infection control procedures.
3. Provide for client privacy.
4. Inquire if the client has any history of the following: problems with neck lumps; neck pain or stiffness; when and how any lumps occurred; previous diagnoses of thyroid problems; and other treatments provided (e.g., surgery, radiation).

ASSESSMENT	NORMAL FINDINGS	DEVIATIONS FROM NORMAL
Neck Muscles		
5. Inspect the neck muscles (sternocleidomastoid and trapezius) for abnormal swellings or masses. Ask the client to hold the head erect.	Muscles equal in size; head centered	Unilateral neck swelling; head tilted to one side (indicates presence of masses, injury, muscle weakness, shortening of sternocleidomastoid muscle, scars)
6. Observe head movement. Ask client to: • Move the chin to the chest. **Rationale:** *This determines function of the sternocleidomastoid muscle.* • Move the head back so that the chin points upward. **Rationale:** *This determines function of the trapezius muscle.* • Move the head so that the ear is moved toward the shoulder on each side. **Rationale:** *This determines function of the sternocleidomastoid muscle.* • Turn the head to the right and to the left. **Rationale:** *This determines function of the sternocleidomastoid muscle.*	Coordinated, smooth movements with no discomfort Head flexes 45° Head hyperextends 60° Head laterally flexes 40° Head laterally rotates 70°	Muscle tremor, spasm, or stiffness Limited range of motion; painful movements; involuntary movements (e.g., up-and-down nodding movements associated with Parkinson's disease) Head hyperextends less than 60° Head laterally flexes less than 40° Head laterally rotates less than 70°

SKILL 1.23   Assessing the Neck (*continued*)

ASSESSMENT	NORMAL FINDINGS	DEVIATIONS FROM NORMAL
7. Assess muscle strength. • Ask the client to turn the head to one side against the resistance of your hand. Repeat with the other side. **Rationale:** *This determines the strength of the sternocleidomastoid muscle.* • Ask the client to shrug the shoulders against the resistance of your hands. **Rationale:** *This determines the strength of the trapezius muscles.*	Equal strength Equal strength	Unequal strength Unequal strength
Lymph Nodes		
8. Palpate the entire neck for enlarged lymph nodes. • Face the client, and bend the client's head forward slightly or toward the side being examined. **Rationale:** *This relaxes the soft tissue and muscles.* • Palpate the nodes using the pads of the fingers. Move the fingertips in a gentle rotating motion. • When examining the submental and submandibular nodes, place the fingertips under the mandible on the side nearest the palpating hand, and pull the skin and subcutaneous tissue laterally over the mandibular surface so that the tissue rolls over the nodes. • When palpating the supraclavicular nodes, have the client bend the head forward to relax the tissues of the anterior neck and to relax the shoulders so that the clavicles drop. Use your hand nearest the side to be examined when facing the client (i.e., your left hand for the client's right nodes). Use your free hand to flex the client's head forward if necessary. Hook your index and third fingers over the clavicle lateral to the sternocleidomastoid muscle ❶. • When palpating the anterior cervical nodes and posterior cervical nodes, move your fingertips slowly in a forward circular motion against the sternocleidomastoid and trapezius muscles, respectively. • To palpate the deep cervical nodes, bend or hook your fingers around the sternocleidomastoid muscle.	Not palpable 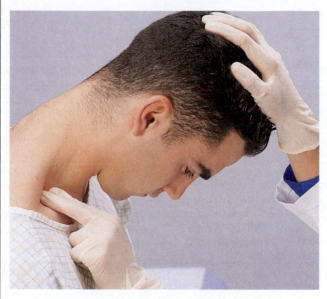 ❶ Palpating the supraclavicular lymph nodes.	Enlarged, palpable, possibly tender (associated with infection and tumors)
Trachea		
9. Palpate the trachea for lateral deviation. Place your fingertip or thumb on the trachea in the suprasternal notch and then move your finger laterally to the left and the right in spaces bordered by the clavicle, the anterior aspect of the sternocleidomastoid muscle, and the trachea.	Central placement in midline of neck; spaces are equal on both sides	Deviation to one side, indicating possible neck tumor; thyroid enlargement; enlarged lymph nodes
10. Document findings in the client record using forms or checklists supplemented by narrative notes when appropriate.		

Developmental Considerations

INFANTS AND CHILDREN

- Examine the neck while the infant or child is lying supine. Lift the head and turn it from side to side to determine neck mobility.

- An infant's neck is normally short, lengthening by about age 3 years. This makes palpation of the trachea difficult.

SKILL 1.24   Assessing the Thorax and Lungs

Delegation

Assessment of the thorax and lungs is not delegated to UAP. However, many aspects of breathing are observed during usual care and may be recorded by individuals other than the nurse. Abnormal findings must be validated and interpreted by the nurse.

Equipment

- Stethoscope
- Skin marker/pencil
- Centimeter ruler

Procedure

1. Prior to performing the procedure, introduce self and verify the client's identity using agency protocol. Explain to the client what you are going to do, why it is necessary, and how he or she can participate. Discuss how the results will be used in planning further care or treatments.
2. Perform hand hygiene and observe other appropriate infection control procedures.
3. Provide for client privacy. In women, drape the anterior thorax when it is not being examined.
4. Inquire if the client has any history of the following: family history of illness, including cancer, allergies, tuberculosis; lifestyle habits such as smoking and occupational hazards (e.g., inhaling fumes); medications being taken; current problems (e.g., swellings, coughs, wheezing, pain).

ASSESSMENT	NORMAL FINDINGS	DEVIATIONS FROM NORMAL
Posterior Thorax		
5. Inspect the shape and symmetry of the thorax from posterior and lateral views. Compare the anteroposterior diameter to the transverse diameter.	Anteroposterior to transverse diameter in ratio of 1:2 Thorax symmetric	Barrel chest; increased anteroposterior to transverse diameter Thorax asymmetric
6. Inspect the spinal alignment for deformities. Have the client stand. From a lateral position, observe the three normal curvatures: cervical, thoracic, and lumbar. • To assess for lateral deviation of the spine (scoliosis), observe the standing client from the rear. Have the client bend forward at the waist and observe from behind.	Spine vertically aligned Spinal column is straight, right and left shoulders and hips are at same height	Exaggerated spinal curvatures (kyphosis, lordosis) Spinal column deviates to one side, often accentuated when bending over Shoulders or hips not even (level)
7. Palpate the posterior thorax. • For clients who have no respiratory complaints, rapidly assess the temperature and integrity of all thorax skin. • For clients who do have respiratory complaints, palpate all areas for bulges, tenderness, or abnormal movements. Avoid deep palpation for painful areas, especially if a fractured rib is suspected. In such a case, deep palpation could lead to displacement of the bone fragment against the lungs.	Skin intact; uniform temperature Thorax intact; no tenderness; no masses	Skin lesions; areas of hyperthermia Lumps, bulges; depressions; areas of tenderness; movable structures (e.g., rib)
8. Palpate the posterior thorax for respiratory excursion (thoracic expansion). Place the palms of both your hands over the lower thorax with your thumbs adjacent to the spine and your fingers stretched laterally ❶. Ask the client to take a deep breath while you observe the movement of your hands and any lag in movement.	Full and symmetric thorax expansion (i.e., when the client takes a deep breath, your thumbs should move apart an equal distance and at the same time; normally the thumbs separate 3 to 5 cm [1½ to 2 in.] during deep inspiration)	Asymmetric and/or decreased thorax expansion

❶ Position of the nurse's hands when assessing posterior respiratory excursion on the posterior thorax.

SKILL 1.24   Assessing the Thorax and Lungs (continued)

ASSESSMENT	NORMAL FINDINGS	DEVIATIONS FROM NORMAL
9. Palpate the thorax for vocal (tactile) **fremitus**, the faintly perceptible vibration felt through the chest wall when the client speaks. • Place the palmar surfaces of your fingertips or the ulnar aspect of your hand or closed fist on the posterior thorax, starting near the apex of the lungs ❷, position A. • Ask the client to repeat such words as "blue moon" or "one, two, three." • Repeat the two steps, moving your hands sequentially to the base of the lungs, through positions B–E in ❷. • Compare the fremitus on both lungs and between the apex and the base of each lung, using either one hand and moving it from one side of the client to the corresponding area on the other side *or* using two hands that are placed simultaneously on the corresponding areas of each side of the thorax.	Bilateral symmetry of vocal fremitus Fremitus is heard most clearly at the apex of the lungs Low-pitched voices of males are more readily palpated than higher-pitched voices of females 	Decreased or absent fremitus (associated with pneumothorax) Increased fremitus (associated with consolidated lung tissue, as in pneumonia) ❷ Areas and sequence for palpating tactile fremitus on the posterior chest.
10. Percuss the thorax. Percussion of the thorax is performed to determine whether underlying lung tissue is filled with air, liquid, or solid material and to determine the positions and boundaries of certain organs. Because percussion penetrates to a depth of 5 to 7 cm (2 to 3 in.), it detects superficial rather than deep lesions ❸. • Ask the client to bend the head and fold the arms forward across the chest. **Rationale:** *This separates the scapula and exposes more lung tissue to percussion.* • Percuss in the intercostal spaces at about 5-cm (2-in.) intervals in a systematic sequence ❹. • Compare one side of the lung with the other. • Percuss the lateral thorax every few inches, starting at the axilla and working down to the eighth rib.	Percussion notes resonate, except over scapula Lowest point of resonance is at the diaphragm (i.e., at the level of the 8th to 10th rib posteriorly) *Note:* Percussion on a rib normally elicits dullness. ❸ Normal percussion sounds on the posterior chest.	Asymmetry in percussion Areas of dullness or flatness over lung tissue (associated with fluid, consolidation of lung tissue, or a mass) ❹ Sequence for posterior chest percussion.
11. Auscultate the thorax using the diaphragm of the stethoscope. **Rationale:** *The diaphragm of the stethoscope is best for transmitting the high-pitched breath sounds.* • Use the systematic zigzag procedure used in percussion. • Ask the client to take slow, deep breaths through the mouth. Listen at each point to the breath sounds during a complete inspiration and expiration. • Compare findings at each point with the corresponding point on the opposite side of the thorax.	Vesicular and bronchovesicular breath sounds	Adventitious breath sounds (e.g., crackles, gurgles, friction rub, wheeze) Absence of breath sounds
12. Inspect breathing patterns (e.g., respiratory rate and rhythm).	Quiet, rhythmic, and effortless respirations	See Table 1–4 for altered breathing patterns and sounds
13. Inspect the costal angle (angle formed by the intersection of the costal margins) and the angle at which the ribs enter the spine.	Costal angle is less than 90°, and the ribs insert into the spine at an approximately 45° angle	Costal angle is widened (associated with chronic obstructive pulmonary disease)
14. Palpate the anterior thorax (see posterior thorax palpation).		

(continued on next page)

SKILL 1.24   Assessing the Thorax and Lungs (continued)

ASSESSMENT	NORMAL FINDINGS	DEVIATIONS FROM NORMAL
15. Palpate the anterior thorax for respiratory excursion. • Place the palms of both your hands on the lower thorax, with your fingers laterally along the lower rib cage and your thumbs along the costal margins ❺. • Ask the client to take a deep breath while you observe the movement of your hands.	Full symmetric excursion; thumbs normally separate 3 to 5 cm (1½ to 2 in.) ❺ Position of the nurse's hands when assessing respiratory excursion on the anterior thorax.	Asymmetric and/or decreased respiratory excursion
16. Palpate tactile fremitus in the same manner as for the posterior thorax and using the sequence shown in ❻. If the breasts are large and cannot be retracted adequately for palpation, this part of the examination is usually omitted.	Same as posterior vocal fremitus; fremitus is normally decreased over heart and breast tissue ❻ Areas and sequence for palpating tactile fremitus on the anterior thorax.	Same as posterior fremitus
17. Percuss the anterior thorax systematically. • Begin above the clavicles in the supraclavicular space, and proceed downward to the diaphragm ❼. • Compare one side of the lung to the other. • Displace female breast to facilitate percussion of the lungs. ❼ Sequence for anterior thorax percussion.	Percussion notes resonate down to the sixth rib at the level of the diaphragm but are flat over areas of heavy muscle and bone, dull on areas over the heart and the liver, and tympanic over the underlying stomach ❽ Flatness over heavy muscles and bones Resonance Cardiac dullness 5th ICS Liver dullness Costal margin Stomach tympany (6th ICS) ❽ Normal percussion sounds on the anterior thorax.	Asymmetry in percussion notes Areas of dullness or flatness over lung tissue
18. Auscultate the trachea.	Bronchial and tubular breath sounds (see normal breath sounds in **Table 1–9** ● and adventitious breath sounds in **Table 1–10** ●)	Adventitious breath sounds
19. Auscultate the anterior thorax. Use the sequence used in percussion, beginning over the bronchi between the sternum and the clavicles.	Bronchovesicular and vesicular breath sounds	Adventitious breath sounds
20. Document findings in the client record using forms or checklists supplemented by narrative notes when appropriate.		

SKILL 1.24 Assessing the Thorax and Lungs (continued)

TABLE 1–9 Normal Breath Sounds

TYPE	DESCRIPTION	LOCATION	CHARACTERISTICS
Vesicular	Soft-intensity, low-pitched, "gentle sighing" sounds created by air moving through smaller airways (bronchioles and alveoli)	Over peripheral lung; best heard at base of lungs	Best heard on inspiration, which is about 2.5 times longer than the expiratory phase (5:2 ratio)
Bronchovesicular	Moderate-intensity and moderate-pitched "blowing" sounds created by air moving through larger airways (bronchi)	Between the scapulae and lateral to the sternum at the first and second intercostal spaces	Equal inspiratory and expiratory phases (1:1 ratio)
Bronchial (tubular)	High-pitched, loud, "harsh" sounds created by air moving through the trachea	Anteriorly over the trachea; not normally heard over lung tissue	Louder than vesicular sounds; have a short inspiratory phase and long expiratory phase (1:2 ratio)

TABLE 1–10 Adventitious Breath Sounds

NAME	DESCRIPTION	CAUSE	LOCATION
Crackles (rales)	Fine, short, interrupted crackling sounds; alveolar rales are high pitched. Sound can be simulated by rolling a lock of hair near the ear. Best heard on inspiration but can be heard on both inspiration and expiration. May not be cleared by coughing.	Air passing through fluid or collapsed smaller air passages or alveoli	Most commonly heard in the bases of the lower lung lobes
Gurgles (rhonchi)	Continuous, low-pitched, coarse, gurgling, harsh, louder sounds with a moaning or snoring quality. Best heard on expiration but can be heard on both inspiration and expiration.	Air passing through narrowed air passages as a result of secretions, swelling, tumors	Loud sounds can be heard over most lung areas but dominate over the trachea and bronchi. May be altered by coughing.
Friction rub	Superficial grating or creaking sounds heard during inspiration and expiration. Not relieved by coughing.	Rubbing together of inflamed pleural surfaces	Heard most often in areas of greatest thoracic expansion (e.g., lower anterior and lateral thorax)
Wheezes	Continuous, high-pitched, squeaky musical sounds. Best heard on expiration. Not usually altered by coughing.	Air passing through a constricted bronchus as a result of secretions, swelling, tumors	Heard over all lung fields

Sample Documentation

6/10/15 0830 Lungs clear to auscultation except for fine crackles both lower lobes. Rarely moves in bed. Assisted to a chair. Reviewed deep breathing exercises. Effective return demonstration.

_____N. Schmidt, RN

Developmental Considerations

INFANTS

- The thorax is rounded; that is, the diameter from the front to the back (anteroposterior) is equal to the transverse diameter. It is also cylindrical, having a nearly equal diameter at the top and the base. This makes it harder for infants to expand their thoracic space.
- To assess tactile fremitus, place your hand over the crying infant's thorax.
- Infants tend to breathe using their diaphragm; assess rate and rhythm by watching the abdomen, rather than the thorax, rise and fall.
- The right bronchial branch is short and angles downward as it leaves the trachea, making it easy for small objects to be inhaled. Sudden onset of cough or other signs of respiratory distress may indicate that the infant has inhaled a foreign object.

CHILDREN

- By about 6 years of age, the anteroposterior diameter has decreased in proportion to the transverse diameter, with a 1:2 ratio present.
- Children tend to breathe more abdominally than thoracically up to age 6.
- During the rapid growth spurts of adolescence, spinal curvature and rotation (scoliosis) may appear. Children should be assessed for scoliosis by age 12 and annually until their growth slows. Curvature greater than 10% should be referred for further medical evaluation.

OLDER ADULTS

- The thoracic curvature may be accentuated (kyphosis) because of osteoporosis and changes in cartilage, resulting in collapse

(continued on next page)

SKILL 1.24   Assessing the Thorax and Lungs (continued)

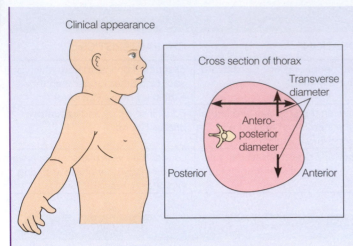

Clinical appearance

Cross section of thorax

Transverse diameter

Antero-posterior diameter

Posterior   Anterior

Configurations of the child's thorax showing anteroposterior diameter and transverse diameter.

of the vertebrae. This can also compromise and decrease normal respiratory effort.

■ Kyphosis and osteoporosis alter the size of the chest cavity as the ribs move downward and forward.

■ The anteroposterior diameter of the thorax widens, giving the person a barrel-chested appearance. This is due to loss of skeletal muscle strength in the thorax and diaphragm and constant lung inflation from excessive expiratory pressure on the alveoli.

■ Breathing rate and rhythm are unchanged at rest; the rate normally increases with exercise but may take longer to return to the preexercise rate.

■ Inspiratory muscles become less powerful, and the inspiratory reserve volume decreases. A decrease in depth of respiration is therefore apparent.

■ Expiration may require the use of accessory muscles. The expiratory reserve volume significantly increases because of the increased amount of air remaining in the lungs at the end of a normal breath.

■ Deflation of the lung is incomplete.

■ Small airways lose their cartilaginous support and elastic recoil; as a result, they tend to close, particularly in basal or dependent portions of the lung.

■ Elastic tissue of the alveoli loses its stretchability and changes to fibrous tissue. Exertional capacity decreases.

■ Cilia in the airways decrease in number and are less effective in removing mucus; older clients are therefore at greater risk for pulmonary infections.

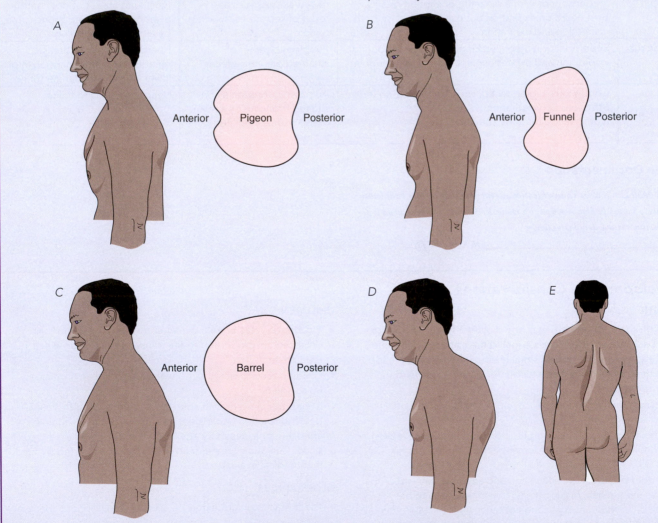

A

Anterior   Pigeon   Posterior

B

Anterior   Funnel   Posterior

C

Anterior   Barrel   Posterior

D

E

Chest deformities: *A*, pigeon chest; *B*, funnel chest; *C*, barrel chest; *D*, kyphosis; *E*, scoliosis.

SKILL 1.25   Assessing the Heart and Central Vessels

Delegation

Assessment of the heart and central vessels is not delegated to UAP. However, many aspects of cardiac function are observed during usual care and may be recorded by individuals other than the nurse. Abnormal findings must be validated and interpreted by the nurse.

Equipment

- Stethoscope
- Centimeter ruler

Procedure

1. Prior to performing the procedure, introduce self and verify the client's identity using agency protocol. Explain to the client what you are going to do, why it is necessary, and how he or she can participate. Discuss how the results will be used in planning further care or treatments.

2. Perform hand hygiene and observe other appropriate infection control procedures.

3. Provide for client privacy.

4. Inquire if the client has any history of the following: family history of incidence of heart disease, high cholesterol levels, high blood pressure, stroke, obesity, congenital heart disease, arterial disease, hypertension, and rheumatic fever and age at which event occurred; client's past history of rheumatic fever, heart murmur, heart attack, varicosities, or heart failure; present symptoms indicative of heart disease (e.g., fatigue, dyspnea, orthopnea, edema, cough, chest pain, palpitations, syncope, hypertension, wheezing, hemoptysis); presence of diseases that affect heart (e.g., obesity, diabetes, lung disease, endocrine disorders); lifestyle habits that are risk factors for cardiac disease (e.g., smoking, alcohol intake, eating and exercise patterns, areas and degree of stress perceived).

ASSESSMENT	NORMAL FINDINGS	DEVIATIONS FROM NORMAL
5. Simultaneously inspect and palpate the precordium for the presence of abnormal pulsations, lifts, or heaves. Locate the valve areas of the heart: • Locate the angle of Louis. It is felt as a prominence on the sternum. • Move your fingertips down each side of the angle until you can feel the second intercostal spaces. The client's right second intercostal space is the aortic area, and the left second intercostal space is the pulmonic area ❶. • From the pulmonic area, move your fingertips down three left intercostal spaces along the side of the sternum. The left fifth intercostal space close to the sternum is the tricuspid or right ventricular area. • From the tricuspid area, move your fingertips laterally 5 to 7 cm (2 to 3 in.) to the left midclavicular line (LMCL) ❷. This is the apical or mitral area, or point of maximal impulse (PMI). If you have difficulty locating the PMI, have the client roll onto the left side to move the apex closer to the chest wall.	No pulsations No pulsations No lift or heave Pulsations visible in 50% of adults and palpable in most PMI in fifth LICS at or medial to MCL Diameter of 1 to 2 cm (⅓ to ½ in.) No lift or heave Aortic pulsations	Pulsations Pulsations Diffuse lift or heave, indicating enlarged or overactive right ventricle PMI displaced laterally or lower (indicates enlarged heart) Diameter over 2 cm (½ in.); indicates enlarged heart or aneurysm Diffuse lift or heave lateral to apex; indicates enlargement or overactivity of left ventricle Bounding abdominal pulsations (e.g., aortic aneurysm)

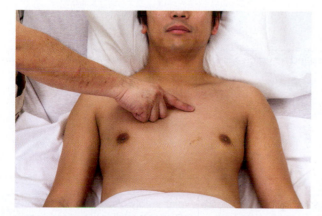

❶ The second intercostal space.

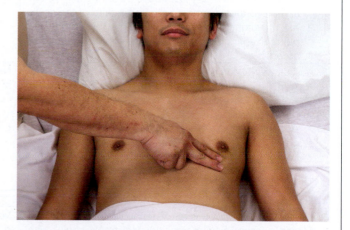

❷ The fifth intercostal space, MCL.

(continued on next page)

SKILL 1.25   Assessing the Heart and Central Vessels (continued)

ASSESSMENT	NORMAL FINDINGS	DEVIATIONS FROM NORMAL
• Inspect and palpate the aortic and pulmonic areas, observing them at an angle and to the side, to note the presence or absence of pulsations. Observing these areas at an angle increases the likelihood of seeing pulsations. • Inspect and palpate the tricuspid area for pulsations and heaves or lifts. • Inspect and palpate the apical area for pulsation, noting its specific location (it may be displaced laterally or lower) and diameter. If displaced laterally, record the distance between the apex and the MCL in centimeters. • Inspect and palpate the epigastric area at the base of the sternum for abdominal aortic pulsations.		
6. Auscultate the heart in all four anatomical sites: aortic, pulmonic, tricuspid, and apical (mitral). Auscultation need not be limited to these areas; the nurse may need to move the stethoscope to find the most audible sounds for each client. • Eliminate all sources of room noise. **Rationale:** *Heart sounds are of low intensity, and other noise hinders the nurse's ability to hear them.* • Keep the client in a supine position with head elevated 30° to 45°. • Use both the diaphragm and the bell to listen to all areas. • In every area of auscultation, distinguish both S$_1$ and S$_2$ sounds. • When auscultating, concentrate on one particular sound at a time in each area: the first heart sound, followed by systole, then the second heart sound, then diastole. Systole and diastole are normally silent intervals. • Later, reexamine the heart while the client is in the upright sitting position. **Rationale:** *Certain sounds are more audible in certain positions.*	S$_1$: Usually heard at all sites Usually louder at apical area S$_2$: Usually heard at all sites Usually louder at base of heart *Systole:* silent interval; slightly shorter duration than diastole at normal heart rate (60 to 90 beats per minute [bpm]) *Diastole:* silent interval; slightly longer duration than systole at normal heart rates S$_3$ in children and young adults S$_4$ in many older adults	Increased or decreased intensity Varying intensity with different beats Increased intensity at aortic area Increased intensity at pulmonic area Sharp-sounding ejection clicks S$_3$ in older adults S$_4$ may be a sign of hypertension
Carotid Arteries		
7. Palpate the carotid artery, using extreme caution. • Palpate only one carotid artery at a time. **Rationale:** *This ensures adequate blood flow through the other artery to the brain.* • Avoid exerting too much pressure and massaging the area. **Rationale:** *Pressure can occlude the artery, and carotid sinus massage can precipitate bradycardia. The carotid sinus is a small dilation at the beginning of the internal carotid artery just above the bifurcation of the common carotid artery, in the upper third of the neck.* • Ask the client to turn the head slightly toward the side being examined. This makes the carotid artery more accessible.	Symmetric pulse volumes Full pulsations, thrusting quality Quality remains same when client breathes, turns head, and changes from sitting to supine position Elastic arterial wall	Asymmetric volumes (possible stenosis or thrombosis) Decreased pulsations (may indicate impaired left cardiac output) Increased pulsations Thickening, hard, rigid, beaded, inelastic walls (indicate arteriosclerosis)
8. Auscultate the carotid artery. • Turn the client's head slightly away from the side being examined. **Rationale:** *This facilitates the placement of the stethoscope.* • Auscultate the carotid artery on one side and then the other. • Listen for the presence of a bruit. If you hear a bruit, gently palpate the artery to determine the presence of a thrill.	No sound heard on auscultation	Presence of bruit in one or both arteries (suggests occlusive artery disease)
Jugular Veins		
9. Inspect the jugular veins for distention while the client is placed in a semi-Fowler's position (15° to 45° angle), with the head supported on a small pillow.	Veins not visible (indicating right side of heart is functioning normally)	Veins visibly distended (indicating advanced cardiopulmonary disease)

SKILL 1.25   Assessing the Heart and Central Vessels (continued)

ASSESSMENT	NORMAL FINDINGS	DEVIATIONS FROM NORMAL
10. If jugular distention is present, assess the jugular venous pressure (JVP). • Locate the highest visible point of distention of the internal jugular vein. Although either the internal or the external jugular vein can be used, the internal jugular vein is more reliable. **Rationale:** *The external jugular vein is more easily affected by obstruction or kinking at the base of the neck.* • Measure the vertical height of this point in centimeters from the sternal angle, the point at which the clavicles meet ❸. • Repeat the preceding steps on the other side.		Bilateral measurements above 3 to 4 cm (1 to 1 ½ in.) are considered elevated (may indicate right-sided heart failure) Unilateral distention (may be caused by local obstruction) Level of the highest visible point of distention The vertical distance between the sternal angle and the highest level of jugular distention Level of the sternal angle External jugular vein Internal jugular vein 15° – 45° ❸ Assessing the highest point of distention of the jugular vein.
11. Document findings in the client record using forms or checklists supplemented by narrative notes when appropriate.		

Developmental Considerations

INFANTS

- Physiological splitting of the second heart sound (S_2) may be heard when the child takes a deep breath and the aortic valve closes a split second before the pulmonic valve. If splitting of S_2 is heard during normal respirations, it is abnormal and may indicate an atrial-septal defect, pulmonary stenosis, or another heart problem.
- Infants may normally have sinus arrhythmia that is related to respiration. The heart rate slows during expiration and increases when the child breathes in.
- Murmurs may be heard in newborns as the structures of fetal circulation, especially the ductus arteriosus, close.

CHILDREN

- Heart sounds may be louder because of the thinner chest wall.

- A third heart sound (S_3), caused as the ventricles fill, is best heard at the apex and is present in about one third of all children.
- The PMI is higher and more medial in children under 8 years old.

OLDER ADULTS

- If no disease is present, heart size remains the same size throughout life.
- Cardiac output and strength of contraction decrease, thus lessening the older person's activity tolerance.
- The heart rate returns to its resting rate more slowly after exertion than it did when the individual was younger.
- S_4 heart sound is considered normal in older adults.
- Extra systoles commonly occur. Ten or more extra systoles per minute are considered abnormal.
- Sudden emotional and physical stress may result in cardiac arrhythmias and heart failure.

SKILL 1.26   Assessing the Peripheral Vascular System

Delegation

Due to the substantial knowledge and skill required, assessment of the peripheral vascular system is not delegated to UAP. However, many aspects of the vascular system are observed during usual care and may be recorded by individuals other than the nurse. Abnormal findings must be validated and interpreted by the nurse.

(continued on next page)

SKILL 1.26   Assessing the Peripheral Vascular System (*continued*)

Equipment

None

Procedure

1. Prior to performing the procedure, introduce self and verify the client's identity using agency protocol. Explain to the client what you are going to do, why it is necessary, and how he or she can participate. Discuss how the results will be used in planning further care or treatments.

2. Perform hand hygiene and observe other appropriate infection control procedures.

3. Provide for client privacy.

4. Inquire if the client has any history of the following: past history of heart disorders, varicosities, arterial disease, and hypertension; lifestyle habits such as exercise patterns, activity patterns and tolerance, smoking, and use of alcohol.

ASSESSMENT	NORMAL FINDINGS	DEVIATIONS FROM NORMAL
Peripheral Pulses		
5. Palpate the peripheral pulses on both sides of the client's body individually, simultaneously (except the carotid pulse), and systematically to determine the symmetry of pulse volume. If you have difficulty palpating some of the peripheral pulses, use a Doppler ultrasound probe.	Symmetric pulse volumes Full pulsations	Asymmetric volumes (indicate impaired circulation) Absence of pulsation (indicates arterial spasm or occlusion) Decreased, weak, thready pulsations (indicate impaired cardiac output) Increased pulse volume (may indicate hypertension, high cardiac output, or circulatory overload)
Peripheral Veins		
6. Inspect the peripheral veins in the arms and legs for the presence and/or appearance of superficial veins when limbs are dependent and when limbs are elevated.	In dependent position, presence of distention and nodular bulges at calves When limbs are elevated, veins collapse (veins may appear tortuous or distended in older people)	Distended veins in the thigh and/or lower leg or on posterolateral part of calf from knee to ankle
7. Assess the peripheral leg veins for signs of phlebitis. • Inspect the calves for redness and swelling over vein sites. • Palpate the calves for firmness or tension of the muscles, the presence of edema over the dorsum of the foot, and areas of localized warmth. **Rationale:** *Palpation augments inspection findings, particularly for greater pigmented people in whom redness may not be visible.* • Push the calves from side to side to test for tenderness. • Firmly dorsiflex the client's foot while supporting the entire leg in extension (Homans test), or have the person stand or walk.	Limbs not tender Symmetric in size	Tenderness on palpation Pain in calf muscles with forceful dorsiflexion of the foot (positive Homans test) Warmth and redness over vein Swelling of one calf or leg No one sign or symptom consistently confirms or excludes presence of phlebitis or a deep venous thrombosis. Pain, tenderness, and swelling are the most predictive (Qaseem et al., 2007)
Peripheral Perfusion		
8. Inspect the skin of the hands and feet for color, temperature, edema, and skin changes.	Skin color pink Skin temperature not excessively warm or cold No edema Skin texture resilient and moist	Cyanotic (venous insufficiency) Pallor that increases with limb elevation Dependent rubor, a dusky red color when limb is lowered (arterial insufficiency) Brown pigmentation around ankles (arterial or chronic venous insufficiency) Cool skin (arterial insufficiency) Marked edema (venous insufficiency) Mild edema (arterial insufficiency) Skin thin and shiny or thick, waxy, shiny, and fragile, with reduced hair and/or ulceration (venous or arterial insufficiency)
9. Assess the adequacy of arterial flow if arterial insufficiency is suspected.		

SKILL 1.26   Assessing the Peripheral Vascular System (continued)

ASSESSMENT	NORMAL FINDINGS	DEVIATIONS FROM NORMAL
Capillary Refill Test		
• Squeeze the client's fingernail and toenail between your fingers sufficiently to cause blanching (about 5 seconds). • Release the pressure, and observe how quickly normal color returns. Color normally returns immediately (less than 2 seconds).	Immediate return of color	Delayed return of color (arterial insufficiency)
Other Assessments		
• Inspect the fingernails for changes indicative of circulatory impairment. See Skill 1.14 on assessment of nails.		
10. Document findings in the client record using forms or checklists supplemented by narrative notes when appropriate.		

Sample Documentation

6/10/15 0830 Legs mottled red bilaterally toes to mid-calf. States "actually looks a bit better." Capillary refill 4 seconds in toes on both feet. Pedal pulses present but weak. Homans test negative. C/o pain in calves after walking 100 feet. _____ N. Schmidt, RN

Client Teaching

- Use the assessment as an opportunity to provide teaching regarding appropriate care of the extremities in those at high risk for or with actual vascular impairment. Educate clients and families regarding skin and nail care, exercise, and positioning to promote circulation.

Developmental Considerations

INFANTS

- Screen for coarctation of the aorta by palpating the peripheral pulses and comparing the strength of the femoral pulses with the radial pulses and apical pulse. If coarctation is present, femoral pulses will be diminished and radial pulses will be stronger.

CHILDREN

- Changes in the peripheral vasculature, such as bruising, petechiae, and purpura, can indicate serious systemic diseases in children (e.g., leukemia, meningococcemia).

OLDER ADULTS

- The overall effectiveness of blood vessels decreases as smooth muscle cells are replaced by connective tissue. The lower extremities are more likely to show signs of arterial and venous impairment because of the more distal and dependent position.
- Peripheral vascular assessment should always include upper and lower extremities' temperature, color, pulses, edema, skin integrity, and sensation. Any differences in symmetry of these findings should be noted.
- Proximal arteries become thinner and dilate.
- Peripheral arteries become thicker and dilate less effectively because of arteriosclerotic changes in the vessel walls.
- Blood vessels lengthen and become more tortuous and prominent. Varicosities occur more frequently.
- In some instances, arteries may be palpated more easily because of the loss of supportive surrounding tissues. Often, however, the most distal pulses of the lower extremities are more difficult to palpate because of decreased arterial perfusion.
- Systolic and diastolic blood pressures increase, but the increase in the systolic pressure is greater. As a result, the pulse pressure widens. Any client with a blood pressure reading above 140/90 should be referred for follow-up assessments.
- Peripheral edema is frequently observed and is most commonly the result of chronic venous insufficiency or low protein levels in the blood (hypoproteinemia).

SKILL 1.27   Assessing Neurovascular Status

Equipment

None

Procedure

1. Assess the swelling in the extremity associated with the injury.
   Rationale: The swelling associated with the injury may constrict blood flow to the distal extremity and pinch the nerves, especially when constriction is present, such as a cast.
2. Assess the extremity distal to the injury for color and temperature and compare to the other extremity.
3. Assess the capillary refill time by pressing on a finger or toe for a couple of seconds, until the skin is blanched. Count how long it takes for blood or color to return to the area pressed. It should take 2 seconds or less.

(continued on next page)

SKILL 1.27 Assessing Neurovascular Status (continued)

4. Assess the extremity for pain and sensation (numbness, tingling, pins and needles sensation) and compare to the other extremity.
5. Consider all the findings simultaneously to complete the neurovascular assessment.
6. The presence of most or all of the following indicates significantly impaired circulation and pressure or injury to the nerve that needs emergency intervention:
   - Pallor or cyanosis

- Pain (moderate to severe)
- Paresthesia (numbness, tingling, or pins and needles sensation)
- Cool or cold temperature
- Capillary refill time greater than 4 seconds.

7. Document the assessment, and repeat it frequently, especially if one or two findings are present. **Rationale:** *If the circulatory and neurological constriction is not detected and promptly relieved, permanent damage to the distal extremity may result.*

SKILL 1.28 Assessing the Breasts and Axillae

Delegation

Assessment of the breasts and axillae is not delegated to UAP. However, individuals other than the nurse may record aspects observed during usual care. Abnormal findings must be validated and interpreted by the nurse.

Equipment

- Centimeter ruler

Procedure

1. Prior to performing the procedure, introduce self and verify the client's identity using agency protocol. Explain to the client what you are going to do, why it is necessary, and how he or she can participate. Inquire whether the client has ever had a clinical breast exam previously. Discuss how the results will be used in planning further care or treatments.

2. Perform hand hygiene and observe other appropriate infection control procedures.
3. Provide for client privacy.
4. Inquire if the client has any history of the following: breast masses and what was done about them; pain or tenderness in the breasts and relation to the woman's menstrual cycle; discharge from the nipple; medication history (some medications, e.g., oral contraceptives, steroids, digitalis, and diuretics, may cause nipple discharge; estrogen replacement therapy may be associated with the development of cysts or cancer); risk factors that may be associated with development of breast cancer (e.g., mother, sister, aunt with breast cancer; alcohol consumption, high-fat diet, obesity, use of oral contraceptives, menarche before age 12, menopause after age 55, age 30 or more at first pregnancy). Inquire if the client performs breast self-examination; technique used and when performed in relation to the menstrual cycle.

ASSESSMENT	NORMAL FINDINGS	DEVIATIONS FROM NORMAL
5. Inspect the breasts for size, symmetry, and contour or shape while the client is in a sitting position.	*Females:* rounded shape; slightly unequal in size; generally symmetric *Males:* breasts even with the chest wall; if obese, may be similar in shape to female breasts	Recent change in breast size; swellings; marked asymmetry
6. Inspect the skin of the breast for localized discolorations or hyperpigmentation, retraction or dimpling, localized hypervascular areas, swelling, or edema ❶. Retraction Lesion ❶ A lesion causing retraction of the skin.	Skin uniform in color (same in appearance as skin of abdomen or back) Skin smooth and intact Diffuse symmetric horizontal or vertical vascular pattern in light-skinned people Striae (stretch marks); moles and nevi	Localized discolorations or hyperpigmentation Retraction or dimpling (result of scar tissue or an invasive tumor) Unilateral, localized hypervascular areas (associated with increased blood flow) Swelling or edema appearing as pig skin or orange peel due to exaggeration of the pores

SKILL 1.28   Assessing the Breasts and Axillae (continued)

ASSESSMENT	NORMAL FINDINGS	DEVIATIONS FROM NORMAL
7. Emphasize any retraction by having the client: • Raise the arms above the head. • Push the hands together, with elbows flexed ❷. • Press the hands down on the hips ❸.	Skin and tissue follow client motion	Retraction or dimpling and skin or underlying tissue does not move freely

❷ Pushing the hands together to accentuate retraction of breast tissue.

❸ Pressing the hands down on the hips to accentuate retraction of the breast tissue. (Southern Illinois University/Science Source)

8. Inspect the areola area for size, shape, symmetry, color, surface characteristics, and any masses or lesions.	Round or oval and bilaterally the same Color varies widely, from light pink to dark brown Irregular placement of sebaceous glands on the surface of the areola (Montgomery tubercles)	Any asymmetry, mass, or lesion
9. Inspect the nipples for size, shape, position, color, discharge, and lesions.	Round, everted, and equal in size; similar in color; soft and smooth; both nipples point in same direction (out in young women and men, downward in older women) No discharge, except from pregnant or breastfeeding females Inversion of one or both nipples that is present from puberty	Asymmetrical size and color Presence of discharge, crusts, or cracks Recent inversion of one or both nipples
10. Palpate the axillary, subclavicular, and supraclavicular lymph nodes ❹ while the client sits with the arms abducted and supported on the nurse's forearm. For palpation of clavicular lymph nodes, use the flat surfaces of all fingertips to palpate the four areas of the axilla: • The edge of the greater pectoral muscle along the anterior axillary line • The thoracic wall in the midaxillary area • The upper part of the humerus • The anterior edge of the latissimus dorsi muscle along the posterior axillary line.	No tenderness, masses, or nodules	Tenderness, masses, or nodules

❹ Location and palpation of the lymph nodes that drain the lateral breast: A, lymph nodes; B, palpating the axilla.

(continued on next page)

SKILL 1.28 Assessing the Breasts and Axillae (*continued*)

ASSESSMENT	NORMAL FINDINGS	DEVIATIONS FROM NORMAL

11. Palpate the breast for masses, tenderness, and any discharge from the nipples. Palpation of the breast is generally performed while the client is supine. **Rationale:** *In the supine position, the breasts flatten evenly against the chest wall, facilitating palpation.* For clients who have a past history of breast masses, who are at high risk for breast cancer, or who have pendulous breasts, examination in both a supine and a sitting position is recommended.
• If the client reports a breast lump, start with the "normal" breast to obtain baseline data that will serve as a comparison to the involved breast.
• To enhance flattening of the breast, instruct the client to abduct the arm and place her hand behind her head. Then place a small pillow or rolled towel under the client's shoulder.
• For palpation, use the palmar surface of the middle three fingertips (held together) and make a gentle rotary motion on the breast.
• Choose one of three patterns for palpation:
  a. Hands-of-the-clock or spokes- on-a-wheel ⑤
  b. Concentric circles ⑥
  c. Vertical strips pattern ⑦.
• Start at one point for palpation, and move systematically to the end point to ensure that all breast surfaces are assessed.
• Pay particular attention to the upper outer quadrant area and the tail of Spence.
	No tenderness, masses, nodules, or nipple discharge	Tenderness, masses, nodules, or nipple discharge
		If you detect a mass, record the following data:
		• *Location:* the exact location relative to the quadrants and axillary tail, or the clock and the distance from the nipple in centimeters
		• *Size:* the length, width, and thickness of the mass in centimeters. If you are able to determine the discrete edges, record this fact
		• *Shape:* whether the mass is round, oval, lobulated, indistinct, or irregular
		• *Consistency:* whether the mass is hard or soft
		• *Mobility:* whether the mass is movable or fixed
		• *Skin over the lump:* whether it is reddened, dimpled, or retracted
		• *Nipple:* whether it is displaced or retracted
		• *Tenderness:* whether palpation is painful

⑤ Hands-of-the-clock or spokes-on-a-wheel pattern of breast palpation.

⑥ Concentric circles pattern of breast palpation.

⑦ Vertical strips pattern for breast palpations.

Start here

ASSESSMENT	NORMAL FINDINGS	DEVIATIONS FROM NORMAL
12. Palpate the areola and the nipples for masses. Compress each nipple to determine the presence of any discharge. If discharge is present, milk the breast along its radius to identify the discharge-producing lobe. Assess any discharge for amount, color, consistency, and odor. Note also any tenderness on palpation.	No tenderness, masses, nodules, or nipple discharge	Tenderness, masses, nodules, or nipple discharge
13. Teach the client the technique of breast self-examination (BSE).		
14. Document findings in the client record using forms or checklists supplemented by narrative notes when appropriate.		

SKILL 1.28   Assessing the Breasts and Axillae (continued)

Client Teaching

Instruct the client to perform the following steps.

Inspection Before A Mirror

Look for any change in size or shape; lumps or thickenings; any rashes or other skin irritations; dimpled or puckered skin; any discharge or change in the nipples (e.g., position or asymmetry). Inspect the breasts in all of the following positions:

- Stand and face the mirror with your arm relaxed at your sides or hands resting on the hips; then turn to the right and the left for a side view (look for any flattening in the side view).
- Bend forward from the waist with arms raised over the head.
- Stand straight with the arms raised over the head and move the arms slowly up and down at the sides. (Look for free movement of the breasts over the chest wall.)
- Press your hands firmly together at chin level while the elbows are raised to shoulder level.

Palpation: Lying Position

- Place a pillow under your right shoulder and place the right hand behind your head. This position distributes breast tissue more evenly on the chest.

- Use the finger pads (tips) of the three middle fingers (held together) on your left hand to feel for lumps.
- Press the breast tissue against the chest wall firmly enough to know how your breast feels. A ridge of firm tissue in the lower curve of each breast is normal.
- Use small circular motions along one arrow in your chosen pattern. Then move your fingers about 2 cm and feel along the next arrow. Repeat this action as many times as necessary until the entire breast is covered.
- Bring your arm down to your side and feel under your armpit, where breast tissue is also located.
- Repeat the exam on your left breast, using the finger pads of your right hand.

Palpation: Standing or Sitting

- Repeat the examination of both breasts while upright with one arm behind your head. This position makes it easier to check the area where a large percentage of breast cancers are found, the upper outer part of the breast and toward the armpit.
- Optional: Do the upright BSE in the shower. Soapy hands glide more easily over wet skin. Report any changes to your healthcare provider promptly.

Developmental Considerations

INFANTS

- Newborns, both boys and girls, up to 2 weeks of age may have breast enlargement and white discharge from the nipples (witch's milk).
- Supernumerary ("extra") nipples infrequently are present along the mammary chain; these may be associated with renal anomalies.

CHILDREN

- Female breast development begins between 9 and 13 years of age and occurs in five stages (Tanner stages). One breast may develop more rapidly than the other, but at the end of development, they are more or less the same size.

  Stage 1: Prepubertal with no noticeable change

  Stage 2: Breast bud with elevation of nipple and enlargement of the areola

  Stage 3: Enlargement of the breast and areola with no separation of contour

  Stage 4: Projection of the areola and nipple

  Stage 5: Recession of the areola by about age 14 or 15, leaving only the nipple projecting.

- Boys may develop breast buds and have slight enlargement of the areola in early adolescence. Further enlargement of

breast tissue (gynecomastia) can occur. This growth is transient, usually lasting about 2 years, resolving completely by late puberty.

- Axillary hair usually appears in Tanner stages 3 or 4 and is related to adrenal rather than gonadal changes.

PREGNANT FEMALES

- Breast, areola, and nipple size increase.
- The areolae and nipples darken; nipples may become more erect; areolae contain small, scattered, elevated Montgomery glands.
- Superficial veins become more prominent, and jagged linear stretch marks may develop.
- A thick yellow fluid (colostrum) may be expressed from the nipples after the first trimester.

OLDER ADULTS

- In the postmenopausal female, breasts change in shape and often appear pendulous or flaccid; they lack the firmness they had in younger years.
- The presence of breast lesions may be detected more readily because of the decrease in connective tissue.
- General breast size remains the same. Although glandular tissue atrophies, the amount of fat in breasts (predominantly in the lower quadrants) increases in most women.

SKILL 1.29   Assessing the Abdomen

Delegation

Assessment of the abdomen is not delegated to UAP. However, signs and symptoms of problems may be observed during usual care and may be recorded by individuals other than the nurse. Abnormal findings must be validated and interpreted by the nurse.

(continued on next page)

SKILL 1.29 Assessing the Abdomen (continued)

Equipment

- Examining light
- Tape measure (metal or unstretchable cloth)
- Water-soluble skin-marking pencil
- Stethoscope

Procedure

1. Prior to performing the procedure, introduce self and verify the client's identity using agency protocol. Explain to the client what you are going to do, why it is necessary, and how he or she can participate. Discuss how the results will be used in planning further care or treatments.
2. Perform hand hygiene and observe other appropriate infection control procedures.
3. Provide for client privacy.
4. Inquire if the client has any history of the following: incidence of abdominal pain; its location, onset, sequence, and chronology; its quality (description); its frequency; associated symptoms (e.g., nausea, vomiting, diarrhea); bowel habits; incidence of constipation or diarrhea (have client describe what client means by these terms); change in appetite, food intolerances, and foods ingested in past 24 hours; specific signs and symptoms (e.g., heartburn, flatulence and/or belching, difficulty swallowing, hematemesis [vomiting blood], blood or mucus in stools, and aggravating and alleviating factors); previous problems and treatment (e.g., stomach ulcer, gallbladder surgery, history of jaundice).
5. Assist the client to a supine position, with the arms placed comfortably at the sides. Place small pillows beneath the knees and the head to reduce tension in the abdominal muscles. Expose the client's abdomen only from the chest to the pubic area to avoid chilling and shivering, which can tense the abdominal muscles.

Sample Documentation

6/10/15 0945 c/o "gassy" pain lower right quadrant. No bowel movement x 48 hrs. Ate 75% regular diet yesterday. Abdomen flat. Active bowel sounds all 4 quadrants. Tympany above umbilicus, dull below. No masses felt on palpation. 30 mL Milk of Magnesia given.

_____ N. Schmidt, RN

ASSESSMENT	NORMAL FINDINGS	DEVIATIONS FROM NORMAL
Inspection of the Abdomen		
6. Inspect the abdomen for skin integrity (refer to the discussion of skin assessment in Skill 1.12).	Unblemished skin Uniform color Silver-white striae (stretch marks) or surgical scars	Presence of rash or other lesions Tense, glistening skin (may indicate ascites, edema) Purple striae (associated with Cushing disease or rapid weight gain and loss)
7. Inspect the abdomen for contour and symmetry: • Observe the abdominal contour (profile line from the rib margin to the pubic bone) while standing at the client's side when the client is supine. • Ask the client to take a deep breath and to hold it. **Rationale:** *This makes an enlarged liver or spleen more obvious.* • Assess the symmetry of contour while standing at the foot of the bed. • If distention is present, measure the abdominal girth by placing a tape around the abdomen at the level of the umbilicus ❶. If girth will be measured repeatedly, use an indelible skin marker to outline the upper and lower margins of the tape placement for consistency of future measurements.	Flat, rounded (convex), or scaphoid (concave) No evidence of enlargement of liver or spleen Symmetric contour ❶ Measuring abdominal girth.	Distended Evidence of enlargement of liver or spleen Asymmetric contour (e.g., localized protrusions around umbilicus, inguinal ligaments, or scars from possible hernia or tumor)
8. Observe abdominal movements associated with respiration, peristalsis, or aortic pulsations.	Symmetric movements caused by respiration Visible peristalsis in very lean people Aortic pulsations in thin people at the epigastric area	Limited movement due to pain or disease process Visible peristalsis in nonlean clients (possible bowel obstruction) Marked aortic pulsations
9. Observe the vascular pattern.	No visible vascular pattern	Visible venous pattern (dilated veins) that is associated with liver disease, ascites, and venocaval obstruction

SKILL 1.29   Assessing the Abdomen (continued)

ASSESSMENT	NORMAL FINDINGS	DEVIATIONS FROM NORMAL
Auscultation of the Abdomen		
10. Auscultate the abdomen for bowel sounds, vascular sounds, and peritoneal friction rubs ❷. Warm the hands and the stethoscope diaphragm and bell. **Rationale:** *Cold hands and a cold stethoscope may cause the client to contract the abdominal muscles, and these contractions may be heard during auscultation.* ❷ Auscultating the abdomen for bowel sounds.		
For Bowel Sounds		
• Use the diaphragm. **Rationale:** *Intestinal sounds are relatively high pitched and best transmitted by the diaphragm. Light pressure with the stethoscope is adequate.* • Ask when the client last ate. **Rationale:** *Shortly after or long after eating, bowel sounds may increase.* They are loudest when a meal is long overdue. Four to 7 hours after a meal, bowel sounds may be heard continuously over the ileocecal valve area while the digestive contents from the small intestine empty through the valve into the large intestine. • Place diaphragm of the stethoscope in each of the four quadrants of the abdomen over the auscultatory sites shown in ❸. • Listen for active bowel sounds—irregular gurgling noises occurring about every 5 to 20 seconds. The duration of a single sound may range from less than a second to more than several seconds. ❸ Sites for auscultating the abdomen. (Copyright ollyy/Shutterstock)	Audible bowel sounds	Hypoactive, i.e., extremely soft and infrequent (e.g., one per minute). Hypoactive sounds indicate decreased motility and are usually associated with manipulation of the bowel during surgery, inflammation, paralytic ileus, or late bowel obstruction Hyperactive/increased, i.e., high-pitched, loud, rushing sounds that occur frequently (e.g., every 3 seconds); also known as borborygmi Hyperactive sounds indicate increased intestinal motility and are usually associated with diarrhea, an early bowel obstruction, or the use of laxatives True absence of sounds (none heard in 3 to 5 minutes) indicates a cessation of intestinal motility
For Vascular Sounds		
• Use the bell of the stethoscope over the aorta, renal arteries, iliac arteries, and femoral arteries. • Listen for bruits.	Absence of arterial bruits	Loud bruit over aortic area (possible aneurysm) Bruit over renal or iliac arteries
Peritoneal Friction Rubs		
• Peritoneal friction rubs are rough, grating sounds like two pieces of leather rubbing together. Friction rubs may be caused by inflammation, infection, or abnormal growths. • To auscultate the splenic site, place the stethoscope over the left lower rib cage in the anterior axillary line, and ask the client to take a deep breath. A deep breath may accentuate the sound of a friction rub area. • To auscultate the liver site, place the stethoscope over the lower right rib cage.	Absence of friction rub	Friction rub

(continued on next page)

SKILL 1.29   Assessing the Abdomen (continued)

ASSESSMENT	NORMAL FINDINGS	DEVIATIONS FROM NORMAL
Percussion of the Abdomen		
11. Percuss several areas in each of the four quadrants to determine presence of tympany (gas in stomach and intestines) and dullness (decrease, absence, or flatness of resonance over solid masses or fluid). Use a systematic pattern: Begin in the lower right quadrant, proceed to the upper right quadrant, the upper left quadrant, and the lower left quadrant ❹.	Tympany over the stomach and gas-filled bowels; dullness, especially over the liver and spleen, or a full bladder 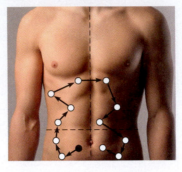 ❹ Systematic percussion sites for all four abdominal quadrants. (Copyright ollyy/Shutterstock)	Large dull areas (associated with presence of fluid or a tumor)
Palpation of the Abdomen		
12. Perform light palpation first to detect areas of tenderness and/or muscle guarding. Systematically explore all four quadrants. Ensure that the client's position is appropriate for relaxation of the abdominal muscles, and warm the hands. **Rationale:** *Cold hands can elicit muscle tension and thus impede palpatory evaluation.*	No tenderness; relaxed abdomen with smooth, consistent tension	Tenderness and hypersensitivity Superficial masses Localized areas of increased tension
Light Palpation		
• Hold the palm of your hand slightly above the client's abdomen, with your fingers parallel to the abdomen. • Depress the abdominal wall lightly, about 1 cm or to the depth of the subcutaneous tissue, with the pads of your fingers ❺. • Move the finger pads in a slight circular motion. • Note areas of tenderness or superficial pain, masses, and muscle guarding. To determine areas of tenderness, ask the client to tell you about them and watch for changes in the client's facial expressions. • If the client is excessively ticklish, begin by pressing your hand on top of the client's hand while pressing lightly. Then slide your hand off the client's and onto the abdomen to continue the examination.	No bulges felt No masses felt 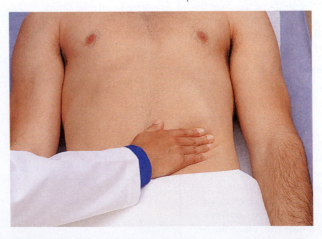 ❺ Light palpation of the abdomen.	Rigid, tender muscles/pain may be due to presence of muscle spasm, inflammation, or infection (peritonitis) Pain or tenderness with quick release of pressure indicates rebound tenderness suggesting peritoneal inflammation If hernia is suspected, have client raise head and shoulders and observe for abdominal bulge

SKILL 1.29   Assessing the Abdomen (continued)

ASSESSMENT	NORMAL FINDINGS	DEVIATIONS FROM NORMAL
Palpation of the Bladder		
13. Palpate the area above the pubic symphysis if the client's history indicates possible urinary retention ❻. 14. Document findings in the client record using forms or checklists supplemented by narrative notes when appropriate.	Not palpable 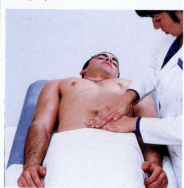 ❻ *Palpating the bladder.*	Distended and palpable as smooth, round, tense mass (indicates urinary retention)

Developmental Considerations

INFANTS

- Internal organs of newborns and infants are proportionately larger than those of older children and adults, so their abdomens are rounded and tend to protrude.
- Umbilical hernias may be present at birth.

CHILDREN

- Toddlers have a characteristic "pot belly" appearance, which can persist until age 3 to 4 years.
- Late preschool and school-age children are leaner than toddlers and have a flat abdomen.
- Peristaltic waves may be more visible than in adults.
- Children may not be able to pinpoint areas of tenderness; by observing facial expressions the examiner can determine areas of maximum tenderness.
- If the child is ticklish, guarding, or fearful, use a task that requires concentration (such as squeezing the hands together) to distract the child, or have the child place his or her hands on yours as you palpate the abdomen, "helping" you to do the exam.

OLDER ADULTS

- The rounded abdomens of older adults are due to an increase in adipose tissue and a decrease in muscle tone.
- The abdominal wall is slacker and thinner, making palpation easier and more accurate than in younger clients. Muscle wasting and loss of fibroconnective tissue occur.
- The pain threshold in older adults is often higher than that of younger adults; major abdominal problems such as appendicitis or other acute emergencies may therefore go undetected.
- Gastrointestinal pain needs to be differentiated from cardiac pain. Gastrointestinal pain may be located in the thorax or abdomen, whereas cardiac pain is usually located in the thorax. However, these relationships are not absolute because cardiac abnormalities may present as gastrointestinal complaints, especially in women. Factors aggravating gastrointestinal pain are usually related to either ingestion or lack of food intake; gastrointestinal pain is usually relieved by antacids, food, or assuming an upright position. Common factors that can aggravate cardiac pain are activity or anxiety. Rest or nitroglycerin relieves cardiac pain.
- Stool passes through the intestines at a slower rate in older adults, and the perception of stimuli that produce the urge to defecate often diminishes.
- Fecal incontinence may occur in older adults who are confused or neurologically impaired.
- Many older adults erroneously believe that the absence of a daily bowel movement signifies constipation. When assessing for constipation, the nurse must consider the client's diet, activity, medications, and characteristics and ease of passage of feces as well as the frequency of bowel movements.
- The incidence of colon cancer is higher among older adults than younger adults. Symptoms include a change in bowel function, rectal bleeding, and weight loss. Changes in bowel function, however, are associated with many factors, such as diet, exercise, and medications.
- Decreased absorption of oral medications often occurs with aging.
- In the liver, impaired metabolism of some drugs may occur with aging.

Setting of Care

- Be sure you have the required equipment on a home visit, including a tape measure and skin-marking pen.
- Use pillows to position the client.
- Undressing the client to perform a complete abdominal examination may not be necessary. Focus the assessment on areas indicated by the history and present complaint.

SKILL 1.30   Assessing the Female Genitals and Inguinal Area

Delegation

Due to the substantial knowledge and skill required, assessment of the female genitals and inguinal lymph nodes is not delegated to UAP. However, individuals other than the nurse may record any aspect of the genital system that is observed during usual care. Abnormal findings must be validated and interpreted by the nurse.

Equipment

- Clean gloves
- Drape
- Supplemental lighting, if needed

Procedure

1. Prior to performing the procedure, introduce self and verify the client's identity using agency protocol. Explain to the client what you are going to do, why it is necessary, and how she can participate. Discuss how the results will be used in planning further care or treatments.
2. Perform hand hygiene, apply gloves, and observe other appropriate infection control procedures.
3. Provide for client privacy. Request the presence of another woman if desired, required by agency policy, or requested by the client.
4. Inquire regarding the following: age of onset of menstruation, date of last menstrual period (LMP), regularity of cycle, duration, amount of daily flow, and whether menstruation is painful; incidence of pain during intercourse; vaginal discharge; number of pregnancies, number of live births, labor or delivery complications; urgency and frequency of urination at night; blood in urine, painful urination, incontinence; history of sexually transmitted infection, past and present.
5. Cover the pelvic area with a sheet or drape at all times when not actually being examined. Position the client supine.

ASSESSMENT	NORMAL FINDINGS	DEVIATIONS FROM NORMAL
6. Inspect the distribution, amount, and characteristics of pubic hair.	There are wide variations; generally kinky in the menstruating adult, thinner and straighter after menopause Distributed in the shape of an inverse triangle	Scant pubic hair (may indicate hormonal problem) Hair growth should not extend over the abdomen
7. Inspect the skin of the pubic area for parasites, inflammation, swelling, and lesions. To assess pubic skin adequately, separate the labia majora and labia minora.	Pubic skin intact, no lesions Skin of vulva area slightly darker than the rest of the body Minimal odor Labia round, full, and relatively symmetric in adult females	Lice, lesions, scars, fissures, swelling, erythema, excoriations, varicosities, or leukoplakia Malodorous discharge; thin, friable labia; protruding uterus
8. Palpate the inguinal lymph nodes ❶. Use the pads of the fingers in a rotary motion, noting any enlargement or tenderness. ❶ Lymph nodes of the groin area.	No enlargement or tenderness.	Enlargement and tenderness
9. Remove and discard gloves. Perform hand hygiene.		
10. Document findings in the client record using forms or checklists supplemented by narrative notes when appropriate.		

Superior or horizontal group

Inferior or vertical group

SKILL 1.30   Assessing the Female Genitals and Inguinal Area (continued)

BOX 1–5   Five Stages of Pubic Hair Development in Females

Stage 1: Preadolescence. No pubic hair except for fine body hair.

Stage 2: Usually occurs at ages 11 and 12. Sparse, long, slightly pigmented curly hair develops along the labia.

Stage 3: Usually occurs at ages 12 and 13. Hair becomes darker in color and curlier and develops over the pubic symphysis.

Stage 4: Usually occurs between ages 13 and 14. Hair assumes the texture and curl of the adult but is not as thick and does not appear on the thighs.

Stage 5: Sexual maturity. Hair assumes adult appearance and appears on the inner aspect of the upper thighs.

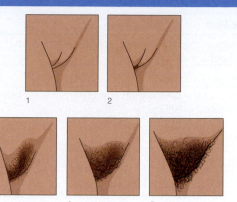

Stages of female pubic hair development.

Developmental Considerations

INFANTS

- Infants can be held in a supine position on the parent's lap with the knees supported in a flexed position and separated.
- In newborns, because of maternal estrogen, the labia and clitoris may be edematous and enlarged, and there may be a small amount of white or bloody vaginal discharge.
- Assess the mons and inguinal area for swelling or tenderness that may indicate the presence of an inguinal hernia.

CHILDREN

- Ensure that you have the parent or guardian's approval to perform the examination and then tell the child what you are going to do. Preschool children are taught not to allow others to touch their "private parts."
- Girls should be assessed for Tanner staging of pubertal development (**Box 1–5 ●**).
- Girls should be referred to a primary care provider for a Papanicolaou (Pap) test if sexually active, or by age 18 years.
- The clitoris is a common site for syphilitic chancres in younger females.

OLDER ADULTS

- Labia are atrophied and flatter in older females.
- The clitoris is a potential site for cancerous lesions in older females.
- The vulva atrophies as a result of a reduction in vascularity, elasticity, adipose tissue, and estrogen levels. Because the vulva is more fragile, it is more easily irritated.
- The vaginal environment becomes drier and more alkaline, resulting in an alteration of the type of flora present and a predisposition to vaginitis. Dyspareunia (difficult or painful intercourse) is also a common occurrence.
- The cervix and uterus decrease in size.
- The fallopian tubes and ovaries atrophy.
- Ovulation and estrogen production cease.
- Vaginal bleeding unrelated to estrogen therapy is abnormal in older women.
- Prolapse of the uterus can occur in older females, especially those who have had multiple pregnancies.

SKILL 1.31   Assessing the Male Genitals and Inguinal Area

Delegation

Due to the substantial knowledge and skill required, assessment of the male genitals and inguinal area is not delegated to UAP. However, individuals other than the nurse may record any aspect of the genital system that is observed during usual care. Abnormal findings must be validated and interpreted by the nurse.

Equipment

- Clean gloves

Procedure

1. Prior to performing the procedure, introduce self and verify the client's identity using agency protocol. Explain to the client what you are going to do, why it is necessary, and how he can participate. Discuss how the results will be used in planning further care or treatments.

2. Perform hand hygiene, apply gloves, and observe other appropriate infection control procedures.

3. Provide for client privacy. Request the presence of another person if desired, required by agency policy, or requested by the client.

4. Inquire regarding the following: usual voiding patterns and changes, bladder control; history of urinary incontinence, frequency, urgency, abdominal pain; symptoms of sexually transmitted infection; swellings that could indicate presence of hernia; family history of nephritis, malignancy of the prostate, or malignancy of the kidney.

5. Cover the pelvic area with a sheet or drape at all times when not actually being examined.

(continued on next page)

SKILL 1.31   Assessing the Male Genitals and Inguinal Area (continued)

ASSESSMENT	NORMAL FINDINGS	DEVIATIONS FROM NORMAL
Pubic Hair		
6. Inspect the distribution, amount, and characteristics of pubic hair.	Triangular distribution, often spreading up the abdomen	Scant amount or absence of hair
Penis		
7. Inspect the penile shaft and glans penis for lesions, nodules, swellings, and inflammation.	Penile skin intact Appears slightly wrinkled and varies in color as widely as other body skin Foreskin easily retractable from the glans penis Small amount of thick white smegma between the glans and foreskin	Presence of lesions, nodules, swellings, or inflammation
8. Inspect the urethral meatus for swelling, inflammation, and discharge. • Compress or ask the client to compress the glans slightly to open the urethral meatus to inspect it for discharge.	Pink and slitlike appearance Positioned at the tip of the penis	Inflammation; discharge Variation in meatal locations (e.g., hypospadias, on the underside of the penile shaft, and epispadias, on the upper side of the penile shaft)
Scrotum		
9. Inspect the scrotum for appearance, general size, and symmetry. • To facilitate inspection of the scrotum during a physical examination, ask the client to hold the penis out of the way. • Inspect all skin surfaces by spreading the rugated surface skin and lifting the scrotum as needed to observe posterior surfaces.	Scrotal skin is darker in color than that of the rest of the body and is loose Size varies with temperature changes (the dartos muscles contract when the area is cold and relax when the area is warm) Scrotum appears asymmetric (left testis is usually lower than right testis)	Discolorations; any tightening of skin (may indicate edema or mass) Marked asymmetry in size
Inguinal Area		
10. Inspect both inguinal areas for bulges while the client is standing, if possible. • First, have the client remain at rest. • Next, have the client hold his breath and strain or bear down as though having a bowel movement. Bearing down may make the hernia more visible.	No swelling or bulges	Swelling or bulge (possible inguinal or femoral hernia)
11. Remove and discard gloves. Perform hand hygiene.		
12. Document findings in the client record using forms or checklists supplemented by narrative notes when appropriate.		

Developmental Considerations

INFANTS

- The foreskin of the uncircumcised infant is normally tight at birth and should not be retracted. It will gradually loosen as the baby grows and is usually fully retractable by 2 to 3 years of age. Assess for cleanliness, redness, or irritation.
- Assess for placement of the urethral meatus.
- Palpate the scrotum to determine if the testes have descended; in the newborn and infant, the testes may retract into the inguinal canal, especially with stimulation of the cremasteric reflex.
- Assess the inguinal area for swelling or tenderness that may indicate presence of an inguinal hernia.

CHILDREN

- Ensure that you have the parent or guardian's approval to perform the examination and then tell the child what you are going to do. Preschool children are taught not to allow others to touch their "private parts."

- In young boys, the cremasteric reflex can cause the testes to ascend into the inguinal canal. If possible have the boy sit cross-legged; this stretches the muscle and decreases the reflex.
- **Table 1–11** ● shows the five Tanner stages of development of pubic hair, penis, and testes/scrotum.

OLDER ADULTS

- The penis decreases in size with age; the size and firmness of the testes decrease.
- Testosterone is produced in smaller amounts.
- More time and direct physical stimulation are required for an older man to achieve an erection, but he can maintain the erection for a longer period before ejaculation than he could at a younger age.
- Seminal fluid is reduced in amount and viscosity.
- Urinary frequency, nocturia, dribbling, and problems with beginning and ending the stream are usually the result of prostatic enlargement.

SKILL 1.31   Assessing the Male Genitals and Inguinal Area (continued)

TABLE 1–11	Tanner Stages of Male Pubic Hair and External Genital Development (12 to 16 Years)		
STAGE	PUBIC HAIR	PENIS	TESTES/SCROTUM
1	None, except for body hair like that on the abdomen	Size is relative to body size, as in childhood	Size is relative to body size, as in childhood
2	Scant, long, slightly pigmented at base of penis	Slight enlargement occurs	Becomes reddened in color and enlarged
3	Darker, begins to curl and becomes more coarse; extends over pubic symphysis	Elongation occurs	Continuing enlargement
4	Continues to darken and thicken; extends on the sides, above and below	Increase in both breadth and length; glans develops	Continuing enlargement; color darkens
5	Adult distribution that extends to inner thighs, umbilicus, and anus	Adult appearance	Adult appearance

SKILL 1.32   Assessing the Anus

Delegation

Assessment of the anus is not delegated to UAP. However, the condition of the anal area may be observed during usual care and may be recorded by individuals other than the nurse. Abnormal findings must be validated and interpreted by the nurse.

Equipment

- Clean gloves

Procedure

1. Prior to performing the procedure, introduce self and verify the client's identity using agency protocol. Explain to the client what you are going to do, why it is necessary, and how he or she can participate. Discuss how the results will be used in planning further care or treatments.

2. Perform hand hygiene, apply gloves, and observe other appropriate infection control procedures for all rectal examinations.

3. Provide for client privacy. Drape the client appropriately to prevent undue exposure of body parts.

4. Inquire if the client has any history of the following: bright blood in stools, tarry black stools, diarrhea, constipation, abdominal pain, excessive gas, hemorrhoids, or rectal pain; family history of colorectal cancer; when last stool specimen for occult blood was performed and the results; and for males, if not obtained during the genitourinary examination, signs or symptoms of prostate enlargement (e.g., slow urinary stream, hesitancy, frequency, dribbling, and nocturia).

5. Position the client in a left lateral or Sims position with the upper leg acutely flexed. A dorsal recumbent position with hips externally rotated and knees flexed may also be used. For males, a standing position while the client bends over the examining table may also be used.

(continued on next page)

SKILL 1.32 Assessing the Anus (continued)

ASSESSMENT	NORMAL FINDINGS	DEVIATIONS FROM NORMAL
6. Inspect the anus and surrounding tissue for color, integrity, and skin lesions. Then, ask the client to bear down as though defecating. Bearing down creates slight pressure on the skin that may accentuate rectal fissures, rectal prolapse, polyps, or internal hemorrhoids. Describe the location of all abnormal findings in terms of a clock, with the 12 o'clock position toward the pubic symphysis.	Intact perianal skin; usually slightly more pigmented than the skin of the buttocks Anal skin is normally more pigmented, coarser, and moister than perianal skin and is usually hairless	Presence of fissures (cracks), ulcers, excoriations, inflammations, abscesses, protruding hemorrhoids (dilated veins seen as reddened protrusions of the skin), lumps or tumors, fistula openings, or rectal prolapse (varying degrees of protrusion of the rectal mucous membrane through the anus)
7. Remove and discard gloves. Perform hand hygiene.		
8. Document findings in the client record using forms or checklists supplemented by narrative notes when appropriate.		

Developmental Considerations

INFANTS

■ Lightly touching the anus should result in a brief anal contraction ("wink" reflex).

CHILDREN

■ Erythema and scratch marks around the anus may indicate a pinworm parasite. Children with this condition may be disturbed by itching during sleep.

OLDER ADULTS

■ Chronic constipation and straining at stool cause an increase in the frequency of hemorrhoids and rectal prolapse.

▶ PHYSICAL ASSESSMENTS FOR THE NEWBORN

For physical assessment of the newborn, see Chapter 16 on reproduction.

▶ CRITICAL THINKING OPTIONS FOR UNEXPECTED OUTCOMES

Not all unexpected outcomes require further nursing intervention; however, many times they do. When the client demonstrates a change in signs/symptoms indicating an emerging problem, the nurse should immediately assess and troubleshoot what is happening. The assessment data must be processed quickly to formulate a hypothesis so the nurse can make a clinical judgment. The nurse then decides how best to resolve the problem and improve the client's situation for a better appropriate outcome.

EXPECTED OUTCOME	PROBLEM SOLVING	NURSING ACTIONS
General Assessment Height and weight are obtained and recorded.	Client's weight varies more than expected from one day to the next.	■ Check time of day weight was measured. ■ Check if same scale was used for both weighings. ■ Check equipment's reliability. ■ Check what clothing or linen was on the client when weighed on both days. ■ Check I&O record for sources of fluid loss or gain. ■ Check MAR for medications that alter fluid balance (e.g., diuretics).
Vital Signs Temperature is within normal range.	Fever develops.	■ Check possible sources of infection and take preventive measures. ■ Notify physician. ■ Employ cooling methods if temperature is dangerously high, such as tepid sponge bath, cool oral fluids, ice packs, or antipyretic drugs. ■ Assess all vital signs.

EXPECTED OUTCOME	PROBLEM SOLVING	NURSING ACTIONS
Temperature is within normal range.	Temperature remains elevated because of bacterial-produced pyrogens.	■ Check for order to obtain culture of possible sources of infection. ■ Give antipyretic drugs as ordered. ■ Decrease room temperature and remove excess covers. ■ Give tepid sponge bath.
	Temperature remains subnormal.	■ Extreme low temperature can cause vasoconstriction; assess for blood clots. ■ Institute measures to promote vasodilation (application of warmth). ■ If extremity is ischemic, monitor that heat source does not exceed body temperature.
Pulse is palpated without difficulty.	Apical, femoral, and carotid pulse are absent.	■ Assess all vital signs and status of the client. ■ Immediately call for the rapid response team. ■ Initiate CPR immediately. ■ Use Doppler device to assess for presence of pulse.
	Peripheral pulse is absent.	■ Assess for other signs and symptoms of circulatory impairment.
Respiratory rate, rhythm, and depth are within normal limits.	Apnea (absence of breathing) occurs, may be intermittent.	■ Assess client for all vital signs and comfort/condition. ■ Begin rescue breathing at the rate of 12 per minute for an adult or 20 per minute for a child
Labored, difficult, or noisy respirations are assessed.	Kussmaul respirations occur (deep and gasping breaths—more than 20 breaths/min).	■ Follow orders to treat for diabetic ketoacidosis, renal failure, or septic shock.
The presence of factors that can alter blood pressure readings is identified.	Blood pressure reading is abnormally high without apparent physiological cause.	■ Check that proper cuff size was used. ■ Check if cuff was not snug. ■ Ask if client has pain, was anxious, or had just exercised. ■ Check blood pressure on both arms. The normal difference from arm to arm is usually about 5 mmHg. ■ Ask client to sit and rest for 15 minutes and then retake blood pressure reading.
Accurate readings are taken by using the correct cuff size and procedure.	Blood pressure cannot be measured on upper extremity due to casts, dialysis shunt, or surgical procedure.	■ Use lower extremity to obtain blood pressures. ■ Be sure to document site where blood pressure reading was obtained.
	Hypotension (systolic pressure less than 90 mmHg) develops.	■ Take all vital signs more frequently until condition has stabilized. ■ Place client in supine position with lower extremities elevated 45°. ■ Assess cause of hypotension, and notify physician. ■ Increase or administer fluids as ordered by physician. ■ Observe postoperative clients for signs of bleeding. ■ Administer oxygen.

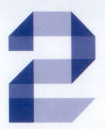 # Caring Interventions

RELATED CONCEPTS

The Biophysical Concepts

The Psychological Concepts

The Social Functioning Concepts

The Developmental Concepts

The Spiritual Concepts

The Health, Wellness, and Illness Concepts

Exemplars

All concepts found in the Individual Domain are related to the Caring Interventions Concept. Throughout all these concepts, cognitive functions of analyzing, interpreting, and making clinical judgments are done to determine priority appropriate caring interventions for best individual client outcomes.

Skills-at-a-Glance

Skills-at-a-Glance *continued*

Because people are usually confined to bed when ill, often for a long period, the bed becomes an important element in the client's life. A place that is clean, safe, and comfortable contributes to the client's ability to rest and sleep and to a sense of well-being. From a holistic perspective, bed-making can be viewed as the preparation of a healing space. Basic furniture in a healthcare facility includes the bed, bedside cabinet, overbed table, one or more chairs, and a storage space for clothing. Most bed units also have a call light, light fixtures, electric outlets, and hygienic equipment in a bedside cabinet. Three types of equipment often installed in an acute care facility are a suction outlet for several kinds of suction, an oxygen outlet for most oxygen equipment, and a sphygmomanometer to measure the client's blood pressure. Some long-term care agencies also permit clients to have personal furniture, such as a television, a chair, and lamps, at the bedside. In the home a client often has personal and medical equipment near the bed.

Personal hygiene is the self-care by which people attend to such functions as bathing, toileting, general body hygiene, and grooming. Hygiene is a highly personal matter determined by various factors, including individual and cultural values and practices. It involves care of the skin, hair, nails, teeth, oral and nasal cavities, eyes, ears, and perineal-genital areas.

Nurses need to determine exactly how much assistance a client needs for hygienic care. Clients may require help after urinating or defecating, after vomiting, and whenever they become soiled, for example, from wound drainage or from profuse perspiration. In addition, culture-specific beliefs and practices influence hygienic care. **Table 2–1** lists factors that influence hygienic practices.

Nurses commonly use the following terms to describe the various types of hygienic care:

- *Early morning care* is provided to clients as they awaken in the morning. This care consists of providing a urinal or bedpan to the client confined to bed, washing the face and hands, and giving oral care.
- *Morning care* is often provided after clients have breakfast, although it may be provided before breakfast. It usually includes providing for elimination needs, a bath or shower,

FACTOR	VARIABLES
TABLE 2–1 Factors That Influence Individual Hygienic Practices	
Culture	North American culture places a high value on cleanliness. Many North Americans bathe or shower once or twice a day, whereas people from some other cultures bathe once a week. Some cultures consider privacy essential for bathing, whereas others practice communal bathing. Body odor is offensive in some cultures and accepted as normal in others.
Religion	Ceremonial washings are practiced by some religions.
Environment	Finances may affect the availability of facilities for bathing. For example, homeless people may not have warm water available; soap, shampoo, shaving lotion, and deodorants may be too expensive for people who have limited resources.
Developmental level	Children learn hygiene in the home. Practices vary according to the individual's age; for example, preschoolers can carry out most tasks independently with encouragement.
Health and energy	Ill people may not have the motivation or energy to attend to hygiene. Some clients who have neuromuscular impairments may be unable to perform hygienic care.
Personal preferences	Some people prefer a shower to a tub bath. People have different preferences regarding the time of bathing (e.g., morning versus evening).

perineal care, and oral, nail, and hair care. Making the client's bed is part of morning care.

- *Hour of sleep care*, or *PM care*, is provided to clients before they retire for the night. It usually involves providing for elimination needs, washing face and hands, giving oral care, and possibly giving a back massage. Some clients prefer bathing in the evening. If possible, the nurse needs to accommodate the client's routine schedule for personal hygiene.

- *As-needed (PRN) care* is provided as required by the client. For example, a client who is diaphoretic (sweating profusely) may need bathing and a change of clothes and linen frequently.

MASSAGE

Massage is a comfort measure that can aid relaxation, promote circulation of blood and lymph, and decrease muscle tension. It may ease anxiety because the physical contact communicates caring. By increasing superficial circulation as well as neurological distraction, pain intensity can be directly reduced as a result of massage. The use of creams, oils, aromatherapy, or liniments may amplify therapeutic potential. Massage is contraindicated in areas of skin breakdown, suspected clots, or infections.

Ironically, nurses in acute care settings seldom use this basic nursing skill. The intensity of the acute care environment and the time demands of high-technology nursing may be contributing factors leading to the disappearance of the back massage. Nurses, however, need to reconsider this simple, effective, traditional skill when research indicates the positive client outcomes.

PERINEAL-GENITAL CARE

Perineal-genital care is also referred to as **perineal care** or **peri-care**. Perineal care as part of the bed bath is embarrassing for many clients. Nurses also may find it embarrassing initially, particularly with clients of the opposite sex. Most clients who require a bed bath from the nurse are able to clean their own perineal area with minimal assistance. The nurse may need to hand a moistened washcloth and soap to the client, rinse the washcloth, and provide a towel.

Because some clients are unfamiliar with terminology for the genitals and perineum, it may be difficult for nurses to explain what is expected. Most clients, however, understand what is meant if the nurse simply says, "I'll give you a washcloth to finish your bath." Older clients may be familiar with the term *private parts*. Whatever expression the nurse uses, it needs to be one that the client understands and one that is comfortable for the nurse to use.

The nurse needs to provide perineal care efficiently and matter of factly. Nurses should wear gloves while providing this care for the comfort of the client and to protect themselves from infection. Skill 2.7 explains how to provide perineal-genital care.

ORAL HYGIENE

Good oral hygiene includes daily stimulation of the gums, mechanical brushing and flossing of the teeth, flushing of the mouth, and regular checkups by a dentist. The nurse is often in a position to help people maintain oral hygiene by helping or teaching them to clean their teeth and oral cavity, by inspecting whether clients (especially children) have done so, or by actually providing mouth care to clients who are ill or incapacitated. The nurse can also be instrumental in identifying problems that require the intervention of a dentist or oral surgeon and arranging a referral.

HAIR CARE

The appearance of the hair often reflects a person's feelings of self-concept and sociocultural well-being. Becoming familiar with hair care needs and practices that may be different from our own is an important aspect of providing competent nursing care to all clients. People who feel ill may not groom their hair as before. A dirty scalp and hair are itchy and uncomfortable, and can have an odor. The hair may also reflect state of health (e.g., excessive coarseness and dryness may be associated with endocrine disorders such as hypothyroidism). Each person has particular ways of caring for hair. Many dark-skinned people need to oil their hair daily because it tends to be dry. Oil prevents the hair from breaking and the scalp from drying. A wide-toothed comb is usually used because finer combs pull and break the hair. Some people brush their hair vigorously before retiring; others comb their hair frequently.

▶ BEDS AND ACTIVITIES OF DAILY LIVING (ADLs)

Expected Outcomes

1. Bed remains clean, dry, and free of wrinkles.
2. Transmission of pathogenic microorganisms is prevented with universal precautions.
3. Bathing and hygiene care are completed without complications.
4. Client's skin, hair, and nails are clean, odor free, and without irritation.
5. Client is comfortable.
6. Eyes and surrounding area are clean and free from crustation.

SKILL 2.1   Changing an Unoccupied Bed

Delegation

Bed-making is usually delegated to unlicensed assistive personnel (UAP). If appropriate, inform the UAP of the proper disposal method for linens that contain drainage. Ask the UAP to inform you immediately if any tubes or dressings become dislodged or removed. Stress the importance of the call light being readily available while the client is out of bed.

Equipment

- Clean gloves, if needed
- Two flat sheets or one fitted and one flat sheet
- Cloth drawsheet (optional)
- One blanket
- One bedspread
- Incontinent pads (optional)
- Pillowcase(s) for the head pillow(s)
- Plastic laundry bag or portable linen hamper, if available

Preparation

- Determine what linens the client may already have in the room. **Rationale:** *Avoids stockpiling of unnecessary extra linens.*

Procedure

1. If the client is in bed, prior to performing the procedure, introduce self and verify the client's identity using agency protocol. Explain to the client what you are going to do, why it is necessary, and how he or she can participate.
2. Perform hand hygiene and observe other appropriate infection control procedures (e.g., clean gloves).
3. Provide for client privacy.
4. Place the fresh linen on the client's chair or overbed table; do not use another client's bed. **Rationale:** *This prevents* **cross-contamination** *(the movement of microorganisms from one client to another) via soiled linen.*
5. Assess and assist the client out of bed using assistive devices (e.g., cane, walker, safety belt) as appropriate. **Rationale:** *This ensures client safety.*
   - Make sure that this is an appropriate and convenient time for the client to be out of bed.
   - Assist the client to a comfortable chair.
6. Raise the bed to a comfortable working height and use good body mechanics to prevent injuries.
7. Apply clean gloves if linens and equipment have been soiled with secretions and/or excretions.
8. Strip the bed (i.e., remove bed linens).
   - Check bed linens for any items belonging to the client, and detach the call bell or any drainage tubes from the bed linen.
   - Loosen all bedding systematically, starting at the head of the bed on the far side and moving around the bed up to the head of the bed on the near side. **Rationale:** *Moving around the bed systematically prevents stretching and reaching and possible muscle strain.*
   - Remove the pillowcases, if soiled, and place the pillows on the bedside chair near the foot of the bed.
   - Fold reusable linens, such as the bedspread and top sheet on the bed, into fourths ❶. First, fold the linen in

half by bringing the top edge even with the bottom edge, and then grasp it at the center of the middle fold and bottom edges. **Rationale:** *Folding linens saves time and energy when reapplying the linens on the bed and keeps them clean.*

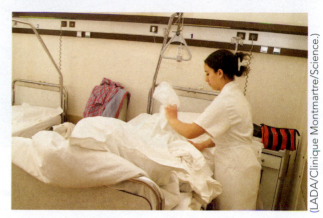

(LADA/Clinique Montmartre/Science.)

❶ Fold reusable linens into fourths when removing them from

- Remove the incontinent pad and discard it if soiled.
- Roll all soiled linen inside the bottom sheet, hold it away from your uniform, and place it directly into the linen hamper, not on the floor ❷. **Rationale:** *These actions are essential to prevent the transmission of microorganisms to the nurse and others.*

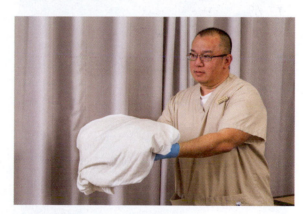

❷ Roll soiled linen inside the bottom sheet and hold away from the body.

- Wipe the mattress with disinfectant if soiled.
- Grasp the mattress securely, using the lugs if present, and move the mattress up to the head of the bed.
- Remove and discard gloves if used. Perform hand hygiene.

9. Apply the bottom sheet and drawsheet.
   - Place the folded bottom sheet with its center fold on the center of the bed ❸. Make sure the sheet is hem-side down for a smooth foundation. Spread the sheet out over the mattress, and allow a sufficient amount of sheet at the top to tuck under the mattress. **Rationale:** *The top of the sheet needs to be well tucked under to remain securely in place, especially when the head of the bed is elevated.* Place the sheet along the edge of the mattress at the foot of the bed and do not tuck it in (unless it is a contour or fitted sheet).

(continued on next page)

SKILL 2.1 Changing an Unoccupied Bed (continued)

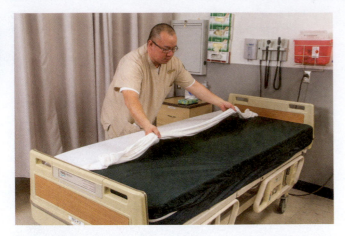

3 Placing the bottom sheet on the bed.

• Miter the sheet at the top corner on the near side **4** **5** and tuck the sheet under the mattress, working from the head of the bed to the foot.

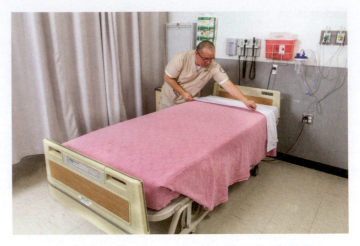

4 Mitered corners help keep bed linens secure.

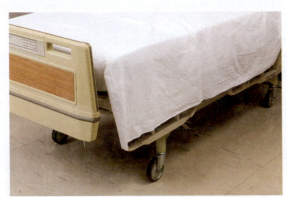

A

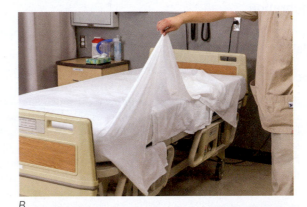

B

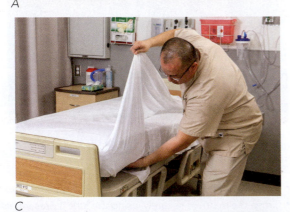

C

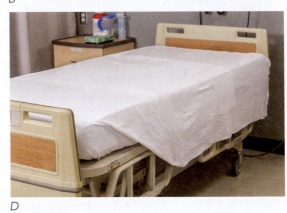

D

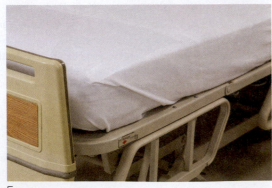

E

5 Mitering the corner of a bed: A, Tuck in the bedcover (sheet, blanket, and/or spread) firmly under the mattress at the bottom or top of the bed. B, Lift the bed cover so that it forms a triangle with the side edge of the bed and the edge of the bedcover is parallel to the end of the bed. C, Tuck the part of the cover that hangs below the mattress under the mattress while holding the triangle up or against the bed. D, Bring the tip of the triangle down toward the floor while the other hand holds the fold of the cover against the side of the mattress. E, Remove the hand and tuck the remainder of the cover under the mattress, if appropriate. The sides of the top sheet, blanket, and bedspread may be left hanging freely rather than tucked in, if desired.

SKILL 2.1　**Changing an Unoccupied Bed** (*continued*)

- If a drawsheet is used, place it over the bottom sheet so that the centerfold is at the centerline of the bed and the top and bottom edges extend from the middle of where the client's back would be on the bed to the area where the midthigh or knee would be ➏. Fanfold the uppermost half of the folded drawsheet at the center or far edge of the bed and tuck in the near edge.

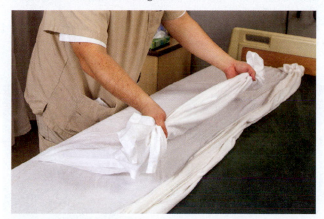

➏ Placing a clean drawsheet on the bed.

- *Optional:* Before moving to the other side of the bed, place the top linens on the bed hem-side up, unfold them, tuck them in, and miter the bottom corners. **Rationale:** *Completing one entire side of the bed at a time saves time and energy.*

10.　Move to the other side and secure the bottom linens.
- Tuck in the bottom sheet under the head of the mattress, pull the sheet firmly, and miter the corner of the sheet.
- Pull the remainder of the sheet firmly so that there are no wrinkles. **Rationale:** *Wrinkles can cause discomfort for the client and breakdown of skin. Tuck the sheet in at the side.*
- Tuck in the drawsheet, if appropriate.

11.　Apply or complete the top sheet, blanket, and spread.
- Place the top sheet, hem-side up, on the bed so that its center fold is at the center of the bed and the top edge is even with the top edge of the mattress.
- Unfold the sheet over the bed.
- *Optional:* Make a vertical or a horizontal toe pleat in the sheet. A toe pleat provides additional room for the client's feet and helps prevent foot drop.
  - a. *Vertical toe pleat:* Make a fold in the sheet 5 to 10 cm (2 to 4 in.) perpendicular to the foot of the bed ➐.
  - b. *Horizontal toe pleat:* Make a fold in the sheet 5 to 10 cm (2 to 4 in.) across the bed near the foot ➑.

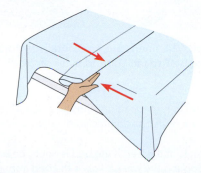

➐ A vertical toe pleat.

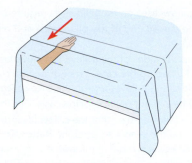

➑ A horizontal toe pleat: Make a fold in the sheet 5 to 10 cm (2 to 4 in.) across the bed near the foot.

Loosening the top covers around the feet after the client is in bed is another way to provide additional space ➒.

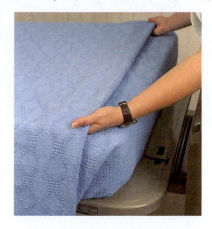

➒ Pleat top linen to allow space for feet.

- Follow the same procedure for the blanket and the spread, but place the top edges about 15 cm (6 in.) from the head of the bed to allow a cuff of sheet to be folded over them.
- Tuck in the sheet, blanket, and spread at the foot of the bed, and miter the corner, using all three layers of linen. Leave the sides of the top sheet, blanket, and spread hanging freely unless toe pleats were provided.
- Fold the top of the top sheet down over the spread, providing a cuff ➓. **Rationale:** *The cuff of sheet makes it easier for the client to pull the covers up.*
- Move to the other side of the bed and secure the top bedding in the same manner.

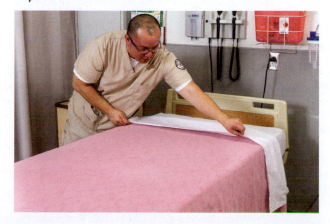

➓ Making a cuff of the top linens.

(*continued on next page*)

SKILL 2.1 Changing an Unoccupied Bed *(continued)*

12. Put clean pillowcases on the pillows as required.
    - Grasp the closed end of the pillowcase at the center with one hand.
    - Gather up the sides of the pillowcase and place them over the hand grasping the case. Then grasp the center of one short side of the pillow through the pillowcase ⑪.
    - With the free hand, pull the pillowcase over the pillow.
    - Adjust the pillowcase so that the pillow fits into the corners of the case and the seams are straight. **Rationale:** *A smoothly fitting pillowcase is more comfortable than a wrinkled one.*
    - Place the pillows appropriately at the head of the bed.

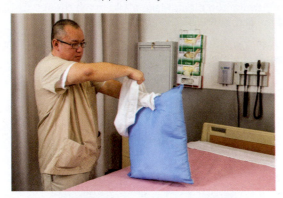

⑪ Method for putting a clean pillowcase on a pillow.

13. Provide for client comfort and safety.
    - Attach the call light so that the client can conveniently reach it. Some call lights have clamps that attach to the sheet or pillowcase. Others are attached by a safety pin. Most beds now have a call light button on the side rail.
    - If the bed is currently being used by a client, either fold back the top covers at one side or fanfold them down to the end of the bed. **Rationale:** *This makes it easier for the client to get into the bed.*
    - Place the bedside cabinet and the overbed table so that they are available to the client.
    - Leave the bed in the high position if the client is returning by stretcher, or place in the low position if the client is returning to bed after being up ambulating or sitting in a chair.

14. Document and report pertinent data.
    - Many agencies use a checklist that indicates if bed linens were changed.
    - Record any nursing assessments, such as the client's physical status and pulse and respiratory rates before and after being out of bed, as indicated.

VARIATION: MAKING A SURGICAL BED

A **surgical bed** is used for the client who is having surgery and will return to bed for the postoperative phase. When making a surgical bed, the linens are horizontally fanfolded to facilitate transfer of the client into the bed. In some agencies, the client is brought back to the unit on a stretcher and transferred to the bed in the room. In other agencies, the client's bed is brought to the surgery suite and the client is transferred there. In the latter situation, the bed needs to be made with clean linens as soon as the client goes to surgery so that it can be taken to the operating room when needed.

- Strip the bed.
- Place and leave the pillows on the bedside chair. **Rationale:** *Pillows are left on a chair to facilitate transferring the client into the bed.*

- Apply the bottom linens as for an unoccupied bed. Place a bath blanket on the foundation of the bed if this is agency practice. **Rationale:** *A flannel bath blanket provides additional warmth.*
- Place the top covers (sheet, blanket, and bedspread) on the bed as you would for an unoccupied bed. Do not tuck them in, miter the corners, or make a toe pleat.
- Make a cuff at the top of the bed as you would for an unoccupied bed. Fold the top linens up from the bottom.
- On the side of the bed where the client will be transferred, fold up the two outer corners of the top linens so they meet in the middle of the bed forming a triangle ⑫.

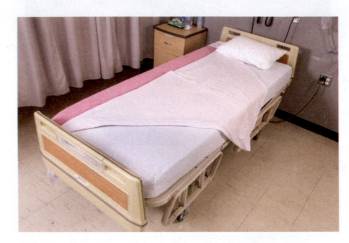

⑫ Fold up the two outer corners of the top linens, forming a triangle.

- Pick up the apex or point of the triangle and fanfold the top linens lengthwise to the side of the bed opposite from where the client will enter the bed ⑬. **Rationale:** *This facilitates the client's transfer into the bed.*

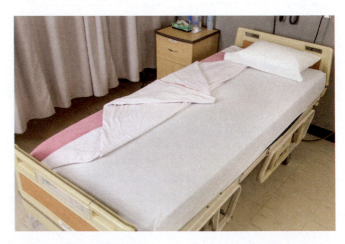

⑬ Surgical bed. The linens are horizontally fanfolded to one side of the bed to facilitate transfer of the client into the bed.

- Leave the bed in high position with the side rails down. **Rationale:** *The high position facilitates the transfer of the client.*
- Lock the wheels of the bed if the bed is not to be moved. **Rationale:** *Locking the wheels keeps the bed from rolling when the client is transferred from the stretcher to the bed.*

SKILL 2.1   Changing an Unoccupied Bed *(continued)*

Practice Guidelines

- Wash hands thoroughly after handling a client's bed linen. Clean gloves need to be used if linens and equipment have been soiled with secretions and/or excretions.
- Hold soiled linen away from uniform.
- Linen for one client is never (even momentarily) placed on another client's bed or on the floor.
- Place soiled linen directly in a portable linen hamper or tucked into a pillowcase at the end of the bed before it is gathered up for disposal.

- Do not shake soiled linen in the air because shaking can disseminate secretions and excretions and the microorganisms they contain.
- When stripping and making a bed, conserve time and energy by stripping and making up one side as much as possible before working on the other side.
- To avoid unnecessary trips to the linen supply area, gather all linen before starting to strip bed.

SKILL 2.2   Changing an Occupied Bed

Evidence-Based Practice

Bed Rails: Best Practices for Fall Prevention

Today about 2.5 million hospital and nursing home beds are in use in the United States. Incidents of clients caught, trapped, entangled, or strangled in beds with rails have been reported. Of these reports, more than half resulted in fatal injury. Most clients involved were frail, older, or confused.

Guidelines to help avoid use of bed rails include the following:

- Use beds that can be raised and lowered close to the floor.
- Keep the bed in the lowest position with wheels locked.

- Use transfer or mobility aids.
- Monitor clients frequently.
- Meet the needs that cause clients to get out of bed: Offer food and fluids, schedule toileting, provide calming interventions, and pain relief.

When bed rails are used, perform an ongoing assessment of the client's physical and mental status.

Data from U.S. Food and Drug Administration (2010).

Delegation

Bed-making is usually delegated to UAP. Inform the UAP to what extent the client can assist or if another person will be needed to assist the UAP. Instruct the UAP about the handling of any dressings and/or tubes of the client and also the need for special equipment (e.g., footboard, heel protectors), if appropriate.

Equipment

- Two flat sheets or one fitted and one flat sheet
- Cloth drawsheet (optional)
- One blanket
- One bedspread
- Incontinent pads (optional)
- Pillowcase(s) for the head pillow(s)
- Plastic laundry bag or portable linen hamper, if available

Preparation

- Determine what linens the client may already have in the room. **Rationale:** *This avoids stockpiling of unnecessary extra linens.*

Procedure

1. Prior to performing the procedure introduce self and verify the client's identity using agency protocol. Explain to the client what you are going to do, why it is necessary, and how he or she can participate.
2. Perform hand hygiene and observe other appropriate infection control procedures. Put on disposable clean gloves if linen is soiled with body fluids.
3. Provide for client privacy.

4. Remove the top bedding.
   - Remove any equipment attached to the bed linen, such as a signal light.
   - Loosen all top linen at the foot of the bed, and remove the spread and the blanket.
   - Leave the top sheet over the client (the top sheet can remain over the client if it is being changed and if it will provide sufficient warmth), or replace it with a bath blanket as follows:
     a. Spread the bath blanket over the top sheet.
     b. Ask the client to hold the top edge of the blanket.
     c. Reaching under the blanket from the side, grasp the top edge of the sheet and draw it down to the foot of the bed, leaving the blanket in place ❶.

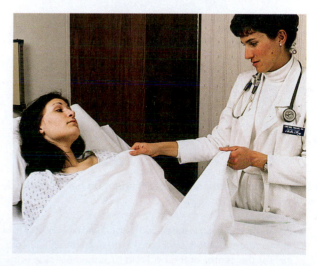

❶ Remove top linen and replace with a bath blanket.

(continued on next page)

SKILL 2.2   Changing an Occupied Bed (continued)

d. Remove the sheet from the bed and place it in the soiled linen hamper.

5. Change the bottom sheet and drawsheet.
   - Raise the side rail that the client will turn toward. **Rationale:** *This protects clients from falling and allows them to support themselves in the side-lying position.* If there is no side rail, have another nurse support the client at the edge of the bed.
   - Assist the client to turn on the side away from the nurse and toward the raised side rail.
   - Loosen the bottom linens on the side of the bed near the nurse.
   - Fanfold the dirty linen (i.e., drawsheet and the bottom sheet) toward the center of the bed as close to and under the client as possible ❷. **Rationale:** *Doing this leaves the near half of the bed free to be changed.*

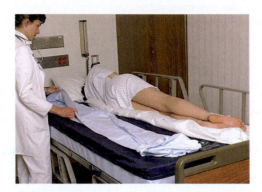

❷ Moving soiled linen as close to the client as possible to make room for clean sheet.

   - Place the new bottom sheet on the bed, and vertically fanfold the half to be used on the far side of the bed as close to the client as possible ❸. Tuck the sheet under the near half of the bed and miter the corner if a contour sheet is not being used.

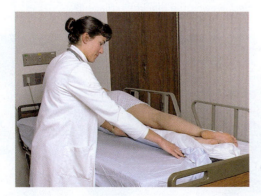

❸ Smooth and tighten new bottom sheet on half of the bed.

   - Place the clean drawsheet on the bed with the center fold at the center of the bed. Fanfold the uppermost half vertically at the center of the bed and tuck the near side edge under the side of the mattress ❹.

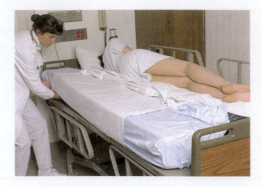

❹ Placing a clean drawsheet on the bed.

   - Assist the client to roll over toward you, over the fanfolded bed linens at the center of the bed, onto the clean side of the bed ❺.

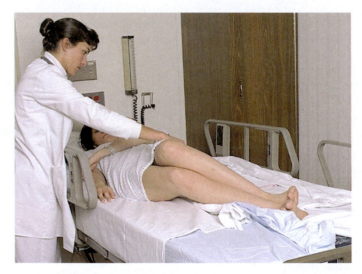

❺ Assist client to roll over to side of bed toward you onto clean linen.

   - Move the pillows to the clean side for the client's use. Raise the side rail before leaving the side of the bed.
   - Move to the other side of the bed and lower the side rail.
   - Remove the used linen and place it in the portable hamper.
   - Unfold the fanfolded bottom sheet from the center of the bed.
   - Facing the side of the bed, use both hands to pull the bottom sheet so that it is smooth and tuck the excess under the side of the mattress.
   - Unfold the drawsheet fanfolded at the center of the bed and pull it tightly with both hands. Pull the sheet in three divisions: (a) Face the side of the bed to pull the middle division, (b) face the far top corner to pull the bottom division, and (c) face the far bottom corner to pull the top division.
   - Tuck the excess drawsheet under the side of the mattress.

6. Reposition the client in the center of the bed.
   - Reposition the pillows at the center of the bed.
   - Assist the client to the center of the bed. Determine what position the client requires or prefers and assist the client to that position.

SKILL 2.2 Changing an Occupied Bed (*continued*)

7. Apply or complete the top bedding.
   • Spread the top sheet over the client and either ask the client to hold the top edge of the sheet or tuck it under the shoulders. The sheet should remain over the client when the bath blanket or used sheet is removed.
   • Complete the top of the bed.

> **CLINICAL ALERT**
> Side rail entrapment, injuries, and deaths do occur. When side rails are used, the nurse must assess the client's physical and mental status and closely monitor high-risk (frail, older, or confused) clients.

8. Ensure continued safety of the client.
   • Raise the side rails. Place the bed in the low position before leaving the bedside.
   • Attach the call light to the bed linen within the client's reach.
   • Put items used by the client within easy reach.
   • Perform hand hygiene.
9. Document. Many agencies use a checklist that indicates if bed linens were changed.

Developmental Considerations

CHILDREN

■ Check if the child has a favorite blanket and if it was brought from home. If so, make sure you replace it on the bed after changing the bed linens.

OLDER ADULTS

■ Because of the older adult's thin, tender, and fragile skin, be sure to check that the linens are dry and free of wrinkles and be especially careful when pulling linens underneath the older client.

Setting of Care

■ If the client needs to remain in bed, determine the caregiver's knowledge and experience with making an occupied bed. The nurse may need to demonstrate how to change the linen.

Emphasize safety for the client and use of correct body mechanics for the caregiver.
■ Assess and discuss with the caregiver the following: need for linens (e.g., incontinence, drainage), available linen supply, and laundry accommodations.

Practice Guidelines

■ Maintain the client in good body alignment. Never move or position a client in a manner that is contraindicated by the client's health. Obtain help if necessary to ensure safety.
■ Move the client gently and smoothly. Rough handling can cause the client discomfort and abrade the skin.
■ Explain what you plan to do throughout the procedure before you do it. Use terms that the client can understand.
■ Use the bed-making time, like the bed bath time, to assess and meet the client's needs.

SKILL 2.3   Providing Morning and Evening Care

Equipment

Disposable cleansing cloth system or towels, washcloth, basin with water and soap
■ Clean linens if needed
■ Dental care items (i.e., toothbrush, toothpaste, dental floss, denture cup, denture cleaner or dentifrice, clean washcloth)
■ Emesis basin, cup
■ Fresh pitcher of water if allowed
■ Skin care lotion if desired
■ Personal care items (e.g., deodorant, skin moisturizers, comb or hairbrush)
■ Bedpan, urinal, toilet paper
■ Miscellaneous supplies as needed (e.g., dressing, special equipment)
■ Clean gloves, if indicated

Preparation

■ Perform hand hygiene.
■ Check two client identifiers.
■ Explain the needs and benefits of evening hygiene care; discuss how the client can be involved. Collect and arrange equipment.

■ Adjust the bed to a comfortable working height, and assist the client into a comfortable position.
■ Ensure privacy.
■ Don gloves if indicated.

Procedure

1. Assess for pain. Medicate as necessary.
2. Offer bedpan or urinal if client is unable to use bathroom. Assist with hand hygiene.
3. If client needs or requests a bath, provide assistance as needed.
4. Assist with mouth and dental care as needed.
   • Place a towel under the client's chin.
   • Apply clean gloves.
   • Moisten the bristles of the toothbrush with tepid water and apply the dentifrice to the toothbrush.
   • Use a soft toothbrush (a small one for a child) and the client's choice of dentifrice.
   • For the client who must remain in bed, place or hold the curved basin under the client's chin, fitting the small curve around the chin or neck.
   • Inspect the mouth and teeth.

(*continued on next page*)

SKILL 2.3   Providing Morning and Evening Care (*continued*)

- Hand the toothbrush to the client, or brush the client's teeth as follows:

  a. Hold the brush against the teeth with the bristles at a 45-degree angle. The tips of the outer bristles should rest against and penetrate under the gingival sulcus ❶. The brush will clean under the sulcus of two or three teeth at one time. **Rationale:** *This sulcular technique removes plaque and cleans under the gingival margins.*

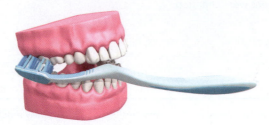

❶ The sulcular technique: Place the bristles at a 45-degree angle with the tops of the outer bristles under the gingival margins.

  b. Move the bristles up and down gently in short strokes from the sulcus to the crowns of the teeth ❷.

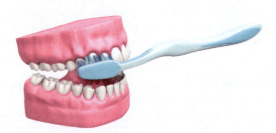

❷ Brushing from the sulcus to the crowns of the teeth.

  c. Repeat until all outer and inner surfaces of the teeth and sulci of the gums have been cleaned.

  d. Clean the biting surfaces by moving the brush back and forth over them in short strokes ❸.

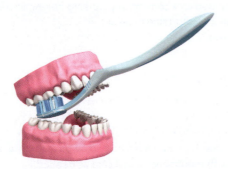

❸ Brushing the biting surfaces.

  e. Brush the tongue gently with the toothbrush. **Rationale:** *Brushing removes bacteria and freshens breath. A coated tongue may be caused by poor oral hygiene, low fluid intake, and side effects of medications. Brushing gently and carefully helps prevent gagging or vomiting.*

- Hand the client the water cup or mouthwash to rinse the mouth vigorously. Then ask the client to spit the water and excess dentifrice into the basin. Some agencies supply a standard mouthwash. Alternatively, a mouth rinse of normal saline can be an effective cleaner and moisturizer.

Rationale: *Vigorous rinsing loosens food particles and washes out already loosened particles.*

- Repeat the preceding step until the mouth is free of dentifrice and food particles.
- Remove the curved basin and help the client wipe the mouth.
- Assist the client to floss independently, or floss the teeth of an alert and cooperative client as follows. Waxed floss is less likely to fray than unwaxed floss; particles between the teeth attach more readily to unwaxed floss than to waxed floss.

  a. Wrap one end of the floss around the third finger of each hand. ❹

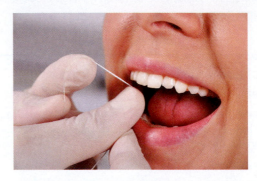

❹ Stretching the floss between the fingers of each hand. (© vetkit)

  b. To floss the upper teeth, use your thumb and index finger to stretch the floss. Move the floss up and down between the teeth. When the floss reaches the gum line, gently slide the floss into the space between the gum and the tooth. Gently move the floss away from the gum with up and down motions (American Dental Association, n.d., Cleaning your teeth). Start at the back on the right side and work around to the back of the left side, or work from the center teeth to the back of the jaw on either side.

  c. To floss the lower teeth, use your index fingers to stretch the floss ❺.

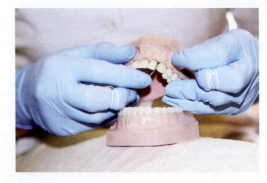

❺ Flossing the teeth, using the fingers to stretch the floss.

- Give the client tepid water or mouthwash to rinse the mouth and a curved basin in which to spit the water.
- Assist the client in wiping the mouth.
- Remove and clean the curved basin.
- Remove and discard gloves. Perform hand hygiene.

5. Remove equipment, extra linens, and pillows, if possible. Remove stockings, ace wraps, and binders.

6. Change dressings. Perform any required procedural techniques.

7. Wash face, hands, and back. Offer back massage in preparation for evening bedtime.

SKILL 2.3 Providing Morning and Evening Care *(continued)*

8. Assist with combing or brushing hair if desired.
9. Replace sequential compression devices, stockings, and binders. Replace soiled linen, or straighten and tuck remaining linen. Fluff pillow and turn cool side next to client.
10. Straighten top linens. Provide additional blankets if desired.
11. Remove any additional equipment. Place call signal and water (if allowed) within client's reach.
12. If evening care, administer sleeping medication if ordered and client requests.
13. Assist client into a comfortable position.
14. Ensure that the client's environment is safe and comfortable.
15. Remove gloves, if used.
16. If care is provided right before sleep, raise upper side rails, place bed in LOW position, and turn lighting to low.
17. Perform hand hygiene.
18. Document care provided.

VARIATION: ARTIFICIAL DENTURES

- Remove the dentures.
  - Apply gloves. **Rationale:** *Wearing gloves decreases the likelihood of spreading infection.*
  - If the client cannot remove the dentures, using the tissue or gauze, grasp the upper plate at the front teeth with your thumb and second finger, and move the denture up and down slightly ❻. **Rationale:** *The slight movement breaks the suction that holds the plate on the roof of the mouth.*

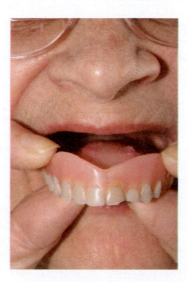

❻ Removing the top dentures by first breaking the suction.

  - Lower the upper plate, move it out of the mouth, and place it in the denture container.
  - Lift the lower plate, turning it so that the left side, for example, is slightly lower than the right, to remove the plate from the mouth without stretching the lips. Place the lower plate in the denture container.
  - Remove a partial denture by exerting equal pressure on the border of each side of the denture, not on the clasps, which can bend or break.
- Clean the dentures.
  - When cleaning dentures, hold them firmly and take care not to drop them ❼. Place a washcloth under them if using a sink. **Rationale:** *A washcloth prevents damage if the dentures are dropped against a hard surface.*

- Using a toothbrush or special stiff-bristled brush, scrub the dentures with the cleaning agent and tepid water. Rinse the dentures with tepid running water. **Rationale:** *Rinsing removes the cleaning agent and food particles.* If the dentures are stained, soak them in a commercial cleaner. Be sure to

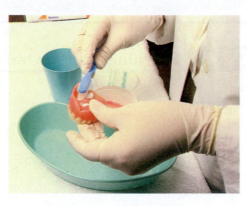

❼ Cleaning the dentures.

follow the manufacturer's directions. To prevent corrosion, dentures with metal parts should not be soaked overnight
- Inspect the dentures and the mouth.
  - Observe the dentures for any rough, sharp, or worn areas that could irritate the tongue or mucous membranes of the mouth, lips, and gums.
  - Inspect the mouth for any redness, irritated areas, or indications of infection.
  - Assess the fit of the dentures. People who have them should see a dentist at least once a year to check the fit and the presence of any irritation to the soft tissues of the mouth. Clients who need repairs to their dentures or new dentures may need a referral for financial assistance.
- Return the dentures to the mouth.
  - Offer some mouthwash and a curved basin to rinse the mouth. If the client cannot insert the dentures independently, insert the plates one at a time. Hold each plate at a slight angle while inserting it, to avoid injuring the lips.

Note: If clients perform self-cleaning of dentures, ensure that dentures are placed in the appropriate container ❽. **Rationale:** *Many older adult clients leave dentures on food trays and risk losing them*

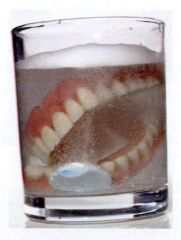

❽ Dentures soaking in solution prior to client self-cleaning.
(© mauritius images GmbH/Alamy)

(continued on next page)

SKILL 2.3 Providing Morning and Evening Care *(continued)*

when food trays are removed. Replacement dentures may not be covered by Medicare.

- Assist the client as needed.
  - Wipe the client's hands and mouth with the towel.
  - If the client does not want to or cannot wear the dentures, store them in a denture container with water. Label the con-

tainer with the client's name and identification number. (Do not place the container on the food tray.)
- Remove and discard gloves. Perform hand hygiene.
- Document all assessments and include any problems such as an irritated area on the mucous membrane.

SKILL 2.4 Providing Special Oral Care for a Client Who is Unconscious or Debilitated

Equipment

- Towel
- Clean gloves
- Curved basin (emesis basin)
- Bite-block to hold the mouth open and teeth apart (optional)
- Toothbrush
- Cup of tepid water
- Dentifrice or denture cleaner
- Tissue or piece of gauze to remove dentures (optional)
- Denture container as needed
- Mouthwash
- Rubber-tipped bulb syringe
- Suction catheter with suction apparatus when aspiration is a concern
- Foam swabs and cleaning solution for cleaning the mucous membranes
- Water-soluble lip moisturizer

Procedure

1. Prior to performing the procedure, if the client is conscious, introduce self and verify the client's identity using agency protocol. Explain to the client and the family what you are going to do and why it is necessary.
2. Perform hand hygiene and observe other appropriate infection control procedures (e.g., clean gloves).
3. Provide for client privacy by drawing the curtains around the bed or closing the door to the room. Some agencies provide signs indicating the need for privacy. **Rationale:** *Hygiene is a personal matter.*
4. Prepare the client.
   - Position the unconscious client in a side-lying position, with the head of the bed lowered. **Rationale:** *In this position, the saliva automatically runs out by gravity rather than being aspirated into the lung. This position also allows for suctioning, if needed. This position is chosen for the unconscious client receiving mouth care. If the client's head cannot be lowered, turn it to one side.* **Rationale:** *The fluid will readily run out of the mouth or pool in the side of the mouth, where it can be suctioned.*
   - Place the towel under the client's chin.
   - Place the curved basin against the client's chin and lower cheek to receive the fluid from the mouth ❶.
   - Apply gloves.
5. Clean the teeth and rinse the mouth.
   - If the client has natural teeth, brush the teeth as described in Skill 2.3. Brush gently and carefully to avoid injuring the gums. If the client has artificial teeth, clean them as described in the *Variation* component of Skill 2.3.
   - Rinse the client's mouth by drawing about 10 mL of water or alcohol-free mouthwash into the syringe and injecting it gently into each side of the mouth. **Rationale:** *If the solu-*

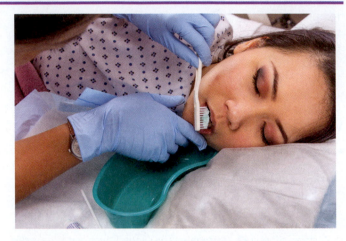

❶ Position of client and placement of curved basin when providing special mouth care.

tion is injected with force, some of it may flow down the client's throat and be aspirated into the lungs.
   - Watch carefully to make sure that all of the rinsing solution has run out of the mouth into the basin. If not, suction the fluid from the mouth. **Rationale:** *Fluid remaining in the mouth may be aspirated into the lungs.*
   - Repeat rinsing until the mouth is free of dentifrice, if used.
6. Inspect and clean the oral tissues.
   - If the tissues appear dry or unclean, clean them with the foam swabs or gauze and cleaning solution following agency policy.
   - Picking up a moistened foam swab, wipe the mucous membrane of one cheek. Discard the swab in a waste container; use a fresh one to clean the next area. **Rationale:** *Using separate applicators for each area of the mouth prevents the transfer of microorganisms from one area to another.*
   - Clean all mouth tissues in an orderly progression, using separate applicators: the cheeks, roof of the mouth, base of the mouth, and tongue.
   - Observe the oral tissues closely for inflammation, dryness, or lesions.
   - Rinse the client's mouth as described in step 5.
7. Ensure client comfort.
   - Remove the basin, and dry around the client's mouth with the towel. Replace artificial dentures, if indicated.
   - Lubricate the client's lips with water-soluble moisturizer. **Rationale:** *Lubrication prevents cracking and subsequent infection.*
8. Remove and discard gloves. Perform hand hygiene.
9. Document assessment of the teeth, tongue, gums, and oral mucosa. Include any problems such as sores or inflammation and swelling of the gums.

SKILL 2.4   Providing Special Oral Care for a Client (continued)

Developmental Considerations

INFANTS

- Most dentists recommend that dental hygiene should begin when the first tooth erupts and be practiced after each feeding. Cleaning can be accomplished by using a wet washcloth or small gauze moistened with water.

CHILDREN

- Beginning at about 18 months of age, brush the child's teeth with a soft toothbrush. Use only a toothbrush moistened with water. Introduce toothpaste later and use one that contains fluoride.
- Frequent snacking on products containing sugar increases the child's risk for developing cavities.

OLDER ADULTS

- Oral care is often difficult for certain older adults to perform due to problems with dexterity or cognitive problems with dementia.
- Most long-term health care facilities have dentists that come on a regular basis to see clients with special needs.

- Dryness of the oral mucosa is a common finding in older adults. Because this can lead to tooth decay, advise clients to discuss it with their dentist or primary care provider.
- Decay of the tooth root is common among older adults. When the gums recede, the tooth root is more vulnerable to decay.
- Promoting good oral hygiene can have a positive effect on older adults' ability to eat.

Setting of Care

- Assess the oral hygiene practices and attitude toward oral hygiene of family members and the client.
- Remind adults to replace their toothbrush every 3 to 4 months and a child's toothbrush more frequently.
- The client with a nasogastric tube or who is receiving oxygen is likely to develop dry oral mucous membranes, especially if the client breathes through the mouth. More frequent oral hygiene will be needed.

SKILL 2.5   Bathing an Adult or Pediatric Client

Delegation

The nurse often delegates the skill of bathing to UAP. However, the nurse remains responsible for assessment and client care. The nurse needs to do the following:

- Inform the UAP of the type of bath appropriate for the client and precautions, if any, specific to the needs of the client.
- Remind the UAP to notify the nurse of any concerns or changes (e.g., redness, skin breakdown, rash) so the nurse can assess, intervene if needed, and document.
- Instruct the UAP to encourage the client to perform as much self-care as appropriate in order to promote independence and self-esteem.
- Obtain a complete report about the bathing experience from the UAP.

Equipment

- Basin or sink with warm water (between 43° and 46°C [110° and 115°F])
- Soap and soap dish
- Linens: bath blanket, two bath towels, washcloth, clean gown or pajamas or clothes as needed, additional bed linen and towels, if required
- Clean gloves, if appropriate (e.g., presence of body fluids or open lesions)
- Personal hygiene articles (e.g., deodorant, powder, lotions)
- Shaving equipment
- Table for bathing equipment
- Laundry bag

Preparation

- Before bathing a client, determine (a) the purpose and type of bath the client needs; (b) self-care ability of the client; (c) any movement or positioning precautions specific to the client; (d) other care the client may be receiving, such as physical therapy or x-rays, in order

to coordinate all aspects of health care and prevent unnecessary fatigue; (e) the client's comfort level with being bathed by someone else; and (f) necessary bath equipment and linens.

- Caution is needed when bathing clients who are receiving intravenous (IV) therapy. Easy-to-remove gowns that have Velcro or snap fasteners along the sleeves may be used. If a special gown is not available, the nurse needs to pay special attention when changing the client's gown after the bath (or whenever the gown becomes soiled). In addition, special attention is needed to reassess the IV site for security of IV connections and appropriate taping around the IV site.
- The nurse should use universal precautions when bathing a client, particularly when performing perineal care. It is not always necessary, however, to wear gloves while providing a bath. The nurse should use clinical judgment when deciding to wear gloves and offer an explanation to the client (Downey & Lloyd, 2008).

Procedure

1. Prior to performing the procedure, introduce self and verify the client's identity using agency protocol. Explain to the client what you are going to do, why it is necessary, and how he or she can participate. Discuss with the client his or her preferences for bathing and explain any unfamiliar procedures to the client.

2. Perform hand hygiene and observe other appropriate infection control procedures (e.g., clean gloves).

3. Provide for client privacy by drawing the curtains around the bed or closing the door to the room. Some agencies provide signs indicating the need for privacy. **Rationale:** *Hygiene is a personal matter.*

4. Prepare the client and the environment.
   - Invite a family member or significant other to participate if desired or requested by the client.
   - Close windows and doors to ensure the room is a comfortable temperature. **Rationale:** *Air currents increase loss of heat from the body by convection.*

(continued on next page)

SKILL 2.5 Bathing an Adult or Pediatric Client (*continued*)

- Offer the client a bedpan or urinal or ask whether the client wishes to use the toilet or commode. **Rationale:** *Warm water and activity can stimulate the need to void. The client will be more comfortable after voiding, and voiding before cleaning the perineum is advisable.*
- Encourage the client to perform as much personal self-care as possible. **Rationale:** *This promotes independence, exercise, and self-esteem.*
- During the bath, assess each area of the skin carefully.

For a Bed Bath

5. Prepare the bed and position the client appropriately.
   - Position the bed at a comfortable working height. Lower the side rail on the side close to you. Keep the other side rail *up*. Assist the client to move near you. **Rationale:** *This avoids undue reaching and straining and promotes good body mechanics, and allows the nurse to wash both sides of the client's body without moving around the bed. It also ensures client safety.*
   - Place a bath blanket over the top sheet. Remove the top sheet from under the bath blanket by starting at the client's shoulders and moving linen down toward the client's feet ❶. Ask the client to grasp and hold the top of the bath blanket while pulling linen to the foot of the bed. **Rationale:** *The bath blanket provides comfort, warmth, and privacy.*

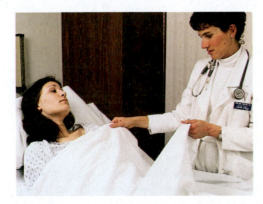

❶ Remove top sheet from under the bath blanket.

Note: If the bed linen is to be reused, place it over the bedside chair. If it is to be changed, place it in the linen hamper, not on the floor. **Rationale:** *Placing used linens in the linen hamper, rather than the floor, prevents the spread of microorganisms.*

- Remove client's gown while keeping the client covered with the bath blanket. Place gown in linen hamper.

6. Make a bath mitt with the washcloth ❷. **Rationale:** *A bath mitt retains water and heat better than a cloth loosely held and prevents the ends of the washcloth from dragging across the skin.*

7. Wash the face. **Rationale:** *Begin the bath at the cleanest area and work downward toward the feet.*
   - Place towel under client's head.
   - Wash the client's eyes with water only and dry them well. Use a separate corner of the washcloth for each eye. **Rationale:** *Using separate corners prevents transmitting microorganisms from one eye to the other.* Wipe from the inner to the outer canthus ❸. **Rationale:** *This prevents secretions from entering the nasolacrimal ducts.*

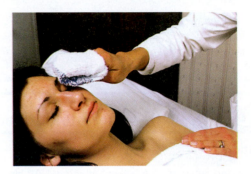

❸ Using a separate corner of the washcloth for each eye, wipe from the inner to the outer canthus.

- Ask whether the client wants soap used on the face. **Rationale:** *Soap has a drying effect, and the face, which is exposed to the air more than other body parts, tends to be drier.*
- Wash, rinse, and dry the client's face, ears, and neck.
- Remove the towel from under the client's head.

8. Wash the arms and hands. (Omit the arms for a partial bath.)
   - Place a towel lengthwise under the arm away from you. **Rationale:** *It protects the bed from becoming wet.*
   - Wash, rinse, and dry the arm by elevating the client's arm and supporting the client's wrist and elbow. Use long, firm strokes from wrist to shoulder, including the axillary area ❹. **Rationale:** *Firm strokes from distal to proximal areas promote circulation by increasing venous blood return.*

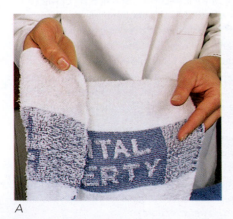 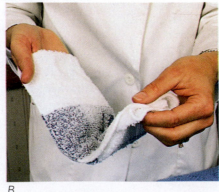 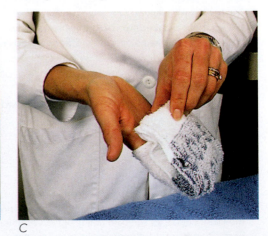

A B C

❷ Making a bath mitt, rectangular method: *A*, Wrap one edge of cloth around palm and fingers; *B*, wrap cloth around hand and anchor with thumb; *C*, tuck far edge of cloth under edge in palm of hand.

SKILL 2.5 Bathing an Adult or Pediatric Client (continued)

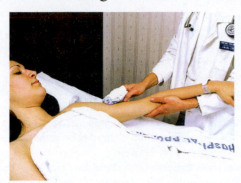

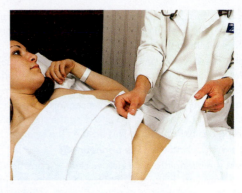

❹ Washing the far arm using long, firm strokes from wrist to shoulder area.

❻ Place the bath towel across the client's chest.

- Apply deodorant or powder if desired. Special caution is needed for clients with respiratory alterations. **Rationale:** *Powder is not recommended due to potential adverse respiratory effects.*
- *Optional:* Place a towel on the bed and put a washbasin on it. Place the client's hands in the basin ❺. **Rationale:** *Many clients enjoy immersing their hands in the basin and washing themselves. Soaking loosens dirt under the nails.* Assist the client as needed to wash, rinse, and dry the hands, paying particular attention to the spaces between the fingers.

10. Wash the legs and feet. (Omit legs and feet for a partial bath.)
    - Expose the leg farthest from you by folding the bath blanket toward the other leg, being careful to keep the perineum covered. **Rationale:** *Covering the perineum promotes privacy and maintains the client's dignity.*
    - Lift leg and place the bath towel lengthwise under the leg. Wash, rinse, and dry the leg using long, smooth, firm strokes from the ankle to the knee to the thigh ❼. **Rationale:** *Washing from the distal to proximal areas promotes circulation by stimulating venous blood flow.*

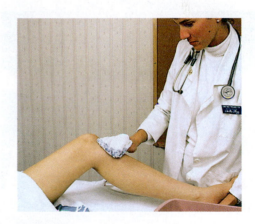

❼ Washing the client's leg.

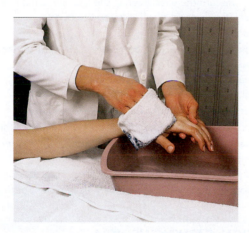

❺ Wash hands by soaking them in a basin.

- Reverse the coverings and repeat for the other leg.
- Wash the feet by placing them in a basin of water ❽.

- Repeat for hand and arm nearest you. Exercise caution if an intravenous infusion is present, and check its flow after moving the arm. Avoid submersing the IV site.

9. Wash the chest and abdomen. (Omit the chest and abdomen for a partial bath. However, the areas under a woman's breast may require bathing if this area is irritated or if the client has significant perspiration under the breasts.)
   - Place the bath towel lengthwise over the chest. Fold the bath blanket down to the client's pubic area. **Rationale:** *This keeps the client warm while preventing unnecessary exposure of the chest* ❻.
   - Lift the bath towel off the chest, and bathe the chest and abdomen with your mitted hand using long, firm strokes. Give special attention to the skin under the breasts and any other skinfolds, particularly if the client is overweight. Rinse and dry well.
   - Replace the bath blanket when the areas have been dried.

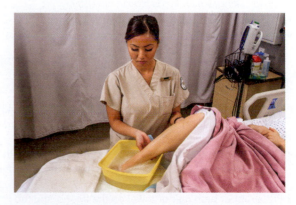

❽ Soaking a foot in a basin.

(continued on next page)

SKILL 2.5 Bathing an Adult or Pediatric Client *(continued)*

- Dry each foot. Pay particular attention to the spaces between the toes. If preferred, wash one foot after that leg before washing the other leg.
- Obtain fresh, warm bathwater now or when necessary. **Rationale:** *Water may become dirty or cold.* Because surface skin cells are removed with washing, the bathwater from dark-skinned clients may be dark, however, this does not mean the client is dirty. Lower the bed and raise the side rails when refilling basin. **Rationale:** *This ensures the safety of the client.*

11. Wash the back and then the perineum 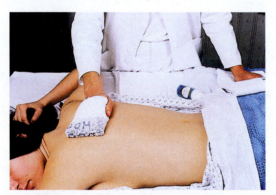.
    - Assist the client into a prone or side-lying position facing away from you. Place the bath towel lengthwise alongside the back and buttocks while keeping the client covered with the bath blanket as much as possible. **Rationale:** *This provides warmth and prevents undue exposure.*
    - Wash and dry the client's back, moving from the shoulders to the buttocks, and upper thighs, paying attention to the gluteal folds. **Rationale:** *Wash from the area of least contamination (the back) to that of greatest (gluteal folds).*
    - Remove and discard gloves if used.
    - Perform a back massage now or after completion of bath (see Skill 4.4).
    - Assist the client to the supine position and determine whether the client can wash the perineal area independently. If the client cannot do so, drape the client and wash the area.

9 Washing the back.

12. Assist the client with grooming aids such as powder, lotion, or deodorant.
    - Use powder sparingly. Release as little as possible into the atmosphere. **Rationale:** *This will avoid irritation of the respiratory tract by powder inhalation. Excessive powder can cause caking, which leads to skin irritation.*
    - Help the client put on a clean gown or pajamas.
    - Assist the client to care for hair, mouth, and nails. Some people prefer or need mouth care prior to their bath.

For a Tub Bath or Shower

13. Prepare the client and the tub.
    - Fill the tub about one third to one half full of water at 43° to 46°C (110° to 115°F). **Rationale:** *Sufficient water is needed to cover the perineal area.*
    - Cover all intravenous catheters or wound dressings with plastic coverings, and instruct the client to prevent wetting these areas if possible.
    - Put a rubber bath mat or towel on the floor of the tub if safety strips are not on the tub floor. **Rationale:** *These prevent slippage of the client during the bath or shower.*

14. Assist the client into the shower or tub.
    - Assist the client taking a standing shower with the initial adjustment of the water temperature and water flow pressure, as needed. Some clients need a chair to sit on in the shower because of weakness. Hot water can cause older adults to feel faint due to vasodilation and decreased blood pressure from positional changes.
    - If the client requires considerable assistance with a tub bath, a hydraulic bathtub chair may be required (see *Variation* section later in this skill).
    - Explain how the client can signal for help, leave the client for 2 to 5 minutes, and place an "Occupied" sign on the door. For safety reasons, do not leave a client with decreased cognition or clients who may be at risk (e.g., history of seizures, syncope).

15. Assist the client with washing and getting out of the tub.
    - Wash the client's back, lower legs, and feet, if necessary.
    - Assist the client out of the tub. If the client is unsteady, place a bath towel over the client's shoulders and drain the tub of water before the client attempts to get out of it. **Rationale:** *Draining the water first lessens the likelihood of a fall. The towel prevents chilling.*

16. Dry the client, and assist with follow-up care.
    - Follow step 12.
    - Assist the client back to his or her bed.
    - Clean the tub or shower in accordance with agency practice, discard the used linen in the laundry hamper, and place the "Unoccupied" sign on the door.

17. Document the following:
    - Type of bath given (i.e., complete, partial, or self-help). This is usually recorded on a flow sheet.
    - Skin assessment, such as excoriation, erythema, exudates, rashes, drainage, or skin breakdown.
    - Nursing interventions related to skin integrity.
    - Ability of the client to assist or cooperate with bathing.
    - Client response to bathing. Also, document the need for reassessment of vital signs if appropriate.
    - Educational needs regarding hygiene.
    - Information or teaching shared with the client or the family.

VARIATION: BATHING USING A HYDRAULIC BATHTUB CHAIR

A hydraulic lift, often used in long-term care or rehabilitation settings, can facilitate the transfer of a client who is unable to ambulate to a tub. The lift also helps eliminate strain on the nurse's back.
- Bring the client to the tub room in a wheelchair or shower chair.
- Fill the tub and check the water temperature with a bath thermometer. **Rationale:** *This avoids thermal injury to the client.*
- Lower the hydraulic chair lift to its lowest point, outside the tub.
- Transfer the client to the chair lift and secure the seat belt **10**.
- Raise the chair lift above the tub.
- Support the client's legs as the chair is moved over the tub. **Rationale:** *This avoids injury to the legs.*
- Position the client's legs down into the water and slowly lower the chair lift into the tub.
- Assist in bathing the client, if appropriate.
- Reverse the procedure when taking the client out of the tub.
- Dry the client and transport him or her to the room.

SKILL 2.5   Bathing an Adult or Pediatric Client (*continued*)

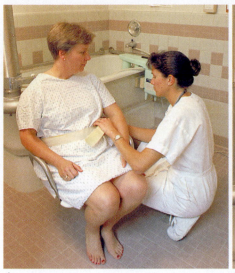
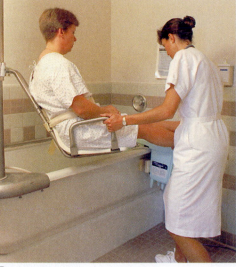
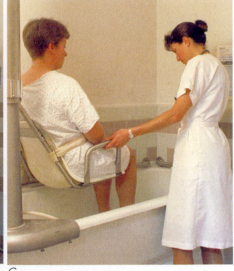

A   *B*   *C*

🔟 *A,* Attach seat belt before swinging chair over the tub. *B,* support client in chair as chair is swung over tub. *C,* Lower chair into tub filled with water.

General Guidelines for Bathing Clients with Dementia

- Focus on the client rather than the task.
  - Evaluate to determine if the client needs pain control before the bath.
  - Time the bath to fit the client's history, preferences, and mood.
  - Cover! Keep the client covered as much as possible to keep him or her warm.
  - Move slowly and let the client know when you are going to move or touch him or her.
  - Use a gentle touch. Use soft cloths. Pat dry rather than rubbing.
  - Consider adapting your methods (e.g., distracting the client with singing while bathing), the environment (e.g., correct size of shower chair, reducing noise, playing music), and the procedure (e.g., consistently assigning same caregiver, inviting family to help).
  - Encourage flexibility in scheduling of the bath based on client's preference.

- Use persuasion, not coercion.
  - Give choices and respond to individual requests.
  - Help the client feel in control.
  - Use a supportive, calm approach and praise the client often.
- Be prepared.
  - Gather everything that you will need for the bath (e.g., towels, washcloths, clothes) before approaching the client.
- Stop when a client becomes distressed. It is not normal to have cries, screams, or protests from the client.
  - Stop what you are doing and assess for causes of the distress.
  - Adjust your approach.
  - Shorten or stop the bath.
  - Try to end on a positive note.
  - Reapproach later to wash critical areas if necessary.
- Ask for help.
  - Talk with others, including the family, about different ways to help make the bath more comfortable for the client.

VARIATION: BATHING USING A DISPOSABLE SYSTEM

Equipment

- Commercial cleansing system
- Bath blanket
- Clean gown
- Disposable bag
- Clean gloves, if appropriate

Preparation

- Obtain package with cleansing cloths. Cloths are premoistened with an aloe and vitamin E formula. **Rationale:** *The cleansing cloths are less drying as they maintain the skin at a pH of 4.7 to 4.9.*
- Heat package in microwave for no more than 45 seconds. Check temperature before applying to skin. **Rationale:** *Increased time could lead to excessive heat and burning of the skin. The commercial system can be used at room temperature.*

- Explain procedure to client. **Rationale:** *This procedure may be new to the client and an explanation is needed to ensure client understands the difference between a bed bath and a bath using a cleansing system. The client may not think he has had a complete bath but only a "sponge bath."*
- Perform hand hygiene.
- Don gloves if there is a risk of contact with body secretions.
- Replace top linen and gown with bath blanket or top sheet if bath blanket not available.

Procedure

- Open package and remove one cloth at a time.
- Remove bath blanket at each site when cleansing with cloth.
- Replace bath blanket when cloth removed. **Rationale:** *To prevent client chilling.*
- Use a new cloth for each section of the body as follows:
  - Face, neck, and chest
  - Right arm and axilla
  - Left arm and axilla

(*continued on next page*)

SKILL 2.5 Bathing an Adult or Pediatric Client (*continued*)

- Perineum
- Right leg
- Left leg
- Back
- Buttocks

■ Discard cloth after cleansing each area. Do not flush down toilet. Rinsing is not required with this system. Replace bath blanket or sheet over each part of the body after it has been cleaned. **Rationale:** *To prevent the client from becoming chilled.*

■ Place clean gown on client.

■ Place client in comfortable position.

■ Discard cloths in appropriate receptacle.

■ Perform hand hygiene.

■ Document bath on flow sheet or nurses' notes.

Evidence-Based Nursing Practice

Bed Bath or Disposable Bed Bath

A study compared the traditional bathing method with the disposable bath method in 100 clients in coma. Its focus was on nurse satisfaction and on costs of the two methods. Fifty clients were bathed with the traditional method and 50 clients with the disposable method. Thirty nurses were interviewed about the two methods.

The nurses expressed a statistically significant preference for the disposable bath method. The disposable method was preferred for both skin softness and ease of administration. By assessing equipment, supplies, and labor, the study determined that the disposable bath system, based on cost of nurses' time, was more cost effective than the traditional bathing method.

Data from Sucre & De Nicola (2009).

VARIATION: BATHING AN INFANT

Equipment

■ Tub or basin filled with warm water 37.8°C (100°F)

■ Two towels

■ Washcloth

■ Suction bulb

■ Mild soap

■ Cotton balls

■ Blanket

■ Clean clothing

■ Clean gloves, if indicated

Preparation

■ Provide a comfortable room environment (i.e., comfortable temperature, lighting.)

■ Check client ID.

■ Perform hand hygiene.

■ Collect necessary equipment, and place articles within reach.

■ Position the bed at a comfortable working height.

■ Place towel, laid out in diamond fashion, on bed next to basin.

■ Don gloves if there is a risk of exposure to body secretions.

Procedure

1. Test water temperature with your wrist or elbow.
2. Lift infant using football hold.

3. Remove all clothing except shirt and diaper.
4. Cover infant with towel or blanket. Never let go of the infant during the bath. **Rationale:** *This is a safety intervention to prevent falls or other injury.*
5. Clean infant's eyes, using a cotton ball moistened with water. Wipe from inner to outer canthus, using a new cotton ball for each eye. **Rationale:** *This procedure prevents water and particles from entering the lacrimal duct.*

> **CLINICAL ALERT**
> Discharge from the eyes may be present for 2 to 3 days due to prophylactic eyedrops administered at birth.

6. Make a mitt with the washcloth.
7. Wash infant's face with water.
8. Suction nose, if necessary, by compressing suction bulb prior to placing it in nostril. **Rationale:** *This prevents aspiration of moisture. Gently release bulb after it is placed in nostril.*
9. Wash infant's ears and neck, paying attention to folds; dry all areas thoroughly. Use mild soap and rinse.
10. Remove shirt or gown.
11. Remove diaper by picking up infant's ankles in your hand.
12. Pick up infant and place feet first into basin or tub. Immerse infant in tub of water only after umbilical cord has healed. Pick up infant by placing your hand and arm around infant, cradling the infant's head and neck in your elbow. Grasp the infant's thigh with your hand. **Rationale:** *The umbilical cord is kept dry to prevent infection.*
13. Wash and rinse the infant's body, especially the skinfolds. *Note:* Some facilities use disposable cleansing systems to bathe neonates and infants. There are four infant-size washcloths for infants up to 25 pounds. The bathing procedure is the same for infants and adults.
14. Wash infant's genitalia.
    - For a female infant: Separate labia and with a cotton ball moistened with soap and water, cleanse downward once on each side. Use a new piece of cotton on each side.
    - For an uncircumcised male infant: Do not force foreskin back. Gently cleanse the exposed surface with a cotton ball moistened with soap and water.
    - For a circumcised male infant: Gently cleanse with plain water.
15. Wrap the infant in a towel and use a football hold when washing an infant's head. Soap your own hands and wash infant's hair and scalp paying attention to the nape of the neck and using a circular motion. Rinse hair and scalp thoroughly. **Rationale:** *Football hold is the most secure for active infants.*
16. Place infant on a clean, dry towel with head facing the top corner and wrap infant.
17. Use the corner of the towel to dry infant's head with gentle, yet firm, circular movements.
18. Replace infant's diaper and redress in a new gown or shirt.
19. Provide comfort by holding the infant for a time following the bath procedure.
20. Perform hand hygiene.

SKILL 2.5 Bathing an Adult or Pediatric Client (*continued*)

Client Teaching

Dry Skin

- Use cleansing creams to clean the skin rather than soap or detergent, which cause drying and, in some cases, allergic reactions.
- Thoroughly rinse soap or detergent, if used, from the skin.
- Bathe less frequently when environmental temperature and humidity are low.
- Increase fluid intake.
- Humidify the air with a humidifier or by keeping a tub or sink full of water.
  - Use moisturizing or emollient creams that contain lanolin, petroleum jelly, or cocoa butter to retain skin moisture.
  - Moisturizers should be applied in the direction of hair growth, after bathing, immediately after the client has patted self dry so there is still moisture in the skin.
- Daily use of a moisturizer is recommended.

Skin Rashes

- Keep the area clean by washing it with a mild soap. Rinse the skin well, and pat it dry.

- To relieve itching, try a tepid bath or soak. Some over-the-counter preparations, such as Caladryl lotion, may help but should be used with full knowledge of the product.
- Avoid scratching the rash to prevent inflammation, infection, and further skin lesions.
- Choose clothing carefully. Too much can cause perspiration and aggravate a rash.

Acne

- Wash the face frequently with soap or detergent and hot water to remove oil and dirt.
- Avoid using oily creams, which aggravate the condition.
- Avoid using cosmetics that block the ducts of the sebaceous glands and the hair follicles.
- Never squeeze or pick at the lesions. This increases the potential for infection and scarring.
- Many treatments are available, some over the counter. Inform the client that it often takes 6 weeks before results are evident (Penzer, 2008).

Developmental Considerations

FACTORS THAT CAN INCREASE RISK OF SKIN BREAKDOWN AND DELAY WOUND HEALING

- Inadequate nutritional intake.
- Compromised immune system.
- Compromised circulatory and respiratory systems.
- Poor hydration.
- Decreased mobility and activity.

SKIN CHANGES WITH AGE

- Delayed cellular migration and proliferation.
- Skin is less effective as a barrier and slow to heal.
- There is increased vulnerability to trauma.
- There is less ability to retain water.
- Geriatric skin is dry (xeroderma) due to decreased endocrine secretion and loss of elastin. This can cause pruritus, which could lead to skin ulceration.
- Increased skin susceptibility to shearing stress leading to blister formation and skin tears.
- There is increased vascular fragility.

NEED FOR ASSESSMENT OF THE SKIN OF OLDER ADULTS

- Decreased temperature, degree of moisture, dryness resulting from decreased dermal vascularity.
- Skin not intact, open lesions, tears, pressure ulcers as a result of increased skin fragility.
- Decreased turgor, dehydration as a result of decreased oil and sweat glands.
- Pigmentation alterations, potential cancer.
- Pruritus—dry skin most common cause because of decreased oil and sweat glands.
- Bruises, scars from increased skin fragility.

BATHING ADAPTATIONS TO MINIMIZE DRYNESS

- Have client take complete bath only twice a week.
- Use superfatted or mild soap or lotions to aid in moisturizing.

- Use tepid, not hot, water.
- Apply emollient (lanolin) to skin after bathing.

INFANTS

- Sponge baths are suggested for the newborn because daily tub baths are not considered necessary. After the bath, the infant should be immediately dried and wrapped. Parents need to be advised that the infant's ability to regulate body temperature has not yet fully developed and newborns' bodies lose heat readily.

CHILDREN

- Encourage a child's participation as appropriate for developmental level.
- Closely supervise children in the bathtub. Do not leave them unattended.

ADOLESCENTS

- Assist adolescents as needed to choose deodorants and antiperspirants. Secretions from newly active sweat glands react with bacteria on the skin, causing a pungent odor.

OLDER ADULTS

- Changes of aging can decrease the protective function of the skin in older adults. These changes include fragile skin, less oil and moisture, and a decrease in elasticity.
- To minimize skin dryness in older adults, avoid excessive use of soap.
- The ideal time to moisturize the skin is immediately after bathing.
- Avoid powder because it causes moisture loss and is a hazardous inhalant. Cornstarch should also be avoided because in the presence of moisture it breaks down into glucose and can facilitate the growth of organisms.
- Protect older adults and children from injury related to hot water burns.

(continued on next page)

SKILL 2.5 Bathing an Adult or Pediatric Client (continued)

Cultural Considerations

DEFINING CLEANLINESS

Cultures define cleanliness in different ways. Cultures and sub-cultures can have varying attitudes around hygiene and cleanliness. For example, some cultures value body cleanliness and the absence of body odor. Some value the use of perfumes, deodorants, and aftershave lotions as a major part of their hygienic care. In other cultures, natural body odor is thought to have sex appeal.

When providing hygienic care for clients, the nurse needs to assess the client's usual pattern of bathing, hygienic products usually used, and cultural rituals and beliefs.

Modesty and bathing rituals and beliefs must be considered in caring for clients. For example, some cultures and religions do not allow members of the opposite sex to see them from the waist to the knees. In other cultures, women have a strong sense of modesty and do not want healthcare workers to see them unclothed.

BIOCULTURAL VARIATIONS IN BODY SECRETIONS

Some individuals have a mild to absent body odor, whereas others may have strong body odor.

- The amount of chloride excreted by sweat glands varies widely.
- Some cultural groups have adapted to their environment and sweat less than others on their trunks and extremities but more on their faces. This adaptation allows for temperature regulation without the need to change clothes because of perspiration.

Source: From *Transcultural Concepts in Nursing Care*, 6th ed. (p. 335), by M. M. Andrews and J. S. Boyle, 2011, Philadelphia, PA: Lippincott Williams & Wilkins.

SKILL 2.6 Changing Gown for Client with an IV

Equipment

Clean gown
Bathing supplies, if needed

Procedure

1. Check client care plan for infusion drip rate, type of solution, and any special considerations.
2. Perform hand hygiene.
3. Identify client using two descriptors.
4. Take equipment to client's room and explain procedure to client.
5. Untie back of gown, and remove gown from unaffected arm.
6. Support arm with IV and slip gown down arm to IV tubing.
7. Place clean gown over client's chest and abdomen.
8. Use tubing clamp to slow infusion to "keep-open" rate and remove tubing from infusion pump if in use.
9. Remove IV bag from hook and slip sleeve over bag, keeping bag above client's arm. **Rationale:** This prevents backflow of blood into tubing. Do not jar or pull tubing. IV tubing may become dislodged and infiltrate into surrounding tissue.
10. Place your hand up through distal end of clean gown sleeve and grasp IV bag. Pull bag and tubing out through clean gown sleeve.
11. Rehang bag on hook, and check to see that infusion is running according to ordered drip rate.
12. Replace tubing into infusion pump, unclamp, and reestablish prescribed infusion flow rate.
13. Guide sleeve of gown up client's arm to shoulder.
14. Assist client to put other arm through remaining sleeve.
15. Tie gown at the back.
16. Check IV infusion rate and IV tubing to determine that solution is flowing unimpeded into client's vein. **Rationale:** Kinks in tubing impede solution flow.
17. Return bed to comfortable position for client.
18. Remove dirty linen from room.
19. Perform hand hygiene.

Note: Most facilities provide "IV gowns" that snap from the shoulder down the sleeve of the gown for ease in removal without disturbing the IV.

SKILL 2.7 Providing Perineal-Genital Care

Delegation

Perineal-genital care can be delegated to UAP; however, if the client has recently had perineal, rectal, or genital surgery, the nurse needs to assess if it is appropriate for the UAP to perform perineal-genital care.

Equipment

Perineal-Genital Care Provided in Conjunction with the Bed Bath

- Bath towel
- Bath blanket

- Clean gloves
- Bath basin with warm water at 43° to 46°C (110° to 115°F)
- Soap
- Washcloth

Special Perineal-Genital Care

- Bath towel
- Bath blanket
- Clean gloves
- Solution bottle, pitcher, or container filled with warm water or a prescribed solution

SKILL 2.7 Providing Perineal-Genital Care (*continued*)

- Bedpan to receive rinse water
- Perineal pad

Preparation

- Determine whether the client is experiencing any discomfort in the perineal-genital area.
- Obtain and prepare the necessary equipment and supplies.

Procedure

1. Prior to performing the procedure, introduce self and verify the client's identity using agency protocol. Explain to the client what you are going to do, why it is necessary, and how he or she can participate, being particularly sensitive to any embarrassment felt by the client.

2. Perform hand hygiene and observe other appropriate infection control procedures (e.g., clean gloves).

3. Provide for client privacy by drawing the curtains around the bed or closing the door to the room. Some agencies provide signs indicating the need for privacy. **Rationale:** *Hygiene is a personal matter.*

4. Prepare the client:
   - Fold the top bed linen to the foot of the bed and fold the gown up to expose the genital area.
   - Place a bath towel under the client's hips. **Rationale:** *The bath towel prevents the bed from becoming soiled.*

5. Position and drape the client and clean the upper inner thighs.
   - Cover the body and legs with the bath blanket positioned so a corner is at the head, the opposite corner at the feet, and the other two on the sides. Drape the legs by tucking the bottom corners of the bath blanket under and then over the inner sides of the legs ❶. **Rationale:** *Minimum exposure lessens embarrassment and helps to provide warmth.* Bring the middle portion of the base of the blanket up and then over the pubic area.

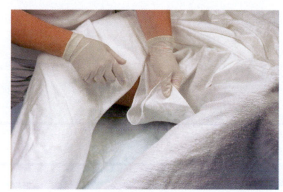

❶ Draping the client for perineal-genital care.

   - Position the female in a back-lying position with the knees flexed and spread well apart.
   - Position the male client in a supine position with knees slightly flexed and hips slightly externally rotated.
   - Apply gloves. Wash and dry the upper inner thighs.

6. Inspect the perineal area.
   - Note particular areas of inflammation, excoriation, or swelling, especially between the labia in females and the scrotal folds in males.
   - Also note excessive discharge or secretions from the orifices and the presence of odors.

7. Wash and dry the perineal-genital area.

For Female Clients

   - Clean the labia majora. Then spread the labia to wash the folds between the labia majora and the labia minora ❷. **Rationale:** Secretions that tend to collect around the labia minora facilitate bacterial growth.

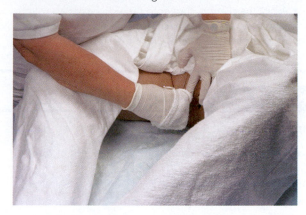

❷ Cleaning the labia.

   - Use separate quarters of the washcloth for each stroke, and wipe from the pubis to the rectum. For menstruating women and clients with indwelling catheters, use clean wipes. Use a clean wipe for each stroke. **Rationale:** *Using separate quarters of the washcloth or new wipes prevents the transmission of microorganisms from one area to the other. Wipe from the area of least contamination (the pubis) to that of greatest (the rectum).*
   - Rinse the area well. You may place the client on a bedpan and use a peri-wash or a solution bottle to pour warm water over the area. Dry the perineum thoroughly, paying particular attention to the folds between the labia. **Rationale:** *Moisture supports the growth of many microorganisms.*

For Male Clients

   - Wash and dry the penis, using firm strokes.
   - If the client is uncircumcised, retract the prepuce (foreskin) to expose the glans penis (the tip of the penis) for cleaning. Replace the foreskin after cleaning and drying the glans penis ❸. **Rationale:** *Retracting the foreskin is necessary to remove the smegma (thick, cheesy secretion) that collects under the foreskin and facilitates bacterial growth. Replacing the foreskin prevents constriction of the penis, which may cause edema.*

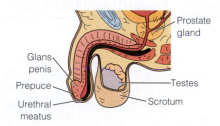

❸ Male genitals.

   - Wash and dry the scrotum. The posterior folds of the scrotum may need to be cleaned when the buttocks are cleaned. **Rationale:** *The scrotum tends to be more soiled than the penis because of its proximity to the rectum; thus it is usually cleaned after the penis.*

8. Inspect perineal orifices for intactness.

(continued on next page)

SKILL 2.7 Providing Perineal-Genital Care (continued)

- Inspect particularly around the urethra in clients with indwelling catheters. **Rationale:** *A catheter may cause excoriation around the urethra.*

9. Clean the natal cleft (between the gluteal folds) and the entire buttocks.
   - Assist the client to turn onto the side facing away from you.
   - Pay particular attention to the anal area and posterior folds of the scrotum in males. Clean the anus with toilet tissue before washing it, if necessary.

- Dry the area well.
- For postdelivery or menstruating females, apply a perineal pad as needed from front to back. **Rationale:** *This prevents contamination of the vagina and urethra from the anal area.*

10. Remove and discard gloves. Perform hand hygiene.
11. Document any unusual findings such as redness, excoriation, skin breakdown, discharge or drainage, and any localized areas of tenderness.

SKILL 2.8 Shaving a Male Client

Equipment

- Safety or electric razor, specific to client's needs or wishes
- Shaving cream
- Aftershave lotion (optional)
- Two towels
- Basin of warm water

Preparation

- Place client in sitting position.
- Perform hand hygiene.
- Place towel over chest and under chin.
- Put up mirror on overbed table.
- Determine how the client usually shaves (i.e., use of safety edge or electric razor; special products).
- Check to see if the client has excessive bleeding tendencies due to pathological conditions (hemophilia) or the use of specific medications (anticoagulants or large doses of aspirin). **Rationale:** *If client is accidentally cut, it could lead to some loss of blood.*

> **CLINICAL ALERT**
>
> According to the hospital policy, be sure to have the electric razor checked for safety aspects. Some hospitals do not allow clients to use their own electric razors.
>
> A beard or a mustache should not be shaved off without the client's consent.

Procedure

1. If using a safety edge razor:
   - Don gloves and apply a warm, moist towel to soften the hair.
   - Apply a thick layer of soap or shaving cream to the shaving area.
   - Holding skin taut, use firm but small strokes in the direction of hair growth.
   - Gently remove soap or lather with a warm, damp towel. Inspect for areas you may have missed.
2. If using electric razor:
   - Use rotating motion of razor and start from lateral aspect of face and move toward chin and upper lip area.
   - Clean razor with brush or remove head and clean facial hair from head of razor.
3. Apply aftershave lotion or powder as desired.
4. Reposition client for comfort if needed.
5. Remove gloves and replace equipment.
6. Perform hand hygiene.

SKILL 2.9 Providing Hair Care

Delegation

Brushing and combing hair, shampooing hair, and shaving facial hair can be delegated to UAP unless the client has a condition in which the procedure would be contraindicated (e.g., cervical spinal injury or trauma). The nurse needs to assess the UAP's knowledge and experience of hair care for clients of other cultures, as appropriate.

Equipment

- Clean brush and comb (A wide-toothed comb may be preferred by some individuals because finer combs pull the hair into knots and may also break the hair.)
- Two bath towels
- Hair oil preparation or other hair care products, as requested by client

Procedure

1. Prior to performing the procedure, introduce self and verify the client's identity using agency protocol. Explain to the client what you are going to do, why it is necessary, and how he or she can participate.
2. Perform hand hygiene and observe other appropriate infection control procedures (e.g., clean gloves).
3. Provide for client privacy by drawing the curtains around the bed or closing the door to the room. Some agencies provide signs indicating the need for privacy. **Rationale:** Hygiene is a personal matter.
4. Position and prepare the client appropriately.
   - Assist the client who can sit to move to a chair. **Rationale:** Hair is more easily brushed and combed when the client is in a sitting position. If health permits, assist a client confined

SKILL 2.9 Providing Hair Care (*continued*)

to a bed to a sitting position by raising the head of the bed. Otherwise, assist the client to alternate side-lying positions, and do one side of the head at a time.

- If the client remains in bed, place a clean towel over the pillow and the client's shoulders. Place it over the sitting client's shoulders. **Rationale:** The towel collects any removed hair, dirt, and scaly material.
- Remove any pins or ribbons in the hair.

5. Remove any mats or tangles gradually.
   - Separate the hair into sections to untangle mats using one's fingers to pull them apart or work them out with repeated brushings to help prevent hair breakage and discomfort. Move fingers in a circular motion starting at the roots and gently moving up to the tip of the hair.
   - If the hair is very tangled, apply hair oil, alcohol, or another oil, such as mineral oil, on the strands to help loosen the tangles as the client indicates. Use a large open-toothed comb to untangle hair in sections as needed. Grasp a small section of hair and, holding the hair at the tip with one hand, start untangling at the tip and work down toward the scalp.

- Dampen the hair with water or use a leave-in conditioner to help loosen tangling in hair.
- Continue to comb out tangles in small sections of hair holding from the tips of the hair in one hand while the other hand stabilizes the scalp. **Rationale:** This avoids scalp trauma.

6. Brush and comb the hair.
   - For short hair, brush and comb one side at a time. Divide long hair into two sections by parting it down the middle from the front to the back. If the hair is very thick, divide the hair into more sections and then into front and back subsections or into several layers.

7. Arrange the hair as neatly and attractively as possible, according to the client's desires.
   - Ask if the client would like the hair braided. **Rationale:** Braiding will decrease tangling; however, the choice is the client's. Position hair clips or fasteners as appropriate and requested by the client.

8. Document assessments made during the procedure and requested nursing care interventions. Daily combing and brushing of the hair are not normally recorded.

SKILL 2.10 Shampooing Hair

Equipment

- Two bath towels
- Washcloth
- Large container for water
- Shampoo
- Conditioner, if desired
- Hair dryer, if allowed by hospital

For Disposable System

- Package containing shampoo cap **1** **2**
- Face or bath towel
- Hair care products, as requested by client
- Comb and/or brush

Note: Ensure that electrical equipment is checked by maintenance department before using. **Rationale:** *This confirms that equipment is grounded and mechanically safe.*

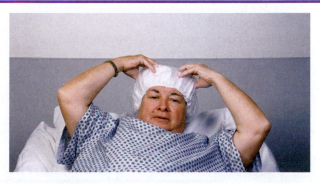

2 Disposable shampoo cap can be used for clients on bed rest.

Preparation

- Determine client's hair care needs.
- Perform hand hygiene.
- Collect and assemble equipment.
- Help client into a comfortable position to perform hair care.

> **CLINICAL ALERT**
> If the client is an older adult, do not press the neck down on the edge of the sink—this position can diminish circulation to the brain and has been reported to be a possible cause of strokes.

- Shampooing the hair can be accomplished in a variety of ways depending on the client's usual routine and physical condition. In many institutions, a physician's order is necessary before shampooing a client's hair.
- If possible, the easiest way to shampoo is to assist the client while he or she is in the shower. Caution should be taken to prevent the client from becoming overly tired or weak while in the shower. (Use shower chair if necessary.)

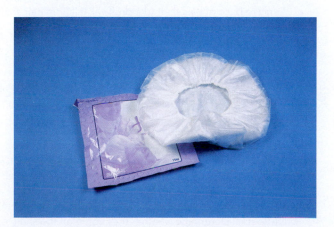

1 Shampoo system activated by microwave.

(continued on next page)

SKILL 2.10 Shampooing Hair (continued)

Procedure

For Routine Hair Care

1. Have all hair care items within reach.
2. Drape a towel over client's shoulders.
3. Brush or comb client's hair from scalp to hair ends, using gentle, even strokes.
   - *Tangled hair:* Use short gentle strokes. Work from end of hair shaft toward scalp. May use conditioner to make combing easier.
   - *Curly hair:* Use wet comb on wet hair (water or oil) for ease of combing.
4. Style hair in a manner suitable to client.
5. Replace hair care items in appropriate place and clean items as needed.
6. Perform hand hygiene.

For Client on a Stretcher

1. Have shampoo items readily available.
2. Position stretcher with head end at sink.
3. Lock wheels on stretcher. **Rationale:** *This prevents the gurney from moving away from the sink.*
4. Pad the edge of the sink with a towel or bath blanket.
5. Move the client's head just beyond the edge of the stretcher. **Rationale:** *To allow water to run off more easily.*
6. Put a pillow or a rolled blanket under the client's shoulders. **Rationale:** *To help elevate and extend the head.*
7. Drape one towel over client's shoulders and around neck. Place another towel within reach.
8. Use a washcloth to protect client's eyes. Wet hair and gently make a lather with shampoo.
9. Rinse thoroughly and repeat if necessary.
10. Towel dry, add conditioner if desired, and rinse again.
11. Using a dry towel, pat hair dry, and wrap turban style to transport back to room.

12. Use hair dryer if available.
13. Style as desired.
14. Replace equipment.
15. Perform hand hygiene.

For Client Using Disposable System

1. Heat shampoo package in microwave for no more than 30 seconds.
2. Perform hand hygiene.
3. Open package and check temperature. **Rationale:** *Clients react to heat at different temperatures; therefore, check the cap temperature with client before placing on client's head.*
4. Place cap on head. Ensure that all hair is contained within the cap. For longer hair, place cap on top of head and then tuck all hair up inside cap.
5. Gently massage cap with hands, 1 to 2 minutes for short hair and 2 to 3 minutes for longer hair. **Rationale:** *This will assist in saturating the hair with the solution. There is no need to rinse hair after using solution.*

> **CLINICAL ALERT**
>
> If hair is tangled, the cap may need to stay on for a longer period of time in order to saturate hair. If blood or other secretions are present on hair, they may need to be removed using the washcloths from the disposable bath system before attempting to shampoo the hair.

6. Remove cap and place in appropriate receptacle.
7. Towel dry hair.
8. Complete hair care according to client's needs and desires.
9. Perform hand hygiene.

Note: Disposable hair care systems provide a quick and easy way to freshen client's hair with minimal client movement.

SKILL 2.11 Identifying and Removing Lice and Nits (Lice Eggs)

Equipment

- Bright lamp/light
- Magnifying glass
- Clean gloves
- Isolation bag
- Nit comb or tongue blade

Procedure

Note: Lice become adult in 17 days. Each louse lays 4 to 8 eggs/day for next 18 days, then dies (each louse lays 100 to 400 eggs). The nits/eggs hatch in 9 days. Adult lice can survive up to 55 hours without a host.

1. Perform hand hygiene. Don clean gloves.
2. Check two forms of client ID, introduce yourself, and explain procedure to client.
3. Position client so head or affected body area is well lighted by lamp.
4. Use fine-tooth comb after removing tangles and comb from roots to end. After each stroke, examine comb for live louse or a viable egg. Use magnifying glass to observe scalp and hair.
   - For live lice:
     Gray-white to reddish brown in color
     2 to –4 mm long; 1 mm wide

Flat body with six clawed legs
Live lice crawl, but do not fly, jump or hop
Feed on blood 3 to 4 times/day.
   - For viable eggs or nymph:
     Tiny and hard
     Yellow to white oval, tear-drop–shaped capsules Attached firmly to base of hair shaft (dandruff will fall from hair shaft when touched)
     Nits hatch after 7 to 10 days
     Nits within 6 mm of scalp are usually viable and indicate an active infestation
     Easier to detect close behind the ears or at the nape of the neck
5. Identify lice or nits:
   - Fine-toothed louse comb: After removing tangles, comb from roots to end with the nit comb. After each stroke, examine comb carefully for signs of lice.
   - Nits present without lice does not indicate there is an active infestation. Assess further: previous treatment, timing, and distance from scalp.
   - Put hair strands between two tongue blades and scrape white specks. Determine whether they come off the shaft easily. Observe base of scalp carefully for tiny lice.

SKILL 2.11   Identifying and Removing Lice and Nits (Lice Eggs) *(continued)*

VARIATION: REMOVING LICE AND NITS

Equipment

- Isolation bags (optional)
- Topical insecticide/pediculicides:
  Permethrin (Nix®, RID)
  Pyrethrin® (A-200, Pronto, Tisit)
  Malathion (Ovice, by prescription)
  Benzyl alcohol (Ulesfia, by prescription)
- Clean linen
- Fine-tooth "nit" comb
- Disinfectant for comb
- Clean gloves
- Towels

Procedure

1. Determine if client is allergic to ragweed or chrysanthemums. **Rationale:** *Pyrethrin is obtained from these plants and cannot be used to treat lice if client has allergic reaction to them.*

> **CLINICAL ALERT**
>
> When using any of the lice treatment products, the nurse needs to check for allergies to ragweed or chrysanthemum flowers. Allergies to ragweed can cause breathing difficulties or an asthmatic attack. Allergies to chrysanthemums can cause pneumonia, muscle paralysis, or death due to respiratory failure.

2. Perform hand hygiene.
3. Don clean gloves. Gloves are used even when completing treatment at home.
4. Remove and bag client's clothing and linens. Client's clothes do not need to be bagged separately and placed in isolation bags if standard precautions are used.
5. Notify physician and other healthcare providers of lice infestation. Begin treatment as ordered by physician.
6. Follow manufacturer's directions for product ordered.
7. Apply lotion, mousse, or gel to scalp and dry hair, beginning at the roots, and extend to the end of the hair shaft. If using shampoo before treatment, be sure to towel dry hair.
8. Leave product on hair for 10 minutes (leave malathion longer, according to directions).
9. Rinse hair thoroughly.
10. Give client a towel to protect eyes and face while applying product and rinsing hair.
11. Comb out nits using a fine-tooth or lice/nit comb. Hair should remain slightly damp while removing nits. If hair dries during combing, dampen slightly with water. **Rationale:** *Combing is the most important step in the process of lice removal, as eggs can be left behind and hatch at a later time.*
12. Disinfect combs and brushes with the shampoo.
13. Remove gloves.
14. Perform hand hygiene.
15. Instruct client, parent, or significant other to check hair and use "nit" comb every 2 to 3 days until lice are gone and to check skin for removal of scabies. (Pruritus may last for 2 weeks after treatment.)
16. Wash clothes and linens that person has used within 48 hours before treatment. **Rationale:** *Head lice rarely survive more than 48 hours off the body.*
17. Place stuffed toys in hot dryer or place in a plastic bag and seal for 2 to 4 weeks.

18. Instruct client or family to vacuum furniture and floors to rid house of lice. **Rationale:** *Head lice need a human host and therefore do not survive long after falling off head.*
19. Administer Bactrim if ordered (usually used with resistant cases). **Rationale:** *Used if multiple treatments have been attempted to rid hair of lice.*
20. Inspect all family members using wet louse comb or magnifying glass in bright light for lice/nits (eggs). Look for tiny nits near scalp, beginning at back of neck and behind ears. Examine small section of hair one at a time. Treat each member infested with lice using the same treatment plan **❶**.
21. Discuss the cause, treatment, and preventive measures regarding lice infestation with client and family.
22. Reinspect hair every 1 to 3 days for signs of reinfestation.
23. Apply second treatment within 7 to 10 days to kill any newly hatched lice.

Note: Nix is the treatment of choice and is an over-the-counter preparation. It is recommended by the American Academy of Pediatrics because of its efficacy and lack of toxicity.

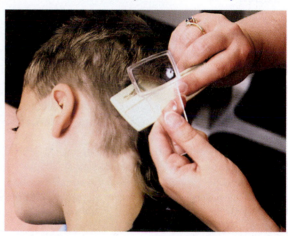

❶ Use magnifying glass when inspecting for head lice.

> **CLINICAL ALERT**
>
> - Do not use near eyes, eyebrows, eyelids, inside nose, mouth, or vagina.
>   If product gets into eyes, immediately flush eyes with water. If child swallows product, immediately contact a poison control center for directions on care.
> - Stop treatment immediately if client complains of breathing difficulties, eye irritation, or skin or scalp irritation.
> - Adverse reactions and side effects may be more frequent and severe in younger clients. Consult with physician about treatment dose. Pediculicides are not effective on some resistant strains of lice.
>
> **Removing Nits from Hair**
> - Part hair into sections; start at top of head and do one section at a time.
> - Lift a 1- to 2-inch-wide strand of hair. Place comb as close to scalp as possible and comb with a firm, even motion away from scalp.
> - Pin back each strand of hair after combing.
> - Clean comb often. Wipe nits away with tissue and discard into a plastic bag. Seal bag and discard to prevent lice from spreading.
> - After combing, thoroughly recheck for lice/nits. Recomb as needed.
> - Check daily for missed lice.

SKILL 2.12 Providing Foot Care

Delegation

Foot care for the *nondiabetic* client can be delegated to UAP. Remind the UAP to notify the nurse of anything that looks out of the ordinary. Review with the UAP the agency policy about cutting or trimming nails.

Equipment

- Wash basin containing warm water
- Pillow
- Moisture-resistant disposable pad
- Towels
- Soap
- Washcloth
- Toenail cleaning and trimming equipment, if agency policy permits
- Lotion or foot powder

Preparation

- Assemble all of the necessary equipment and supplies if nails need trimming and agency policy permits.

Procedure

1. Prior to performing the procedure, introduce self and verify the client's identity using agency protocol. Explain to the client what you are going to do, why it is necessary, and how he or she can participate.
2. Perform hand hygiene and observe other appropriate infection control procedures (e.g., clean gloves).
3. Provide for client privacy by drawing the curtains around the bed or closing the door to the room. Some agencies provide signs indicating the need for privacy. **Rationale:** *Hygiene is a personal matter.*
4. Prepare the equipment and the client.
   - Fill the washbasin with warm water at about 40° to 43°C (105° to 110°F). **Rationale:** *Warm water promotes circulation, comforts, and refreshes.*
   - Assist the ambulatory client to a sitting position in a chair, or the bed-bound client to a supine or semi-Fowler's position.
   - Place a pillow under the bed client's knees, if not contraindicated. **Rationale:** *This provides support and prevents muscle fatigue.*
   - Place the washbasin on the moisture-resistant pad at the foot of the bed for a bed client or on the floor in front of the chair for an ambulatory client ❶.
   - For a bed client, pad the rim of the washbasin with a towel. **Rationale:** *The towel prevents undue pressure on the skin.*
5. Wash the foot and soak it.
   - Place one of the client's feet in the basin and wash it with soap, paying particular attention to the interdigital areas. Prolonged soaking is generally not recommended for clients with diabetes or individuals with peripheral vascular disease. **Rationale:** *Prolonged soaking may remove natural skin oils, thus drying the skin and making it more susceptible to cracking and injury.*
   - Rinse the foot well to remove soap. **Rationale:** *Soap irritates the skin if not completely removed.*
   - Rub calloused areas of the foot with the washcloth. **Rationale:** *This helps remove dead skin layers.*

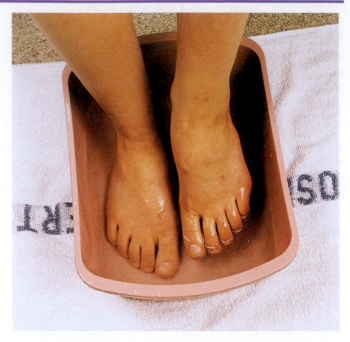

❶ Place towel on floor in front of client and place feet in basin for soaking.

- If the nails are brittle or thick and require trimming, replace the water and allow the foot to soak for 10 to 20 minutes. **Rationale:** *Soaking softens the nails and loosens debris under them.*
- Clean the nails as required with an orange stick. **Rationale:** *This removes excess debris that harbors microorganisms.*
- Remove the foot from the basin and place it on the towel.

6. Dry the foot thoroughly and apply lotion or foot powder.
   - Blot the foot gently with the towel to dry it thoroughly, particularly between the toes. **Rationale:** *Harsh rubbing can damage the skin. Thorough drying reduces the risk of infection.*
   - Apply lotion or lanolin cream to the foot but not between the toes. **Rationale:** *This lubricates dry skin and keeps the area between the toes dry.*

   or

   - Apply a foot powder containing a nonirritating deodorant if the feet tend to perspire excessively. **Rationale:** *Foot powders have greater absorbent properties than regular bath powders; some also contain menthol, which makes the feet feel cool.*

7. If agency policy permits, trim the nails of the first foot while the second foot is soaking.
   - See the discussion on nails in the accompanying Nail Care box for the appropriate method to use for trimming nails. Note that in many agencies, toenail trimming requires a primary care provider's order or is contraindicated for clients with diabetes mellitus, toe infections, and peripheral vascular disease, unless performed by a podiatrist, general practice physician, or advanced practice provider such as a nurse practitioner.

8. Document any foot problems observed.
   - Foot care is not generally recorded unless problems are noted.
   - Record any signs of inflammation, infection, breaks in the skin, corns, troublesome calluses, bunions, and pressure areas. This is of particular importance for clients with peripheral vascular disease and diabetes.

SKILL 2.12   Providing Foot Care *(continued)*

Client Teaching

- Wash the feet daily, and dry them well, especially between the toes.
- When washing, inspect the skin of the feet for breaks or red or swollen areas. Use a mirror if needed to visualize all areas.
- To prevent burns, check the water temperature before immersing the feet.
- Cover the feet, except between the toes, with creams or lotions to moisten the skin. Lotion will also soften calluses. A lotion that reduces dryness effectively is a mixture of lanolin and mineral oil.
- To prevent or control an unpleasant odor due to excessive foot perspiration, wash the feet frequently and change socks and shoes at least daily. Special deodorant sprays or absorbent foot powders are also helpful.
- File the toenails rather than cutting them to avoid skin injury. File the nails straight across the ends of the toes. If the nails are too thick or misshapen to file, consult a podiatrist.
- Wear clean stockings or socks daily. Avoid socks with holes or darns that can cause pressure areas.
- Wear comfortable, well-fitting shoes that neither restrict the foot nor rub on any area; rubbing can cause corns and calluses. Check worn shoes for rough spots in the lining. Break in new

shoes gradually by increasing the wearing time 30 to 60 minutes each day.
- Avoid walking barefoot, because injury and infection may result. Wear slippers in public showers and in change areas to avoid contracting athlete's foot or other infections.
- Several times each day exercise the feet to promote circulation. Point the feet upward, point them downward, and move them in circles.
- Avoid wearing constricting garments such as knee-high elastic stockings, and avoid sitting with the legs crossed at the knees, which may decrease circulation.
- When the feet are cold, use extra blankets and wear warm socks rather than using heating pads or hot water bottles, which may cause burns. Test bathwater before stepping into it.
- Wash any cut on the foot thoroughly, apply a mild antiseptic, and notify the primary care provider.
- Avoid self-treatment for corns or calluses. Pumice stones and some callus and corn applications are injurious to the skin. Do not cut calluses or corns. Consult a podiatrist or primary care provider first.
- Notify the primary care provider if you notice abnormal sores or drainage, pain, or changes in temperature, color, and sensation of the foot.

Nail Care

- Check the agency's policy regarding nail care. Often, podiatrists must be consulted for clients with diabetes.
- To provide nail care, the nurse needs a nail cutter or sharp scissors, a nail file, an orange stick to push back the cuticle, hand lotion or mineral oil to lubricate any dry tissue around the nails, and a basin of water to soak the nails if they are particularly thick or hard.
- One hand or foot is soaked, if needed, and dried. Then, the nail is cut or filed straight across beyond the end of the finger or toe. Avoid trimming or digging into nails at the lateral corners. **Rationale:** Trimming toes at the corners predisposes the client to ingrown toenails.
- Clients who have diabetes or circulatory problems should have their nails filed rather than cut. Inadvertent injury to tissues can occur if scissors are used.
- After the initial cut or filing, the nail is filed to round the corners and the nurse cleans under the nail. Fingernails are trimmed straight across.
- Gently push back the cuticle, taking care not to injure it.
- The next finger or toe is cared for in the same manner.
- Any abnormalities, such as an infected cuticle or inflammation of the tissue around the nail, are recorded and reported.

SKILL 2.13   Providing Routine Eye Care

Equipment

- Small basin
- Water or normal saline solution
- Washcloth or cotton balls
- Clean gloves

Preparation

- Determine client's eye care needs, and obtain physician's order if needed.
- Explain necessity for and method of eye care to client. Discuss how client can assist you.
- Collect necessary equipment.
- Perform hand hygiene and don gloves.

Procedure

1. Use water or saline solution at room temperature.
2. Using the washcloth or cotton balls moistened in water or saline, gently wipe each eye from the inner to outer canthus. Use separate cotton ball or corner of washcloth for each eye.

Rationale: *To prevent cross-contamination from one eye to the other.*
3. If crusting is present, gently place a warm, wet compress over eye(s) until crusting is loosened.
4. Dispose of used supplies and return basin to appropriate area.
5. Remove and discard gloves.
6. Perform hand hygiene.

> **CLINICAL ALERT**
>
> **Eye Care for Comatose Client**
> - Use a dropper to instill a sterile ophthalmic solution (liquid tears, saline, methylcellulose) every 3 to 4 hours as ordered by physician **Rationale:** *To prevent corneal drying and ulceration.*
> - Keep client's eyes closed if blink reflex is absent. If eye pads or patches are used, explain their purpose to client's family. Do not tape eyes shut. **Rationale:** *Corneal abrasions and drying occur when eyes lose blink reflex.*
> - Remove gloves and perform hand hygiene.
> - Remove patch and evaluate condition of eye every 4 hours.

SKILL 2.14 Removing and Cleaning Contact Lenses

Equipment

- Towel
- Contact lens container
- Commercially prepared cleaning solution
- Commercially prepared disinfecting solution
- Commercially prepared rinsing and storing solution
- Enzymatic agent (protein remover)
- Clean gloves

Procedure

1. Place client in semi-Fowler's position, and place a towel under the client's chin.
2. Perform hand hygiene and don gloves.
3. Place the tip of your thumb across the lower lid below its margin.
4. Place the tip of the forefinger of the same hand on the upper lid above its margin.
5. Spread eyelids apart as wide as possible and locate outer edges of soft lens which should appear as a rim around outer edge of iris.
6. Place thumb and forefinger directly on soft lens.
7. Gently remove soft lens from surface of eyeball by squeezing lens between thumb and fingertip. To remove rigid lens, place thumb on lower eyelid and index finger on upper lid. Press gently against eyeball to release suction; lens is released as eyelids meet lens edge. Catch lens in your hand. **Rationale:** *Corneas are avascular and the use of contact lenses interrupts flow of oxygen into cornea. Removing lenses for a period of time allows oxygen to reach the cornea, thus preventing corneal complications.*
8. Release eyelids.
9. Place lens in palm of hand or place disposable lenses in trash. Disposable lenses are not to be cleaned or reused. Lens cleaners are not available for these lenses.
10. Place 2 to 3 drops of cleaning solution on lens.
11. Clean lens thoroughly by rubbing between fingertip and palm of hand of 20 to 30 seconds.

12. Rinse lens thoroughly with sterile saline solution or rinsing solution. Use only lens cleaning system recommended by ophthalmologist. Do not interchange cleaning solution systems.
13. Place lens in disinfecting solution according to physician directions. Time varies from hours to 1 full day. **Rationale:** *This destroys microorganisms on lenses.*
14. Rinse lens thoroughly with rinsing solution.
15. Repeat procedure on second lens.
16. Use enzyme tablet or solution according to physician orders, usually weekly. **Rationale:** *This removes stubborn protein and lipids.*
17. Clean lens container daily and leave open to dry. Replace as directed by physician, either weekly or monthly.
18. Remove gloves and perform hand hygiene.

Note: A suction cup can be placed gently against lens for easy removal of lens. Squeeze suction cup with dominant hand, place on lens, open finger slightly to create suction between lens and cup. Rock lens gently to remove it.

Client Teaching

Instruct the client in the following safety issues:

- Notify physician immediately if eyes are red, not comfortable, or you can't see clearly.
- Use only rinsing solution, not saliva, to wet lenses.
- Use only commercially prepared saline solution or rinsing solution to cleanse lenses.
- Do not interchange types of lens cleaning systems.
- Maintain lens care regimen prescribed by physician.
- Put on makeup before inserting lens.
- Use appropriate type of lenses for their intended use. Do not use daily-wear lenses at night or disposable lenses more than once.
- Do not allow soft lenses to dry out.
- Contact lens wearers should be instructed to carry appropriate identification on type and care for specific lens he or she wears.

SKILL 2.15 Removing, Cleaning, and Inserting a Hearing Aid

Delegation

A nurse can delegate the task of caring for a hearing aid to the UAP. It is important, however, for the nurse to first determine that the UAP knows the correct way to care for a hearing aid. Inform the UAP to report the presence of ear inflammation, discomfort, excess wax, or drainage to the RN.

Equipment

- Client's hearing aid
- Soap, water, and towels or a damp cloth
- Pipe cleaner or toothpick (optional)
- New battery (if needed)

Procedure

1. Prior to performing the procedure, introduce self and verify the client's identity using agency protocol. Explain to the client what you are going to do, why it is necessary, and how he or she can participate.
2. Perform hand hygiene and observe other appropriate infection control procedures (e.g., clean gloves).
3. Provide for client privacy by drawing the curtains around the bed or closing the door to the room. Some agencies provide signs indicating the need for privacy. **Rationale:** *Hygiene is a personal matter.*
4. Remove the hearing aid.

SKILL 2.15   Removing, Cleaning, and Inserting a Hearing Aid (continued)

- Turn the hearing aid off and lower the volume. The on/off switch may be labeled "O" (off), "M" (microphone), "T" (telephone), or "TM" (telephone/microphone). **Rationale:** *The batteries continue to run if the hearing aid is not turned off.*
- Remove the earmold by rotating it slightly forward and pulling it outward.
- If the hearing aid is not to be used for several days, remove the battery. **Rationale:** *Removal prevents corrosion of the hearing aid from battery leakage.*
- Store the hearing aid in a safe place and label with client's name. Avoid exposure to heat and moisture. **Rationale:** *Proper storage prevents loss or damage.*

5. Clean the earmold.
   - Detach the earmold if possible. Disconnect the earmold from the *receiver of a body* hearing aid or from the hearing aid case of behind-the-ear and eyeglass hearing aids where the tubing meets the hook of the case. Do not remove the earmold if it is glued or secured by a small metal ring. **Rationale:** *Removal facilitates cleaning and prevents inadvertent damage to the other parts.*
   - If the earmold is detachable, soak it in a mild soapy solution. Rinse and dry it well. Do not use isopropyl alcohol. **Rationale:** *Alcohol can damage the hearing aid.*
   - If the earmold is not detachable or is for an in-the-ear aid, wipe the earmold with a damp cloth.
   - Check that the earmold opening is patent. Blow any excess moisture through the opening or remove debris (e.g., earwax) with a pipe cleaner or toothpick.
   - Reattach the earmold if it was detached from the rest of the hearing aid.

6. Insert the hearing aid.
   - Determine from the client if the earmold is for the left or the right ear.
   - Check that the battery is inserted in the hearing aid. Turn off the hearing aid, and make sure the volume is turned all the way down. **Rationale:** *A volume that is too loud is distressing.*
   - Inspect the earmold to identify the ear canal portion. Some ear molds are fitted for only the ear canal and concha; others are fitted for all the contours of the ear. The canal portion, common to all, can be used as a guide for correct insertion.
   - Line up the parts of the earmold with the corresponding parts of the client's ear.
   - Rotate the earmold slightly forward, and insert the ear canal portion.
   - Gently press the earmold into the ear while rotating it backward.

- Check that the earmold fits snugly by asking the client if it feels secure and comfortable.
- Adjust the other components of a behind-the-ear or body hearing aid.
- Turn the hearing aid on, and adjust the volume according to the client's needs.

7. Correct problems associated with improper functioning.
   - If the sound is weak or there is no sound:
     a. Ensure that the volume is turned high enough.
     b. Ensure that the earmold opening is not clogged.
     c. Check the battery by turning the hearing aid on, turning up the volume, cupping your hand over the earmold, and listening. A constant whistling sound indicates the battery is functioning. If necessary, replace the battery. Be sure that the negative (–) and positive (+) signs on the battery match those where indicated on the hearing aid.
     d. Ensure that the ear canal is not blocked with wax, which can obstruct sound waves.
   - If the client reports a whistling sound or squeal after insertion:
     a. Turn the volume down.
     b. Ensure that the earmold is properly attached to the receiver.
     c. Reinsert the earmold.

8. Document pertinent data.
   - The removal and the insertion of a hearing aid are not normally recorded.
   - Report and record any problems the client has with the hearing aid.

Setting of Care

- People who need a hearing aid may not wear one because they view the hearing aid as a stigma of old age.
- It is important for the client who has just purchased a hearing aid to know that it often takes weeks or even months to adjust to the hearing aid. At first, the sounds will seem shrill as they start hearing high-frequency sounds that had been forgotten. Remind them that it is a hearing aid, not a hearing cure. Encourage them to not give up.
- The client needs to adjust to the hearing aid gradually by increasing the amount of time each day until the aid can be worn for a full day.
- Encourage clients to purchase their hearing aids from a company that has a minimum warranty of a 30-day return policy.
- Emphasize the importance of maintaining the hearing aid, that is, having it cleaned and checked regularly.

▶ MEDICATION ADMINISTRATION

Expected Outcomes

1. Client's MAR is current with physician's orders.
2. Rationale for medication administration is clear.
3. Medication is administered according to the "six rights."
4. Medications remain controlled and safe.
5. Sign-out documentation for medications is accurate.

SKILL 2.16   Preparing for Medication Administration

Equipment

- Reference resource (e.g., *Physicians' Desk Reference*, pharmacology textbook, drug handbook)
- Calculator (if indicated)
- Medication administration record (MAR)
- Client's chart

Procedure

1. Check physician's orders and client's MAR for medications client is to receive (drug, dosage, route of administration, time intervals).
2. Identify any unfamiliar drugs.
3. Research unfamiliar drugs using appropriate reference:
   a. Generic and trade name
   b. Drug classification and major uses
   c. Pharmacologic actions
   d. Safe dosage, route, and time of administration
   e. Side effects; adverse reactions
   f. Nursing implications
   g. Complete client teaching as needed.

CLINICAL ALERT

Individual drugs are designed to be administered by a specific route—be sure to check drug labels for appropriate route of administration.

4. Review client's record for allergies, lab data, any factor (e.g., NPO status, planned procedures) that contraindicates administration of ordered medications.
5. Check client's daily MAR with previous day's MAR every 24 hours for each drug's dosage, route, and time to be given. **Rationale:** *Pharmacy produces each daily MAR sheet. Any new medication, discontinued medication, or altered dosage must be identified and verified with the physician's orders.*
6. Validate carefully that the MAR is consistent with the physician's most recent order for each medication. **Rationale:** *Some medication dosages are adjusted on a daily basis. Errors in transmission of intentions may occur between physician, pharmacy, and client's MAR.*
7. Perform hand hygiene.
8. Take medication to client's room.
9. Open medication cart; take out client's medication drawer.
10. Starting at the top of the medication record, check each medication in order against the medication packages in the drawer. Alternately, obtain client's medication from the automated dispensing system.
11. Retrieve medication to be given and compare drug label with MAR. **Rationale:** *This is a safety check to ensure the right medication is given.*
12. Inspect label for expiration date, and ensure that medication is indicated for ordered route of administration. **Rationale:** *Different preparations of the same medication are used for different routes of administration.*

13. Determine if any calculation is necessary to prepare the correct dosage.
14. Calculate client's dosage based on strength of medication, if indicated. Have another nurse double check your calculation. (See page 122 for formulas.)
15. Prepare medication as indicated for nonparenteral or parenteral route, checking drug label before, during, and after preparation.

Evidence-Based Nursing Practice

Medication Administration Errors

It is difficult to get accurate measurements of how often preventable adverse drug events (ADEs) occur. One study estimated 380,000 preventable ADEs in hospitals each year, another estimated 450,000, and the researchers believe that both are likely to be underestimates.

The numbers are equally disturbing in other settings. One study calculates, for example, that 800,000 preventable ADEs occur each year in long-term care facilities. Another finds that outpatient Medicare clients incur 530,000 preventable ADEs each year. And, the evidence suggests that both of these numbers are likely to be underestimates as well. Furthermore, none of these studies includes errors of omission—failures to prescribe medication in cases where it should be. Taking all of these numbers into account, the researchers conclude that at least 1.5 million preventable ADEs occur in the United States each year.

Data from National Academy of Sciences, Institute of Medicine (2006).

LEGAL ALERT

Transcription Error and Reconciliation Failure: *Robert Ferguson v. Baptist Health System, Inc.,* 2005

Robert Ferguson brought a medical malpractice action against Baptist after experiencing drug toxicity due to a medication (Dilantin) transcription error on the part of the pharmacist and failure on the part of the nurse to conduct reconciliation between the MAR entry and the physician's order. The physician's order was for Dilantin, 300 milligrams "PO QHS." The MAR was generated by pharmacy for Dilantin, 300 milligrams, "t.i.d." The agency policy dictated that any time a new medication order was entered, the nurse initially undertaking to administer the medication was responsible for comparing the MAR to the actual order to "reconcile" the two. In this case, the pharmacy error was not detected by the reconciliation process. Subsequent erroneous doses were administered, but none of the nurses administering the Dilantin detected the error "due to the fact that there were no additional checks, balances, or other safeguards in place to prevent the repetition of the error." No one ever checked the original physician's order "despite the unusually large amount of Dilantin being administered." None of the nurses suspected that Ferguson's symptoms represented Dilantin toxicity. Ferguson was awarded compensatory damages and punitive damages.

SKILL 2.17   Administering Medication Protocol

Equipment

- Prepared medication
- Gloves (if indicated)
- Stethoscope and sphygmomanometer, if indicated

Procedure

1. Check client's name and room number against the medication record and lock the medication cart before entering client's room, if cart is used ❶. **Rationale:** *Locking the cart is a safety measure.*

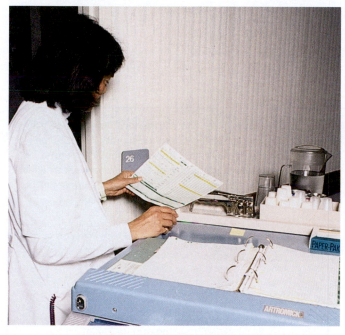

❶ Check client's name and room number against medication record.

2. Check client's identity band and ask client to state name and birth date ❷.

> **CLINICAL ALERT**
>
> Use at least two client identifiers other than room number when administering medications or providing treatments (e.g., stated name and birth date or hospital number).

3. Provide for client privacy.
4. Explain procedure and purpose of medication to client.
5. Assist client to appropriate position for medication administration.
6. Check client's vital signs if indicated before administering medication. **Rationale:** *Medication's effects may cause hemodynamic instability if client's vital signs are at the high or low extreme of normal.*
7. Perform hand hygiene and don gloves if indicated. **Rationale:** *Parenteral and enteral medication administration may require the use of gloves.*

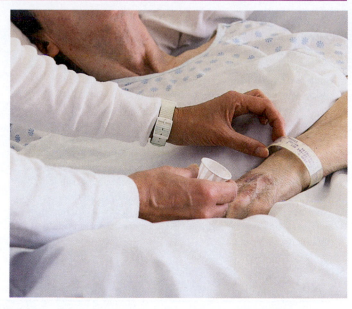

❷ Check client's identification band and ask client to state name and birth date.

8. Administer medication according to route procedure and adhering to the "six rights" of medication administration.
9. Dispose of equipment appropriately; then remove gloves, if used, and wash your hands.
10. Record administered medications in client's record; the time, medication given, dosage, and route (including site of injection); and any relevant assessment findings.

> **CLINICAL ALERT**
>
> **Reporting Actual or Potential Error**
>
> Report any actual or potential error (e.g., sound-alike/look-alike drug names, confusion over abbreviations) to the Institute for Safe Medication Practices at 1-800-FAIL-SAF(E) or complete the form at www.ismp.org/orderforms/reporterrortoISMP.asp. All communications are kept confidential. This agency publicizes warnings and notices in response to submitted information to help alert other professionals to potentially dangerous medication pitfalls.
>
> *Source:* Pump up the volume—Tips for increasing error reporting. (2009). *Nurse Advise-ERR, 7*(7), 1–3.
>
> **National Patient Safety Goals**
>
> All Joint Commission–accredited agencies must have protocols developed for documenting and reconciling medications across the continuum (admission, transfer, discharge). A list of the client's home medications is compared with the admitting medication orders. Upon transfer, medications being taken are compared with orders in the new unit. Upon discharge, medications taken in the hospital are compared to the discharge medi-

(continued on next page)

SKILL 2.17   Administering Medication Protocol *(continued)*

cation orders. Verification, clarification, and reconciliation of discrepancies help prevent adverse drug events throughout the client's hospitalization.

The Joint Commission's Hospital National Patient Safety Goals guideline for 2014 identifies specific safety goals related to medication administration.

One priority prevention action is to make sure all medications, solutions, and their containers are appropriately labeled in all client-care settings. Another focus on medication safety is to prevent errors during anticoagulant therapy including the physician's order, accurate medication preparation, and correct administration to the right client. A final measure to improve medication safety is accuracy in communicating about client's medications to other appropriate care providers, like during a hand-off report, shift report, or transfer report of client to another appropriate nurse, unit, or facility.

Evidence-Based Nursing Practice

Medication Errors—A Growing Problem

Medication errors originate across the spectrum of care: prescribing, 39%; transcribing, 17%; dispensing, 11%; and administering, 38%. Nurses must identify errors before administering medications: both the mistakes of others, and their own.

Data from Cohen (2008).

Medication Safety Measures

- Accurately and completely reconcile the client's medications across the continuum of care.
- Keep all medicines in locked carts or cabinets.
- Limit access to and use special safeguards with "high-alert" drugs (those causing significant client harm if used in error; e.g., hypoglycemic, anticoagulant, anesthetic agents, narcotics, paralytic agents, chemotherapy drugs, certain cardiac drugs). This list is periodically updated by the Institute for Safe Medication Practices (ISMP).
- Keep narcotics in double-locked cabinets or PYXIS. Count all narcotics with oncoming staff at the end of each shift.
- Separate topical medications from parenteral or oral medications.
- Clearly label all prepared medication containers (syringes, medicine cups, solutions). Check with another nurse (1) mathematical calculations for dosages and (2) dispensed/prepared "high-alert" drugs and those for high-risk clients (e.g., insulin, anticoagulants, concentrated electrolytes, digoxin, and hemodynamic agents if not premixed).
- Do not leave any medication at client's bedside unless there is a specific physician's order to do so.
- Report any errors in drug administration to charge nurse and client's physician immediately. Monitor the client closely for adverse effects. Document the drug given, and complete a written variance report.
- Provide complete instructions to clients regarding medication to be used at home.

Cultural Considerations

Some genetic factors may result in predispositions for medical conditions in different populations. An example of a genetic factor that differs among ethnic groups is the potential of a predisposition for African American clients to have high blood pressure. Some scientists attribute this to earlier generations living in hot, dry African locations becoming salt-sensitive, resulting in higher levels of sodium in their bodies. Because of the higher levels of sodium, the extracellular fluid volume is increased causing hypertension. Current generations could manifest this genetic sodium factor. The nurse should obtain a list of each client's current medications as well as any alternative therapies used so that possible untoward interactions can be prevented.

Source: Harvard Health Publishing, 2015, Race and ethnicity: Clues to your heart disease risk? https://www.health.harvard.edu/heart-health/race-and-ethnicity-clues-to-your-heart-disease-risk.

The Six Rights

- **Right medication.** Compare medication container label to the medication administration record (MAR) three times (when obtaining the medication, when preparing the medication, and after preparation). Note medication expiration date. Know action, dosage, and method of administration. Know side effects of the medication and any allergies the client might have.
- **Right client.** Check the room and bed number and client's identity band. Validate correct client with two identifiers other than room number (e.g., stated name and date of birth).
- **Right time.** Medication given 30 to 45 minutes before or after time ordered is acceptable (according to agency policy).
- **Right method or route of administration.** If a change in route is indicated, request new orders from physician.
- **Right dose.** Validate calculations of divided doses with another nurse. Have another nurse double-check your preparation of insulin, potassium chloride, morphine, hydromorphone HCl, heparin, and warfarin sodium (Joint Commission high-alert drugs). Know the usual dose and question any dose outside safe range.
- **Documentation.** After administration, documentation may be considered to be the sixth right. The nurse should document the name of the drug, the dose and route, time administered, and the client's response to the medication administered.

SKILL 2.17 Administering Medication Protocol (continued)

Seven Parts of Medication Orders

- Client's name
- Date medication was ordered
- Name of medication
- Medication dosage
- Route of administration and any special instruction for administration
- Time and frequency medication is to be given
- Signature of individual ordering the drug

Common communication breakdowns leading to medication errors include:

- Unapproved or unclear abbreviations
- Illegible writing
- Misplaced or unnoticed decimals (e.g., .2 rather than 0.2)
- "Verbal orders"
- Incomplete orders

See **Table 2–2** ● for abbreviations.

The Joint Commission (2011) has identified certain abbreviations that are associated with frequent errors in medication administration. Their website keeps a list of abbreviations that should not be used. For example, the word "unit" should always be spelled out, because its abbreviations (u, U) can be misread. The abbreviations Q.D. (every day) and Q.O.D. (every other day) are often mistaken for each other. Therefore, the Joint Commission recommends writing out "daily" or "every other day."

Orders with zero should be written with special care. For a full unit (e.g., 1 mg), avoid the "trailing zero" (**do not write** 1.0 mg). If the trailing zero is used and the decimal point is not seen, 10 mg might be administered instead of 1 mg.

If the ordered amount of medication is less than one unit (e.g., seven-tenths of a milligram), it is important to include a zero before the decimal (0.7 mg). Otherwise, the amount may be read as 7 mg, resulting in administration of ten times the ordered dose.

TABLE 2–2 List of Abbreviations and Symbols

aa	of each	NPO	nothing by mouth
a.c.	before meals	oz	ounce
ad lib.	freely, as desired	p.c.	after meals
BID	twice each day	per	by, through
c̄	with	PO	by mouth
C	carbon	prn, or PRN	whenever necessary
Ca	calcium	q.h.	every hour
Cl	chlorine	q.i.d.	four times each day
dr or Z	dram	q.s.	as much as required, quantity sufficient
et	and	q2h	every 2 hours
GI	gastrointestinal	q3h	every 3 hours
gt or gtt	drop(s)	q4h	every 4 hours
H_2O	water	RX	treatment, "take thou"
H_2O_2	hydrogen peroxide	s̄	without
IM	intramuscular	STAT	immediately
K	potassium	TID	three times each day
lb or #	pound	tsp	teaspoon
m	meter	°	degree
mcg	microgram	–	minus, negative, alkaline reaction
mEq	milliequivalent	+	plus, positive, acid reaction
mg	milligram	%	percent
mL	milliliter	v	Roman numeral 5
mmol	millimole	vii	Roman numeral 7
Na	sodium	ix	Roman numeral 9
NA	not applicable	xiii	Roman numeral 13
NG	nasogastric		

SKILL 2.18   Using the Narcotic Control System

Equipment

- Medication record sheet
- Narcotic sign-out sheet
- Medication

Procedure

For Client Administration

1. Check client's medication sheet for narcotic order.
2. Check dose and time last narcotic was administered.

3. Unlock and open narcotic drawer, and find appropriate narcotic container.
4. Count the number of pills, ampules, or prefilled cartridges in container.
5. Check the narcotic sign-out sheet, and check that the number of narcotics in drawer matches the number on specific narcotic sign-out sheet. **Rationale:** *Laws on controlled substances require careful monitoring of narcotics.*
6. Correct any discrepancy before proceeding with narcotic administration.
7. Sign out for the narcotic on the narcotic sheet after taking narcotic out of drawer ❶.

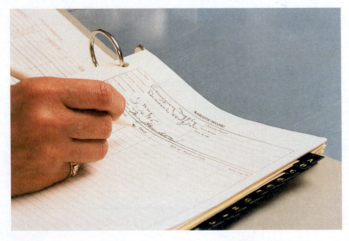

❶ Sign on specific narcotic sign-out sheet after taking narcotic out of drawer.

8. Lock drawer after dispensing medication ❷.
9. Administer medication according to specific oral or parenteral procedure.
10. Document narcotic on client's medication record according to usual procedure. Include client's pain rating (e.g., 8/10) and sedation level before and after narcotic administration according to agency policy.

For Unit Narcotic Stock

11. Check narcotic counts every 8 hours. One off-going and one on-coming *licensed* nurse must check the narcotics together. The number on each narcotic sign-out sheet must match the number of that particular narcotic remaining in the drawer.

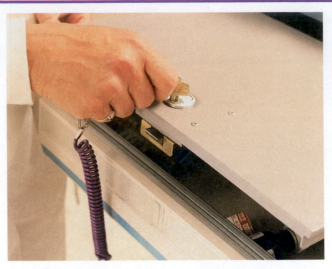

❷ Lock narcotic drawer after removing medication. Keep key with you at all times.

12. Explore any discrepancy in stock and recorded dispensed narcotic numbers. **Rationale:** *Counts must balance. It is the nurse's responsibility to account for all controlled substances dispensed.*
13. Licensed nurses cosign the narcotic record if the count is accurate.

SKILL 2.19   Using an Automated Dispensing System

Equipment

- Automated dispensing system (e.g., PYXIS)
- Client's medication record

Procedure

1. Touch the screen to activate the system.
2. Enter your ID code number and user password or scanned fingerprint ❶. **Rationale:** *This process controls access to medications.*

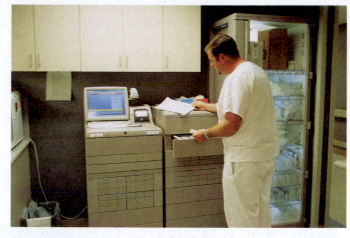

❷ Validate that client's MAR matches selected medications and dose on screen.

7. Type in quantity (#) of doses desired if indicated by a range of possible doses ordered.
8. Enter a witness ID/scan (by another nurse) to validate wasted medication (if partial dose is needed).
9. Remove the medication from the automated delivery system.
10. Close drawer/storage door, and exit the system.
11. Prepare medication and administer according to route.

Note: Certain medications (e.g., cough syrup and other client-specific multiple-dose medications) may be dispensed by pharmacy and placed in the client's medication drawer rather than being accessed through the automated system.

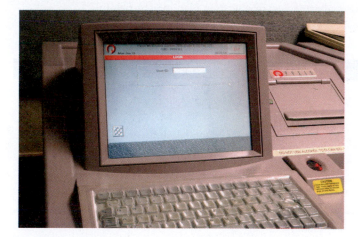

❶ User ID and a password or scanned fingerprint control access to medications.

3. From the main menu, select command on medication management station (e.g., *remove, waste, return*).
4. Select client's room number, medication, and name and additional identifiers (e.g., *birth date, hospital number*).
5. Touch/select medication desired from client's displayed list of ordered medications.
6. Validate that client's medication record matches selected medication and dose on monitor screen ❷.

CLINICAL ALERT

The usual checks and balances between nurses and pharmacists may be bypassed with automated dispensing systems, increasing the risk for medication errors.

Dispensing Medications— Safe Practices

- No technology system eliminates the risk for error.
- Never become complacent about what technology can do to support safe practice.
- No computer has your ability to think critically, to understand whether an ordered drug is appropriate for your client.
- Technology (e.g., bar codes) increases the amount of time spent administering medications, but does reduce time spent in documentation.

▶ HOME SETTING: ADMINISTERING MEDICATIONS

Ambulatory and Community Settings Administering Medications

The nurse should instruct the client to:

- Learn the names of the medications as well as their actions and possible adverse effects. Carry a complete list of all prescriptions, OTC medications, and home remedies at all times.
- Keep all medications out of reach of children and pets.
- If using a syringe to administer the medication to an infant or child, remove and dispose of the plastic cap that fits on the end of the syringe. Infants and small children have been known to choke on these caps.

- Take the medications only as prescribed. Know which medications need to be taken on an empty stomach and which can be taken with food/meals.
- Immediately consult the nurse, pharmacist, or primary care provider about any problems with the medication.
- Always check the medication label to make sure the correct medication is being taken.
- Request labels printed with larger type on medication containers if there is difficulty reading the label.
- Check the expiration date and discard outdated medications. Previously, most people discarded old medicines by flushing

them down the toilet. The Environmental Protection Agency (EPA) no longer recommends this. Inform clients to check with their local government. Many cities and towns have household hazardous waste facilities where old medicines can be disposed. Expired medications may be placed in the trash if the following precautions are used: Keep the medication in the original container and mark out the person's name. Add a nontoxic but bad-tasting product (e.g., cayenne pepper, mustard) to the container to keep individuals or animals from eating it. Place in a sturdy container, tape the container shut, and have this container be the last thing put in the garbage can.

■ Ask the pharmacist to substitute childproof caps with ones that are more easily opened, as necessary.

■ If a dose or more is missed, do not take two or more doses; ask the pharmacist or primary care provider for directions.

■ Do not crush or cut a tablet or capsule without first checking with the primary care provider or pharmacist. Doing so may affect the medication's absorption.

■ Never stop taking the medication without first discussing it with the primary care provider.

■ Always check with the pharmacist before taking any nonprescription medications. Some OTC medications can interact with the prescribed medication. Additionally, the nurse can set up a medication plan to assist clients and family members to remember a schedule. Weekly pill containers (available at pharmacies) or a written plan may be helpful.

▶ MEDICATION PREPARATION

Expected Outcomes

1. Dosage calculations are accurate.
2. Medications are prepared using safe procedures.
3. Medications are accurately labeled.
4. Complications of medication administration are prevented.

SKILL 2.20 Calculating Dosages

Equipment

■ Orders for dosage of medication needed
■ Dosage of medication on hand

Procedure

1. To calculate oral dosages, use the following formula, noting that D and H must be in same unit of measure:

$$\frac{D}{H} = X$$

where

D = dose desired
H = dose on hand
X = dose to be administered.

Example: Give 500 mg of ampicillin sodium when the dose on hand is in capsules containing 250 mg.

$$\frac{500 \text{ mg}}{250 \text{ mg}} = 2 \text{ capsules}$$

2. To calculate dose when in liquid form, use the following formula:

$$\frac{D}{H} \times Q = X$$

where

D = dose desired
H = dose on hand

Q = quantity
X = amount to be administered.

Example: Give 375 mg of ampicillin when it is supplied as 250 mg/5 mL.

$$\frac{375 \text{ mg}}{250 \text{ mg}} \times 5$$

$$1.5 \times 5 = 7.5 \text{ mL}$$

3. To calculate parenteral dosages, use the following formula:

$$\frac{D}{H} \times Q = X$$

Example: Give client 40 mg gentamicin C complex sulfate. On hand is a multidose vial with a strength of 80 mg/2 mL.

$$\frac{40}{80} \times 2 = 1 \text{ mL}$$

4. To calculate dosages for infants and children using body surface area (BSA), use the following formula:

$$\frac{BSA}{1.7 \times \text{adult dose}} = \text{pediatric dose}$$

5. To calculate dosages for infants and children using Clark's weight rule:

$$\text{Child's dose} = \frac{\text{child's wt. in lbs.}}{150} \times \text{adult dose}$$

6. Check your calculations before drawing up the medications.

SKILL 2.21 Preparing Medications from Ampules

Delegation

Preparing medications from ampules involves knowledge and use of sterile technique. Therefore, these skills are not delegated to UAP.

Equipment

■ Client's medication administration record (MAR) or computer printout
■ Ampule of sterile medication

SKILL 2.21 Preparing Medications from Ampules *(continued)*

- File (if ampule is not scored) and small gauze square or plastic ampule opener
- Antiseptic swabs
- Syringe
- Needle for administering the medication
- Filter needle or straw for withdrawing medication from the ampule

Preparation

- Check the MAR.
- Check the label on the ampule carefully against the MAR to make sure that the correct medication is being prepared.
- Follow the three checks for administering medications. Read the label on the medication (1) when it is taken from the medication cart, (2) before withdrawing the medication, and (3) after withdrawing the medication.
- Organize the equipment.

Procedure

1. Perform hand hygiene and observe other appropriate infection control procedures (e.g., clean gloves).
2. Prepare the medication ampule for drug withdrawal.
   - Flick the upper stem of the ampule several times with a fingernail. **Rationale:** *This will bring all medication down to the main portion of the ampule.*
   - Use an ampule opener, or place a piece of gauze or an unopened alcohol wipe between your thumb and the ampule neck or around the ampule neck, and break off the top by bending it toward you to ensure the ampule is broken away from yourself and others ❶. **Rationale:** *The gauze*

> **CLINICAL ALERT**
> Small fragments of glass can be released when the ampule is broken open. Use an ampule opener when possible. This device covers the section of the ampule that is broken and prevents small pieces of glass from being scattered.

protects the fingers from the broken glass, and any glass fragments will spray away from the nurse.
   - Dispose of the top of the ampule in the sharps container.
3. Withdraw the medication.
   - Place the ampule on a flat surface.
   - Attach the filter needle or straw to the syringe. **Rationale:** *The filter needle or straw prevents glass particles from being withdrawn with the medication.*
   - Remove the cap from the filter needle or straw and insert the needle into the center of the ampule. If not using a filter needle or straw, do not touch the rim of the ampule with the needle tip or shaft. **Rationale:** *This will keep the needle sterile. Withdraw all of the drug.*
   - Hold the ampule slightly on its side, if necessary, to obtain all of the medication ❷.

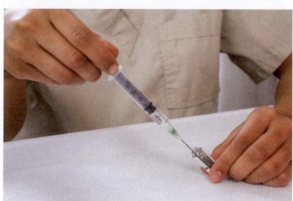

A

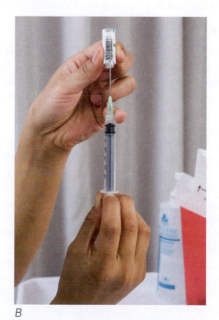

B

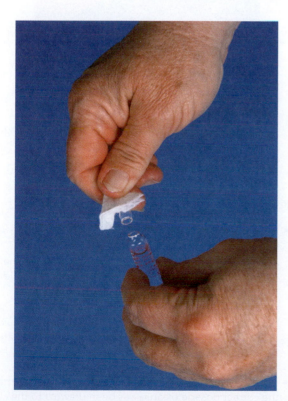

❶ Breaking the neck of an ampule using an unopened alcohol wipe.

❷ Withdrawing medication: *A,* from an ampule on a flat surface; *B,* from an inverted ampule.

(continued on next page)

SKILL 2.21 Preparing Medications from Ampules (continued)

- Tap syringe barrel below bubbles to dislodge air bubbles to hub of syringe.
- Eject air with syringe in an upright position. If amount of solution is overdrawn, invert syringe and remove excess solution to the medical waste (black box) receptacle. **Rationale:** *Appropriate waste disposal is mandated by the EPA.*
- Dispose of the filter needle or straw by placing it in a sharps container **3**.
- Replace the filter needle or straw with a regular needle, tighten the cap at the hub of the needle, and push solution into the needle, to the prescribed amount.
- Label the syringe with medication name and dosage drawn up in the syringe. **Rationale:** *This can be used to do a last medication check for accuracy before administering the medication to client.*

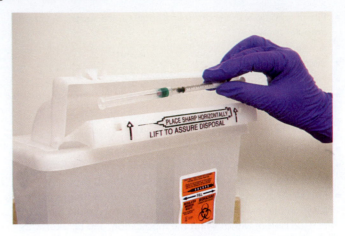

3 Discard syringe in biohazard container following use.

SKILL 2.22 Preparing Medications from Vials

Delegation

Preparing medications from vials involves knowledge and use of sterile technique. Therefore, these techniques are not delegated to UAP.

Equipment

- Client's MAR or computer printout
- Vial of sterile medication
- Antiseptic swabs
- Safety needle and syringe
- Filter needle (check agency policy)
- Sterile water or normal saline, if drug is in powdered form

Procedure

1. Perform hand hygiene and observe other appropriate infection control procedures (e.g., clean gloves).
2. Prepare the medication vial for drug withdrawal.
   - Mix the solution, if necessary, by rotating the vial between the palms of the hands, not by shaking. **Rationale:** *Some vials contain aqueous suspensions, which settle when they stand. In some instances, shaking is contraindicated because it may cause the mixture to foam.*
   - Remove the protective cap, or clean the rubber cap of a previously opened vial with an antiseptic wipe by rubbing in a circular motion. **Rationale:** *The antiseptic cleans the rubber cap and reduces the number of microorganisms.*
3. Withdraw the medication.
   - Attach a filter needle, as agency practice dictates, to draw up premixed liquid medications from multidose vials. **Rationale:** *Using the filter needle prevents any solid particles from being drawn up through the needle.*
   - Ensure that the needle is firmly attached to the syringe.
   - Remove the cap from the needle, then draw up into the syringe the amount of air equal to the volume of the medication to be withdrawn.
   - Carefully insert the needle into the upright vial through the center of the rubber cap, maintaining the sterility of the needle.
   - Inject the air into the vial, keeping the bevel of the needle above the surface of the medication **1**. **Rationale:** *The air*

will allow the medication to be drawn out easily because negative pressure will not be created inside the vial. The bevel is kept above the medication to avoid creating bubbles in the medication.

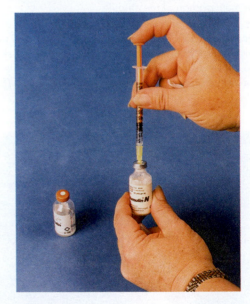

1 Injecting air into a vial.

- Withdraw the prescribed amount of medication using either of the following methods:
  a. Hold the vial down (i.e., with the base lower than the top), move the needle tip so that it is below the fluid level, and withdraw the medication **2**.

  or

  b. Invert the vial, ensure the needle tip is below the fluid level, and gradually withdraw the medication **3**. **Rationale:** *Keeping the tip of the needle below the fluid level prevents air from being drawn into the syringe.*
- Hold the syringe and vial at eye level to determine that the correct dosage of drug has been drawn into the syringe. Eject air remaining at the top of the syringe into the vial.

SKILL 2.22   Preparing Medications from Vials *(continued)*

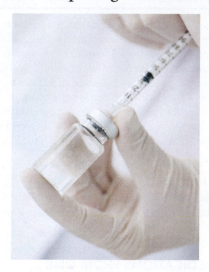

2 Withdrawing a medication from a vial that is held with the base down. © PhotoAlto/Alamy

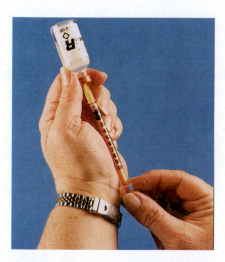

3 Withdrawing a medication from an inverted vial.

- When the correct volume of medication plus a little more (e.g., 0.25 mL [in case of air bubbles]) is obtained, withdraw the needle from the vial, and replace the cap over the needle using the one-hand scoop method, thus maintaining its sterility and preventing possible needlestick injuries **4**.

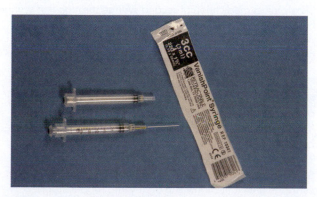

4 Healthcare facilities must use safety needles to conform to needlestick safety legislation.

- If necessary, gently tap the syringe barrel with a finger or pen while holding the syringe with the needle end pointing up to dislodge any air bubbles present in the syringe. Carefully and slowly expel the air and any excess medication from the syringe, maintaining the "needle up" position. **Rationale:** *The tapping motion will cause the air bubbles to rise to the top of the syringe where they can be ejected out of the syringe. Sometimes when ejecting the air bubbles, the resulting amount of medication is less than ordered. Drawing up a little extra medication, as in the previous step, helps avoid this.*
- If giving an injection, replace the filter needle, if used, with a regular or safety needle of the correct gauge and length. Eject air from the new needle.
- Label the syringe with medication name and dosage drawn up in the syringe. **Rationale:** *This can be used to do a last medication check for accuracy before administering the medication to the client.*

CLINICAL ALERT
Change needle after withdrawing medication from ampule or vial.

Federal needlestick safety legislation **requires** healthcare facilities to implement devices that protect against accidental needlesticks.

VARIATION: PREPARING AND USING MULTIDOSE VIALS

- Read the manufacturer's directions.
- Withdraw an equivalent amount of air from the vial before adding the diluent, unless otherwise indicated by the directions.
- Add the amount of sterile water or saline indicated in the directions.
- If a multidose vial is reconstituted, label the vial with the date and time it was prepared, the amount of drug contained in each milliliter of solution, and your initials. **Rationale:** *Time is an important factor to consider in the expiration of these medications.*
- Once the medication is reconstituted, store it in a refrigerator or as recommended by the manufacturer.

CLINICAL ALERT
If multiple-use vials are opened, they should be marked with the date and time the container is entered and nurse's initials. Consult the product label or package insert to determine if refrigeration is necessary. Unless contamination is suspected, the Centers for Disease Control and Prevention (CDC) recommends that the vial be discarded either when empty or on the expiration date set by the manufacturer.

Reconstituting Powdered Medication
- Insert needle into upright powdered medication vial.
- Remove the amount of air equal to desired quantity of diluent; this provides space for the diluent.
- Inject diluent into upright powdered medication vial.
- Remove needle and cover with guard.
- Rotate powdered medication vial with diluent between palms. Do not shake vial because shaking creates air bubbles and may cause difficulty withdrawing medication dose.
- Withdraw medication from vial.

Delegation

Mixing medications in one syringe involves knowledge and use of aseptic technique. Therefore, this procedure is not delegated to UAP.

Equipment

- Client's MAR or computer printout
- Two vials of medication; one vial and one ampule; two ampules; or one vial or ampule and one cartridge
- Antiseptic swabs
- Sterile syringe and safety needle or insulin syringe and needle (if insulin is being given, use a small-gauge hypodermic needle, e.g., #26 gauge.)
- Additional sterile subcutaneous or intramuscular safety needle (optional)

Preparation

- Check the MAR.
- Check the label on the medications carefully against the MAR to make sure that the correct medication is being prepared.
- Follow the three checks for administering medications. Read the label on the medication (1) when it is taken from the medication cart, (2) before withdrawing the medication, and (3) after withdrawing the medication.
- Before preparing and combining the medications, ensure that the total volume of the injection is appropriate for the injection site.
- Organize the equipment.

Procedure

1. Perform hand hygiene and observe other appropriate infection control procedures (e.g., clean gloves).
2. Prepare the medication ampule or vial for drug withdrawal.
   - Inspect the appearance of the medication for clarity. Note, however, that some medications are always cloudy. **Rationale:** *Preparations that have changed in appearance should be discarded.*
   - If using insulin, thoroughly mix the solution in each vial prior to administration. Rotate the vials between the palms of the hands. **Rationale:** *Mixing ensures an adequate concentration and thus an accurate dose. Shaking insulin vials can make the medication frothy, making precise measurement difficult.*
   - Clean the tops of the vials with antiseptic swabs.
3. Withdraw the medications.

MIXING MEDICATIONS FROM TWO VIALS

- Take the syringe and draw up a volume of air equal to the volume of medications to be withdrawn from both vials A and B.
- Inject a volume of air equal to the volume of medication to be withdrawn into vial A. Make sure the needle does not touch the solution. **Rationale:** *This prevents cross-contamination of the medications.*
- Withdraw the needle from vial A and inject the remaining air into vial B.
- Withdraw the required amount of medication from vial B. **Rationale:** *The same needle is used to inject air into and withdraw medication from the second vial. It must not be contaminated with the medication in vial A.*
- Using a newly attached sterile needle, withdraw the required amount of medication from vial A. Avoid pushing the plunger

because that will introduce medication B into vial A. If using a syringe with a fused needle, withdraw the medication from vial A. The syringe now contains a mixture of medications from vials A and B. **Rationale:** *With this method, neither vial is contaminated by microorganisms or by medication from the other vial.* Be careful to withdraw only the ordered amount and not to create air bubbles. **Rationale:** *The syringe now contains two medications, and an excess amount cannot be returned to the vial. See also the variation later in this skill.*

CLINICAL ALERT

Check appropriate text or consult agency pharmacist to ensure compatibility of medications before combining in a syringe for injection.

MIXING MEDICATIONS FROM ONE VIAL AND ONE AMPULE

- First prepare and withdraw the medication from the vial. **Rationale:** *The ampule does not require the addition of air prior to withdrawal of the drug because it is an open container.*
- Then withdraw the required amount of medication from the ampule.

MIXING MEDICATIONS FROM ONE CARTRIDGE AND ONE VIAL OR AMPULE

- First ensure that the correct dose of the medication is in the cartridge. Discard any excess medication and air.
- Draw up the required medication from the vial or ampule into the cartridge. Note that when withdrawing medication from a vial, an equal amount of air must first be injected into the vial.
- If the total volume to be injected exceeds the capacity of the cartridge, use a syringe with sufficient capacity to withdraw the desired amount of medication from the vial or ampule, and transfer the required amount from the cartridge to the syringe.

For Combining Medications Using Alternative Method

- Draw up ordered dose from each vial or ampule into two separate syringes. First syringe must be able to hold entire volume of combined medications.
- Remove needle from first syringe.
- Pull back plunger of first syringe to allow space for volume of second medication to be added.
- Insert needle of second syringe into hub of first syringe.
- Slowly inject medication of second syringe through first syringe hub, then withdraw needle.
- Attach new needle to first syringe.
- Discard needles and second syringe.

For Preparing Prefilled Medication Cartridge Syringe

- Hold barrel of cartridge syringe (e.g., Tubex) in one hand and pull back on plunger with other hand.
- Insert prefilled medication cartridge, needle first, into cartridge barrel.
- Twist cartridge syringe flange clockwise until it is secure.
- Screw plunger rod onto screw at bottom of medication cartridge until it fits firmly and tightly into rubber stopper.
- Remove needle guard and any air bubbles.
- Determine if dosage in cartridge is greater than required amount. If so, invert Tubex and gently expel excess medication,

SKILL 2.23 Mixing Medications Using One Syringe *(continued)*

being careful to maintain sterility of needle. **Rationale:** *If perma-nent needle is contaminated, the cartridge becomes contaminated and must be discarded.*

- Replace needle guard, using scoop method.

VARIATION: MIXING INSULINS

The following is an example of mixing 10 units of regular insulin and 30 units of NPH insulin, which contains protamine.

- Inject 30 units of air into the NPH vial and withdraw the needle. (There should be no insulin in the needle.) The needle should not touch the insulin .

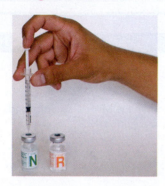

1 Mixing two types of insulin.

- Inject 10 units of air into the regular insulin vial and immediately withdraw 10 units of regular insulin **3**. Always withdraw the regular insulin first. **Rationale:** *This minimizes the possibility of the regular insulin becoming contaminated with the additional protein in the NPH.*
- Reinsert the needle into the NPH insulin vial and withdraw 30 units of NPH insulin **4**. (The air was previously injected into the vial.) Be careful to withdraw only the ordered amount and not to create air bubbles. If excess medication has been drawn up, discard the syringe and begin the procedure over again. **Rationale:** *The syringe now contains two medications, and an excess amount cannot be returned to the vial because the syringe*

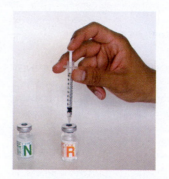

2   **3**

contains regular insulin, which, if returned to the NPH vial, would dilute the NPH with regular insulin. The NPH vial would not provide accurate future dosages of NPH insulin.

By using this method, you avoid adding NPH insulin to the regular insulin.

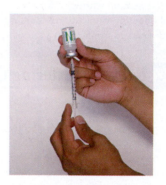

4

CLINICAL ALERT

One way to determine which insulin to withdraw first is to remember the saying "Clear before cloudy." (Regular insulin is clear and NPH is cloudy due to the proteins in the insulin.)

Sites for Injections

INTRADERMAL INJECTIONS

- Injection sites: inner aspect of forearm or scapular area of back; upper chest, medial thigh.
- Purpose: to test for antigens (tubercle bacillus, allergens).
- Amount injected: ranges from 0.01 to 0.1 mL.
- Absorption rate: slow.

SUBCUTANEOUS INJECTIONS

- Injection sites: fatty tissue of abdomen, lateral and posterior aspects of upper arm or thigh, scapular area of back, upper ventrodorsal gluteal areas.
- Purpose: for medications that are absorbed slowly.
- Amount injected: variable—no more than 2 mL. If repeated doses are necessary, alter site accordingly.

INTRAMUSCULAR INJECTIONS

- Purpose: to promote rapid absorption of the drug; to provide an alternate route when drug is irritating to subcutaneous tissues.
- Amount injected: variable—may be large amount of fluid. If more than 5 mL for adult or 3 mL for child and 1 mL for infant, divide dose into two syringes.

- Absorption rate: depends on circulatory state of client.
- Injection sites:

VENTROGLUTEAL INJECTION SITE

(Preferred site for IM injection for all clients over age 7 months.)

1. Place client in side-lying position.
2. Use right hand for left anterior hip, or left hand for right anterior hip.
3. Identify greater trochanter and place palm at site.
4. Keep palm on greater trochanter and point index finger toward client's anterior superior iliac spine and fan out other three fingers.
5. Form "V" area with index finger separated from other three fingers.
6. Inject medication at 90-degree angle within "V" area.

VASTUS LATERALIS INJECTION SITE

1. Place client in supine position with thigh exposed.
2. Identify greater trochanter and lateral femoral condyle.
3. Using middle third and anterior lateral aspect of thigh, select site.

(continued on next page)

SKILL 2.23   Mixing Medications Using One Syringe *(continued)*

4. Inject medication directly into muscle at 90-degree angle.

DELTOID INJECTION SITE (SOLUTION MUST BE NONIRRITATING)
1. Expose client's upper arm.
2. Deltoid site is two fingerbreadths below acromion process.
3. Place left hand on acromion process and right index finger two fingerbreadths below.
4. Inject limited medication volume (0.5 to 1 mL) in deltoid IM site at 90-degree angle.

SELECTING THE APPROPRIATE-SIZE NEEDLE
- Intradermal injections: 1 mL tuberculin syringe with short bevel, 25–27 gauge, 3/8–1/2 inch needle.
- Subcutaneous injections: 0.5–3 mL syringe with 25–27 gauge, 1/2–5/8 inch needle.
- Intramuscular injections: 1–5 mL syringe with needle gauge and length appropriate for muscle site and fat thickness; deltoid muscle requires 23–25 gauge, 5/8–1 inch needle; needle sizes for the vastus lateralis and gluteus muscles vary from 18 to 23 gauge, with needle lengths from 1 to 1 1/2 inches.

▶ COMMON MEDICATION ROUTES

Expected Outcomes

1. Client takes medication without difficulty.
2. Desired local effect of medication occurs without side effects.
3. Client self-administers medication according to instructions.
4. Documentation on the MAR is accurate and current.
5. Medication therapeutic effect is achieved.

SKILL 2.24   Administering Oral Medications

Delegation

In acute care settings, administration of oral/enteral medications is performed by the nurse and is not delegated to unlicensed assistive personnel (UAP). The nurse can inform the UAP of the intended therapeutic effects and/or specific side effects of the medication and request the UAP to report specific client observations to the nurse for follow-up. In some states, trained UAP may administer certain medications to stable clients in long-term care settings. It is important, however, for the nurse to remember that the medication knowledge of the UAP is limited and *assessment and evaluation of the effectiveness of the medication remain the responsibility of the nurse.*

Equipment

- Dispensing system
- Disposable medication cups: small paper or plastic cups for tablets and capsules, waxed or plastic calibrated medication cups for liquids
- MAR or computer printout
- Pill crusher/cutter
- Straws to administer medications that may discolor the teeth or to facilitate the ingestion of liquid medication for certain clients
- Drinking glass and water or juice
- Soft foods such as applesauce or pudding to use for crushed medications for clients who may choke on liquids

Preparation

- Know the reason why the client is receiving the medication, the drug classification, contraindications, usual dosage range, side effects, and nursing considerations for administering and evaluating the intended outcomes for the medication.
- Check the MAR.
- Check for the drug name, dosage, frequency, route of administration, and expiration date for administering the medication, if appropriate. **Rationale:** *Orders for certain medications*

(e.g., narcotics, antibiotics) expire after a specified time frame and need to be reordered by the primary care provider.

- If the MAR is unclear or pertinent information is missing, compare the MAR with the prescriber's most recent written order.
- Report any discrepancies to the charge nurse or the prescriber, as agency policy dictates.
- Verify the client's ability to take medication orally.
- Determine whether the client can swallow, is NPO, is nauseated or vomiting, has gastric suction, or has diminished or absent bowel sounds.
- Organize the supplies. **Rationale:** *Organization of supplies saves time and reduces the chance of error.*
- Gather the MAR(s) for each client so that medications can be prepared for one client at a time.

SAFETY ALERT

2014 National Patient Safety Goal (NPSG) for Using Medicines Safely

The Joint Commission's process for using medicines safely is as follows:

- *Before a procedure,* label medicines that are not labeled. For example, medicines in syringes, cups and basins. Do this in the area where medicines and supplies are set up.
- Take extra care with patients who take medicines to thin their blood.
- Record and pass along correct information about a patient's medicines. Find out what medicines the patient is taking. Compare those medicines to new medicines given to the patient. Make sure the patient knows which medicines to take when he or she is at home. Tell the patient it is important to have an up-to-date list of medicines to give the physician every time he or she has an appointment..

SKILL 2.24 Administering Oral Medications *(continued)*

Procedure

1. Perform hand hygiene and observe other appropriate infection control procedures (e.g., clean gloves).
2. Unlock the dispensing system.
3. Obtain appropriate medication.
   - Read the MAR and take the appropriate medication from the shelf, drawer, or refrigerator. The medication may be dispensed in a bottle, box, or unit-dose package.
   - Compare the label of the medication container or unit-dose package against the order on the MAR or computer printout **1**. **Rationale:** *This is a safety check to ensure that the right medication is given.* If these are not identical, recheck the prescriber's written order in the client's chart. If there is still a discrepancy, check with the nurse in charge or the pharmacist.

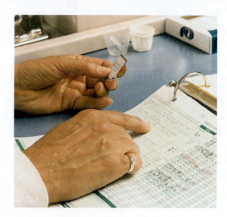

1 Compare the medication label to the MAR.

   - Check the expiration date of the medication. Return expired medications to the pharmacy. **Rationale:** *Outdated medications are not safe to administer.*
   - Use only medications that have clear, legible labels. **Rationale:** *This ensures accuracy.*
4. Prepare the medication.
   - Calculate the medication dosage accurately.
   - Prepare the correct amount of medication for the required dose, without contaminating the medication. **Rationale:** *Aseptic technique maintains drug cleanliness.*
   - While preparing the medication, recheck each prepared drug and container with the MAR again. **Rationale:** *This second safety check reduces the chance of error.*

Tablets or Capsules

   - Place packaged unit-dose capsules or tablets directly into the medicine cup. Do not remove the medication from the package until at the bedside. **Rationale:** *The wrapper keeps the medication clean. Not removing the medication facilitates identification of the medication in the event the client refuses the drug or assessment data indicate to hold the medication. Unopened unit-dose packages can usually be returned to the medication cart.*
   - If using a stock container, pour the required number into the bottle cap, and then transfer the medication to the disposable cup without touching the tablets.
   - Keep narcotics and medications that require specific assessments, such as pulse measurements, respiratory rate or depth, or blood pressure, separate from the others. **Rationale:** *This reminds the nurse to complete the needed*

assessment(s) in order to decide whether to give the medication or to withhold the medication if indicated.

   - Break only scored tablets if necessary to obtain the correct dosage. Use a cutting or splitting device if needed **2**. Check agency policy as to whether unused portions of a medication are to be discarded.

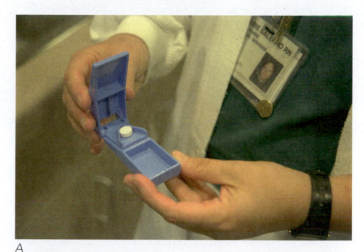

A

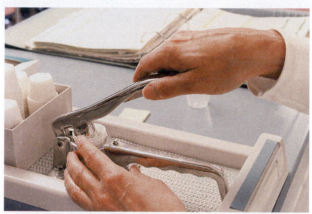

B

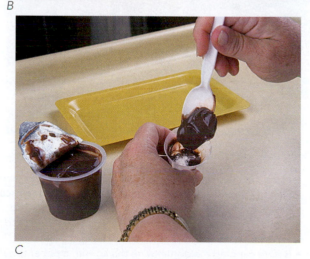

C

2 *A,* If partial dose is ordered, place table in pill cutter to be cut in half. *B,* Place pill in crusher to crush tablet, or pulverize/crush pill in unit-dose container. *C,* Mix pulverized medication (or powder from opened capsule) carefully in small amount of soft food (pudding, jelly, applesauce). A cutting device can be used to divide tablets.

(continued on next page)

SKILL 2.24 Administering Oral Medications (*continued*)

- If the client has difficulty swallowing, check if the medication can be crushed. Some drug handbooks have an appendix that lists the "Do Not Crush" medications. The Institute for Safe Medication Practices (2010) provides on its Web site an updated list of medications that should not be crushed. Some medications that should not be crushed include time-released and enteric-coated medications. An example of tablets that should not be crushed is oxycodone (OxyContin), a long-acting narcotic that normally lasts 12 hours after administration. Tablet disruption may cause a potentially fatal overdose of oxycodone. If it is acceptable, crush the tablets to a fine powder with a pill crusher or between two medication cups. Then, mix the powder with a small amount of soft food (e.g., custard, applesauce).

> **CLINICAL ALERT**
> Check with the pharmacy before crushing tablets. Sustained-action, enteric-coated, buccal, or sublingual tablets should not be crushed.

Liquid Medication

- Thoroughly mix the medication before pouring. Discard any medication that has changed color or turned cloudy. Remove the cap and place it upside down on the countertop. **Rationale:** *This avoids contaminating the inside of the cap.*
- Hold the bottle so the label is next to the palm of the hand and pour the medication away from the label ❸. **Rationale:** *This prevents the label from becoming soiled and illegible as a result of spilled liquids.*

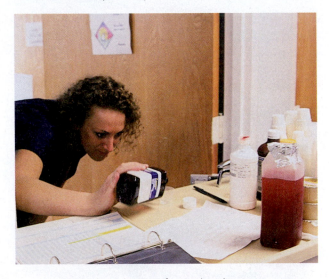

❸ Pouring a liquid medication from a bottle.

- Place the medication cup on a flat surface at eye level and fill it to the desired level, using the *bottom* of the **meniscus** (crescent-shaped upper surface of a column of liquid) to align with the container scale ❹. **Rationale:** *This method ensures accuracy of measurement.*
- Before capping the bottle, wipe the lip with a paper towel. **Rationale:** *This prevents the cap from sticking.*
- When giving small amounts of liquids (e.g., <5 mL), prepare the medication in a sterile syringe without the needle or in a specially designed oral syringe. Label the syringe with the name of the medication and the route (PO). **Rationale:** *Any oral solution removed from the original container and placed into a syringe should be labeled to avoid medica-*

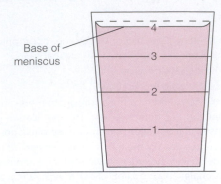

Base of meniscus

❹ The bottom of the curved meniscus is the measuring guide.

tions being given by the wrong route (e.g., IV). This practice facilitates client safety and avoids tragic errors.

- Keep unit-dose liquids in their package and open them at the bedside.

Oral Narcotics

- If an agency uses a manual recording system for controlled substances, check the narcotic record for the previous drug count and compare it with the supply available. Some medications, including narcotics, are kept in plastic containers that are sectioned and numbered.
- Remove the next available tablet and drop it in the medicine cup.
- After removing a tablet, record the necessary information on the appropriate narcotic control record and sign it.

Note: Computer-controlled dispensing systems allow access only to the selected drug and automatically record its use.

All Medications

- Place the prepared medication and MAR together on the medication cart.
- Recheck the label on the container before returning the bottle, box, or envelope to its storage place. **Rationale:** *This third check further reduces the risk of error.*
- Avoid leaving prepared medications unattended. **Rationale:** *This precaution prevents potential mishandling errors.*
- Lock the medication cart before entering the client's room. **Rationale:** *This is a safety measure because medication carts must not be left open when unattended.*
- Check the room number against the MAR if agency policy does not allow the MAR to be removed from the medication cart. **Rationale:** *This is another safety measure to ensure that the nurse is entering the correct client room.*

5. Introduce self and verify the client's identity using agency protocol. **Rationale:** *This ensures that the right client receives the medication.*
6. Provide for client privacy.
7. Prepare the client.
   - Assist the client to a sitting position or, if not possible, to a side-lying position. **Rationale:** *These positions facilitate swallowing and prevent aspiration.*
   - If not previously assessed, take the required assessment measures, such as pulse and respiratory rates or blood pressure. Take the apical pulse rate before administering digitalis preparations. Take blood pressure before giving antihypertensive drugs. Take the respiratory rate prior to

SKILL 2.24 Administering Oral Medications (continued)

administering narcotics. **Rationale:** *Narcotics depress the respiratory center.* If any of the findings are above or below the predetermined parameters, consult the primary care provider before administering the medication.

8. Explain the purpose of the medication and how it will help, using language that the client can understand. Include relevant information about effects; for example, tell the client receiving a diuretic to expect an increase in urine output. **Rationale:** *Information can facilitate acceptance of and compliance with the therapy.*

9. Administer the medication at the correct time.
   - Take the medication to the client within 30 minutes before or after the scheduled time.
   - Give the client sufficient water or preferred juice to swallow the medication. Before using juice, check for any food and medication incompatibilities. **Rationale:** *Fluids ease swallowing and facilitate absorption from the gastrointestinal tract.* Liquid medications other than antacids or cough preparations may be diluted with 15 mL (1/2 oz) of water to facilitate absorption.
   - If the client is unable to hold the pill cup, use the pill cup to introduce the medication into the client's mouth, and only give one tablet or capsule at a time. **Rationale:** *Putting the cup to the client's mouth maintains the cleanliness of the nurse's hands. Giving one medication at a time eases swallowing.*
   - If an older child or adult has difficulty swallowing, ask the client to place the medication on the back of the tongue before taking the water. **Rationale:** *Stimulation of the back of the tongue produces the swallowing reflex.*
   - If the medication has an objectionable taste, ask the client to suck a few ice chips beforehand, or give the medication with juice, applesauce, or bread if there are no contraindications. **Rationale:** *The cold temperature of the ice chips will desensitize the taste buds, and juices or bread can mask the taste of the medication.*
   - If the client says that the medication you are about to give is different from what the client has been receiving, do not give the medication without first checking the original order. **Rationale:** *Most clients are familiar with the appearance of medications taken previously. Unfamiliar medications may signal a possible error.*

   - Stay with the client until all medications have been swallowed. **Rationale:** *The nurse must see the client swallow the medication before the drug administration can be recorded. The nurse may need to check the client's mouth to ensure that the medication was swallowed and not hidden inside the cheek.* A primary care provider's order or agency policy is required for medications left at the bedside.

10. Document each medication given.
    - Record the medication given, dosage, time, any complaints or assessments of the client, and your signature.
    - If medication was refused or omitted, record this fact on the appropriate record; document the reason, when possible, and the nurse's actions according to agency policy.

11. Dispose of all supplies appropriately.
    - Replenish stock (e.g., medication cups) and return the cart to the appropriate place.
    - Discard used disposable supplies.

Cultural Considerations

Cultural and genetic factors affect how a client reacts to medications. Cultural acceptance factors include values and beliefs, educational level, previous experiences, family influence, and physician–client relationship.

Physiological rhythms, use of alcohol, and stress may either inhibit or accelerate drug biodynamics. The concomitant use of "natural" remedies can also alter the client's response to drug therapy.

One genetic factor noted to differ among ethnic groups is variation in metabolic pathways that may accelerate or slow drug metabolism. It is also thought that the pathophysiology of various disease states may differ among populations based on genetic determination. For example, African American clients respond differently to different antihypertensives than do Caucasians. African American respond better to diuretics than they do to beta-blockers and angiotensin-converting enzyme (ACE) inhibitors for hypertension.

Source: The New York Times, 2017, High Blood Pressure Medications, http://www.nytimes.com/health/guides/disease/hypertension/medications.html.

SKILL 2.25 Administering Medications by Enteral Tube

Delegation

The administration of medications through an enteral tube is performed by the nurse and is not delegated to UAP. The nurse can inform the UAP of the intended therapeutic effects and/or specific side effects of the medication and request the UAP to report specific client observations to the nurse for follow-up.

Equipment

- Medication to be administered
- Disposable medication cups: small paper or plastic calibrated medication cups for liquids
- 60-mL syringe with catheter tip for large-bore tube or Luer-Lok tip for small-bore tube
- Pill crusher for medications that need to be crushed

- Tongue blade or straw to stir dissolved medication
- pH test strip
- Warm water to dissolve crushed medications
- Tap water (room temperature) or sterile water or normal saline for flushing tube (check agency policy)
- Emesis basin
- Clean gloves
- MAR or computer printout

Preparation

- Know the reason why the client is receiving the medication, the drug classification, contraindications, usual dosage range, side effects, and nursing considerations for administering and evaluating the intended outcomes for the medication.
- Check the MAR.

(continued on next page)

SKILL 2.25 Administering Medications by Enteral Tube (continued)

- Check the MAR for the drug name, dosage, frequency, route of administration, and expiration date for administration of the medication, if appropriate. **Rationale:** *Orders for certain medications (e.g., narcotics, antibiotics) expire after a specified time frame and need to be reordered by the primary care provider.*
- If the MAR is unclear or pertinent information is missing, compare the MAR with the prescriber's most recent written order.
- Report any discrepancies to the charge nurse or the prescriber, as agency policy dictates.
- Organize the supplies. **Rationale:** *Organization of supplies saves time and reduces the chance of error.*
- Gather the MAR(s) for each client so that medications can be prepared for one client at a time.

Procedure

1. Introduce self and verify the client's identity using agency protocol. **Rationale:** *This ensures that the right client receives the medication.*
2. Perform hand hygiene and observe other appropriate infection control procedures (e.g., clean gloves).
3. Provide for client privacy.
4. Prepare the client.
   - Assist the client to a Fowler's position in bed or a sitting position in a chair. If a sitting position is contraindicated, a slightly elevated right side-lying position is acceptable. **Rationale:** *These positions enhance gravitational flow and prevent aspiration of fluid into the lungs.*
   - If not previously assessed, take the required assessment measures, such as pulse and respiratory rates or blood pressure. Take the apical pulse rate before administering digitalis preparations. Take blood pressure before giving antihypertensive drugs. Take the respiratory rate prior to administering narcotics. **Rationale:** *Narcotics depress the respiratory center.* If any of the findings are above or below the predetermined parameters, consult the primary care provider before administering the medication.
5. Prepare medications for appropriate administration by enteral tube (e.g., use liquids or crush and dissolve tablets). Calculate medication dosage accurately.
6. Explain the purpose of the medication and how it will help, using language that the client can understand. Include relevant information about effects; for example, tell the client receiving an analgesic to expect a decrease in pain. **Rationale:** *Information can facilitate acceptance of and compliance with the therapy.*
7. Apply clean gloves.
8. If client is receiving a continuous tube feeding, press the "Hold" button on the enteric feeding pump ❶. **Rationale:** *Pausing or holding the pump temporarily stops the administration of the tube feeding.*
9. Disconnect tubing that is being used for suction or feeding from gastric tube. Place cap on end of tubing. **Rationale:** *Putting a cap on the end of the tubing prevents contamination.*
10. Assess tube placement.
11. Pinch or fold over the gastric tube ❷. **Rationale:** *Pinching or folding over the tubing prevents gastric contents from flowing out of the tube.*
12. Gently aspirate all the stomach contents and measure the residual volume ❸.

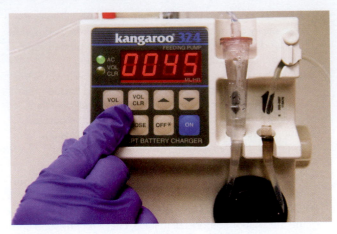

❶ Pausing the enteral feeding pump prior to administering medication by pressing the "Hold" button.

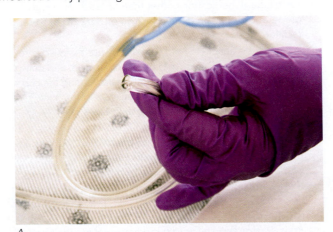

A

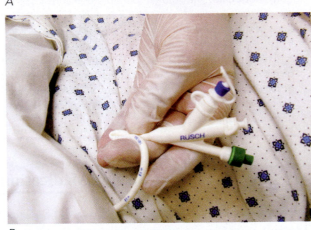

B

❷ Pinching or folding over *A*, a nasogastric tube, and *B*, a gastrostomy tube.

13. Return residual back to stomach. **Rationale:** *Returning the residual prevents loss of fluids and electrolytes.* Pinch or fold over the gastric tube and remove the syringe.
    - Check agency policy if residual volume is greater than 100 mL.
14. Administer the medication(s).
    - Remove the plunger from the syringe and connect the syringe to a pinched or folded over tube. **Rationale:** *Pinching or folding over the tube prevents excess air from entering the stomach and causing distention.*

SKILL 2.25   Administering Medications by Enteral Tube (*continued*)

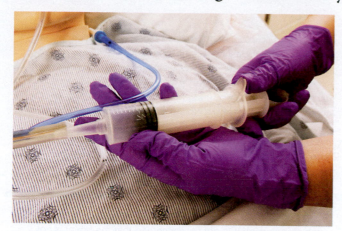

3 Gently aspirate for residual volume prior to medication administration.

- Put 30 mL of water into the syringe barrel to flush the tube before administering the first medication. Raise or lower the barrel of the syringe to adjust the flow as needed. Pinch or clamp the tubing before all of the water is instilled. **Rationale:** *This prevents excess air from entering the stomach.*
- Pour liquid or dissolved medication into syringe barrel and allow to flow by gravity into enteral tube.
- If administering more than one medication, flush with between 5-15 mL of tap water between each medication.
- After administering the last medication, flush the tube with 30 mL of tap water. **Rationale:** *Flushing clears the tube and*

prevents clogging of the tube (American Society for Parenteral and Enteral Nutrition, 2009).

- Pinch or fold over the gastric tube and reconnect to tubing for continuous tube feeding. If the client was previously connected to suction, keep the gastric tube clamped for 20 to 30 minutes after giving the medication. **Rationale:** *Keeping the tube clamped for that time will help ensure that the medication is absorbed before restarting the suction.*
- Remove and discard gloves. Perform hand hygiene.

15. Document each medication given.
   - Record the medication given, dosage, time, any complaints or assessments of the client, and your signature.
   - If medication was refused or omitted, record this fact on the appropriate record; document the reason, when possible, and the nurse's actions according to agency policy.
   - Record fluid intake accurately if client is on intake and output.
16. Dispose of all supplies appropriately.
   - Replenish stock (e.g., medication cups) and return cart to the appropriate place.
   - Discard used disposable supplies.

> **CLINICAL ALERT**
> Consult with pharmacist before deciding to alter the form of *any* medication. Have pharmacist substitute liquid form of medication if available, or substitute a short-acting formulation that can be safely crushed for administration. Contact the physician for a substitute medication if formulation alternatives are unavailable.

SKILL 2.26   Administering Sublingual Medications

Equipment

- Sublingual medication (e.g., nitroglycerin tablets in a dark bottle). (Tablets lose potency when exposed to light; opened bottle should be replaced in 3 months.)

or

- Nitrolingual aerosol spray in canister

Preparation

- Prepare the medications.
- Assess vital signs if administering sublingual nitroglycerin. (*Systolic BP should not be lower than 90 mmHg.*)
- Place client in a sitting position.

Procedure

1. Follow steps for preparing and administering oral medications, *except:*
   - Explain that client must not swallow drug or eat, smoke, or drink until medication is completely absorbed.
   - Ask client to place tablet under the tongue or to hold tongue up so tablet can be placed under tongue **1**. **Rationale:** *This ensures that absorption will be rapid and complete due to the vast network of capillaries in this area.*

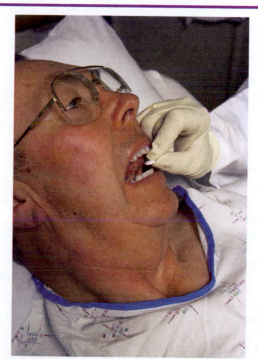

1 Sublingual medication is placed under client's tongue for rapid absorption.

(*continued on next page*)

SKILL 2.26   Administering Sublingual Medications *(continued)*

- *Alternate:* Hold Nitrolingual canister vertically with spray opening as close to mouth as possible. Deliver 1 or 2 metered sprays onto or under tongue, then have client close mouth immediately. Tell client not to inhale medication.

2. Evaluate client for drug action and possible side effects (e.g., headache).

> ### CLINICAL ALERT
> Assess client's chest discomfort: quality, location, radiation, intensity, duration and precipitating factors. When administering rapid-acting (sublingual) nitroglycerin, monitor client's response and vital signs. If chest discomfort is not relieved in 5 minutes, notify physician. Obtain order for opiate analgesic (morphine sulfate), ECG, ST segment monitoring, and cardiac markers. No more than three doses of nitroglycerin should be administered in a 15-minute period because of potential hypotensive effect (BP ≤90 mmHg) or bradycardia (HR ≤50) as this would preclude adequate dosage of morphine sulfate for pain control.

Evidence-Based Nursing Practice

Guidelines—Nitroglycerin Tablets

The National Library of Medicine at the National Institutes of Health advises clients who have been previously prescribed nitroglycerin to follow the prescriber's instructions carefully. In the event of chest discomfort/pain, common guidelines are as follows:

- Sit down and take one dose of nitroglycerin when an attack begins. Do not chew or swallow nitroglycerin tablets. Instead, place the tablet under the tongue or between the cheek and gum and wait for it to dissolve. The tablet may cause burning or tingling as it dissolves. This is normal but is not a sign that the tablet is working. Do not be concerned that the tablet is not working if there is no burning or tingling.

- If symptoms do not improve much or if they worsen, take a second dose after 5 minutes have passed and a third dose 5 minutes after the second dose. Call for emergency medical help right away if chest pain has not gone away completely 5 minutes after you take the third dose. (Some care providers will instruct clients to call for emergency help if symptoms are not relieved or worsen after the first dose.)

Data from National Library of Medicine, National Institutes of Health (2014).

SKILL 2.27   Administering Ophthalmic Medications

Delegation

Due to the need for assessment, interpretation of client status, and use of sterile technique, ophthalmic medication administration is not delegated to UAP.

Equipment

- Clean gloves
- Sterile absorbent sponges soaked in sterile normal saline
- Medication
- Sterile eye dressing (pad) as needed and paper tape to secure it

For an Irrigation, Add:

- Irrigating solution (e.g., normal saline) and irrigating syringe or tubing
- Dry sterile absorbent sponges
- Moisture-resistant towel
- Basin (e.g., emesis basin)

Preparation

- Check the medication administration record (MAR).
- Check for the drug name, dose, and strength. Also confirm the prescribed frequency of the instillation and which eye is to be treated.
- Check client allergy status.
- If the MAR is unclear or pertinent information is missing, compare it with the most recent primary care provider's written order.
- Report any discrepancies to the charge nurse or primary care provider, as agency policy dictates.

- Know the reason why the client is receiving the medication, the drug classification, contraindications, usual dose range, side effects, and nursing considerations for administering and evaluating the intended outcomes of the medication.

Procedure

1. Compare the label on the medication tube or bottle with the medication record and check the expiration date. **Rationale:** *Outdated medications are not safe to administer.*
2. If necessary, calculate the medication dosage.
3. Introduce self and explain to the client what you are going to do, why it is necessary, and how he or she can participate. The administration of an ophthalmic medication is not usually painful. Ointments are often soothing to the eye, but some liquid preparations may sting initially. Discuss how the results will be used in planning further care or treatments.
4. Perform hand hygiene and observe other appropriate infection control procedures (e.g., clean gloves).
5. Provide for client privacy.
6. Prepare the client.
   - Prior to performing the procedure, verify the client's identity using agency protocol. **Rationale:** *This ensures that the right client receives the right medication.*
   - Assist the client to a comfortable position, usually lying.
7. Clean the eyelid and the eyelashes.
   - Apply clean gloves.
   - Use sterile cotton balls moistened with sterile irrigating solution or sterile normal saline, and wipe from the inner

SKILL 2.27 Administering Ophthalmic Medications (*continued*)

canthus to the outer canthus. **Rationale:** *If not removed, material on the eyelid and lashes can be washed into the eye. Cleaning toward the outer canthus prevents contamination of the other eye and the lacrimal duct.*

8. Administer the eye medication.
   - Check the ophthalmic preparation for the name, strength, and number of drops if a liquid is used. **Rationale:** *Checking medication data is essential to prevent a medication error.* Draw the correct number of drops into the shaft of the dropper if a dropper is used. If ointment is used, discard the first bead. **Rationale:** *The first bead of ointment from a tube is considered to be contaminated.*
   - Instruct the client to look up to the ceiling. Give the client a dry sterile absorbent sponge. **Rationale:** *The person is less likely to blink if looking up. While the client looks up, the cornea is partially protected by the upper eyelid. A sponge is needed to press on the nasolacrimal duct after a liquid instillation to prevent systemic absorption or to wipe excess ointment from the eyelashes after an ointment is instilled.*
   - Expose the lower conjunctival sac by placing the thumb or fingers of your nondominant hand on the client's cheekbone just below the eye and gently drawing down the skin on the cheek. If the tissues are edematous, handle the tissues carefully to avoid damaging them. **Rationale:** *Placing the fingers on the cheekbone minimizes the possibility of touching the cornea, avoids putting any pressure on the eyeball, and prevents the person from blinking or squinting.*
   - Holding the medication in the dominant hand, place hand on client's forehead to stabilize hand. Approach the eye from the side and instill the correct number of drops onto the outer third of the lower conjunctival sac. Hold the dropper 1 to 2 cm (0.4 to 0.8 in.) above the sac ❶. **Rationale:** *The client is less likely to blink if a side approach is used. When instilled into the conjunctival sac, drops will not harm the cornea as they might if dropped directly on it. The dropper must not touch the sac or the cornea.*

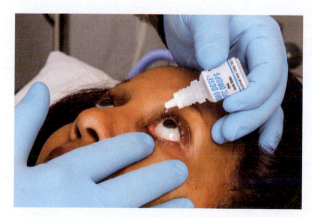

❶ Instilling eye drops into the lower conjunctival sac

or

   - Holding the tube above the lower conjunctival sac, squeeze 2 cm (0.8 in.) of ointment from the tube into the lower conjunctival sac from the inner canthus outward.
   - Instruct the client to close the eyelids but not to squeeze them shut. **Rationale:** *Closing the eye spreads the medication over the eyeball. Squeezing can injure the eye and push out the medication.*

   - For liquid medications, press firmly or have the client press firmly on the nasolacrimal duct for at least 30 seconds ❷. **Rationale:** *Pressing on the nasolacrimal duct prevents the medication from running out of the eye and down the duct, preventing systemic absorption.*
   - Remove and discard gloves. Perform hand hygiene.

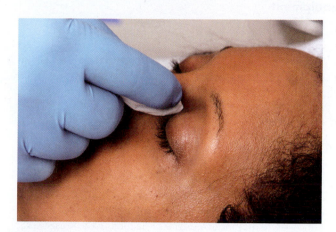

❷ Pressing on the eye's nasolacrimal duct

VARIATION: EYE IRRIGATION

- Place absorbent pads under the head, neck, and shoulders. Place an emesis basin next to the eye to catch drainage. Some eye medications cause systemic reactions such as confusion or a decrease in heart rate and blood pressure if the eyedrops go down the nasolacrimal duct and get into the systemic circulation.
- Expose the lower conjunctival sac. Or, to irrigate in stages, first hold the lower lid down, then hold the upper lid up. Exert pressure on the bony prominences of the cheekbone and beneath the eyebrow when holding the eyelids. **Rationale:** *Separating the lids prevents reflex blinking. Exerting pressure on the bony prominences minimizes the possibility of pressing the eyeball and causing discomfort.*
- Fill and hold the eye irrigator about 2.5 cm (1 in.) above the eye. **Rationale:** *At this height the pressure of the solution will not damage the eye tissue, and the irrigator will not touch the eye.*
- Irrigate the eye, directing the solution onto the lower conjunctival sac and from the inner canthus to the outer canthus. **Rationale:** *Directing the solution in this way prevents possible injury to the cornea and prevents fluid and contaminants from flowing down the nasolacrimal duct.*
- Irrigate until the solution leaving the eye is clear (no discharge is present) or until all the solution has been used.
- Instruct the client to close and move the eye periodically. **Rationale:** *Eye closure and movement help to move secretions from the upper to the lower conjunctival sac.*
- Clean and dry the eyelids as needed. Wipe the eyelids gently from the inner to the outer canthus to collect excess medication.
- Remove and discard gloves. Perform hand hygiene.
- Apply an eye pad if needed, and secure it with paper eye tape.
- Assess the client's response immediately after the instillation or irrigation and again after the medication should have acted.
- Document all relevant assessments and interventions. Include the name of the drug or irrigating solution, the strength, the number of drops if a liquid medication, the time, and the response of the client.

SKILL 2.28 Administering Otic Medications

Delegation

Due to the need for assessment, interpretation of client status, and use of sterile technique, otic medication administration is not delegated to UAP.

Equipment

- Clean gloves
- Cotton-tipped applicator
- Correct medication bottle with a dropper
- Flexible rubber tip (optional) for the end of the dropper, which prevents injury from sudden motion, for example, by a disoriented client
- Cotton fluff

For an Irrigation, Add:

- Moisture-resistant towel
- Basin (e.g., emesis basin)
- Irrigating solution at 37°C (98.6°F) temperature, about 500 mL (16 oz) or as ordered **Rationale:** *A solution that is not at body temperature may induce dizziness* (Jacobs, 2008; Kraszewski, 2008).
- Container for the irrigating solution
- Syringe (rubber bulb or Asepto syringe is frequently used)

Preparation

- Check the medication administration record (MAR).
- Check for the drug name, strength, number of drops, and prescribed frequency.
- Check client allergy status.
- If the MAR is unclear or pertinent information is missing, compare it with the most recent primary care provider's written order.
- Report any discrepancies to the charge nurse or primary care provider, as agency policy dictates.
- Know the reason why the client is receiving the medication, the drug classification, contraindications, usual dose range, side effects, and nursing considerations for administering and evaluating the intended outcomes of the medication.

Procedure

1. Compare the label on the medication container with the medication record and check the expiration date. **Rationale:** *Outdated medications are not safe to administer.*
2. If necessary, calculate the medication dosage.
3. Introduce self and explain to the client what you are going to do, why it is necessary, and how he or she can participate. The administration of an otic medication is not usually painful. Discuss how the results will be used in planning further care or treatments.
4. Perform hand hygiene and observe other appropriate infection control procedures (e.g., clean gloves).
5. Provide for client privacy.
6. Prepare the client.
   - Prior to performing the procedure, verify the client's identity using agency protocol. **Rationale:** *This ensures that the right client receives the right medication.*
   - Assist the client to a comfortable position for eardrop administration, usually lying with the ear being treated uppermost.

7. Clean the pinna of the ear and the meatus of the ear canal.
   - Apply gloves if infection is suspected.
   - Use cotton-tipped applicators and solution to wipe the pinna and auditory meatus. **Rationale:** *This removes any discharge present before the instillation so that it won't be washed into the ear canal.* Ensure that applicator does *not* go into the ear canal. **Rationale:** *This avoids damage to tympanic membrane or wax becoming impacted within the canal.*
8. Administer the ear medication.
   - Warm the medication container in your hand, or place it in warm water for a short time. **Rationale:** *This promotes client comfort and prevents nerve stimulation and pain.*
   - Partially fill the ear dropper with medication.
   - Straighten the auditory canal. Pull the pinna upward and backward for clients over 3 years of age. **Rationale:** *The auditory canal is straightened so that the solution can flow the entire length of the canal.*
   - Instill the correct number of drops along the side of the ear canal.
   - Press gently but firmly a few times on the tragus of the ear (the cartilaginous projection in front of the exterior meatus of the ear). **Rationale:** *Pressing on the tragus assists the flow of medication into the ear canal.*
   - Ask the client to remain in the side-lying position for about 5 minutes. **Rationale:** *This prevents the drops from escaping and allows the medication to reach all sides of the canal cavity.*
   - Insert a small piece of cotton fluff loosely at the meatus of the auditory canal for 15 to 20 minutes. Do not press it into the canal. **Rationale:** *The cotton helps retain the medication when the client is up. If pressed tightly into the canal, the cotton would interfere with the action of the drug and the outward movement of normal secretions.*

VARIATION: EAR IRRIGATION

- Explain that the client may experience a feeling of fullness, warmth, and, occasionally, discomfort when the fluid comes in contact with the tympanic membrane.
- Assist the client to a sitting or lying position with head tilted toward the affected ear. **Rationale:** *The solution can then flow from the ear canal to a basin.*
- Place the moisture-resistant towel around the client's shoulder under the ear to be irrigated, and place the basin under the ear to be irrigated.
- Fill the syringe with solution.

or

- Hang up the irrigating container, and run solution through the tubing and the nozzle. **Rationale:** *Solution is run through to remove air from the tubing and nozzle.*
- Straighten the ear canal.
- Insert the tip of the syringe into the auditory meatus, and direct the solution gently upward against the top of the canal. **Rationale:** *The solution will flow around the entire canal and out at the bottom. The solution is instilled gently because strong pressure from the fluid can cause discomfort and damage the tympanic membrane.*
- Continue instilling the fluid until all the solution is used or until the canal is cleaned, depending on the purpose of the irrigation. Take care not to block the outward flow of the solution with the syringe.

SKILL 2.28 Administering Otic Medications (*continued*)

- Assist the client to a side-lying position on the affected side. **Rationale:** *Lying with the affected side down helps drain the excess fluid by gravity.*
- Place a cotton fluff in the auditory meatus to absorb the excess fluid.
- Remove and discard gloves. Perform hand hygiene.
- Assess the client's response and the character and amount of discharge, appearance of the canal, discomfort, and so on,

immediately after the instillation and again when the medication is expected to act. Inspect the cotton ball for any drainage.

- Document all nursing assessments and interventions relative to the procedure. Include the name of the drug or irrigating solution, the strength, the number of drops if a liquid medication, the time, and the response of the client.

SKILL 2.29 Administering Nasal Medications

Delegation

Due to the need for assessment and interpretation of client status, nasal medication administration is not delegated to UAP.

Equipment

- Tissues
- Clean gloves
- Correct medication bottle with a dropper

Preparation

- Check the MAR.
- Check for the drug name, strength, and number of drops. Also confirm the prescribed frequency of the instillation and which side of the nose is to be treated.
- Check client allergy status.
- If the MAR is unclear or pertinent information is missing, compare it with the most recent primary care provider's written order.
- Report any discrepancies to the charge nurse or primary care provider, as agency policy dictates.
- Know the reason why the client is receiving the medication, the drug classification, contraindications, usual dose range, side effects, and nursing considerations for administering and evaluating the intended outcomes of the medication.

Procedure

1. Compare the label on the medication container with the medication record and check the expiration date. **Rationale:** *Outdated medications are not safe to administer.*
2. If necessary, calculate the medication dosage.
3. Introduce self and explain to the client what you are going to do, why it is necessary, and how he or she can participate ❶ ❷. The administration of nasal medication is not usually painful. Discuss how the results will be used in planning further care or treatments.
4. Perform hand hygiene and observe other appropriate infection control procedures (e.g., clean gloves).
5. Provide for client privacy.
6. Prepare the client.
   - Prior to performing the procedure, verify the client's identity using agency protocol. **Rationale:** *This ensures that the right client receives the right medication.*
7. Assist the client to a comfortable position.
   - To treat the opening of the eustachian tube, have the client assume a back-lying position. **Rationale:** *The drops will flow into the nasopharynx, where the eustachian tube opens.*

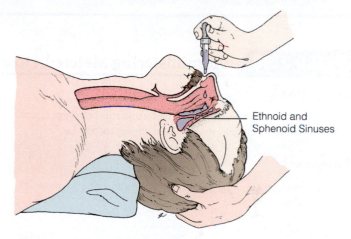

Ethnoid and Sphenoid Sinuses

❶ Instruct client to tilt head backwards and place dropper inside nares when instilling nose drops.

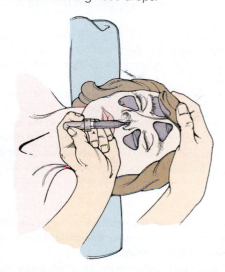

❷ Tilt client's head back for nose drops to reach maxillary and frontal sinuses.

- To treat the ethmoid and sphenoid sinuses, have the client assume a back-lying position with the head over the edge of the bed or a pillow under the shoulders so that the head is tipped backward.
- To treat the maxillary and frontal sinuses, have the client assume the same back-lying position, with the head turned toward the side to be treated. If only one side is to be treated, be sure the client is positioned so that the correct side is accessible. If the client's head is over the edge of the bed, support it with your hand so that the neck muscles are not strained.

(continued on next page)

SKILL 2.29 Administering Nasal Medications (*continued*)

8. Administer the medication.
   - Apply clean gloves.
   - Draw up the required amount of solution into the dropper.
   - Hold the tip of the dropper just above the nostril, and direct the solution laterally toward the midline of the superior concha of the ethmoid bone as the client breathes through the mouth. Do not touch the mucous membrane of the nares. **Rationale:** *If the solution is directed toward the base of the nasal cavity, it will run down the eustachian tube. Touching the mucous membrane with the dropper could damage the membrane and cause the client to sneeze.*
   - Repeat for the other nostril if indicated.

   - Ask the client to remain in the position for 5 minutes. **Rationale:** *The client remains in the same position to help the solution come in contact with all of the nasal surface or flow into the desired area.*
   - Discard any remaining solution in the dropper, and dispose of soiled supplies appropriately.
   - Remove and discard gloves. Perform hand hygiene.
9. Document all nursing assessments and interventions relative to the procedure. Include the name of the drug or irrigating solution, the strength, the number of drops if a liquid medication, the time, and the response of the client.

SKILL 2.30 Administering Metered-Dose Inhaler Medications

Delegation

Due to the need for assessment and interpretation of client status, inhaled medication administration is not delegated to UAP.

Equipment

- Metered-dose nebulizer with medication canister and extender if indicated

Preparation

- Check the MAR.
- Check for the drug name, strength, and prescribed frequency.
- Check client allergy status.
  - If the MAR is unclear or pertinent information is missing, compare it with the most recent primary care provider's written order.
  - Report any discrepancies to the charge nurse or primary care provider, as agency policy dictates.
  - Know the reason why the client is receiving the medication, the drug classification, contraindications, usual dose range, side effects, and nursing considerations for administering and evaluating the intended outcomes of the medication.

Procedure

1. Compare the label on the medication container with the MAR and check the expiration date. **Rationale:** *Outdated medications are not safe to administer.*
2. Introduce self and explain to the client what you are going to do, why it is necessary, and how he or she can participate. Discuss how the results will be used in planning further care or treatments.
3. Perform hand hygiene and observe other appropriate infection control procedures (e.g., clean gloves).
4. Provide for client privacy.
5. Prepare the client.
   - Prior to performing the procedure, verify the client's identity using agency protocol. **Rationale:** *This ensures that the right client receives the right medication.*
   - Explain that this nebulizer delivers a measured dose of drug with each push of the medication canister, which fits into the top of the nebulizer.

6. Instruct the client to use the metered-dose nebulizer as follows:

Metered-Dose Inhaler (MDI)
   - Ensure that the canister is firmly and fully inserted into the inhaler.
   - Remove the mouthpiece cap. Holding the MDI upright, shake the inhaler vigorously for 3 to 5 seconds to mix the medication evenly.
   - Exhale comfortably (as in a normal full breath).
   - Hold the inhaler with the canister on top and the mouthpiece at the bottom.
     a. Hold the MDI 2 to 4 cm (1 to 2 in.) from the open mouth.
     or
     b. Put the mouthpiece far enough into the mouth with its opening toward the throat such that the lips can tightly close around the mouthpiece.

Metered-Dose Inhaler with Spacer
   - Insert the MDI mouthpiece into the spacer.
   - Holding the inhaler and spacer, shake vigorously for 3 to 5 seconds to mix the medication evenly.
   - An MDI with a spacer or extender is always placed in the mouth.
7. Administer the medication.
   - Press down *once* on the MDI canister (which releases the dose) and inhale slowly (for 3 to 5 seconds) and deeply through the mouth.
   - Hold your breath for 10 seconds or as long as possible. **Rationale:** *This allows the aerosol to reach deeper airways.*
   - Remove the inhaler from or away from the mouth.
   - Exhale slowly through *pursed* lips. **Rationale:** *Controlled exhalation keeps the small airways open during exhalation.*
8. Repeat the inhalation if ordered. Wait 1 to 2 minutes between inhalations of bronchodilator medications. **Rationale:** *The first inhalation has a chance to work and the subsequent dose reaches deeper into the lungs.*
   - Many MDIs contain steroids for an anti-inflammatory effect. Prolonged use increases the risk of fungal infections in the mouth, indicating a need for attentive mouth care.
   - Following use of the inhaler, rinse mouth with water and spit it out. **Rationale:** *Rinsing the mouth removes any remaining medication and reduces irritation and risk of*

SKILL 2.30 Administering Metered-Dose Inhaler Medications (continued)

infection. Swallowing the rinse water could increase the chance of the medication entering the bloodstream and causing adverse reactions (Bower, 2005).

- Clean the MDI mouthpiece, and spacer if appropriate, daily. Use mild soap and water, rinse it, and let it air dry before reusing.
  - Store the canister at room temperature. Avoid extremes of temperature.
  - Report adverse reactions such as restlessness, palpitations, nervousness, or rash to the primary care provider.
9. Document all nursing assessments and interventions relative to the procedure. Include the name of the drug, the strength, the time, and the response of the client.

CLINICAL ALERT

If two inhalers are to be used, the bronchodilator medication (which opens the airways) should be given prior to other medications. A mnemonic to help remember this is B before C (i.e., bronchodilator before corticosteroid).

Check inhaler medication label for number of actuations (propellant-driven medication doses, e.g., 200). Have client maintain a record of actuations and discard after the number indicated. Final puffs may be nothing but propellant, which would not dilate airways in an emergency situation.

Inhaled steroids may not be correctly used by clients because they do not associate these medications with immediate symptom relief. The bronchodilators act to open the airways in the short term. However, it is the inhaled steroids that act as "chemical Band-Aids" to keep airway inflammation under control.

Evidence-Based Nursing Practice

MDI Canister Actuations—Client Monitoring

A study evaluated how clients determined that their MDI canisters were empty. Of the clients studied, 74% did not know how many actuations were in their canisters and used their MDIs until they could no longer "hear" the medication when actuating. Additionally, while 78% knew to shake the canister before actuating, only half did so. The conclusion was that clients are likely to use the medication for up to twice the intended duration, using canisters with no active ingredients more than 50% of the time. The authors concluded that dose counters appear to be the only practical solution.

Data from Rubin & Durotoye (2004).

Spacer with MDI versus Nebulizer in Children with Asthma

The Medical College in Ayub, Abbottabad, Pakistan, performed a study to determine which of two management processes showed evidence of being best practice in acute asthma attack in children. The two methods in use were the MDI plus spacer and the nebulizer. Using the outcomes of time to clinical improvement and duration of hospital stay, the group studied 54 children whose asthma ranged from mild to life threatening. One group received medication (salbutamol) via an MDI plus spacer and the other received it via a nebulizer. Results showed that there was no major difference between the two groups, but that MDI plus spacer was better for treatment of several acute asthma attacks in children. The study supported evidence that the MDI plus spacer is at least as effective as a nebulizer in the management of acute asthma in children.

Data from Fayaz, Sultana, & Rai (2009).

SKILL 2.31 Administering Dry Powder Inhaled (DPI) Medication

Equipment

- Dry powder capsule intended for oral inhalation
- Medication package insert (instructions)
- Handheld inhalation device intended for medication to be given

Preparation

- See Skill 2.30 on administering metered-dose inhaler medications.
- Review medication package insert instructions.
- Perform hand hygiene.

Procedure

1. Take dry powder capsule package and inhalation device to client's room.
2. Check client's identity band, and ask client to state name and birth date.
3. Provide for client privacy.
4. Explain procedure and purpose to client.
5. Assist client to a sitting position.
6. Remove capsule from package, peeling back foil cover to expose only one capsule. **Rationale:** *Capsules should be used immediately; unused capsules exposed to air may lose effectiveness.*

7. Open the outer cap of inhaler device (pull cap upward).
8. Open the mouthpiece.
9. Insert the capsule into center of chamber of the inhalation device ❶.

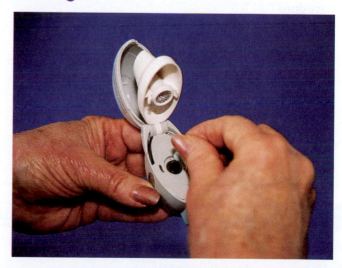

❶ Insert capsule into center of chamber of the inhalation device.

(continued on next page)

SKILL 2.31   Administering Dry Powder Inhaled (DPI) Medication *(continued)*

10. Hold the device upright, and, leaving the outer cap open, close mouthpiece/lid firmly until a click is heard. Leave the outer cap open.
11. Press the side-mounted piercing button in completely, then release. **Rationale:** *The piercing button punctures the capsule, allowing medication to be released upon inhalation.*
12. Have the client breathe out completely.
13. Have the client keep his or her head in an upright position and place lips tightly round the mouthpiece.
14. Have client breathe slowly and deeply with sufficient energy to hear the medication capsule vibrate. **Rationale:** *As long as the capsule rattles, the client's inhalation is fast enough.*

Note: Some DPIs require a fast initial inhalation to activate the medication distribution.

15. Have the client hold the deep breath as long as comfortable, then return to normal breathing.
16. Have client repeat steps 12 through 15 if indicated in medication package insert. **Rationale:** *Repeating the steps may be necessary to get the full dose of medication.*
17. Open mouthpiece and discard remaining capsule. Document.
18. Close mouthpiece and outer cap and store at client's bedside.
19. Clean unit only as necessary, using warm water and allowing device to air dry thoroughly before next use. **Rationale:** *No cleaning agents should be used and the device should not be wet when used.*

SKILL 2.32   Administering Medications by Nonpressurized (Nebulized) Aerosol (NPA)

Equipment

- Nebulizer medication chamber
- T-piece, mouthpiece, or mask
- Corrugated tubing
- Airflow tubing
- Prescribed medication (e.g., bronchodilator)
- Prescribed diluent (normal saline)
- Wall source (or other source) for compressed air, or oxygen with flowmeter

Preparation

- Review medication preparation protocol.
- Perform hand hygiene.
- Dilute medication as ordered and place in nebulizer chamber.
- Attach one end of tubing to compressed air source.
- Attach other end of tubing to nozzle at side or bottom of nebulizer.
- Keep nebulizer chamber vertical, and connect top of chamber to mask or T-piece sidearm.
- Hold mouthpiece in its protective cover, and attach to one end of T-piece.
- Attach corrugated tubing to other end of T-piece.

Procedure

1. Turn on air or oxygen (8 L/min) source, and observe for mist flow.
   - If the client is receiving 3 L/min or less of oxygen therapy, deliver aerosolized medications with compressed air (yellow wall outlet).
   - If the client is receiving 4 L/min or more of oxygen therapy, deliver the aerosol medication with the oxygen flowmeter (green wall outlet) set at 8 L/min.
2. Have client place mouthpiece in mouth and close lips ❶.
3. Instruct client to breathe normally in and out of mouthpiece or mask.

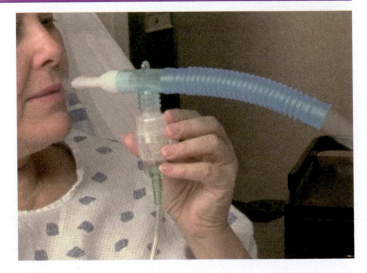

❶ Nonpressurized aerosol (NPA) treatment in progress.

4. Have client take a deep breath and hold for several seconds, then exhale slowly every 3 to 5 breaths. (Treatment is complete when all medication is used and no mist is seen.)
5. Turn power (air or O_2 flow) off, and unplug compressor (if used), or reset prescribed O_2 flow rate.
6. Clean mouthpiece, and place equipment in plastic bag at bedside. (Dispose of and replace components according to agency policy.) Document.

> **CLINICAL ALERT**
> The plastic containers with respiratory medications for nebulizers are similar to the plastic containers for single-dose eyedrops. Both products have the drug name molded into the plastic, but it is difficult to see.

SKILL 2.33   Administering Topical Medications

Equipment

- Medication container (tube or jar)
- Soap and water to cleanse skin
- Clean gloves
- Tongue blade
- Gauze or transparent dressing (as indicated)
- Tape
- Pen (to label dressing, if indicated)

SKILL 2.33 Administering Topical Medications (continued)

Preparation

- Review medication preparation protocol.

Procedure

1. Take medication container and dressing supplies to client's room.
2. Check room and bed number against client's record and check client's identity band, asking client to state name and birth date.
3. Provide for client privacy.
4. Explain procedure and purpose to client.
5. Perform hand hygiene and don clean gloves.

> **CLINICAL ALERT**
> Systemic absorption of topical medication from open lesions can result in toxic reactions.

6. Cleanse skin site with soap and water and dry thoroughly.
7. Squeeze medication from tube or use a tongue blade to take cream/ointment from medication container.
8. Spread small quantity of medication smoothly and evenly with gloved hand over client's skin following direction of hair follicles. **Rationale:** *Gloves facilitate smooth application.*
9. Apply dressing if indicated ❶. **Rationale:** *Dressing may ensure that medication is not rubbed off.*

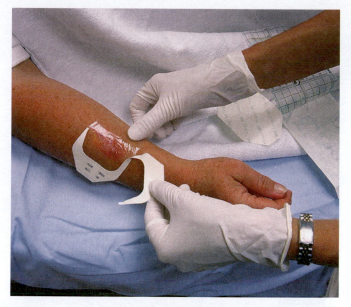

❶ Apply dressing; then label with date, time, and initials.

10. Label dressing with date, time, and your initials.
11. Remove gloves and perform hand hygiene.
12. Check that client is comfortable.
13. Return medication container to storage area. Document.

SKILL 2.34 Applying a Transdermal Medication Patch

Equipment

- Medication patch or tube
- Gloves
- Premeasured medication administration paper
- Soap and water
- Clear plastic wrap (optional)
- Tape and pen for labeling dressing

Preparation

- Review physician's order and medication preparation protocol.
- Obtain transdermal patch or premeasured paper that accompanies medication tube.
- Carefully read the manufacturer's directions for application. **Rationale:** *Directions as well as application areas of the body differ.*

> **CLINICAL ALERT**
> - Never cut a transdermal patch. Doing so releases the entire dose of medication to the client at once. Overdose and accidental death may occur.
> - Manufacturers' directions for application of transdermal agents differ significantly. Body temperature and blood flow to different regions influence the suggested application site. Always adhere to the manufacturer's specific guidelines and precautions when administering these systems.

Procedure

1. Take medication to client's room, and check room and bed number against medication record.
2. Check client's identity band, and ask client to state name and birth date.
3. Provide for client privacy.
4. Perform hand hygiene.
5. Don gloves. **Rationale:** *Gloves prevent you from absorbing transdermal medication* ❶.
6. Alternate areas with each dose of medication to prevent skin irritation. Remove previous medicated paper/patch, fold patch in half with sticky side in, and discard in biohazard box.
7. Cleanse area before applying new dose at another site.
8. Place prescribed medication directly on paper (usually 1/2- to 1-in. strip).
9. Apply medicated paper to clean, dry, hairless, intact skin.
10. Use paper to spread medication paste over a 2-in. area. Secure paper with tape or cover medicated area with plastic wrap and tape.
11. For patch, remove protective covering and immediately apply patch to clean, dry, hairless, intact skin.
12. Press patch with palm for 30 seconds to attain a good seal.
13. Remove gloves and perform hand hygiene.
14. Label patch or paper with date, time, and your initials. Dispose of waste appropriately. Document care.
15. Return medication tube to appropriate storage area.

(continued on next page)

SKILL 2.34 Applying a Transdermal Medication Patch (continued)

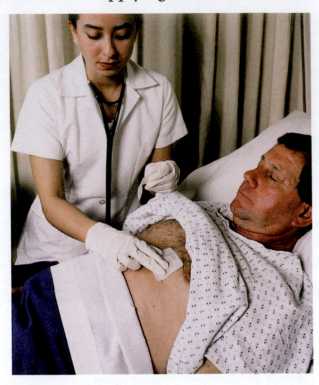

CLINICAL ALERT

The use of heating pads or hot tubs can increase the absorption rate of transdermal medications. The nonadhesive backing of some drug patches contains metal that may not be visible. These may become heated during MRI and can cause second-degree burns. Warnings may be missing from patch labels. Patches should be removed before MRI. Self-improvement patches purporting to deliver herbs or other substances (marketed on TV or the Internet) are not FDA regulated. Counterfeit patches also endanger clients. Refer clients to the FDA Web site for more information.

Dispose of used transdermal patch by folding sticky sides together and discarding in medical waste receptacle to protect others from exposure to medication. Do not flush used patches down the toilet because trace amounts of the drug may appear in treated water.

❶ Wear gloves to prevent drug absorption through fingertips.

SKILL 2.35   Administering Vaginal Medications

Delegation

Due to the need for assessments and interpretation of client status, vaginal medication administration is not delegated to UAP.

Equipment

- Drape
- Correct vaginal suppository or cream
- Applicator for vaginal cream
- Clean gloves
- Lubricant for a suppository
- Disposable towel
- Clean perineal pad

For an Irrigation, Add:

- Moisture-proof pad
- Vaginal irrigation set (these are often disposable) containing a nozzle, tubing, clamp, and a container for the solution
- Irrigating solution (the solution should be warmed to a temperature of 37.8° to 43.3°C [100°F to 110°F] if not specified, to minimize discomfort caused by cooler solutions.)

Preparation

- Check the MAR.
- Check for the drug name, strength, and prescribed frequency.
- Check client allergy status.
- If the MAR is unclear or pertinent information is missing, compare it with the most recent primary care provider's written order.

- Report any discrepancies to the charge nurse or primary care provider, as agency policy dictates.
- Know the reason why the client is receiving the medication, the drug classification, contraindications, usual dose range, side effects, and nursing considerations for administering and evaluating the intended outcomes of the medication.

Procedure

1. Compare the label on the medication container with the medication record and check the expiration date. **Rationale:** *Outdated medications are not safe to administer.*
2. If necessary, calculate the medication dosage.
3. Introduce self and explain to the client what you are going to do, why it is necessary, and how she can participate. Explain to the client that a vaginal instillation is normally a painless procedure, and in fact may bring relief from itching and burning if an infection is present. Many people feel embarrassed about this procedure, and some may prefer to perform the procedure themselves if instruction is provided. Discuss how the results will be used in planning further care or treatments.
4. Perform hand hygiene and observe other appropriate infection control procedures (e.g., clean gloves).
5. Provide for client privacy.
6. Prepare the client.
   - Prior to performing the procedure, verify the client's identity using agency protocol. **Rationale:** *This ensures that the right client receives the right medication.*
   - Ask the client to void. **Rationale:** *If the bladder is empty, the client will have less discomfort during the treatment,*

SKILL 2.35   Administering Vaginal Medications (continued)

and the possibility of injuring the vaginal lining is decreased.
- Assist the client to a back-lying position with the knees flexed and the hips rotated laterally.
- Drape the client appropriately so that only the perineal area is exposed.

7. Prepare the equipment.
    - Unwrap the suppository, and put it on the opened wrapper.

or

- Fill the applicator with the prescribed cream, jelly, or foam. Directions are provided with the manufacturer's applicator.

8. Assess and clean the perineal area.
    - Apply gloves. **Rationale:** *Gloves prevent contamination of the nurse's hands from vaginal and perineal microorganisms.*
    - Inspect the vaginal orifice, note any odor or discharge from the vagina, and ask about any vaginal discomfort.
    - Provide perineal care to remove microorganisms. **Rationale:** *This decreases the chance of moving microorganisms into the vagina.*

9. Administer the vaginal suppository, cream, foam, jelly, or irrigation.

Suppository

- Lubricate the rounded (smooth) end of the suppository, which is inserted first. **Rationale:** *Lubrication facilitates insertion.*
- Lubricate your gloved index finger.
- Expose the vaginal orifice by separating the labia with your nondominant hand.
- Insert the suppository about 8 to 10 cm (3 to 4 in.) along the posterior wall of the vagina, or as far as it will go. **Rationale:** *The posterior wall of the vagina is about 2.5 cm (1 in.) longer than the anterior wall because the cervix protrudes into the uppermost portion of the anterior wall.*
- Ask the client to remain lying in the supine position for 5 to 10 minutes following insertion. The hips may also be elevated on a pillow. **Rationale:** *This position allows the medication to flow into the posterior fornix after it has melted.*

Vaginal Cream, Jelly, or Foam

- Gently insert the applicator about 5 cm (2 in.).
- Slowly push the plunger until the applicator is empty.
- Remove the applicator and place it on the towel. **Rationale:** *The applicator is put on the towel to prevent the spread of microorganisms.*
- Discard the applicator if disposable or clean it according to the manufacturer's directions.

- Ask the client to remain lying in the supine position for 5 to 10 minutes following the insertion.

Irrigation

- Place the client on a bedpan.
- Clamp the tubing. Hold the irrigating container about 30 cm (12 in.) above the vagina. **Rationale:** *At this height, the pressure of the solution should not be great enough to injure the vaginal lining.*
- Run fluid through the tubing and nozzle into the bedpan. **Rationale:** *Fluid is run through the tubing to remove air and to moisten the nozzle.*
- Insert the nozzle carefully into the vagina ❶. Direct the nozzle toward the sacrum, following the direction of the vagina.

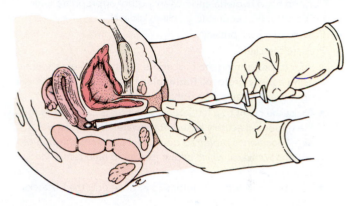

❶ Insert vaginal suppository at least 5 cm (2 in.) into vaginal canal using applicator as shown.

- Insert the nozzle about 7 to 10 cm (3 to 4 in.), start the flow, and rotate the nozzle several times. **Rationale:** *Rotating the nozzle irrigates all parts of the vagina.*
- Use all of the irrigating solution, permitting it to flow out freely into the bedpan.
- Remove the nozzle from the vagina.
- Assist the client to a sitting position on the bedpan. **Rationale:** *Sitting on the bedpan will help drain the remaining fluid by gravity.*

10. Ensure client comfort.
    - Dry the perineum with tissues as required.
    - Apply a clean perineal pad if there is excessive drainage.

11. Remove and discard gloves. Perform hand hygiene.

12. Document all nursing assessments and interventions relative to the skill. Include the name of the drug or irrigating solution, the strength, the time, and the response of the client.

SKILL 2.36   Administering Rectal Medications

Delegation

Due to the need for assessment and interpretation of client status, rectal medication administration is not delegated to UAP.

Equipment

- Correct suppository
- Clean glove
- Lubricant

Preparation

- Check the MAR.
- Check for the drug name, strength, and prescribed frequency.
- Check client allergy status.
    - If the MAR is unclear or pertinent information is missing, compare it with the most recent primary care provider's written order.
    - Report any discrepancies to the charge nurse or primary care provider, as agency policy dictates.

(continued on next page)

SKILL 2.36 Administering Rectal Medications (continued)

- Know the reason why the client is receiving the medication, the drug classification, contraindications, usual dose range, side effects, and nursing considerations for administering and evaluating the intended outcomes of the medication.

Procedure

1. Compare the label on the medication container with the medication record and check the expiration date. **Rationale:** *Outdated medications are not safe to administer.*
2. Introduce self and explain to the client what you are going to do, why it is necessary, and how he or she can participate. Discuss how the results will be used in planning further care or treatments.
3. Perform hand hygiene and observe other appropriate infection control procedures (e.g., clean gloves).
4. Provide for client privacy.
5. Prepare the client.
   - Prior to performing the procedure, verify the client's identity using agency protocol. **Rationale:** *This ensures that the right client receives the right medication.*
   - Assist the client to a left lateral or left Sims' position, with the upper leg acutely flexed. **Rationale:** *The left lateral Sims' position is preferred because it positions the sigmoid colon downward, which allows gravity to help retain the suppository.*
   - Fold back the top bedclothes to expose only the buttocks.
6. Prepare the equipment.
   - Unwrap the suppository, and leave it on the opened wrapper.
   - Apply glove on the hand used to insert the suppository. **Rationale:** *The glove prevents contamination of the nurse's hand by rectal microorganisms and feces.*
   - Lubricate the smooth, rounded end of the suppository, or see the manufacturer's instructions. **Rationale:** *The smooth, rounded end is inserted first. Lubrication prevents anal friction and tissue damage on insertion.*
   - Lubricate the gloved index finger.
7. Insert the suppository.
   - Ask the client to breathe through the mouth. **Rationale:** *This usually relaxes the external anal sphincter.*
   - Insert the suppository gently into the anus, rounded end first (or according to the manufacturer's instructions) and along the wall of the rectum with the gloved index finger ❶. For an adult, insert the suppository 10 cm (4 in.) or after passing the sphincter. **Rationale:** *The rounded end facilitates insertion. The suppository needs to be placed along the wall of the rectum, rather than amid feces, in order to be absorbed effectively.*

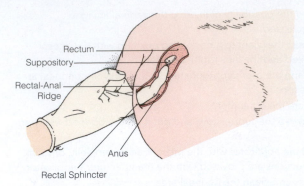

❶ Insert rectal suppository beyond the anal rectal ridge to ensure it is retained.

- Withdraw the finger. Press the client's buttocks together for a few minutes. **Rationale:** *This helps minimize any urge to expel the suppository.*
- Remove the glove by turning it inside out and discard. **Rationale:** *Turning the glove inside out contains the rectal microorganisms and prevents their spread.*
- Perform hand hygiene.
- Ask the client to remain flat or in the left lateral position for at least 5 minutes. **Rationale:** *This helps prevent expulsion of the suppository. The suppository should be retained at least 30 to 40 minutes or according to manufacturer's instructions.*
- If the client has been given a laxative suppository, place the call light within easy reach to summon assistance for the bedpan or toilet.

8. Document all nursing assessments and interventions relative to the procedure. Include the type of suppository given/name of the drug, the time it was given, the amount of time it was retained if it was expelled, the results or effects, and the response of the client.

Developmental Considerations

INFANTS/CHILDREN

- Obtain assistance to immobilize an infant or young child. **Rationale:** *This prevents accidental injury due to sudden movement during the procedure.*
- For a child under 3 years, the nurse should use the gloved fifth finger for insertion. After this age, the index finger can usually be used.
- For a child or infant, insert a suppository 5 cm (2 in.) or less.

► PARENTERAL ROUTES

Expected Outcomes

1. Safe technique prevents self-harm when administering parenteral injections.
2. Injection is as painless as possible.
3. Injection is administered without complications.
4. Medication is infused over appropriate time span.
5. IV piggyback medication is compatible with IV solution.

SKILL 2.37 Administering Intradermal Injections

Equipment

- Medication (e.g., 0.1 mL purified protein derivative antigen for tuberculin testing)
- Unit dose (1-mL) tuberculin syringe with a 3/8- to 1/2-in., 25- to 27-gauge needle
- Antimicrobial wipes
- Gauze pads
- Clean gloves (if indicated)
- Pen to mark injection site

Procedure

1. Take prepared injection to client's room, checking room and bed number against client's medication record.
2. Check client's identity band and ask client to state name and birth date.
3. Explain procedure and purpose to client.
4. Perform hand hygiene and don gloves if exposure anticipated.
5. Select lesion-free injection site on undersurface, upper third of forearm for skin testing.
6. Cleanse area with antimicrobial wipe and allow to dry.
7. Remove needle guard.
8. Grasp the client's dorsal forearm to gently pull the skin taut on ventral forearm.
9. Holding syringe almost parallel to skin, insert needle at a 10- to 15-degree angle with bevel facing up, about 1/8 in. **1**. Needle point should be visible under skin. DO NOT ASPIRATE.
10. Inject medication slowly, observing for a wheal (blister) formation and blanching at the site **2**. **Rationale:** *This indicates that the medication was injected within the dermis. If no wheal develops, injection was given too deeply.*
11. Withdraw needle at same angle as inserted. Pat area gently with dry gauze pad but DO NOT MASSAGE. **Rationale:** *Massaging could disperse medication.*
12. Activate needle safety feature and discard syringe unit in puncture proof container.
13. Mark injection site with pen for future assessment.

> **CLINICAL ALERT**
> For tuberculin testing, instruct client to return and have the site checked by the healthcare provider in 48 to 72 hours.

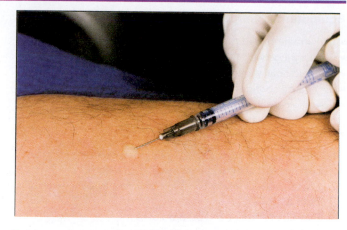

2 Inject solution to form wheal on skin.

14. Return client to comfortable position.
15. Dispose of gloves and perform hand hygiene.
16. Record site and antigen in client's record.

Evidence-Based Nursing Practice

Needlestick Injuries

In a 2008 study of more than 700 nurses' views, researchers found that safety concerns influence the decisions made by the vast majority of nurses (87%) about the type of nursing they do; 74% say they would not consider working for an employer that does not provide safety syringes.

Of nurses interviewed, 64% of nurses report being accidentally stuck by a needle while working. The three principal causes account for two thirds (66%) of the problem:

- While giving an injection: 28%
- Before activating the safety feature: 19%
- During disposal of nonsafety device: 19%.

Other causes of accidental needlestick injury were a sharp left on a surface by a coworker, an action of a coworker, and during activation of the safety feature.

Although 71% of U.S. nurses state they are familiar with the Needlestick Safety and Prevention Act of 2001, the majority (62%) said they would benefit from more information about needlestick injury prevention.

Data from *Nursing World* (2008).

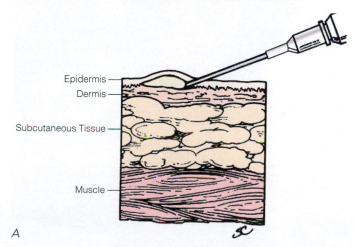

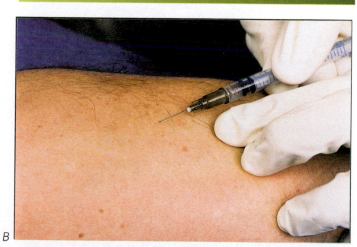

1 A, Insert needle at a 15-degree angle just under the epidermis for intradermal injection. B, Insert needle with bevel up for intradermal injection.

SKILL 2.38   Administering Subcutaneous Injections

Equipment

- Nonirritating medication
- 3-mL syringe with 1/2- to 5/8-in. needle (usually 25 to 27 gauge)
- Antimicrobial wipes
- Dry gauze sponge
- Clean gloves if indicated

Procedure

1. Take prepared injection to client's room, checking room and bed number against client's medication record.
2. Check client's identity band and ask client to state name and birth date.
3. Explain procedure and purpose to client.
4. Perform hand hygiene and don gloves.

5. Select fatty site for injection (e.g., abdomen, avoiding 5 cm [2-in.] radius around umbilicus), alternating sites for each injection ❶. **Rationale:** *This prevents repeated trauma to tissue.*
6. Cleanse area with antimicrobial wipe.
7. Remove needle guard.
8. Use thumb and forefinger and gently grasp loose area ("pinch an inch") of fatty tissue on appropriate site (e.g., posterior-lateral aspect, middle third of arm) ❷. **Rationale:** *This ensures insertion of medication within subcutaneous tissue, not muscle.*

Note: This action is not necessary when there is substantial fatty tissue.

9. Hold syringe like a dart between the thumb and forefinger.
10. Insert needle at a 45- or 90-degree angle. A 90-degree angle is used more commonly due to short needles on prepackaged syringes ❸. **Rationale:** *Angle varies with the amount of subcutaneous tissue, selected site, and needle length.*
11. Continue to hold tissue and aspirate by pulling back on plunger with thumb of dominant hand. If no blood appears, administer injection. If blood appears, then prepare a new injection. **Rationale:** *Blood indicates needle has entered a blood vessel. Injecting the drug IV may be dangerous.*
12. Inject medication slowly, 10 sec/mL.
13. Wait 10 seconds to prevent leakback, then withdraw needle quickly and activate needle safety feature.
14. Release tissue and massage area with dry gauze sponge (if indicated). **Rationale:** *Massaging area aids absorption.*
15. Discard needle/syringe unit in puncture-proof container.
16. Return client to position of comfort.
17. Discard gloves and perform hand hygiene.
18. Record medication and site used.

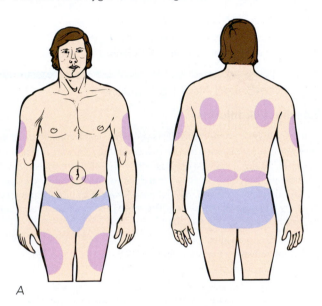

A

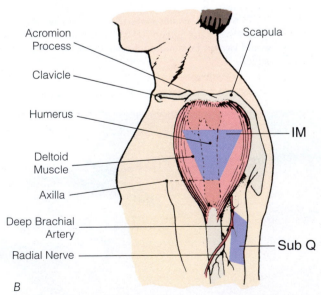

Acromion Process
Clavicle
Humerus
Deltoid Muscle
Axilla
Deep Brachial Artery
Radial Nerve
Scapula
IM
Sub Q

B

❶ A, Sites for subcutaneous injections given routinely. (Avoid umbilicus area.) Abdomen site preferred for insulin injection because absorption is more predictable. B, Use upper shaded triangle for IM injection in upper arm; use lower shaded area for subcutaneous injection.

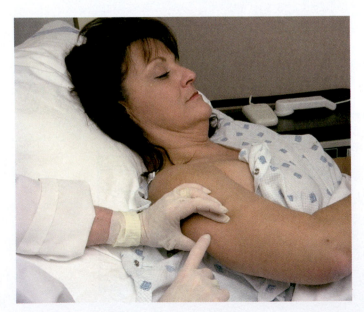

❷ Select site on lateral aspect of mid-upper arm for subcutaneous injection.

SKILL 2.38 Administering Subcutaneous Injections *(continued)*

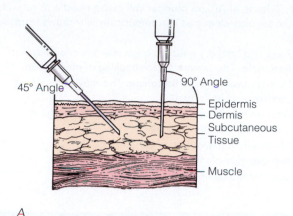

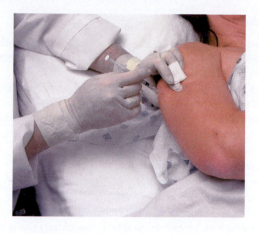

A *B*

③ *A*, Insert needle at 45- or 90-degree angle into tissue for subcutaneous injection. *B*, Insert needle at 45- or 90-degree angle, using short needle for subcutaneous injection.

Gloving Protocol for Injections

The CDC has no regulations concerning the wearing of gloves during injections. OSHA recommends that gloves are not necessary when administering IM or subcutaneous injections, as long as bleeding that could result in hand contact with blood (or other potentially infectious material) is not anticipated.

The practice of whether or not to wear gloves for subcutaneous or IM injections is in transition. Therefore, each hospital policy should dictate gloving protocol for injections.

If wearing gloves for mass inoculations, nurses must change gloves between clients and perform hand hygiene. Therefore, nurses may choose not to wear gloves in these situations.

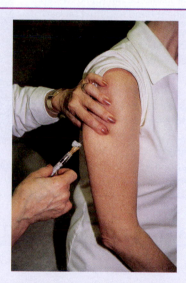
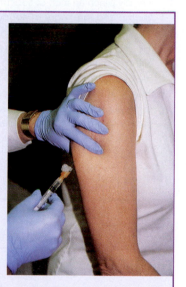

SKILL 2.39 Administering Subcutaneous Anticoagulants (Heparin, LMWH, Arixtra)

Equipment

- Heparin in vial (*carefully note units per milliliter*)
- 1-mL tuberculin syringe or unit-dose syringe with small (1/2- to 5/8-in., 25- to 27-gauge) needle

or

- Low-molecular-weight heparin (LMWH) or Arixtra in prefilled syringe
- Antimicrobial swabs
- Dry gauze sponge
- Gloves if indicated

Preparation

- Review process for providing injections.
- Double-check heparin calculated dose with another nurse.

CLINICAL ALERT

Heparin is available in a variety of strengths (e.g., vials of 1,000, 2,500, 5,000, 10,000, 25,000 units/mL). *Carefully* check vial units per milliliter before drawing into syringe and have another nurse double-check your calculations and prepared injection.

Subcutaneous injection of LMWH or Arixtra involves low doses that help prevent clot formation but do not alter blood coagulation studies and do not require coagulation monitoring as does unfractionated heparin.

- Place client in supine position.
- Perform hand hygiene.

Note: To avoid loss of drug, do not clear prefilled syringe needle of air before injecting LMWH or Arixtra

(continued on next page)

SKILL 2.39 Administering Subcutaneous Anticoagulants (*continued*)

Procedure

1. Check client's record for site of previous injection. **Rationale:** *Injections should be rotated to prevent local postinjection complications.*
2. Take prepared injection to client's room, and check room and bed number against client's MAR.
3. Check client's identity band, and ask client to state name and birth date.
4. Provide for client privacy.
5. Explain procedure and purpose to client.
6. Don gloves (if indicated).
7. Assist client to supine position.
8. Select site on client's lower abdomen (at least two finger-breadths from umbilicus) or select area of fatty tissue above iliac crest. **Rationale:** *Anticoagulants should not be administered IM or in the extremities.*
9. Avoid ecchymotic area or lesions.
10. Cleanse site gently with antimicrobial swab, and allow to dry.
11. Gently pinch an inch of subcutaneous tissue (fat roll) between thumb and forefinger of nondominant hand and hold fat pad throughout injection.
12. Hold syringe between thumb and forefinger of dominant hand and insert full length of needle into skinfold at a 90-degree angle.
13. Inject medication slowly without aspirating first. Press prefilled syringe plunger rod firmly as far as it will go. **Rationale:** *Aspiration can rupture small vessels and increase risk of bleeding into tissue.*
14. Wait 10 seconds before gently withdrawing needle at same angle in which it entered skin. **Rationale:** *This allows medication to absorb into tissue and minimizes bruising.*

Note: Release of Arixtra plunger will cause needle to retract into the security sleeve as it automatically withdraws from the skin.

15. Press and hold dry gauze sponge over injection site. **Rationale:** *This prevents back-tracking of medication.*
16. Do not massage area. **Rationale:** *This may cause tissue damage and bruising.*
17. Activate needle safety feature and discard syringe in puncture-proof container ❶.
18. Return client to position of comfort.
19. Remove gloves and perform hand hygiene.
20. Document injection.

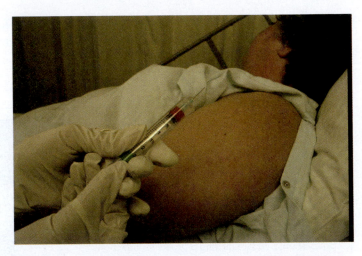

❶ After activating needle safety feature, dispose of syringe in sharps container.

SKILL 2.40 Administering Intramuscular (IM) Injections

Equipment

- Medication vial or ampule
- 3-mL syringe with 5/8- to 1 1/2-in. (18- to 25-gauge) needle, depending on the muscle site and fat thickness
- Antimicrobial swab
- Dry gauze sponge
- Gloves if indicated

Preparation

See the Medication Preparation section of this chapter.

Procedure

1. Check client's record for site of previous IM injections. **Rationale:** *IM injections should be rotated to prevent local postinjection complications.*
2. Take prepared injection to client's room. Check room number against client's MAR.
3. Check client's identity band, and ask client to state name and birth date.
4. Provide for client privacy.
5. Explain procedure to client.
6. Perform hand hygiene and don gloves if indicated.
7. Select injection site, identifying bony landmarks. Consider client's size, amount and viscosity of medications being injected. Alternate sites each time injections are given.

Evidence-Based Nursing Practice

Choosing the Right Needle Size

For injections into the deltoid muscle of the arm, use a 22- to 25-gauge needle. Choose the injection site and needle length appropriate to the adult's body mass:

- Male or female less than 130 lb: 5/8 to 1 in. *Note:* Use a 5/8-in. needle *only* if the skin is stretched tight, subcutaneous tissue is not bunched, and injection is made at a 90-degree angle.
- Female 130–200 lb or male 130–260 lb: 1–1½ in.
- Female 200+ lb or male 260+ lb: 1½ in.

Data from Immunization Action Coalition (2009).

8. Cleanse area with antimicrobial swab and allow to dry.
9. Spread skin taut between thumb and forefinger (grasping muscle is acceptable in pediatric and geriatric clients with less fatty tissue) to ensure needle placement in muscle belly.

SKILL 2.40 Administering Intramuscular (IM) Injections *(continued)*

10. Insert needle at a 90-degree angle to the muscle, using a quick, darting motion ❶. **Rationale:** *This angle facilitates medication reaching muscle.*

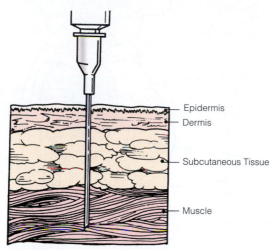

❶ Insert needle at 90-degree angle for IM injections into muscle.

11. Pull back on plunger for 5 to 10 seconds; if blood returns, discard and prepare a new injection. **Rationale:** *The appearance of blood indicates needle has entered a blood vessel, and medication injected directly into bloodstream may be dangerous.*

12. Inject medication slowly. **Rationale:** *This allows time for medication to disperse through tissue.*

13. Hold needle in place for 10 seconds to prevent leakback. Then withdraw needle and massage area with dry gauze sponge.

14. Activate needle safety feature.

15. Dispose of syringe/needle unit in puncture-proof container.

16. Return client to comfortable position.

17. Discard gloves and perform hand hygiene.

18. Chart medication and site of injection.

VARIATION: VENTROGLUTEAL INJECTION SITE ❷ ❸ ❹

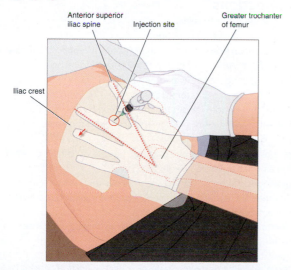

❷ Overlay of hand shows area of injection into ventrogluteal site for IM injections (client's right side). Copyright (© SPL/Custom Medical Stock Photo—All rights reserved).

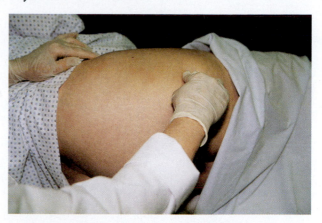

❸ Locate greater trochanter and anterior superior iliac spine.

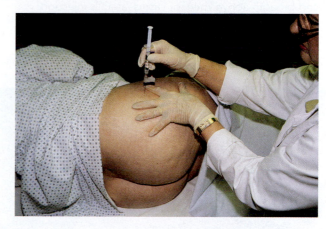

❹ Place palm at trochanter and index finger at anterior superior iliac spine; fan remaining fingers posteriorly.

VARIATION: VASTUS LATERALIS INJECTION SITE ❺ ❻ ❼ ❽

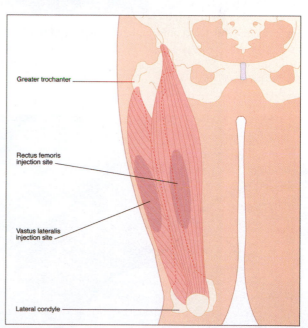

❺ Shaded area indicates site location for vastus lateralis injection. (Copyright © SPL/Custom Medical Stock Photo—All rights reserved).

(continued on next page)

SKILL 2.40   Administering Intramuscular (IM) Injections *(continued)*

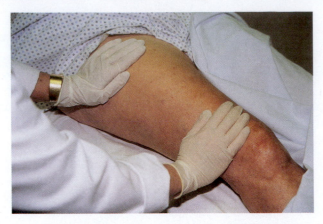

6 Select site one hand-breadth below greater trochanter and 1 hand-breadth above knee for vastus lateralis injection.

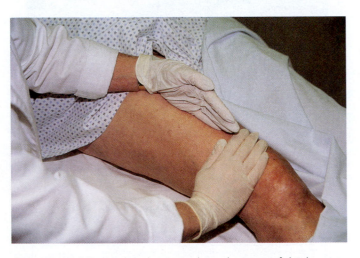

7 Site is middle third and anterior lateral aspect of thigh.

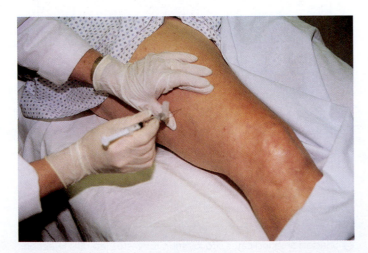

8 Inject medications at 90-degree angle directly into muscle.

VARIATION: DELTOID IM INJECTION SITE **9** **10**

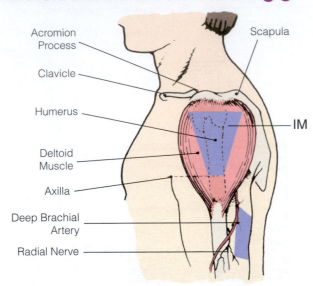

Acromion Process
Clavicle
Humerus
Deltoid Muscle
Axilla
Deep Brachial Artery
Radial Nerve
Scapula
IM

9 Locate deltoid site on outer lateral aspect of upper arm.

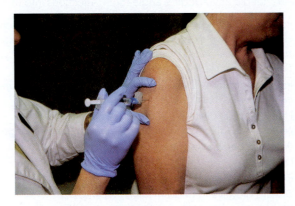

10 Inject medication into deltoid area site.

Techniques for Minimizing Pain During IM Injections

- Encourage client to relax.
- Use a new needle for injection.
- Place client on side with upper knee flexed for ventrogluteal injection.
- Have client place hand on hip to relax deltoid muscle.
- Avoid injecting into sensitive or hardened tissue.
- Apply pressure to site for 10 seconds before injecting.
- Ensure that needle length reaches muscle for IM injection.
- Prevent antiseptic from clinging to needle during insertion by waiting until skin prep is dry.
- Reduce puncture pain by "darting" needle quickly into muscle.
- Use as small a gauge needle as possible.
- Inject medication slowly (10 seconds per mL).
- Hold needle in place for 10 seconds after injecting medication to prevent leakback.
- Maintain grasp on syringe; do not move needle once inserted.
- Withdraw needle quickly after injection.
- Use Z-track technique (see Skill 2.41).
- EMLA cream, a topical anesthetic, may be applied 30 to 40 minutes prior to injection.

SKILL 2.41 Using the Z-Track Method

Equipment

- Syringe
- 2-in. needle for injection
- Medication
- Antimicrobial swabs
- Dry gauze sponge
- Gloves

Preparation

- Review the Medication Preparation section of this chapter.

Procedure

1. Use filter needle to draw up prescribed medication into syringe.
2. Attach new 2-in. sterile needle to syringe. **Rationale:** *A new needle prevents introducing medication that could be irritating to tissue. A long needle allows medication to go deep into the muscle.*

> **CLINICAL ALERT**
>
> Irritating medications such as Vistaril must not be administered subcutaneously, or tissue necrosis may result. Such medications should be administered intramuscularly in the ventrogluteal site using the Z-track method.
>
> If client is obese, use a 2- to 3-in. needle so that medication is absorbed into muscle (not fat) tissue and blood level of drug is achieved.
>
> The Z-track method prevents medication from leaking into the "track" of the needle; it is recommended for administering medications into the ventrogluteal or vastus lateralis sites.

3. Take medication to client's room; check room number against MAR.
4. Check client's identity band, and ask client to state name and birth date.
5. Provide for client privacy.
6. Explain procedure and purpose to client.
7. Perform hand hygiene and don gloves (if indicated).
8. Position client for ventrogluteal or vastus lateralis injection.
9. Cleanse site with antimicrobial swab.
10. Pull skin 1 to 1 1/2 in. laterally away from injection site. **Rationale:** *This tissue displacement creates a track that keeps medication from seeping into subcutaneous tissue.*
11. Maintain displacement and insert needle at a 90-degree angle 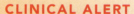. Aspirate by pulling back on plunger (5 to 10 seconds) to see if needle is in blood vessel. If so, discard and prepare new injection.

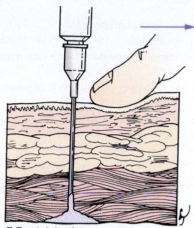

Z-Track Injection

1 Z-track injection: Maintaining displacement, insert needle at 90-degree angle. Aspirate by pulling back on plunger, checking to see if needle is in blood vessel. If blood is aspirated, discard and prepare new injection.

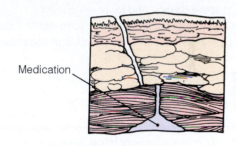

Medication

2 Z-track injection, after displacement released. Method is used to prevent backflow of medications into subcutaneous tissue.

12. Inject medication slowly (10 sec/mL) and wait 10 seconds to prevent leakback, keeping skin taut **2**. **Rationale:** *Permits muscle relaxation and absorption of medication.*
13. Withdraw needle and release retracted skin. **Rationale:** *Lateral tissue displacement interrupts needle track and seals medication in the muscle when the tissue is released.*
14. Apply light pressure with dry gauze sponge. Do not massage. **Rationale:** *Massage may disperse medication into subcutaneous tissue and cause tissue irritation.*
15. Activate needle safety feature.
16. Return client to a position of comfort and safety.
17. Discard gloves and equipment in appropriate area.
18. Perform hand hygiene.
19. Document administration of medications in the medication record.

SKILL 2.42 Adding Medications to Intravenous Fluid Containers

Delegation

Adding medications to IV fluid containers involves the application of nursing knowledge and critical thinking. The nurse does not delegate this procedure to UAP. However, the nurse can inform the UAP of the intended therapeutic effects and/or specific side effects of the medication(s) in the IV and direct the UAP to report specific client observations to the nurse for follow-up.

(continued on next page)

SKILL 2.42 Adding Medications to Intravenous Fluid Containers (continued)

Equipment

- Client's MAR or computer printout
- Correct sterile medication
- Diluent for medication in powdered form (see manufacturer's instructions)
- Correct solution container, if a new one is to be attached
- Antiseptic swabs
- Sterile syringe of appropriate size (e.g., 5 or 10 mL) and a 1- to 1 ½-in., 20- or 21-gauge sterile safety needle if not using a needleless system
- IV additive label

Preparation

- Check the medication administration record.
- Check the label on the medication carefully against the MAR to make sure that the correct medication is being prepared.
- Follow the three checks for administering medications. Read the label on the medication (1) when it is taken from the medication cart, (2) before withdrawing the medication, and (3) after withdrawing the medication.
- Confirm that the dosage and route are correct.
- Verify which infusion solution is to be used with the medication.
- Consult a pharmacist, if required, to confirm compatibility of the drugs and solutions being mixed.
- Organize the equipment.

Procedure

1. Perform hand hygiene and observe other appropriate infection control procedures (e.g., clean gloves).
2. Prepare the medication ampule or vial for drug withdrawal. Check the agency's practice for using a filter needle to withdraw premixed liquid medications from multidose vials or ampules.
3. Add the medication.

To New IV Container

- Locate the injection port. Clean the port with the antiseptic or alcohol swab. **Rationale:** *This reduces the risk of introducing microorganisms into the container when the needle is inserted.*
- Remove the needle cap from the syringe, insert the needle through the center of the injection port, and inject the medication into the bag. Activate the needle safety device. Mix the medication and solution by gently rotating or slowly inverting the bag or bottle several times. **Rationale:** *This should disperse the medication throughout the solution.*

- Complete the IV additive label with the client's name and room number (if appropriate), name and dose of medication, date, time, and nurse's initials. Attach it on the bag or bottle. **Rationale:** *This documents that medication has been added to the solution. The label should be easy to read when the bag is hanging.*
- Clamp the IV tubing. Remove the spike from the current IV container, taking care not to touch anything with the exposed spike. Place the used IV container in a sink or basin temporarily while attaching the new IV container. Spike the bag or bottle with IV tubing and hang the IV. If no IV infusion was running, be sure to fully flush the IV solution through the new tubing and verify that no air bubbles are present in the tubing prior to connecting to the IV access. **Rationale:** *Clamping prevents rapid infusion of the solution.*
- Regulate infusion rate as ordered. Often a controller device such as an IV pump is used to ensure accurate rate of infusion.

To an Existing Infusion

- Determine that the IV solution in the container is sufficient for adding the medication. **Rationale:** *Sufficient volume is necessary to dilute the medication adequately.*
- Confirm the desired dilution of the medication, that is, the amount of medication per milliliter of solution.
- Close the infusion clamp. **Rationale:** *This prevents the medication from infusing directly into the client as it is injected into the bag or bottle.*
- Wipe the medication port with the alcohol or disinfectant swab. **Rationale:** *This reduces the risk of introducing microorganisms into the container when the needle is inserted.*

Remove the needle cover from the medication syringe.

- While supporting and stabilizing the bag with your thumb and forefinger, carefully insert the syringe needle through the port and inject the medication. **Rationale:** *The bag is supported during the injection of the medication to avoid punctures.* If the bag is too high to reach easily, lower it from the IV pole. Activate the needle safety device.
- Remove the bag from the pole and gently rotate or invert the bag. **Rationale:** *This will mix the medication and solution.* Rehang the container and regulate the flow rate, making sure that no air has entered the tubing during the procedure. **Rationale:** *This establishes the correct flow rate.*
- Complete the medication label and apply to the IV container.

4. Dispose of the equipment and supplies according to agency practice. **Rationale:** *This prevents inadvertent injury to others and the spread of microorganisms.*
5. Document the medication(s) on the appropriate form in the client's record.

SKILL 2.43 Administering Intermittent Intravenous Medication Using a Secondary Set

Delegation

The administration of intermittent IV medications involves the application of nursing knowledge and critical thinking. Check the state's nurse practice act to verify the scope of practice for the LPN/LVN as it relates to IV medication administration. Agency policy also must be checked and followed. This skill is not delegated to UAP. The nurse, however, can inform the UAP of the intended therapeutic effects and/or specific side effects of the medication

and direct the UAP to report specific client observations to the nurse for follow-up.

Equipment

- Client's MAR or computer printout
- 50- to 250-mL infusion bag with medication (most medication infusion bags are prepared by the pharmacist)

SKILL 2.43 Administering Intermittent Intravenous Medication *(continued)*

- Secondary administration set
- Antiseptic swabs
- Sterile needle if system is not needleless
- Tape
- Sterile needle or needleless adapter, syringe, and saline if medication is incompatible with the primary infusion

Preparation

- Check the MAR.
  - Check the label on the medication carefully against the MAR to make sure that the correct medication is being prepared.
  - Confirm that the dosage is correct.
  - Ensure medication compatibility with primary infusion solution.
  - Consult a pharmacist, if required, to confirm compatibility of the drugs and solutions being mixed.
- Organize the equipment.
- Remove medication bag from the refrigerator 30 minutes before administration, if appropriate.

Procedure

1. Perform hand hygiene and observe other appropriate infection control procedures (e.g., clean gloves).
2. Provide for client privacy.
3. Prepare the client.
   - Prior to performing the procedure, introduce self and verify the client's identity using agency protocol. **Rationale:** *This ensures that the right client receives the right medication.*
   - If not previously assessed, take the appropriate assessment measures necessary for the medication.
4. Explain the purpose of the medication and how it will help, using language that the client can understand. Include relevant information about the effects of the medication. **Rationale:** *Information can facilitate acceptance of and compliance with the therapy.*
5. Assemble the secondary infusion:
   - Close clamp on secondary infusion tubing. Spike the secondary medication infusion bag and fully flush the tubing, making sure no air is trapped in the tubing. Do not allow more than one or two drops of the solution to exit the tubing to ensure that the client receives the full dose of medication.
   - Hang the secondary container at or above the level of the primary infusion. Use the extension hook to lower the primary infusion if a piggyback setup is required. Some infusion pumps do not require this.
   - Attach the needleless cannula to the tubing.
   - Attach appropriate label to the secondary tubing. *Secondary tubing is usually changed every 24 to 48 hours. Check agency policy.*
   - If the secondary tubing remains from a prior medication administration, attach a new needleless cannula. **Rationale:** *Changing the needleless cannula will reduce the risk of transmission of microorganisms.*

> **CLINICAL ALERT**
> Each IV medication bag requires its own secondary tubing. Medication from the IV infusion bag remains in the secondary tubing. It is important, therefore, when hanging subsequent IV infusion bags to hang the same medication on the same secondary tubing. This avoids the mixing of incompatible medications.

6. Attach the secondary infusion to the primary infusion.
   - Clean the Y-port on the primary IV line with an antiseptic swab. Clean the **primary port** (the port furthest from the client) for a piggyback alignment and the **secondary port** (the port closest to the client) for a tandem setup.
   - If the medication is *not* compatible with the primary infusion, temporarily discontinue the primary infusion. Flush the primary line with a sterile saline solution before attaching the secondary set. To flush the line, wipe the port with an antiseptic swab, clamp the primary line, and, using a sterile syringe and needleless adapter, instill sufficient sterile saline solution through the port to flush any primary fluid out of the infusion tubing.
   - Insert the needleless cannula of the secondary line into the primary tubing port.
7. Back prime the secondary tubing if primary and secondary fluids are compatible.
   - Lower the medication infusion bag below the primary IV bag.
   - Open the clamp of the medication bag.
   - Allow the solution from the primary IV bag to backfill the secondary IV tubing and one third to one half of the secondary tubing chamber. **Rationale:** *This method of priming the secondary tubing allows for no loss of medication.*
   - Clamp the secondary IV tubing.
   - Hang the secondary IV bag on the IV pole.
8. Program the IV pump for the infusion rate of the IV medication bag.
9. Unclamp the secondary IV tubing and check that the secondary solution is infusing.
10. After infusion of the secondary IV medication bag, regulate the rate of the primary solution by adjusting the clamp or IV pump infusion rate. Some infusion pumps will do this automatically.
11. Leave the secondary bag and tubing in place for future administration or discard as appropriate.
12. Document relevant data.
    - Record the date, time, medication, dose, route, and solution; assessment of the IV site, if appropriate; and the client's response.
    - Record the volume of fluid of the medication infusion bag on the client's intake and output record.

VARIATION: USING A SALINE LOCK

Intermittent infusion devices may be attached to an intravenous catheter to allow medications to be administered intravenously without requiring a continuous intravenous infusion. The device may also have a port at one end of the lock and a needleless injection cap at the other end with the extension tubing between the two ends.

- Prepare two normal saline prefilled syringes (1 mL each).
- Spike the medication bag with minidrip (60 gtt/mL) IV tubing.
- Attach the needleless adapter to the tubing, prime the tubing, and close the clamp.
- Clean the needleless injection port of the saline lock with an antiseptic swab. Open the saline lock clamp, if appropriate.
- Insert first saline syringe into the port and gently aspirate to check for patency. Flush slowly noting any resistance, swelling, pain, or burning. **Rationale:** *This ensures placement of IV in vein.*
- After connecting the IV tubing to the injection port of the lock, administer the medication regulating the drip rate to allow medication to infuse for appropriate time period. Macrodrip (10

(continued on next page)

SKILL 2.43 Administering Intermittent Intravenous Medication (*continued*)

to 20 gtt/mL) tubing may also be used if using an IV pump to regulate the flow.

- When the medication has been infused, disconnect the IV tubing maintaining sterility of the end of the IV tubing. Insert the second saline syringe into the port and gently flush the saline lock. **Rationale:** *This clears the tubing and maintains patency.* Clamp the saline lock after flushing, if appropriate.
- Dispose of syringes in the appropriate container.

VARIATION: ADDING A MEDICATION TO A VOLUME-CONTROL INFUSION

- Withdraw the required dose of the medication into a syringe.
- Ensure that there is sufficient fluid in the volume-control fluid chamber to dilute the medication. Generally, at least 50 mL of

fluid is used. Check the directions from the drug manufacturer or consult the pharmacist.

- Close the inflow to the fluid chamber by adjusting the upper roller or slide clamp above the fluid chamber; also ensure that the clamp on the air vent of the chamber is open.
- Clean the medication port on the volume-control fluid chamber with an antiseptic swab.
- Inject the medication into the port of the appropriately filled volume-control set (i.e., the ordered amount of solution).
- Gently rotate the fluid chamber until the fluid is well mixed.
- Regulate the flow by adjusting the lower roller clamp below the fluid chamber.
- Attach a medication label to the volume-control fluid chamber.
- Document relevant data and monitor the client and the infusion.

SKILL 2.44 Administering Intravenous Medications Using IV Push

Delegation

The administration of intravenous medication via IV push involves the application of nursing knowledge and critical thinking. This procedure is not delegated to UAP. The nurse, however, can inform the UAP of the intended therapeutic effects and/or specific side effects of the medication and direct the UAP to report specific client observations to the nurse for follow-up.

Note: Administration of IV push medications varies by state nurse practice acts. For example, some states may allow the RN to delegate certain medications to be given by an LPN/LVN, whereas other states may allow only the RN to administer IV push medications. Nurses need to know their scope of practice according to their state's nurse practice act and agency policies.

Equipment

- Client's MAR
- Medication in a prefilled syringe, vial, or ampule
- Sterile syringe (3 to 5 mL) (to prepare the medication)
- Sterile needles, 2.5 cm (1 in.), 21 to 25 gauge (needle is not needed if using a needleless system)
- Antiseptic swabs
- Watch with a digital readout or second hand
- Clean gloves

IV Push for an IV Lock

- Client's MAR
- Medication in a prefilled syringe, vial, or ampule
- Sterile syringe (3 to 5 mL) (to prepare the medication)
- Sterile syringe (3 mL) (for the saline or heparin flush)
- Vial of preservative-free normal saline to flush the IV catheter or vial of heparin flush solution or both depending on agency practice. **Rationale:** *These maintain the patency of the IV lock. Saline is frequently used for peripheral locks.*
- Sterile needles (21 gauge) (needle is not needed if using a needleless system)
- Antiseptic swabs
- Watch with a digital readout or second hand
- Clean gloves

Preparation

- Check the MAR.
- Check the label on the medication carefully against the MAR to make sure that the correct medication is being prepared.
- Follow the three checks for correct medication and dose. Read the label on the medication (1) when it is taken from the medication cart, (2) before withdrawing the medication, and (3) after withdrawing the medication.
- Calculate medication dosage accurately and the recommended delivery rate (e.g., 20 mg over 1 minute).
- Confirm that the route is correct.
- Organize the equipment.

Procedure

1. Perform hand hygiene and observe other appropriate infection control procedures (e.g., clean gloves).
2. Prepare the medication.

Existing Line

- Prepare the medication according to the manufacturer's direction. **Rationale:** *It is important to have the correct dose and the correct dilution.*

IV Lock

- Flushing with saline:
  a. Prepare two syringes, each with 1 mL of sterile normal saline.
- Flushing with heparin (if indicated by agency policy) and saline:
  a. Prepare one syringe with 1 mL of heparin flush solution (if indicated by agency policy).
  b. Prepare two syringes with 1 mL each of sterile, normal saline.
  c. Draw up the medication into a syringe.

3. Put a small-gauge needle on the syringe if using a needle system.
4. Perform hand hygiene and apply clean gloves. **Rationale:** *This reduces the transmission of microorganisms and reduces the likelihood of the nurse's hands contacting the client's blood.*

SKILL 2.44 Administering Intravenous Medications Using IV Push (continued)

5. Provide for client privacy.
6. Prepare the client.
   - Prior to performing the procedure, introduce self and verify the client's identity using agency protocol. **Rationale:** *This ensures that the right client receives the right medication.*
   - If not previously assessed, take the appropriate assessment measures necessary for the medication. If any of the findings are above or below the predetermined parameters, consult the primary care provider before administering the medication.
7. Explain the purpose of the medication and how it will help, using language that the client can understand. Include relevant information about the effects of the medication. **Rationale:** *Information can facilitate acceptance of and compliance with the therapy.*
8. Administer the medication by IV push.

IV Lock with Needle

- Clean the injection port with the antiseptic swab. **Rationale:** *This prevents microorganisms from entering the circulatory system during needle insertion.*
- Insert the needle of the syringe containing normal saline through the center of the injection port and aspirate for blood. **Rationale:** *The presence of blood confirms that the catheter or needle is in the vein. In some situations, blood will not return even though the lock is patent.* Flush the lock by injecting saline using the push-pause method (a rapid succession of push-pause-push-pause movements exerted on the plunger of the syringe barrel). **Rationale:** *This creates a turbulence within the catheter lumen that causes a swirling effect to remove any debris (e.g., blood or medication) attached to the catheter lumen (Phillips, 2010, p. 351).*
- Remove the needle and syringe. Activate the needle safety device.
- Clean the lock's injection port with an antiseptic swab. **Rationale:** *This prevents the transfer of microorganisms.*
- Insert the needle of the syringe containing the prepared medication through the center of the injection port.
- Inject the medication slowly at the recommended rate of infusion. Use a watch or digital readout to time the injection. Observe the client closely for adverse reactions. Remove the needle and syringe when all medication has been administered. **Rationale:** *Injecting the drug too rapidly can have a serious untoward reaction.*
- Activate the needle safety device.
- Clean the injection port of the lock.
- Attach the second saline syringe, and inject 1 mL of saline. **Rationale:** *The saline injection flushes the medication through the catheter and prepares the lock for heparin if this medication is used. Heparin is incompatible with many medications.*
- If heparin is to be used, insert the heparin syringe and inject the heparin slowly into the lock.

IV Lock with Needleless System

- Clean the injection port of the lock.
- Insert syringe containing normal saline into the injection port. Flush the lock by injecting saline using the push-pause method (a rapid succession of push-pause-push-pause movements exerted on the plunger of the syringe barrel).

Rationale: *This creates a turbulence within the catheter lumen that causes a swirling effect to remove any debris (e.g., blood or medication) attached to the catheter lumen (Phillips, 2010, p. 351).*
- Remove the syringe.
- Insert the syringe containing the medication into the port.
- Inject the medication following the precautions described previously.
- Withdraw the syringe.
- Repeat injection of 1 mL of saline.

Existing Line

- Identify the injection port closest to the client. Some ports have a circle indicating the site for needle insertion. **Rationale:** *An injection port must be used because it is self-sealing. Any puncture to the plastic tubing will cause a leak.*
- Clean the port with an antiseptic swab.
- Stop the IV flow by closing the clamp or pinching the tubing above the injection port.
- Connect the syringe to the IV system.
  a. Needle system:
     - Hold the port steady.
     - Insert the needle of the syringe that contains the medication through the center of the port. **Rationale:** *This prevents damage to the IV line and to the diaphragm of the port.*
  b. Needleless system:
     - Remove the cap from the needleless syringe. Connect the tip of the syringe directly to the port.
     - Inject the medication at the ordered rate. Use the watch or digital readout to time the medication administration. **Rationale:** *This ensures safe drug administration because a too rapid injection could be dangerous.*
- After injecting the medication, withdraw the needle and activate the needle safety device. For a needleless system, detach the syringe and attach a new sterile cap to the port.
- Release the clamp or tubing. Resume IV flow as ordered.
9. Dispose of equipment according to agency practice. **Rationale:** *This reduces needlestick injuries and the spread of microorganisms.*
10. Remove and dispose of gloves. Perform hand hygiene.
11. Observe the client closely for adverse reactions.
12. Determine agency policy about recommended times for changing the IV lock. Some agencies advocate a change every 48 to 72 hours for peripheral IV devices.
13. Document all relevant information.
    - Record the date, time, drug, dose, and route; client response; and assessments of infusion or heparin lock site if appropriate.

VARIATION: POSITIONING A CHILD FOR INJECTIONS OR INTRAVENOUS ACCESS

Preparation

- Determine if the parent wants to be present during an uncomfortable procedure or to be available after the procedure to comfort the child.

(continued on next page)

SKILL 2.44 Administering Intravenous Medications Using IV Push *(continued)*

- When the parent wishes to be present, discuss the parent's role (e.g., holding the child or providing distraction or comfort during the procedure).
- Make sure the person positioning and holding the child (parent or other assistant) clearly understands what body parts must be held still and how to do this safely.

Procedure

Supine Position

1. Place the child in a supine position on a bed or stretcher. **Rationale:** *This position allows the child to see what is happening so that some of the child's fear is reduced.*
2. Have the parent, a nurse, or an assistant lean over the child to restrain the child's body and extend the extremity to be used for access or injection. **Rationale:** *The nurse's body provides a source of human contact as well as securing the child so that the procedure can be done quickly.*

Sitting Position

1. Have the child sit on the parent's or assistant's lap with his or her legs held firmly between the assistant's legs.
2. The child's arm closest to the adult can be wrapped around the back of the parent's or assistant's waist.
3. Have the parent or assistant hold the child firmly against the chest, wrapping arms around the child's upper body ❶. Hold firmly but gently, ensuring that the child has chest expansion allowing for normal breathing. **Rationale:** *This hugging position adds comfort as well as security so the procedure can be done quickly.*

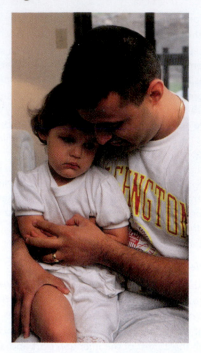

❶ The child should be restrained by the parent or assistant during intramuscular injections. Alternatively, the child's arm closest to the adult can be wrapped around the adult's waist, leaving just the other arm in front to immobilize. The leg not used for the injection is securely located between the adult's legs. Be certain that the child can breathe freely during restraining procedures.

▶ CRITICAL THINKING OPTIONS FOR UNEXPECTED OUTCOMES

Not all unexpected outcomes require further nursing intervention; however, many times they do. When the client demonstrates a change in signs/symptoms indicating an emerging problem, the nurse should immediately assess and troubleshoot what is happening. The assessment data must be processed quickly to formulate a hypothesis so the nurse can make a clinical judgment. The nurse then decides how best to resolve the problem and improve the client's situation for a better appropriate outcome.

EXPECTED OUTCOME	PROBLEM SOLVING	NURSING ACTIONS
Beds and Activities of Daily Living Bed remains clean, dry, and free of wrinkles.	Clients refuse to have bed made.	■ Assess reason for refusal. Client may be in pain or does not want to be disturbed. ■ Offer to make the bed at a later time. ■ Change only the pillowcase and drawsheet, if client allows. ■ Beds do not need to be changed unless soiled or damp, so allow client's independence, if possible.
Transmission of pathogenic microorganisms is prevented with universal precautions.	Cross-contamination occurs from improper linen disposal.	■ Provide adequate linen hampers for the nursing personnel. ■ Attend in-service education programs on infection control.
Client's skin, hair, and nails are clean, odor free, and without irritation.	Client's skin becomes irritated from linen or begins to break down.	■ Obtain hypoallergenic linen. ■ Place therapeutic mattress under client. ■ Provide skin care with appropriate lotion.
Bathing and hygiene care are completed without complications.	Even with increased oral hygiene, client still has odorous breath.	■ Use antiseptic mouthwash between oral hygiene care. ■ Notify the physician, as this could be a symptom of systemic disease. ■ Obtain dental consultation to check for presence of dental caries or gum disease. ■ Examine client's nutritional intake. Absent nutrients or imbalanced intake of fats, protein, or carbohydrates can result in bad breath.

EXPECTED OUTCOME	PROBLEM SOLVING	NURSING ACTIONS
Client is comfortable.	Client complains of extreme oral mucosal irritation or sensitivity.	■ Request physician's order for one of the following solutions: 　■ Saline solutions: for soothing, cleansing rinses 　■ Anesthetic solutions: to dull extreme pain in the oral cavity 　■ Effervescent solutions (e.g., hydrogen peroxide or ginger ale) to loosen and remove debris from the mouth 　■ Coating solutions (e.g., Maalox) to protect irritated surfaces 　■ Antibacterial–antifungal rinses (e.g., nystatin [Mycostatin]) to prevent the spread of organisms that cause thrush.
Bathing and hygiene care are completed without complications.	Client needs care after oral surgery or oral trauma.	■ Oral care following surgery or trauma is always ordered by physician. 　No oral hygiene care should be attempted until physician has clearly defined the specific care. ■ Suctioning equipment should always be present. ■ Assessment of client's head, face, neck, and general status is critical at this time.
	Client is unwilling to accept a complete bed bath.	■ Respect client's wishes and use other opportunities for assessment. ■ Have client wash hands, face, and genitals. You should wash back and give back care. Re-explain the purpose of the bath to the client and request client participation.
Client's skin, hair, and nails are clean, odor free, and without irritation.	Client has foul odor even after perineal care.	■ Obtain order for sitz bath. ■ Request order for medicated solution. ■ Request culture of discharge so the appropriate treatment can be instituted.
Client is comfortable.	Shaving is difficult and painful for the client.	■ Place warm towels on area to be shaved for 15 minutes. ■ Apply more shaving cream. ■ Ensure that razor is sharp.
Eyes and surrounding area are clean and free from crusting.	Eyelids become crusted from exudate.	■ Place warm, moist washcloth across eyes and leave in place for several minutes. ■ Moisten cotton applicator stick with sterile saline and gently twist the applicator stick over crusted surface to assist in removing crust.
Medication Administration Rationale for medication administration is clear.	Medication or dosage on MAR does not fit client's clinical picture.	■ Compare new MAR with previous MAR. ■ Compare new MAR with recent physician's orders. ■ Discuss concerns with agency protocol. ■ Contact physician for clarification.
Sign-out documentation for medications is accurate.	Medication sign-out sheet does not correspond to remaining stock.	■ Check with other nurses who may have dispensed stock medication. ■ Check MARs for unclaimed stock that may have been administered. ■ Complete discrepancy report if sign-out sheets and stock cannot be reconciled.
Medication is administered according to the "six rights."	Client receives wrong medication.	■ Document the medication administered on client's MAR. ■ Monitor client closely for potential undesired effects and document findings. ■ Notify client's physician and document. ■ Complete anonymous variance report according to agency policy. ■ Always check two client identifiers before administering medication.
Medication Preparation Dosage calculations are accurate.	Nurse is unsure of dosage calculation.	■ Utilize helpful calculation formulas. ■ Use a calculator. ■ Request that another nurse check calculation or conversion. ■ Seek agency pharmacist's assistance.

(continued on next page)

EXPECTED OUTCOME	PROBLEM SOLVING	NURSING ACTIONS
Complications of medication administration are prevented.	Client has an allergic or anaphylactic response to medication.	<ul><li>Immediately stop or hold medication.</li><li>Notify physician at once; prepare to administer epinephrine to dilate bronchi and support blood pressure.</li><li>If reaction is severe: Keep client flat in bed with head elevated. Take vital signs every 10–15 min; stay with client. Assess for hypotension or respiratory distress. Establish airway, if necessary. Have emergency equipment available. Provide psychological support to client to alleviate fears. Record type and progression of reactions.</li></ul>
Client takes medication without difficulty.	Client has difficulty swallowing medication.	<ul><li>Offer water before administering oral medication.</li><li>Crush medications if appropriate and administer mixed with food such as applesauce, pudding or jelly.</li><li>Consult pharmacist to dispense same medication in liquid form.</li><li>If difficulty continues, consult physician for altered route of medication delivery (rectal, parenteral).</li><li>Request swallow study.</li></ul>
	Client is nauseated and oral medications have not been taken.	<ul><li>Hold medication. Notify physician for antiemetic medication order and alternate route for administering necessary medications.</li><li>Administer antiemetic if ordered, then administer medication when client's nausea is relieved.</li></ul>
Medication therapeutic effect is achieved.	Client's discomfort is not relieved with sublingual nitroglycerin.	<ul><li>Check bottle for expiration date—potency is lost 3 months after opening bottle.</li><li>Administer second tablet in 5 min. If discomfort continues, administer opiate analgesic, call rapid response team, notify physician, and obtain stat ECG.</li><li>Administer no more than three tablets/sprays in a 15-min period.</li><li>Monitor for blood pressure effect. Hold medication if systolic BP is less than 90 mmHg.</li><li>Consult with physician for blood test for possible myocardial injury and need for continuous cardiac monitoring.</li></ul>
	Client fails to have BM after laxative suppository administration.	<ul><li>Reassess abdomen and check client for rectal fecal impaction.</li><li>Consult with physician to order oil-retention enema or cleansing enema.</li><li>Teach client ways to prevent constipation.</li></ul>
Desired local effect of medication is achieved without undesired side effects.	Client states that breathing has not improved after using inhaler.	<ul><li>Place client in Fowler's position. Validate that MDI/spacer/NPA device is functioning properly (e.g., canister shaken before use.)</li><li>Check number of actuations left in MDI canister.</li><li>Validate that client's lips have tight fit around MDI mouthpiece so mist is inhaled.</li><li>Instruct client to hold breath 10 sec after MDI use and to wait 2 min between puffs.</li></ul>
	Client using MDI reports painful white patches in mouth.	<ul><li>Instruct client to use spacer with MDI steroid medication.</li><li>Instruct client to rinse mouth with water and expectorate after administering MDI steroid.</li><li>Notify physician of findings.</li></ul>

EXPECTED OUTCOME	PROBLEM SOLVING	NURSING ACTIONS
Parenteral Routes Injection is administered without complications.	Ecchymosis occurs following heparin injection.	■ Rotate injection site. Do not inject medication into ecchymotic area. ■ Do not aspirate before injection or massage site following needle withdrawal. ■ Do not pinch tightly when forming fat pad in preparation for injection site. ■ Apply ice to area before injecting heparin.
	Medication is administered using wrong parenteral route.	■ Notify physician; medications may need to be administered to reverse the action of the medication. ■ Monitor client's response closely and report adverse findings immediately. ■ Medication administered IM or IV rather than subcutaneous route leads to faster absorption rates; therefore an assessment must be done to determine effects. (IV administration has immediate action.) ■ Complete unusual occurrence report according to agency policy.
	Client has allergic or anaphylactic response to medication.	■ Call rapid response team immediately. ■ Maintain a patent airway and follow ABCs of emergency care. ■ Notify client's physician. ■ Document incident; place allergy alert bracelet on client. ■ Complete unusual occurrence report according to agency policy.
Injection is as painless as possible.	Client experiences pain with IM injection.	■ Use Z-track method for ventrogluteal or vastus lateralis sites to prevent medication from leaking into subcutaneous tissue. ■ Use new needle for injection. ■ Inject medication slowly (10 sec/mL) to allow medication to diffuse. ■ Hold needle in place for 10 sec after injection. ■ Use a dry gauze sponge to apply pressure to site after withdrawing needle.
IV piggyback medication is compatible with IV solution.	Solution in primary IV tubing is incompatible with medication to be administered via secondary piggyback solution.	■ Turn primary infusion off. ■ Before administering medication, flush primary tubing with solution compatible with medication (e.g., normal saline). ■ Hang a separate solution compatible with medication and run through line to flush during drug administration.

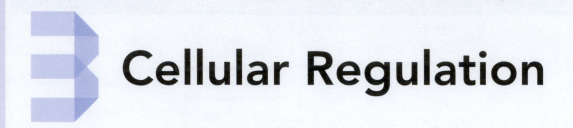

Cellular Regulation

RELATED CONCEPTS

The Concept of Cellular Regulation

Exemplar 2.1
  Cancer

Exemplar 2.2
  Anemia

Exemplar 2.5
  Leukemia

Exemplar 2.8
  Sickle Cell Disease

The Concept of Perfusion

Exemplar 16.5
  Disseminated Intravascular Coagulation

Exemplar 16.12
  Shock

Skills-at-a-Glance

The body strives to maintain homeostasis through both passive and active regulatory processes. Cellular regulation describes the many processes that occur within individual cells. Sometimes cells may develop abnormally in shape or at an extremely high rate, resulting in conditions that threaten the homeostasis of the body. Blood supports many of these processes and is vital for survival. Extreme changes in the quality of blood components or in the quantity of blood volume can lead to life-threatening conditions. This chapter includes nursing skills relative to supporting cellular regulation and perfusion processes.

Expected Outcomes

1. Priority considerations for client safety and comfort will be given during a bone marrow biopsy for best client outcomes in avoiding complications postprocedure.
2. Client is prepared psychologically and physically for procedure.
3. Specimens from studies sent to laboratory according to facility policy, in appropriate container, and in a timely manner.
4. Transfusions of blood or blood products will be done utilizing best evidence safety protocols to avoid errors and minimize occurrence of adverse reactions for best client outcomes.
5. Client's blood deficiency is corrected.
6. Transfusion reaction does not occur.

SKILL 3.1   Assisting with Bone Marrow Aspiration

A common type of diagnostic study is the **biopsy**. A biopsy is a procedure whereby tissue is obtained for examination. Biopsies are performed on many different types of tissues, for example, bone marrow, liver, breast, lymph nodes, and lung.

A bone marrow biopsy is the removal of a specimen of bone marrow for laboratory study. The biopsy is used to detect specific diseases of the blood, such as pernicious anemia and leukemia. The bones of the body commonly used for a bone marrow biopsy are the sternum, iliac crests, anterior or posterior iliac spines, and proximal tibia in children. The *posterior superior iliac crest* is the preferred site with the client placed prone or on the side ❶.

After injecting a local anesthetic, a small incision may be made with a scalpel to avoid tearing the skin or pushing skin into the bone marrow with a needle. The primary care provider then introduces a bone marrow needle with stylet into the red marrow of the spongy bone ❷.

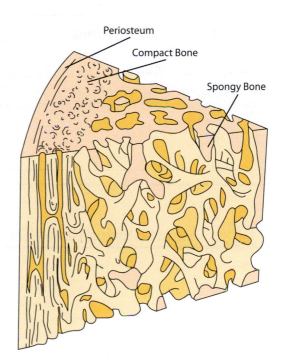

❷ A cross section of a bone.

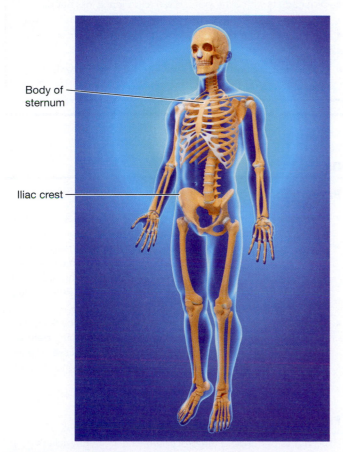

❶ The sternum and the iliac crests are common sites for a bone marrow biopsy.
© Science Photo Library/Alamy

Once the needle is in the marrow space, the stylet is removed and a 10-mL syringe is attached to the needle. The plunger is withdrawn until 1 to 2 mL of marrow has been obtained. The primary care provider replaces the stylet in the needle, withdraws the needle, and places the specimen in test tubes and/or on glass slides. The nurse places a small sterile dressing over the puncture site. Nursing actions to assist with bone marrow biopsy are provided in **Table 3–1** ●.

(continued on next page)

SKILL 3.1 Assisting with Bone Marrow Aspiration (continued)

TABLE 3–1 Assisting with Bone Marrow Aspiration

PROCEDURE	BEFORE THE PROCEDURE	DURING THE PROCEDURE	AFTER THE PROCEDURE
Bone marrow biopsy	Prepare the client: ■ Explain the procedure. The client may experience pain when the marrow is aspirated and hear a crunching sound as the needle is pushed through the cortex of the bone. The procedure usually takes 15–30 minutes. Explain when and where the procedure will occur, who will be present, and which site will be used. ■ Help the client assume a supine position (with one pillow if desired) for a biopsy of the sternum (sternal puncture) or a prone position for a biopsy of either iliac crest. Fold the bedclothes back or drape the client to expose the area. ■ Administer a sedative as ordered.	Monitor and support the client throughout: ■ Describe the steps of the procedure as needed and provide verbal support. ■ Observe the client for pallor, diaphoresis, and faintness due to bleeding or pain. Place a small sterile dressing over the site of the puncture after the needle is withdrawn. ■ Some agency protocols recommend applying direct pressure over the site for 5–10 minutes to prevent bleeding. Assist with preparing specimens as needed.	Monitor the client: ■ Assess for discomfort and bleeding from the site. The client may experience some tenderness in the area. Bleeding and hematoma formation need to be assessed for several days. Report bleeding or pain to the nurse in charge. ■ Provide an analgesic as needed and ordered. Document all relevant information: ■ Include date and time of the procedure; the primary care provider's name; and any nursing assessments and interventions. Document any specimens obtained. Transport the specimens to the laboratory.

Developmental Considerations

CHILDREN

■ Young clients need emotional support due to the pain and pressure associated with this procedure.

■ Young clients may require gentle restraint to prevent movement during the procedure.

OLDER ADULTS

■ Older adults with osteoporosis will experience less needle pressure.

■ Ask the client to empty the bladder for comfort before the procedure.

■ Provide pillows and blankets to help older adults remain comfortable during the procedure.

SKILL 3.2 Administering Blood Transfusions

Delegation

Due to the need for sterile technique and technical complexity, blood transfusion is not delegated to UAP. The nurse must ensure that the UAP knows what complications or adverse signs can occur and should be reported to the nurse. In some stages, only RNs can administer blood or blood products.

Equipment

■ Unit of whole blood, packed RBCs, or other component
■ Blood administration set
■ IV pump, if needed
■ 250 mL normal saline for infusion
■ IV pole
■ Venipuncture start kit containing a 18- to 20-gauge needle or catheter (if one is not already in place) or, if the blood is to be administered quickly, a larger catheter
■ Alcohol swabs
■ Tape
■ Clean gloves

Preparation

■ If the client has an intravenous solution infusing, check whether the IV catheter and solution are appropriate to administer blood. The preferred IV catheter size is #18 to #20 gauge, and the solution *must* be normal saline. Dextrose (which causes lysis of RBCs), Ringer solution, medications, and other additives, and hyperalimentation solutions are incompatible. Refer to step 5 below if the infusing solution is not compatible.

■ If the client does not have an IV solution infusing, check agency policies. In some agencies an infusion must be running before the blood is obtained from the blood bank. In this case, you will need to perform a venipuncture on a suitable vein and start an IV infusion of normal saline.

Procedure

1. Prior to performing the procedure, check the physician's order, introduce self and verify the client's identity using agency protocol. Ensure signed consent is in record. Explain to the client what you are going to do and why. Instruct the

SKILL 3.2 Administering Blood Transfusions (continued)

client to report promptly any sudden chills, nausea, itching, rash, dyspnea, back pain, or other unusual symptoms. .

2. Provide for client privacy and prepare the client.
   - Assist the client to a comfortable position, either sitting or lying. Expose the IV site but provide for client privacy.
3. Perform hand hygiene and observe other appropriate infection control procedures.
4. Prepare the infusion equipment.
   - Ensure that the blood filter inside the drip chamber is suitable for the blood components to be transfused. Attach the blood tubing to the blood filter, if necessary. **Rationale:** *Blood filters have a surface area large enough to allow the blood components through easily but are designed to trap clots.*
   - Apply gloves.
   - Close all the clamps on the Y-set: the main flow rate clamp and both Y-line clamps.
   - Insert the piercing pin (spike) into the saline solution.
   - Hang the container on the IV pole about 1 m (39 in.) above the venipuncture site.
5. Prime the tubing.
   - Open the upper clamp on the normal saline tubing, and squeeze the drip chamber until it covers the filter and one third of the drip chamber above the filter.
   - Tap the filter chamber to expel any residual air in the filter.
   - Open the main flow rate clamp, and prime the tubing with saline.
   - Close both clamps.
6. Start the saline solution.
   - If an IV solution incompatible with blood is infusing, stop the infusion and discard the solution and tubing according to agency policy.
   - Attach the blood tubing primed with normal saline to the intravenous catheter.
   - Open the saline and main flow rate clamps and adjust the flow rate. Use only the main flow rate clamp to adjust the rate.
   - Allow a small amount of solution to infuse to make sure there are no problems with the flow or with the venipuncture site. **Rationale:** *Infusing normal saline before initiating the transfusion also clears the IV catheter of incompatible solutions or medications.*
7. Obtain the correct blood component for the client.
   - Check the order with the requisition.
   - Check the requisition form and the blood bag label with a laboratory technician or according to agency policy. Specifically, check the client's name, identification number, blood type (A, B, AB, or O) and Rh group, the blood donor number, and the expiration date of the blood. Observe the blood for abnormal color, clumping, gas bubbles, and extraneous material. Return outdated or abnormal blood to the blood bank.
   - With another nurse (most agencies require an RN), verify the following before initiating the transfusion (Phillips, 2010, p. 747):
     - *Order:* Check the blood or component against the primary care provider's written order.
     - *Client identification:* The name and identification number on the client's identification band must be identical to the name and number attached to the unit of blood.

   - *Unit identification:* The unit identification number on the blood container, the transfusion form, and the tag attached to the unit must agree.
   - *ABO and Rh type:* The ABO group and Rh type on the primary label of the donor unit must agree with those recorded on the transfusion form.
   - *Expiration:* The expiration date and time of the donor unit should be verified as acceptable.
   - *Compatibility:* The interpretation of compatibility testing must be recorded on the transfusion form and on the tag attached to the unit.
   - If any of the information does not match *exactly*, notify the charge nurse and the blood bank. Do not administer blood until discrepancies are corrected or clarified.
   - Sign the appropriate form with the other nurse according to agency policy.
   - Make sure that RBCs are left at room temperature for no more than 30 minutes before starting the transfusion. Agencies may designate different times at which the blood must be returned to the blood bank if it has not been started. **Rationale:** *As blood components warm, the risk of bacterial growth increases.* If the start of the transfusion is unexpectedly delayed, return the blood to the blood bank within 30 minutes. Do **not** store blood in the unit refrigerator. **Rationale:** *The temperature of unit refrigerators is not precisely regulated and the blood may be damaged.*
8. Prepare the blood bag.
   - Invert the blood bag gently several times to mix the cells with the plasma. **Rationale:** *Rough handling can damage the cells.*
   - Expose the port on the blood bag by pulling back the tabs [1].
   - Insert the remaining Y-set spike into the blood bag.
   - Suspend the blood bag.
9. Establish the blood transfusion.
   - Close the upper clamp below the IV saline solution container.
   - Open the upper clamp below the blood bag. The blood will run into the saline-filled drip chamber. If necessary, squeeze the drip chamber to reestablish the liquid level with the drip chamber one third full. (Tap the filter to expel any residual air within the filter.)
   - Readjust the flow rate with the main clamp.
   - Remove and discard gloves. Perform hand hygiene.
10. Observe the client closely for the first 15 minutes.
    - It is recommended that transfusions of RBCs be started at 5 mL/min for the first 15 minutes of the transfusion. **Rationale:** *This small amount is enough to produce a severe reaction but small enough that the reaction could be treated successfully* (Phillips, 2010, p. 749).
    - Note adverse reactions, such as chilling, nausea, vomiting, skin rash, or tachycardia. **Rationale:** *The earlier a transfusion reaction occurs, the more severe it tends to be. Promptly identifying such reactions helps to minimize the consequences.*
    - Remind the client to call a nurse immediately if any unusual symptoms are felt during the transfusion such as chills, nausea, itching, rash, dyspnea, or back pain.
    - If any of these reactions occur, report these to the nurse in charge, and take appropriate nursing action.

(continued on next page)

SKILL 3.2 Administering Blood Transfusions (continued)

11. Document relevant data.
    - Record starting the blood, including vital signs, type of blood, blood unit number, sequence number (e.g., #1 of three ordered units), site of the venipuncture, size of the needle, and drip rate.
12. Monitor the client.
    - Fifteen minutes after initiating the transfusion (or according to agency policy), check the vital signs. If there are no signs of a reaction, establish the required flow rate. Most adults can tolerate receiving one unit of blood in 1½ to 2 hours. Do not transfuse a unit of blood for longer than 4 hours.
    - Assess the client, including vital signs, every 30 minutes or more often, depending on the health status and agency policy. If the client has a reaction and the blood is discontinued, send the blood bag to the laboratory for investigation of the blood.
13. Terminate the transfusion.
    - Apply clean gloves.
    - If no infusion is to follow, clamp the blood tubing. Check agency protocol to determine if the blood component bag needs to be returned or if the blood bag and tubing can be disposed of in a biohazard container. The IV line can be discontinued or capped with an adapter, or a new infusion line and solution container may be added. If another transfusion is to follow, clamp the blood tubing and open the saline infusion arm. A new blood administration set is to be used with each component (Phillips, 2010, p. 751).
    - If the primary IV is to be continued, flush the maintenance line with saline solution. Disconnect the blood tubing system and reestablish the intravenous infusion using new tubing. Adjust the drip to the desired rate. Often a normal saline or other solution is kept running in case of delayed reaction to the blood.
    - Measure vital signs.
14. Follow agency protocol for appropriate disposition of the used supplies.
    - Discard the administration set according to agency practice.
    - Dispose of blood bags and administration sets.
      a. On the requisition attached to the blood unit, fill in the time the transfusion was completed and the amount transfused.
      b. Attach one copy of the requisition to the client's record and another to the empty blood bag if required by agency policy.
      c. Agency policy generally involves returning the bag to the blood bank for reference in case of subsequent or delayed adverse reaction.
    - Remove and discard gloves. Perform hand hygiene.
15. Document relevant data.
    - Record completion of the transfusion, the amount of blood absorbed, the blood unit number, and the vital signs. If the primary intravenous infusion was continued, record connecting it. Also record the transfusion on the IV flow sheet and intake and output record.

Sample Documentation

4/21/15 1420 c/o feeling warm, headache, & backache. Skin flushed. T 102.6°F, BP 140/90 mmHg, P 112 bpm, R 28/min. Approximately 50 mL PRBCs infused over past 20 minutes. Infusion stopped. Tubing changed, NS infusing at 15 mL/h. Blood & admin. tubing sent to blood bank. Dr. Riley notified. _____ C. Jones, RN

SKILL 3.3 Administering Blood Components

Equipment

- Blood component
- Appropriate IV administration kit
- Filter, if indicated
- Clean gloves

Procedure

1. Check physician's orders and client's signed consent for transfusion.
2. Obtain blood component and administration set.
3. Introduce self, explain the procedure, and verify client's identity.
4. Perform hand hygiene and don gloves.
5. Follow directions for proper administration of the solution.
6. Identify rate at which blood component should infuse.
7. Document procedure and client response.

Modified Blood Products

In addition to the usual blood components such as platelets and cryoprecipitate, modified blood products are becoming more popular. Washed, irradiated, or leukocyte-removed blood is being used for clients at risk because of multiple transfusions or a weakened immune system. Testing for cytomegalovirus and matching RBC or human leukocyte antigens is also done to ensure safe transfusions.

Note, however, that when infusing a blood product that has undergone leukocyte reduction, it still must be filtered again through a standard blood administration set in order to trap cellular debris that may have accumulated since the original filtration.

▶ CRITICAL THINKING OPTIONS FOR UNEXPECTED OUTCOMES

Not all unexpected outcomes require further nursing intervention; however, many times they do. When the client demonstrates a change in signs/symptoms indicating an emerging problem, the nurse should immediately assess and troubleshoot what is happening. The assessment data must be processed quickly to formulate a hypothesis so the nurse can make a clinical judgment. The nurse then decides how best to resolve the problem and improve the client's situation for a better appropriate outcome.

EXPECTED OUTCOME	PROBLEM SOLVING	NURSING ACTIONS
Priority considerations for client safety and comfort will be given during a bone marrow biopsy for best client outcomes in avoiding complications postprocedure.	Bleeding occurs from puncture site after bone marrow aspiration.	■ Apply direct pressure until pressure dressing can be applied. ■ Monitor amount of blood loss. ■ Monitor vital signs ■ Notify physician.
Client is prepared psychologically and physically for procedure.	Client very apprehensive and refuses procedure at last minute.	■ Identify reasons for anxiety and attempt to allay fears. ■ Notify physician and ask if he or she wants to cancel or postpone test to later time. Do not attempt to "talk client into it." ■ Discuss use of sedation during procedure.
Transfusion reaction does not occur.	Transfusion reaction occurs.	■ Stop blood administration and begin infusion of normal saline to keep IV open. ■ Check transfusion reaction form for appropriate nursing intervention. ■ Complete all relevant nursing actions.
Transfusions of blood or blood products will be done utilizing best evidence safety protocols to avoid errors and minimize occurrence of adverse reactions for best client outcomes.	Blood does not flow through tubing.	■ Check client's IV site and gauge of catheter (at least 18 or 20 gauge). ■ Gently agitate blood bag to mix blood cells with the anticoagulant. ■ Raise blood bag higher on IV pole. Squeeze flexible tubing to promote blood flow. ■ Adjust clamp on tubing. As the blood passes over the filter, more blood microaggregates clog the filter and slow drip rate. ■ Replace tubing. ■ Utilize an infusion pump, especially if administering blood through a small catheter.
	Potential circulatory overload occurs.	■ Monitor symptoms: sudden dyspnea, tachypnea, tachycardia, chest discomfort, distended neck veins, moist crackles and rales, restlessness, sudden increase in blood pressure. ■ Stop transfusion and place client in Fowler's position. ■ Start oxygen at 2 L/min per nasal cannula. ■ Be prepared for ECG and chest x-ray. ■ Be prepared to administer Lasix and morphine sulfate.

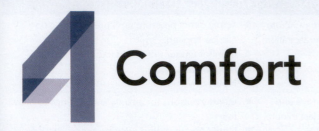

Comfort

RELATED CONCEPTS

Skills-at-a-Glance

Comfort interventions are done to ease a client's physical or psychological distress or pain. A client's pain experience is dependent on many variables that individualize it to the client; for example, an acute process versus a chronic condition, a high versus a low pain threshold, and the use of alternative therapies for pain management. Comfort may be obtained with nonpharmacologic and pharmacologic approaches, or a combination of both. This chapter includes a variety of interventions to meet a client's need for comfort based on the individual's preferences, ability to participate, and effectiveness.

▶ ACUTE/CHRONIC PAIN MANAGEMENT

Expected Outcomes

1. Pain is controlled through nonpharmacologic methods such as massage, relaxation techniques, or TENS.
2. Client is satisfied with level of pain control.
3. Client receives adequate pain medications; pain level does not interfere with ambulation, getting out of bed, etc.
4. Client's anxiety level is lowered in relation to pain.
5. Client is able to identify and alleviate stress caused by mental concerns.

SKILL 4.1 Assessing the Client in Pain

Delegation

The nurse is responsible for the initial and regular reassessment of pain. As the fifth vital sign, it may be that unlicensed assistive personnel (UAP) most frequently assess clients for pain if they are responsible for vital signs. After the assessment and in collaboration with the client, the nurse can discuss and delegate the performance of appropriate comfort measures to UAP. For example, the UAP may reposition the client at regular intervals, give the client a back massage, or provide rest periods. Emphasize to the UAP the importance of reporting any changes in the client's pain to the nurse.

Equipment

- Pain assessment flow sheet ❶
- Pain rating scale

Preparation

- Identify those factors that may cause the client to be in pain. For example, does the client have a prior history of low back pain or diabetic neuropathy? Has the client had a major surgical procedure? Has the client experienced recent trauma? Note the client's baseline vital signs.

Procedure

1. Prior to performing the procedure, introduce self and verify the client's identity using agency protocol. Explain to the client what you are going to do, why it is necessary, and how he or she can participate. Discuss how the results will be used in planning further care or treatments.
2. Perform hand hygiene and observe other appropriate infection control procedures.
3. Provide for client privacy.
4. Assess client's perception of pain. For clients experiencing acute or severe pain, the nurse may focus on the first three aspects of the assessment—determining location, intensity,

and quality—and quickly follow with an intervention. Clients with less severe or chronic pain can usually provide a more detailed description and the nurse can obtain a comprehensive pain assessment.

- *Location:* Ask the client to place a mark on the figure on the pain assessment flow sheet or form, if appropriate. If there is more than one area of pain, use letters (e.g., A, B, C) to differentiate among the various sites. If the client is unable or unwilling to mark the figure, ask the client to tell you where the pain is located. Follow up by asking the client to point to the painful site with one finger. **Rationale:** *This will help verify if the verbal description and the location are the same.*
- *Intensity:* Ask the client to rate the pain using the appropriate scale per agency policy.
- *Quality:* Ask the client, "What words would you use to describe your pain?" **Rationale:** *Although this question may be difficult for the client to answer, the assessment is most accurate when the client provides the description.*
- *Onset, duration, and recurrence:* This assessment can include such questions as "How long have you been having pain?" "Have you noticed any activity (e.g., swallowing, eating, stress, urinating, exertion) that increases or decreases the pain?" "How long does the pain last?" "How often does the pain occur?" "Is the pain better or worse at certain times of the day or night?"
- *Manner of expressing pain:* Observe for behavioral cues such as grimacing, crying, or a change in body posture ❷. **Rationale:** *Learning how a client expresses pain is particularly important for the client who cannot communicate or is very young, very old, or unable to hear.*
- *Precipitating factors:* Ask what causes or increases the pain. **Rationale:** *Knowledge of those activities can both help prevent the pain from occurring and, sometimes, help determine the cause.*

(continued on next page)

Sunrise Hospital and Medical Center & Sunrise Children's Hospital
Pain Management Flow Sheet

SR-1420 (6/00)

Patient's stated pain level goal: _____

*Monitoring Guidelines outlined on back of form

Mode of Administration

A-PO opioid and nonopioid medications
B-PCA Infuser Basal with Patient Control
C-Continuous Infusion
D-Epidural Infuser Continuous Basal Only
E-Epidural Infuser Basal & Patient Control
F-Intermittent IV/IM Injection
G-Transdermal opioids
H-On-QPump
I-Per Rectum

Level of Pain Assessment Scales

Faces Pain Rating Scale

0 ...... 2 ...... 4 ...... 6 ...... 8 10

1-10 Pain Scale

No pain or pain relieved   Worst pain imaginable

0-10 Sum Scale

0 - - - - - - - - - - - - 10

A. Vocal
0 = Positive/ETT
1 = Whimpers
2 = Crying
3 = Screaming

C. Facial
0 = Smiling
1 = Neutral
2 = Frown/grimace
3 = Clenched teeth

B. Body Movement
0 = Moves easily
1 = Neutral shifting
2 = Tense/flailing limbs

D. Touching (localizing)
0 = Notouching
1 = Reaching/patting
2 = Grabbing

Location of Pain:

Right   Left

Left   Right

Frequency of Pain:
A = No pain.
B-Z = Use letters to mark location of pain on graph
0 = Occasional   F = Frequent   C = Constant

Type of Pain:
A = Burning   D = Sharp   G = Isolated
B = Stabbing   E = Shooting   H = Other
C = Radiating   F = Dull

Arousal Score:
0 = Alert   1 = Medically sedated/ETT
2 = Drowsy   3 = Somnolent
                   4 = Asleep

Non-Pharmacologic Interventions:
C = Cold   P = Pacifier
D = Distraction   PO = Positioning
H = Heat   R = Relaxation
HO = Holding   RO = Rocking
I = Imagery   S = SecurityObject
M = Massage   T = TensUnit
MU = Music   O = Other

Analgesia Order:
1 = Increase in dosage/rate
2 = Decrease in doseage/rate
3 = Extra bolus
4 = PRN medication for break-through pain
5 = Discontinue

Reason for Analgesia Order:
1 = Unrelieved pain
2 = Decreased arousal/neuroscore
3 = Side effects (See below)
4 = Discontinue therapy/change to oral route
5 = Adverse drug reactions
(Document all adverse drug reactions in Nsg notes and complete an ADR report)

Side Effects:
0 = None
A = Anxiety   N = Nausea
C = Confused   R = Respiratory Depression
Co = Constipation U = Urinary Rentention
I = Itching   V = Vomiting

Sensory Function   Epidural Only
0 = Moves all extremities well
1 = Unable to move all extremities well

Motor Function   Epidural Only
0 = Able to feel tactile pressure
1 = Unable to feel tactile pressure

Neuro Score: Epidural Only
0 = No numbness, no weakness
1 = Medically sedated/ETT
2 = Numbness without weakness
3 = Numbness and weakness

Catheter Site: Epidural Only
1 = No redness, drainage, inflammation or swelling
2 = Red, inflamed
3 = Visable clear drainage
4 = Visable purulent drainage
5 = Visable serosanguinous/sanguinous drainage
6 = Swelling

Catheter Integrity Upon Removal: Epidural Only
1 = Catheter tip visually intact
2 = Catheter NOT visually intact-See Nsg Notes

Date											
Time											
Initials											
Mode of Admin											
Level of Pain											
Location of Pain											
Frequency of Pain											
Type of Pain											
Arousal Score											
Non-Pharm. Intervent.											
Analgesia Order											
Reason for Order											
Side Effects											
Adverse Effects (Y/N)											
Sensory Function Epidural Only											
Motor Function Epidural Only											
Neuro Score Epidural Only											
Catheter Site Epidural Only											
Cath Integrity Epidural Only											
O2 Saturation											
Respirations											
Pulse											
Blood Pressure											
See Nursing Notes (Y/N)											

Initials	Signature			

Patient Identification Label

1 Pain management flow sheet. Children's Hospital. Courtesy of Aprille Ciaverella, RN, and Lori Townsend, RN, at Sunrise Hospital and Medical Center and Sunrise Children's Hospital, Las Vegas, Nevada.

SKILL 4.1   Assessing the Client in Pain *(continued)*

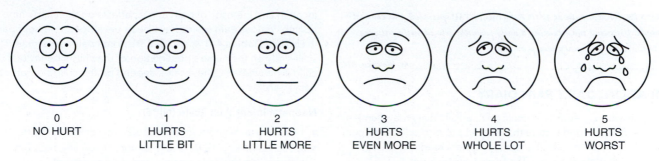

0	1	2	3	4	5
NO HURT	HURTS LITTLE BIT	HURTS LITTLE MORE	HURTS EVEN MORE	HURTS WHOLE LOT	HURTS WORST

Explain to the person that each face is for a person who feels happy because he has no pain (hurt) or sad because he has some or a lot of pain. Face 0 is very happy because he doesn't hurt at all. Face 1 hurts just a little bit. Face 2 hurts a little more. Face 3 hurts even more. Face 4 hurts a whole lot. Face 5 hurts as much as you can imagine, although you don't have to be crying to feel this bad. Ask the person to choose the face that best describes how he is feeling.

Rating scale is recommended for individuals age 3 years of age and older.

Brief word instructions: Point to each face using the words to describe the pain intensity. Ask the child to choose the face that best describes own pain and record the appropriate number.

② The FACES rating scale. From Hockenberry MJ, Wilson D: Wong's essentials of pediatric nursing, 9th ed., St. Louis, 2013, Mosby. Used with permission. Copyright Mosby.

- *Alleviating factors:* Ask questions such as "What makes the pain go away or lessen?" "What methods of relief have you tried?" "How long did you use them?" "How effective were they?" **Rationale:** *Asking these questions can assist the nurse and the client to determine if some of the methods (such as listening to music or relaxation) can continue to be used while at the healthcare facility.*
- *Associated symptoms:* Ask if there are any other symptoms (e.g., nausea, vomiting, dizziness) that occur prior to, with, or after the pain. **Rationale:** *These symptoms may relate to the onset of the pain or may result from the presence of the pain.*
- *Effects of pain:* Explore the client's feelings and the effect the pain has on the client's life. This is particularly important for the client with chronic pain. **Rationale:** *Assessing the areas of sleep, appetite, physical activity, relationships, emotions, and concentration provides the nurse with information about the level of the client's functioning on a daily basis.*
- *Other comments:* Ask if there is any other information that would be helpful for the primary care providers and nurses to know. Emphasize that you want to work with the client and family to get the best control of the pain.

5. Assess physiological response to pain. Note blood pressure, pulse rate, respiratory rate, skin color, and presence of diaphoresis. **Rationale:** *Signs of sympathetic nervous system stimulation (fight or flight) may be present with acute pain; however, clients with chronic pain may not have physical signs because of CNS adaptation.*
6. Assess affected body part, if appropriate. **Rationale:** *Additional assessment may provide additional information about the pain and possible intervention.*
7. Document findings of the pain assessment and include the intervention(s) and the client's response to the interventions. **Rationale:** *Thorough assessment and documentation assists the nurse to gain insights into the nature and pattern of the client's pain and ensures continuity of care. Maintaining a pain management flow sheet (see ①) will clarify and communicate each client's pain experience to enhance effective pain relief efforts. In settings where a pain management flow sheet is not used, data can be documented in the client record as in the following Sample Documentation section.*

Sample Documentation

7/22/15 0900 Admitted for elective foot surgery. c/o dull, throbbing, continuous pain in right cheek and jaw area radiating to right shoulder. Rates pain at 6/10. States pain began 6 months ago. Holding jaw throughout interview, became teary when describing negative effects on sleep, mood, and daily functioning. Associates onset with stress at work, and states she has been clenching her teeth throughout the day and grinding her teeth during sleep. States pain seems worse today with anxiety about surgery. Reports that Advil and heating pad relieve pain temporarily. Given moist heat pack to use now and relaxation breathing demonstrated with client participation. _____ *M. Blaszko, RN*

CLINICAL ALERT

Perception is reality. The client's self-report of pain is what must be used to determine pain intensity. The nurse is obligated to record the pain intensity as reported by the client. By challenging the believability of the client's report, the nurse is undermining the therapeutic relationship and preventing the fulfillment of advocacy and helping people with pain, which is called for in the American Nurses Association's Standards of Professional Performance for Pain Management Nursing.

(Sample Documentation continued on next page)

SKILL 4.1   Assessing the Client in Pain (continued)

7/22/15 0930 Rates pain at 1/10. Referrals to TMJ specialist and counseling made. Discussed maintaining a daily pain diary to identify patterns and to share with primary care provider.

——————————————————————M. Blaszko, RN

VARIATION: DAILY PAIN DIARY

For clients who experience chronic pain, a daily diary may illuminate pain patterns and factors that exacerbate or mediate the pain experience. In home care, the family or other caregiver can be taught to complete the diary. The record can include:

- Time or onset of pain and activity or situation preceding pain
- Relevant data (e.g., weather conditions the client deems significant)
- Physical pain character (quality) and intensity level (1–10)
- Emotions experienced and intensity level (0–10)
- Use of analgesics or other relief measures
- Duration of pain
- Time spent in relief activities and effectiveness of these activities.

VARIATION: CHILD PAIN ASSESSMENT

Pain is considered the fifth vital sign, and every child has the right to be assessed for pain and receive pain management. The goal of pain assessment is to provide accurate information about the location and intensity of pain and its effects on the child's functioning. Various pain scales have been developed to assess pain in children (**Tables 4–1** ● and **4–2** ●). Some pain assessment scales rely on the nurse's observation of the child's behavior if the child is nonverbal. Other scales depend on the child's report of pain intensity.

Neonatal Infant Pain Scale (NIPS)

- Use in preterm and term infants up to 6 weeks after birth.
- Observe the infant's facial expression, cry quality, breathing pattern, arm and leg position, and state of arousal.

FLACC Pain Scale

- This scale is designed to measure acute pain in infants and young children following surgery or while sleeping.
- FLACC is an acronym for the five categories that are assessed: face, legs, activity, cry, and consolability.
- Use until the child is able to self-report pain with another pain scale.

Oucher Scale

- Use in children between 3 and 7 years of age. Select the scale that matches the child's ethnic background—Caucasian, African American, or Hispanic.
- The child selects the face that matches his or her level of pain ❸. The older child can select a number between 0 and 10.

TABLE 4–1   Neonatal Infant Pain Scale (NIPS)

CHARACTERISTIC	SCORING CRITERIA
Facial Expression	
0 = Relaxed muscles	■ Restful face with neutral expression
1 = Grimace	■ Tight facial muscles; furrowed brow, chin, and jaw (*Note:* At low gestational ages, infants may have no facial expression.)
Cry	
0 = No cry	■ Quiet, not crying
1 = Whimper	■ Mild moaning, intermittent cry
2 = Vigorous cry	■ Loud screaming, rising, shrill, and continuous (*Note:* Silent cry may be scored if infant in intubated, as indicated by obvious facial movements.)
Breathing Patterns	
0 = Relaxed	■ Relaxed, usual breathing pattern maintained
1 = Change in breathing	■ Change in breathing, irregular, faster than usual, gagging, or holding breath
Arm Movements	
0 = Relaxed/restrained	■ Relaxed, no muscle rigidity, occasional random (with soft restraints) movements of the arms
1 = Flexed/extended	■ Tense, straight arms; rigid; or rapid extension and flexion
Leg Movements	
0 = Relaxed/restrained	■ Relaxed, no muscle rigidity, occasional random (with soft restraints) movements of legs
1 = Flexed/extended	■ Tense, straight legs; rigid; or rapid extension and flexion
State of Arousal	
0 = Sleeping/awake	■ Quiet, peaceful, sleeping; or alert and settled
1 = Fussy	■ Alert and restless or thrashing; fussy

Source: Data from Lawrence et al. (1993) and Morrow (2010).

SKILL 4.1   Assessing the Client in Pain *(continued)*

TABLE 4–2   FLACC Behavioral Pain Assessment Scale

CATEGORIES	SCORING		
	0	1	2
Face	No particular expression or smile	Occasional grimace or frown; withdrawn, disinterested	Frequent to constant frown, clenched jaw, quivering chin
Legs	Normal position or relaxed	Uneasy, restless, tense	Kicking or legs drawn up
Activity	Lying quietly, normal position, moves easily	Squirming, shifting back and forth, tense	Arched, rigid, or jerking
Cry	No cry (awake or asleep)	Moans or whimpers; occasional complaint	Crying steadily, screams or sobs; frequent complaints
Consolability	Content, relaxed	Reassured by occasional touching, hugging, or being talked to; distractible	Difficult to console or comfort

How to Use the FLACC

In clients who are awake: Observe for 1 to 5 minutes or longer. Observe legs and body uncovered. Reposition client or observe activity. Assess body for tenseness and tone. Initiate consoling interventions if needed.

In clients who are asleep: Observe for 5 minutes or longer. Observe body and legs uncovered. If possible, reposition the client. Touch the body and assess for tenseness and tone.

Face
- Score 0 if the client has a relaxed face, makes eye contact, shows interest in surroundings.
- Score 1 if the client has a worried facial expression, with eyebrows lowered, eyes partially closed, cheeks raised, mouth pursed.
- Score 2 if the client has deep furrows in the forehead, closed eyes, an open mouth, deep lines around nose and lips.

Legs
- Score 0 if the muscle tone and motion in the limbs are normal.
- Score 1 if client has increased tone, rigidity, or tension; if there is intermittent flexion or extension of the limbs.
- Score 2 if client has hypertonicity, the legs are pulled tight, there is exaggerated flexion or extension of the limbs, tremors.

Activity
- Score 0 if the client moves easily and freely, normal activity or restrictions.
- Score 1 if the client shifts positions, appears hesitant to move, demonstrates guarding, a tense torso, pressure on a body part.
- Score 2 if the client is in a fixed position, rocking; demonstrates side-to-side head movement or rubbing of a body part.

Cry
- Score 0 if the client has no cry or moan, awake or asleep.
- Score 1 if the client has occasional moans, cries, whimpers, sighs.
- Score 2 if the client has frequent or continuous moans, cries, grunts.

Consolability
- Score 0 if the client is calm and does not require consoling.
- Score 1 if the client responds to comfort by touching or talking in 30 seconds to 1 minute.
- Score 2 if the client requires constant comforting or is inconsolable.

Whenever feasible, behavioral measurement of pain should be used in conjunction with self-report. When self-report is not possible, interpretation of pain behaviors and decisions regarding treatment of pain require careful consideration of the context in which the pain behaviors are observed.

Interpreting the Behavioral Score
Each category is scored on the 0–2 scale, which results in a total score of 0–10.

0 = Relaxed and comfortable   **4–6 =** Moderate pain
1–3 = Mild discomfort   **7–10 =** Severe discomfort or pain or both

Source: From Merkel, S. I., Voepel-Lewis, T., Shayevitz, J. R., & Malviya, S. (1997). The FLACC: A behavioral scale for scoring postoperative pain in young children. *Pediatric Nursing, 23*(3), 293–297. The FLACC scale was developed by Sandra Merkel, MS, RN, Terri Voepel-Lewis, MS, RN, and Shobha Malviya, MD, at C. S. Mott Children's Hospital, University of Michigan Health System, Ann Arbor, MI. Used with permission.

(continued on next page)

SKILL 4.1   Assessing the Client in Pain (continued)

10 —   10 —   10 —   10 —
9 —   9 —   9 —   9 —
8 —   8 —   8 —   8 —
7 —   7 —   7 —   7 —
6 —   6 —   6 —   6 —
5 —   5 —   5 —   5 —
4 —   4 —   4 —   4 —
3 —   3 —   3 —   3 —
2 —   2 —   2 —   2 —
1 —   1 —   1 —   1 —
0 —   0 —   0 —   0 —

A   B   C   D

③ Oucher Scale 3–7 years.

Note: In the form presented in this book, the Oucher is for educational purposes only and cannot be used for client care. *A*, The Caucasian version of the Oucher, developed and copyrighted by Judith E. Beyer, RN, Ph.D., 1983. *B*, The African American version of the Oucher, developed and copyrighted by Mary J. Denyes, RN, Ph.D., and Antonio M. Villarruel, RN, Ph.D., 1990. Cornelia P. Porter, RN, Ph.D., and Charlotta Marshall, RN, MSN, contributed to the development of the scale. *C*, The Hispanic version of the Oucher, developed and copyrighted by Antonio M. Villarruel, RN, Ph.D., and Mary J. Denyes, RN, Ph.D., 1990. *D*. The Asian version of the Oucher, developed and copyrighted by C. H. Yeh, RN, Ph.D., and C. H. Wang, BNS, 2003. http://www.oucher.org.

Developmental Considerations

INFANT

- Giving an infant, particularly a very-low-birth-weight infant, a water and sucrose solution administered through a pacifier is effective in reducing pain during procedures that may be painful, but should not replace anesthetic or analgesic medications when indicated.

CHILD

- Distract the child with toys, books, or pictures.
- Hold the child to console and promote comfort.
- Explore misconceptions about pain and correct in understandable "concrete" terms. Be aware of how your explanations may be misunderstood. For example, telling a child that surgery will not hurt because the child will be "put to sleep" will be very upsetting to a child who knows of an animal that was "put to sleep."
- Children can use their imagination during guided imagery. To use the "pain switch," ask the child to imagine a pain switch (even give it a color) and tell them to visualize turning the switch off in the area where there is pain. A "magic glove" or "magic blanket" is an imaginary object that the child applies on areas of the body (e.g., hand, thigh, back, hip) to lessen discomfort.

OLDER ADULTS

- Promote the client's use of pain control measures that have worked in the past for the client.

- Spend time with the client and listen carefully.
- Clarify misconceptions. Encourage independence whenever possible.
- Carefully review the treatment plan to avoid drug–drug, food–drug, or disease–drug interactions.

Setting of Care

CLIENT

- *Level of knowledge:* Pharmacologic and nonpharmacologic pain relief measures selected; adverse effects and measures to counteract these effects; warning signs to report to primary care provider.
- *Self-care abilities for analgesic administration:* Ability to use analgesics appropriately; physical dexterity to take pills or to administer intravenous medications and to store medications safely; ability to obtain prescriptions or over-the-counter medications at the pharmacy.

FAMILY

- *Caregiver availability, skills, and willingness:* Primary and secondary individuals able and willing to assist with pain management; shopping if the client has restricted activity; ability to comprehend selected therapies (e.g., infusion pumps, imagery, massage, positioning, and relaxation techniques) and perform them or assist the client with them as needed.

SKILL 4.1   Assessing the Client in Pain (continued)

- *Family role changes and coping:* Effect on financial status, parenting and spousal roles, sexuality, social roles.

COMMUNITY

- *Resources:* Availability of and familiarity with resources such as supplies, home health aide, or financial assistance.

Cultural Considerations

CLIENTS IN PAIN

A priority responsibility for the nurse caring for a client in pain is to obtain assessment data to give meaning to the client's self-report of the pain experience. Client self-report is the most reliable indicator of the presence and level of pain. Obtaining this data helps the nurse make decisions about nonpharmacologic and pharmacologic interventions for treating the client's pain. As an advocate, the nurse can then evaluate the client's response to these different measures and make further recommendations for control of pain relief.

Individual behaviors in response to pain have been noted with clients of all ages. How they react and respond to various pains and pain intensities depends on many factors including the individual's experience of pain, history of pain, health beliefs, and cultural customs. The nurse must always seek to understand the individual client's experience of pain. There are multiple resources available for the nurse to gain insight and understanding of the pain experience.

To provide sensitive care of individual clients for best outcomes:

- Use a standard measure (such as a 0 to 10 scale for intensity) when asking about pain. These standard measures can help avoid undertreatment or overtreatment of pain if the nurse does not know the client's usual method of pain expression. They can also help overcome the tendency to try and guess if the client is having pain based on the terms of pain expression or requests for pharmacologic intervention.
- Accept the client's thoughts and feelings about pain. The meaning of pain varies among people. For some people, pain is an expected part of life; in others it may be associated with punishment for life choices. Do not judge or argue with how the client responds to pain.
- Identify and support the client's methods of coping with pain, whether that is spiritual (offering up suffering in prayer), social (having multiple family members participate in care), or stoic (quietly accepting the pain).
- Regularly evaluate the effect of treatment on the pain and on client's overall well-being. The client's satisfaction with how pain is being managed is often more important than the exact number of that pain on the pain scale. Participation in the plan of care enhances the client's sense of control and strengthens the nurse-client relationship.

AVOIDING STEREOTYPES

Healthcare personnel working in a variety of settings maintain that pain is a culturally influenced phenomenon. How pain is experienced and expressed varies by cultural group. For example, some cultures (such as Italians and Jewish people) encourage open expression of feelings like pain, whereas others (the stoic English, Irish, and Chinese) believe that pain is something to be ignored or endured in silence. This was demonstrated by Zborowski's study conducted in the 1950s. Although these general conclusions may lead to stereotyping, it is important to consider the impact of the individual's culture in the assessment of pain level.

Source: Spector, R. (2012). *Cultural diversity in health and illness* (8th ed.). Upper Saddle River, NJ: Prentice Hall Health.

VARIATIONS IN EXPRESSION OF PAIN

Expressions of pain vary from one individual to another individual. Here are some common expressions about pain, thoughts, beliefs, and behaviors that a nurse can assess and explore further with the client to determine if pain relief intervention is needed:

- May believe pain and suffering is a part of life and is to be endured.
- May believe that enduring pain is a sign of strength.
- May believe that prayer and laying on of hands will free a person from suffering and pain.
- May believe that pain is "God's will."
- May deny or avoid dealing with the pain until it becomes unbearable.
- May tend to view pain as a part of life.
- May question "Why is God doing this to me?"
- May view pain as an indicator of the seriousness of an illness.
- May be loud and outspoken in expressions of pain. This is a socially learned way to cope and it is important for the nurse to not judge or disapprove.
- May value silence when having pain.
- May be quiet when in pain to avoid causing dishonor to their family.
- May be quiet and less expressive verbally and nonverbally.
- May tolerate a high level of pain.
- May become stoic (minimal verbal and nonverbal expressions) in response to pain.
- May refuse pain medication.
- May be calm when in pain to bring oneself to a higher state of being.
- May not request pain medication and tolerate pain until physically disabled.
- May be considered a private matter and reserved for immediate family only, not for health professionals.
- May not want to be a bother by asking for something for pain.
- May lead to conflicting perceptions between the client, the family members, and the nurse regarding the client's pain relief.
- May desire to remain with pain as a means to punish themselves for some thought or action.
- May be scared of becoming addicted to pain relief medication if receiving it too often.

SKILL 4.2   Teaching Controlled Breathing

Procedure

1. Instruct client to sit so that his or her back is well supported, with spine straight but not rigid ❶.
2. Have client place feet flat on floor and place hands on legs.
3. If client is lying down, have him or her place hands at sides.
4. Suggest client find a comfortable position, close eyes, and take a deep, slow breath through nostrils.
5. Continue giving the client the following instructions:
   - Extend your abdominal muscles.

(continued on next page)

SKILL 4.2   Teaching Controlled Breathing *(continued)*

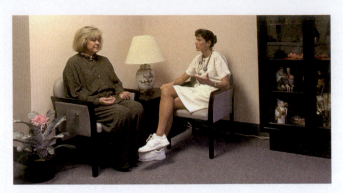

1 Find a quiet room to teach the relaxation process.

- Hold your breath for the count of four. Then very slowly release the air through slightly parted lips, making a whoosh sound.
- When you think that all the air is out, hold your stomach in to push out even more air.
- Repeat this breathing pattern several times so that your body relaxes.

- Breathe in through your nostrils to the count of four—1-2-3-4. Hold it—1-2-3-4—and slowly expel the breath all the way out, slowly releasing the air through your mouth.
- As the air goes out, feel all of the tension drain out with it.
- Now double the count, and breathe in slowly, filling your lungs all the way to the top to the count of eight. 1-2-3-4-5-6-7-8. Hold it—1-2-3-4—and now slowly release the breath—5-6-7-8.
- Again breathe in slowly to the count of 10 and count for the client—1-2-3-4-5-6-7-8-9-10. Hold it to the count of eight—1-2-3-4-5-6-7-8—and slowly release the air through your mouth to the count of 10: 1-2-3-4-5-6-7-8-9-10. Pause.
- Continue with your regular breathing pattern, letting your lungs breathe for you.

6. Stop the process by having the client open his or her eyes. Document teaching and client response.

> **CLINICAL ALERT**
>
> If you are motivated to learn complementary and alternative medicine (CAM) techniques, numerous classes are available. In fact, to implement certain CAM therapies such as Reiki, therapeutic touch, acupressure, or acupuncture, you will need specialized classes/training.

SKILL 4.3   Teaching Progressive Muscle Relaxation

Delegation

Noninvasive pain management techniques can be delegated to UAP if they have experience using the technique and are comfortable doing so. The nurse is responsible for assessing the client's willingness to participate in the relaxation or imagery exercise. The nurse instructs UAP to report the client's response to the nurse.

Equipment

- A printed relaxation script that an individual can read until the client learns the technique. Many are available online and through stress management resource books and tapes.
- CD player or iPod (optional). CD or iPod could be used to provide the script for the exercise or for the playing of background music.

Preparation

- Allow 10 to 15 minutes of uninterrupted time for the session. Ensure that the environment is private, quiet, and at a temperature that suits the client. The client should have an empty bladder. **Rationale:** *Interruptions or distractions interfere with the client's ability to achieve full relaxation. Once clients learn how to use this technique, they will be able to do it in less than 5 minutes as part of self-care and ongoing stress management.*

Evidence-Based Nursing Practice

Stress Response

The stress response is a physical "fight-or-flight" reaction of the body. Although it began as a survival mechanism, it can also be triggered by other "threatening" events (a work deadline, job worries, even sitting at a traffic light). Stressors can trigger a cascade of stress hormones that produce physiological changes. The heart beats faster, breath quickens, muscles tense, and beads of sweat appear.

Over the years, researchers have determined that prolonged stress has various detrimental effects on the body. These include high blood pressure, atherosclerosis, brain changes that may contribute to anxiety, depression, and addiction. They may also contribute to obesity directly (causing people to eat more) or indirectly (decreasing sleep and exercise).

Many people find that they can counter the stress response using techniques to elicit a relaxation response. These include deep abdominal breathing, repetition of a word, imagining oneself in a peaceful place, prayer, yoga, or other meditative techniques.

In one study, researchers at Massachusetts General Hospital conducted a double-blind, randomized controlled trial of 122 patients with hypertension, ages 55 and older. Half performed relaxation response training and the other half received information about blood pressure control. After 8 weeks, more than half of those using the relaxation response had reduced their systolic blood pressure by more than 5 mmHg. This "passed" them to the phase of the study in which they could reduce their dosage of blood pressure medication. In the second phase, half were able to eliminate at least one blood pressure medication, in contrast to the control group, in which only 19% could eliminate a medication.

Overall, a combined approach to stress reduction is recommended long term, including relaxation techniques, exercise, and support groups or cognitive therapy.

Data from *Harvard Mental Health Letter* (2011).

Procedure

1. Prior to performing the procedure, introduce self and verify the client's identity using agency protocol. Explain to the client what you are going to do, why it is necessary, and how he or she can participate.
2. Perform hand hygiene and observe other appropriate infection control procedures.
3. Provide for client privacy.
4. Prepare the client:
   - Tell the client how progressive muscle relaxation works.
   - Provide a rationale for the procedure. **Rationale:** *It has been noted that muscular tension accompanies most stress*

SKILL 4.3   Teaching Progressive Muscle Relaxation (*continued*)

states. *By aiming to reduce muscle tension, the negative effects of stress on the mind–body can be lessened.*

- Ask the client to identify the stressors operating in the client's life and the reactions to these stressors. **Rationale:** *Awareness is important as the client learns how to cope effectively.*
- Demonstrate the method of tensing and relaxing groups of muscles and have client do it with you. It is easy to start with making fists—tensing the muscles with 100% effort the first time, and then with only 50% effort the second time. **Rationale:** *Demonstration and initial practice enables the client to understand the progression of muscle relaxation more clearly.*
- Assist the client to a comfortable position.

5. If music is to be used, select music that is instrumental, calming, neutral, and unfamiliar to the client. **Rationale:** *Music should not be recognizable and should not intentionally elicit memories or emotion. In this way, the music will enhance relaxation. Classical music can sometimes be too "busy" and may evoke memories and emotion that could be distracting for the client.*
   - Ensure that all body parts are supported and the joints slightly flexed with no strain or pull on the muscles (e.g., arms and legs should not be crossed). **Rationale:** *Assuming a position of comfort facilitates relaxation.*

6. Encourage the client to begin slow, deep diaphragmatic or abdominal breathing to rest the mind and begin relaxing the body. Inhaling through the nose and exhaling through the mouth (pursed lips are best) slows down the breath and enhances relaxation.

7. Instruct the client to tense and then relax each group of muscles starting from the head and moving down the body. Use a tone of voice throughout the exercise that invites participation rather than directs.
   - The following script suggestions are just one way of doing the technique:
     a. Take in a deep breath, and close eyes tightly shut, furrowing your brows and wrinkling your forehead. Hold this contraction with the most effort you can, and then release as you exhale slowly. Again, take a breath and contract these same muscles with half the effort you used last time. Hold, hold, and now release with your breath, feeling the tension leave your body as a soothing wave of relaxation flows over your head and face. . . . You could keep your eyes softly closed throughout this exercise. . . .
     b. You might want to clench your jaw as you breathe in, feeling the muscles in your cheeks and throat and base of your tongue tightening as you hold, hold, and then release. You could repeat this contraction as you inhale, and hold with less tension this time, and then release as you exhale, allowing all of these muscles to soften, allowing your teeth to rest just slightly apart.
     c. Next, pull your shoulders up toward your ears as you take a full and gentle breath in and hold as tightly as you can. Now relax and release your shoulders with your breath, allowing a soothing wave of relaxation to flow into your neck and shoulder area. This time hunch your shoulders up with only half the effort you used last time . . . hold it . . . and release, allowing any tension to run down your arms and through your hands and out the tips of your fingers. . . .
     d. Next, you could inhale and make tight fists of both hands and hold these fists as strongly as you can. Release your fists and your breath. Take another breath

in and make fists again, this time with less effort . . . hold . . . and release, allowing tension to leave your hands, being replaced with softness.
     e. Now we can focus on the arms. As you breathe in, think about contracting the muscles of the arms, perhaps making fists again, and feeling the entire length of your arms tightening and flexing. Hold, hold, and release, feeling the tension leaving your arms and flowing out through your hands and fingertips. This time breathe in and tighten your arms with less effort, and then release with your breath, feeling a sense of comfort and peace as the tension leaves you now.
     f. You could focus on your abdominal muscles, and pull them in tightly as if to button your navel onto the front of your spine. You may even notice tension in your back muscles, and hold this as tightly as you can. Exhale and release all of these muscles, feeling as if a band of tightness around your midsection is being released. Breathe in and tense this abdominal and low back band of muscles again. Hold more gently this time and then release, exhaling slowly. Enjoy the feelings as your muscles become relaxed and loose.
     g. You could inhale deeply and flex your hip and buttock muscles, feeling yourself lift as the muscles contract. Hold, and then release as you exhale. This time, flex these muscles a bit more gently, aware of the peace that is flowing throughout your body as you continue to relax.
     h. You could inhale and flex your heels away from your body as you pull your toes hard, hard toward your face. Hold this, feeling your calf and thigh muscles flexing as well, and then release as you exhale. Inhale again and this time press your toes away from your face and feel the tension throughout the entire length of your leg once again. You can repeat this with less effort, and feel the whole body relax and release.
   - Encourage the client to breathe slowly and deeply during the entire procedure. **Rationale:** *Quiet, full, slow breathing with an emphasis on prolonged exhalation elicits a parasympathetic response that is the opposite of the fight-or-flight response.*
   - Speak in a calm voice that encourages relaxation and coach the client to mentally focus on each muscle group being addressed. **Rationale:** *By suggesting rather than directing throughout the process, you avoid triggering any underlying control issues in the client.*

8. Ask the client to state whether any tension remains after all muscle groups have been tensed and relaxed.
   - Repeat the procedure for muscle groups that are not relaxed.

9. Terminate the relaxation exercise slowly by counting from 1 to 3, suggesting that the client will feel calm and alert.
   - Ask the client to move the body slowly: first the hands and feet, then arms and legs, and finally the head and neck.

10. Remind the client that this technique can be used any time the client needs to release tension or wants to feel more relaxed.

11. Document the client's response to the exercise.

Sample Documentation

7/20/15 2300 Reports "mild" headache, 1–2/10 on pain scale. Also expressing anxiety about recent diagnosis, having difficulty falling asleep. Progressive muscle relaxation taught using relaxation music as a background. Participated fully, stated "headache is gone." Asleep when nurse returned with sleep med. Sleep med held. _____ B. Montgomery, RN

SKILL 4.4   Providing a Back Massage

Delegation

The nurse can delegate this skill to UAP; however, the nurse should first assess for UAP's comfort and ability, any contraindications, and client willingness to participate.

Equipment

- Lotion
- Towel for excess lotion

Preparation

- Determine (1) previous assessments of the skin, (2) special lotions to be used, and (3) positions contraindicated for the client. Arrange for a quiet environment with no interruptions to promote maximum effect of the back massage.

Procedure

1. Prior to performing the procedure, introduce self and verify the client's identity using agency protocol. Explain to the client what you are going to do, why it is necessary, and how he or she can participate. Encourage the client to give you feedback as to the amount of pressure you are using during the back rub.

2. Perform hand hygiene and observe other appropriate infection control procedures.

3. Provide for client privacy.

4. Prepare the client.
   - Assist the client to move to the near side of the bed within your reach and adjust the bed to a comfortable working height. **Rationale:** *This prevents back strain.*
   - Establish which position the client prefers. The prone position is recommended for a back rub. The side-lying position can be used if a client cannot assume the prone position.
   - Expose the back from the shoulders to the inferior sacral area. Cover the remainder of the body. **Rationale:** *This prevents chilling and minimizes exposure.*

5. Massage the back 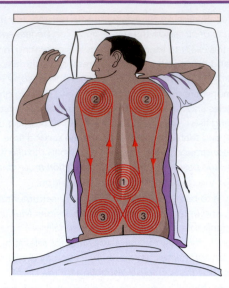.
   - Pour a small amount of lotion onto the palms of your hands and hold it for a minute. The lotion bottle can also be placed in a bath basin filled with warm water. **Rationale:** *Back rub preparations tend to feel uncomfortably cold to people. Warming the solution facilitates client comfort.*
   - Using your palm, begin in the sacral area using smooth, circular strokes.
   - Move your hands up the center of the back and then over both scapulae.
   - Massage in a circular motion over the scapulae.
   - Move your hands down the sides of the back.

❶ One suggested pattern for a back massage.

   - Massage the areas over the right and left iliac crests. Massage the back in an orderly pattern using a variety of strokes and appropriate pressure.
   - Apply firm, continuous pressure without breaking contact with the client's skin.
   - Repeat above for 3 to 5 minutes, obtaining more lotion as necessary.
   - While massaging the back, assess for skin redness and areas of decreased circulation.
   - Pat dry any excess lotion with a towel.

6. Document that a back massage was performed and the client's response. Record any unusual findings.

Sample Documentation

6/22/15 1400 Reports aching, intermittent back pain. Wincing and grimacing when attempting to move in bed. Rates pain at 4–5 on 0–10 scale. States uses massage to help relieve pain when at home. Back massaged. Stated the massage helped him "to relax." Lights dimmed and door to room closed.
_____ *M. Black, RN*

1430 Rates pain at 1–2/10. States feels "much more comfortable." Moving in bed with ease. _____ *M. Black, RN*

Evaluation

Compare the client's current response to his or her previous response. Is there a positive client outcome such as increased relaxation and decrease in pain and anxiety as a result of the back massage?

SKILL 4.5   Assisting with Guided Imagery

Preparation

- Allow 10 to 15 minutes for this process. Provide a private, comfortable, quiet environment free of distractions. Ensure thermal comfort and make sure the client has an empty bladder. **Rationale:** *Comfort and freedom from distractions are necessary for the client to relax and focus on the exercise.*

Procedure

1. Prior to performing the procedure, introduce self to the client and verify the client's identity using agency protocol. Explain to the client what you are going to do, why it is necessary, and how he or she can participate. Explain the rationale and benefits of imagery. Ask the client about the goals for the session. Imagery can pro-

SKILL 4.5   Assisting with Guided Imagery (*continued*)

vide relaxation and feelings of empowerment, lead to creative problem solving, and facilitate healing. The content used will vary depending on the client's goals. Many books, tapes, and CDs are available for those who want to learn more about this powerful technique. **Rationale:** *The client is an active participant in an imagery exercise and can offer direction for the session.*

2. Perform hand hygiene and observe other appropriate infection control procedures.

3. Provide for client privacy.

4. Assist the client to a comfortable position.
   - Assist the client to a reclining position and ask the client to close the eyes. **Rationale:** *A position of comfort can enhance the client's focus during the imagery exercise.*

5. Implement actions to induce relaxation.
   - Speak clearly in a calming and neutral tone of voice. **Rationale:** *Positive voice coaching can enhance the effect of imagery. A shrill or loud voice can distract the client from the image.*
   - Ask the client to take slow, full diaphragmatic/abdominal breaths and to relax all muscles. Use progressive muscle relaxation exercises as needed to assist the client to achieve total relaxation.
   - Guide the client through relaxation breathing and then through muscle relaxation. Then begin to guide the client toward a most beautiful or peaceful place. The client may have been to this place before or may be imagining this place. Do *not* impose your own suggestions as to where they might be. Clients know where they want and need to go! Slowly guide them to approach and then finally enter the place. Prompt them to use all of their senses as they look around the place, listen to the sounds of the place, feel the air, feel what's underfoot, and smell the fragrances of the place. Have them find and move toward a safe spot where they can rest for awhile.
   - While clients are in their safe spot, you can assist them to do some work. For example, if they need stress management or pain relief, they can picture themselves (from the safety of this, their very safe spot) in a potentially tense situation. Then have them inhale and exhale slowly three times, saying to

themselves "relax, relax, relax" with each exhalation. For internal healing work, encourage the client to focus on a meaningful image of power and use it to control the specific problem. Or, the client can be educated beforehand to use anatomical and physiological imagery for her own healing. These kinds of goals are facilitated with some prior preparation on the part of the nurse and client, and many resources exist to prepare people for this work. Ask the client to use all the senses when practicing imagery. **Rationale:** *Using all the senses enhances the client's benefit from imagery. Clients may be asked to assign a color to their pain, and then identify a color signifying "no pain." Then they can use imagery to change the color of their pain to the "no-pain color."*

6. Take the client out of the image by suggesting that it is time for the client to leave this most beautiful and safe place. Suggest that the client can return at any time desired and that her breathing will lead the way.
   - Slowly count from 1 to 3, suggesting that it is time for the client to leave this most beautiful and safe place. Suggest that the client come back into the here and now. Tell the client that she will feel rested and refreshed when she opens her eyes on 3.
   - Remain until the client is alert. If the client remains in a trancelike state, simply repeat that she will wake up on the number 3 and count to three again. No harm will occur if the client stays "asleep." You can allow her to remain so, or gently touch her to facilitate awakening.

7. Following the experience, ask the client to describe the physical and emotional feelings elicited by the imagery session. The meanings images have for the individual client can be very helpful in the therapeutic process. Direct the client to explore the response to images because this enables the client to modify the imagery for future sessions.

8. Encourage the client to practice the imagery technique.
   - Imagery is a technique that can be done independently by the client once the client knows how.

9. Document the client's response to the exercise, noting signs of increased relaxation and reduced anxiety.

SKILL 4.6   Teaching Bedtime Strategies to Promote and Regulate Sleep

Healthy individuals need to learn the importance of sleep in maintaining active and productive lifestyles. They need to learn (1) the conditions that promote sleep and those that interfere with sleep, (2) safe use of sleep medications, (3) effects of other prescribed medications on sleep, (4) effects of their disease states on sleep, and (5) importance of long periods of uninterrupted sleep. The nurse can provide tips for promoting sleep. When the session is complete, the nurse documents teaching and notes client response.

Client Teaching

Promoting Sleep

- If you have difficulty falling asleep or staying asleep, it is important to establish a regular bedtime and wake-up time for all days of the week to enhance your biological rhythm. A short daytime nap (e.g., 15 to 30 minutes), particularly among older adults, can be restorative and not interfere with nighttime sleep. A younger person with insomnia should not nap.
- Establish a regular, relaxing bedtime routine before sleep such as reading, listening to soft music, taking a warm bath, or doing some other quiet activity you enjoy.
- Avoid dealing with office work or family problems before bedtime.
- Get adequate exercise during the day to reduce stress, but avoid excessive physical exertion at least 3 hours before bedtime.

- Use the bed for sleep or sexual activity, so that you associate it with sleep. Take work material, computers, and TVs out of the bedroom. Lying awake, tossing and turning, will strengthen the association between wakefulness and lying in bed (many people with insomnia report falling asleep in a chair or in front of the TV but having trouble falling asleep in bed).
- When you are unable to sleep, get out of bed, go into another room, and pursue some relaxing activity until you feel drowsy.

Environment

- Create a sleep-conducive environment that is dark, quiet, comfortable, and cool. Keep noise to a minimum; block out extraneous

(continued on next page)

SKILL 4.6 Teaching Bedtime Strategies to Promote and Regulate Sleep *(continued)*

noise as necessary with white noise from a fan, air conditioner, or white noise machine. Music is not recommended as studies have shown that music promotes wakefulness because it is interesting and people will pay attention to it.

■ Sleep on a comfortable mattress and pillows.

Diet

■ Avoid heavy meals 2 to 3 hours before bedtime.
■ Avoid alcohol and caffeine-containing foods and beverages (e.g., coffee, tea, chocolate) at least 4 hours before bedtime. Caffeine can interfere with sleep. Both caffeine and alcohol act as diuretics, creating the need to void during sleep time.

■ If a bedtime snack is necessary, consume only light carbohydrates or a milk drink. Heavy or spicy foods can cause gastrointestinal upsets that disturb sleep.

Medications

■ Use sleeping medications only as a last resort. Use OTC medications sparingly because many contain antihistamines that cause daytime drowsiness.
■ Take analgesics before bedtime to relieve aches and pains.
■ Consult with your healthcare provider about adjusting other medications that may cause insomnia.

Developmental Considerations

CHILDREN

Learning to sleep alone without the parent's help is a skill that all children need to master. Regular bedtime routines and rituals such as reading a book help children learn this skill and can prevent sleep disturbance. Some sleep disturbances seen in children include the following:

■ *Trained night feeder:* Infants who are fed during the night and fed until they fall asleep and then put into bed, or infants who have a bottle left with them in their bed learn to expect and demand middle-of-the-night feedings. Infants who are growing well do not need night feeding after about 4 months of age. Infants who are failing to thrive may need feeding at night.

■ *Sleep refusal:* Many toddlers and young children are resistant to settling down to sleep. This sleep refusal may be due to not being tired, anxiety about separation from the parent, stress (e.g., a recent move), lack of a regular sleep routine, the child's temperament, or changes in sleep arrangements (e.g., move from a crib to a "big" bed).

■ *Night terrors:* Night terrors are partial awakenings from non-REM, stage III or IV sleep. They are usually seen in children 3 to 6 years of age. The child may sleepwalk, or may sit up in bed screaming and thrashing about. They usually cannot be wakened, but should be protected from injury, helped back to bed, and soothed back to sleep. Babysitters should be alerted to the possibility of a night terror occurring. Children do not remember the incident the next day, and there is no indication

of a neurological or emotional problem. Excessive fatigue and a full bladder may contribute to the problem. Having the child take an afternoon nap and empty the bladder before going to sleep at night may be helpful.

ADULTS

■ New jobs, pregnancy, and babies are common examples of situations that often disrupt the sleep of a young adult.
■ The sleep patterns of middle-aged adults can be disrupted if they are taking care of older parents and/or chronically ill partners in the home.

OLDER ADULTS

The quality of sleep is often diminished in older adults. Some of the leading factors that often are influential in sleep disturbances include the following:

■ Side effects of medications
■ Gastroesophageal reflux disease
■ Respiratory and circulatory disorders, which may cause breathing problems or discomfort
■ Pain from arthritis, increased stiffness, or impaired immobility
■ Nocturia
■ Depression
■ Loss of life partner and/or close friends
■ Confusion related to delirium or dementia.

SKILL 4.7 Managing a TENS Unit

Delegation

The assessment for and application of a transcutaneous electrical nerve stimulation (TENS) unit requires specialized knowledge and problem solving. It is important for the nurse to understand how this method of pain management works. In an acute care health setting, the nurse would not delegate the skill of managing a TENS unit to UAP. A TENS unit is often ordered for home use and the nurse is responsible for teaching the client or caregiver how to safely and effectively use the device.

Equipment

■ TENS unit
■ Bath basin with warm water
■ Soap

■ Washcloth
■ Towel
■ Conduction cream, gel, or water (see manufacturer's instructions)
■ Hypoallergenic tape

Procedure

1. Prior to performing the procedure, check physician's order, introduce self and verify the client's identity. Explain to the client what you are going to do, why it is necessary, and how he or she can participate. The TENS unit may not completely eliminate pain but should reduce pain to a level that allows the client to rest more comfortably and/or carry out everyday activities.

2. Perform hand hygiene and observe other appropriate infection control procedures.

SKILL 4.7   Managing a TENS Unit *(continued)*

3. Provide for client privacy.
4. Prepare the equipment.
   - Insert the battery into the TENS unit to test its functioning.
   - With the TENS unit off, plug the lead wires into the battery-operated unit at one end, leaving the electrodes at the other end.
5. Clean the application area.
   - Wash, rinse, and dry the designated area with soap and water. **Rationale:** *This reduces skin irritation and facilitates adhesion of the electrodes to the skin for a longer period of time.*
6. Apply the electrodes to the client.
   - If the electrodes are not pre-gelled, moisten them with a small amount of water or apply conducting gel. (Consult the manufacturer's instructions.) **Rationale:** *This facilitates electrical conduction.*
   - Place the electrodes on a clean, unbroken area of skin. Choose the area according to the location, nature, and origin of the pain.
   - Ensure that the electrodes make full surface contact with the skin. Tape all sides evenly with hypoallergenic tape. **Rationale:** *This prevents an inadvertent burn.*
7. Turn the unit on.
   - Ascertain that the amplitude control is set at level 0.
   - Slowly increase the intensity of the stimulus (amplitude) until the client notes a slight increase in discomfort.
   - When the client notes discomfort, slowly decrease the amplitude until the client notes a pleasant sensation. Once this has been achieved, keep the TENS unit set at this level to maintain blockage of the pain sensation. Most clients select frequencies between 60 and 100 Hz.
8. Monitor the client.
   - If the client complains of itching, pricking, or burning, explore the following options:
     a. Turn the pulse-width dial down.
     b. Check that the entire electrode surface is in contact with the skin.
     c. Increase the distance between the electrodes.
     d. Select another type of electrode suitable for the model of TENS unit in use.
     e. Discontinue the TENS and consider the possibility of another brand of TENS.

- If the sensation of the stimulus is unpleasant, too intense, or distracting, turn down both the amplitude and pulse-width dial.
- If the client complains of headache or nausea during application or use, turn down both the amplitude and the pulse-width dial. Repositioning of the electrodes may also be helpful.
- If further troubleshooting is not effective, discontinue use of the TENS unit and notify the primary care provider.

9. After the treatment:
   - Turn off the controls and unplug the lead wires from the control box.
   - Clean the electrodes according to the manufacturer's instructions. Clean the client's skin with soap and water.
   - Replace the used battery pack with a charged battery. Begin recharging the used battery.
   - If continuous therapy is used, remove the electrode patches and inspect the skin at least once daily.
10. Provide client teaching.
    - Review instructions for use with the client and verify that the client understands.
    - Have the client demonstrate the use of the TENS unit and verbalize ways to troubleshoot if headache, nausea, or unpleasant sensations occur.
    - Instruct the client not to submerge the unit in water but instead to remove and reapply it after bathing.
11. Document all relevant information.
    - Record the date and time TENS therapy was initiated, the location of electrode placement and status of skin in that area, the character and quality of the pain, settings of TENS unit used, side effects experienced, and the client's response.

Sample Documentation

7/30/15 1100 Reports sharp pain in right hip that radiates down back of right leg. Rates pain at 3/10, and achieves some relief with positional changes that take weight off of hip. TENS applied over lateral aspect of right hip at 70 Hertz. _____M. Johnstone, RN

7/30/15 1110 Reports nausea. Frequency reduced to 60 Hertz; nausea resolved. _____M. Johnstone, RN

7/30/15 1140 TENS discontinued. Rates pain at 0–1/10. No c/o nausea. skin intact. _____M. Johnstone, RN

Setting of Care

TENS units are frequently ordered for home use to relieve chronic pain. Instruct the client or caregiver on:

- How to use and care for the TENS equipment.
- How to troubleshoot if side effects or problems occur and who to call if the equipment malfunctions.
- Where and how to obtain supplies needed for the TENS unit.
- How to remove the electrodes daily and check for skin breakdown at the electrode sites.
- Teach client to keep a pain diary to monitor pain onset, activity before pain, pain intensity, use of analgesics or other relief measures, and so on.

- Instruct client to contact a healthcare professional if planned pain control measures are ineffective.
- Teach the use of preferred and selected nonpharmacologic techniques such as relaxation, guided imagery, distraction, music therapy, massage, and so on (**Table 4–3 ●**).
- Instruct the client to use pain control measures before the pain becomes severe.
- Inform the client of the effects of untreated pain.
- Provide appropriate information about how to access community resources, home care agencies, and associations that offer self-help groups and educational materials.

(continued on next page)

SKILL 4.7   Managing a TENS Unit (continued)

TABLE 4–3   Nonpharmacologic Approaches to Pain

PHYSICAL METHODS	ADVANTAGES
TENS—stimulating skin with mild electric current—provides pain relief by blocking pain impulses to the brain	Noninvasive method Higher level of activity Studies show more effective for postoperative pain Gives staff confidence they can assist client with pain Choice for chronic pain
Acupuncture—ancient Chinese form of treating diseases and pain through insertion and manipulation of needles at specific points on the body	Insertion of thin needles is not painful to the client Pain-relieving capacity extends beyond actual procedure Method may provide relief when no other method works
Biofeedback—electric monitoring device that feeds back effect of behavior so client can control internal processes (e.g., heartbeat)	Noninvasive method Completely controlled by client Promotes stress reduction as well as pain relief After mastery, instruments are not needed to achieve result
Vibration or massage—hands-on manipulation of muscles or electrical form of massage (vibration)	Noninvasive method—electrically alleviates pain by numbness or paresthesia or through touch Increases circulation and endorphins to area Relaxes muscles and reduces tension on nerves and promotes relaxation Useful only for light to moderate pain
Cold therapy—cold wraps, gel packs, cold therapy, ice massage; do not use on irradiated tissue or when clients have peripheral vascular disease	Relieves pain faster than heat therapy Numbs nerves and decreases inflammation and spasms Effective for nerve, abdominal, and lower back pain Alters pain threshold Decreases tissue injury response
Heat therapy—hot wraps, dry heat, moist heat; do not use on irradiated tissue or tumors	Noninvasive method Decreases pain by reducing inflammation Promotes relaxation of muscles Increases vasodilation and blood flow to area Facilitates clearance of tissue toxins and fluids
Counterirritants—mentholated ointments or lotions (Ben-Gay or Icy Hot)	May contain salicylates (reduces inflammation) but dangerous if client has potential bleeding problems May be irritating to the skin—potential skin breakdown
Acupressure application—based on the ancient Chinese method of acupuncture, this method involves using specific points located on meridians at various places on the body	Noninvasive method Redirection of energy flow through pressure on meridian points Reduces pain and increases endorphins
Chiropractic adjustment	Manipulation of muscles and realignment of spinal column Nerve function is restored Structural integrity and balance are restored
COGNITIVE–BEHAVIORAL METHODS	ADVANTAGES
Relaxation—body relaxation of muscles used with imagery, therapist instruction	Relaxes tense muscles and reduces stress Effective in reducing pain Easy to learn and implement techniques for self-mastery Reduces fear and anxiety connected to pain
Imagery—visualization technique of forming sensory images, or seeing in the "mind's eye" an image that distracts from the sensation of pain	Effective in reducing pain Client can control use and timing of technique Reduces high-level anxiety connected to pain
Deep breathing—techniques using breath to control pain	Effective in reinforcing body relaxation and visualization Reduces pain through breath control; increases oxygen utilization
Hypnosis—creating a state of altered consciousness so that client is susceptible to instruction	Effective with a client who is suggestive and who experiences tension and anxiety accompanying pain

SKILL 4.8   Managing Pain with a PCA Pump

Delegation

Initiating and maintaining a PCA pump requires application of nursing knowledge, aseptic technique, critical thinking, and administration of a controlled substance and, therefore, is not delegated to UAP. The nurse can inform UAP of the intended therapeutic effects and specific side effects of the medication and direct UAP to report specific client observations (e.g., unrelieved pain) to the nurse for follow-up. UAP must not administer a dose (push the button) for the client.

SKILL 4.8 Managing Pain with a PCA Pump (continued)

Equipment

- PCA pump and appropriate tubing
- Operational manual for specific pump to be used
- Alcohol swab

Preparation

- Before initiating PCA therapy, determine factors that may contra-indicate use (e.g., impaired mental status, impaired respiratory status), the amount of narcotic specified by the order, bolus and continuous infusion dosage parameters, and type of primary fluid.
- Calculate:
  - The initial bolus dose based on the number of milligrams of drug per milliliter of fluid
  - The dose per intermittent bolus delivery
  - The 4-hour lockout drug limit.
- Check the medication administration record (MAR):
- Check the label on the medication carefully against the MAR to make sure that the correct medication is being prepared.
- Organize the equipment.

Procedure

1. Prior to performing the procedure, check physician's order, introduce self and verify the client's identity. Explain to the client the purpose and operation of the PCA, why it is necessary, and how he or she can participate.
2. Perform hand hygiene and observe other appropriate infection control procedures.
3. Provide for client privacy.
4. Prepare the client.
   - If not previously assessed, take baseline vital signs. If any of the findings are above or below the predetermined parameters, consult the primary care provider before administering the medication.
5. Set up the PCA infusion line according to the manufacturer's instructions.
   - Attach needleless adapter to end of PCA tubing.
   - Prime the PCA tubing.
   - Clamp the tubing. **Rationale:** *This prevents accidental bolusing and flushing of the primary line with the narcotic.*
   - Place the medication syringe in the PCA machine according to the operational instructions.
6. Connect the PCA infusion line to the primary fluid line.
   - Cleanse injection port of primary IV with alcohol swab.
   - Connect the PCA tubing to the primary fluid line at the injection port closest to the client.
7. Deliver the loading dose, as prescribed.
   - Set the pump for a lockout time of zero minutes.
   - Set the volume to be delivered based on calculated dosage volume for the loading dose.
   - Inject the loading dose by pressing the loading dose control button.
8. Set the safety parameters for the infusion on the PCA pump according to the manufacturer's instructions. For example:
   - Dose volume limits. **Rationale:** *This will limit the amount of drug that the client can receive when the client pushes the control button.*
   - Lockout interval between each dose. The lockout interval is generally between 5 and 15 minutes. **Rationale:** *This sets the minimum time that must elapse before the client can receive another dose of the drug. Lockout time is based on the usual onset of the IV narcotic and the assessment of the client.*
   - Dosage limit. Set the dosage limit (usually 1 or 4 hours) as specified on the orders. **Rationale:** *This is an additional safety feature to limit the amount of medication delivered.*
9. Lock the machine.
   - Close the door on the pump.
   - Look for any digital cues or alarms that may indicate the machine is not set, and make corrections as needed.
   - Lock the machine with the key.
10. Begin the infusion.
    - Place the client control button within reach.
11. Monitor the client.
    - Monitor the status of the client every 2 hours during the first 24 to 36 hours of infusion and regularly thereafter, depending on the client's health and agency protocol.
12. Monitor the infusion.
    - Observe the IV site for signs of infiltration and phlebitis.
    - Inspect the tubing for kinks that may occlude the line.
    - Note the total number of doses and milligrams received.
13. Document all relevant information.
    - Record the initiation of PCA, the dose setting, the doses received, pain intensity, and all assessments. See agency protocol for specific guidelines.

▶ HEAT AND COLD APPLICATION

Expected Outcomes

1. Bleeding and edema formation are minimized.
2. Client reports decrease in pain.
3. Inflammation is enhanced.
4. Target core body temperature is achieved.
5. Client has no adverse responses to therapy (arrhythmias, bleeding, shivering, afterdrop or rebound hyperthermia).

Heat and cold are applied to the body to promote comfort and the repair and healing of tissues. The form of thermal application generally depends on its purpose. Cold applied to a body part draws heat from the area; heat, of course, warms the area. The application of heat or cold produces physiological changes in the temperature of the tissues, size of the blood vessels, capillary blood pressure, capillary surface area for exchange of fluids and electrolytes, and tissue metabolism. The duration of the application also affects the response. See **Table 4–4** ● for a summary of the physiological effects of heat and cold, **Table 4–5** ● for selected indications for the use of heat and cold, and **Table 4–6** ● for correct temperatures for heat and cold applications.

TABLE 4–4   Physiological Effects of Heat and Cold

HEAT	COLD
Vasodilation	Vasoconstriction
Increases capillary permeability	Decreases capillary permeability
Increases cellular metabolism	Decreases cellular metabolism
Increases inflammation	Slows bacterial growth, decreases inflammation
Sedative effect	Local anesthetic effect

TABLE 4–5   Selected Indications for the Use of Heat and Cold

INDICATION	EFFECT OF HEAT	EFFECT OF COLD
Muscle spasm	Relaxes muscles and increases their contractility.	Relaxes muscles and decreases their contractility.
Inflammation	Increases blood flow, softens exudates.	Vasoconstriction decreases capillary permeability, decreases blood flow, slows cellular metabolism.
Pain	Relieves pain, possibly by promoting muscle relaxation, increasing circulation, and promoting psychological relaxation and a feeling of comfort; acts as a counterirritant.	Decreases pain by slowing nerve conduction rate and blocking nerve impulses; produces numbness, acts as a counterirritant, increases pain threshold.
Joint contracture	Reduces contracture and increases joint range of motion by allowing greater distention of muscles and connective tissue.	
Joint stiffness	Reduces joint stiffness by decreasing viscosity of synovial fluid and increasing tissue distensibility.	
Traumatic injury		Decreases bleeding by constricting blood vessels; decreases edema by reducing capillary permeability.

TABLE 4–6   Temperatures for Hot and Cold Applications

DESCRIPTION	TEMPERATURE	APPLICATION
Very cold	Below 15°C (59°F)	Ice bags
Cold	15–18°C (59–65°F)	Cold pack
Cool	18–27°C (65–80°F)	Cold compresses
Tepid	27–37°C (80–98°F)	Alcohol sponge bath
Warm	37–40°C (98–104°F)	Warm bath, aquathermia pads
Hot	40–46°C (104–115°F)	Hot soak, irrigations, hot compresses
Very hot	Above 46°C (above 115°F)	Hot water bags for adults

Variables Affecting Physiological Tolerance to Heat and Cold

- *Body part:* The back of the hand and foot are not very temperature sensitive. In contrast, the inner aspect of the wrist and forearm, the neck, and the perineal area are temperature sensitive.
- *Size of the exposed body part:* The larger the area exposed to heat and cold, the lower the tolerance.
- *Individual tolerance:* The very young and the very old generally have the lowest tolerance. Individuals who have neurosensory impairments may have a high tolerance, but the risk of injury is greater.
- *Length of exposure:* People feel hot and cold applications most while the temperature is changing. After a period of time, tolerance increases.
- *Intactness of skin:* Injured skin areas are more sensitive to temperature variations.

Contraindications to the Use of Heat and Cold Therapies

Determine the presence of any conditions contraindicating the use of heat:

- *The first 24 hours after traumatic injury:* Heat increases bleeding and swelling.
- *Active hemorrhage:* Heat causes vasodilation and increases bleeding.
- *Noninflammatory edema:* Heat increases capillary permeability and edema.
- *Localized malignant tumor:* Because heat accelerates cell metabolism and cell growth and increases circulation, it may accelerate metastases (secondary tumors).
- *Skin disorder that causes redness or blisters:* Heat can burn or cause further damage to the skin.

Determine the presence of any conditions contraindicating the use of cold:

- *Open wounds:* Cold can increase tissue damage by decreasing blood flow to an open wound.

- *Impaired circulation:* Cold can further impair nourishment of the tissues and cause tissue damage. In clients with Raynaud disease, cold increases arterial spasm.
- *Allergy or hypersensitivity to cold:* Some clients have an allergy to cold that may be manifested by an inflammatory response, for example, erythema, hives, swelling, joint pain, and occasional muscle spasm. Some react with a sudden increase in blood pressure, which can be hazardous if the person is hypertensive.

Determine the presence of any conditions indicating the need for special precautions during heat and cold therapy:

- *Neurosensory impairment:* Individuals with sensory impairments are unable to perceive that heat is damaging the tissues and are at risk for burns, or they are unable to perceive discomfort from cold and are unable to prevent tissue injury.
- *Impaired mental status:* Individuals who are confused or have an altered level of consciousness need monitoring and supervision during applications to ensure safe therapy.
- *Impaired circulation:* Individuals with peripheral vascular disease, diabetes, or congestive heart failure lack the normal ability to dissipate heat via the blood circulation, which puts them at risk for tissue damage with heat applications. Cold applications are contraindicated for these people.
- *Open wounds:* Tissues around an open wound are more sensitive to heat and cold.

Developmental Considerations

Older adult clients are more susceptible to injury from heat and cold therapy as a result of physiological changes or medical conditions:

- The epidermal cells are replaced more slowly in older adults.
- Skin in older adults is thin and contains less moisture.
- Older adults have a reduced sensitivity to pain, and therefore may not feel untoward effects of heat and cold treatment.
- Temperature should be reduced when using heat therapy because older adult client's skin burns more easily.

Vital signs and frequent assessment may be necessary during heat and cold therapy, because vasodilation from heat or vasoconstriction from cold can cause changes in cardiac function and blood pressure:

- Peripheral circulation may be compromised due to atherosclerosis or microvascular disease.
- Sensation in distal extremities may be impaired in older adult clients with neuropathy due to diabetes.
- Older adults may take medications that decrease sweating (anticholinergics for Parkinson's) or increase heat production (CNS stimulants or lithium).
- Serious infections may not elicit a febrile response.
- The temperature threshold for sweating is higher in the older adult client and the ability to mount a metabolic response to temperature loss is limited.
- Living conditions and financial limitations may not afford adequate environmental control.
- Hemodynamic responses to heat/cold therapies may be more unpredictable.

SKILL 4.9   Applying Dry Heat Measures

Delegation

Application of certain heat measures (e.g., baths) may be delegated to unlicensed assistive personnel (UAP) if they meet the general criteria for delegation (see Chapter 1). Sometimes, heat is applied as a component of wound care. However, in all cases, assessment of the client and the determination that the measure is safe to employ are the responsibility of the nurse. UAP may observe the area being treated during usual care and must report abnormal findings to the nurse. Abnormal findings must be validated and interpreted by the nurse.

Equipment

- Hot water bottle (bag)
  - Hot water bottle with a stopper
  - Cover
  - Hot water and a thermometer
- Electric heating pad
  - Electric pad and control
  - Cover (waterproof if there will be moisture under the pad when it is applied)
  - Gauze ties (optional)
- Aquathermia pad
  - Pad
  - Distilled water
  - Control unit
  - Cover
  - Gauze ties or tape (optional)
- Disposable hot pack
  - One or two commercially prepared disposable hot packs

Preparation

- Test all equipment for proper functioning and integrity (lack of leaks) before taking it to the client if possible.

Procedure

1. Prior to performing the procedure, introduce self and verify the client's identity using agency protocol. Explain to the client what you are going to do, why it is necessary, and how he or she can participate. Discuss how the results will be used in planning further care or treatments.
2. Perform hand hygiene and observe other appropriate infection control procedures.
3. Provide for client privacy.
   - Expose only the area to be treated.
4. Apply the heat.

CLINICAL ALERT

Heat transfers more quickly than cold therapy. Do not allow the client to lie on a "constant heat source" such as a heating pad or aquathermia pad.

Contraindications to heat therapies include acute injury or inflammation, recent or potential hemorrhage, deep venous thrombophlebitis, impaired circulation, impaired sensation, and impaired mentation.
   When treating an area where skin is not intact, cover lesion with sterile gauze and insulating barrier before applying heat.

Do not apply heat to an edematous area until the reason for edema has been determined.

(continued on next page)

SKILL 4.9 Applying Dry Heat Measures *(continued)*

VARIATION: HOT WATER BOTTLE

(Most Commonly Used in the Home Setting)

- Measure the temperature of the water. Follow agency practice for the appropriate temperature. The following temperatures are commonly used:
  a. 46° to 52°C (115° to 125°F) for a healthy adult
  b. 40° to 46°C (104° to 115°F) for a debilitated or unconscious adult.
- Fill the hot water bottle about two thirds full.
- Expel the air from the bottle. **Rationale:** *Air remaining in the bottle prevents it from molding to the body part being treated.*
- Secure the stopper tightly.
- Hold the bottle upside down, and check for leaks.
- Dry the bottle.
- Wrap the bottle in a towel or hot water bottle cover ❶.

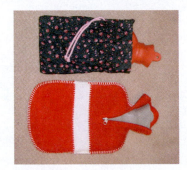

❶ Hot water bottle and cloth covers.

- Apply the bottle to the body part using pillows to support it if necessary.

VARIATION: ELECTRIC HEATING PAD

(Most Commonly Used in the Home Setting)

- Ensure that the body area is dry. **Rationale:** *Electricity in the presence of moisture can conduct a shock.*
- Check that the electric pad is functioning properly. The cord should be free from cracks, wires should be intact, heating components should not be exposed, and temperature distribution over the pad should be even.
- Place the cover on the pad. Some models have waterproof covers to be used when the pad is placed over a moist dressing. **Rationale:** *Moisture could cause the pad to short circuit and burn or shock the client.*
- Plug the pad into the electric socket.
- Set the control dial for the correct temperature.
- After the pad has heated, place the pad over the body part to which heat is being applied.
- Use gauze ties instead of safety pins to hold the pad in place, if needed. **Rationale:** *A pin might strike a wire, damaging the pad and giving an electric shock to the client.*

VARIATION: AQUATHERMIA PAD (ALSO CALLED A K-PAD)

- Fill the unit ❷ with distilled water until it is two thirds full. The unit will warm the water, which circulates through the pad.
- Secure the lid.
- Regulate the temperature with the key if it has not been preset. Normal temperature is 40° to 46°C (104° to 115°F). Check the manufacturer's instructions.

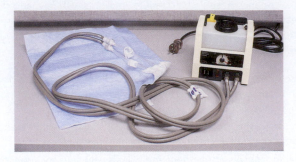

❷ An aquathermia heating unit and pad.

- Cover the pad with a towel or pillowcase.
- Plug in the unit.
- Check for any leak or malfunctions of the pad before use.
- Use tape or gauze ties to hold the pad in place. Never use safety pins. They can cause leakage.
- If unusual redness or pain occurs, discontinue the treatment, and report the client's reaction.

VARIATION: DISPOSABLE HOT PACK

- Microwave, strike, squeeze, or knead the pack according to the manufacturer's directions.
- Note the manufacturer's instructions about the length of time that heat is produced.
- Depending on the type of pack, wrap in a towel or enclose in a cover prior to application.

5. Give the client the following instructions:
   - Do not insert any sharp, pointed object (e.g., a pin) into the bottle, pack, or pad.
   - Do not lie directly on the bottle or pad. **Rationale:** *The surface below the object promotes heat absorption instead of normal heat dissipation.*
   - To prevent injury, avoid adjusting the heat higher than specified. **Rationale:** *The degree of heat felt shortly after application will decrease, because the body's temperature receptors quickly adapt to the temperature. This adaptive mechanism can lead to tissue injury if the temperature is adjusted higher.*
   - Call the nurse if any discomfort is felt.
6. Leave the heat in place for only the designated time to avoid the rebound phenomenon, usually 30 minutes. Check the application and skin area after 5 to 10 minutes to be sure the skin is intact.
7. Document the application of the heat and the client's response in the client record, using forms or checklists supplemented by narrative notes when appropriate.

Developmental Considerations

INFANTS/CHILDREN

- The temperature of water in a hot water bottle should be 40.5° to 46°C (105° to 115°F) for a child under 2 years of age.

OLDER ADULTS

- Use special care in assessing the area to be treated and in evaluating the effects of the treatment because older adults have many conditions that predispose them to injury with heat measures.

SKILL 4.10   Applying Compresses and Moist Packs

Delegation

Application of unsterile compresses or packs may be delegated to UAP if they meet the general criteria for delegation. However, in all cases, assessment of the client and the determination that the measure is safe to employ are the responsibility of the nurse. UAP may observe the area being treated during usual care and must report abnormal findings to the nurse. Abnormal findings must be validated and interpreted by the nurse.

Equipment

Use sterile equipment and supplies for an open wound.

Compress

- Disposable gloves or sterile gloves (for an open wound)
- Solution at the strength and temperature specified by the primary care provider or the agency
- Container for the solution
- Thermometer
- Gauze squares
- Cotton applicator sticks
- Petroleum jelly
- Insulating towel
- Plastic wrap
- Ties (e.g., roller gauze or masking tape)
- Hot water bottle or aquathermia pad (optional)

or

- Ice bag (optional)
- Sterile dressing, if required

Moist Pack

- Clean gloves
- Flannel pieces or towel packs
- Hot-pack machine for heating the packs

or

- Basin of water with some ice chips
- Cotton applicator sticks
- Petroleum jelly
- Insulating material (e.g., flannel or towels)
- Plastic wrap
- Hot water bottle (optional)

or

- Ice bag (optional)
- Sterile dressing, if required

Preparation

- If possible, perform care so that the application of the compress or pack will not need to be interrupted for other activities such as toileting.

Procedure

1. Prior to performing the procedure, introduce self and verify the client's identity using agency protocol. Explain to the client what you are going to do, why it is necessary, and how he or she can participate. Discuss how the results will be used in planning further care or treatments.
2. Perform hand hygiene and observe other appropriate infection control procedures.
3. Provide for client privacy.
   - Expose only the area to be treated.
4. Prepare the client.
   - Assist the client to a comfortable position.
   - Expose the area for the compress or pack.
   - Provide support for the body part requiring the compress or pack.
   - If indicated, apply clean gloves, and remove the wound dressing. Remove and discard gloves. Perform hand hygiene.
5. Moisten the compress or the pack.
   - Place the gauze in the solution.

or

   - Heat the flannel or towel in a steamer, or chill it in the basin of water and ice chips.
6. Protect the surrounding skin as indicated.
   - If a wound is exposed, apply petroleum jelly to the skin surrounding the wound, not on the wound or open areas of the skin, using a cotton applicator stick. **Rationale:** *Jelly protects the skin from possible burns, maceration, and the irritating effects of some solutions.*
7. Apply the moist compress or pack.
   - Wring out the gauze compress so that the solution does not drip from it. For a sterile compress, use sterile forceps or sterile gloves to wring out the gauze.
   - Apply the gauze lightly and gradually to the designated area and, if tolerated by the client, mold the compress close to the body. **Rationale:** *Air is a poor conductor of cold or heat, and molding excludes air.*

or

   - Wring out the flannel (for a sterile pack, use sterile gloves).
   - Apply the flannel to the body area, molding it closely to the body part.
8. Immediately insulate and secure the application.
   - Cover the gauze or flannel quickly with a dry towel and a piece of plastic wrap. **Rationale:** *This step helps maintain the temperature of the application and thus its effectiveness.*
   - Secure the compress or pack in place with gauze ties or tape.
   - *Optional:* Apply a hot water bottle, aquathermia pad, or ice bag over the plastic wrap to maintain the heat or cold.
9. Monitor the client.
   - Assess the client for discomfort at 5- to 10-minute intervals. If the client feels any discomfort, assess the area for erythema, numbness, maceration, or blistering.
   - For applications to large areas of the body, note any change in the pulse, respirations, and blood pressure.
   - In the event of unexpected reactions, terminate the treatment and report to the nurse in charge.
10. Remove the compress or pack at the specified time.
    - Compresses and packs with an external heat or cold source on top may remain in place 1 to 2 hours. Without external heat or cold, they need to be changed every few minutes.
    - Apply a sterile dressing if one is required.
11. Document the application of the compress or pack and the client's response in the client record using forms or checklists supplemented by narrative notes when appropriate.

SKILL 4.11 Assisting with a Sitz Bath

Equipment

- Disposable sitz bath with tubing and bag
- Warm water (40° to 43°C [104° to 109°F]) *Note:* Cold temperature may be indicated for client's situation.
- Towels for drying
- Thermometer
- Clean gloves

Preparation

- Verify physician's order for sitz bath, duration and frequency of treatments.
- Raise toilet seat and place sitz bath basin with "FRONT" facing the front of the toilet bowl ❶.

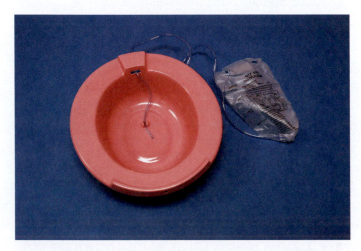

❶ Individual disposable sitz bath units are used for infection control purposes.

- Fill basin with warm water (40° to 43°C [104° to 109°F]) one half to two thirds full
- Close flow tubing clamp.
- Open top of plastic bag and fill with hot water (40° to 43°C [104° to 109°F]).
- Hang bag at a level higher than the sitz basin so that fluid will flow by gravity.
- Insert tubing through front or rear entry hole in sitz bath, then snap or secure tubing into channel or "eye" in bottom of basin.
- Perform hand hygiene.

Procedure

1. Identify client by checking the client's identity band and asking client to state name and birth date.
2. Explain procedure and rationale for sitz bath.
3. Assist client to treatment area with accessible call bell.
4. Provide privacy by placing sign on door.
5. Check to ensure that temperature of thermotherapy water is 40.5° to 43.3°C (105° to 110°F). *Note:* Most hospitals control water temperature so that it will not exceed 43.3°C (110°F).
6. Assist client to sit in sitz bath for 15 to 20 minutes.
7. Maintain water temperature by continually adding water of appropriate temperature to bag. *Note:* Overflow will drain into toilet through openings in back of basin.
8. Upon completion, assist client to dry area and allow client to sit briefly to allow normalization of blood pressure and to prevent hypotension upon standing. **Rationale:** *Orthostatic hypotension may occur with rapid position change following warm sitz bath due to vasodilation.*
9. Don clean gloves, empty and rinse client's sitz basin, and store in convenient location for future use.
10. Discard soiled linen.
11. Perform hand hygiene. Document action and client response.

SKILL 4.12 Providing Tepid Sponges

Equipment

- Water or other coolant at prescribed temperature
- Basin or tub
- Washcloth and towels
- Bath blanket
- Electric fan
- Automated blood pressure unit
- Core temperature thermometer, cable, and module to monitor

Preparation

- Review order for cooling method.
- Gather equipment and bring to client's room.
- Check two forms of client ID and introduce yourself.
- Provide privacy and explain procedure.
- Perform hand hygiene.
- Establish continuous core temperature monitoring (rectal, esophageal, bladder, or pulmonary artery), if indicated.
- Establish ongoing blood pressure and cardiac monitoring.

Procedure

1. Remove client's clothing to allow for cooling and observation. Use bath blanket for privacy.
2. Monitor skin color and vital signs every 15 to 30 minutes during cooling. Immerse washcloths or material for sponging in ordered solution, generally 21° to 27°C (70° to 81°F). **Rationale:** *Cool application reduces heat by conduction.*
3. Wring out excess solution and place cloths on neck, axillae, groin. **Rationale:** *The vascularity of these areas promotes cooling.*
4. Depending on type of bath, change cloths every 5 minutes. **Rationale:** *This prevents cloths from warming and losing effectiveness.*

CLINICAL ALERT

Do not immerse the client in cold or ice slush. Resulting peripheral vasoconstriction will impair body cooling and induce shivering, which produces heat.

SKILL 4.12 Providing Tepid Sponges (*continued*)

5. Cool the ambient temperature to 20° to 22°C (68° to 72°F). **Rationale:** *This enhances therapy by convection and evaporation.*

6. Direct a warm fan onto client to promote evaporation. **Rationale:** *This enhances cooling by evaporation.*

7. Assess client for early signs of shivering (ECG tremor artifact, palpable jaw line "hum," or trapezius muscle tension).

8. Stop treatment if client has early signs of shivering and notify physician. **Rationale:** *Shivering raises core temperature, defeating purpose of cooling intervention.* The physician may order a narcotic or benzodiazepine for sedation.

9. Monitor client's temperature frequently. When temperature has decreased to desired level, dry skin and replace light covering over client; reposition for comfort. **Rationale:** *A thin client will cool faster than one with more subcutaneous fat.*

10. Continue to monitor vital signs, cardiac rhythm, I&O, and electrolytes.

11. Provide fluids and a high-calorie diet. **Rationale:** *Increased temperatures increase metabolic rate.*

12. Place clothes in linen hamper and return equipment to utility or storage area.

13. Perform hand hygiene. Document action and client response.

SKILL 4.13 Using a Neonatal Incubator/Infant Radiant Warmer

Equipment

- Radiant warmer with skin probe and temperature gel patch to secure probe to infant's skin
- Bedding and positioning aids appropriate for bed and infant

Preparation

- Check physician's order. Follow manufacturer's operating instructions for safety. (Several different radiant warmers/infant care centers are available ❶ ❷.)

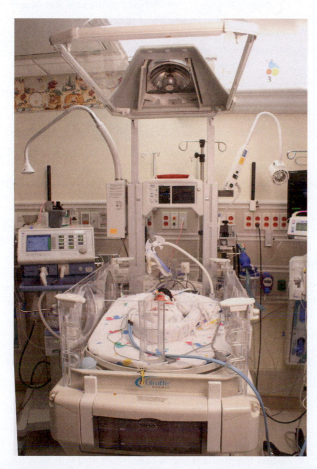

❶ Giraffe bed in radiant warmer mode, offering quick and easy access to the critically ill neonate.

- Check caster locks to make certain that each is in locked position.
- Adjust bed to desired position.
- Plug cord into three-prong receptacle.
- Turn power switch on; bed will take approximately 30 seconds to power up.
- Set bed to manual control mode for desired temperature. **Rationale:** *This allows bed to warm up prior to placing infant on bed.*

Procedure

1. Plug temperature probe into bed. **Rationale:** *To obtain a digital recording of the infant's skin temperature.*

2. Place infant on bed, then set bed to skin control mode.

3. Attach skin probe with polished surface over a location of fatty tissue on infant's body, avoiding any bony prominence.

4. Attach temperature gel patch to secure probe to infant's skin; do not use adhesive tape. **Rationale:** *To prevent skin irritation. The infant's skin is very thin and fragile.*

5. Allow 3 to 5 minutes for probe to reach infant's temperature.

6. Monitor placement of skin probe:
   - Validate appropriate skin temperature reading. **Rationale:** *If reading is not at desired temperature, probe may need to be repositioned.*
   - Inspect infant's skin under probe at regular intervals. **Rationale:** *Infant's skin is delicate and irritates easily.*
   - Change probe location if irritation begins to appear.

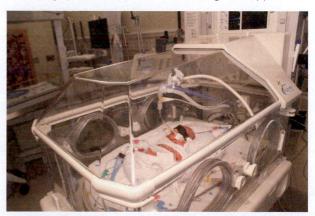

❷ Giraffe bed in incubator mode, offering a quiet, neutral thermal environment.

SKILL 4.14   Applying Dry Cold Measures

Delegation

Application of certain cold measures (e.g., cooling baths) may be delegated to UAP if they meet the general criteria for delegation. However, in all cases, assessment of the client and the determination that the measure is safe to employ are the responsibility of the nurse. UAP may observe the area being treated during usual care and must report abnormal findings to the nurse. Abnormal findings must be validated and interpreted by the nurse.

Equipment

- Ice bag, collar, glove, or cold pack
- Ice chips
- Protective covering
- Roller gauze, a binder or a towel, and tape

Procedure

1. Prior to performing the procedure, introduce self and verify the client's identity using agency protocol. Explain to the client what you are going to do, why it is necessary, and how he or she can participate. Discuss how the results will be used in planning further care or treatments.
2. Perform hand hygiene and observe other appropriate infection control procedures.
3. Provide for client privacy.
   - Expose only the area to be treated, and provide warmth to avoid chilling.
4. Prepare the client.
   - Assist the client to a comfortable position, and support the body part requiring the application.
5. Apply the cold measure.

Evidence-Based Nursing Practice

Postoperative Cold Versus Cold-Plus-Compression Therapy

A randomized, prospective clinical trial evaluated the effectiveness of cryotherapy with or without intermittent pneumatic compression after arthroscopic ACL reconstructive surgery. Clients used therapy at least 30 minutes three times a day. Results were compared preoperatively and at 1, 2, and 6 weeks after surgery.

The study measured compliance, use of pain medications, swelling (girth), and quality of life and knee scores. During weeks 1 and 2, patients with compressive cryotherapy had 100% compliance; the control group had 83% compliance. At 6 weeks, 83.3% of the compression and cryotherapy group had discontinued all pain medication. In contrast, just 27.8% of the control group (5 of 18 people) had discontinued all pain medication.

Data from Waterman et al. (2012).

VARIATION: ICE BAG, COLLAR, OR GLOVE

- Fill the device one half to two thirds full of crushed ice. **Rationale:** *Partial filling makes the device more pliable so that it can be molded to a body part.*

- Remove excess air by bending or twisting the device. **Rationale:** *Air inflates the device so that it cannot be molded to the body part.*
- Insert the stopper securely into an ice bag or collar, or tie a knot at the open end of a glove. **Rationale:** *This prevents leakage of fluid when the ice melts.*
- Hold the device upside down, and check it for leaks.
- Cover the device with a soft cloth cover, if it is not already equipped with one. **Rationale:** *The cover absorbs moisture that condenses on the outside of the device. It is also more comfortable for the client.*
- Hold the device in place with roller gauze, ties, a binder, or a towel. Secure with tape as necessary.

CLINICAL ALERT

Never apply a fully cooled reusable cold pack directly to the skin; also, do not overinsulate the area.

Bony areas (knee, ankle, elbow) usually require half the treatment time that fatty areas require. Superficial nerves at these joint sites are especially vulnerable to cold-induced neuropathy, especially if cold is combined with compression.

Crushable chemical packs should be used as the last resort because they are not as cold nor do they last as long as crushed ice.

Do not apply an instant chemical pack to the face and never use pins to secure pack. Leakage of chemical contents can cause serious injury. If contents are exposed to skin, immediately flush with copious amounts of water and notify physician.

- Frozen gel packs and crushed ice packs using ice frozen in a refrigerator or freezer ($-16°$ to $-19°C$ [$3°$ to $-2°F$]) should not be applied directly to the skin.
- Packs with ice from an ice machine ($-1°C$ [$30°F$]) do not require insulation.
- During cryotherapy, erythema will occur.
- The client will experience four stages of cold progression: cold/stinging/burning/numbness.
- Discontinue therapy upon numbness.

VARIATION: DISPOSABLE COLD PACK

- Strike, squeeze, or knead the cold pack according to the manufacturer's instructions. **Rationale:** *The action activates the chemical reaction that produces the cold.*
- Cover with a soft cloth cover if the pack does not have a cover. Most commercially prepared cold packs have soft outer coverings to permit application directly to the body part.

6. Instruct the client as follows:
   - Remain in position for the duration of the treatment.
   - Call the nurse if discomfort is felt.
7. Monitor the client during the application.
   - Assess the client in terms of comfort and skin reaction (e.g., pallor, mottled appearance) as frequently as necessary for the client's safety (e.g., every 5 to 10 minutes).

SKILL 4.14   Applying Dry Cold Measures *(continued)*

Check more often if client has had previous negative responses to applications and or client has difficulty reporting problems.

- Report untoward reactions and remove the application.

8. Leave the cold in place for only the designated period of time. **Rationale:** *Avoid the rebound phenomenon and the harmful effects of prolonged cold.*

9. Document the application of the cold and the client's response in the client record using forms or checklists supplemented by narrative notes when appropriate.

Sample Documentation

3/30/15 2245 Rt foot and ankle swollen toes to lower calf. Reports pain is 7/10. Moves toes and ankle, pedal pulses present. Skin warm, no bruising or wounds noted. Padded ice pack applied x10 minutes. Reports pain 5/10. _____ P. Wilder, RN

SKILL 4.15   Using a Cooling Blanket

Evidence-Based Nursing Practice

Hypothermia and Stroke Outcome

A 2010 report supported by the NIH National Institute of Neurological Disorders and Stroke supported the neuroprotective role of hypothermia in clients with cardiac arrest and some pediatric clients with hypoxic brain insult. The study states that hypothermia is a protectant against brain ischemia, but that its effect in hemorrhagic stroke is less clear. Early clinical studies show that hypothermia may have some feasibility in clients with stroke, but it must be weighed against potential negative sequelae such as pneumonia and possible reduction in thrombolytic efficacy. The report recommends further exploration of combining hypothermia with other neuroprotectants and modern reperfusion therapies. It also suggests there may be a role for newer, less invasive cooling methods that include pharmacologic cooling strategies.

Data from Midori & Hemmen (2010).

Equipment

- Thermal (heating/cooling) unit
- Sterile or distilled water
- Low-reading (below 34.4°C [94°F]) thermometer: rectal probe and lubricant, esophageal probe, urinary retention catheter, or pulmonary artery catheter with cable and module for continuous core temperature monitoring, depending on thermometer used
- Clean gloves
- Disposable thermal (cooling) blanket
- One sheet or thin blanket
- Covering for client
- Four towels to wrap client's lower arms and legs
- Tape
- Lower extremity (or foot) compression wraps
- Sphygmomanometer and stethoscope or automated BP monitoring equipment
- Continuous ECG monitoring (if indicated)
- Supplemental oxygen therapy equipment

Preparation

- Check physician's orders for desired client temperature.
- Identify medications client has received (narcotic, sedative).

- Gather equipment and take to client's room.
- Connect power cord to grounded outlet.
- Ensure that reservoir (sterile or distilled water) level is adequate.
- Perform hand hygiene.
- Introduce self. Check client's identity band and have client state name and birth date.
- Provide privacy and explain procedure.
- Obtain baseline vital signs.

Procedure

1. Place the cooling blanket on bed, and connect it to the temperature control unit machine. **Rationale:** *The cooling blanket increases heat transfer from client and reduces body temperature by conduction.*
   - Push the tubing tab to insert male tubing connector of the cooling pad into inlet opening. Release the tab.
   - Repeat connection using the outlet opening.
   - Turn the unit ON by pushing power switch.
   - Enter client's target temperature set point.
2. Place a sheet or a thin bath blanket over the cooling blanket.
3. Place client on the cooling blanket.
4. Apply leg or foot compression wraps. **Rationale:** *This helps to prevent thrombus formation and reduces edema.*
5. Wrap client's lower arms and hands and lower legs and feet (and scrotum if indicated) in towels and tape to secure. **Rationale:** *This prevents stimulation of skin thermoreceptors that initiate shivering.*
6. Establish continuous core temperature monitoring.
7. Set the master temperature control to either automatic or manual operation. **Rationale:** *There are two separate temperature controls, one for automatic and one for manual operation.*

For Automatic Control

- Don clean gloves.
- If using rectal thermometer probe, digitally examine client's rectum to determine it is empty of stool. **Rationale:** *Rectal temperature probe must make contact with mucosa.*
- Insert lubricated temperature probe into client's rectum 2 inches.
- If using bladder retention catheter with integrated temperature probe, determine that urine output is at least 20 mL/hr. **Rationale:** *Probe actually measures urine temperature.*

(continued on next page)

SKILL 4.15   Using a Cooling Blanket *(continued)*

- Set temperature control at the desired temperature (fluid temperature set point).
- Turn automatic mode light on and press "START." **Rationale:** *The pad fluid temperature will adjust automatically to bring client's temperature to a selected set point.*
- Check that the pad temperature limits are set as ordered.

For Manual Control

- Observe that the *manual* mode light is on.
- Monitor the fluid set point, which indicates temperature of pad. **Rationale:** *This ensures pad temperature is maintained at desired level.*

8. Set the temperature control to 37°C, and begin lowering temperature 1°C every 30 minutes to 1 hour as tolerated to prevent shivering, until 33° or 34°C or set temperature is reached. **Rationale:** *Blanket will cool client to set temperature independent of client's temperature. Gradual cooling helps prevent shivering.*

9. Monitor client's temperature. **Rationale:** *To prevent excessive cooling.*

10. Assess client every 15 minutes for early signs of shivering: ECG muscle tremor artifact, jaw line "hum," or trapezius muscle tension.

11. If early signs of shivering occur, discontinue therapy and notify physician or refer to agency hypothermia protocol. **Rationale:** *Shivering causes an increase in core temperature, thus defeating the purpose of treatment. Shivering imposes a heavy metabolic burden and increases oxygen demand.*

Mild	32°–37°C (89.6°–98.6°F)
Moderate	28°–32°C (82.4°–89.6°F)
Severe	20°–28°C (68.0°–82.4°F)

12. Monitor vital signs every 15 to 30 minutes during therapy. **Rationale:** *Bradycardia may occur. Blood pressure usually remains elevated due to vasoconstriction.*

13. Monitor ECG for possible arrhythmias. **Rationale:** *Potassium shifts into cells with induced hypothermia.*

14. Monitor client's serum glucose. **Rationale:** *Insulin levels are decreased with induced hypothermia. Glucose levels may rise with shivering. An insulin drip may be necessary to maintain glucose at 80 to 130 mg/dL.*

15. Turn and deep-breathe client every 1 to 2 hours. **Rationale:** *Hypothermia reduces carbon dioxide production with possible resultant hypoventilation.*

16. Monitor client's skin condition and bony prominences every 2 hours. **Rationale:** *Client is at risk for pressure ulcers when skin temperature is lowered.*

17. Turn off unit when client's temperature is 1° to 3°C above desired temperature. **Rationale:** *Cooling will continue upon discontinuation of therapy.*

18. Monitor vital signs every 15 minutes during rewarming.

19. Observe for edema. **Rationale:** *Hypothermia causes fluid shift into the interstitium.*

20. Clean and return reusable equipment to appropriate area and dispose of blanket.

21. Monitor client's vital signs frequently after discontinuation of treatment. **Rationale:** *Overshoot hypothermia may occur.*

22. Make client comfortable.

23. Perform hand hygiene. Document relevant information.

> **CLINICAL ALERT**
>
> The effectiveness and safety of cooling blankets for treatment of fever are poorly demonstrated. They may be dangerous in some instances. Use of a cooling blanket is discouraged except for environmental hyperthermia.

▶ END-OF-LIFE CARE

Expected Outcomes

1. Client is able to progress through stages of grief with support of family and nursing staff.
2. Client's cultural beliefs are considered throughout the dying process.
3. Client's dignity is maintained while completing postmortem care.
4. Client's relatives are supported by staff during grief process.
5. Appropriate procedures are carried out for organ donations.

Nurses may interact with dying clients and their families or caregivers in a variety of settings, from fetal demise (death of an unborn child), to the adolescent victim of an accident, to the older adult client who finally succumbs to a chronic illness. Death can be viewed as a person's final opportunity to experience life in ways that bring significance and fulfillment. The nurse's role is to provide or facilitate physical, emotional, and spiritual care of the dying client and the client's family.

Caring for the dying and the bereaved (those individuals mourning the dead) is one of the nurse's most complex and challenging responsibilities, bringing into play all skills needed for holistic physiological and psychosocial care. This chapter emphasizes physical care. It is beyond the scope of this chapter to address in detail theoretical concepts such as grief and grieving or legal aspects such as the process of organ donation and living wills. The reader is referred to a fundamentals or concepts book for additional material.

> **CLINICAL ALERT**
>
> The goal of care for the dying client changes from curative to palliative care. Helping the client achieve a measure of comfort and knowing that family members and significant others are being supported during this process is a comfort for the client.

SKILL 4.16   Meeting the Physiological Needs of the Client Who Is Dying

Delegation

Comfort measures and supportive care strategies for care of clients at the end of life are often delegated to UAP. The nurse reviews with the UAP those measures and strategies needed for a specific client. UAPs must inform the nurse if the client appears in unanticipated or unrelieved distress.

Equipment

Needed equipment depends on the specific comfort measures being provided. Items may include medications, linens, and hygiene supplies.

Preparation

■ The physiological needs of people who are dying are related to a slowing of body processes and to homeostatic imbalances. Interventions include providing personal hygiene measures; controlling pain; relieving respiratory difficulties; assisting with movement, nutrition, hydration, and elimination; and providing measures related to sensory changes.

Clinical Manifestations

Impending Clinical Death

Loss of Muscle Tone

■ Relaxation of the facial muscles (e.g., the jaw may sag)
■ Difficulty speaking
■ Difficulty swallowing and gradual loss of the gag reflex
■ Decreased activity of the gastrointestinal tract, with subsequent nausea, accumulation of flatus, abdominal distention, and retention of feces, especially if narcotics or tranquilizers are being administered
■ Possible urinary and rectal incontinence due to decreased sphincter control
■ Diminished body movement

Slowing of the Circulation

■ Diminished sensation
■ Mottling and cyanosis of the extremities
■ Cold skin, first in the feet and later in the hands, ears, and nose (the client, however, may feel warm if there is a fever)
■ Slower and weaker pulse
■ Decreased blood pressure

Changes in Respirations

■ Rapid, shallow, irregular, or abnormally slow respirations
■ Noisy breathing, referred to as the death rattle, due to collecting of mucus in the throat
■ Mouth breathing, dry oral mucous membranes

Sensory Impairment

■ Blurred vision
■ Impaired senses of taste and smell
■ Various consciousness levels may exist just before death. Some clients are alert, whereas others are drowsy, stuporous, or comatose. Hearing is thought to be the last sense lost.

Procedure

1. Prior to performing the procedure, introduce self and verify the client's identity using agency protocol. Explain to the client what you are going to do, why it is necessary, and how he or she can participate.

2. Perform hand hygiene and observe other appropriate infection control procedures.

3. Provide for client privacy depending on the specific interventions.

4. Perform bathing/hygiene.
   • Provide frequent baths and linen changes if diaphoretic, incontinent, or need for odor control. **Rationale:** *Dying individuals may have wounds, fever, or loss of sphincter control, which can be both uncomfortable when substances are left on the skin and cause distressing smells.*
   • Give mouth care as needed for dry mouth, to remove secretions, and to provide comfort.
   • Apply moisturizing creams and lotions for dry skin, and moisture-barrier skin preparations for incontinent clients.
   • Cleanse skin areas around wounds or areas that collect wound drainage.

5. Provide pain control.
   • Pain control is essential to enable clients to maintain some quality in their life and their daily activities, including eating, moving, and sleeping. Many drugs have been used to control the pain associated with terminal illness: morphine, heroin, methadone, and alcohol.
   • Usually the primary care provider determines the dosage, but the client's opinion should be considered; the client is the one ultimately aware of personal pain tolerance and fluctuations of internal states. Because primary care providers usually prescribe a range for the dosage of pain medication, nurses use their own judgment as to the specific amount and frequency of pain medication needed to provide client relief.
   • Because of decreased blood circulation, if analgesics cannot be administered orally, they are given by intravenous infusion, sublingually, or rectally, rather than subcutaneously or intramuscularly. **Rationale:** *Subcutaneous or intramuscular injections given to clients with impaired circulation will not reach the desired receptors and, thus, will be ineffective.*
   • Clients on narcotic pain medications also require implementation of a protocol to treat opioid-induced constipation.
   • Under periods of stress, the brain releases endorphins, morphine-like substances that modulate pain perception. Although studied primarily in animal models and in near-death experiences, some scientists believe that large amounts of endorphins may be released at the time of death. This could explain the seemingly peaceful sense of dissociation from the reality of pain, floating outside the body, seeing a tunnel, or moving toward the light that is expressed by some individuals.

6. Provide respiratory support.
   • For clients with difficulty clearing their own airway, place in Fowler's position if conscious, lateral position if unconscious. **Rationale:** *Fowler's position makes breathing easier. The lateral position allows secretions to drain out rather than entering the client's airway.*
   • Perform oral throat suctioning as needed, especially for conscious clients who express discomfort.

(continued on next page)

SKILL 4.16   Meeting the Physiological Needs of the Client Who Is Dying (continued)

- Apply nasal oxygen for hypoxic clients. **Rationale:** *Supplemental oxygen may relieve the signs and symptoms of oxygen deprivation such as confusion.*
- Anticholinergic medications (e.g., atropine, hyoscine hydrobromide) may be indicated to help dry secretions. Note that noisy respirations, sometimes referred to as the *death rattle*, are believed to be more distressing to those who have to listen to the sounds than the condition is for the dying client.
- For clients who have air hunger (the sensation of needing to breathe), open windows or use a fan to circulate air. Morphine may be indicated in an acute episode.

7. Assist with movement.
   - Assist client out of bed periodically, if client is able.
   - Regularly change client's position.
   - Support client's position with pillows, blanket rolls, or towels as needed.
   - Elevate client's legs when sitting up.
   - Implement pressure ulcer prevention program and use pressure-relieving surfaces as indicated.

8. Provide nutrition and hydration as indicated.
   - Administer antiemetics to treat nausea.
   - Encourage favorite foods as tolerated.
   - Support family members who may be very concerned that their loved one is not eating or drinking sufficiently or who believe that failure to push nutrition signifies giving up and failure.
   - In some states, a feeding tube cannot be removed from a person in a persistent vegetative state (PVS) without a prior directive from the client, but in other states the removal is allowed at the family's request or with a physician's order.
   - Teach family that clients with dehydration and alterations in electrolytes at the end of life may not be experiencing discomfort. In addition, dehydration actually reduces secretions and the need for elimination.

9. Assist with elimination.
   - For constipation, provide dietary fiber as tolerated or stool softeners or laxatives as needed.
   - Perform meticulous skin care in response to incontinence of urine or feces.
   - Keep the bedpan, urinal, or commode chair within easy reach and the call light within reach for assistance with elimination.
   - Use absorbent pads under incontinent clients; change linen as often as needed.
   - Urinary catheterization may be performed, if necessary.
   - Keep the room as clean and odor free as possible.

10. Be aware of sensory changes.
    - Check the client's preference for a light or dark room. Position to be able to view the television, favorite items or photos, or a window as desired.
    - Hearing is not diminished; speak clearly and do not whisper. Use music as desired.
    - Touch sensation is diminished, but client will feel pressure of touch.
    - Provide gown, clothing, and bedding that feels and looks as the client prefers.
    - Facilitate client interaction with others as desired. This may require flexing agency rules regarding visiting hours or presence of pets. Advocate for the client as much as possible about these.
    - Implement a pain management protocol if indicated; medicate for other sensory alterations such as itching.

11. Family members should be encouraged to participate in the physical care of the dying person as much as they wish to and are able. The nurse can suggest they assist with bathing, speak or read to the client, and hold hands. The nurse must not, however, have specific expectations for family members' participation. Those who feel unable to care for or be with the dying person also require support from the nurse and from other family members. They should be shown an appropriate waiting area if they wish to remain nearby.

12. Consider how routine care should be modified based on the dying client. Often vital signs are measured less frequently, blood and other laboratory tests are no longer performed, and active, invasive, or expensive treatment measures (such as antibiotics for infection) are suspended. Caring for dying clients who have agreed to organ donation can also be complex in terms of determining which medications, treatments, or equipment must be continued until the time for harvesting the organs has arrived.

13. Document all client care, especially the effectiveness of symptom management activities.

Sample Documentation

12/20/15 23:30

S	*"I am so tired. Please don't make me turn right now. Could you give me some ice chips?"*
O	*Lotion and massage to reachable back and extremities. Repositioned slightly to shift weight off bony prominences. Ice chips given and placed within reach.*
A	*Care modified to support dying client autonomy.*
P	*Turn q3h instead of q2h if the client prefers. Reinforce need to assess and treat dependent skin areas. Assess need for analgesics before each turn. Request pressure-reducing mattress.*

————————————————————————————— S. Amber, RN

Client Teaching

Caregivers of a dying person need ongoing support and ongoing teaching as the client's condition changes. Some of these teaching needs include:

- Ways to feed the client when swallowing becomes difficult
- Ways to transfer and reposition the client safely
- Ways to communicate if verbalization becomes more difficult

- Nonpharmacologic methods of pain control
- Comfort measures, such as frequent oral care and frequent repositioning
- Person to contact for different sources of support (e.g., respite care, pharmacies that deliver to the home, information about interpreting changes in the client's condition).

SKILL 4.16 Meeting the Physiological Needs of the Client Who Is Dying (continued)

Setting of Care

CARING FOR THE DYING

People facing death may need help accepting that they have to depend on others. Some dying clients require only minimal care; others need continuous attention and services. People need help, well in advance of death, in planning for the period of dependence. They need to consider what will happen and how and where they would like to die.

A major factor in determining whether a person will die in a healthcare facility or at home is the availability of willing and able caregivers. If the dying person wishes to be at home, and family or others can provide care to maintain symptom control, the nurse should facilitate a referral to outpatient hospice services. Hospice staff and nurses will then conduct a full assessment of the home and care providers' skills.

Although the original hospice was a freestanding facility, according to the National Hospice and Palliative Care Organization (2012), the largest segment of hospice care in the United States is delivered in the home (41.6% of hospice cases). The hospice concept is also implemented in hospice centers (26.1% of cases), palliative care areas in acute care hospitals (7.4% of cases), and designated locations within long-term care facilities (24.9% of cases). Most insurance policies, including Medicare, cover hospice services. In 2011, more than 44% of all deaths in the United States occurred under hospice care.

Cultural Considerations

Kawaga-Singer and Blackhall (2001), in an article title "Negotiating Cross-Cultural Issues at the End of Life," stated that culture is an important part of how everyone understands their world and how this impacts their decisions, especially on healthcare issues. This includes healthcare professionals as well. Culture influences the way people make meaning out of illness and dying; therefore, it also influences how they utilize the medical community at the end of life. Each individual has a perspective that is also influenced by factors such as personal psychology, gender, and life experiences. Wide variations in beliefs and behaviors exist within any ethnic population. This leads us to realize that each client needs to be treated individually. Healthcare professionals must not influence clients with their own beliefs or cultures. Failure to take the client's cultural background seriously means we fail to understand the values held by the client.

Lack of cultural competence and skills can lead to inappropriate clinical outcomes and poor interaction with clients and families at a very crucial point in their end-of-life process. Addressing and respecting cultural differences will increase trust, leading to a more satisfactory end-of-life process for both the client and the family.

Data from Kagawa-Singer & Blackhall (2001).

CULTURAL DIVERSITY AT THE END OF LIFE

Every ten years, a census is done in the United States to identify percentages of cultural diversity in the population. These statistics can be used to monitor trends of growth in the various cultural groups of people that live in the United States. With the makeup of the United States showing changes every ten years according to census results, healthcare workers must become more aware of how cultural factors influence clients' reactions to serious illness and how they make decisions and cope with end-of-life issues. There are three basic dimensions in end-of-life treatment that vary culturally: communications regarding "bad news," locus of decision-making, and attitudes toward advance directives and end-of-life care.

Sometimes healthcare workers conceal adverse diagnoses from clients, believing that it is disrespectful, impolite, or even harmful to share them with the clients. Decisions on end-of-life care are most often made by the family or the family in consultation with the physician, not the clients. Advance directives are usually not completed by some clients because they have a distrust of the United States healthcare system.

SKILL 4.17 Performing Postmortem Care

Evidence-Based Nursing Practice

Critical Care Family Needs

Truog and colleagues (2001) identified 10 important needs of families with critically ill dying family members:

1. To be with the person.
2. To be helpful to the dying person.
3. To be informed of the dying person's changing condition.
4. To understand what is being done to the client and why.
5. To be assured of the client's comfort.
6. To be comforted.
7. To ventilate emotions.
8. To be assured that their decisions were right.
9. To find meaning in the dying of their loved one.
10. To be fed, hydrated, and rested.

Davidson (2009) reviewed studies of critical care interventions to determine whether clear, effective strategies had been identified to assist the family members of critical care clients. Family members of ICU patients need to be able to see the client, and they need information, support, assurance, and comfort. The research determined that nurses can help via a structured approach to providing family support and that certain interventions, such as looking back to clarify what has happened and including the family in care, may be helpful. In particular, personal individualized interaction with the family may improve family outcomes and ability to adapt to the critical illness. The report suggests, however, that while various interventions have been studied, conclusive data are not yet available and further research is required to validate findings.

Data from Truog et al. (2001) and Davidson (2009).

(continued on next page)

SKILL 4.17 Performing Postmortem Care *(continued)*

Delegation

Postmortem care can be delegated to UAPs after the activities described above have been completed so that the UAP knows what tubes or other medical devices can be removed or other special care provided.

Equipment

- Shroud or other linens used by the agency to wrap the body
- Washcloths, towels
- Absorbent pads
- Clean gloves and any other personal protective equipment as indicated by the client's condition
- Patient gown (if the family will be viewing the body)
- Bags for personal belongings and the medical record document used to record transfer of the belongings and valuables

Preparation

- Consider whether more than one person is needed to perform the postmortem care since turning the body is involved. For caregivers who are performing postmortem care for the first time, it is especially advised that at least two caregivers work together to provide the care.
- Postmortem care can be time consuming. Arrange for someone to cover the caregiver's other clients during this time.

Procedure

1. Observe appropriate infection control procedures. Apply clean gloves.
2. Because the deceased person's family often wants to view the body immediately after death, and because it is important that the deceased appear natural and comfortable, nurses need to position the body, place dentures in the mouth, and close the eyes and mouth before rigor mortis sets in.
   - Normally the body is placed in a supine position with the arms either at the sides, palms down, or across the abdomen.
   - After blood circulation has ceased, the red blood cells break down, releasing hemoglobin, which discolors the surrounding tissues. This discoloration, referred to as **livor mortis**, appears in the lowermost or dependent areas of the body. One pillow is placed under the head and shoulders to prevent blood from discoloring the face by settling in it.
   - Close the eyelids and hold in place for a few seconds so they remain closed.
   - Dentures are usually inserted to help give the face a natural appearance. The mouth is then closed.

   If the body will be viewed in the hospital:
   - Place a clean gown on the client, and comb the hair.
   - Adjust the top bed linens neatly to cover the client to the shoulders.
   - Provide tissues, soft lighting, and chairs for the family.
   - Remove all equipment, soiled linen, and supplies from the bedside.

3. Some agencies require that all tubes in the body remain in place; in other agencies, tubes may be cut to within 2.5 cm (1 in.) of the skin and taped in place; in others, all tubes may be removed. In some cases, if a central IV line is in place, it may be left to assist with the process of preserving the body (embalming). Use the same careful handling you would use with a living body. **Rationale:** *As the body cools, the skin loses its elasticity and can easily be broken when removing dressings and adhesive tape.*
4. Soiled areas of the body are washed; however, a complete bath is not necessary, because the body will be washed by the mortician (also referred to as an undertaker), a person trained in care of the dead.
5. Absorbent pads are placed under the buttocks to take up any feces and urine released because of relaxation of the sphincter muscles.
6. Remove all jewelry, except a wedding band in some instances, which is taped to the finger.
7. The deceased's wrist identification tag is left on. After the body has been viewed by the family, additional identification tags are applied. **Rationale:** *Mislabeling can create legal problems if the body is inappropriately identified and prepared incorrectly for burial or a funeral.*
8. Wrap the body in a **shroud**, a large piece of plastic or cotton material used to enclose a body after death ❶. Apply identification to the outside of the shroud ❷.
   - If the dentures were placed in the mouth for the viewing, secure the jaw with a strap or remove them so they do not fall out as the mouth muscles relax.
   - Remove and discard gloves. Perform hand hygiene.

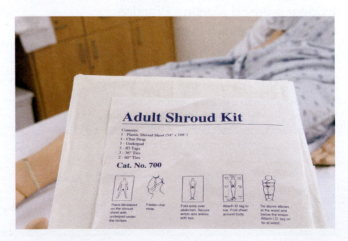

❶ Shroud contents.

SKILL 4.17 Performing Postmortem Care *(continued)*

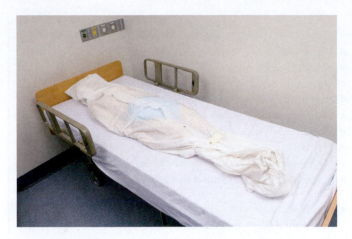

❷ A body wrapped in a shroud.

9. Take the body to the morgue if arrangements have not been made to have a mortician pick it up from the client's room. Nurses have a duty to handle the deceased with dignity and to label the body appropriately. **Rationale:** *Mishandling can cause emotional distress to survivors.*

10. Document the postmortem care in the client record and on forms designed for this purpose. Include what items were removed from the body, whether the body was viewed by the family, and whether the body was taken to the morgue or picked up from the room.

Developmental Considerations

CHILDREN

- Children's responses to death or loss depend on the messages they get from adults and others around them as well as their understanding of death. When adults are able to cope effectively with a death, they are more likely to be able to support children through the process.
- Comprehension of death evolves as the person develops.
- *From infancy to 5 years:* The child does not understand concept of death. An infant's sense of separation forms basis for later understanding of loss and death. They believe death is reversible, a temporary departure, or sleep.
- *Ages 5 to 9 years:* Child understands that death is final. Believes own death can be avoided. Associates death with aggression or violence. Believes wishes or unrelated actions can be responsible for death.
- *Ages 9 to 12 years:* Child understands death as the inevitable end of life. Begins to understand own mortality, expressed as interest in afterlife or as fear of death.
- *Ages 12 to 18 years:* Adolescent fears a lingering death. May fantasize that death can be defied, acting out defiance through reckless behaviors (e.g., dangerous driving, substance abuse). Seldom thinks about death, but views it in religious and philosophic terms. May seem to reach "adult" perception of death but be emotionally unable to accept it. May still hold concepts from previous developmental stages.
- One of the saddest situations is that of parents who experience the death of a child. They will likely feel shock, disbelief, and many other emotions. The nurse supports the parents by giving concrete and specific information about the child's condition, arranging for the parents to be close to the child as often as they desire, and facilitating parent participation in the child's care (Ball & Bindler, 2012). The challenges of providing "competent, compassionate, and consistent care that meets [the] physical, emotional, and spiritual needs" of dying children and their families has been well described in a report by the Institute of Medicine (Field & Behrman, 2003), which is available to read free online.

OLDER ADULTS

- Older adults who are dying often have a need to know that their lives had meaning. An excellent way to assure them of this is to make audiotapes or videotapes of them telling stories of their lives. This gives the client a sense of value and worth and also lets him or her know that family members and friends will also benefit from it. Doing this with children and grandchildren often eases communication and support during this difficult time.
- Older adults fear prolonged illness and see death as having multiple meanings (e.g., freedom from pain, or reunion with already deceased family members).

Three Out of Four Older Adults Die of Heart Disease, Cancer, or Stroke

- Heart disease is the leading cause of death in older adults, although it has declined since 1968.
- Death rates from cancer have decreased, but lung cancer has increased in women.
- Death statistics for people in the 65- to 74-year-old age group reveal that heart disease accounted for 38% of deaths; cancer for 30%.
- Two thirds of hospice clients are over 65 years of age.

Death in The Life Cycle

- In American culture, the obsession with youth often results in denial of death as a natural phase of the life cycle, and death is not considered a positive process.
- Older adults may see death as an end of suffering and loneliness.
- Death is usually not feared if the person has lived a long and fulfilled life, having completed all developmental tasks.
- Spiritual beliefs or philosophy of life are important.

(continued on next page)

SKILL 4.17   *Performing Postmortem Care* (*continued*)

Cultural Considerations

DEATH RITUALS VARY FROM ONE CULTURE TO ANOTHER
There may be cultural customs, beliefs, and rituals surrounding the deceased client's body care. The dying person may have already let the nurse know of any requests about this and family can contribute input or guidance. As appropriate and practical, the nurse should try to support the client and family requests. Here are some common examples relative to clients and families:

CLIENTS

- May prefer to die in the hospital.
- May believe it is bad luck to die at home.
- May have no rituals associated with care of the body.
- May prefer dying at home.
- May be fatalistic when faced with a terminal illness and death.

FAMILIES

- May not openly anticipate death or grieve for a dying person.
- May gather in the hospital.
- May practice special rituals after death, such as washing the body and all orifices.
- May care for the client at home until death is imminent, then bring
- the client to the hospital.
- May lose trust in the healthcare system if a DNR option is offered them.

- May avoid contact with the dying client.
- May want to be present 24 hours a day.
- May believe that dying at home brings bad luck.
- May consider death a family affair.
- May believe the spirit will get lost if death occurs in the hospital.
- May not want to talk about dying and death.
- May believe eating and playing games in the hospital are OK.
- May need nurse's support in their beliefs.
- May bring healers to attend to the spiritual health of the dying client.
- May feel obligated to visit frequently.
- May want a family member to always be with the dying client.
- May wrap the body and not allow a mortuary to prepare the body.
- May avoid all contact with the body.
- May believe organ donation is generally not practiced.
- May believe organ donation is the honorable thing to do.
- May believe or not believe in cremation.
- May believe the body should be kept intact.
- May believe organ donation is not done out of respect for the body.
- May not openly grieve for a dying client.

▶ CRITICAL THINKING OPTIONS FOR UNEXPECTED OUTCOMES

Not all unexpected outcomes require further nursing intervention; however, many times they do. When the client demonstrates a change in signs/symptoms indicating an emerging problem, the nurse should immediately assess and troubleshoot what is happening. The assessment data must be processed quickly to formulate a hypothesis so the nurse can make a clinical judgment. The nurse then decides how best to resolve the problem and improve the client's situation for a better appropriate outcome.

EXPECTED OUTCOME	PROBLEM SOLVING	NURSING ACTIONS
Acute/Chronic Pain Management Client is able to identify and alleviate stress caused by mental concerns.	Client moves into the stage of exhaustion, and stress becomes dangerous to health.	■ Immediately take measures to remove stressors through medication, complete rest, and so forth. ■ Implement specific stress-reducing measures, such as relaxation processes, visualization, and biofeedback.
Pain is controlled through nonpharmacologic methods such as massage, relaxation techniques, or TENS.	Client cannot focus on relaxation technique.	■ Start with very simple breathing techniques and progress slowly to relaxation.
Client is satisfied with level of pain control.	Client experiences pain, asks about alternative measures for relief.	■ Cold therapy may be an option, or heat/cold alternating therapy as counterirritants; these therapies alter nerve transmission. ■ Assess if application is too hot. ■ Ensure that temperature is not over 43.3°C (110°F) if heating pad is used.
Heat and Cold Application Noninflammatory edema is reduced.	Swelling is not reduced with heat therapy.	■ Ensure that acute inflammation is not present, because heat therapy will not reduce swelling (exudate) due to acute tissue injury. ■ Support venous return by elevating the part.
Client reports decrease in pain.	Client complains pain from local edema is increasing.	■ Elevate extremity above level of heart. ■ Ensure that body surface is sufficiently covered with cold application to cause vasoconstriction. ■ Check that area is not overinsulated.

EXPECTED OUTCOME	PROBLEM SOLVING	NURSING ACTIONS
Bleeding and edema formation are minimized.	Bleeding/bruising continues in spite of local cold applications.	■ Reassess area for possible "bleeders," which may require cautery or ligation by the physician. ■ Apply pressure to site to stop bleeding. ■ Assess pulse distal to bleed.
Client has no adverse responses to therapy (arrhythmias, bleeding, shivering, afterdrop or rebound hyperthermia).	Client begins to shiver.	■ Stop the procedure or warm the solution a few degrees (or both). ■ Monitor temperature because shivering causes an increase in the metabolic rate, leading to an increase in heat production. ■ Monitor temperature every 15 minutes to detect additional temperature decrease. ■ Contact physician for medication order (narcotic or sedative agent). ■ Provide supplemental oxygen therapy.
Target core body temperature is achieved.	Cooling blanket does not function properly.	■ Check that plug is connected to the outlet. ■ Check that the fluid level is sufficient and that unit freezing has not occurred. ■ Check that the thermistor probe is properly connected. ■ Check that the cool limit on the pad is not set too high.
End-of-Life Care Postmortem care is completed, maintaining client's dignity.	Client is not identified properly when sent to the morgue.	■ Check client's identity band and shroud label before releasing client to mortician. ■ Request another nurse to check labels.
Appropriate procedures are carried out for organ donations.	Donated organs are needed.	■ Provide support to family members and an opportunity to ask questions. ■ Obtain signatures for consent form. (Kidneys should be removed within 1 hour after death. Eyes should be removed within 6–24 hours after death.) ■ Examine reverse side of driver's license, or remind the charge nurse to call mortician if burial plans have been made previously, to check on permission for organ donation through a living will.

5 Digestion

Skills-at-a-Glance

Eating food is an everyday action that allows humans to consume nutrients. Digestion is the process that breaks the food down physically and chemically on a molecular level into these nutrients so they can be absorbed into the body and utilized for energy, movement, growth, and systems performing specific actions. Healthy digestion requires all gastrointestinal components and related organs to be able to function to support this process. Physical factors that may impede healthy digestion include changes in stomach acid production, food allergens, certain medications, anatomical variations, foods that irritate the lining of the gastrointestinal tract, and an imbalance of pathogenic bacteria.

Digestion is also affected strongly by psychosocial factors. An upset stomach may be caused by an emotional state or interpersonal experience. Stressors can affect an individual physically; sustained stress levels can trigger higher cortisol production, leading to increased central fat deposition. Stress can also play a role in poor digestion when people eat too fast, swallow bites that are too large, or eat as way to relax or feel comforted.

This chapter includes skills nurses can use to assist clients in identifying risk factors for dietary management and healthy digestion, implementing stress management strategies to improve eating habits, using lifestyle and behavioral modification strategies to help maintain therapeutic diets, and using enteric contact precautions to prevent transmission of pathogenic microorganisms through vomitus or fecal material.

Expected Outcomes

1. Healthy digestion will be supported by utilizing stress reduction and relaxation strategies focused on the eating experience for best client outcomes.
2. Clients with chronic digestive disorders will make lifestyle and behavioral changes to maintain best digestion outcomes.
3. The client on a therapeutic diet will modify eating habits and behaviors to provide daily allowance of nutrients needed while following specific dietary guidelines.
4. Transmission of pathogenic microorganisms through vomitus or fecal material will be avoided by using enteric contact precautions.

SKILL 5.1   Stress Reduction Strategies for Mealtimes

Equipment

None required

Procedure

1. Identify the client and introduce self. State the topic of the interview (discussing stress-reducing strategies for mealtimes).
2. Provide privacy. **Rationale:** *A quiet environment will allow greater focus. Discussion of food and eating habits may be embarrassing for clients.*
3. Obtain dietary data. Dietary data includes the client's usual eating patterns and habits; food preferences, allergies, and intolerances; frequency, types, and quantities of foods consumed; and social, economic, ethnic, or religious factors influencing nutrition. Factors may include, but are not limited to, living and eating companions, ability to purchase and prepare food, availability of refrigeration, and the effect of ethnicity on food choices. Four possible methods for collecting dietary data are:
   - **24-hour food recall:** The nurse asks the client to recall all of the food and beverages the client consumes during a typical 24-hour period when at home. The data obtained are then generally evaluated according to the federal government's MyPlate nutrition guide to judge overall adequacy.
   - **Food frequency record:** This is a checklist that indicates how often general food groups or specific foods are eaten. Frequency may be categorized as times/day, times/week, times/month, or frequently, seldom, never. This record provides information about the types of foods eaten but not the quantities. When specific foods or nutrients are suspected of being deficient or excessive, the healthcare professional may use a selective food frequency that focuses, for example, on fat, fruit, vegetable, or fiber intake.

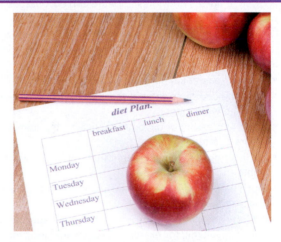

❶ Sample food diary. (*Source:* Ivan1981Roo/Shutterstock)

   - **Food diary ❶:** This is a detailed record of measured amounts (portion sizes) of all food and fluids a client consumes during a specified period, usually 3–7 days.
   - **Diet history:** This comprehensive, time-consuming assessment of a client's food intake involves an extensive interview by a nutritionist or dietitian. Medical and psychosocial factors are assessed to evaluate their impact on nutritional requirements, food habits, and choices. Data obtained are analyzed by computer and translated into caloric and nutrient intake. Results are compared with the Dietary Reference Intakes (DRIs) that are appropriate for the client's age, gender, and condition.

4. Identify normal mealtime patterns as well as patterns that might be more relaxed. **Rationale:** *This will help to determine whether patterns exist that might contribute to digestive upset. Excessive noise; eating while feeling pressured or angry; and eating while standing, riding in a car, or engaged in another activity can affect how much and how an individual eats.*

(continued on next page)

SKILL 5.1   Stress Reduction Strategies for Mealtimes (*continued*)

- Encourage client to name specific elements of a relaxed eating experience. **Rationale:** *This will provide concrete steps the client can take to create a healthy eating environment.*

5. Identify foods that trigger digestive upset. Certain foods are difficult or impossible for some people to digest. This inability results in digestive upsets and, in some instances, the passage of watery stools. Foods that may cause problems include:
   - Excessive sugar (can cause diarrhea)
   - Gas-producing foods, such as cabbage, onions, cauliflower, bananas, and apples
   - Laxative-producing foods, such as bran, prunes, figs, chocolate, and alcohol
   - Constipation-producing foods, such as cheese, pasta, eggs, and lean meat.

6. Teach the importance of regular eating habits. **Rationale:** *Irregular eating can create irregular bowel activity. Individuals who eat at the same times every day usually have a regularly timed, physiological response to the food intake and a regular pattern of peristaltic activity in the colon. This, in turn, leads to a more comfortable digestive tract at meals.*

7. Identify foods that are healthful and appealing. **Rationale:** *Thinking of foods one wants (instead of foods one is "not allowed to have") promotes appetite and encourages positive thinking about food consumption.*

8. Discuss ways of focusing (being mindful of the process) when eating and of having a positive mealtime experience. Some possible methods are:
   - Identify healthful, familiar food that you like.
   - Take small portions and eat them slowly, putting the fork down between bites.
   - Avoid unpleasant or uncomfortable activities immediately before or after a meal.
   - Eat in a tidy, clean environment that is free of unpleasant sights and odors.
   - Brush teeth before mealtime. This improves the client's ability to taste.
   - Address any illness symptoms that depress appetite before mealtime; for example, take an analgesic for pain or an antipyretic for a fever or allow rest for fatigue.
   - Reduce psychological stress. Do not eat while discussing difficult topics or arguing.

VARIATION: SERVING A FOOD TRAY

Setting up a food tray for a client provides an opportunity to reduce stressors at mealtimes. The nurse should check that the foods and liquids on the tray are included in the client's specific diet. The client may need assistance in opening packaged utensils, condiments, liquids, and so forth. The food may need to be cut up, seasoned, or warmed up for the client. The client needs to be comfortable, which can mean taking care of toileting needs, providing hygiene for hands and face, and positioning the client to support eating.

Equipment

- Completed diet slip
- Diet tray
- Overbed table
- Utensils
- Protective covering (e.g., towel)

Preparation

- Check client's chart for physician's diet order.
- Obtain dietary consult, if necessary, to meet client's needs.
- Elicit food preferences of the client.
- Check all diet trays before serving to ensure the diet provided is the one ordered.
- Ensure that hot food is hot and cold food is cold.
- Keep food trays attractive. Avoid spilling liquids on tray.
- Assist client to empty bladder (if needed) and perform hand hygiene.
- Remove unpleasant objects from area.

Procedure

1. Identify client by checking identification band and having client state name and birth date.
2. Perform hand hygiene and assist client to do so.
3. Assist client to sit in a chair, or elevate the head of the bed to 90 degrees.
4. Place protective covering over client's chest.
5. Place food tray on overbed table and adjust the table so client can see the food.
6. Assist client as needed (cut meat, open containers).
7. Leave call light in client's reach and check on client periodically.
8. Reposition tray table at bedside when meal is completed.
9. Assist client with hand and oral hygiene if desired.
10. Position client for comfort.
11. Note percentage and type of food eaten.
12. Remove food tray from room.
13. Document percentage and type of food eaten and, if indicated, amount of liquid intake on I&O record.
14. Perform hand hygiene.

CLINICAL ALERT

Clients sensitive to latex have the potential for serious allergic reactions to some plant proteins. Cross-reactivity to latex has been shown with foods such as avocado, banana, papaya, chestnuts, kiwi, potatoes, and tomatoes. Clients with allergies to these foods may have a latex allergy and vice versa.

VARIATION: TEACHING RELAXATION STRATEGIES FOR MEALTIME

- Encourage client to sit for a moment before eating, closing eyes and taking two or three relaxed breaths, or simply focusing on the environment and the food. **Rationale:** *Mindfulness (a state of awareness about the present time and situation) helps an individual be able to eat slowly and chew food thoroughly.*
- Teach about managing stress through diet:
  - Certain foods and drug substances (caffeine, alcohol, sugar, junk foods, preservatives, tobacco) act as potent stressors on our bodies. Avoidance of highly stimulating foods can provide relief to the digestive tract.
  - Consuming high-stress foods results in negative body changes, such as hypertension, high cholesterol, labile blood sugar levels, and a rapid, bounding pulse rate.

SKILL 5.1   Stress Reduction Strategies for Mealtimes (*continued*)

- Consuming a low-stress diet results in more energy and stamina to cope with stress. Teach client that a low-stress diet includes reducing saturated fat and limiting protein intake to 10%–15% of consumed calories. Remainder of intake should be raw or barely cooked vegetables, fruits, whole grains, nuts, low-fat dairy products, and plenty of liquids. Eliminate sodas, caffeine products, and most alcohol. Exclude refined sugars and carbohydrates and convenience or processed foods.
- Encourage the use of vitamin supplements if needed: vitamin C, B-complex, mineral supplements. Assist client to examine diet and the use of vitamin and mineral supplements. **Rationale:** *There is much controversy today over whether the average American consumes a diet that provides enough of the essential nutrients to prevent disease*

and aging. Some say that if you follow the federal MyPlate nutrition guide, you do not need supplements. Others say that food today (unless you are eating a majority of organic/ natural foods) is so deficient in nutrients that you cannot sustain a healthy diet. More and more research is showing that diet/nutrition is a major contributor to health and the prevention of disease.

- Encourage the client, whether eating or performing other activities, to be aware of signals of stress (anger, anxiety, eating disorders, fatigue, and restlessness) that might affect the eating environment. **Rationale:** *Awareness of these stress sensations can help the client make conscious responses to deal with the sources of the stress sensations; awareness is necessary in order to alter unhealthy habits and patterns of response.*
- Document teaching and client response.

SKILL 5.2   Eating Modifications with Chronic Digestive Disorders

Equipment

None required

Procedure

1. Identify the client and introduce self. State the topic of the interview (discussing eating modifications).
2. Provide for client privacy. **Rationale:** *A quiet environment will allow greater focus.*
3. Assess for the foods that cause digestion disturbances for the client. Keep a low-key, professional tone when discussing the need for dietary changes. **Rationale:** *Thinking about changing eating habits may be difficult for clients.*

4. Engage the client in developing eating modifications related to chronic digestive disorders. Help client identify lifestyle and behavioral changes that will be needed. **Rationale:** *Lifestyle and behavioral changes require full involvement on the client's part. The nurse helps prepare the client to take the initiative and assume responsibility for his or her own health. The role of the nurse and physician is to guide clients to various healthcare options.*
5. Help the client identify indicators of stress so that sources of stress can be resolved or at least set aside before eating.
6. Document relevant information.

Signals of Stress

- Digestion disturbances—acid, nausea, gas, cramps, colitis
- Eating disorders—compulsive eating, loss of appetite
- Disorganization
- Skin eruptions—rash, hives, itching, eczema, acne
- Sexual difficulties—impotence, low libido (desire), nonorgasmic
- Elimination disorders—diarrhea, constipation, vaginitis
- Alcohol and drug abuse

Developmental Considerations

Nutrition

CHILDREN

- Children learn eating habits from their parents. It is the parents' responsibility to be good nutritional role models, both in terms of what they eat and how they incorporate food into their lifestyle.
- During the preschool and early school-age years, children learn lifelong eating habits. It is the parents' responsibility to provide the child with adequate amounts of nutritious foods in an environment that is relaxed and comfortable for eating. It is the child's responsibility to decide what and how much of the nutritious foods to eat. Parents should be counseled that eating can become a source of conflict if the parent tries to tell the child

what and how much to eat, or if the child tries to tell the parent what foods should be eaten. Children's access to "junk food" should be limited, but completely forbidding a food may also create conflict.

- Although adolescents who are vegetarians are at risk for some nutritional deficits, the diet of adolescents who eat eggs, milk products, and, on occasion, non–red meat is more healthful than that of their red-meat-eating peers (Grant et al., 2008).

ADULTS

- For many years, the World Health Organization has recommended weekly iron folic acid supplementation for sexually active women of fertile age worldwide to prevent fetal birth defects.

OLDER ADULTS

Most older adults take several medications as a result of having an increase in the number of chronic illnesses. Considerations for potential problems include:

- Some foods interact adversely or decrease the effectiveness of certain medications, such as foods high in vitamin K and the anticoagulant Coumadin. Older adults should not change their diet significantly without consulting a healthcare provider because a drug dosage may have been based on the older adult's previous dietary intake.

(*continued on next page*)

SKILL 5.2 Eating Modifications with Chronic Digestive Disorders (*continued*)

- Some medications increase appetite, such as glucocorticoids.
- Some medications decrease appetite by their actions or by causing an unpleasant taste.
- Certain tablets should not be crushed to be given by mouth or by gastric tubes, such as enteric-coated or slow-release medications.

Conditions such as neuromuscular disorders and dementia can make it difficult for older adults to eat or to be fed. Safety should always be a priority concern with attention paid to prevent aspiration. All healthcare personnel and family caregivers should be taught proper techniques to reduce this risk. Effective techniques include:

- Use the chin-tuck method when feeding clients with dysphagia. Having them flex the head toward the chest when swallowing decreases the risk of aspiration into the lungs.

- Use foods of prescribed consistency. Many older adults can swallow foods with a thicker consistency more easily than thin liquids.
- Try to focus on food preferences—the family can help provide this information.
- Try to maintain mealtime as a positive social occasion with conversations and extra attention to having a pleasant environment.

Economic factors may influence older adults' nutritional status if they cannot afford food, especially if a prescribed diet requires expensive supplements. Inexpensive or convenience foods such as canned soups are often high in fat and sodium.

SKILL 5.3 Managing a Therapeutic Diet

Assisting Clients with Special Diets

Alterations in a client's diet are often needed to treat a disease process such as diabetes mellitus, to prepare for a special examination or surgery, to increase or decrease weight, to restore nutritional deficits, or to allow an organ to rest and promote healing. It is a skill to know how to live on a special diet. Clients need to learn how to do this successfully. Diets are modified in one or more of the following aspects: texture, kilocalories, specific nutrients, seasonings, or consistency.

Hospitalized clients who do not have special needs eat the regular (standard or house) diet, a balanced diet that supplies the metabolic requirements of a sedentary person (about 2,000 kilocalories [Kcal]). Most agencies offer clients a daily menu from which to select their meals for the next day; others provide standard meals to each client on the general diet. Diets that are modified in consistency are often given to clients before and after surgery or to promote healing in clients with gastrointestinal distress. These diets include clear liquid, full liquid, soft, and diet as tolerated. In some agencies, clients who have had gastrointestinal surgery are not permitted red-colored liquids or candy because, if vomited, the color may be confused with blood.

For clients with chronic digestive disorders, therapeutic diets may be ordered. Clients may be required to restructure their lives and eating patterns in order to promote health. Instruction and emotional support are important elements in achieving a successful outcome.

Healthy People 2020 addresses many areas that need attention in our nation to promote improved health in the population. One of the priorities of action is a focus on correcting the alarming trend toward overweight/obesity.

Documentation for Modified Therapeutic Diets

- Type of diet provided
- Client's daily weight
- Intake and output
- Client's understanding of dietary restriction
- Any client or family teaching provided
- Nutritional consult requested
- Client's tolerance of diet progression
- Community agency referral offered

LIFESTYLE AND BEHAVIORAL MODIFICATION STRATEGIES TO HELP MAINTAIN COMMON THERAPEUTIC DIETS

Therapeutic Diet	Modification Strategies
Restricting dietary protein	a. Decrease protein allowance to 0.5–0.6 g/kg/day (predialysis). b. Limit high-protein foods, such as eggs, meat, milk, and milk products.
Restricting dietary fat	a. Restrict total fat to less than 30% of calories, restrict saturated fat to 7% of calories, and reduce cholesterol to 200 mg/day. b. Higher percentage may be allowed if saturated and trans fats are substituted with monosaturated fats found primarily in plant products (olive oil, canola oil, avocados, pecans, almonds); use low-fat or nonfat products; increase intake of fruits and vegetables, whole grains, legumes, and seeds. c. Limit high-cholesterol foods found in animal products, such as egg yolk, red meat, shellfish, organ meats, bacon, and pork. d. Avoid such foods as gravies, fatty meat and fish, cream, fried foods, rich pastries, whole-milk products, cream soups, salad and cooking oils, nuts, and chocolate.

SKILL 5.3   Managing a Therapeutic Diet (continued)

Therapeutic Diet	Modification Strategies
Restricting mineral nutrients (sodium, potassium)	a. Restrict salt in cooking or at the table. May prohibit any product containing sodium, such as soda bicarbonate. b. Be aware of sodium content of some medications (e.g., antacids).
Providing consistent carbohydrate diets	a. Refined or simple sugars are limited. b. Counting grams of carbohydrates and using the glycemic index (describes how much blood glucose level rises with a specific food when compared with an equivalent amount of glucose) are nutritional tools for managing diabetes. c. Equal (consistent) amount of carbohydrate is provided at each meal to ease management of blood sugars. d. Restricted foods are simple carbohydrates; for example, juices, white sugar, white rice, and white flour.
Providing nutrient-enhanced diets	1. *High-iron diet:* 　a. Include foods high in iron content, such as meats (especially organ meats), egg yolks, seafood (especially shellfish), and plant-based sources such as whole-wheat products, leafy vegetables, nuts, dried fruit, and legumes. 　b. Vitamin C enhances absorption of plant-based iron. 2. *High-calcium diet:* 　a. Increase normal adult intake of 1 g/day to 1.5 g/day for postmenopausal female. 　b. Use *fortified* low-fat and nonfat dairy products, fruit juices, and oatmeals. 　c. If lactose intolerant, use leafy green vegetables and nonliquid dairy products (cheese, yogurt) or lactose-free dairy products, fish products, and almonds.
Postoperative diet progression	a. *Clear liquid diet:* 1,000–1,500 mL/day of liquid foods such as water, tea, broth, gelatin, and pulp-free juices or clear carbonated beverages. b. *Full liquid diet:* Includes any food that is liquid at room temperature—clear liquids, milk and milk products, custards, puddings, creamed soups, sherbet, ice cream, and any fruit juice. c. *Surgical soft diet:* Includes items in a full liquid diet plus pureed vegetables, eggs (not fried), milk, cheese, fish, fowl, tender beef, veal, potatoes, and cooked fruit. Include foods that are easy to chew and digest and limited in fiber; do not include gas-formers. d. *General diet:* Take into consideration food tolerances and preferences.
Bland diet	a. Have frequent, small feedings during active stress periods. b. Establish regular meals and food patterns when condition permits.
Mechanical soft diet	a. Eat foods that can be easily digested. Allows variations in tastes that are not allowed on a soft diet (chili beans).
Pureed diet	a. Mash, mince, or grind foods. b. Do not mix all pureed food together or feed out of one bowl or dish. Try to keep foods separate and eat alternately, with dessert last.
Blenderized liquid diet	a. Blenderize food and liquid to a liquid form.

Client Teaching

Healthy Nutrition

- Discuss importance of properly fitted dentures and dental care.
- Discuss safe food preparation and preservation techniques as appropriate.
- Discuss the purpose of the diet.
- Discuss allowed and excluded foods.
- Explain the importance of reading food labels when selecting packaged foods.
- Include family or significant others in the discussions.
- Reinforce information provided by the dietitian or nutritionist as appropriate.
- Discuss herbs and spices as alternatives to salt and substitutes for sugar.
- Discuss physiological, psychological, and lifestyle factors that predispose to weight changes.
- Discuss ways to adapt eating practices by using smaller plates, taking smaller servings, chewing each bite a specified number of times, and putting fork down between bites.
- Discuss ways to control the desire to eat by taking a walk, drinking a glass of water, or doing slow deep-breathing exercises.
- Discuss stress reduction techniques.
- Provide information about available community resources (e.g., weight-loss groups, Meals-on-Wheels, dietary counseling, exercise programs, self-help groups).
- Discuss factors contributing to inadequate nutrition and weight changes.
- Discuss ways to manage, minimize, or alter the factors contributing to malnourishment.

Teaching Parents Dietary Management

For Infants

- Encourage parents to provide only breast milk or formula until the infant reaches the age of 6 months. **Rationale:** *Breast milk provides all of an infant's needs and is associated with some benefits*

(continued on next page)

SKILL 5.3 Managing a Therapeutic Diet *(continued)*

(reduced incidence of allergies, diarrhea) and some protection (transmission of mother's immunities). Feeding an infant only formula for the first 6 months helps prevent childhood obesity.

- Give feedings when the infant cries for food, not by the clock.
- Introduce one food at a time, starting with foods with low allergy potential, such as rice cereal.
- Do not lay the baby down to sleep with a bottle. **Rationale:** *Any liquid other than water can cause tooth decay, even in erupting teeth. Oral health has a great impact on digestion.*

For Toddlers

- Teach parents about potential for choking and about what foods to avoid.
- Offer a variety of finger foods from all food groups but do not be concerned about quantity. Provide small portions. **Rationale:** *Toddlers may have a very low intake due to slower growth during this period.*
- Make foods available at meal and snack times only. Do not force food intake. **Rationale:** *This helps to prevent tantrums related to eating times.*
- Encourage involvement in snack preparation. **Rationale:** *Even at an early age, children can begin to learn about good nutrition. Involvement in preparation provides a teaching time.*
- Do not use food as a bribe.

For School-Age Children

- Teach parents that habits formed in early years will affect their children for life. It is important to give them information about good food choices and to help them participate in healthy practices.
- Provide nutritious foods following the federal government's MyPlate nutrition guide. Provide small portions.
- Recognize children's likes and dislikes. Do not force children to eat foods they dislike, but do not limit family intake to their limited choices.

For Teens

- Recognize the importance of peer pressure.
- Encourage teens planning a party or gathering to find healthful choices that will appeal to their age group.
- Engage teens in making decisions about meal planning.
- Help overweight teens to think of rewards other than food and provide positive reinforcement that is not food (e.g., a movie, a manicure).
- Provide healthful foods and avoid criticism during mealtimes.

SKILL 5.4 Using Enteric Contact Precautions

Enteric precautions are isolation practices designed to prevent transmission of pathogens through contact with fecal matter and vomitus. The Centers for Disease Control and Prevention has issued guidelines for various precautions. Guidelines for enteric precautions are shown in **Table 5–1** ●.

Donning Personal Protective Equipment (PPE) Utilizing Standard Precautions

Equipment

- Disposable gloves
- Gown
- Mask
- Protective eyewear (goggles or face shield)

Procedure

1. Wash hands using nonantimicrobial soap and dry.
2. Put on gown by placing one arm at a time through sleeves. Wrap gown around body so it covers clothing completely. **Rationale:** *Gowns are worn when it is likely that personal clothing will come in contact with blood, body fluids (e.g., vomitus), secretions, and excretions (e.g., fecal material).*
3. Bring waist ties from back to front of gown or tie in back, according to hospital policy. **Rationale:** *This will ensure that all personal clothing is covered by the gown, preventing accidental contamination.*
4. Tie gown at neck or adhere Velcro strap to gown.
5. Don goggles or face shield to avoid being splashed. **Rationale:** *Eye protection is worn when contact with*

blood or body fluids (e.g., vomitus or fecal material) is anticipated.

6. Don disposable gloves. **Rationale:** *Gloves prevent contamination of hands when there is contact with blood, body fluids (e.g., vomitus), secretions, or excretions (e.g., fecal material).*
7. Place all contaminated articles and trash in leakproof hazard bags.
8. Place clients at risk for contaminating the environment in a private room with separate bathroom facilities.

VARIATION: REMOVING PPE UTILIZING STANDARD PRECAUTIONS

Equipment

- Linen hamper
- Garbage bag

Procedure

- Untie string of gown at waist. **Rationale:** *Any surface below waist level is considered contaminated; therefore, the strings at the waist are untied before removing gloves.*
- Remove first glove by turning it inside out and placing the rolled-up glove in the second hand. Remove second glove by slipping one finger under glove edge and pulling glove off. Dispose of both gloves in garbage bag.
- Untie gown at neck. **Rationale:** *The back of the neck is considered clean and the tie should not be touched with contaminated gloves.*

SKILL 5.4   Using Enteric Contact Precautions *(continued)*

TABLE 5–1   CDC Guidelines for Enteric Contact Precautions

PATHOGEN	TYPE OF PRECAUTION	CONSIDERATIONS
Gastroenteritis	S	Use contact precautions for diapered or incontinent persons for the duration of illness or to control institutional outbreaks for gastroenteritis caused by all of the agents below.
Adenovirus	S	Use contact precautions for diapered or incontinent persons for the duration of illness or to control institutional outbreaks.
Cholera (*Vibrio cholerae*)	S	Use contact precautions for diapered or incontinent persons for the duration of illness or to control institutional outbreaks.
Clostridium difficile	C	Discontinue antibiotics if appropriate. Do not share electronic thermometers. Ensure consistent environmental cleaning and disinfection. Hypochlorite solutions may be required for cleaning if transmission continues. Hand washing with soap and water preferred because of the absence of sporicidal activity of alcohol in waterless antiseptic hand rubs.
Escherichia coli		
Enteropathogenic O157:H7 and other Shiga toxin–producing strains	S	Use contact precautions for diapered or incontinent persons for the duration of illness or to control institutional outbreaks.
Other species	S	Use contact precautions for diapered or incontinent persons for the duration of illness or to control institutional outbreaks.
Noroviruses	S	Use contact precautions for diapered or incontinent persons for the duration of illness or to control institutional outbreaks. Individuals who clean areas heavily contaminated with feces or vomitus may benefit from wearing masks since virus can be aerosolized from these body substances; ensure consistent environmental cleaning and disinfection with focus on restrooms even when apparently unsoiled. Hypochlorite solutions may be required when there is continued transmission. Alcohol is less active, but there is no evidence that alcohol antiseptic hand rubs are not effective for hand decontamination. Cohorting of affected clients to separate airspaces and toilet facilities may help interrupt transmission during outbreaks.
Rotavirus	C	Ensure consistent environmental cleaning and disinfection and frequent removal of soiled diapers. Prolonged shedding may occur in both immunocompetent and immunocompromised children and older adults.
Salmonella species (including *S. typhi*)	S	Use contact precautions for diapered or incontinent persons for the duration of illness or to control institutional outbreaks.
Shigella species (bacillary dysentery)	S	Use contact precautions for diapered or incontinent persons for the duration of illness or to control institutional outbreaks.

S = standard precautions; C = contact precautions.
Source: Siegel, J. D., Rhinehart, E., Jackson, M., Chiarello, L., & the Healthcare Infection Control Practices Advisory Committee (2007). *2007 Guideline for isolation precautions: Preventing transmission of infectious agents in healthcare settings.* Retrieved from Centers for Disease Control website.

- Take off gown by pulling down from shoulders, turn gown inside out, and pull arms out of gown. **Rationale:** *The inside of the gown is not considered contaminated and, therefore, if it accidentally touches your uniform, it will not be contaminated.*
- Dispose of gown in linen hamper. If disposable, place in garbage bag.
- Remove protective eyewear.
- Wash hands thoroughly using a nonantimicrobial soap and dry.

▶ CRITICAL THINKING OPTIONS FOR UNEXPECTED OUTCOMES

Not all unexpected outcomes require further nursing intervention; however, many times they do. When the client demonstrates a change in signs/symptoms indicating an emerging problem, the nurse should immediately assess and troubleshoot what is happening. The assessment data must be processed quickly to formulate a hypothesis so the nurse can make a clinical judgment. The nurse then decides how best to resolve the problem and improve the client's situation for a better appropriate outcome.

EXPECTED OUTCOMES	PROBLEM SOLVING	NURSING ACTIONS
Healthy digestion will be supported by utilizing stress reduction and relaxation strategies focused on the eating experience for best client outcomes.	■ Client refuses to acknowledge that stress is affecting his or her eating patterns.	■ Attempt to elicit feelings of client before giving information about the role and effect of stress on one's eating habits. ■ Refer client to resources, articles, and knowledgeable persons who can discuss the effect of stress and the importance of eliminating stressors before, during, and after eating.
Clients with chronic digestive disorders will make lifestyle and behavioral changes to maintain best digestion outcomes.	■ Client moves into the stage of exhaustion, and overeating (or under-eating) from stress becomes dangerous to health.	■ Immediately take measures to remove stressors through medication, complete rest, calm/quiet environment, and so forth. ■ Implement specific stress-reducing measures, such as relaxation processes, visualization, and biofeedback.
	■ Client does not adhere to diet.	■ Elicit client's feelings to determine reason for non-adherence. ■ Check method of diet preparation and administration to see if it is attractive and appealing. ■ Ensure that environment is conducive to eating. ■ Notify dietitian to discuss diet with client.
The client on a therapeutic diet will modify eating habits and behaviors to provide daily allowance of nutrients needed while following specific dietary guidelines.	■ Client with sodium-restricted diet states that food has no taste.	■ Recommend use of lemon, herbs, and spices to add flavor to foods. ■ Encourage client to avoid processed foods, frozen entrees, salty snacks. ■ Inform client that salt craving decreases over time with change in diet. ■ Consult physician for recommendation of potassium-containing salt substitute.
	■ Client states that fat is fat and all fats are to be avoided in preference to carbohydrates.	■ Suggest client remove all visible fat from and limit intake of red meats. ■ Encourage client to substitute poultry (skin removed) and fish for red meat. ■ Limit intake of butter, salad dressings, and trans fat (partially hydrogenated) products. ■ Use low-fat or nonfat products. ■ Increase intake of fruits, vegetables, and legumes.
	■ Postmenopausal client has lactose intolerance but is concerned about need for increased calcium to prevent osteoporosis.	■ Consult with registered dietitian. ■ Encourage intake of nonliquid dairy products (yogurt, cheese) or lactose-free dairy products. ■ Suggest intake of leafy vegetables, canned fishes. ■ Teach that calcium carbonate supplements are best absorbed. ■ Recommend calcium carbonate supplement in low dose (500 mg or less) several times/day for better absorption and efficacy.
Prevention of the transmission of pathogenic microorganisms through vomitus or fecal material will be avoided by using enteric contact precautions.	■ Outbreak of disease occurs in isolation environment.	■ Identify cause of outbreak, and contact the infection control practitioner for consultation. ■ Examine handwashing and infection control practices among staff. ■ Attend educational program on isolation techniques to increase awareness of appropriate procedures.

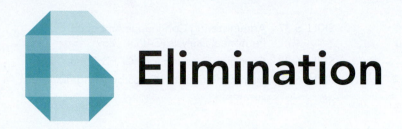

6 Elimination

RELATED CONCEPTS

Skills-at-a-Glance

(continued on next page)

Skills-at-a-Glance *(continued)*

▶ ASSESSMENT: COLLECTING SPECIMENS

Elimination from the urinary tract is usually taken for granted. Only when a problem arises do most people become aware of their urinary habits and any associated symptoms. The nurse's role in urinary elimination may be to (1) assist the client with urinary control, (2) obtain a urine specimen (voided or catheterized), or (3) establish bladder emptiness through catheterization.

Expected Outcomes

1. Client understands purpose of test.
2. Client is able to follow procedure of collection when appropriate.
3. Specimen collected is adequate for testing.

SKILL 6.1   Collecting a Routine Urine Specimen

Delegation

UAP may be assigned to collect a routine urine specimen. Provide the UAP with clear directions on how to instruct the client to collect his or her own urine specimen or how to correctly collect the specimen for the client who may need to use a bedpan or urinal.

Equipment

- Clean gloves as needed
- Clean bedpan, urinal, or commode for clients who are unable to void directly into the specimen container
- Wide-mouthed specimen container
- Completed laboratory requisition
- Completed specimen identification label

Preparation

- Obtain needed equipment.
- Determine if the client requires supervision or assistance in the bathroom. Clients who are seriously ill, physically incapacitated, or disoriented may need to use a bedpan or urinal in bed. A fracture bedpan may be needed for a client with a hip fracture.

Procedure

1. Prior to performing the procedure, introduce self and verify the client's identity using agency protocol. Explain to the client what you are going to do, why it is necessary, and how he or she can participate. Discuss how the results will be used in planning further care or treatments. Give ambulatory clients the following information and instructions:
   - Explain the purpose of the urine specimen and how the client can assist.
   - Explain that all specimens must be free of fecal contamination, so voiding needs to occur at a different time from defecation.
   - Instruct clients to discard the toilet tissue in the toilet or in a waste bag rather than in the bedpan. **Rationale:** *Tissue in the specimen makes laboratory analysis more difficult.*
2. Perform hand hygiene and observe other appropriate infection control procedures such as using gloves when handling specimen containers.
   - Give the client the specimen container, and direct the client to the bathroom to void into it.
3. Provide for client privacy.
4. Assist clients who are seriously ill, physically incapacitated, or disoriented. Provide required assistance in the bathroom, or help the client to use a bedpan or urinal in bed. Direct client to void in the container.
5. Ensure that the specimen is sealed and the container clean.
   - Put the lid tightly on the container. **Rationale:** *This prevents spillage of the urine and contamination of other objects.*
   - If the outside of the container has been contaminated by urine, apply clean gloves and clean it with soap and water. **Rationale:** *This prevents the spread of microorganisms.*
   - Remove and discard gloves. Perform hand hygiene.
6. Label and transport the specimen to the laboratory, using appropriate biohazard specimen bags or containers.
   - Ensure that the specimen label and the laboratory requisition have the correct information on them. Attach them securely to the specimen container. **Rationale:** *Inappropriate identification of the specimen can lead to errors of diagnosis or therapy for the client.*
   - Arrange for the specimen to be taken immediately to the laboratory or placed in a refrigerator. **Rationale:** *Urine deteriorates relatively rapidly from bacterial contamination when left at room temperature; specimens should be analyzed immediately after collection. If the urine specimen is delayed from reaching the lab by more than 1 hour, a new specimen may be needed.*
7. Document the collection of the specimen on the client's chart. Include the date and time of collection and the appearance and odor of the urine.

SKILL 6.1   Collecting a Routine Urine Specimen (*continued*)

Developmental Considerations

INFANTS

- The process for cleaning the perineal area and the urethral opening is similar to the process for an adult. A specimen bag, however, is used to collect the urine specimen. The specimen bag has an adhesive backing that attaches to the skin. After the infant has voided a desired amount, gently remove the bag from the skin.
- If you are having trouble obtaining a bagged urine specimen from an infant, try cutting a hole in the diaper (front for a boy and middle for a girl) and pulling part of the bag through. You can see when urine is collected without having to untape the diaper.

> **CLINICAL ALERT**
>
> When applying the urine bag on girls, begin by placing the bag below the vaginal opening and then allow it to adhere to the labia. For boys, be sure the bag adheres to the scrotum and that the scrotum is not inside the bag's opening.

CHILDREN

- When collecting a routine urine specimen, explain the procedure in simple, nonmedical terms to the child and ask the child to void using a potty chair or a bedpan placed inside the toilet.

- Give the child a clean specimen container to play with.
- Allow a parent to assist the child, if possible. The child may feel more comfortable with a parent.

OLDER ADULTS

- For a clean-catch urine specimen, an older adult may have difficulty controlling the stream of urine.
- An older female adult with arthritis may have difficulty holding the labia apart during the collection of a clean-catch urine specimen.

Setting of Care

- Assess the client's ability and willingness to collect a timed urine specimen. If poor eyesight or hand tremors are a problem, suggest using a clean funnel to pour the urine into the container.
- Always wash hands well with warm, soapy water before and after collecting urine samples.
- Always wear gloves if handling another person's urine.
- The home should have a refrigerator or other method for cooling the urine samples. Tell the client to keep the specimen container in a plastic or paper bag in the refrigerator, separate from other refrigerator contents. The client may also use a cooler with ice.

SKILL 6.2   Collecting a Timed Urine Specimen

- Determine the client's ability to understand instructions and to provide urine samples independently. Are there any fluid or dietary requirements associated with the test?
- Are there any medication restrictions or requirements for the test?

Delegation

UAP may be assigned to assist in the collection of a timed urine specimen. Provide clear directions about the collection procedure, proper storage of the specimen container, and the importance of saving all of the client's urine to avoid the need to restart the collection process.

Equipment

- Appropriate specimen containers with or without preservative in accordance with the specific test
- Completed specimen identification labels
- Completed laboratory requisition
- Bedpan or urinal
- Sign on or near the bed indicating the specific times for urine collection
- Clean gloves, as needed
- Ice-filled container if a refrigerator is not available

Preparation

- Obtain a specimen container with preservative (if indicated) from the laboratory. Label the container with identifying

information for the client, the test to be performed, time started, and time of completion.
- Provide a clean receptacle for collecting urine (bedpan, commode, or toilet collection device).
- Post signs in the client's chart, Kardex, room, and bathroom alerting personnel to save all urine during the specified time.

Procedure

1. Prior to performing the procedure, introduce self and verify the client's identity using agency protocol. Explain to the client what you are going to do, why it is necessary, and how he or she can participate. Discuss how the results will be used in planning further care or treatments. Give the client the following information and instructions:
   - The purpose of the test and how the client can assist.
   - When the specimen collection will begin and end. (For example, a 24-hour urine test commonly begins at 0700 hours and ends at the same hour the next day.)
   - That all urine must be saved and placed in the specimen containers once the test starts.
   - That the urine must be free of fecal contamination and toilet tissue.
   - That each specimen must be given to the nursing staff immediately so that it can be placed in the appropriate specimen bottle.
2. Perform hand hygiene and observe other appropriate infection control procedures.

(*continued on next page*)

SKILL 6.2 Collecting a Timed Urine Specimen (*continued*)

3. Provide for client privacy.
4. Start the collection period.
   - Ask the client to void in the toilet or bedpan or urinal. *Discard* this urine (check agency procedure), and document the time the test starts with this discarded specimen. Collect all subsequent urine specimens, including the one specimen collected at the end of the period.
   - Ask the client to ingest the required amount of liquid for certain tests or to restrict fluid intake. Follow the test directions.
   - Intake and output should be implemented and documented.
   - Instruct the client to void all subsequent urine into the bedpan or urinal and to notify the nursing staff when each specimen is provided. Some tests require voiding at specified times.
   - Label the specimen containers sequentially (e.g., first specimen, second specimen, third specimen) if separate specimens are required.
5. Collect all of the required specimens.
   - Place each specimen into the appropriately labeled container. For some tests, each specimen is not kept separately but is poured into a large bottle.
     Note: All urine specimens must be collected for timed collections. If one voiding is missed, the timed urine collection may need to be restarted and the lab notified.
   - If the outside of the specimen container is contaminated with urine, apply gloves and clean it with soap and water. **Rationale:** *Cleaning prevents the transfer of microorganisms to others.*

- Ensure that each specimen is refrigerated throughout the timed collection period. If not refrigerated, specimens are often kept on ice. Preservative may be used. **Rationale:** *Refrigeration or another form of cooling prevents bacterial decomposition of the urine.*
- Measure the amount of each urine specimen if required.
- Ask the client to provide the last specimen 5 to 10 minutes before the end of the collection period.
- Inform the client that the test is completed.
- Remove the signs and the specimen equipment from the client's unit and bathroom.
- Remove and discard gloves. Perform hand hygiene.
6. Cover and send entire specimen with proper requisition to the lab.
7. Document all relevant information.
   - Record the starting time of the test, the name of the test, and completion of the specimen collection on the client's chart. Include the date and specific time. In addition, if indicated for the specific test, note the time each urine specimen was collected, the volume of each specimen, the appearance of the urine, and other relevant data such as fluid intake or restrictions.

CLINICAL ALERT

Note any dietary restrictions or medication precautions in preparation for 24-hour urine collection.

SKILL 6.3 Collecting a Urine Specimen for Culture and Sensitivity by the Clean-Catch Method

Delegation

UAP may perform the collection of a clean-catch or midstream urine specimen. It is important, however, that the nurse inform the UAP how to instruct the client in the correct process for obtaining the specimen. Proper cleansing of the urethra should be emphasized to avoid contaminating the urine specimen.

Equipment

Equipment used varies from agency to agency. Some agencies use commercially prepared disposable clean-catch kits. Others use agency-prepared sterile trays. Both prepared trays and kits generally contain the following items:

- Clean gloves
- Antiseptic towelettes
- Sterile specimen container
- Specimen identification label

In addition, the nurse needs to obtain the following:
- Completed laboratory requisition form
- Urine receptacle, if the client is not ambulatory
- Basin of warm water, soap, washcloth, and towel for the nonambulatory client

Preparation

- Collect the necessary equipment needed for the collection of the specimen. Use visual aids, if available, to assist the client to understand the midstream collection technique.

Procedure

1. Prior to performing the procedure, introduce self and verify the client's identity using agency protocol. Explain to the client that a urine specimen is required, give the reason, and explain the method to be used to collect it. Discuss how the results will be used in planning further care or treatments.
2. Perform hand hygiene and observe other appropriate infection control procedures.
3. Provide for client privacy.
4. For an ambulatory client who is able to follow directions, instruct the client on how to collect the specimen.
   - Direct or assist the client to the bathroom.
   - Ask the client to wash and dry the genitals and perineal area with soap and water. **Rationale:** *Washing the perineal area reduces the number of skin and transient bacteria, decreasing the risk of contaminating the urine specimen.*
   - Ask the client if he or she is sensitive to any antiseptic or cleansing agents. **Rationale:** *This will avoid unnecessary irritation of the genitals or perineum.*
   - Instruct the client on how to clean the urinary meatus with antiseptic towelettes. **Rationale:** *The antiseptic further reduces bacterial contamination of the urinary meatus and the risk of contaminating the specimen.*

   For Female Clients
   - Use each towelette only once. Clean the perineal area from front to back and discard the towelette ❶. Use all towelettes provided (usually two or three).

SKILL 6.3   Collecting a Urine Specimen for Culture and Sensitivity (*continued*)

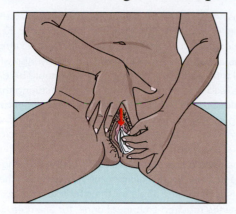

1 Cleansing the female urinary meatus. Spread the labia minora with one hand and with the other hand, cleanse perineal area from front to back.

> **Rationale:** *Cleaning from front to back cleans the area of least contamination to the area of greatest contamination.*

For Male Clients
- If uncircumcised, retract the foreskin slightly to expose the urinary meatus.
- Using a circular motion, clean the urinary meatus and the distal portion of the penis **2**. Use each towelette only once, then discard. Clean several inches down the shaft of the penis. **Rationale:** *This cleans from the area of least contamination to the area of greatest contamination.*

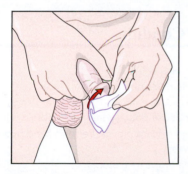

2 Cleansing the male urinary meatus. Retract the foreskin if needed. Using a towelette, cleanse the urinary meatus by moving in a circular motion from center of the urethral opening around the glans and down the distal portion of the shaft of the penis.

5. For a client who requires assistance, prepare the client and equipment.
   - Apply clean gloves.
   - Wash the perineal area with soap and water, rinse, and dry.
   - Assist the client onto a clean commode or bedpan. If using a bedpan or urinal, position the client as upright as allowed or tolerated. **Rationale:** *Assuming a normal anatomical position for voiding facilitates urination.*
   - Remove and discard gloves. Perform hand hygiene.
   - Open the clean-catch kit, taking care not to contaminate the inside of the specimen container or lid. Place the lid in the upright position. **Rationale:** *It is important to maintain sterility of the specimen container to prevent contamination of the specimen.*

- Apply clean gloves.
- Clean the urinary meatus and perineal area as described in step 4.

6. Collect the specimen from a nonambulatory client or instruct an ambulatory client on how to collect it.
   - Instruct the client to start voiding. **Rationale:** *Bacteria in the distal urethra and at the urinary meatus are cleared by the first few milliliters of urine expelled.*
   - Place the specimen container into the midstream of urine and collect the specimen, taking care not to touch the container to the perineum or penis. **Rationale:** *It is important to avoid contaminating the interior of the specimen container and the specimen itself.*
   - Collect urine in the container.
   - Cap the container tightly, touching only the outside of the container and the cap. **Rationale:** *This prevents contamination or spilling of the specimen.*
   - If necessary, clean the outside of the specimen container with disinfectant. **Rationale:** *This prevents transfer of microorganisms to others.*
   - Remove and discard gloves. Perform hand hygiene.

7. Label the specimen and transport it to the laboratory.
   - Ensure that the specimen label is attached to the specimen cup, not the lid, and that the laboratory requisition provides the correct information. Place the specimen in a plastic bag that has a biohazard label on it. Attach the requisition securely to the bag. **Rationale:** *Inaccurate identification or information on the specimen container can result in errors of diagnosis or therapy.*
   - Arrange for the specimen to be sent to the laboratory immediately. **Rationale:** *Bacterial cultures must be started immediately before any contaminating organisms can grow, multiply, and produce false results.*

8. Document pertinent data.
   - Record collection of the specimen, any pertinent observations of the urine such as color, odor, or consistency, and any difficulty in voiding that the client experienced.
   - Indicate on the lab slip if the client is taking any current antibiotic therapy or if the client is menstruating.

Sample Documentation

6/15/15 0800 Informed of MD order for clean-catch urine for C&S. Instructed how to perform. Stated she understood. Urine specimen cloudy. States she continues to have burning on urination. Urine specimen sent to lab. Antibiotic started per MD orders _____ T. Sanchez, RN

VARIATION: OBTAINING A URINE SPECIMEN FROM A CLOSED DRAINAGE SYSTEM

Sterile urine specimens can be obtained from closed drainage systems by inserting a sterile needle attached to a syringe through a drainage port in the tubing. Aspiration of urine from catheters can be done only with self-sealing rubber catheters—not plastic, silicone, or Silastic catheters. When self-sealing rubber catheters are used, the needle is inserted just above the location where the catheter is attached to the drainage tubing. The area from which to obtain urine may be marked by a patch on the catheter. Closed drainage urinary systems now have needleless ports, which avoids use of a needle to obtain a sample **3**. This protects the nurse from

(*continued on next page*)

SKILL 6.3   Collecting a Urine Specimen for Culture and Sensitivity *(continued)*

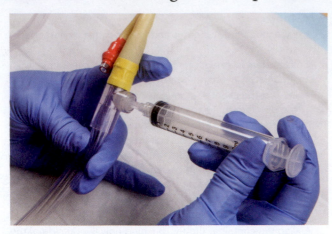

3 Obtaining a urine specimen from a retention catheter using a needleless port.

a needlestick injury and maintains the integrity and sterility of the catheter system by eliminating the need to puncture the tubing.

The needleless port accepts a Luer-Lok syringe. Position the syringe perpendicular to the center of the port and insert, twist, and lock into the port. When the specimen is obtained and the syringe removed, the port seals itself.

To collect a specimen from a Foley (retention) catheter or a drainage tube, follow these steps:

- Apply clean gloves.

- If there is no urine in the catheter, clamp the drainage tubing at least 8 cm (3 in.) below the sampling port for about 30 minutes. **Rationale:** *This allows fresh urine to collect in the catheter.*
- Wipe the area where the needle or Luer-Lok syringe will be inserted with a disinfectant swab. The site should be distal to the tube leading to the balloon to avoid puncturing this tube. **Rationale:** *Disinfecting the needle insertion site removes any microorganisms on the surface of the catheter, thereby avoiding contamination of the needle and the entrance of microorganisms into the catheter.*
- Insert the needle at a 30- to 45-degree angle. This angle of entrance facilitates self-sealing of the rubber. Insert the Luer-Lok syringe at a 90-degree angle for the needleless port.
- Withdraw the required amount of urine, for example, 3 mL for a urine culture or 10 mL for a routine urinalysis.
- Unclamp the catheter.
- Transfer the urine to the specimen container. If a sterile culture tube is used, make sure the needle or syringe (depending on the system) does not touch the outside of the container.
- Discard the syringe and needle or syringe (depending on the system) in an appropriate sharps container.
- Cap the container.
- Remove and discard gloves. Perform hand hygiene.
- Label the container, and send the urine to the laboratory immediately for analysis or refrigeration.
- Record collection of the specimen and any pertinent observations of the urine on the appropriate records.

SKILL 6.4   Obtaining a Urine Specimen from an Ileal Conduit

Equipment

- Sterile catheter kit
- Prep solution
- Sterile saline or water
- Underpad
- New urinary pouch
- Supplies necessary to apply new pouch
- Bath blanket, towels
- Clean gloves
- Soap and water
- Pitcher of water and glass
- Biohazard bag

Preparation

- Check physician's orders and client care plan.
- Gather equipment.
- Perform hand hygiene.
- Explain procedure to client.
- Provide privacy.
- Place bath blanket over client's chest and position top covers over lower abdomen.
- Place towels around stoma. **Rationale:** *Urine will leak around catheter.*
- Don gloves.

Procedure

1. Open sterile packages.
2. Remove pouch or snap pouch off wafer flange.
   Note: Do not use pouch contents to obtain urine specimen.
3. Remove and discard gloves. Perform hand hygiene and don sterile gloves.
4. Place sterile drape over stoma.
5. Remove lid from specimen container, and place end of catheter into container.
6. Apply lubricant to catheter.
7. Use forceps to pick up cotton ball and prep stoma with solution and rinse with sterile saline or water.
8. Insert tip of catheter into stoma approximately 4 cm (1.5 in.) **1**.

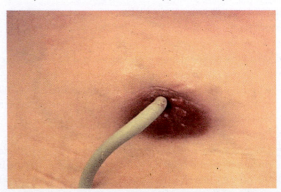

1 A catheter is used to obtain a specimen from an ileal conduit.

SKILL 6.4   Obtaining a Urine Specimen from an Ileal Conduit (continued)

9. When urine specimen is obtained (usually not more than 5 to 25 mL), remove catheter. If no urine obtained, have client drink water.
10. Return lid to specimen container and apply label.
11. If wafer removed, wash and dry peristomal area.

12. Replace pouch or apply new pouch.
13. Remove and discard gloves. Perform hand hygiene.
14. Place specimen container in biohazard bag and send specimen to lab immediately or refrigerate.
15. Document actions.

SKILL 6.5   Performing Urine Tests

Delegation

Urine testing may be performed by UAP. It is important for the UAP to understand the specific specimen collection procedure and report the results of the test to the nurse. Inform the UAP to save the urine sample to allow the nurse to repeat the test if necessary.

Equipment

For All Tests

- Clean gloves

For Specific Gravity

- Multiple-test dipstick that has a separate reagent area for specific gravity

For Urine pH

- Dipstick or litmus paper (red or blue)

For Glucose

- Reagent tablet or reagent test strip
- Appropriate color chart
- Clean test tube and a dropper, if a tablet is used

For Ketone Bodies

- Reagent tablet or dipstick

For Occult Blood

- Reagent strip

Preparation

- Use a fresh urine sample.
- Determine the appropriate equipment and testing product for the client.
- Follow the manufacturer's instructions.

Procedure

1. Prior to performing the procedure, introduce self and verify the client's identity using agency protocol. Explain to the client what you are going to do, why it is necessary, and how he or she can participate. Discuss how the results will be used in planning further care or treatments.
2. Perform hand hygiene and observe other appropriate infection control procedures.
3. Provide for client privacy.

4. To measure specific gravity:
   - Apply clean gloves and place dipstick into the urine specimen.
   - Observe the color and compare it to a standardized color chart on the bottle.
5. To measure pH:
   - Apply a glove and dip a strip of either red or blue litmus paper into the urine specimen.
   - Observe the color of the litmus paper and compare it to a standardized color chart on the bottle. The blue litmus paper, more commonly used, remains blue if the urine is alkaline and turns red if it is acidic. The red litmus paper remains red in the presence of acidic urine and turns blue if the urine is alkaline. Whichever litmus strip is used, red always indicates acidic urine and blue always indicates alkaline urine.
6. To test for glucose:
   - Obtain a freshly voided specimen. Most agencies require a **second-voided specimen**: Ask the client to void, and in 30 minutes to void again, providing a specimen for the test this time. **Rationale:** *A second-voided specimen more accurately reflects the present condition of the body. Urine that has accumulated in the bladder (e.g., overnight) reflects the condition of the body at the time the urine was produced (e.g., 0300 hours).*
   - To carry out the test, apply gloves and follow the directions specified by the manufacturer. If Clinitest tablets are used, be careful not to touch the bottom of the test tube because it becomes extremely hot when the tablet boils in the presence of urine and water.
7. To test for ketone bodies:
   - Apply a glove and place one or two drops of urine on a reagent tablet (e.g., an Acetest tablet) or dip a reagent test strip (e.g., Ketostix) into the urine.
   - Observe and compare the results with the appropriate color chart to determine the quantity of ketones present.
8. To test for occult blood:
   - Apply a glove, and dip the reagent strip (e.g., Hemastix) into a sample of urine.
   - Compare the color change with a color chart in the same manner as with other reagent strips.
9. For all tests:
   - Discard the urine following the tests. Clean the equipment with soap and water.
   - Remove and discard gloves. Perform hand hygiene.
10. Document the results in accordance with the product used and agency practice.

SKILL 6.6   Using a Bladder Scanner

Equipment

- Ultrasound BladderScan device
- Ultrasound conducting gel
- Tissues

Preparation

- Check physician's order to evaluate client's bladder.
- Identify client by checking the client's identity band and asking client to state name and birth date.
- Explain procedure and purpose.
- If female, ask client if she has had a hysterectomy or is pregnant. If a hysterectomy is not documented, and settings are not adjusted appropriately, results may be inaccurate. **Rationale:** *Scanner is not indicated for pregnant clients.*
- Provide for client privacy.
- Determine time and amount of last void or assist client to empty bladder if residual volume is to be evaluated.
- Determine that client does not have an indwelling catheter. **Rationale:** *Scanner reflects off the catheter bulb, giving an echo reading.*
- Perform hand hygiene and observe other appropriate infection control procedures.
- Place client flat and supine, and palpate client's bladder to locate appropriate site.

Procedure

1. Turn the device on and press "SCAN."
2. Apply conducting gel to scanner head.
3. Select MALE or FEMALE mode on scan unit. Select *MALE MODE* if female client has had a hysterectomy.
4. Fanfold linens to expose client's suprapubic area.
5. Place head of scanner 3 cm (1 in.) above client's symphysis pubis, directed toward the bladder, and align the icon ❶.

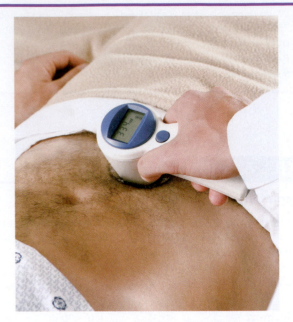

❶ Handheld portable ultrasound bladder scanner.

6. Press scan head button and hold scanner still until a beep is heard.
7. Scan until bladder image is lined up on cross-hairs.
8. Take several scans at different angles and press "DONE" when finished.
9. Press "PRINT" for a printout of client's bladder volume in milliliters.
10. Wipe gel from client's skin.
11. Reposition client for comfort.
12. Wipe ultrasound probe with antiseptic solution.
13. Perform hand hygiene.
14. Document actions.

SKILL 6.7   Obtaining and Testing Stool Specimens

Delegation

UAP may obtain and collect stool specimen(s). The nurse, however, needs to consider the collection process before delegating this task. For example, a random stool specimen collected in a specimen container may be delegated, but a stool culture requiring a sterile swab in a test tube should be done by the nurse. Use of an incorrect collection technique can cause inaccurate test results.

The task of obtaining and testing a stool specimen for occult blood may be performed by UAP. It is important that the nurse instruct the UAP to tell the nurse if blood is detected and/or if the test is positive. In addition, the stool specimen should be saved to allow the nurse to repeat the test.

Equipment

Collecting a Stool Specimen

- Clean bedpan or bedside commode
- Clean gloves
- Cardboard or plastic specimen container (labeled) with a lid or, for stool culture, a sterile swab in a test tube, as policy dictates
- Two tongue blades
- Paper towel
- Completed laboratory requisition

Testing the Stool for Occult Blood

- Clean bedpan or bedside commode
- Clean gloves
- Two tongue blades
- Paper towel
- Test product

Preparation

- Assemble the needed equipment. Post a sign in the client's bathroom if a timed specimen is required (e.g., "Save All Stools").

SKILL 6.7   Obtaining and Testing Stool Specimens *(continued)*

Procedure

1. Prior to performing the procedure, introduce self and verify the client's identity using agency protocol. Explain to the client what you are going to do, why it is necessary, and how he or she can participate. Discuss how the results will be used in planning further care or treatments. Give ambulatory clients the following information and instructions:
   - The purpose of the stool specimen and how the client can assist in collecting it.
   - To defecate in a clean bedpan or bedside commode.
   - To not contaminate the specimen, if possible, with urine or menstrual discharge.
   - To void before the specimen collection.
   - To not place toilet tissue in the bedpan after defecation, because contents of the paper can affect the laboratory analysis.
   - To notify the nurse as soon as possible after defecation, particularly for specimens that need to be sent to the laboratory immediately after collection.

2. Perform hand hygiene and observe other appropriate infection control procedures.
   - When obtaining stool samples (i.e., when handling the client's bedpan, when transferring the stool sample to a specimen container, and when disposing of the bedpan contents), the nurse follows medical aseptic technique meticulously.

3. Provide for client privacy.

4. Assist clients who need help.
   - Assist the client to a bedside commode or a bedpan placed on a bedside chair or under the toilet seat in the bathroom.
   - Apply gloves to prevent hand contamination, and clean the client as required. Inspect the skin around the anus for any irritation, especially if the client defecates frequently and has liquid stools.

5. Transfer the required amount of stool to the stool specimen container.
   - Use one or two tongue blades to transfer some or all of the stool to the specimen container, taking care not to contaminate the outside of the container. The amount of stool to be sent depends on the purpose for which the specimen is collected. Usually, 2.5 cm (1 in.) of formed stool or 15 to 30 mL of liquid stool is adequate. For some timed specimens, however, the entire stool passed may need to be sent. Visible pus, mucus, or blood should be included in the sample.
   - For a culture, dip a sterile swab into the specimen, preferably where purulent fecal matter is present in the feces. Place the swab in a sterile test tube using sterile technique.
   - For a fecal occult blood test (FOBT) using the traditional Hemoccult test, see step 7.
   - Wrap the used tongue blades in a paper towel before disposing of them in a waste container. **Rationale:** *These measures help prevent the spread of microorganisms through contact with other articles.*
   - Place the lid on the container as soon as the specimen is in the container. **Rationale:** *Putting the lid on immediately prevents the spread of microorganisms.*

6. Ensure client comfort.
   - Empty and clean the bedpan or commode, and return it to its place.
   - Remove and discard the gloves. Perform hand hygiene.

7. Label and send the specimen to the laboratory.
   - Ensure that the specimen label and the laboratory requisition have the correct information on them and are securely attached on the specimen container. **Rationale:** *Inappropriate identification of the specimen can lead to errors of diagnosis or therapy for the client.*
   - Ensure that specimens are placed in appropriate biohazard containers or specimen bags.
   - Arrange for the specimen to be taken to the laboratory. Specimens to be cultured or tested for parasites need to be sent immediately. If this is not possible, follow the directions on the specimen container. In some instances, refrigeration is indicated because bacteriological changes take place in stool specimens left at room temperature. Never place a stool specimen in a refrigerator that contains food or medication. **Rationale:** *This prevents contamination of "clean" items with "dirty" items. It also follows OSHA standards for biohazard materials.*

FOBT Using the Hemoccult Test

- Apply clean gloves.
- Follow the manufacturer's directions. For example:
  - For a Hemoccult slide, smear a thin layer of feces over the circle inside the envelope, and drop reagent solution onto the smear ❶ A and B.

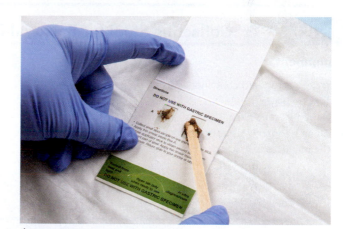

A

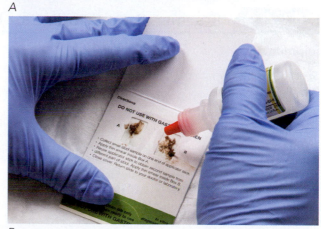

B

❶ *A,* Opening the front cover of a Hemoccult slide and applying a thin smear of feces on the slide. *B,* Opening the flap on the back of the slide and applying two drops of developing fluid over each smear.

(continued on next page)

SKILL 6.7 Obtaining and Testing Stool Specimens (continued)

- Note the reaction. For all tests, a blue color indicates a positive result, that is, the presence of occult blood.
- Remove and discard gloves. Perform hand hygiene.
8. Document all relevant information.
    - Record the collection of the specimen on the client's chart. Include the date and time of the collection and all nursing assessments (e.g., color, odor, consistency, and amount of feces); presence of abnormal constituents, such as blood or mucus; results of test for occult blood if obtained; discomfort during or after defecation; status of perianal skin; any bleeding from the anus after defecation.
    - For an FOBT, record the type of test product used and the reaction.

Developmental Considerations

INFANTS

- To collect a stool specimen for an infant, the stool is scraped from the diaper, being careful not to contaminate the stool with urine.

CHILDREN

- A child who is toilet trained should be able to provide a fecal specimen, but may prefer being assisted by a parent.
- When explaining the procedure to the child, use words appropriate for the child's age rather than medical terms. Ask the parent what words the family normally uses to describe a bowel movement.

OLDER ADULTS

- Older adults may need assistance if serial stool specimens are required.

Setting of Care

- Ask the client or caregiver to call when the stool specimen is obtained. If a laboratory test is needed, the home health nurse can pick up the specimen or a family member may take it to the laboratory.
- Place the stool specimen inside a plastic biohazard bag. Carry the bag in a sealed container marked "Biohazard" and take it to the laboratory promptly. Do not expose the specimen to extreme temperatures in the car.

SKILL 6.8 Collecting Stool for Bacterial Culture

Equipment

- Waxed cardboard container with cover
- Tongue blade
- Label for container
- Clean bedpan or bedside commode
- Clean gloves

Procedure

1. Don clean gloves before collecting stool specimen.

2. Collect exudate, mucus, and blood with all specimens.
3. Place a small amount of feces in a waxed cardboard container (if entire specimen is not needed).
4. Remove and discard gloves. Perform hand hygiene.
5. Send entire specimen to the laboratory immediately after collection. If there is any delay, the specimen must be iced.
6. Report and calculate on the basis of daily output any stool specimens that are to undergo chemical analysis.

SKILL 6.9 Teaching Parents to Test for Pinworms

Equipment

- Specimen container with paddle
- Clean gloves

Procedure

1. Explain procedure to child and parent.
   Note: This test is rarely done or seen in hospital settings, so if pinworms are suspected, the parents can be taught how to obtain a specimen at home.
2. Parents may choose to wear clean gloves.
3. Instruct parents to make collection upon arising in the morning before bathing, cleansing, or passing a bowel movement. *Note:* For very active children, specimens may be collected a few hours after going to bed, while the child is sleepy and more cooperative. **Rationale:** *Pinworms, when present, migrate out of the anus to lay eggs during sleep.*

4. Remove cap in which is inserted a plastic paddle with one side coated with a nontoxic, adhesive material. This side is marked "sticky side." Do not touch this side with fingers.
5. Separate buttocks and press the sticky side against several areas around anus using moderate pressure.
6. Replace the paddle in tube. Be sure there is no stool on paddle.
7. Label container with client's full name, medical record number, and date.
8. Keep specimen at room temperature until all specimens are collected (on consecutive days). Return all tubes to the physician.
9. Document teaching and client understanding.

CLINICAL ALERT

After treatment (drug of choice is mebendazole) and to prevent reinfection, use meticulous cleaning practices and teach parents of the child to do the same.

SKILL 6.10   Collecting Stool for Ova and Parasites

Equipment

- Waxed cardboard or plastic container with cover
- Tongue blade
- Label for container
- Clean bedpan or bedside commode
- Clean gloves

Procedure

1. Follow the steps for collecting a stool specimen in Skill 6.7. Don clean gloves to collect stool specimen **1**.

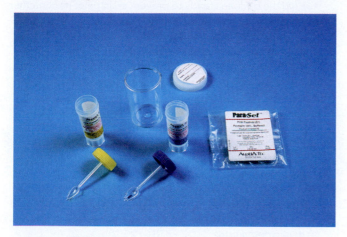

1 Equipment necessary for collecting ova and/or parasite specimen.

2. Collect exudate, mucus, and blood with all specimens.
   - Place stool into container (with a preservative fluid).
   - Mash the specimen in the container until mixed well with preservative. **Rationale:** *Parasites thrive in this type of medium.*
3. Replace and tighten cup. Shake the contents until mixed well.
4. Keep loose fluid specimens at body temperature to be examined within 30 minutes. **Rationale:** *Organisms must be seen in their active stages. Loose, fluid stools are likely to contain trophozoites or intestinal amoebas and flagellates. Well-formed or semiformed stool specimens do not usually need to be maintained at body temperature or be examined quickly even though they may contain ova or a cystic form of parasites.*
5. Collect complete stools after purgative medications are administered. **Rationale:** *When the presence of tapeworms is suspected, all stools must be examined in their entirety in order to find the head of the parasite.*
6. Do not give barium, oil, and laxatives containing heavy metals that interfere with the extraction process for 7 days before stool examination. **Rationale:** *Ova or cysts are not revealed in the presence of these materials.*
7. Use only normal saline solution or tap water if an enema must be administered to collect specimens. Do not use soap suds or other substances.
8. Do not contaminate the specimen with urine as it kills amoeba.
9. Collect three random, normally passed stool specimens to ensure accurate test results.
10. Provide air freshener, if needed.
11. Document relevant information.

▶ BLADDER INTERVENTIONS

Expected Outcomes

1. Client voids 200 to 500 mL of urine without discomfort or difficulty.
2. Skin irritation does not occur with condom catheter use.
3. Suprapubic catheter remains intact.
4. Client remains free of urinary tract infection.
5. Client demonstrates self-care skills.
6. Peristomal skin remains intact and healthy.

SKILL 6.11   Assisting with a Bedpan

Delegation

UAP commonly assist clients with bedpans. The nurse must determine if the specific client has unique needs that would require special training of the UAP in the use of the bedpan. Ensure that personnel are aware of any specimens that need to be collected. Abnormal findings must be validated and interpreted by the nurse.

Equipment

- Clean bedpan and cover
- Toilet tissue
- Basin of water, soap, washcloth, and towel
- Equipment for a specimen if required
- Clean gloves
- Disposable absorbent pad

Preparation

- Adjust the bed to a height appropriate to prevent back strain.
- Elevate the rail on the opposite side of the bed. **Rationale:** *This prevents the client from falling and provides a hand grasp for the client if needed.*

Procedure

1. Prior to performing the procedure, introduce self to the client and verify the client's identity using agency protocol. Explain to the client what you are going to do, why it is necessary, and how he or she can participate.

(continued on next page)

SKILL 6.11   Assisting with a Bedpan (continued)

CLINICAL ALERT

Individuals (especially children) may use very different terms for a bowel movement. The nurse may need to try several different common words before finding one the client understands.

2. Perform hand hygiene and observe other appropriate infection control procedures.

3. Apply clean gloves.

4. Provide for client privacy.

5. Prepare the client.
   - For clients who can assist by raising their buttocks, fold down the top bed linen on the near side to expose the hip, and adjust the gown so that it will not fall into the bedpan. **Rationale:** *A pie fold of the top bed linens exposes the client minimally and facilitates placement of the bedpan.*
   - For clients who cannot raise their buttocks onto and off a bedpan, fold the top bed linens down to the hips.

6. Place client on the bedpan.
   - For clients who can lift their buttocks:
     a. Ask the client to flex the knees, rest their weight on the back and the heels, and then raise the buttocks. The client can use a trapeze, if present, or grasp the side rail for support. Assist the client to lift the buttocks by placing the hand nearest the person's head palm up under the lower back, resting the elbow on the mattress, and using the forearm as a lever. **Rationale:** *Use of appropriate body mechanics by both client and nurse prevents unnecessary muscle strain and exertion.*
     b. Place the absorbent pad on the bed where the bedpan will be located. Position a regular bedpan under the buttocks with the narrow end toward the foot of the bed and the buttocks resting on the smooth, rounded rim. Place a slipper (fracture) pan with the flat end under the client's buttocks. **Rationale:** *Improper placement of the bedpan can cause skin abrasion to the sacral area and spillage of the bedpan's contents.*
   - For clients who cannot lift their buttocks:
     a. Assist the client to a side-lying position.
     b. Place the bedpan against the buttocks with the open rim toward the foot of the bed.
     c. Smoothly roll the client onto the bedpan while holding the bedpan against the buttocks.

7. Elevate the head of the bed to a semi-Fowler's position. **Rationale:** *This position relieves strain on the client's back and permits a more normal position for elimination.* Recheck the position of the bedpan because it may have been repositioned while the head of the bed was being raised.

   - If the person is unable to assume a semi-Fowler's position, place a small pillow under the back, or help the client to another comfortable position.

8. Replace the top bed linen.

9. Provide the client with toilet tissue, raise the side rail, lower the bed height, and ensure that the call light is readily accessible. Ask the client to signal when finished. Leave only when, in your judgment, it is safe to do so. **Rationale:** *Having necessary items within reach prevents falls.*

Removing a Bedpan

10. Return the bed to the position used when giving the bedpan.
    - Hold the bedpan steady to prevent spillage of its contents.
    - Cover the bedpan, and place it on an adjacent chair with a pad or towel under it. **Rationale:** *Covering the bedpan reduces offensive odors and reduces the client's embarrassment.*

11. Assist the client with any needed hygienic measures.
    - Wrap toilet tissue several times around the gloved hand, and wipe the person from the pubic area to the anal area, using one stroke for each piece of tissue. **Rationale:** *Cleaning in this direction—from the less soiled area to the more soiled area—helps prevent the spread of microorganisms.*
    - Place the soiled tissue in the bedpan.
    - Wash the anal area with soap and water as indicated, and thoroughly dry the area. **Rationale:** *Adequate washing and drying prevents skin abrasion and excessive accumulation of microorganisms.*
    - Remove the disposable absorbent pad or replace the drawsheet if it is soiled.
    - Offer the client materials to wash and dry the hands. **Rationale:** *Hand washing following elimination is a practice that helps prevent the spread of microorganisms.*

12. Attend to any unpleasant odors in the environment.
    - Spray the air with an air freshener as needed unless contraindicated because of respiratory problems, or allergies, or because it is offensive. **Rationale:** *Elimination odor can be embarrassing to clients and visitors alike. However, sprays may be harmful to people with respiratory problems, and some perfume sprays are offensive to some people.*

13. Attend to the used bedpan.
    - Acquire a specimen if required. Place it in the appropriately labeled container.
    - Empty and clean the bedpan. Provide a clean bedpan cover, if necessary, before returning it to the client's unit.
    - Remove and discard gloves. Perform hand hygiene.

14. Document findings (e.g., color, odor, amount, and consistency of feces) in the client record using forms or checklists supplemented by narrative notes when appropriate.

SKILL 6.12   Assisting with a Urinal

In preparing to assist the client with the use of a urinal, determine if there are any restrictions in positioning the client. Inquire whether the client has used a urinal previously. If so, determine if the client has any unique needs related to the use of the urinal. Locate the client's urinal.

Delegation

Assisting the client with a urinal is often delegated to UAP. Ensure that UAP are aware of any specimens that need to be collected. The nurse must validate and interpret abnormal findings.

SKILL 6.12 Assisting with a Urinal (continued)

Equipment

- Clean urinal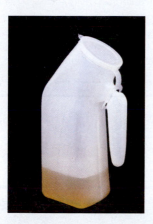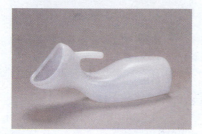
- Toilet tissue
- Equipment for specimen if required
- Clean gloves

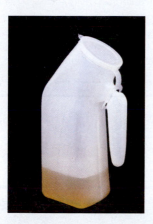

① Male urinal. Copyright James E. Knopf/Shutterstock

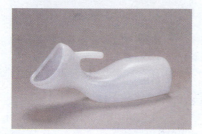

② Female urinal.

Preparation

- Assist the client to an appropriate position.
- Both males and females confined to bed may prefer a semi-Fowler's position, or the male may prefer a standing position at the side of the bed if health permits.

Procedure

1. Prior to performing the procedure, introduce self and verify the client's identity using agency protocol. Explain to the client what you are going to do, why it is necessary, and how he or she can participate.
2. Perform hand hygiene and observe other appropriate infection control procedures.
3. Provide for client privacy.
4. Assist the client with using the urinal:
   - Offer the urinal so that the client can position it independently.
     or
   - Place the urinal between the client's legs with the handle uppermost so that urine will flow into it.
   - Leave the signal cord within reach of the person. **Rationale:** The client can then call for assistance if required.
   - Leave for 2 to 3 minutes or until the client signals.
     or
   - Remain if the client needs support to stand at the bedside or other assistance.
5. Assist the client with removing the urinal as needed.
   - Apply clean gloves. Remove the urinal.
   - If wet, wipe the area around the urethral orifice with a tissue. Dry the perineum.
   - Change the linens or pad under the client if wet.
   - Provide the client with hand wipes, a dampened washcloth, or water, soap, and a towel to wash and dry hands.
6. Attend to the urine as required.
   - Measure the urine if the client is on monitored intake and output, and transfer a specimen to the appropriate container if required.
   - Empty and rinse out the urinal, and return it to the bedside unit. If the male client prefers, the urinal may be hung on the side rail by its handle for easy access. Perform hand hygiene.
   - Remove and discard gloves. Perform hand hygiene.
7. Document findings in the client record using forms or checklists supplemented by narrative notes when appropriate. Record the amount of urine, if it was measured, and all assessment data (e.g., cloudy urine, reddened perineum).

Sample Documentation

4/22/15 1320 Assisted with use of urinal due to arm in cast. Voided 450 mL dark yellow, clear, odorless urine. Specimen to lab for UA. Encouraged to drink more fluids; ice water and juice placed at bedside. Client verbalizes agreement to increase intake. _____ K. Clark, R.N.

Developmental Considerations

INFANTS

- Babies have no conscious control, and the urine is released after a small amount accumulates in the bladder.

CHILDREN

- In children, 50 to 200 mL stimulates stretch receptors in the bladder.
- Urinary control normally takes place between 2 and 4 1/2 years of age. Boys are usually slower than girls in developing this control.

- Teaching proper perineal hygiene can reduce infection. Girls should learn to wipe from front to back and wear cotton underwear. **Rationale:** *Wiping from front to back prevents stool or vaginal secretions from contaminating the urethral meatus. Wearing cotton underwear is recommended over nylon because it "breathes" and is less likely to support bacterial growth.*
- Teach children and parents that they should go to the bathroom as soon as the sensation to void is felt and not try to hold the urine in.

(continued on next page)

SKILL 6.12 Assisting with a Urinal (*continued*)

OLDER ADULTS

- Bladder capacity decreases in older adults, as does ability to completely empty the bladder.
- Decreased muscle tone may lead to nocturia, frequency, and increased residual.
- Altered cognition may lead to incontinence since it prevents the person from understanding the need to urinate and the actions needed to perform the activity.
- Many older men have enlarged prostate glands, which can inhibit complete emptying of the bladder. This often results in

urinary retention and urgency, which sometimes causes incontinence.

- Women past menopause have decreased estrogen, which results in a decrease in perineal tone and support of bladder, vagina, and pelvic tissues. This often results in urgency and stress incontinence and can even increase the incidence of urinary tract infections (UTIs).
- Increased stiffness and pain in joints, previous joint surgery, and neuromuscular problems can impair mobility and often make it difficult to get to the bathroom.

SKILL 6.13 Assisting a Client to the Commode

Equipment

- Commode with locking wheels or rubber-tipped legs
- Toilet tissue
- Nurse's call bell
- Slippers
- Bath blanket

Procedure

1. Place commode at foot of bed. Be sure to lock wheels on commode if needed.
2. Place slippers on client.
3. Raise head of bed to facilitate moving client to edge of bed.
4. Move client to edge of bed and assist to a sitting position at edge of bed. Instruct client to place feet flat on floor.
5. Stand directly in front of client, blocking client's toes with your feet and client's knees with your knees. **Rationale:** *Prevents client from buckling knees.*
6. Flex your knees.
7. Place your arms securely around client's waist. **Rationale:** *Stabilizes client for transfer.*
8. When starting to transfer, avoid bending at the waist. **Rationale:** *Prevents back strain.*
9. Instruct client to push self off bed and support his or her own weight.
10. Straighten your knees and hips as you raise client to standing position.
11. Pivot client in front of commode ❶. Instruct client to grasp arm rest on farthest side.
12. Lower client onto commode, using correct body mechanics (flexing your hip and knees but not your back) to ensure client is securely positioned on commode.
13. Place toilet tissue within easy reach.
14. Cover client with bath blanket for warmth and privacy.
15. Place call bell within easy access of client.
16. Provide privacy by closing curtains and shutting door.
17. Perform hand hygiene.
18. Assist client back to bed.
19. Empty and clean commode.
20. Perform hand hygiene.

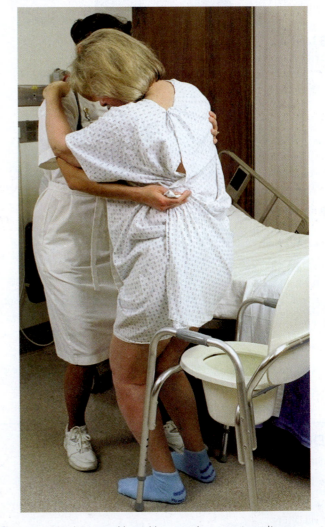

❶ Pivot with client and bend knees when seating client.

Sample Documentation

Document the amount, color, appearance, and odor of urine; techniques effective in stimulating voiding; equipment used (e.g., commode, bedpan), and type of support needed for transfer to commode.

SKILL 6.13   Assisting a Client to the Commode (*continued*)

Cultural Considerations

Some cultures incorporate the participation of family members to provide personal care, particularly assistance with using a bedpan or bedside commode, to maintain modesty. The nurse should ask clients about their personal preferences for assistance with personal care to maintain their modesty.

SKILL 6.14   Applying an External Urinary Device

- Discuss the use of external urinary devices with the client and/or family. Research has shown that condom catheters may be more comfortable and cause fewer UTIs than indwelling catheters (Chung et al., 2008; Martelly-Kebreau & Farren, 2009).
- Determine if the client has had an external catheter previously and any difficulties with it.
- Perform any procedures that are best completed without the catheter in place; for example, weighing the client would be easier without the tubing and bag.

Delegation

Applying a condom catheter may be delegated to UAP. However, the nurse must determine if the specific client has unique needs such as impaired circulation or latex allergy that would require special training of the UAP in the use of the condom catheter. Abnormal findings must be validated and interpreted by the nurse.

Equipment

- Condom sheath of appropriate size: small, medium, large, extra-large (Use the manufacturer's size guide as indicated. Use latex-free silicone for clients with latex allergies. Use self-adhering condoms, or those with Velcro, or other external securing device.) ❶

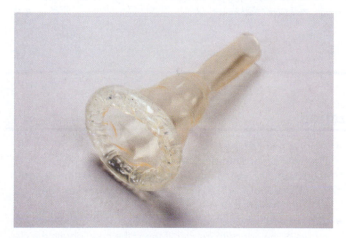

❶ An external or condom catheter.

- Leg drainage bag if ambulatory or urinary drainage bag with tubing
- Clean gloves
- Basin of warm water and soap
- Washcloth and towel

Preparation

- Assemble the leg drainage bag or urinary drainage bag for attachment to the condom sheath.

- If the condom supplied is not rolled onto itself, roll the condom outward onto itself to facilitate easier application. On some models, an inner flap will be exposed. This flap is applied around the urinary meatus to prevent the reflux of urine.

Procedure

1. Prior to performing the procedure, introduce self and verify the client's identity using agency protocol. Explain to the client what you are going to do, why it is necessary, and how he can participate.

CLINICAL ALERT

Use of an external urine collection system is recommended for incontinent men without urine retention. These devices are comfortable, and there is less chance of a urinary tract infection than with indwelling catheters.

2. Perform hand hygiene and observe other appropriate infection control procedures.
3. Position the client in either a supine or a sitting position. Provide for client privacy.
   - Drape the client appropriately with the bath blanket, exposing only the penis.
4. Apply clean gloves.
5. Inspect and clean the penis.
   - Clean the genital area and dry it thoroughly. **Rationale:** *This minimizes skin irritation and excoriation after the condom is applied.*
6. Apply and secure the condom.
   - Roll the condom smoothly over the penis, leaving 2.5 cm (1 in.) between the end of the penis and the rubber or plastic connecting tube ❷. **Rationale:** *This space prevents irritation of the tip of the penis and provides for full drainage of urine.*

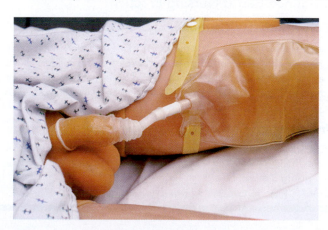

❷ The condom rolled over the penis.

(*continued on next page*)

SKILL 6.14   Applying an External Urinary Device *(continued)*

- Secure the condom firmly, but not too tightly, to the penis. Avoid catching pubic hair if possible. Some condoms have an adhesive inside the proximal end that adheres to the skin of the base of the penis. Many condoms are packaged with special fixation material. If neither is present, use a strip of flexible self-adhesive tape or Velcro around the base of the penis over the condom. Ordinary tape is contraindicated because it is not flexible and can stop blood flow.

7. Securely attach the urinary drainage system.
   - Make sure that the tip of the penis is not touching the condom and that the condom is not twisted. **Rationale:** *A twisted condom could obstruct the flow of urine.*
   - Attach the urinary drainage system to the condom.
   - Remove and discard gloves. Perform hand hygiene.
   - If the client is to remain in bed, attach the urinary drainage bag to the bed frame.
   - If the client is ambulatory, attach the bag to the client's leg **3**. **Rationale:** *Attaching the drainage bag to the leg helps control the movement of the tubing and prevents twisting of the thin material of the condom appliance at the tip of the penis.*

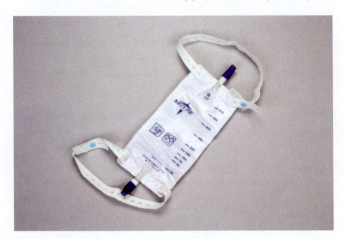

3 Urinary drainage leg bag.

8. Teach the client about the drainage system.
   - Instruct the client to keep the drainage bag below the level of the condom and to avoid loops or kinks in the tubing. Instruct the client to report pain, irritation, swelling, or wetness/leaking around the penis to healthcare personnel.

9. Inspect the penis 30 minutes following the condom application and at least every 4 hours. Check for urine flow. Document these findings.
   - Assess the penis for swelling and discoloration. **Rationale:** *This indicates that the condom is too tight.*
   - Assess urine flow if the client has voided. Normally, some urine is present in the tube if the flow is not obstructed.

10. Change the condom as indicated and provide skin care. In most settings, the condom is changed daily.
    - Remove the flexible tape or Velcro strip, apply clean gloves, and roll off the condom.
    - Wash the penis with soapy water, rinse, and dry it thoroughly.
    - Assess the foreskin for signs of irritation, swelling, and discoloration.
    - Apply a new condom.
    - Remove and discard gloves. Perform hand hygiene.

11. Document in the client record using forms or checklists supplemented by narrative notes when appropriate. Record the application of the condom, the time, and pertinent observations, such as irritated areas on the penis.

Sample Documentation

4/22/15 2245 Condom catheter applied for the night per client request. Glans clean, skin intact. Catheter attached to bedside collection bag. Instructed to notify staff if pain, irritation, swelling, or wetness/leaking occurs. Verbalized that he would. _____ L. Chan, R.N.

SKILL 6.15   Performing Urinary Catheterization

Evidence-Based Nursing Practice

Foley Catheter Cautions

Some studies have shown that the standard Foley catheter with a solitary drainage hole at its tip (1.5 cm above the base of the balloon) allows residual urine to accumulate. This may lead to inaccurate measurement of urine output and may increase risk for urinary tract infections.
Source: Fallis (2005).

Intermittent Catheterization Preferred

CDC guidelines state that intermittent catheterization is preferable to indwelling urethral or suprapubic catheters in clients with bladder emptying dysfunction.
Source: Centers for Disease Control and Prevention (2009).

- Allow adequate time to perform the catheterization. Although the entire procedure can require as little as 15 minutes, several sources of difficulty could result in a much longer time period. If possible, this procedure should not be performed just prior to or after the client eats.
- Some clients may feel uncomfortable being catheterized by nurses of the opposite gender. If this is the case, obtain the client's permission. Also consider whether agency policy requires or encourages having a person of the client's same gender present for the procedure.

Delegation

Due to the need for sterile technique and detailed knowledge of anatomy, insertion of a urinary catheter is not delegated to UAP.

Equipment

- Sterile catheter of appropriate size (An extra catheter should also be at hand.)

SKILL 6.15   Performing Urinary Catheterization (continued)

> **CLINICAL ALERT**
> Recommended urinary catheter sizes for children:
>
> Infant: 4–5 French
>
> Toddler and preschooler: 6–8 French
>
> School-age child: 6–10 French
>
> Adolescent: 8–14 French

Catheterization Kit ❶ or Individual Sterile Items

- Sterile gloves
- Waterproof drape(s)
- Antiseptic solution
- Cleansing balls
- Forceps
- Water-soluble lubricant
- Urine receptacle
- Specimen container

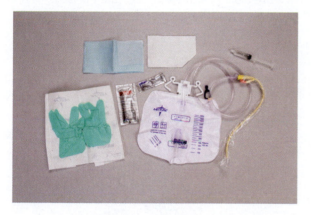

❶ Catheter insertion kit for a straight catheterization.

For an Indwelling Catheter

- Syringe prefilled with sterile water in amount specified by catheter manufacturer ❷
- Collection bag and tubing
- 5 to 10 mL 2% Xylocaine gel or water-soluble lubricant for urethral injection (if agency permits)
- Clean gloves
- Supplies for performing perineal cleansing
- Bath blanket or sheet for draping the client
- Adequate lighting (Obtain a flashlight or lamp if necessary.)

Preparation

- If using a catheterization kit, read the label carefully to ensure that all necessary items are included.
- Apply clean gloves and perform routine perineal care to cleanse the meatus from gross contamination. For women, use this time to locate the urinary meatus relative to surrounding structures.
- Remove and discard gloves. Perform hand hygiene.

Procedure

1. Prior to performing the procedure, check physician's order, introduce self and verify the client's identity using agency protocol. Explain to the client what you are going to do, why it is necessary, and how he or she can participate.

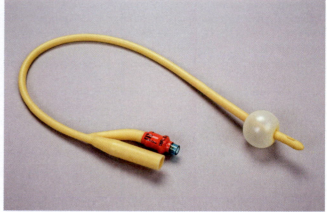

A

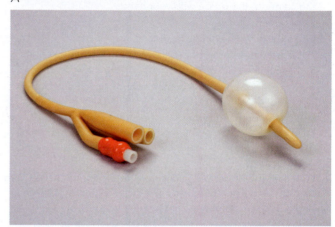

B

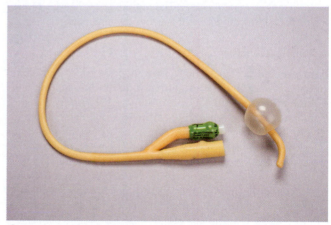

C

❷ A, A retention (Foley) catheter with the balloon inflated. B, Three-way Foley catheter, often used for continuous bladder irrigation. C, Coudé catheter tip.

2. Perform hand hygiene and observe other appropriate infection control procedures.
3. Provide for client privacy.
4. Place the client in the appropriate position and drape all areas except the perineum.
   - *Female:* supine with knees flexed, feet about 2 feet apart, and hips slightly externally rotated, if possible
   - *Male:* supine, thighs slightly abducted or apart

(continued on next page)

SKILL 6.15 Performing Urinary Catheterization (*continued*)

5. Establish adequate lighting. Stand on the client's right if you are right-handed, on the client's left if you are left-handed.

6. If using a collecting bag and it is not contained within the catheterization kit, open the drainage package and place the end of the tubing within reach. **Rationale:** *Because one hand is needed to hold the catheter once it is in place, open the package while two hands are still available.*

7. If agency policy permits, apply clean gloves and inject 10 to 15 mL Xylocaine gel or water-soluble lubricant into the urethra of the male client (Lo, 2008). Wipe the underside of the penile shaft to distribute the gel up the urethra. Wait at least 5 minutes for the gel to take effect before inserting the catheter.

8. Remove and discard gloves. Perform hand hygiene.

9. Open the catheterization kit. Place a waterproof drape under the buttocks (female) or penis (male) without contaminating the center of the drape with your hands.

10. Apply sterile gloves.

11. Organize the remaining supplies:
    * Saturate the cleansing balls with the antiseptic solution.
    * Open the lubricant package.
    * Remove the specimen container and place it nearby with the lid loosely on top.

12. Attach the prefilled syringe to the indwelling catheter inflation hub. Apply agency policy regarding pretesting of the balloon. *Note:* Silicone catheter balloons should not be pretested.

13. Lubricate the catheter 2.5 to 5 cm (1 to 2 in.) for females, 15 to 17.5 cm (6 to 7 in.) for males and place it with the drainage end inside the collection container.

14. If desired, place the fenestrated drape over the perineum, exposing the urinary meatus.

15. Cleanse the meatus. *Note:* The nondominant hand is considered contaminated once it touches the client's skin.

For Female Clients

■ Use your nondominant hand to spread the labia so the meatus is visible. Establish firm but gentle pressure on the labia. The antiseptic may make the tissues slippery, but the labia must not be allowed to return over the cleaned meatus. (*Note:* Location of the urethral meatus is best identified during the cleansing process.) Pick up a cleansing ball with the forceps in your dominant hand and wipe one side of the labia majora in an anteroposterior direction. Use great care that wiping the client does not contaminate this sterile hand. Use a new ball for the opposite side. Repeat for the labia minora ❸ ❹. Use the last ball to cleanse directly over the meatus.

For Male Clients

■ Use your nondominant hand to grasp the penis just below the glans. If necessary, retract the foreskin. Hold the penis firmly upright, with slight tension. **Rationale:** *Lifting the penis in this manner helps straighten the urethra.* Pick up a cleansing ball with the forceps in your dominant hand and wipe from the center of the meatus in a circular motion around the glans to the base. Use great care that wiping the client does not contaminate this sterile hand. Use a new ball and repeat three more times. The antiseptic may make the tissues slippery but the foreskin must not be allowed to return over the cleaned meatus nor the penis be dropped.

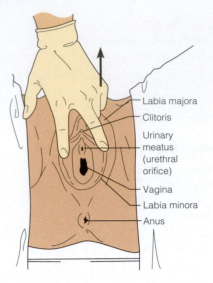

❸ To expose the urinary meatus, separate the labia minora and retract the tissue upward.

Labia majora
Clitoris
Urinary meatus (urethral orifice)
Vagina
Labia minora
Anus

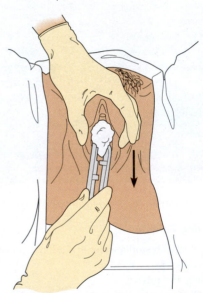

❹ When cleaning the labia minora, move the swab downward.

16. Insert the catheter.
    * Grasp the catheter firmly 5 to 7.5 cm (2 to 3 in.) from the tip. Ask the client to take a slow deep breath and insert the catheter as the client exhales. Slight resistance is expected as the catheter passes through the sphincters. If necessary, twist the catheter or hold pressure on the catheter until the sphincter relaxes.
    * Advance the catheter 5 cm (2 in.) farther after the urine begins to flow through it. **Rationale:** *This is to be sure it is fully in the bladder, will not easily fall out, and the balloon is into the bladder completely.* For male clients, some experts recommend advancing the catheter to the "Y" bifurcation of the catheter (Villanueva & Hemstreet, 2008). Check your agency's policy.
    * If the catheter accidentally contacts the labia or slips into the vagina, it is considered contaminated and a new, sterile catheter must be used. The contaminated catheter may be left in the vagina until the new catheter is inserted to help avoid mistaking the vaginal opening for the urinary meatus.

SKILL 6.15   Performing Urinary Catheterization (*continued*)

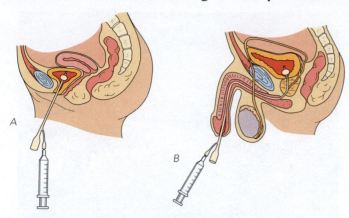

A

B

⑤ Placement of catheter and inflated balloon: *A*, female client; *B*, male client.

17. Hold the catheter with the nondominant hand.
18. For an indwelling catheter, inflate the retention balloon with the designated volume.
    - Without releasing the catheter (and, for females, without releasing the labia), hold the inflation valve between two fingers of your nondominant hand while you attach the syringe (if not left attached earlier when testing the balloon) and inflate with your dominant hand. If the client complains of discomfort, immediately withdraw the instilled fluid, advance the catheter further, and attempt to inflate the balloon again.

- Pull gently on the catheter until resistance is felt to ensure that the balloon has inflated and to place it in the trigone of the bladder **⑤**.

CLINICAL ALERT

Catheter-associated urinary tract infection (CAUTI) is the most common type of healthcare-associated infection.

Chronic irritation and inflammation of bladder mucosa due to long-term (over 8 months) presence of an indwelling catheter (urethral or suprapubic) is associated with an increased risk for bladder cancer.

19. Collect a urine specimen if needed. For a straight catheter, allow 20 to 30 mL to flow into the bottle without touching the catheter to the bottle. For an indwelling catheter preattached to a drainage bag, a specimen may be taken from the bag this initial time only.
20. Allow the straight catheter to continue draining into the urine receptacle. If necessary (e.g., an open system), attach the drainage end of an indwelling catheter to the collecting tubing and bag.
21. Examine and measure the urine. In some cases, only 750 to 1,000 mL of urine are to be drained from the bladder at one time. Check agency policy for further instructions if this should occur.
22. Remove the straight catheter when urine flow stops. For an indwelling catheter, secure the catheter tubing to the thigh for female clients or the upper thigh or abdomen for male clients with enough slack to allow usual movement **⑥**. The

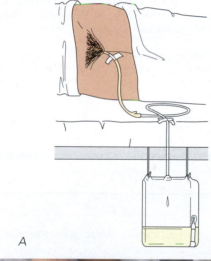

A

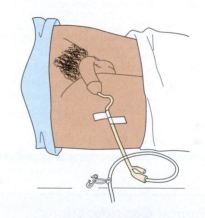

B

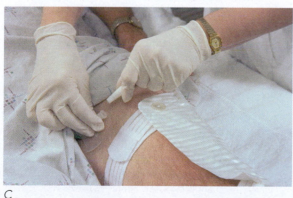

C

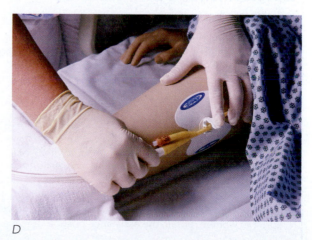

D

⑥ Tape the catheter to the *A*, inside of a female's thigh or *B*, thigh or abdomen of a male client. *C*, A Velcro catheter securement device *D*, A dissolvable, adhesive device with a swivel clamp to hold the urinary catheter in place.

(*continued on next page*)

SKILL 6.15   Performing Urinary Catheterization (continued)

Society of Urologic Nurses and Associates and the CDC recommend proper securement to prevent movement and urethral trauma (Gray, 2008; Newman, 2007; Willson et al., 2009). A manufactured catheter-securing device should be used to secure the catheter tubing to the client. **Rationale:** *This prevents unnecessary trauma to the urethra* (Dumont & Wakeman, 2010). Next hang the bag below the level of the bladder. No tubing should fall below the top of the bag **7**.

23. Wipe any remaining antiseptic or lubricant from the perineal area. Replace the foreskin if retracted earlier. Return the client to a comfortable position. Instruct the client on positioning and moving with the catheter in place.

24. Discard all used supplies in appropriate receptacles.

25. Remove and discard gloves. Perform hand hygiene.

26. Document the catheterization procedure, including catheter size and results, in the client record using forms or checklists supplemented by narrative notes when appropriate.

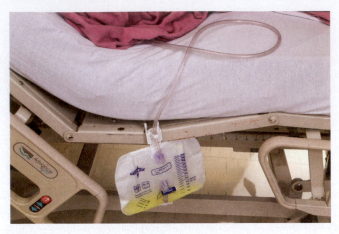

7 Correct position for urine drainage bag and tubing.

Sample Documentation

2/24/15 0530 Client agreed to insertion of indwelling catheter for pre-op as per orders. #16 Foley with 10-mL balloon inserted without difficulty, secured to thigh, connected to straight drainage. Immediate return of 100 mL pale, clear yellow urine. _____ G, Hampton, R.N.

Client Teaching

Urinary Catheterization

For indwelling catheters, instruct the client to:

- Never pull on the catheter.
- Keep the catheter tubing attached to the leg using a catheter securing device.
- Ensure that there are no kinks or twists in the tubing.
- Keep the urine drainage bag below the level of the bladder.
- Report signs and symptoms of UTI including burning, urgency, abdominal pain, cloudy urine; in older adults, confusion may be an early sign.
- Maintain adequate oral intake of fluids.

Clients who have indwelling catheters for lengthy periods of time need to have the catheter and bag changed at regular intervals. Changing equipment once a month is often the standard, although agency policy may differ. Inform the client of this routine.

Also, issues of sexuality must be discussed with clients who have indwelling catheters at home. Nurses who are not familiar or comfortable with providing the client this information must request another healthcare provider to assume this responsibility.

Developmental Considerations

INFANTS/CHILDREN

- Adapt the size of the catheter for pediatric clients.
- Ask a family member to assist in holding the child during catheterization, if appropriate.

OLDER ADULTS

- Obtaining consent and cooperation from older adults may take longer than with younger clients.
- When catheterizing older adults, be very attentive to problems of limited movement, especially in the hips. Arthritis, or previous hip or knee surgery, may limit the movement of older adults and cause discomfort. Modify the position (e.g., side-lying) as needed to perform the procedure safely and comfortably. For women, obtain the assistance of another nurse to flex

and hold the client's knees and hips as necessary or place her in a modified Sims' position.

- If the female meatus cannot be visualized, insert a gloved finger into the vagina and press gently upward. **Rationale:** *This action may straighten the urethra and make the meatus visible* (Villanueva & Hemstreet, 2008).

Setting of Care

- Clients with spinal cord injuries who are unable to stimulate voiding may use intermittent straight catheterization every few hours. The client or another caregiver can perform this procedure once taught by a nurse. Often, the client will use clean rather than sterile technique and reuse equipment since the microorganisms to which the client is exposed are his or her own.

SKILL 6.15 Performing Urinary Catheterization (continued)

- For intermittent self-catheterization, instruct the client to:
  - Follow instructions for clean technique.
  - Wash hands well with warm water and soap prior to handling equipment or performing catheterization.
  - Monitor for signs and symptoms of UTIs including burning, urgency, abdominal pain, and cloudy urine; in older adults, confusion may be an early sign.
  - Ensure adequate oral intake of fluids.
  - After each catheterization, assess the urine for color, odor, clarity, and the presence of blood.
  - Wash reusable catheters thoroughly with soap and water after use, dry, and store in a clean place.
- For ambulatory clients, those in the home, or those in wheelchairs who have indwelling catheters, modifications are needed in securing the catheter and maintaining the collection bag below bladder level. A leg bag may substitute for a hanging bag for those who are upright.
- Discuss with the client and family ways to minimize UTIs in those requiring frequent catheterization. Increasing fluid intake and urine acidification by drinking cranberry juice is an example. Also discuss modifications in hygiene and sexual intercourse that may be indicated for individuals with indwelling catheters.
- Teach the client and family when and how to empty the collection bag and to assess the urine for signs of infection, bleeding, or other complications.
- Clients with an indwelling catheter should take a shower rather than a tub bath. **Rationale:** *Sitting in a tub allows bacteria easier access into the urinary tract.*

SKILL 6.16 Performing Catheter Care and Removal

If the catheter requires changing, an entire new system with collecting bag must be used.

Evidence-Based Nursing Practice

Reminder Reduces Urinary Catheterization Use

A study demonstrated that catheter use could be decreased if physicians received automatic computerized (or written) reminders that their clients had catheters and how long they had been in place. Because urinary catheters are a major source of healthcare-associated infection, they should be used for as brief a time as possible.

Source: Saint et al. (2005).

Cranberry for Urinary Tract Infection Prophylaxis

There is some evidence to support the use of cranberry juice and cranberry supplements for the prevention of urinary tract infections (UTIs). Cranberry may be used as an adjunct in treating UTIs, but it is not effective as a first-line treatment. Because cranberry juice or supplements are safe, it is reasonable to recommend moderate use as prophylaxis against UTI.

Source: Mayo Clinic (2013b).

Delegation

Routine care of the client with an indwelling catheter may be delegated to UAP. Abnormal findings must be validated and interpreted by the nurse. Removal of an indwelling catheter may be performed by UAP according to agency policy, provided they have been thoroughly trained in the procedure and are aware of conditions that could arise that require the assistance of a nurse.

Equipment

- Clean gloves, 3 pairs
- Washcloth, soap, and towels

For Catheter Removal

- Paper towel or waste receptacle
- Luer-Lok or slip-tip syringe at least as large as the size of the retention balloon (printed on the inflation port)

Preparation

- Determine an appropriate time for catheter care or removal, and client's knowledge and need for teaching.

Procedure

1. Prior to performing the procedure, check physician's order, introduce self and verify the client's identity using agency protocol. Explain to the client what you are going to do, why it is necessary, and how he or she can participate. Discuss how the results will be used in planning further care or treatments.
2. Perform hand hygiene and observe other appropriate infection control procedures.
3. Provide for client privacy.
4. Prepare the client.
   - Ask the client to assume a back-lying position.
   - Obtain a sterile urine specimen if ordered or recommended by agency protocol.
5. Perform catheter care.
   - Apply clean gloves.
   - Wash the urinary meatus and the proximal catheter with soap and water. Dry gently.
   - Remove and discard gloves. Perform hand hygiene.

(continued on next page)

SKILL 6.16   Performing Catheter Care and Removal (continued)

6. Empty the collection bag at least every 8 hours and whenever close to half full.
   - Apply clean gloves.
   - Obtain the graduated container used for measuring urine for that client.
   - Place a paper towel on the floor below the bag.
   - Remove the end of the drainage tube from its protective housing on the collection bag without touching the end.
   - Point the tube into the container and release the clamp.
   - After the bag is completely emptied, cleanse the end of the tube according to agency policy (e.g., with an alcohol swab), clamp the tube, and replace it into the protective housing.
   - Note the volume and characteristics of the urine. Empty the container into the toilet if the urine does not need to be saved.
   - Rinse the container and return it to its storage location.
   - Remove and discard gloves. Perform hand hygiene.
7. To remove the catheter:
   - Place a towel or receptacle between the client's legs.
   - Detach the catheter from where it has been secured to the client's skin.
   - Apply clean gloves.
   - Insert the hub of the syringe into the inflation tube of the catheter.
   - Withdraw all the fluid from the balloon ❶ ❷. **Rationale:** *This will permit the balloon to deflate.* If not all fluid can be removed, report this fact to the nurse in charge before proceeding. *Do not pull* the catheter while the balloon is inflated. **Rationale:** *The urethra may be injured if the inflated balloon is pulled through it.*

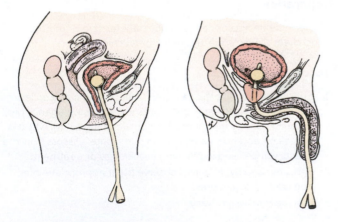

❶ Balloon must be deflated before removing to prevent damage to urethra.

   - Gently withdraw the catheter, observe for intactness, and place in the towel or waste receptacle. **Rationale:** *If the catheter is not intact, parts may remain in the bladder. Report this immediately to the nurse in charge or primary care provider.*
   - Wash and dry the perineal area.

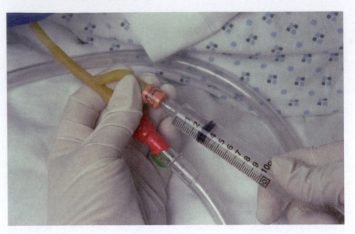

❷ Insert syringe hub into balloon port and withdraw fluid from retention catheter balloon.

CLINICAL ALERT
Do not aspirate balloon vigorously. Doing so may collapse inflation lumen and prevent balloon deflation.

8. Measure the urine in the drainage bag (see step 6 above).
9. Discard all used supplies in appropriate receptacles,
10. Remove and discard gloves. Perform hand hygiene.
11. Document the procedure and assessment data.
    - Record the time the catheter was removed; the intactness of the catheter; and the amount, color, and clarity of the urine.
12. Determine time of first voiding and the amount voided over the first 8 hours. Compare this with the fluid intake. **Rationale:** *When the fluid output is considerably less than the fluid intake, the bladder may be retaining urine.* If urine retention is suspected, scan or palpate the bladder for fullness. Use noninvasive methods to encourage voiding such as allowing the client to hear running water or placing the client's hand in water. Notify the primary care provider if the client has not voided in 8 hours (or another interval specified by policy) because the client may need to be recatheterized. Record the voiding or other action taken.

Sample Documentation

7/3/15 1015 Foley removed intact after aspirating balloon for 10 mL fluid without difficulty. Moderate amount white sediment noted around catheter tip. Peri care provided. Skin intact and without lesions. Taught to continue goal intake of fluids of 150 mL/hour. Verbalized agreement. _____ S. Brown, RN

7/3/15 1645 Up to BR. Voided 600 mL amber urine. C/o slight burning at start of urination. States will continue fluid intake. Dr. Wertz notified of burning on urination. _____ S. Brown, RN

SKILL 6.17 Performing Bladder Irrigation

Before irrigating a catheter or bladder, check (1) the **reason** for the irrigation; (2) the **order** authorizing the continuous or intermittent irrigation (in most agencies, a primary care provider's order is required); (3) the type of sterile **solution**, the amount, and strength to be used, and the rate (if continuous); and (4) the type of **catheter** in place. If these are not specified on the client's chart, check agency protocol.

Delegation

Due to the need for sterile technique, urinary irrigation is generally not delegated to UAP. If the client has continuous irrigation, the UAP may care for the client and note abnormal findings. These must be validated and interpreted by the nurse.

Equipment

- Clean gloves, 2 pairs
- Retention catheter in place
- Drainage tubing and bag (if not in place)
- Drainage tubing clamp
- Antiseptic swabs
- Sterile receptacle
- Sterile irrigating solution warmed or at room temperature (Label the irrigant clearly with the words *Bladder Irrigation,* including the information about any medications that have been added to the original solution, and the date, time, and nurse's initials.)
- Infusion tubing
- IV pole

Procedure

1. Prior to performing the procedure, introduce self and verify the client's identity using agency protocol. Explain to the client what you are going to do, why it is necessary, and how he or she can participate. The irrigation should not be painful or uncomfortable. Discuss how the results will be used in planning further care or treatments.
2. Perform hand hygiene and observe other appropriate infection control procedures.
3. Provide for client privacy.
4. Apply clean gloves.
5. Empty, measure, and record the amount and appearance of urine present in the drainage bag. Discard urine and gloves. **Rationale:** *Emptying the drainage bag allows more accurate measurement of urinary output after the irrigation is in place or completed. Assessing the character of the urine provides baseline data for later comparison.*
6. Prepare the equipment.
   - Perform hand hygiene.
   - Connect the irrigation infusion tubing to the irrigating solution and flush the tubing with solution, keeping the tip sterile. **Rationale:** *Flushing the tubing removes air and prevents it from being instilled into the bladder.*
   - Apply clean gloves and cleanse the port with antiseptic swabs.
   - Connect the irrigation tubing to the input port of the three-way catheter.
   - Connect the drainage bag and tubing to the urinary drainage port if not already in place.
   - Remove and discard gloves. Perform hand hygiene.

7. Irrigate the bladder.
   - For closed continuous bladder irrigation using a three-way catheter, open the clamp on the urinary drainage tubing (if present) ❶. **Rationale:** *This allows the irrigating solution to flow out of the bladder continuously.*
     a. Apply clean gloves.
     b. Open the regulating clamp on the irrigating fluid infusion tubing and adjust the flow rate as prescribed by the primary care provider or to 40 to 60 drops per minute if not specified.
     c. Assess the drainage for amount, color, and clarity. The amount of drainage should equal the amount of irrigant entering the bladder plus expected urine output. Empty the bag frequently so that it does not exceed half full.

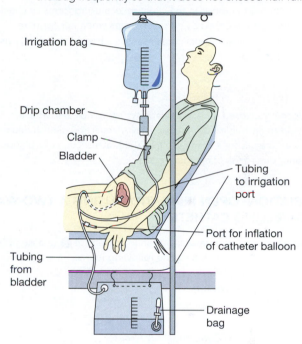

❶ A continuous bladder irrigation (CBI) setup.

   - For closed intermittent irrigation, determine whether the solution is to remain in the bladder for a specified time.
     a. If the solution is to remain in the bladder (a bladder irrigation or instillation), close the clamp to the urinary drainage tubing. **Rationale:** *Closing the flow clamp allows the solution to be retained in the bladder and in contact with bladder walls.*
     b. If the solution is being instilled to irrigate the catheter, open the flow clamp on the urinary drainage tubing. **Rationale:** *Irrigating solution will flow through the urinary drainage port and tubing, removing mucous shreds or clots.*
     c. If a three-way catheter is used, open the flow clamp to the irrigating fluid infusion tubing, allowing the specified amount of solution to infuse. Then close the clamp on the infusion tubing.
     or
     a. If a two-way catheter is used, connect an irrigating syringe with a needleless adapter to the injection port on the drainage tubing and instill the solution.

(continued on next page)

SKILL 6.17   Performing Bladder Irrigation *(continued)*

    b. After the specified period the solution is to be retained has passed, open the drainage tubing flow clamp and allow the bladder to empty.

    c. Assess the drainage for amount, color, and clarity. The amount of drainage should equal the amount of irrigant entering the bladder plus expected urine output.

- Remove and discard gloves. Perform hand hygiene.

8. Assess the client and the urinary output.
   - Assess the client's comfort.
   - Apply clean gloves.
   - Empty the drainage bag and measure the contents. Subtract the amount of irrigant instilled from the total volume of drainage to obtain the volume of urine output.
   - Remove and discard gloves. Perform hand hygiene.

9. Document findings in the client record using forms or checklists supplemented by narrative notes when appropriate.
   - Note any abnormal constituents such as blood clots, pus, or mucous shreds.

> ### CLINICAL ALERT
> Opening a closed urinary drainage system is indicated as a last resort to reestablish catheter patency. Manual irrigation should be done carefully for a client with transurethral resection of a bladder tumor due to risk of bladder rupture.

VARIATION: OPEN IRRIGATION USING A TWO-WAY INDWELLING CATHETER

- Assemble the equipment. Use an irrigation set ② or assemble individual items, including the following items:
  - Clean gloves
  - Disposable water-resistant towel
  - Sterile irrigating solution
  - Sterile basin
  - Sterile 30- to 50-mL irrigating syringe
  - Antiseptic swabs
  - Sterile protective cap for drainage tubing
- Prepare the client (see steps 1 through 5 of main procedure for catheter irrigation).
- Prepare the equipment.
  - Perform hand hygiene.
  - Using aseptic technique, open supplies and pour the irrigating solution into the sterile basin or receptacle. **Rationale:** *Aseptic technique is vital to reduce the risk of instilling microorganisms into the urinary tract during the irrigation.*
  - Place the disposable water-resistant towel under the catheter.

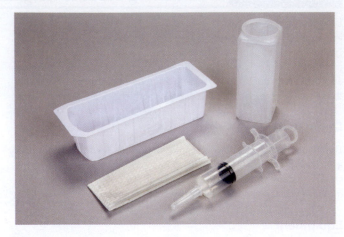

② An irrigation set.

- Apply clean gloves.
- Disconnect catheter from drainage tubing and place the catheter end in the sterile basin. Place the sterile protective cap over end of drainage tubing. **Rationale:** *The end of the drainage tubing will be considered contaminated if it touches bed linens or skin surfaces.*
- Draw the prescribed amount of irrigating solution into the syringe, maintaining the sterility of the syringe and solution.
- Irrigate the bladder.
  - Insert the tip of the syringe into the catheter opening.
  - Gently and slowly inject the solution into the catheter at approximately 3 mL per second. In adults, about 30 to 40 mL generally is instilled for catheter irrigations; 100 to 200 mL may be instilled for bladder irrigation or instillation. **Rationale:** *Gentle instillation reduces the risks of injury to bladder mucosa and of bladder spasms.*
  - Remove the syringe and allow the solution to drain back into the basin.
  - Continue to irrigate client's bladder until the total amount to be instilled has been injected or when fluid returns are clear and/or clots are removed.
  - Remove protective cap from drainage tube and wipe with antiseptic swab.
  - Reconnect catheter to drainage tubing.
  - Remove and discard gloves. Perform hand hygiene.
  - Assess the drainage for amount, color, and clarity. The amount of drainage should equal at least the amount of irrigant entering the bladder plus any urine that may have been dwelling in the bladder.
- Assess the client and the urinary output and document the procedure as in steps 8 and 9 above.

SKILL 6.18   Maintaining Continuous Bladder Irrigation

Equipment

- Irrigating solution (2,000 mL sterile normal saline, or less than drainage bag volume) as prescribed
- IV tubing with roller clamp
- IV pole
- Antiseptic swabs
- Clean gloves

Procedure

1. Check physician's orders and client care plan.
2. Note if client has triple lumen indwelling catheter and drainage bag ❶.
3. Identify client by checking the client's identity band and asking client to state name and birth date.

SKILL 6.18 Maintaining Continuous Bladder Irrigation *(continued)*

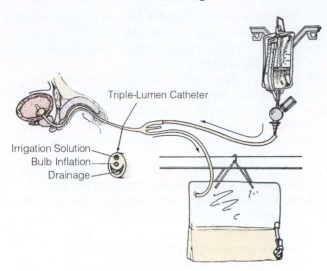

❶ Maintain continuous bladder irrigation by using a triple-lumen catheter for procedure.

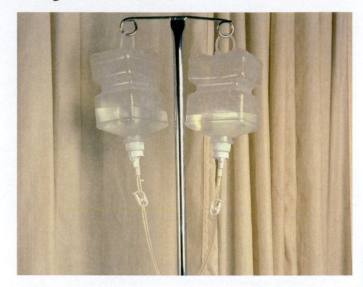

❷ Hang irrigating solution on IV pole at height of 60 to 90 cm (24 to 36 in.) above bladder.

4. Explain procedure to client and provide privacy.
5. Perform hand hygiene and don clean gloves.
6. Remove protective covering from spike on tubing, and insert spike into insertion port of solution container. Use aseptic technique.
7. Hang irrigating solution container on IV pole and prime tubing. Height of pole is usually 60 to 90 cm (24 to 36 in.) above bladder ❷.
    *   Remove protective cover from end of tubing using aseptic technique.
    *   Open roller clamp, and allow irrigating solution to run through tubing until all air is expelled. **Rationale:** *This prevents air from entering bladder and causing discomfort.*
    *   Close roller clamp.
8. Connect tubing to catheter irrigating (indwell) lumen using aseptic technique.
9. Check for patency of catheter; ensure there are no clots or foreign bodies that may obstruct catheter.
10. Remove and discard gloves. Perform hand hygiene and don new gloves.

11. Adjust drip rate of irrigating solution by adjusting the clamp on the tubing to increase or decrease based on urine outflow color.
    *   Infuse continuously to keep urine drainage pink to clear.
    *   When drainage is dark red or contains tissue or blood clots, increase drip rate. **Rationale:** *Increased drip rate will clear the drainage and flush out debris and clots.*
    *   Change irrigation solution bottle using aseptic technique.
12. Check for bladder distention or abdominal pain. Note urine color.
13. Monitor urine output at least every hour to observe patency of system.
14. Empty drainage bag as needed. Subtract amount of irrigant infused from total output to obtain urine output and record.
15. Maintain catheter traction if taped to thigh. **Rationale:** *This promotes venous hemostasis.*
16. Remove and discard gloves. Perform hand hygiene. Document care.

    Note: Procedure is done to flush clots and debris from bladder after prostatic surgery and to prevent catheter obstruction and promote patency. Immediately report bright red urine outflow, because this indicates an arterial bleed.

SKILL 6.19 Providing Suprapubic Catheter Care

Equipment

*   Closed drainage system, including Foley catheter tubing and bag
*   Catheter clamp and plug
*   Dry sterile dressing and tape if ordered
*   Cleansing solution
*   Clean gloves
*   Sterile gloves

Preparation

*   Check physician's orders and client care plan.
*   Identify client by checking the client's identity band and asking client to state name and birth date and explain purpose of catheter.

*   Describe procedure for continuous or intermittent urinary drainage.
*   Perform hand hygiene and observe other appropriate infection control procedures.
*   Provide for client privacy.

Procedure

1. Observe catheter for patency. **Rationale:** *The most common problem with suprapubic catheters is occlusion with sediment or clots.*
    *   *First 24 hours:* Check the catheter every hour to detect possible obstruction. Urine output should be in excess of 30 mL/hr.

(continued on next page)

SKILL 6.19 Providing Suprapubic Catheter Care (continued)

- *Second day:* Check the catheter every 8 hours.
- *Third day:* Check the catheter when the catheter is unclamped.
2. Maintain a closed drainage system. Do not open system to irrigate or obtain urine sample.
3. Observe for signs of urinary tract infection (color, odor, presence of sediment).
4. Keep the dressing dry around site of insertion. Apply a new dressing, maintaining sterile technique, every morning and as necessary.
   - Place bed in high position.
   - Perform hand hygiene and don clean gloves.
   - Remove old dressing, discard gloves, and dispose in appropriate container.
   - Perform hand hygiene and open sterile supplies.
   - Open cleansing solution and pour over sterile gauze.
   - Don sterile gloves.
   - Assess skin surrounding suprapubic catheter.
   - Cleanse area with cleansing solution. Allow to dry.
   - Apply sterile dressing and secure with tape ❶.
   - Remove gloves and supplies and discard in appropriate container.
   - Perform hand hygiene.
   - Replace bed in low position.

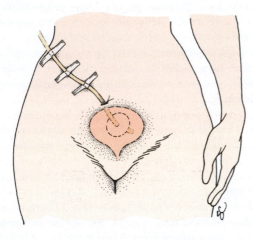

❶ Tape catheter and connect to a closed system.

5. Perform clamping protocol according to physician orders for intermittent urinary drainage.
   - Explain the clamping procedure and ask client to help monitor the clamping.
   - Instruct client to report if he or she feels fullness in the bladder during clamping.
   - Don clean gloves.
   - Clamp the catheter.
6. Empty the drainage bag or remove drainage tubing from catheter, maintaining aseptic technique.

- Place drainage tubing in sterile package to maintain sterility.
- Place catheter plug in catheter end.
- Remove and discard gloves. Perform hand hygiene.
- Record urine output on I&O record.
- Leave the catheter clamped or plugged for 3 to 4 hours depending on client's level of comfort and physician's orders.
7. At 3- to 4-hour intervals, or when client feels bladder fullness, ask client to void normally. Perform hand hygiene and don clean gloves to measure the urine and record output on I&O bedside record.
8. Immediately after client voids, unclamp catheter and leave unclamped for 5 minutes, collecting the residual urine.
   - Measure the residual urine following unclamping of the catheter.
   - Reclamp catheter.
   - Remove gloves and perform hand hygiene.
   - If ordered, send a urine specimen to laboratory after the first clamping. **Rationale:** *Specimen is used to check for presence of microorganisms.*
9. Repeat clamping protocol every 3 to 4 hours according to physician orders. The catheter may be open to drainage from bedtime until 6 a.m.
10. When the client is voiding normally, clamp the catheter throughout the night in preparation for its removal.
11. When the client's residual urine output is less than 100 mL or retains less than 20% of residual urine on two successive checks, notify the physician for removal of the catheter.
12. Cleanse insertion area with antimicrobial swab.
13. Deflate balloon and remove catheter, if order written for nurse to remove.
14. Perform hand hygiene and don clean gloves.
15. Apply a 2 × 2 sterile dressing over the insertion site.
16. Dispose of the catheter in biohazard bag.
17. Remove gloves and perform hand hygiene.
18. If the client is discharged from the hospital with the catheter, provide the following teaching for home care:
    - Instruct the client to drink one glass of fluid every hour while awake.
    - Instruct client to follow clamping procedure when awake or as instructed by physician.
    - Instruct the client to leave the catheter open to the drainage system at night. (Drainage system may be urinary tubing and bag or leg bag.)
    - Tell client to notify physician if dysuria occurs when voiding or if urine becomes cloudy, odorous, or has sediment.

Documentation

Document time catheter clamped; length of time clamped; client's ability to void spontaneously; client's feelings of fullness; time specimen sent to laboratory; color, amount, and odor of urine obtained; and color, amount, and odor of residual urine.

SKILL 6.20 Performing Urinary Ostomy Care

Review the client's record to determine the type of urinary diversion. Determine when the device was last changed and any pertinent findings at that time. Generally, a urinary diversion appliance adheres to the client's skin for 3 to 5 days.

Delegation

Due to the complexity of the procedure, the need for assessment skills, and use of aseptic technique, changing a urostomy device is

SKILL 6.20 Performing Urinary Ostomy Care *(continued)*

not delegated to UAP. However, aspects of ostomy function are observed during usual care and may be recorded by individuals other than the nurse. Abnormal findings must be validated and interpreted by the nurse.

Equipment

- One- or two-piece urinary pouch ①
- Tail closure clamp

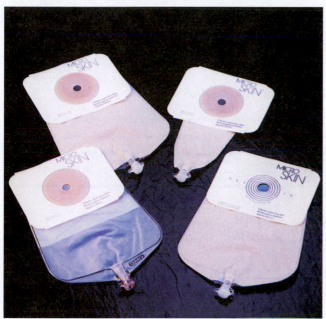

A

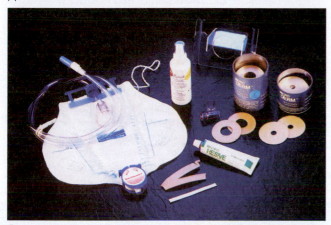

B

① *A*, One-piece urostomy system. *B*, Urostomy supplies. (Courtesy of Cymed Ostomy Company)

- Clean gloves
- Cleaning materials, including tissues, warm water, mild soap (optional), cotton balls, washcloth or gauze pads, towel
- Skin barrier/prep (gel, liquid, powder, or film)
- Stoma measuring guide
- Pen or pencil and scissors
- Deodorant liquid drops (optional)
- Bedpan or graduated cylinder

Preparation

- Determine the need for an appliance change.
- Assess the used appliance for leakage of urine. **Rationale:** *Urine irritates the peristomal skin.*
- Ask the client about any discomfort at or around the stoma. **Rationale:** *A burning sensation may indicate breakdown beneath the faceplate of the pouch.*
- Assess the fullness of the pouch. **Rationale:** The weight of an overly full bag may loosen the faceplate and separate it from the skin, causing the urine to leak and irritate the peristomal skin.
- If there is pouch leakage or discomfort at or around the stoma, change the appliance.
- Select an appropriate time to change the appliance.
- Avoid times close to meals or visiting hours. **Rationale:** *Ostomy odor may reduce appetite or embarrass the client.*

Procedure

1. Prior to performing the procedure, introduce self and verify the client's identity using agency protocol. Explain to the client what you are going to do, why it is necessary, and how he or she can participate. Discuss how the results will be used in planning further care or treatments. Changing an ostomy appliance should not cause discomfort, but it may be distasteful to the client. Communicate acceptance and support to the client. It is important to change the appliance competently and quickly. Include support individuals as appropriate.
2. Perform hand hygiene and observe other appropriate infection control procedures.
3. Provide for client privacy.
4. Assist the client to a comfortable sitting or lying position in bed or a sitting or standing position in the bathroom. **Rationale:** *Lying or standing positions may facilitate smoother pouch application.*
5. Empty and remove the ostomy appliance. *Note:* Because urine flows continuously, if the stoma can be measured for the new appliance with the appliance in place, perform step 8 first. This can usually be accomplished if the pouch is thin or transparent enough to fit the measuring guide snugly over the stoma while it is in place.
   - Apply clean gloves.
   - Empty the pouch through the bottom opening into a bedpan or graduated cylinder. **Rationale:** *Emptying before removing the pouch prevents spillage of urine onto the client's skin.*
   - Peel the bag off slowly while holding the client's skin taut. **Rationale:** *Holding the skin taut minimizes client discomfort and prevents abrasion of the skin.*
   - Place tissue or gauze pad over the stoma, and change as needed. **Rationale:** *This absorbs urine seepage from the stoma.*
6. Clean and dry the peristomal skin and stoma.
   - Use warm water, mild soap (optional), and damp cotton balls, gauze, or a washcloth and towel to clean the skin and stoma. Check agency practice on the use of soap. **Rationale:** *Soap is sometimes not advised because it can be irritating to the skin.*
   - Dry the area thoroughly by patting with a towel or cotton balls. **Rationale:** *Excess rubbing can abrade the skin.*

(continued on next page)

SKILL 6.20 Performing Urinary Ostomy Care (continued)

7. Assess the stoma and peristomal skin.
   - Inspect the stoma for color, size, shape, and bleeding.
   - Inspect the peristomal skin for any redness, ulceration, or irritation. Transient redness after removal of adhesive is normal.
8. Prepare and apply the new pouch.
   - Use the guide to measure the size of the stoma.
   - On the backing of the skin barrier, trace a circle the same size as the stomal opening.
   - Cut out the traced stoma pattern to make an opening in the skin barrier. Make the opening no more than 0.3 cm (1/8 in.) larger than the stoma. **Rationale:** *This allows space for the stoma to expand slightly when functioning and minimizes the risk of urine contacting peristomal skin.*
   - Remove the backing to expose the sticky adhesive side of the barrier. The backing can be saved and used as a pattern when making an opening for future skin barriers.
   - Apply the peristomal skin barrier to the faceplate of the ostomy appliance or around the stoma depending on the manufacturer's recommendations. Skin barrier powder may be used on irritated skin, but Skin-Prep liquid may not be applied to irritated skin.

- Center the faceplate over the stoma, and gently press it onto the client's skin, smoothing out any wrinkles or bubbles. Hold in place for about 30 seconds. **Rationale:** *The heat and pressure help activate the adhesives in the skin barrier.*
- Remove the air from the pouch. **Rationale:** *Removing the air helps the pouch lie flat against the abdomen.*
- *Optional:* Place approximately 10 drops of deodorant in the pouch.
- Close the pouch by turning up the bottom a few times, fan-folding its end lengthwise, and securing it with a tail closure clamp or replacing the drainage outlet cap (see ❶).
- Discard all used supplies in appropriate receptacles.
- Remove and discard gloves, and perform hand hygiene.
9. Document findings in the client record using forms or checklists supplemented by narrative notes when appropriate.

Sample Documentation

8/31/15 0900 Urostomy bag changed due to slight leakage. Had been in place for 6 days. No redness or irritation around stoma. Stoma pink, bled a few drops when washed. Client states home care RN changes the appliance when home. _____M. Earl, RN

SKILL 6.21 Applying a Urinary Diversion Pouch

Equipment

- One- or two-piece urinary pouch with skin barrier, flange, and spigot at bottom of pouch to empty urine
- Items to clean stoma (e.g., soft cloth or gauze sponges) and warm water
- Plastic bag for disposal of used equipment
- Gauze for drying skin and for wicking stoma
- Underpad to protect bedding
- Scissors if indicated
- Protective barriers such as skin prep, skin gel, or protective barrier film if necessary
- Stoma measuring guide
- Clean gloves

Preparation

- Check physician's order and client care plan. Pouch should be changed every 3 to 7 days.
- Gather equipment.
- Perform hand hygiene.
- Identify client by checking the client's identity band and asking client to state name and birth date and explain procedure.
- Provide for client privacy.
- Place client in a position that promotes visualization and self-care.
- Place protective pad under client.
- Place bath blanket over client's chest and position top covers over lower abdomen without impeding client's visualization of procedure.

Procedure

1. Don clean gloves.

2. Empty, then remove entire ostomy appliance by pushing the skin gently away from the appliance and peeling the appliance downward. Discard in plastic bag.
3. Wash stoma and peristomal skin with warm water and soap if needed, rinse well, and pat skin dry. **Rationale:** *Chemical or perfumed wipes can irritate skin or may interfere with pouch seal. Note: Stoma may bleed slightly when wiped.*
4. Check stoma for healing; it should be bright but not dark red and moist, and raised 1.3 to 2.5 cm (0.5 to 1 in.) above skin surface (or may be flush). Check for mucocutaneous separation ulceration, encrustation, and signs of infection, skin sensitivities, or allergies.
5. Check skin surrounding stoma to ensure urine has not been draining under the wafer, causing skin irritation.
6. Prepare new urinary pouch ❶. Place gauze over stoma to prevent urine from oozing onto skin. A wick can be placed in stoma, if needed. **Rationale:** *To keep urine from contact with skin during pouch change.* Measure stoma site with measuring guide, unless pouch has precut opening.

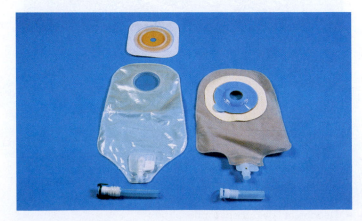

❶ One-piece and two-piece urinary diversion pouches.

SKILL 6.21   Applying a Urinary Diversion Pouch *(continued)*

7. Trace size of stoma on wafer and cut 1/16 to 1/8 in. larger than size ❷. **Rationale:** *This small opening prevents leakage of effluent onto skin; however, the size is large enough to prevent pressure on the stoma from the wafer rubbing on skin.*

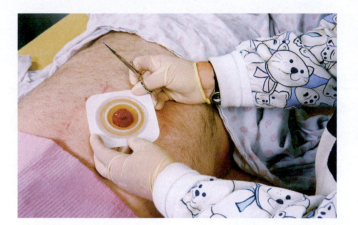

❷ Cut wafer opening slightly larger than stoma.

8. Apply protective barrier (only if indicated) to skin surrounding stoma or to wafer ❸. Do not use lotion. **Rationale:** *Protective barriers contain alcohol and cause burning, and may interfere with seal. In addition, barrier must be removed with adhesive remover.*

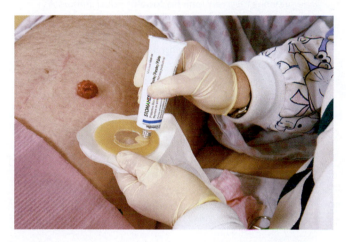

❸ Apply protective barrier paste to wafer only if indicated.

9. Let site dry thoroughly ❹.
10. Remove paper from adhesive on wafer of one- or two-piece appliance.
11. Remove wick and center wafer over stoma; apply to dry skin, starting at bottom, and working up around stoma. Press wafer on skin for 3 minutes ❺. **Rationale:** *To promote adherence to skin.* If two-piece pouch, attach pouch to wafer flange.

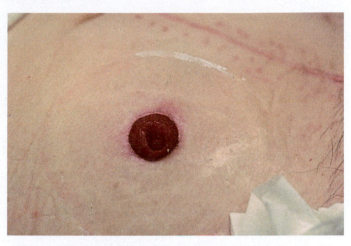

❹ Cleanse stoma and peristomal skin; dry thoroughly.

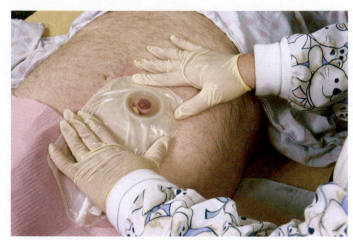

❺ Apply pouch and press firmly to facilitate seal.

12. Remove air from clean pouch and close spout. Attach pouch to gravity drainage bag only while client is in bed. Empty pouch when one third full.
13. Discard equipment in appropriate receptacle.
14. Remove and discard gloves. Perform hand hygiene.
15. Document the procedure.

> **CLINICAL ALERT**
>
> Thin plastic tubes (stents) may be placed in each ureter during surgery. These exit stoma and remain in place for up to 10 days. They serve to maintain patency until swelling has subsided at ureteroileal anastomosis site (6 to 10 days). Their presence and length of exposure should be documented. The surgeon should be notified when they wash out into collection pouch.

▶ BOWEL INTERVENTIONS

Elimination of the waste products of digestion from the body is essential to health. The excreted waste products are referred to as feces or stool. Defecation is the expulsion of feces from the anus and rectum. It is also called a bowel movement. The frequency of defecation is highly individual, varying from several times per day to two or three times per week. The amount defecated also varies from person to person. When peristaltic waves move the feces into the sigmoid colon and the rectum, the sensory nerves in the rectum are stimulated and the individual becomes aware of the need to defecate.

Expected Outcomes

1. Clients experience increased comfort and relief from abdominal distention.
2. Enema administered without difficulty.
3. Relief obtained from fecal impaction or constipation.
4. Pouch remains intact without leakage for 3 to 5 days.
5. Pouching system provides maximal skin protection.
6. Client gradually assumes an active role in applying the pouch.
7. Client's skin remains free of erythema, excoriation, and infection.

SKILL 6.22 Developing a Regular Bowel Routine

Evidence-Based Nursing Practice

Management of Constipation in Older Adults

Constipation is a very common disorder, and its prevalence increases with age, as reported by 26% of women and 16% of men ages 65 years and older. In people over age 84, the incidence increases to 34% and 26%, respectively.

There are three types of constipation, and treatment may vary by type:

- Functional constipation is the term used when clients experience small, hard stools that are difficult to pass. There may be abdominal pain or discomfort that is relieved with evacuation. Intestinal transit times and pelvic function studies are normal.
- Pelvic floor constipation—difficult or inadequate expulsion of stool—is due to faulty coordination of the abdominal and pelvic floor muscles, altered perineal descent, or structural abnormalities.
- Slow transit constipation (colonoparesis) involves some degree of partial paralysis in the colon resulting from dysfunction of the colonic nerves, smooth muscle, or both.

Effective management can occur with (1) education about diet and exercise and (2) use of certain techniques, such as timing of evacuation, breathing, and positioning on the toilet. Fiber supplements in water may improve consistency and weight of stool in some clients, but in others (such as clients with severe pelvic floor dysfunction), high-fiber supplements may have a negative effect. Therefore, knowing the primary cause of constipation is an important factor is establishing effective treatment.

Data from Mayo Clinic (2013a).

Equipment

- Clean gloves, 1 or 2 pairs
- Lubricant
- Bedpan or commode
- Absorbent pad
- Specific enema if ordered
- Washcloth and towel

Preparation

- Check physician's orders and client care plan.
- Identify client by checking the client's identity band and asking client to state name and birth date and explain procedure.
- Identify time of day client usually evacuates bowels.
- Evaluate diet, exercise, and former use of medications for bowel evacuation.

- Administer the following drugs as ordered:
  a. Stool softener (Colace, Dialose, DCS, Coloxyl) daily
  b. Bulk former (Metamucil or FiberCon)—daily to TID
  c. Mild laxative (Senokot, Doxidan, Dulcolax) 8 hours before program
  d. Suppository (glycerin or Dulcolax) just before digital stimulation.
- Perform hand hygiene.

Procedure

1. Don gloves. You may want to double-glove to prevent contamination if glove tears.
2. Perform digital stimulation one half hour after dinner or breakfast or according to client's time schedule for evacuation (see previous intervention). **Rationale:** *Food stimulates bowel activity.*
3. Place client on toilet or commode. (Use bedpan if client is on bed rest.) **Rationale:** *Assuming normal posture for bowel movement facilitates evacuation.*
4. Encourage client to contract abdominal muscles or bend forward while bearing down. **Rationale:** *Increases abdominal pressure and helps evacuate the bowel.*
5. Remove and discard gloves. Perform hand hygiene.
6. Provide privacy and sufficient time for evacuation.
7. Don gloves.
8. Wash and dry perineal area if client is unable to do so.
9. Remove and discard gloves.
10. Place client in wheelchair or bed and position for comfort.
11. Perform hand hygiene. Document actions and client response.
12. Wean client away from suppositories and laxatives when spontaneous bowel movements occur with digital stimulation.

Client Teaching

Good bowel training programs include:

- Initiation of defecation on demand with digital stimulation and abdominal massage
- Evacuation at same time each day; best time is 20 to 40 minutes after a meal
- Proper diet, increased fiber and fluids
- Daily physical exercise regimen
- Client and family education

SKILL 6.22 Developing a Regular Bowel Routine (continued)

Developmental Considerations

Preventing Constipation

OLDER ADULTS

- Assess constipation by obtaining the client's history, including information regarding the amount of fluid intake, food ingested, and dietary fiber.
- Review medications associated with an increased risk of developing constipation; screen for polypharmacy.

- Identify bowel patterns using a bowel diary.
- Increase fluids to 1500 to 2000 mL/day; minimize caffeine and alcohol intake.
- Promote regular consistent toileting.
- Tailor physical activity to client's physical abilities.

Source: Registered Nurses Association of Ontario (2005).

SKILL 6.23 Inserting a Rectal Tube

Equipment

- Rectal tube: size 22 to 24 straight (French) for adults and size 12 to 18 French for children
- Small plastic bag or stool specimen container
- Hypoallergenic paper tape
- Water-soluble lubricant
- Bed protector
- Clean gloves, 2 pairs
- Washcloth and towel

Procedure

1. Check physician's orders and client care plan.
2. Perform hand hygiene.
3. Gather equipment.
4. Identify client by checking the client's identity band and asking client to state name and birth date and explain the procedure.
5. Provide privacy. Place client on left side in a recumbent position and drape. **Rationale:** *This position facilitates insertion of tube following the normal curve of rectum and sigmoid colon.*
6. Place bed protector under client.
7. Tape the plastic bag around the distal end of the rectal tube or insert the tube into the stool specimen container.
8. Vent the upper side of the plastic bag to prevent inflation.
9. Don gloves.
10. Lubricate the proximal end of the rectal tube with water-soluble lubricant.
11. Gently separate buttocks, and ask client to take in a deep breath. **Rationale:** *Taking a deep breath relaxes the anal sphincter and prevents tissue trauma during tube insertion.* Gently insert the tube into the client's rectum, past the external and internal anal sphincters (2 to 4 in. in adults, 1 to 3 in. in children). Do not force the rectal tube ❶.
12. With adults, gently tape the tube in place, using hypoallergenic paper tape. With children, hold the tube in place manually.

CLINICAL ALERT
Rectal tubes should not be used to manage diarrhea, only for removal of flatus.

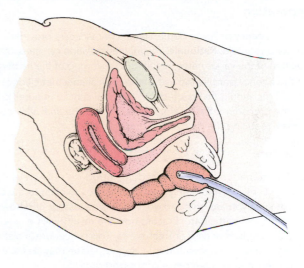

❶ Insert rectal tube past the external and internal anal sphincters.

13. Remove and discard gloves. Perform hand hygiene.
14. Take client's pulse. **Rationale:** *Alterations in pulse rate can indicate a vagal stimulation and the rectal tube may need to be removed. This can occur particularly in a client with a cardiac condition.*
15. Leave the tube in place no longer than 20 minutes. **Rationale:** *Prolonged stimulation of the anal sphincter may result in a loss of the neuromuscular response. The prolonged presence of a catheter may cause pressure necrosis of the mucosal surface.*
16. Don gloves.
17. Remove the tube and provide perianal care.
18. Help the client assume a comfortable position.
19. Clean the tubing, and replace in bathroom if to be reused. Remove and discard the plastic bag.
20. Instruct client that chewing gum, sucking on candy, drinking liquids through a straw, carbonated beverages, and smoking tend to promote the swallowing of air and increase abdominal distention.
21. Remove and discard gloves. Perform hand hygiene. Document care and client response.

SKILL 6.24 Removing a Fecal Impaction

Delegation

Due to the potential results of stimulation of the vagus nerve during the procedure, digital removal of an impaction is generally not delegated to UAP.

Equipment

- Bath blanket
- Disposable absorbent pad
- Bedpan and cover
- Toilet tissue
- Clean gloves
- Lubricant
- Soap, water, and towel
- Topical lidocaine (if agency permits)

Preparation

- Check agency policy to determine if a primary care provider's order is required. **Rationale:** *Rectal manipulation can cause stimulation of the vagus nerve, resulting in a slowing of the heart rate.*
- If the agency permits the use of the topical anesthetic lidocaine, 1 to 2 mL should be inserted into the anal canal 5 minutes prior to the procedure. **Rationale:** *This will numb the anal and rectal areas, reducing the pain of the procedure.*

Procedure

1. Prior to performing the procedure, introduce self and verify the client's identity using agency protocol. Explain to the client what you are going to do, why it is necessary, and how he or she can participate. Discuss how the results will be used in planning further care or treatments. This procedure is distressing, tiring, and uncomfortable, so the person may desire the presence of another nurse or support person.
2. Perform hand hygiene and observe other appropriate infection control procedures.
3. Apply clean gloves.
4. Provide for client privacy.
5. Assist the client to a right or left lateral or Sims' position with the back toward you. **Rationale:** *When the person lies on the right side, the sigmoid colon is uppermost; thus, gravity can aid removal of the feces. Positioning on the left side allows easier access to the sigmoid colon.*
6. Place the disposable absorbent pad under the client's hips, and arrange the top bed linen to ensure that it falls obliquely over the hips, exposing only the buttocks.
7. Place the bedpan and toilet tissue nearby on the bed or a bedside chair.

8. Lubricate the gloved index finger. **Rationale:** *Lubricant reduces resistance by the anal sphincter as the finger is inserted.*
9. Remove the impaction. Have the client take slow, deep breaths during the procedure. Ensure the client does not hold their breath. **Rationale:** *Holding the breath can stimulate a vagal response.*
   - Gently insert the index finger into the rectum, moving toward the umbilicus.
   - Gently massage around the stool. **Rationale:** *Gentle action prevents damage to the rectal mucosa. A circular motion around the rectum dislodges the stool, stimulates peristalsis, and relaxes the anal sphincter.*
   - Work the finger into the hardened mass of stool to break it up ①. If you cannot break up the impaction with one finger, insert two fingers and try to break up the impaction scissor style.

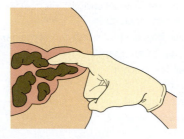

① Digital removal of fecal impaction.

   - Work the stool down to the anus, remove it in small pieces, and place them in the bedpan.
   - Carefully continue to remove as much fecal material as possible; at the same time, assess for bleeding or signs of pallor, feelings of faintness, shortness of breath, perspiration, or changes in pulse rate. Terminate the procedure if these occur. **Rationale:** *Manual stimulation could result in mucosal damage, excessive vagal nerve stimulation, and subsequent cardiac arrhythmia.*
   - Assist the client to a position on a clean bedpan, commode, or toilet. **Rationale:** *Digital stimulation of the rectum may induce the urge to defecate.*
10. Assist the client with hygienic measures as needed.
    - Wash the rectal area with soap and water and dry gently.
    - Remove and discard gloves. Perform hand hygiene.
11. Document the results of the procedure in the client record using forms or checklists supplemented by narrative notes when appropriate.

Developmental Considerations

OLDER ADULTS

- Fecal impaction is not uncommon with older adult clients due to decreased mobility and exercise, dietary habits, and tendency to overuse enemas and laxatives.
- Encourage clients to decrease use of laxatives and enemas, increase fluid intake and fiber in diet, and increase exercise.

Dehydration resulting from inadequate fluid intake leads to constipation and fecal impaction.

- To select the proper ostomy appliance for an older adult, the nurse must determine if the client has any physical limitations that could influence the type of appliance needed. These limitations include poor vision, use of only one hand, arthritis, and inability to perform cleaning and pouching procedure.

SKILL 6.25 Administering an Enema

Before administering an enema, determine that there is a primary care provider's order. At some agencies, a primary care provider must order the kind of enema and the time to give it, for example, the morning of an examination. At other agencies, enemas are given at the nurses' discretion (i.e., as necessary on a PRN order). In addition, determine the presence of kidney or cardiac disease that contraindicates the use of a hypotonic solution.

Delegation

Administration of some enemas may be delegated to UAP. However, the nurse must ensure the personnel are competent in the use of standard precautions. Abnormal findings such as inability to insert the rectal tip, client inability to retain the solution, or unusual return from the enema must be validated and interpreted by the nurse.

Equipment

- Disposable linen-saver pad
- Bath blanket
- Bedpan or commode
- Clean gloves
- Water-soluble lubricant if tubing not prelubricated
- Paper towel

Large-Volume Enema

- Solution container with tubing of correct size and tubing clamp
- Correct solution, amount, and temperature

Small-Volume Enema

- Prepackaged container of enema solution with lubricated tip

Preparation

- Lubricate about 5 cm (2 in.) of the rectal tube (some commercially prepared enema sets already have lubricated nozzles). **Rationale:** *Lubrication facilitates insertion through the sphincter and minimizes trauma.*
- Run some solution through the connecting tubing of a large-volume enema set and the rectal tube to expel any air in the tubing, then close the clamp. **Rationale:** *Air instilled into the rectum, although not harmful, causes unnecessary distention.*

Procedure

1. Prior to performing the procedure, introduce self and verify the client's identity using agency protocol. Explain to the client what you are going to do, why it is necessary, and how he or she can participate. Discuss how the results will be used in planning further care or treatments. Indicate that the client may experience a feeling of fullness while the solution is being administered. Explain the need to hold the solution as long as possible.
2. Perform hand hygiene and observe other appropriate infection control procedures.
3. Apply clean gloves.
4. Provide for client privacy.
5. Assist the adult client to a left lateral position, with the right leg as acutely flexed as possible ❶ and the linen-saver pad under the buttocks. Place bed protector under client and bedpan or commode within reach. **Rationale:** *This position facilitates the flow of solution by gravity into the sigmoid and*

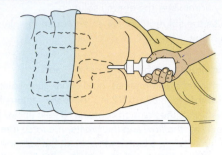

❶ Assuming a left lateral position for an enema. Note the commercially prepared enema.

descending colon, which are on the left side. Having the right leg acutely flexed provides for adequate exposure of the anus.

6. Insert the enema tube.
   - For clients in the left lateral position, lift the upper buttock. **Rationale:** *This ensures good visualization of the anus.*
   - Insert the tube smoothly and slowly into the rectum, directing it toward the umbilicus ❷. **Rationale:** *The angle follows the normal contour of the rectum. Slow insertion prevents spasm of the sphincter.*

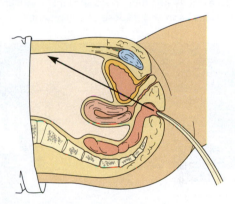

❷ Inserting the enema tube following the direction of the rectum.

   - Insert the tube 7 to 10 cm (3 to 4 in.). **Rationale:** *Because the anal canal is about 2.5 to 5 cm (1 to 2 in.) long in the adult, insertion to this point places the tip of the tube beyond the anal sphincter into the rectum.*
   - If resistance is encountered at the internal sphincter, ask the client to take a deep breath, then run a small amount of solution through the tube. **Rationale:** *This relaxes the internal anal sphincter.*
   - Never force tube or solution entry. If instilling a small amount of solution does not permit the tube to be advanced or the solution to freely flow, withdraw the tube. Check for any stool that may have blocked the tube during insertion. If present, flush it and retry the procedure. You may also perform a digital rectal examination to determine if there is an impaction or other mechanical blockage. If resistance persists, end the procedure and report the resistance to the primary care provider and nurse in charge.

(continued on next page)

SKILL 6.25 Administering an Enema *(continued)*

7. Slowly administer the enema solution.
   - Raise the solution container, and open the clamp to allow fluid flow.
   or
   - Compress a pliable container by hand.
   - During most low enemas, hold or hang the solution container no higher than 30 cm (12 in.) above the rectum. **Rationale:** *The higher the solution container is held above the rectum, the faster the flow and the greater the force (pressure) in the rectum. During a high enema, hang the solution container about 45 cm (18 in.).* **Rationale:** *The fluid must be instilled farther to clean the entire bowel.* See agency protocol.
   - Administer the fluid slowly. If the client complains of fullness or pain, lower the container or use the clamp to stop the flow for 30 seconds, and then restart the flow at a slower rate. **Rationale:** *Administering the enema slowly and stopping the flow momentarily decreases the likelihood of intestinal spasm and premature ejection of the solution.*
   - If you are using a plastic commercial container, roll it up as the fluid is instilled. This prevents subsequent suctioning of the solution ❸. After all the solution has been instilled or when the client cannot hold any more and feels the desire to defecate (the urge to defecate usually indicates that sufficient fluid has been administered), close the clamp and remove the enema tube from the anus.
   - Place the enema tube in a disposable towel as you withdraw it. Clean and dispose of equipment.

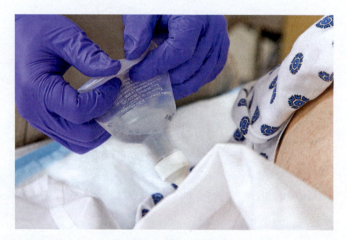

❸ Rolling up a commercial enema container.

8. Encourage the client to retain the enema.
   - Ask the client to remain lying down. **Rationale:** *It is easier for the client to retain the enema when lying down than when sitting or standing, because gravity promotes drainage and peristalsis.*
   - Request that the client retain the solution for the appropriate amount of time, for example, 5 to 10 minutes for a cleansing enema or at least 30 minutes for a retention enema.
9. Assist the client to defecate.
   - Assist the client to a sitting position on the bedpan, commode, or toilet. A sitting position facilitates the act of defecation.
   - Ask the client who is using the toilet not to flush it. The nurse needs to observe the feces.
   - If a specimen of feces is required, ask the client to use a bedpan or commode.
10. Remove and discard gloves. Perform hand hygiene.
11. Document the type and volume, if appropriate, of enema given. Describe the results.

Sample Documentation

8/2/2015 1000. States last BM five days ago. Abdomen distended and firm. Bowel sounds hypoactive. Fleet's enema given per order resulting in large amount of firm brown stool. States he "feels better."
_____ *M. Lopez, RN*

VARIATION: ADMINISTERING AN ENEMA TO AN INCONTINENT CLIENT

Occasionally a nurse needs to administer an enema to a client who is unable to control the external sphincter muscle and thus cannot retain the enema solution for even a few minutes. In that case, after the rectal tube is inserted, the client assumes a supine position on a bedpan. The head of the bed can be elevated slightly, to 30 degrees if necessary for easier breathing, and pillows support the client's head and back.

VARIATION: ADMINISTERING A RETURN-FLOW ENEMA

For a return-flow enema, the solution (100 to 200 mL for an adult) is instilled into the client's rectum and sigmoid colon. Then the solution container is lowered so that the fluid flows back out through the rectal tube into the container, pulling the flatus with it. The inflow–outflow process is repeated five or six times (to stimulate peristalsis and the expulsion of flatus), and the solution is replaced several times during the procedure if it becomes thick with feces.

Document type of solution; length of time solution was retained; the amount, color, and consistency of the returns; and the relief of flatus and abdominal distention in the client record using forms or checklists supplemented by narrative notes when appropriate.

SKILL 6.26 Administering a Retention Enema

Equipment

- Commercially prepared disposable oil retention enema (adult: 150–200 mL oil; child: 75–100 mL oil)
- Water-soluble lubricant
- Bedpan or commode
- Bed protector
- Skin care items (e.g., soap, water, towels)
- Clean gloves

SKILL 6.26   Administering a Retention Enema (*continued*)

Preparation

- Check physician's order.
- Identify and prepare client as for any enema.
- Provide for client privacy.
- Gather equipment—disposable oil retention enema is administered like a small enema. Read directions on enema container.

Procedure

1. Explain steps of procedure to client.
2. Raise bed to HIGH position.
3. Perform hand hygiene and don gloves.
4. Place bed protector on bed.
5. Warm the prepared enema container with solution. **Rationale:** *Warming the enema solution to body temperature is beneficial to stimulate the rectal mucosa. Cold solutions should be avoided as they may cause cramping.*

6. Expose anal opening, and gently insert rectal tube tip of container 7.5 to 10 cm (3 to 4 in.). Commercially prepared enemas are prelubricated.
7. Squeeze contents slowly, and empty entire amount into rectum.
8. Keep container compressed and remove rectal tube gently. **Rationale:** *To prevent solution from being drawn back into container.*
9. Lower bed.
10. Discard equipment and gloves, following standard precautions. Perform hand hygiene.
11. Explain to client that oil should be retained for 30 to 60 minutes before it is expelled. **Rationale:** *Purpose of enema is to soften stool.*
12. A cleansing enema may need to be given to remove oil and stimulate defecation.
13. Don gloves and provide hygienic care if needed. Discard washcloth and towel in laundry.
14. Remove and discard gloves. Perform hand hygiene.
15. Document actions and client response.

Developmental Considerations

INFANTS/CHILDREN

- Provide a careful explanation to the parents and child before the procedure. An enema is an intrusive procedure and therefore threatening.
- The enema solution should be isotonic (usually normal saline). Some hypertonic commercial solutions (e.g., Fleet phosphate enema) can lead to hypovolemia and electrolyte imbalances. In addition, the osmotic effect of the enema may produce diarrhea and subsequent metabolic acidosis.
- Infants and small children do not exhibit sphincter control and need to be assisted in retaining the enema. The nurse administers the enema while the infant or child is lying with the buttocks over the bedpan, and the nurse firmly presses the buttocks together to prevent the immediate expulsion of the solution. Older children can usually hold the solution if they understand what to do and are not required to hold it for too long a period. It may be necessary to ensure that the bathroom is available for an ambulatory child before starting the procedure or to have a bedpan ready.
- The enema solution needs to be warmed before giving to the child.
- Large-volume enemas consist of 50 to 200 mL in children less than 18 months old; 200 to 300 mL in children 18 months to 5 years; and 300 to 500 mL in children 5 to 12 years old.
- Careful explanation is especially important for the preschool child.
- For infants and small children, the dorsal recumbent position is frequently used. Position them on a small padded bedpan with support for the back and head. Secure the legs by placing a

diaper under the bedpan and then over and around the thighs. Place the underpad under the client's buttocks to protect the bed linen, and drape the client with the bath blanket.
- Insert the tube 5 to 7.5 cm (2 to 3 in.) in a child and only 2.5 cm (1 in.) in an infant.
- For children, lower the height of the solution container appropriately for the age of the child. See agency protocol.
- To assist a small child in retaining the solution, apply firm pressure over the anus with tissue wipes, or firmly press the buttocks together.

OLDER ADULTS

- Older adults may fatigue easily.
- Older adults may be more susceptible to fluid and electrolyte imbalances. Use tap water enemas with great caution.
- Monitor the client's tolerance during the procedure, watching for vagal episodes (e.g., slow pulse) and dysrhythmias.
- Protect older adults' skin from prolonged exposure to moisture.
- Assist older clients with perineal care as indicated.

Setting of Care

Teach the caregiver or client the following:

- To make saline solution, mix 1 teaspoon of table salt with 500 mL of tap water.
- Use enemas only as directed. Do not rely on them for regular bowel evacuation.
- Prior to administration, make sure a bedpan, commode, or toilet is nearby.

SKILL 6.27   Applying a Fecal Ostomy Pouch

Equipment

- One- or two-piece transparent ostomy pouch with adhesive wafer
- Warm water and mild soap
- Soft cloths
- Bath blanket
- Plastic bag for pouch disposal
- Tail closure or night adapter for pouch
- Clean gloves

(*continued on next page*)

SKILL 6.27   Applying a Fecal Ostomy Pouch (continued)

- Graduate or bedpan
- Measuring guide
- Tissues
- Ostomy scissors and dark marking pen

Preparation

- Check client care plan and identify client by checking the client's identity band and asking client to state name and birth date.
- Determine exact supplies client uses ❶ A–D.
- Gather equipment.
- Explain procedure to client.
- Provide for client privacy.
- Raise bed to high position.
- Perform hand hygiene and don gloves.

Procedure

1. Place bath blanket over client. Place absorbent pad or towels under client. **Rationale:** *To protect bed from spillage.*

2. Observe placement of stoma. **Rationale:** *To determine normal amount of output and consistency. (Immediately after surgery, all stomas will have very liquid stool and high flatus output.)*

> **CLINICAL ALERT**
> To promote the client's self-esteem and body image, be aware of your own body language. Even subtle changes in the way you look at the stoma could indicate disgust or disapproval and an altered self-esteem could result.

3. Empty old pouch into graduated container, bedpan, or toilet.
4. Remove old pouch by pushing against skin as you pull backing from skin and discard in plastic bag. Save tail closure on bottom of pouch.
5. Measure output, if ordered.

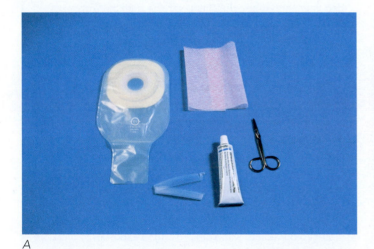

A

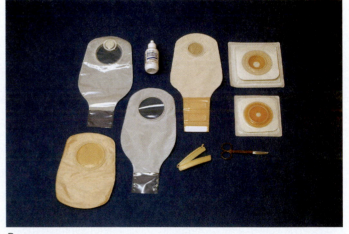

B

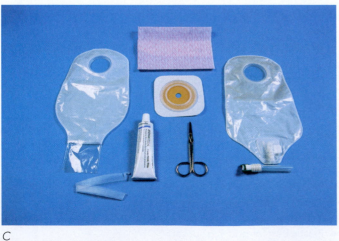

C

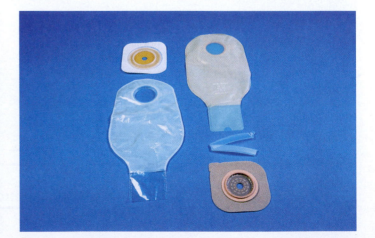

D

❶ A, Supplies needed to change one-piece pouches; B, fabric pouches, convexity faceplates, pouch with filter; C, supplies needed to change two-piece pouches; D, two-piece fecal pouches.

SKILL 6.27   Applying a Fecal Ostomy Pouch (continued)

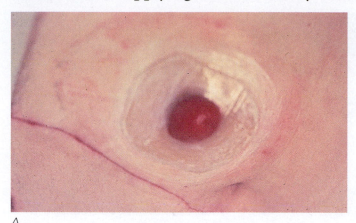
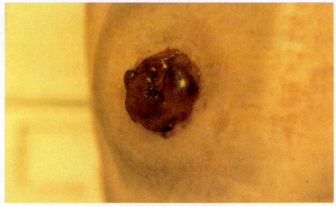

A   *B*

② *A*, Viable stoma; *B*, nonviable parastomal hernia.

6. Clean skin and stoma gently with warm water and soft cloth. **Rationale:** *Oily substances can interfere with pouch adhesive. If adhesive doesn't come off, leave it on the skin. If you pick at it, the peristomal skin can be damaged.*

7. Dry skin well with soft cloth. Keep tissues available if stoma functions while pouch is off.

8. Observe skin; it should be free of erythema or excoriation. The stoma is assessed for changes in size, ulceration, and color (stoma should be moist, pink, or beefy red) **②** *A* and *B*. Notify the physician if stoma is black, blue, or purple. This indicates a nonviable stoma.

9. Measure stoma at the base with measuring guide.

10. Trace measured pattern on pouch.

11. Cut pouch to pattern, making sure opening is large enough (at least 1/8 in.) to encircle stoma without pushing on edges. **Rationale:** *No skin should appear between the pouch edge and the stoma.*

12. If using a two-piece pouch, snap the wafer and pouch together.

13. Remove paper from skin barrier on pouch and save it. **Rationale:** *This may be used as a pattern for next pouch change.*

14. Apply a ring of skin barrier paste to opening on pouch.

15. Apply Stomahesive powder to denuded skin only.

16. Remove paper from outer ring.

17. Center and apply pouch to clean and dry skin. Smooth edges of adhesive to skin. **Rationale:** *If adhesive is wrinkled,*

it may result in leakage from pouch. To promote optimum wear of the pouch, warm the adhesive by placing your gloved hand over the adhesive and gently hold it over the site for 1/2 to 1 minute. **Rationale:** *This will activate the adhesive in the skin barrier.*

18. Pouches can be applied over an incision. **Rationale:** *Incisions are sealed within 24 hours of surgery.*

19. Close and secure end of pouch with tail closure.
    - Ensure bowed end is next to body. **Rationale:** *This provides a better fit to body, and prevents outpouching of clamp through clothing.*
    - Lay hook on top of bag and fold bag 1 in. over end of pouch.
    - Squeeze clamp together to close.

20. Remove soiled pouch and tissues from bedside.

21. Remove and discard gloves. Perform hand hygiene.

22. Position client for comfort. Return bed to low position.

23. Put away supplies and reorder as necessary.

24. Document relevant information.

> **CLINICAL ALERT**
>
> Clients with ostomies will need a nutritional consult and a written dietary guide. They need to limit the amount of hard-to-digest foods for at least the first 2 to 3 weeks postop. Also, limiting gas-producing foods will prevent gas-forming odors.

Changing One-Piece Fecal Ostomy Pouch ③—⑬

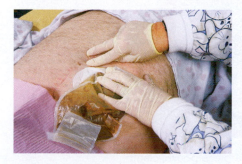
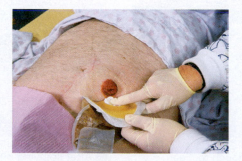
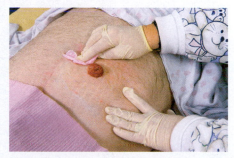

③ Starting at upper corner, remove old pouch.

④ As you remove old pouch, push against skin while pulling down on pouch.

⑤ Clean skin with warm water; dry well.

(continued on next page)

SKILL 6.27 Applying a Fecal Ostomy Pouch (continued)

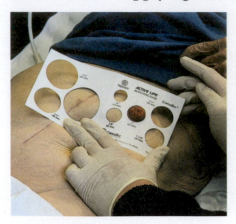

6 Measure stoma size.

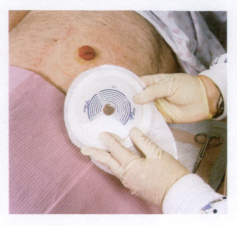

7 Remove plastic covering from one-piece pouch.

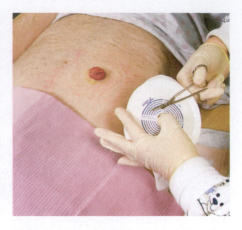

8 Cut pouch opening to exact size of stoma.

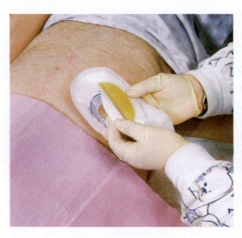

9 Remove paper from inner wafer. Save pattern for future pouch changes.

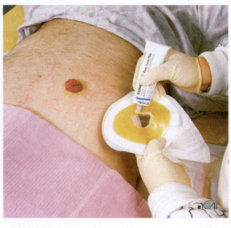

10 Apply ring of paste to opening on pouch.

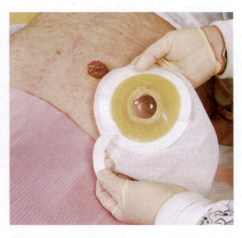

11 Remove paper from outer adhesive ring of pouch.

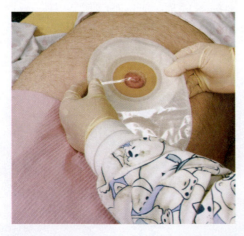

12 Center and apply pouch to clean, dry skin.

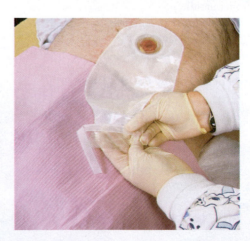

13 After applying one-piece pouch, clamp bottom of pouch.

SKILL 6.27   Applying a Fecal Ostomy Pouch (*continued*)

Applying Two-Piece Fecal Ostomy Pouch 🔟 *A–L*

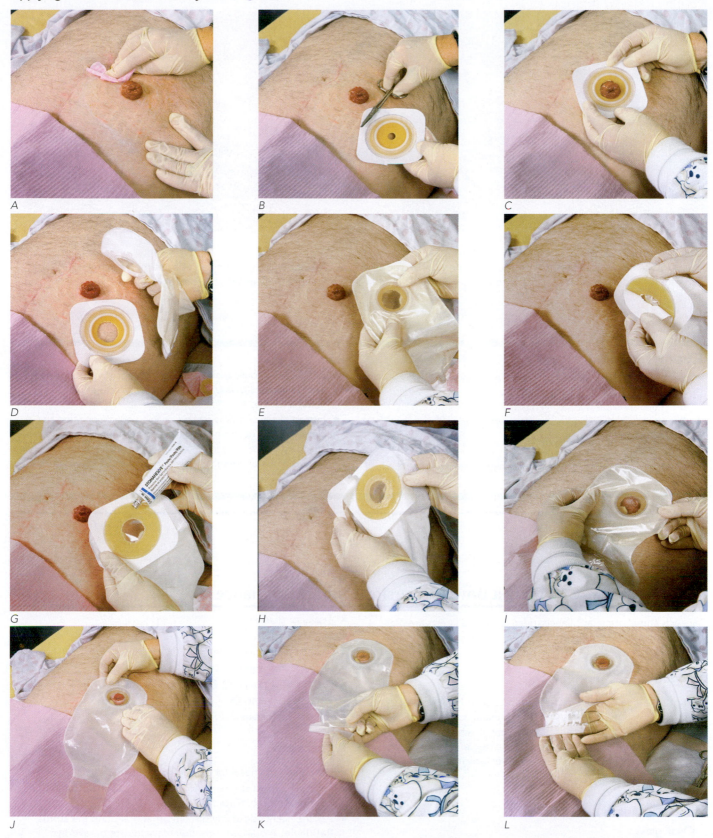

🔟 *A,* Clean and dry skin thoroughly before applying two-piece pouch. *B,* Cut opening of a two-piece pouch to exact size of stoma. *C,* Check size of opening to ensure proper fit. *D,* Snap pouch onto wafer when using a two-piece pouch. *E,* Check for secure fit by tugging at bottom of pouch. *F,* Remove paper from inner barrier. *G,* Apply paste to inner circle of wafer. *H,* Remove paper from outer adhesive ring. *I,* Center pouch over stoma and press onto skin. *J,* Secure adhesive to skin. *K,* Clamp bottom of pouch. *L,* Check that clamp is secure.

(*continued on next page*)

SKILL 6.27   Applying a Fecal Ostomy Pouch (*continued*)

Loop Colostomy with Rod/Rod Removed ⑮ *A and B*

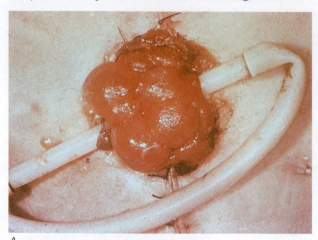

A

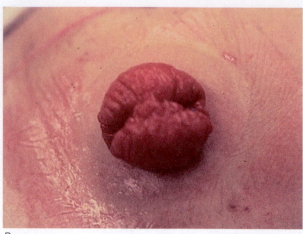

B

⑮ *A*, loop of bowel is brought onto the abdomen and is supported by a plastic rod. *B*, two openings are made in the colostomy. Proximal loop is functional and discharges fecal material. Distal end is nonfunctional and discharges only mucus.

Client Teaching

- Empty pouch when one third full of stool or flatus.
  a. Empty into toilet.
  b. Pouch should last for 3 to 4 days.
- Rinse pouch using room temperature water and a rubber ear syringe (squirt into pouch).
- Use pouch deodorant if desired.
- Empty each morning and last thing at night even if not one third full.

- Check seal on daily basis for tight fit; change if needed.
- Instruct client to always carry a supply of ostomy equipment for emergency use.
- Instruct client on emptying and cleaning pouch, opening and closing clamp, observing and cleaning peristomal area, and changing pouch.
- Have client return demonstration until able to perform activities correctly.

SKILL 6.28   Changing a Bowel Diversion Ostomy Appliance

Review features of the appliance to ensure that all parts are present and functioning correctly.

Delegation

Care of a *new* ostomy is not delegated to UAP. However, aspects of ostomy function are observed during usual care and may be recorded by individuals other than the nurse. Abnormal findings must be validated and interpreted by the nurse. In some agencies, UAP may remove and replace well-established ostomy appliances.

Equipment

- Clean gloves
- Bedpan
- Moisture-proof bag (for disposable pouches)
- Cleaning materials, including warm water, mild soap (optional), washcloth, towel

- Tissue or gauze pad
- Skin barrier (optional)
- Stoma measuring guide
- Pen or pencil and scissors
- New ostomy pouch ❶ ❷ with optional belt ❸
- Tail closure clamp ❹
- Deodorant for pouch (optional)

Preparation

- Determine the need for an appliance change.
- Assess the used appliance for leakage of stool. **Rationale:** *Stool can irritate the peristomal skin.*
- Ask the client about any discomfort at or around the stoma. **Rationale:** *A burning sensation may indicate breakdown beneath the faceplate of the pouch.*
- Assess the fullness of the pouch. **Rationale:** *The weight of an overly full bag may loosen the skin barrier and separate it from the skin, causing the stool to leak and irritate the peristomal skin.*

SKILL 6.28 Changing a Bowel Diversion Ostomy Appliance *(continued)*

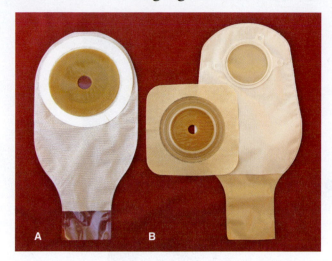

1 *A*, One-piece ostomy appliance of pouching system; *B*, two-piece ostomy or pouching system. (Courtesy of Hollister, Inc.)

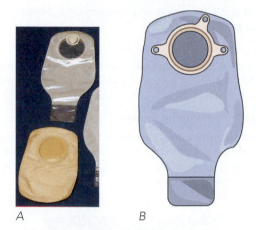

2 *A*, Closed pouch; *B*, drainable pouch.

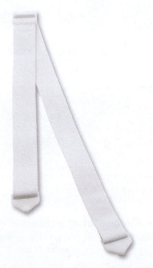

3 Adjustable ostomy belt. (Courtesy of Hollister, Inc.)

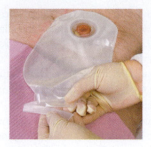

4 Applying a pouch clamp.

- If there is pouch leakage or discomfort at or around the stoma, change the appliance.
- Select an appropriate time to change the appliance:
  - Avoid times close to mealtimes or visiting hours. **Rationale:** *Ostomy odor and stool may reduce appetite or embarrass the client.*
  - Avoid times immediately after meals or the administration of any medications that may stimulate bowel evacuation. **Rationale:** *It is best to change the pouch when drainage is least likely to occur.*

Procedure

1. Prior to performing the procedure, introduce self and verify the client's identity using agency protocol. Explain to the client what you are going to do, why it is necessary, and how he or she can participate. Discuss how the results will be used in planning further care or treatments. Changing an ostomy appliance should not cause discomfort, but it may be distasteful to the client. Communicate acceptance and support to the client. It is important to change the appliance competently and quickly. Include support individuals as appropriate.
2. Perform hand hygiene and observe other appropriate infection control procedures.
3. Apply clean gloves.
4. Provide for client privacy preferably in the bathroom, where clients can learn to deal with the ostomy as they would at home.
5. Assist the client to a comfortable sitting or lying position in bed or preferably a sitting or standing position in the bathroom. **Rationale:** *Lying or standing positions may facilitate smoother pouch application (i.e., avoid wrinkles).*
6. Unfasten the belt if the client is wearing one.
7. Empty the pouch and remove the ostomy skin barrier.
   - Empty the contents of a drainable pouch through the bottom opening into a bedpan or toilet. **Rationale:** *Emptying before removing the pouch prevents spillage of stool onto the client's skin.*
   - If the pouch uses a clamp, do not throw it away because it can be reused.
   - Assess the consistency, color, and amount of stool.

(continued on next page)

SKILL 6.28 Changing a Bowel Diversion Ostomy Appliance (continued)

- Peel the skin barrier off slowly, beginning at the top and working downward, while holding the client's skin taut. **Rationale:** *Holding the skin taut minimizes client discomfort and prevents abrasion of the skin.*
- Discard the disposable pouch in a moisture-proof bag.

8. Clean and dry the peristomal skin and stoma **5**.
   - Use toilet tissue to remove excess stool.
   - Use warm water, mild soap (optional), and a washcloth to clean the skin and stoma. Check agency practice on the use of soap. **Rationale:** *Soap is sometimes not advised because it can be irritating to the skin.* If soap is allowed, do not use deodorant or moisturizing soaps. **Rationale:** *They may interfere with the adhesives in the skin barrier.*
   - Dry the area thoroughly by patting with a towel. **Rationale:** *Excess rubbing can abrade the skin.*

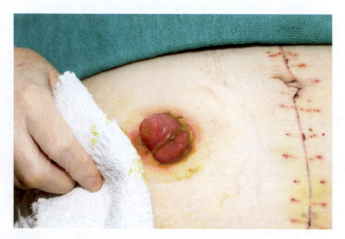

5 Cleaning the skin. (Copyright PavleMarjanovic/Shutterstock.)

9. Assess the stoma and peristomal skin.
   - Inspect the stoma for color, size, shape, and bleeding.
   - Inspect the peristomal skin for any redness, ulceration, or irritation. Transient redness after the removal of adhesive is normal.

10. Place a piece of tissue or gauze over the stoma, and change it as needed. **Rationale:** *This absorbs any seepage from the stoma while the ostomy appliance is being changed.*

11. Prepare and apply the skin barrier (peristomal seal).
   - Use the guide to measure the size of the stoma **6**.
   - On the backing of the skin barrier, trace a circle the same size as the stomal opening.
   - Cut out the traced stoma pattern to make an opening in the skin barrier **7**. Make the opening no more than 0.3 to 0.6 cm (1/8 to 1/4 in.) larger than the stoma. **Rationale:** *This allows space for the stoma to expand slightly when functioning and minimizes the risk of stool contacting peristomal skin.*

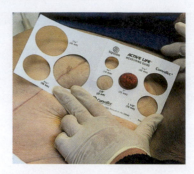

6 A guide for measuring the stoma.

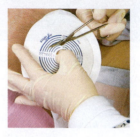

7 The nurse is making a stoma opening on a disposable one-piece pouch.

- Remove the backing to expose the sticky adhesive side. The backing can be saved and used as a pattern when making an opening for future skin barriers.

For a One-Piece Pouching System

- Center the one-piece skin barrier and pouch over the stoma, and gently press it onto the client's skin for 30 seconds **8 9**. **Rationale:** *The heat and pressure help activate the adhesives in the skin barrier.*

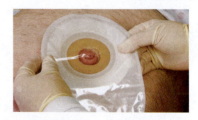

8 Centering the skin barrier over the stoma.

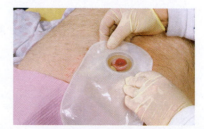

9 Pressing the skin barrier of a disposable one-piece pouch for 30 seconds to activate the adhesives in the skin barrier.

SKILL 6.28   Changing a Bowel Diversion Ostomy Appliance (continued)

For a Two-Piece Pouching System

- Center the skin barrier over the stoma and gently press it onto the client's skin for 30 seconds.
- Remove the tissue over the stoma before applying the pouch.
- Snap the pouch onto the flange or skin barrier wafer.
- For drainable pouches, close the pouch according to the manufacturer's directions.
- Remove and discard gloves. Perform hand hygiene.

12. Document the procedure in the client record using forms or checklists supplemented by narrative notes when appropriate. Report and record pertinent assessments and interventions. Report any increase in stoma size, change in color indicative of circulatory impairment, and presence of skin irritation or erosion. Record on the client's chart discoloration of the stoma, the appearance of the peristomal skin, the amount and type of drainage, the client's reaction to the procedure, the client's experience with the ostomy, and skills learned by the client.

Sample Documentation

8/3/2015 0900 Colostomy bag changed. Moderate to large amount of semi-formed brown stool. Stoma reddish color. No redness or irritation around stoma.

Client looked at stoma today and started asking questions about how she will be able to change the pouch when she is home. Asked if she would like to do the next changing of the pouch. Stated "yes." _____ G. Hsu, RN

VARIATION: EMPTYING A DRAINABLE POUCH

- Empty the pouch when it is one third to one half full of stool or gas. **Rationale:** *Emptying the pouch before it is overfull helps avoid breaking the seal with the skin, resulting in stool coming in contact with the skin.*
- While wearing gloves, hold the pouch outlet over a bedpan or toilet. Lift the lower edge up.
- Unclamp or unseal the pouch.
- Drain the pouch. Loosen feces from sides by moving fingers down the pouch.
- Clean the inside of the tail of the pouch with a tissue or a premoistened towelette.
- Apply the clamp or seal the pouch.
- Dispose of used supplies.
- Remove and discard gloves. Perform hand hygiene.
- Document the amount, consistency, and color of stool.

Practice Guidelines
Irrigating a Colostomy

- Fill the solution bag with 500 mL of warm (body temperature) tap water or other solution as ordered.
- Hang the solution bag on an IV pole so that the bottom of the container is at the level of the client's shoulder, or 30 to 45 cm (12 to 18 in.) above the stoma.
- Attach the colon catheter securely to the tubing.
- Open the regulator clamp, and run fluid through the tubing to expel air from it. Close the clamp until ready for the irrigation.
- Provide for client privacy.
- Perform hand hygiene. Don clean gloves.
- Assist the client who must remain in bed to a side-lying position. Place a disposable pad on the bed in front of the client, and place the bedpan on top of the disposable pad, beneath the stoma. Assist an ambulatory client to sit on the toilet or on a commode in the bathroom.
- Remove the colostomy bag and dispose of used pouch in a plastic bag.
- Center the irrigation drainage sleeve over the stoma and attach it snugly. Direct the lower, open end of the drainage sleeve into the bedpan or between the client's legs into the toilet.
- Lubricate the tip of the stoma cone or colon catheter with a water-soluble lubricant.
- Using a rotating motion, insert the catheter or stoma cone through the opening in the top of the irrigation drainage sleeve and gently through the stoma. Insert a catheter only 7 cm (3 in.); insert a stoma cone just until it fits snugly. Use of a stoma cone avoids the risk of perforating the bowel.
- Open the tubing clamp, and allow the fluid to flow into the bowel. If cramping occurs, stop the flow until the cramps subside and then resume the flow.
- After all the fluid is instilled, remove the catheter or cone and allow the colon to empty, usually 10 to 15 minutes.
- Cleanse the base of the irrigation drainage sleeve, and seal the bottom with a drainage clamp, following the manufacturer's instructions.
- Encourage an ambulatory client to move around for about 30 minutes to completely empty the colon.
- Empty and remove the irrigation sleeve.
- Clean the area around the stoma, and dry it thoroughly.
- Apply skin barrier and colostomy appliance as needed.

(continued on next page)

SKILL 6.28   Changing a Bowel Diversion Ostomy Appliance (continued)

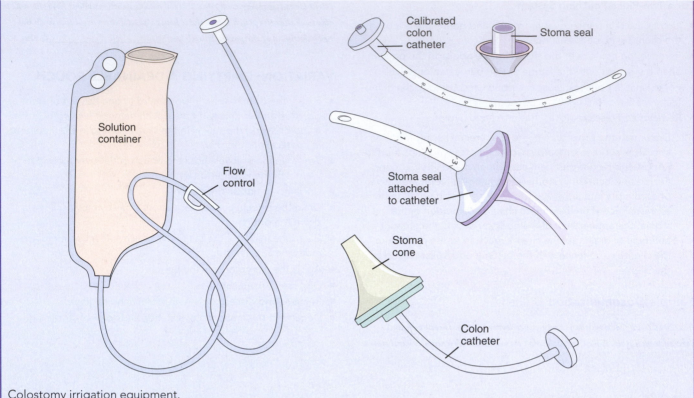

Colostomy irrigation equipment.

Setting of Care

- Provide the client with the names and phone numbers of a wound ostomy continence nurse, supply vendor, and other resource people to contact when needed. Provide pertinent Internet resources for information and support.
- Inform the client of signs to report to a healthcare provider, such as peristomal redness, skin breakdown, and changes in stomal color.
- Provide client and family education regarding care of the ostomy and appliance when traveling.

- Educate the client and family regarding infection control precautions, including proper disposal of used pouches since these cannot be flushed down a toilet.
- Younger clients may have special concerns about odor and appearance. Provide information about ostomy care and community support groups. A visit from someone who has had an ostomy under similar circumstances may be helpful.

▶ DIALYSIS

Expected Outcomes

1. Dialysis proceeds without complication (excess fluids and wastes removed from blood).
2. Vascular access site remains patent.
3. Client demonstrates self-care after teaching.

SKILL 6.29   Assisting with Peritoneal Dialysis Catheter Insertion

Anuria (lack of urine production), oliguria (inadequate urine production), and both acute and chronic renal failure can occur as a result of kidney disease, severe heart failure, burns, and shock. These conditions can be fatal if some other means is not used to remove the body waters. Dialysis is the technique by which blood

is filtered for the removal of these wastes and excess fluid. When hemodialysis is used, intravascular needles or catheters are inserted directly into blood vessels so that the blood can be removed from the body, cycled through machines that filter the blood, and then returned to the body.

SKILL 6.29   Assisting with Peritoneal Dialysis Catheter Insertion (continued)

Delegation

Assisting with peritoneal catheter insertion is a sterile procedure and not delegated to UAP.

Equipment

- Sterile gloves, masks, caps, goggles, and gowns for primary care provider, nurse, and anyone assisting; mask for client
- Sterile peritoneal dialysis set:
  - Peritoneal catheter
  - Local anesthetic (e.g., lidocaine), 25-gauge 5/8-in. needle, and 3-mL syringe
  - Alcohol sponges
  - Scalpel with a blade
  - Precut gauze to place around the catheter
  - Drape
  - Transfer set
  - Protective transfer set cap
  - Sutures, needles, and needle driver
  - Trocar (the sharp, needle-like instrument used to make a hole in body tissues)
  - Connector
  - 4 × 4 gauze square
  - Specimen container
  - Antiseptic ointment (e.g., povidone-iodine or mupirocin)
- 10-mL syringe and 1.5-in. needle
- Scissors
- Skin preparation/dressing set:
  - Chlorhexidine gluconate 2%, povidone-iodine, or other disinfecting solution
  - Razor and blade or scissors
  - Gauze sponges
  - Nonallergenic tape

Preparation

- Although the primary care provider will have already done initial client and family teaching, the nurse reinforces key elements. Review the technique of peritoneal dialysis and its purpose with the client and family.
- Explain that since the kidneys are not functioning properly, this procedure will rid the blood and body of excess wastes and fluid that are normally excreted by the kidneys.
- Explain that inserting the trocar (which is the primary care provider's responsibility) may be uncomfortable. The discomfort can be reduced by the client tensing the abdominal muscles as if for a bowel movement.
- Explain that the purpose of the masks, gowns, gloves, and caps is to reduce the possibility of contaminating the site during insertion. Then explain that the client will also need to wear a mask for the same reason.

Procedure

1. Prior to performing the procedure, introduce self and verify the client's identity using agency protocol. Explain to the client what your role will be, why it is necessary, and how he or she can participate. Remind the client that additional teach-

ing will be done at the time of the actual peritoneal dialysis treatment.
2. Perform hand hygiene and observe other appropriate infection control procedures throughout the various phases of the procedure. Assist the client with use of the mask.
3. Provide for client privacy.
4. Prepare the client.
   - Ask the client to urinate before the procedure. In some cases, bowel cleansing is also done prior to catheter insertion. **Rationale:** *Emptying the bladder and bowels moves them away from the peritoneal wall and lessens the danger that they will be punctured by the trocar.*
   - Administer analgesics and prophylactic antibiotics if ordered.
   - Assist the client to a supine position, and arrange the bedding to expose the area around the umbilicus. **Rationale:** *The insertion site is usually in the midline just below the umbilicus.*
5. Prepare the solution and the tubing.
6. Implement surgical aseptic practices and body fluid precautions according to agency protocol.
   - Apply masks. **Rationale:** *Applying masks prior to breaking the seals on the packages reduces the chance of contamination.*
   - Apply cap, gown, and goggles.
   - Open the dialysis set and any sterile supplies not part of the set.
   - Apply sterile gloves.
7. Assist the primary care provider as needed during and after the catheter insertion.
   - Ensure that the transfer set that has been connected to the catheter is securely capped.
   - Cover the catheter site with antiseptic ointment and precut sterile gauze, and tape the occlusive dressing in place.
   - Remove and discard gloves. Perform hand hygiene.
8. Administer prophylactic antibiotics as ordered. The medication can be administered 30 to 60 minutes prior to (preferred) or immediately following catheter insertion. **Rationale:** *A single dose of a first- or second-generation cephalosporin is recommended to reduce wound and exit site infections* (Perakis et al., 2009).
9. Recheck vital signs. Report to the primary care provider if significantly different from baseline.
10. Document findings in the client record using forms or checklists supplemented by narrative notes when appropriate. Record the date and time of the procedure, client's response, and appearance of exit site and dressing.

Sample Documentation

5/19/15 1430 Double-cuff coiled Tenckhoff peritoneal catheter inserted in right lower quadrant by Dr. Novar under local anesthesia using sterile technique throughout. Postinsertion VS consistent with baseline. Catheter taped to abdominal skin. Dry, sterile, occlusive dressing applied to exit site. _____ U. Schmidt, RN

SKILL 6.30 Conducting Peritoneal Dialysis Procedures

Delegation

Conducting peritoneal dialysis procedures is not delegated to UAP. However, the client's status is observed during usual care and may be recorded by individuals other than the nurse. Abnormal findings must be validated and interpreted by the nurse.

Equipment

For Infusing the Dialysate

- Container of peritoneal solution at body temperature, of the amount and kind ordered by the primary care provider (Bags range in size from 1 to 3 liters.)
- IV pole
- Sterile peritoneal dialysis administration set (separate or combined pieces):
  - Y connector
  - IV-type tubing for dialysate
  - Drainage bag with tubing
- Sterile transfer set cap
- Dialysis log or flow sheet
- Clean gloves
- Mask and goggles
- Povidone-iodine swabs or other antiseptic per agency protocol. (Some agencies recommend a sterile bowl and antiseptic for soaking the transfer set tubing.)

For Changing the Catheter Site Dressing

- Sterile gloves and masks (gowns and goggles as needed)
- Sterile cotton-tipped applicators
- Chlorhexidine gluconate, povidone-iodine solution, or soap and water as specified by agency protocol
- Povidone-iodine ointment
- Precut sterile 2 × 2 gauze or slit transparent occlusive dressing
- Nonallergenic tape

Preparation

- Determine when the last dressing change was performed. Following initial catheter insertion, the dressing is not changed for several days to allow for stabilization of the catheter exit site. Subsequently, the dressing should be changed when wet, soiled, loose, or at intervals specified by agency policy.

Procedure

1. Prior to performing the procedure, check physician's order, introduce self and verify the client's identity using agency protocol. Explain to the client what you are going to do, why it is necessary, and how he or she can participate. Discuss how the results will be used in planning further care or treatments.
2. Perform hand hygiene and observe other appropriate infection control procedures.
3. Provide for client privacy.
4. Prepare the solution and the tubing.
   - Examine the label on the container and the expiration date. Examine the dialysate solution. It should be clear and the seals unbroken.
   - Warm the dialysate using an approved warmer (not a microwave oven) to at least body temperature. **Rationale:** *Warmed solution enhances exchange and is more comfortable for the client.*
   - Following agency policy for the required technique, add any prescribed medication to the dialysate solution. This may require soaking the injection port of the bag in antiseptic solution. Heparin is sometimes added. **Rationale:** *This prevents the accumulation of fibrin in the catheter.*
   - Apply the mask and spike the solution container. Close the clamp, and hang the container on the IV pole.
   - Prime the tubing: Remove the protective cap and hold the tubing over a cup or basin. Maintain the sterility of the end of the tubing and the cap. Open the clamp and let the fluid run through the tubing, removing all bubbles. Close the tubing clamp. **Rationale:** *This rids the tubing of air that could enter the peritoneal cavity, causing discomfort and preventing free drainage outflow.*
5. Connect the solution to the catheter.
   - Apply clean gloves, mask, and goggles.
   - Free the catheter end from the dressing if necessary.
   - Cleanse or soak the transfer set that connects to the Y connector with povidone-iodine or other specified disinfectant for the time listed in the agency protocol (usually 5 minutes). If tubing is not already attached, remove the cap from the transfer set and attach the Y connector and end of the tubing from the solution to the catheter.
   - Connect the drainage receptacle to the outflow tubing if not preattached. Close the outflow tubing clamp.
   - If necessary, cover the catheter site with the precut sterile gauze, and tape the dressing in place. Minimize handling of the catheter.
   - Remove and discard gloves. Perform hand hygiene.
6. Infuse the peritoneal dialysate.
   - Open the clamp on the inflow tubing so that the dialysate can flow into the peritoneal cavity for the time specified by the order. If no rate is specified, the client can usually tolerate a steady open flow.
   - Observe the client for any signs of discomfort, particularly respiratory distress or abdominal pain.
   - After the fluid has infused, clamp the inflow tubing. **Rationale:** *With the tubing clamped, air will not enter the peritoneal cavity.*
   - Leave the fluid in the cavity for the designated time.
7. Ensure client comfort and safety.
   - Assist the client into a comfortable position.
   - Monitor the client's vital signs.
   - Periodically assess the client's comfort during the dwell time.
8. Remove the fluid.
   - Unclamp the outflow tubing, and permit the fluid to drain into the drainage bag by gravity for about 30 minutes.
   - If the fluid does not drain freely, assist the client to change position, or raise the head of the bed. If specified, drain only the amount ordered.
9. Assess the outflow fluid.
   - Observe the appearance of the outflow fluid. **Rationale:** *A cloudy pink-tinged or blood-tinged return may indicate peritonitis (infection/inflammation of the peritoneal cavity). During the first two to four exchanges following insertion of the peritoneal dialysis catheter, the return may be blood tinged but should quickly progress to a straw-color return.*
   - Apply clean gloves.
   - Measure the amount of outflow fluid, and discard the fluid and used supplies in an appropriate area.

SKILL 6.30 Conducting Peritoneal Dialysis Procedures *(continued)*

10. Calculate the fluid balance for each exchange.
    - Compare the amount of outflow fluid with the amount of solution infused for each exchange.
    - If more fluid was infused than removed, the client's fluid balance is positive (+); if more fluid was removed than infused, the fluid balance is negative (−).
      Example:
      + 2,000 mL dialysate solution infused
      − 1,500 mL fluid returned in drainage bag
      = 500 mL balance for this exchange
    - Repeat steps for each exchange.
11. Calculate the cumulative fluid balance at least every 24 hours. The cumulative fluid balance should be negative.
    - Add the balance from each exchange (from step 10) to the total exchange balance:
      Example:

Previous cumulative exchange balance	+500 mL
Present exchange balance	−700 mL
Cumulative exchange balance	−200 mL

12. Check the dressing at the catheter site if present.
    - Assess the dryness or wetness of the dressing. **Rationale:** *The dressing should remain dry during dialysis.*
    - To change the catheter site dressing, use the equipment listed above and follow correct technique for assessing and changing the dressing. Do not forcibly remove crusts or scabs. **Rationale:** *This may irritate skin and increase the risk of exit site infection.* Dressings may not be necessary for well-healed insertion sites.

13. If another bag is not to be infused at this time, or after the infusion of the new bag, disconnect the catheter from the tubing, and cover the end of the catheter with a new sterile cap. **Rationale:** *This allows the catheter to remain in place between each of the exchanges without contamination of the catheter.*
14. Remove and discard gloves. Perform hand hygiene.
15. Document findings in the client record using forms or checklists supplemented by narrative notes when appropriate. Include the time during which the fluid infused, the exchange number, dialysate and additives used, details of the exchange balance, color of outflow solution from client, client's response, appearance of the catheter exit site and dressing, and client's weight before and after the set of exchanges (daily). These may be written in the nurse's notes or on a flowchart.

Sample Documentation

5/20/15 0830 First 1 L dialysate infused over 20 minutes thru PD catheter. VS unchanged, no complaints of discomfort. Insertion site dressing clean & ≈dry. _____ S. Everley, RN

5/20/15 1330 VS stable, dressing dry & intact. 950 mL pink-tinged fluid returned from PD catheter by gravity flow over 20 minutes. PD bag #2, 1 L, infused in 15 minutes. Ambulated in hall independently. _____ S. Everley, RN

Setting of Care

Most clients undergoing peritoneal dialysis perform these procedures themselves at home. The nurse performs initial teaching and documents that the client and family are knowledgeable and able to demonstrate the techniques involved. In addition, the nurse assists with arrangements for all equipment and supplies that the client requires for home care.

For clients using CAPD, the empty dialysate solution bag can be left attached to the catheter during dwelling and is then used as the drainage bag. A special belt that stabilizes the catheter and holds the administration set between uses is available.

Teach the client and family:

- Store supplies in a clean, cool, dry place.
- Examine the solution for any signs of contamination before using it.
- Warm the dialysate for about 1 hour using a heating pad that has been checked for appropriate temperature.
- Hang dialysate bag at approximately shoulder height for infusion. Assist the client with obtaining an IV pole or other hanging device.
- Perform thorough hand hygiene and wear a surgical mask when changing tubing.
- Record weight and dialysis fluid balance daily or as ordered. Weight should be measured after draining the dialysate, and on the same scale, at the same time of day, and wearing similar clothing each time.
- Report any signs of peritonitis:
  - Fever.
  - Nausea or vomiting.
  - Redness or pain around the exit site.

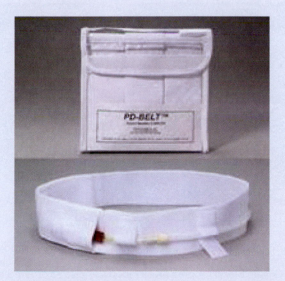

Peritoneal dialysis belt with tubing pouch stored in place.

SKILL 6.31   Providing Hemodialysis

Equipment

- Dialyzer (types are hollow fiber or cellulose acetate)
- 1000-mL bag of 0.9% normal saline IV solution
- Machine blood lines
- Fistula needles, 15/16 gauge, 1 to 1.5 in. in length
- Sterile gauze pads, alcohol swabs, and povidone-iodine or ChloraPrep swabs
- Two 3-mL syringes
- Two 20-mL syringes
- Drape
- Client mask
- Hemostats, cannula clamps
- Tape
- Sterile gloves and clean gloves
- Gown
- Protective goggles and face mask or visor shield
- 12-mL syringe
- Heparin solution 1,000 units/mL
- Hemastix

Preparation

- Check physician's order. Introduce self and identify client. Perform hand hygiene, following infection control measures, and verify client's identity. Provide privacy. Provide comfort and safety for client and self.
- Obtain dialysate bath composition as ordered.
- Set up 1000-mL IV of normal saline using IV tubing in blood line set.
- Load heparin pump (e.g., 8 mL heparin) per manufacturer's instructions. **Rationale:** *Heparin is added to system just before blood enters dialyzer to prevent clotting. The clotting mechanism is activated when blood moves outside body and is in contact with foreign substances.*
- Check location of nearest emergency power outlet. **Rationale:** *To maintain electric current if routine power fails.*
- Test dialysis machine ❶ for presence of bleach with Hemastix. **Rationale:** *This detects presence of caustic agents that could result in client complications.*

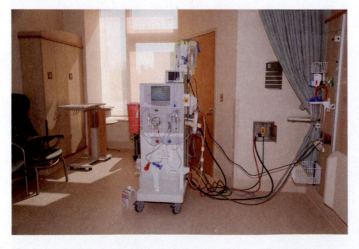

❶ Hemodialysis unit used to treat renal failure clients.

- Prime dialyzer and arterial and venous blood lines with saline.
- Hang additional IV solution of saline. **Rationale:** *Saline infusions must be available immediately for rapid reversal of hypotension or discontinuation of dialysis.*

- Connect pressure monitor lines to both arterial and venous drip chambers. **Rationale:** *This monitors the amount of hydrostatic pressure exerted on blood in the ultrafiltration process used to extract fluid throughout dialysis treatment.*
- Set the alarm pressures, both high and low.
- Connect air leak detector to venous drip chamber.
- Test all machine alarms: venous and arterial pressure, air detector, and blood leak detector.
- Connect arterial and venous lines for recirculation with adapter, and turn blood pump to 200 mL/min.
- Document alarm checks in dialysis log.

CLINICAL ALERT

When a hemodialysis client is hospitalized:

1. Place an identifying bracelet on access arm.
2. Post safety precautions at head of bed (e.g., "Do not use access arm for blood pressure or venipuncture" and "Fluid restriction specified").
3. Notify dialysis specialty nurse of client's admission to hospital.

Procedure

For AV Fistula or Graft

1. Place blood line at the same level as the bed.
2. Don mask and gown. Put on goggles, and perform hand hygiene.
3. Don clean gloves, and remove dressing, if used. Remove and discard gloves and perform hand hygiene.
4. Don sterile gloves.
5. Clean access site using ChloraPrep or alcohol swab, then povidone–iodine swab. Using a circular motion, cleanse from needle insertion site outward. Allow to dry. **Rationale:** *Cleansing occurs from cleanest to dirtiest area preventing contamination of the site.*
6. Insert needles into fistula or graft ❷. Tape securely to extremity.

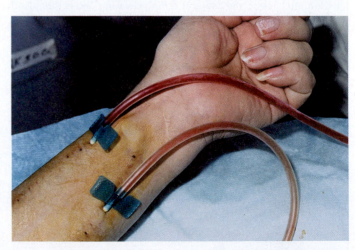

❷ Arterial and venous needles placed in graft for hemodialysis.

7. Obtain blood for predialysis blood samples as ordered by the physician. (Usually electrolytes, hematocrit, clotting time, etc.)
8. After blood is drawn for lab work, heparin bolus should be given to client according to physician's order—start heparin pump at ordered rate.

SKILL 6.31 Providing Hemodialysis *(continued)*

9. Prime the extracorporeal circuit with blood.
   - Connect arterial tubing of the blood line to client's arterial site.
   - Connect venous tubing.
   - Unclamp venous blood line.
   - Unclamp arterial blood line.
   - Clamp saline infusion line. Remove gloves and perform hand hygiene.
10. Note time of dialysis initiation.
11. Tape all connections securely; secure blood tubing to client's extremity.
12. Set alarm pressures, both high and low.
13. Establish blood flow rate (usually 200 to 400 mL/min) and the dialysate rate of 500 mL/hr. **Rationale:** *These flow rates allow the imbalances in fluids and electrolytes to be corrected rapidly (3 to 4 hours per run and 2 to 3 times/week).*
14. Ensure that access connections are visible.
15. Check client's blood pressure and pulse once dialysis has been initiated, then every 30 minutes unless otherwise indicated.
16. Assess client at least every 30 minutes for vital signs and potential complications.
17. Administer any ordered medication through the venous line. **Rationale:** *Medication infuses into client, not machine.*
18. Turn heparin infusion off during the last 30 to 60 minutes or as ordered.
19. Document procedure and client response.

The Hemodialysis Process

Hemodialysis works by removing blood from the client's arterial access site (graft, fistula, or catheter). It travels through a blood pump and an arterial pressure monitor to a dialyzer (filter). In the dialyzer, the blood is separated from the dialysate by a synthetic semipermeable membrane. The dialysate (bath) runs against the blood flowing on the opposite side of the semipermeable membrane leading to osmosis, diffusion, and ultrafiltration. Fluid, electrolytes, and toxins are removed from the blood. The blood then flows from the dialyzer through a tubing system to the client's venous access site. Fluid is removed through the use of hydrostatic pressure applied to the blood and a negative hydrostatic pressure applied to the dialysate bath. The difference between these two pressures is termed *transmembrane pressure* and this results in the process of ultrafiltration.

Blood Flow for Dialysis

An adequate vascular access should permit blood flow to the dialyzer of 200 to 400 mL/min. Optimal blood access and blood flow to the dialyzer influences dialysis efficiency.

Safety Precautions for Fistula or Graft

- Feel for vibration (thrill) over access site regularly.
- Do not measure blood pressure on extremity.
- Do not perform venipuncture in extremity.
- Counsel client not to wear constrictive clothing on extremity.
- Counsel client to avoid lying on extremity.
- Avoid carrying heavy loads with access extremity.
- Immediately report swelling, discoloration, drainage, or coldness, numbness, or weakness of hand.

Assessing Arteriovenous Fistula

- Perform hand hygiene.
- Position client's arm so fistula is easily accessed.
- Palpate the area to feel for thrill (vibration). This indicates arterial to venous blood flow and fistula patency.
- Auscultate with a stethoscope to detect a bruit (swishing noise). This indicates a patent fistula.
- Palpate pulses distal to fistula to check circulation.
- Observe capillary refill in extremity digits.
- Assess for numbness, tingling, coldness, pallor, or alternation in sensation in digits of fistula extremity.
- Assess for signs and symptoms of infection: redness, edema, soreness, warmth, or increased temperature.

Note: Vascular access promotes more efficient removal and replacement of blood during dialysis, resulting in fewer complications. Vascular access should be prepared weeks or months before using it for dialysis. This will stabilize the graft site and ensure adequate blood flow when used for dialysis.

Cultural Considerations

- African Americans have a more rapid decline in glomerular filtration rate than do Caucasians.
- Hypertensive African Americans have decreased renal excretion of sodium, making sodium restriction an important factor in treatment.
- Hypertension, diabetes, and end-stage renal disease (ESRD) are three to four times more common in African Americans and American Indians than in Caucasians.

SKILL 6.32 Providing Ongoing Care of a Hemodialysis Client

Procedure

1. Limit fluid intake to prescribed amount (e.g., 1,500 mL/day).
2. Maintain individualized diet as prescribed: high-quality protein 1.1 g/kg ideal body wt/day; sodium 70 mEq/day; potassium, average 70 mEq/day.
3. Check blood pressure for hypertension/hypotension; check temperature for possible infection.
4. Auscultate heart and lung sounds for signs of fluid overload (pulmonary edema and pericarditis).
5. Provide access site care.
6. Observe mental status—indicative of fluid and electrolyte imbalance.
7. Administer Epogen, if ordered, to improve hemoglobin level (given at time of dialysis).
8. Encourage regular rest periods.
9. Weigh daily to assess fluid accumulation.
10. Use antibacterial soap and lotion to bathe. **Rationale:** *This decreases risk of staphylococcal infections.*

(continued on next page)

SKILL 6.32   Providing Ongoing Care of a Hemodialysis Client (continued)

11. Determine that client understands when and how to take medications (e.g., Tums with meals).
12. Provide continued emotional support.
    - Allow for expression of feelings about change in body image and role performance.
    - Encourage expression of fears.
    - Encourage caregiver support.
    - Give support for required change in lifestyle.
13. Instruct client to prevent obstruction to blood flow on fistula arm.
14. Document care and client response.

Note: Dialysis adequacy is improved with increased prescription, conversion of catheters to grafts or fistulas, and by not shortening treatments.

Evidence-Based Nursing Practice
Survival Rate in Clients Receiving Hemodialysis

A 10-year follow-up retrospective study was conducted on 120 clients with end-stage renal disease (ESRD). The study was done to examine whether there was a difference in survival rates among those receiving dialysis treatments during the morning versus those receiving them in the afternoon. Previous studies had indicated that morning treatments could increase survivability rate.

The cases of 60 clients in each category were reviewed. The mean survival rates of clients receiving hemodialysis in the morning and those receiving it in the afternoon were not statistically different. The unadjusted 5-year survival rate for clients on morning-shift hemodialysis was 87.3% versus 86.4% for clients on afternoon-shift hemodialysis. The study concluded that survival rates of clients receiving hemodialysis are not affected by treatment in the morning versus the afternoon.

Source: Kim et al. (2012).

SKILL 6.33   Terminating Hemodialysis

Equipment

- Clean gloves
- Gown
- Goggles
- Mask
- Nonsterile pads
- Tubing clamps

Procedure

1. Don gloves, gown, goggles, and protective mask.
2. Remove tape and dressing to visualize needle insertion site.
3. Place pads under connectors.
4. Open IV of normal saline to return blood on the arterial side of tubing.
5. Start blood pump at 200 mL/min.
6. Return venous blood.
7. Clamp lines.
8. Remove needles according to unit protocol and apply pressure to sites ❶ ❷ ❸.

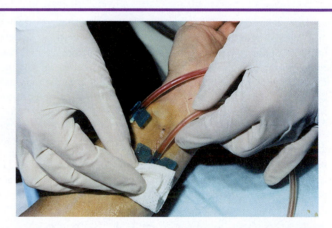

❷ Remove arterial and venous needles, using needle safety shields.

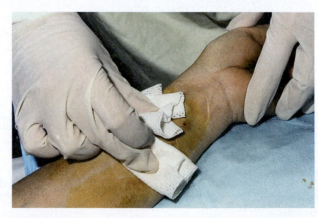

❸ Apply pressure over needle site for 5 to 10 minutes.

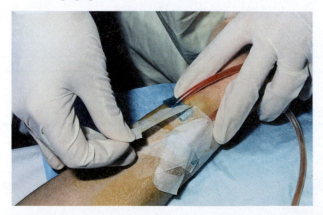

❶ Carefully remove tape from needle sites when terminating dialysis.

9. Apply sterile dressing to needle sites maintaining aseptic technique. **Rationale:** *Sepsis is the primary cause of client death for acute renal failure clients.*
10. Remove and discard protective gear. Perform hand hygiene.
11. Measure and document postdialysis vital signs and weight.

SKILL 6.34 Maintaining Central Venous Dual-Lumen Dialysis Catheter (DLC)

Equipment

- Heparin, 1,000 units/mL
- Sterile normal saline for injection
- Betadine spray
- Sterile 4 ×4 gauze pads
- Sterile transparent occlusive dressings if indicated
- Tape
- Luer-Lok catheter caps
- Nonsterile drape
- Two 3-mL syringes
- Two 20-mL syringes
- Clean gloves
- Two masks
- Sterile gloves

Preparation

- Identify self and client. Perform hand hygiene.
- Fill two 20-mL syringes with 20 mL each of normal saline, and two 3-mL syringes with 3 mL of 1,000 units/mL heparin.
- Mask client and self, and don clean gloves.
- Place drape under catheter lumens.
- Remove gauze wrap from lumens, if present, and discard in appropriate receptacle.
- Remove and discard gloves. Perform hand hygiene.

Procedure

1. Open sterile supplies.
2. Holding corner of 4 × 4 gauze, place under catheter lumens.
3. Spray lumens with Betadine and allow to dry.
4. Don sterile gloves.
5. Remove old lumen caps.
6. Use 4 × 4 gauze to pick up new caps and place on lumens.
7. Unclamp and inject 20 mL saline solution into each lumen using positive pressure technique.
8. Inject 3 mL heparin into each catheter using positive pressure technique.
9. Reclamp lumens.
10. Remove old dressing, and discard in biohazard receptacle ❶.

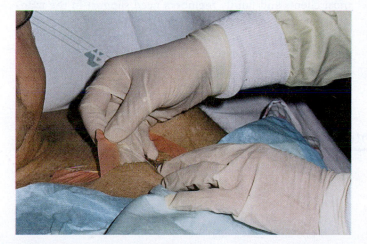

❶ Maintain sterility while carefully removing dressing from dual-lumen catheter.

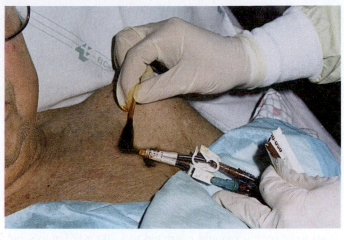

❷ Cleanse catheter insertion site with antimicrobial swabs.

11. Cleanse area surrounding catheter with antimicrobial swabs ❷.
12. Place sterile transparent dressing over catheter insertion site.

Note: Provide catheter site care after each dialysis treatment. Dressing is not required after permanent catheter site epithelializes around catheter (about 2 weeks).

13. If desired, wrap lumens in gauze and tape. **Rationale:** *To prevent skin irritation from lumen clamps.*
14. Dispose of equipment in biohazard receptacle.
15. Remove and discard gloves and mask. Perform hand hygiene.
16. Monitor daily and document signs of infection, bleeding, or displacement of catheters ❸.

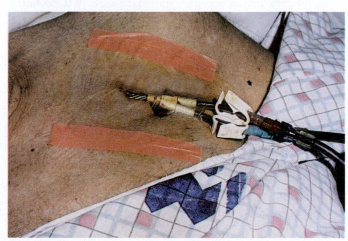

❸ Monitor frequently for signs of infection, bleeding, or catheter displacement.

CLINICAL ALERT

Central venous dual-lumen dialysis catheter (DLC) maintenance (heparin "pack" and site dressing) is performed *only* by the nephrology nurse after a dialysis treatment. These catheters are not maintained the way CVADs are. Instead, they are "packed" with undiluted heparin after dialysis, then "unpacked" (3 mL blood withdrawn from catheter) before the next dialysis treatment.

> **▶ HOME CARE**

Expected Outcomes

1. Client uses clean technique with self-care interventions.
2. Client with an ostomy utilizes appropriate appliances and supplies to maintain bowel or bladder elimination.

▶ URINARY ELIMINATION

Home care clients who require assistance with emptying their bladders are usually placed on intermittent clean catheterization protocols rather than having an indwelling catheter. This procedure assists in preventing penoscrotal abscess formation, overwhelming infection, and altered body image. Fluid intake needs to be monitored and restricted to 1,500 mL/day to avoid bladder distention. If spontaneous voiding returns, frequency of catheterizations can be extended to every 12 hours and discontinued when the residual urine is consistently less than 100 mL in 24 hours.

When an indwelling catheter is used, nurses must be aware that it may lead to urinary tract infection (UTI). The nurse must teach the client and family to observe for signs and symptoms of UTI and sepsis. They should note odor, color, and consistency of the urine. Catheter changes are the responsibility of the nurse and are usually performed once a month. Encouraging fluids becomes a major role assumed by family members and monitored by the nurse. Urinary antiseptics are adjunctive measures when catheterizations are required.

Home care dialysis is common in many areas of the country. The principles and procedures are similar to those in a hospital or free-standing dialysis unit. The major change is the advent of portable dialysis methods such as continuous ambulatory peritoneal dialysis (CAPD) and continuous cycling peritoneal dialysis (CCPD). These procedures allow individuals to participate in a normal lifestyle. However, use of these methods requires monitoring by the nurse and specific teaching of the essential components to prevent complications and promote health. Peritoneal dialysis (PD) reflects more normal kidney function than hemodialysis. Fluid and electrolytes are removed gradually and, therefore, clients have fewer complications with blood pressure alterations and disequilibrium syndrome. PD has fewer dietary and fluid restrictions, allowing clients to lead a

more normal life. PD also provides the client with a more flexible schedule, allowing him or her to work, travel, and participate in activities. One major restriction, besides ensuring the ordered number of exchanges each day, is the monthly appointment at the dialysis center for lab work and consultation with the physician or nurse.

The catheter is placed in a dependent position in the peritoneal cavity to minimize the chance of catheter obstruction or erosion into other abdominal organs. The catheter is placed outside of the abdomen to decrease infections. Several devices are placed around the catheter to prevent fluid leaks from the peritoneal cavity. These devices impede the migration of bacteria.

There are three types of PD: continuous ambulatory peritoneal dialysis (CAPD), continuous cycling peritoneal dialysis (CCPD), and intermittent peritoneal dialysis (IPD). The two most common types for home care clients are CAPD and CCPD.

▶ BOWEL ELIMINATION

The actual care of clients requiring interventions for altered bowel elimination is basically the same for hospitalized clients as home care clients. Equipment may be slightly different, but it is similar enough to make it easy to teach clients and family members to perform the skills.

A major responsibility of the nurse is to provide client and family education in the care and management of the ostomy, bowel elimination interventions, and how to administer an enema. At the time of discharge from the hospital, most clients and family members need support in the management of an ostomy. The home care nurse will need to not only demonstrate and evaluate the performance and outcome of the ostomy care, but will also need to provide emotional support.

| **SKILL 6.35** | Using Clean Technique for Intermittent Self-Catheterization |

Equipment

- Straight catheters in clean container, plastic bag, or wrapped in aluminum foil
- Washcloth, soap, water
- Water-soluble lubricant (e.g., K-Y, Surgilube)
- Plastic bags
- Basin or container
- Mirror

Procedure

1. Attempt to urinate. If unable to do so, continue to follow these steps.
2. Perform hand hygiene and gather equipment. (Keep equipment in one large container.)
3. Assume sitting position on bed or commode. (Place plastic under towel if bed is used.)
4. Insert the catheter.

SKILL 6.35   Using Clean Technique for Intermittent Self-Catheterization (continued)

For Female Clients
- Separate labia with one hand while cleaning with soap and water front to back with other hand.
- Position mirror to visualize urinary meatus.
- Remove catheter from container (plastic bag or aluminum foil).
- Lubricate end of catheter with water-soluble lubricant and place other end in container to catch urine.
- While holding labia apart with one hand, insert catheter about 8 cm (3 in.) or until urine flows.

For Male Clients
- Retract the foreskin, if present, and wash tip of penis with soap and water.
- Remove catheter from container (plastic bag or aluminum foil).

- Lubricate the first 7 to 10 in. of catheter with water-soluble lubricant. Place other end in container to catch urine.
- Hold penis at right angle to body, keeping foreskin retracted. Insert catheter 7 to 10 in. into penis or until urine begins to flow. Then insert catheter 1 in. farther.

5. Press down with abdominal muscles to promote bladder emptying.
6. Pinch off catheter after all urine has drained and withdraw gently, holding tip of catheter upright.
7. Wash and dry perineal area.
8. Wash catheter in warm, soapy water.
9. Rinse with clear water and dry outside with paper towel.
10. Place in plastic bag for storage.
11. Use catheters for 2 to 4 weeks and then discard.
12. Perform hand hygiene.

SKILL 6.36   Teaching Suprapubic Catheter Care

Equipment

- Catheter plug and clamp
- Closed drainage system
- Sterile dressings if necessary
- Clean gloves
- Receptacle to drain urine from drainage bag
- Normal saline solution or mild soap and water
- White vinegar
- Applicator sticks
- 4 × 4 gauze pads
- Paper tape

Procedure

1. Instruct client to gather equipment for specific skill to be done. Then provide the following instructions for the client.
   - Perform hand hygiene and don gloves.
   - Clean around catheter site with normal saline solution or mild soap and water. Use applicator sticks to remove material from around catheter opening.
   - Ensure catheter is not pulling on exit site. Tape catheter to skin so a gentle curve is present to prevent tugging on catheter.
   - Empty catheter bag. Some clients use leg bags. Empty into container and then dispose of contents in toilet or, if removing bag, empty directly into toilet.

   - Clean drainage bags with warm water and soap every day or two. Place one teaspoon of vinegar in rinse water to reduce odor.
   - Replace catheter bag on catheter.
   - Remove and discard gloves. Perform hand hygiene.
2. Instruct client in bladder testing.
   - Wash hands and catheter connections with soap and water.
   - Clamp the suprapubic tube so it does not drain. Use catheter plug or clamp.
   - Have client attempt to void when client feels urge to urinate. Measure amount of urine.
   - Unclamp the suprapubic tube immediately after voiding; empty urine into container and measure residual urine amount.
   - Instruct client to keep a log of each voiding and residual amount.
   - Call physician with findings when residual amount is less than 20% voided amount. Usually, this amount is about 60 mL. Usually, the suprapubic tube is removed when client is able to urinate without complications.
3. Instruct client to monitor carefully for signs of urinary tract infection and notify physician immediately. Check for bladder pain, confusion, bleeding, temperature over 37.8°C (100°F), chills, cloudy urine, drainage or edema around the suprapubic tube. Document teaching and client response.

SKILL 6.37   Administering Continuous Ambulatory Peritoneal Dialysis (CAPD)

Equipment

- Sterile dialysate solution, 1 to 2 bags, warmed
- Heating pad
- Transfer set, either Y-set tubing or straight, and cap
- Disconnect cap (FlexiCap or MiniCap)
- Hook on wall of room used for dialysis
- Clamp
- Paper towels
- Low stool or table
- Intake and output record

- Sterile gloves, 2 pairs
- Mask
- Antibacterial soap
- Cleansing solution for catheter
- Medication, if ordered

Preparation

- Check physician's order.
- Perform hand hygiene thoroughly, dry using paper towel.
- Obtain container of sterile dialysate.

(continued on next page)

SKILL 6.37 Administering Continuous Ambulatory Peritoneal Dialysis (CAPD) *(continued)*

- Check that strength and amount of solution are accurate as ordered.
- Take equipment to clean area for assembly.

Procedure

For Draining Fluid

1. Perform hand hygiene and don clean gloves. **Rationale:** *This is an infection control precaution for caregivers when there is potential contact with blood or body fluids.*
2. Don mask.
3. Uncap catheter maintaining aseptic technique.
4. Attach sterile bag and transfer set to catheter for draining dialysate.
5. Place bag on low stool or table below level of client's abdomen. **Rationale:** *This position allows fluid to drain by gravity from client's peritoneal cavity.*
6. Unclamp tubing.
7. Allow fluid to drain into bag from abdomen until flow ceases, approximately, 10 to 20 minutes.
8. Reclamp tubing.
9. Examine drainage for discoloration or cloudiness. **Rationale:** *Change in color may indicate presence of infection; the presence of a white gelatin-like material indicates shredding of the peritoneal lining's old skin; an increase in this fibrin indicates potential peritonitis.*
10. Disconnect tubing from drainage bag while maintaining aseptic technique. Unscrew catheter from tubing and attach disconnect cap, according to clinic's instruction. **Rationale:** *The glucose in the dialysate solution predisposes the client to infections.*
11. Weigh drainage bag on scale. Effluent should weigh at least 4.5 pounds. This is equal to 2 liters of fluid. **Rationale:** *To ensure all fluid is drained from abdomen.*
12. Dispose of effluent into toilet.
13. Double bag tubing and drainage bag. Place biohazardous label on bag. Discard by placing in biohazardous container. Tubing is usually disposed of following each exchange.
14. Remove and discard gloves and mask. Perform hand hygiene.
15. Check blood pressure and pulse. **Rationale:** *Rapid fluid shift may cause hypotension.*

Note: Disconnect cap disinfects dialysis tubing between exchanges.

For Infusing Dialysate

1. Warm dialysate. The bag can be encased in a heating pad for 1 hour. DO NOT PLACE IN MICROWAVE. **Rationale:** *Microwave heating will produce uneven heating and can cause burning in the client.*
2. Perform hand hygiene for 3 minutes with antibacterial soap. **Rationale:** *To prevent contamination.*
3. Gather equipment. Don gloves.
4. Open plastic wrap on dialysate solution and inspect solution bag for expiration date and color and consistency of dialysate. Assess bag for possible leaks.
5. Add medications as ordered. Maintain sterile technique during this step. **Rationale:** *Some clients add routine drugs to dialysate, such as insulin.*
6. Connect tubing to dialysate bag by removing protective cover from port and spiking into dialysate bag. Maintain sterility throughout this step. Each manufacturer has a slightly different mechanism for connecting the tubing and bag. Follow manufacturer's directions. (See the Transfer Sets box.)
7. Hang new dialysate bag on hook, which is positioned above client at shoulder height.
8. Open clamp and adjust height to ensure inflow of solution by gravity over a 10- to 20-minute period.
9. Clamp tubing.
10. Discard empty dialysate bag or place in a holding pouch at client's waist, according to type of transfer set being used.
11. Allow fluid to remain in peritoneal cavity approximately 4 hours.
12. Remove and discard gloves. Perform hand hygiene.
13. Repeat procedure four times daily, the last time at bedtime, allowing fluid to remain in peritoneal cavity overnight.
14. Ensure that client and caregiver are knowledgeable in strict aseptic technique.
15. Instruct client to notify physician if there is evidence of infection.
16. Document findings for physician at each visit.

Transfer Sets

Transfer sets consist of tubing that connects a bag of dialysate solution to a catheter. Two types are currently being used for CAPD.

STRAIGHT TUBING

Straight tubing stays connected to the catheter. For each exchange, the "free" end is connected to the solution. With this type of transfer set, the empty bag from solution is rolled up and worn under clothing. That bag is then unrolled, placed on the floor, and used to drain dialysate from the abdomen. After draining is completed, tubing is disconnected from the straight transfer set and a new solution bag and tubing are connected to the catheter.

Y-SET TUBING

This type of tubing is disconnected between exchanges. The base of the Y is connected to the catheter. One branch of the Y is con-

nected to a new bag of solution and the other to an empty bag. The base of the Y is closed and a small amount of solution is drained from the full bag into the empty bag. This is done to rid the transfer set of any bacteria that might be in the tubing. The branch that leads to the empty bag is then closed and the solution flows into the abdomen. Once the solution bag is empty, the Y-set is disconnected from the catheter. This removes the need to wear the bag around the waist while solution is in abdomen. The catheter is then reconnected to the Y-set and solution is drained into an empty bag to discard. A new bag of solution is hung and the process continues. The Y-set is filled with disinfectant when not in use. The disinfectant is flushed out with the used dialysate. The Y-set can be reused for several months.

SKILL 6.38 Changing Dressing for a CAPD Client

Equipment

- Dressing according to facility policy
- Antimicrobial swabs or sterile 4 × 4 dressings and Betadine solution
- Tape
- Sterile gloves, 2 pairs
- Forceps (optional)
- Povidone iodine ointment
- 4 × 4 gauze pads and precut drain dressings
- Warm soapy water, if needed

Procedure

1. Perform hand hygiene.
2. Don sterile gloves.
3. Remove old dressing with sterile gloves.
4. Remove any dried blood or drainage with warm, soapy water.
5. Saturate 4 × 4 dressings with Betadine solution or use swabs and clean skin around catheter, moving in concentric circles from the catheter site outward. Remove crusted material, if present.
6. Inspect site for infection (erythema, edema, warmth, exudate).
7. Apply povidone-iodine ointment to catheter site using sterile dressings.
8. Change gloves.
9. Place two precut drain dressings over catheter site, and tape dressing. **Rationale:** *Dressings are secured to prevent infection at site.*
10. Remove and discard gloves. Perform hand hygiene.
11. Document actions and client response.

SKILL 6.39 Instructing Client in Colostomy Irrigation

Equipment

- Solution container with 1000 mL warm water
- Irrigating tubing with cone
- Clean gloves, 3 pairs
- Irrigating sleeve cut long enough to reach water level in toilet
- Items to clean skin and stoma (e.g., washcloths or gauze sponges)
- Plastic bag for disposal of used pouch
- Clean pouch and closure device
- Skin barriers
- Water-soluble lubricant
- Hook near toilet

Procedure

1. Instruct client in benefits of relaxing and taking periodic deep breaths.
2. Perform hand hygiene and don clean gloves.
3. Remove and dispose of used pouch in plastic bag.
4. Clean stoma and skin with warm water and soft cloth. Assess skin for signs of irrigation or breakdown.
5. Apply irrigation sleeve to peristomal skin, and place belt around waist.
6. Fill container with 1000 mL lukewarm water (500 mL for first irrigation). **Rationale:** *Lukewarm water temperature is 40 to 43°C (105° to 110°F). This temperature prevents injury from hot solutions and cramping from cold solutions.*
7. Suspend container on bathroom hook at level of client's shoulders (no higher than 18 in. above stoma).
8. Open roller clamp and allow solution to run through tubing; close clamp. **Rationale:** *This removes air from tubing and prevents discomfort for client.*
9. Assist client to sit on toilet or on chair in front of toilet.
10. Place sleeve between client's thighs and direct end into toilet.
11. Lubricate cone tip with water-soluble lubricant.
12. Position cone in sleeve by placing through top opening. If cone cannot be inserted easily, do not force it.
13. Hold cone snugly against stoma. **Rationale:** *This prevents back flow of solution.*
14. Open roller clamp on tubing and allow water to run through cone while inserting cone into stoma.
15. Instill solution (750 to 1,000 mL) over 5 to 10 minutes. **Rationale:** *The container height and rate of water flow affects results obtained.* If client complains of feeling light-headed or has vertigo, take pulse and stop instillation. **Rationale:** *These are symptoms of a vagal response.*
16. Clamp tubing briefly if cramping occurs.
17. Remove cone and close off or fold over top of sleeve.
18. Remain seated until most stool and solution return, usually 10–15 minutes.
19. Remove gloves and discard.
20. Rinse sleeve with water, dry bottom of sleeve, and close end of sleeve.
21. Ask client to wear sleeve in this manner for 30–60 minutes while proceeding with other activities. **Rationale:** *Allows time for expelling solution or feces and prevents accidental evacuation.* Then have client remove, clean, and store sleeve.
22. Instruct client to cleanse skin and stoma with warm water and dry thoroughly. Teach client how to apply skin barriers and clean pouch.
23. Place discarded supplies in client's trash. Remove gloves and perform hand hygiene.
24. Document teaching and client response.

▶ CRITICAL THINKING OPTIONS FOR UNEXPECTED OUTCOMES

Not all unexpected outcomes require further nursing intervention; however, many times they do. When the client demonstrates a change in signs/symptoms indicating an emerging problem, the nurse should immediately assess and troubleshoot what is happening. The assessment data must be processed quickly to formulate a hypothesis so the nurse can make a clinical judgment. The nurse then decides how best to resolve the problem and improve the client's situation for a better appropriate outcome.

EXPECTED OUTCOME	PROBLEM SOLVING	NURSING ACTIONS
Collecting a Specimen Client is able to follow procedure of collection when appropriate.	Client is embarrassed by having to give stool specimen.	■ Place a bedpan or other collection device under the toilet seat in bathroom to obtain specimen. ■ If client is confined to bed, pull sheets over client's legs and draw curtains around the bed until procedure is completed. ■ If odor occurs from passage of stool, spray room with air freshener.
Specimen collected is adequate for test.	Client passes liquid stools.	■ Determine if part of entire specimen is required for test. ■ Obtain a plastic container with a cover and several large cotton swabs. Dip cotton swabs into the liquid stool. Place swabs in plastic container. After procedure, pay close attention to skin care. A protective ointment may be necessary to protect skin from liquid stools.
Bladder Interventions Client voids 200 to 500 mL of urine without discomfort or difficulty.	Unable to void on bedpan.	■ Run water in sink. ■ Massage the lower abdomen. ■ Place a hot washcloth on the abdomen. ■ Pour warm water over the perineum with client positioned on toilet or bedpan. ■ Give client a sitz bath after obtaining an order.
	Catheter cannot be inserted into male client.	Obtain new catheter kit and follow these actions: ■ Hold penis vertical to client's body, insert lidocaine gel. ■ Insert catheter while applying slight traction by gently pulling upward on the shaft of the penis ■ If resistance encountered, rotate catheter, increase traction, and lower angle of penis ■ Ask client to cough. ■ Try using a Coudé or 12 Fr catheter (some facilities require a physician's order for this type of catheter)
Skin irritation does not occur with condom catheter use.	Penis becomes reddened with condom catheter use.	■ Remove condom. ■ Notify wound care specialist/physician for topical medication order. ■ Apply adult brief and change frequently until problem resolves. ■ Make sure penis is clean and dry and protective coating is applied before condom application. ■ Clip rolled portion of condom to prevent constriction at base of penis.
Suprapubic catheter remains intact.	Suprapubic catheter becomes dislodged.	■ Place sterile dressing over catheter insertion site; do not attempt to replace catheter. ■ Notify physician. ■ Obtain new catheter to prepare for insertion by physician.
Client remains free of urinary tract infection.	Client develops urinary tract infection	■ Note signs and symptoms of UTI: cloudy malodorous urine with sediment, bladder discomfort/spasms, elevated temperature. ■ Notify physician to obtain order for urinalysis and antimicrobial therapy. ■ Increase fluid intake to at least 2 to 3 L/day (unless contraindicated). ■ Maintain continuous urine drainage per suprapubic catheter.
Pouching system does not leak.	Pouching system leaks.	■ Check area for crease or dip in skin, which allows urine to pool and leak out. ■ Fill in dip area with skin barrier to prevent pooling. ■ Apply belt to improve fit. ■ Apply another type of pouch (e.g., convex). ■ Change more frequently if leak is due to dissolving of skin barrier—or use different barrier. ■ Advise client to avoid using soaps or wipes to clean area because they interfere with pouch adhesion.
Client demonstrates self-care skills.	Client is unable to manage own urinary diversion.	■ Simplify pouch procedure if possible. ■ Provide detailed instruction in more simplified manner. ■ Include caregiver in teaching to assist and support client. ■ Refer client to home health agency for follow-up care.
Bowel Interventions Relief obtained from fecal impaction or constipation.	When digital stimulation is performed, client exhibits reflex spasm that prevents stool expulsion.	■ Apply local anesthetic around rectum and anus, if ordered. ■ Wait for spasm to relax, and then proceed with stimulation.
	Client exhibits signs and symptoms of vagal response during removal of fecal impaction.	■ Immediately discontinue procedure. ■ Place client in shock position. ■ Monitor vital signs every 5–15 min until condition is stable. ■ Notify physician of findings and request medication order for antispasmodic such as atropine. ■ Be prepared for "Code" situation, even though it is not likely to occur.

EXPECTED OUTCOME	PROBLEM SOLVING	NURSING ACTIONS
Relief obtained from fecal impaction or constipation.	Fecal impaction is not relieved.	■ Check orders for oil retention enema. ■ Check catheter size needed. ■ Obtain order for and use digital stimulation and manual extraction of feces if not contraindicated by diagnosis of cardiac or neurological involvement.
Client experiences increased comfort and relief from abdominal distention.	Effective bowel evacuation program is not established.	■ Ask dietitian for altered diet (including more fruits and vegetables). ■ Check if contraindication exists for increasing fluids to 3,000 mL daily. ■ Obtain order from the physician to administer a different stool softener and bulk former or increase dosage. ■ Have client increase physical activity, especially exercise of the abdominal muscles if not contraindicated by condition. ■ Ensure that client begins bowel training program one half hour after a meal.
	Client complains of severe and sudden abdominal pain, nausea, and distention.	■ Remove tubing, and notify physician immediately of possible perforation. (This is an uncommon complication.) ■ Assess vital signs. If you suspect cardiac dysrhythmias, remove bedpan and notify physician immediately. ■ Be prepared to administer emergency drugs, such as atropine. ■ If an IV is not in place, start an IV of 5% dextrose in water (D_5W) using a large-bore needle for emergency use.
Enema is administered without difficulty.	Client expels solution prematurely.	■ Calm and ease client's distress by reassuring him or her as you clean the equipment. ■ Place bedpan under client. Place client in semi-Fowler's position with knees flexed. ■ Hold the rectal tube in client's rectum between thighs. Slow the water flow, and continue with the enema.
Client's skin remains free of erythema, excoriation, and infection.	Stoma becomes ulcerated or cut.	■ Examine pouching system to see if opening of pouch may be cutting into stoma. ■ Recut opening to exact size of stoma.
	Peristomal skin complications occur.	■ Evaluate cause of leakage. ■ Be sure pouch is cut to correct size. ■ Measure stoma at each pouch change for 4–6 weeks. Size will change as edema subsides. ■ Measure stoma at base. ■ May need to fill any creases around stoma with skin barrier paste. ■ Apply thin layer of ostomy powder over area and seal with an alcohol-free coating. ■ May need to use secondary skin barrier like Eakin seal. ■ May need to attach belt to minimize lateral leakage. ■ Change to a product like Durahesive that swells around stoma, preventing leakage. It holds up well to liquid output. ■ Be sure pouch is emptied before it is over one third full of stool or flatus, since an overfull pouch can break seal of pouch. ■ Pouches should not be changed more than once daily.
Dialysis Dialysis proceeds without complication (excess fluids and wastes removed from blood.)	Hypotension occurs during dialysis.	■ Administer normal saline, concentrated saline bolus, or albumin into extracorporeal circuit. ■ Place client in shock position if tolerated. ■ Consider using smaller volume dialyzer, less ultrafiltration, or intermittent normal saline doses to maintain BP in future dialysis sessions. ■ Consider possible dialyzer reaction or myocardial infarction; notify physician for further assessment/diagnostic testing.
Vascular access site remains patent.	Client states hand feels weak; neither thrill nor bruit can be assessed in fistula or graft.	■ Notify physician of potential clotting of fistula/graft (declotting should be attempted ASAP). ■ Prepare to possibly send client to radiology for vascular procedure. ■ Review safety precautions to prevent constriction of blood flow in access extremity.
Client demonstrates self-care after teaching.	Client gains 7 pounds between dialysis sessions; blood pressure is elevated.	■ Assess client's understanding of fluid restriction (1,500 mL/day); advise of hidden fluid in certain foods (ice cream, watermelon, etc.). ■ Encourage client to control blood sugar (if diabetic) to help relieve thirst; decrease salt intake, but avoid salt substitute (KCl). ■ Encourage client to weigh daily.
Home Care Client with an ostomy utilizes appropriate appliances and supplies to maintain bowel or bladder elimination.	Client not coping with altered body image.	■ Refer to United Ostomy Associations of America, the Crohn's and Colitis Foundation of America, American Cancer Society, or the local enterostomal therapy nurse.

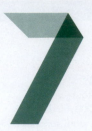

Fluids and Electrolytes

In good health, a delicate balance of fluids, electrolytes, acids, and bases maintains the body. This balance, or **homeostasis**, depends on multiple physiological processes that regulate fluid intake and output, as well as the movement of water and the substances dissolved in it among body compartments.

Measurement and recording of all fluid intake and output (I&O) during a 24-hour period provide important data about the client's fluid and electrolyte balance. **Tables 7–1** ● and **7–2** ● show the average daily fluid intake and output for an adult, respectively.

Input in children is measured as for adults, recording the fluids delivered to the child through parenteral or oral routes in milliliters.

Output is a measurement of what is expelled, drained, secreted, or suctioned from the body. Output sources include urine, stool, vomitus, sweat, drainage from wounds, and nasogastric suction. Output for infants can be measured by weighing the diaper. Output for older children can be measured as for adults with a graduated cylinder and recorded in milliliters.

Accurate measurement of I&O is documented for many adults and children, such as those receiving IV fluids or certain medications, after major surgery, and those with serious infections, renal disease or kidney damage, congestive heart failure, diabetes mellitus, dehydration or hypovolemia, or severe thermal burns.

Expected Outcomes

1. Client's intake and output are maintained within expected parameters of 200 to 300 mL of each other.
2. Fluid intake is at least 2,600 mL unless contraindicated by diagnosis.
3. Output is maintained at 30 mL or more per hour.

TABLE 7–1   Average Daily Fluid Intake for an Adult

SOURCE	AMOUNT (mL)
Oral fluids	1,200–1,500
Water in foods	1,000
Water as by-product of food metabolism	200
Total	2,400–2,700

TABLE 7–2   Average Daily Fluid Output for an Adult

SOURCE	AMOUNT (mL)
Urine	1,400–1,500
Insensible losses	
Lungs	350–400
Skin	350–400
Sweat	100
Feces	100–200
Total	2,300–2,600

SKILL 7.1   Monitoring Intake and Output

Delegation

Measurement and recording of normal oral fluid intake or urinary and gastrointestinal output may be delegated to UAP. Measurement of parenteral fluid intake and output from wounds and tubes generally is not delegated to UAP.

Equipment

- Graduated measuring containers
- I&O records
- Signs to post in room indicating that the client requires I&O recording

Preparation

- Three clinical measurements of fluid balance that the nurse can initiate independently are daily weights, vital signs, and fluid I&O.
- Assessing fluid I&O is an ongoing process that requires the nurse to have measuring devices and methods of recording easily accessible. Most agencies have a form for recording incremental I&O, usually a bedside record on which the nurse lists all items measured and the quantities per shift. These values will then be transferred onto the permanent chart record in the appropriate place (often on the vital signs record).

CLINICAL ALERT

Hourly urine output of less than 30 mL/hr for 2 consecutive hours or 24-hour urine output of less than 500 mL can indicate dehydration or internal bleeding and can result in acute renal failure.

Use client's own graduated receptacle when measuring output. Change gloves and perform hand hygiene between each client. The Centers for Disease Control and Prevention (CDC) calls for decontamination of hands after removing gloves. Gloves should also be changed and hands decontaminated when moving from a contaminated body site to a clean one on the same client.

Procedure

1. Prior to conducting the examination, introduce self and verify the client's identity using agency protocol. Explain to the client what you are going to do, the reason for the examination, and how he or she can participate. Discuss how the findings will be used in planning further care or treatments.
2. Perform hand hygiene and observe other appropriate infection control procedures.
3. If necessary, record on the Kardex or nursing care plan that the client's I&O are to be measured, including when they

(continued on next page)

SKILL 7.1   Monitoring Intake and Output (continued)

should be totaled. In many cases, fluid balance is summed every shift and then totaled for the entire previous 24 hours. In extremely acute situations, the client's I&O may be evaluated hourly so that changes in treatment can be implemented immediately.

4. *Recording intake:* Clients who wish to be involved in recording fluid intake measurements need to be taught how to compute the values and what to measure.

   - Record each fluid item taken, specifying the time and type of fluid. All of the following fluids need to be recorded:
   - *Oral fluids:* Includes water, milk, juice, soft drinks, coffee, tea, cream, soup, and any other beverages. Include water taken with medications. To assess the amount of water taken from a water pitcher, measure what remains and subtract this amount from the volume of the full pitcher. Then refill the pitcher.
   - *Ice chips:* Record the fluid as approximately one half the volume of the ice chips. For example, if the ice chips fill a cup holding 200 mL and the client consumed all of the ice chips, the volume consumed would be recorded as 100 mL.
   - *Foods that are or tend to become liquid at room temperature:* These include ice cream, sherbet, custard, and gelatin. Do not measure foods that are pureed, because purees are simply solid foods prepared in a different form.
   - *Tube feedings:* Remember to include the amount of water flush following medication administration, at the end of intermittent feedings, or during continuous feedings.
   - *Parenteral fluids:* The exact amount of intravenous fluid administered is to be recorded. Blood transfusions and fluids used to flush medications are included.
   - *Intravenous medications:* Intravenous medications that are prepared with solutions such as normal saline (NS) and are administered as an intermittent or continuous infusion must also be included (e.g., ceftazidime 1 g in 50 mL of sterile water). Most intravenous medications are mixed in 50 to 100 mL of solution.
   - *Catheter or tube irrigants:* If the fluid used to irrigate urinary catheters, nasogastric tubes, and intestinal tubes or remaining after peritoneal dialysis is not aspirated after instillation, the remaining fluid volume must be measured and recorded.

5. *Recording output:* Inform clients, family members, and all caregivers that accurate measurements of the client's fluid intake and output are required, explaining why and emphasizing the need to use a bedpan, urinal, commode, or in-toilet collection device (unless a urinary drainage system is in place). Instruct the client not to put toilet tissue into the container with urine. Clients who wish to be involved in recording their own fluid output measurements need to be taught how to handle the fluids and to compute the values.

   - To measure fluid output, measure the following fluids (remember to observe appropriate infection control precautions):
   - *Urinary output:* Following each voiding, pour the urine into a measuring container, observe the amount, and record it and the time of voiding on the I&O form ❶. For clients with retention catheters, empty the drainage bag into a measuring container at the end of the shift (or at prescribed times if output is to be measured more often). Sometimes, urine output is measured hourly. If the client is incontinent of urine, estimate and record these outputs. For example, for a client who is incontinent, the nurse

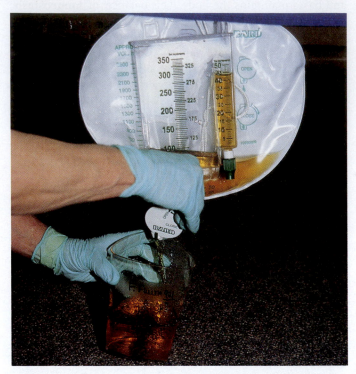

❶ Empty urinal, bedpan, or Foley drainage bag into client's individual (labeled) graduate and record amount of urine.

might record "Incontinent × 3" or "Drawsheet soaked in 12-in. diameter." A more accurate estimate of the urine output of clients who are incontinent may be obtained by first weighing diapers or incontinent pads that are dry, and then subtracting this weight from the weight of the soiled items. Each gram of weight left after subtracting is equal to 1 mL of urine. If urine is frequently soiled with feces, the number of voidings may be recorded rather than the volume of urine.

   - *Vomitus and liquid feces:* The amount, appearance, and type of fluid and the time need to be specified.
   - *Tube drainage, such as gastric or intestinal drainage:* The amount, appearance, and type of fluid and the time need to be specified.
   - *Wound drainage and draining fistulas:* Wound drainage may be recorded by documenting the type and number of dressings or linen saturated with drainage or by measuring the exact amount of drainage collected in a vacuum drainage system (e.g., Hemovac) or gravity drainage system.

6. Document in the client record using forms or checklists supplemented by narrative notes when appropriate. Fluid intake and output measurements are totaled at the end of the shift (every 8 to 12 hours), and the totals are recorded in the client's permanent record. Usually the staff on night shift totals the amounts of I&O recorded for each shift and records the 24-hour total. Check agency policy.

CLINICAL ALERT

Check all drainage receptacles such as Foley bag and NG canister at the beginning of each shift to ensure they were emptied from the previous shift and that there has not been excessive drainage.

SKILL 7.1   Monitoring Intake and Output (*continued*)

Client Teaching

- Consume six to eight glasses of water daily.
- Avoid excess amount of fluids high in salt.
- Limit caffeine and alcohol intake because they have a diuretic effect.
- Increase fluid intake before, during, and after strenuous exercise, particularly when the environmental temperature is high, and replace lost electrolytes from excessive perspiration as needed with commercial electrolyte solutions.
- Learn about and monitor side effects of medications that affect fluid balance (e.g., diuretics) and ways to handle side effects.
- Recognize possible risk factors for fluid imbalance such as prolonged or repeated vomiting, frequent watery stools, or inability to consume fluids because of illness.
- Seek prompt professional health care for notable signs of fluid imbalance such as sudden weight gain or loss, decreased urine volume, swollen ankles, shortness of breath, dizziness, or confusion.

Monitoring Fluid Intake and Output

- Teach and provide the rationale for monitoring fluid intake and output to the client and family as appropriate. Include how to use a commode or collection device ("hat") in the toilet, how to empty and measure urinary catheter drainage, and how to count or weigh diapers.
- Instruct and provide the rationale for regular weight monitoring to the client and family. Weigh at the same time of day, using the same scale and with the client wearing the same amount of clothing.
- Educate and provide the rationale to the client and family on when to contact a healthcare professional, such as in the cases of a significant change in urine output; any change of 2 kg (5 lb) or more in a 1- to 2-week period; prolonged episodes of vomiting, diarrhea, or inability to eat or drink; dry, sticky mucous membranes; extreme thirst; swollen fingers, feet, ankles, or legs; difficulty breathing, shortness of breath, or rapid heartbeat; and changes in behavior or mental status.

Maintaining Fluid Intake

- Establish a 24-hour plan for ingesting the fluids. Generally, half of the desired total volume is given during the day, and the other half is divided between the evening and night, with most of that ingested during the evening. For example, if 2,500 mL is to be ingested in 24 hours, the plan may specify 7 a.m.–3 p.m.: 1,500 mL; 3 p.m.–11 a.m.: 700 mL; and 11 p.m.–7 a.m.: 300 mL. Try to avoid the ingestion of large amounts of fluid immediately before bedtime to prevent the need to urinate during sleeping hours.
- Set short-term outcomes that the client can realistically meet. Examples include ingesting a glass of fluid every hour while awake or a pitcher of water by 12 noon.
- Explain to the client the reason for the required intake and the specific amount needed.
- Identify fluids the client likes and make available a variety of those items, including fruit juices, soft drinks, and milk (if allowed). Remember that beverages such as coffee and tea have a diuretic effect, so their consumption should be limited.

- Help clients to select foods that tend to become liquid at room temperature (e.g., gelatin, ice cream, sherbet, custard), if these are allowed.
- Encourage clients when possible to participate in maintaining the fluid intake record. This assists them to evaluate the achievement of desired outcomes.
- Be alert to any cultural implications of food and fluids. Some cultures may restrict certain foods and fluids and view others as having healing properties.

Helping Clients Increase Fluid Intake

- Teach family members the rationale for the importance of offering fluids regularly to clients who are unable to meet their own needs because of age, impaired mobility or cognition, or other conditions such as impaired swallowing due to a stroke.
- For clients who are confined to bed, supply appropriate cups, glasses, and straws to facilitate appropriate fluid intake and keep the fluids within easy reach.
- Make sure fluids are served at the appropriate temperature: hot fluids heated and cold fluids chilled.

Helping Clients Restrict Fluid Intake

- Explain the reason for the restricted intake and how much and what types of fluids are permitted orally. Many clients need to be informed that ice chips, gelatin, and ice cream, for example, are considered fluid.
- Help the client decide the amount of fluid to be taken with each meal, between meals, before bedtime, and with medications.
- Identify fluids or fluid-like substances the client likes and make sure that these are provided, unless contraindicated. A client who is allowed only 200 mL of fluid for breakfast, for example, should receive the type of fluid the client favors.
- Set short-term goals that make the fluid restriction more tolerable. For example, schedule a specified amount of fluid at one or two hourly intervals between meals. Some clients may prefer fluids only between meals if the food provided at mealtime helps relieve thirst.
- Place allowed fluids in small containers such as a 4-ounce juice glass to allow the perception of a full container.
- Periodically offer the client ice chips as an alternative to water, because ice chips when melted are approximately half of the frozen volume.
- Provide frequent mouth care and rinses to reduce the thirst sensation.
- Instruct the client to avoid ingesting or chewing salty or sweet foods (hard candy or gum), because these foods tend to produce thirst. Sugarless gum may be an alternative for some clients.

Referrals

- Make appropriate referrals to home health or community social services for assistance with resources such as intravenous infusions and access, enteral feedings, and homemaker or home health aide services to help with ADLs.
- Provide a list of sources for supplies such as commodes, catheters and drainage bags, measuring devices, tube feeding formulas, and electrolyte replacement drinks.

(*continued on next page*)

SKILL 7.1   Monitoring Intake and Output (continued)

Developmental Considerations

INFANTS AND CHILDREN

Infants are at high risk for fluid and electrolyte imbalance because

- Their immature kidneys cannot concentrate urine.
- They have a rapid respiratory rate and proportionately larger body surface area than adults, leading to greater insensible losses through the skin and respirations.
- They cannot express thirst, nor actively seek fluids.

Vomiting and/or diarrhea in infants and young children can lead quickly to electrolyte imbalance. Oral rehydration therapy (ORT) with electrolyte solutions such as Pedialyte should be used to restore fluid and electrolyte balance in mild to moderate dehydration. Prompt treatment with ORT can prevent the need for IV therapy and hospitalization. Even if the child is vomiting, small sips of ORT can be helpful.

OLDER ADULTS

Older adults are at high risk for fluid and electrolyte imbalance because of decreases in:

- Thirst sensation
- Ability of the kidneys to concentrate urine
- Intracellular fluid and total body water
- Response to body hormones that help regulate fluid and electrolytes.

Other factors that may influence fluid and electrolyte balance in older adults are:

- Use of diuretics for hypertension and heart disease
- Decreased intake of food and water, especially in older adults with dementia or who are dependent on others to feed them and offer them fluids
- Preparations for diagnostic tests that include being NPO for long period of time, laxatives, or contrast dyes
- Impaired renal function, for example in older adults with diabetes.

All of these conditions increase older adults' risk for fluid and electrolyte imbalance, particularly under conditions that tax the normal compensatory mechanisms, such as a fever, influenza, surgery, or heat exposure. The change can happen quickly and become serious in a short time. Astute observations and quick actions by the nurse can help prevent serious consequences. A change in mental status may be the first symptom of impairment and must be further evaluated to determine the cause.

Setting of Care

Assess for the following:

CLIENT

- Risk factors for imbalance: the client's age, medications required such as diuretic therapy or corticosteroids, and presence of chronic diseases such as diabetes, heart disease, lung disease, or dementia
- Self-care abilities for maintaining fluid intake: mobility; ability to swallow, to access fluids and respond to thirst
- Current level of knowledge (as appropriate) about any fluid restrictions, actions and side effects of prescribed medications, regular weight monitoring, gastric tube care and enteral feedings, and parenteral fluids and nutrition

FAMILY

- Caregiver availability, skills, and responses: availability and willingness to assume responsibility for care, knowledge and ability to provide assistance with maintaining adequate intake of fluids, knowledge of risk factors and early warning signs of problems
- Family role changes and coping: effect on financial status, parenting and spousal roles, social roles

▶ INTRAVENOUS THERAPY

Expected Outcomes

1. Fluid and electrolyte needs are met.
2. IV catheter inserted at appropriate site without difficulty.
3. IV fluids infuse at prescribed rate without complications.
4. IV catheter type/size and equipment are appropriate for client.
5. Fluids are administered without adverse effects.
6. IV site remains clean without signs of infection or infiltration.
7. IV is converted to a saline lock and is functioning properly.
8. Central vascular line is properly placed without complication.
9. Central vascular line remains patent and free of infection.
10. CVP monitoring guides fluid management.
11. Central vascular catheter dressing is changed without complications.
12. Access cap is replaced maintaining sterile technique.
13. IV catheter maintains patency with use of CLC 2000 device.
14. Catheter site remains free of infection.
15. Blood samples are obtained without difficulty.
16. Infusions of medications or fluids are accomplished without difficulty.

SKILL 7.2   Establishing Intravenous Infusions

Many clients require administration of fluids or medications directly into the vascular system through **intravenous** (within or into the vein) devices. Nurses provide a significant amount of this type of therapy both in the hospital and in ambulatory settings and must have substantial knowledge and skill to practice according to safety standards. Changes in principles and practice of intravenous (IV) therapy are always occurring and, therefore, continuing education regarding IV therapy is an ongoing nursing responsibility.

SKILL 7.2   Establishing Intravenous Infusions (continued)

CLINICAL ALERT

Peripheral IVs should be started using aseptic technique. IVs started without proper asepsis, for example, in an emergency or outside the hospital, should be replaced at the earliest opportunity, and within 24 hours.

Do not shave the venipuncture site. Shaving can facilitate the development of infection through the multiplication of organisms in resulting microabrasions. Hairy sites can be clipped with scissors.

Some agencies allow only certified IV therapists to perform venipuncture.

Meticulous care must be used to insert the winged-tipped needle because these needles lead to majority of reported needlestick injuries.

All tape placed under transparent dressings should be sterile. Check facility policy before securing IV site. Some hospitals do not allow tape under the transparent dressing.

Source: Intravenous Nurses Society, Standard 49, 2006.

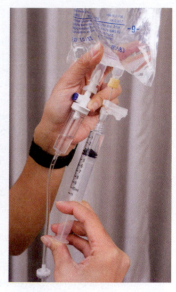

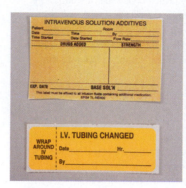

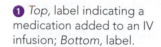

1 *Top*, label indicating a medication added to an IV infusion; *Bottom*, label.

2 Inserting a medication through the injection port of an infusing container.

Delegation

Due to the use of sterile technique, IV infusion therapy is not delegated to UAP. UAP may care for clients receiving IV therapy, and the nurse must ensure that the UAP knows how to perform routine tasks such as bathing and positioning without disturbing the IV. The UAP should also know what complications or adverse signs, such as leakage, should be reported to the nurse.

Equipment

- Clean gloves
- Infusion set
- Sterile parenteral solution
- Labels for IV tubing and container
- IV pole
- Nonallergenic tape
- Electronic infusion device or pump, as determined by the nurse

Preparation

- If possible, select a time to establish the infusion that is convenient for the client. Unless initiating IV therapy is urgent, provide any scheduled care before initiation to minimize excessive movement of the affected limb.
- Make sure that the client's clothing or gown can be removed over the IV apparatus if necessary. Many agencies provide special gowns that open over the shoulder and down the sleeve for easy removal.

Procedure

1. Prior to performing the procedure, check physician's order, introduce self and verify the client's identity using agency protocol. Explain to the client what you are going to do, why it is necessary, and how he or she can participate. If possible, explain how long the infusion will need to remain in place.
2. Perform hand hygiene and observe other appropriate infection control procedures.
3. Apply a medication label to the solution container if a medication was added **1 2**.

- In many agencies, medications and labels are applied in the pharmacy; if they are not, apply the label so it can be read easily when the container is hanging up.
4. Apply a timing strip to the solution container.
   - Mark the strip to indicate the anticipated fluid level at hourly intervals.
   - The timing strip may be applied at the time the infusion is started. Follow agency practice. See discussion of regulating infusion flow rates.
5. Open and prepare the infusion set.
   - Remove tubing from the container, and straighten it out.
   - Slide the tubing clamp along the tubing until it is just below the drip chamber to facilitate its access.
   - Close the clamp.
   - Leave the ends of the tubing covered with the plastic caps until the infusion is started. **Rationale:** *This will maintain the sterility of the ends of the tubing.*
6. Spike the solution container.
   - Expose the insertion site of the bag or bottle by removing the protective cover.
   - Remove the cap from the spike, and insert the spike into the insertion site of the bag or bottle **3**.

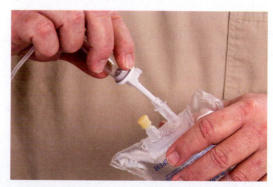

3 Inserting the spike.

(continued on next page)

SKILL 7.2 Establishing Intravenous Infusions (continued)

7. Hang the solution container on the pole.
   - Adjust the pole so that the container is suspended about 1 m (3 ft) above the client's head. **Rationale:** *This height is needed to enable gravity to overcome venous pressure and facilitate flow of the solution into the vein.*
8. Partially fill the drip chamber with solution.
   - Squeeze the chamber gently until it is half full of solution ❹. **Rationale:** *The drip chamber is partly filled with solution to prevent air from moving down the tubing.*
9. Prime the tubing as described below. The term *prime* means "to make ready," but in common use refers to flushing the tubing to remove air.
   - Remove the protective cap, and hold the tubing over a container. Maintain the sterility of the end of the tubing and the cap.
   - Release the clamp, and let the fluid run through the tubing until all bubbles are removed. Tap the tubing if necessary with your fingers to help the bubbles move. **Rationale:** *The tubing is primed to prevent the introduction of air into the client. Air bubbles smaller than 0.5 mL usually do not cause problems in peripheral lines.*
   - Reclamp the tubing, and replace the tubing cap, maintaining sterile technique.
   - For caps with air vents, do not remove the cap when priming this tubing. **Rationale:** *The flow of solution through the tubing will cease when the cap is moist with one drop of solution.*
   - If an infusion control pump or controller is being used, follow the manufacturer's directions for inserting the tubing and setting the infusion rate.
10. Disconnect the used tubing or remove the cap on an intermittent device.
    - Apply clean gloves.
    - Place a sterile swab under the hub of the catheter. **Rationale:** *This absorbs any leakage that might occur when the tubing is disconnected.*
    - Clamp the tubing. With the fourth or fifth finger of the nondominant hand, apply pressure to the vein above the end of the catheter. **Rationale:** *This helps prevent blood from coming out of the IV catheter during the change of tubing.*
    - Holding the hub of the catheter with the nondominant hand, remove the tubing or cap with the dominant hand, using a twisting and pulling motion. **Rationale:** *Holding the catheter firmly but gently maintains its position in the vein.*
    - Place the end of the used tubing or cap in a basin or other receptacle.

VARIATION: STARTING AN INFUSION ON A CENTRAL LINE

- Apply clean gloves and mask.
- Clean the junction of the catheter and tubing or cap with antiseptic, as required by agency protocol. **Rationale:** *This prevents the transfer of microorganisms from the client's skin to the open catheter hub when it is detached; it also decreases the number of microorganisms at the catheter–tubing junction.*
- Clamp the catheter and disconnect the tubing or cap, using a twisting, pulling motion. If the catheter does not have a clamp, ask the client to perform the Valsalva maneuver (that is, to take a deep breath and bear down) and to turn the head

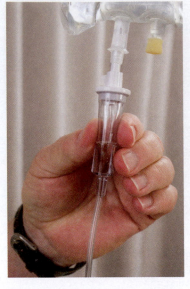

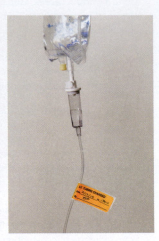

❹ Squeezing the drip chamber.   ❺ Tubing labeled with date, time, and nurse's initials.

away while you detach the tubing or cap. **Rationale:** *Performance of the Valsalva maneuver increases intrathoracic pressure, which reduces the risk of air entering the catheter. Turning the head to the side reduces the chances of contaminating the equipment.*

11. Connect the new tubing, and establish the infusion.
    - Continue to hold the catheter and grasp the new tubing with the dominant hand.
    - Remove the protective tubing cap and, maintaining sterility, insert the tubing end securely into the IV catheter hub.
    - Open the clamp to start the solution flowing.
12. Ensure appropriate infusion flow.
    - Remove and discard gloves. Perform hand hygiene.
    - Apply a padded arm board to splint the joint, as needed.
    - Adjust the infusion rate of flow according to the order.
13. Label the IV tubing.
    - Label the tubing with the date and time of attachment and your initials ❺. This labeling may also be done when the container is set up. **Rationale:** *The tubing is labeled to ensure that it is changed at regular intervals (i.e., every 24 to 96 hours according to agency policy).*

CLINICAL ALERT
The CDC has not established a recommendation for hang time of IV fluids. Follow hospital policy and change fluids accordingly.

14. Loop the tubing and secure it with tape to the client's skin. **Rationale:** *Looping and securing the tubing prevent the weight of the tubing or any movement from pulling on the IV catheter.*
15. Document all assessments and interventions.
    - Record the infusion in the client's chart. Some agencies provide a special form for this purpose ❻. Include the date and time of beginning the infusion; amount and type of solution used, including any additives (e.g., kind and amount of medications); container number; flow rate; and the client's general response.

SKILL 7.2   Establishing Intravenous Infusions *(continued)*

Division of Nursing
Oakland, California 94609

VENIPUNCTURE

DATE	TIME	SITE CODE	TYPE / GAUGE NEEDLE	INIT.	DC DATE	INIT.

CODES

SITE LOCATION:

RH	HAND	LH	HAND
RF	FOREARM	LF	FOREARM
RA	ANTECUBITAL	LA	ANTECUBITAL
RU	UPPER ARM	LU	UPPER ARM
RS	SUBCLAVIAN	LS	SUBCLAVIAN
RJ	JUGULAR	LJ	JUGULAR
RL	LEG	LL	LEG
VA	VASCULAR ACCESS		

SITE CONDITION:
A. PATENT WITHOUT REDNESS OR SWELLING
   OCCLUSIVE DRESSING INTACT
B. PATENT WITH MILD REDNESS AND/OR SWELLING
   OCCLUSIVE DRESSING INTACT
C. DRAINAGE (SEE NOTE)
D. DISLODGED / OCCLUDED
E. INFILTRATED
F. OCCLUSIVE DRESSING CHANGED

I.V. ORDERS

DATE ORDERED	INITIALS TRANS.	CHECK	SOLUTION / ADDITIVE(S)	INFUSION RATE	DURATION

I.V.'s ADMINISTERED

DATE	TIME	INIT.	SITE LOC.	BOTTLE NUMBER	SOLUTION / ADDITIVE(S)	SHIFT	AMOUNT ABSORBED	AMOUNT REMAINING	TIME TUBING CHANGE	SITE COND.	TOTAL INFUSED
						0600					
						1400					
						2200					
						0600					
						1400					
						2200					
						0600					
						1400					
						2200					
						0600					
						1400					
						2200					
						0600					
						1400					
						2200					
						0600					
						1400					
						2200					

SIGN.

INIT.	SIGNATURE / TITLE	INIT.	SIGNATURE / TITLE	INIT.	SIGNATURE / TITLE

SUMMIT MEDICAL CENTER

Intravenous Therapy Record

AFFIX PATIENT
I.D. LABEL HERE

MPN-105 86-6105-0

6 IV flow record.

SKILL 7.3 Performing Venipuncture with All Variations

Before preparing the infusion, first **verify the primary care provider's order** indicating the type of solution, the amount to be administered, and the rate of flow or time over which the infusion is to be completed.

Prior to venipuncture, consider how long the client is likely to have the IV, the kind of fluids to be infused, and medications the client will be receiving or is likely to receive intravenously. These factors may affect choice of vein and catheter size. Review the client record regarding previous venipuncture and client allergies (e.g., to tape or povidone-iodine). Note any difficulties encountered and how they were resolved **1** – **9**.

Delegation

Due to the need for knowledge of anatomy and use of sterile technique, IV infusion therapy is not delegated to unlicensed assistive personnel (UAP). UAP may care for clients receiving IV therapy, and the nurse must ensure that the UAP knows how to perform routine tasks such as bathing and positioning without disturbing the IV. The UAP should also know what complications or adverse signs, such as leakage, should be reported to the nurse. In many states, an LPN or LVN with special IV therapy training may start IV infusions. Check the applicable state's nurse practice act.

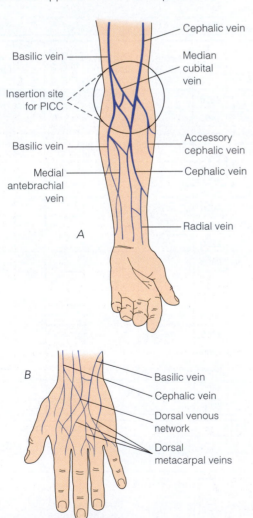

1 Commonly used venipuncture sites of the *A*, arm; *B*, hand. Part A also shows the site used for a peripherally inserted central catheter (PICC).

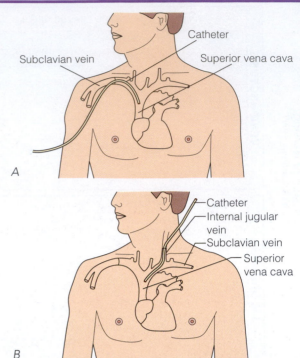

2 Central venous catheters with *A*, subclavian insertion; *B*, left jugular vein insertion.

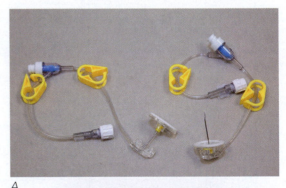

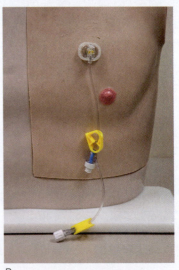

3 *A*, An implantable venous access device and a Huber needle with extension tubing; *B*, device shown on model.

SKILL 7.3   **Performing Venipuncture with All Variations** (*continued*)

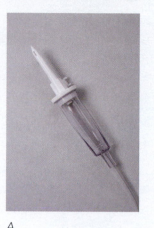

④ A plastic intravenous fluid container.

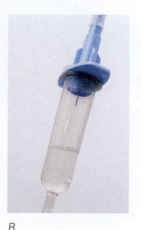

A   *B*

⑥ Infusion set spikes and drip chambers: *A,* nonvented macrodrip; *B,* nonvented microdrip.

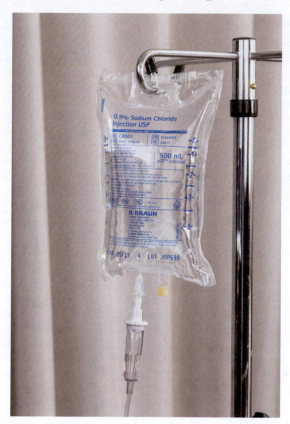

Protector cap for insertion spike

Spike connector for fluid container

Connector to IV catheter

Drip chamber

Secondary port

Clamp

Secondary port

Clamp

⑤ A standard IV administration set.

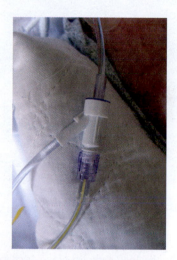

A

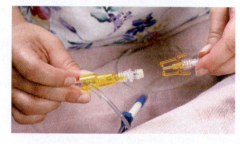

B

⑦ Needleless cannulas used to connect the tubing of secondary sets to primary tubing: *A,* threaded cannula; *B,* lever-lock cannula. (*Source for A: © Slaven MD/Custom Medical Stock Photo.*)

Equipment

Substitute appropriate supplies if the client has tape, antiseptic, or latex allergies.

- Nonallergenic tape
- Clean gloves
- Tourniquet
- Antiseptic swabs such as 10% povidone-iodine or 2% chlorhexidine gluconate (CHG) with alcohol or 70% isopropyl alcohol (CHG is the preferred agent [Phillips, 2010].)

(*continued on next page*)

SKILL 7.3 Performing Venipuncture with All Variations (continued)

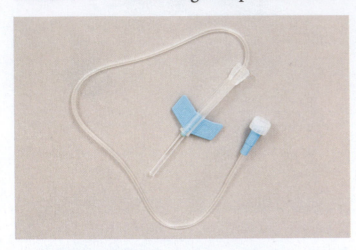

8 A butterfly IV needle.

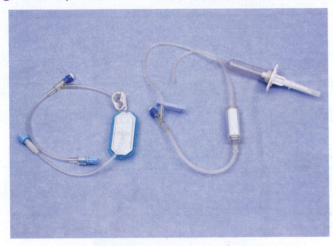

9 Two types of IV filters.

- IV catheter (Choose an IV catheter of the appropriate type and size based on the size of the vein and the purpose of the IV. A 20- to 22-gauge catheter is indicated for most adults. Always have an extra catheter and ones of different sizes available.)
- Sterile gauze dressing or transparent semipermeable membrane (TSM) dressing (preferred)
- Stabilization device
- Splint, if required
- Towel or bed protector
- Local anesthetic (optional and per agency policy)

Preparation

- If possible, select a time to perform the venipuncture that is convenient for the client. Unless initiating IV therapy is urgent, provide any scheduled care before insertion to minimize excessive movement of the affected limb. **Rationale:** *Moving the limb after insertion could dislodge the catheter.*
- Make. sure the client's clothing or gown can be removed over the IV apparatus if necessary. Some agencies provide special gowns that open over the shoulder and down the sleeve for easy removal.
- Visitors or family members may be asked to leave the room if desired by the nurse or the client.

Procedure

1. Prior to performing the procedure, introduce self and verify the client's identity using agency protocol. Explain to the client what you are going to do, why it is necessary, and how he or she can participate. Venipuncture can cause discomfort for a few seconds, but there should be no ongoing pain after insertion. If possible, explain how long the IV will need to remain in place and how it will be used.
2. Perform hand hygiene and observe other appropriate infection control procedures.
3. Prepare the client.
   - Assist the client to a comfortable position, either sitting or lying. Expose the limb to be used but provide for client privacy.
4. Select the venipuncture site.
   - Use the client's nondominant arm, unless contraindicated (e.g., mastectomy, fistula for dialysis). Identify possible venipuncture sites by looking for veins that are relatively straight. The vein should be palpable, but may not be visible, especially in clients with dark skin. Consider the catheter length; look for a site sufficiently distal to the wrist or elbow where the tip of the catheter will not be at a point of flexion. **Rationale:** *Sclerotic veins may make initiating and maintaining the IV difficult. Joint flexion increases the risk of irritation of vein walls by the catheter.*
   - Check agency protocol about shaving if the site is very hairy. Shaving is not recommended. **Rationale:** *Shaving has the potential to cause microabrasions, which can increase the risk of infection.*
   - Place a towel or bed protector under the extremity to protect linens (or furniture if in the home).
5. Dilate the vein.
   - Place the extremity in a dependent position (lower than the client's heart). **Rationale:** *Gravity slows venous return and distends the veins. Distending the veins makes it easier to insert the IV properly.*
   - Apply a tourniquet firmly 15 to 20 cm (6 to 8 in.) above the venipuncture site if the blood pressure is within normal range **10**. If the client has hypertension, place the tourniquet higher on the arm. If the client is hypotensive, move the tourniquet closer to the venipuncture site (Phillips, 2010, p. 322). Explain that the tourniquet will feel tight. **Rationale:** *The tourniquet must be tight enough to obstruct venous flow but not so tight that it occludes arterial flow. Obstructing arterial flow inhibits venous filling. If a radial pulse can be palpated, the arterial flow is not obstructed.*

Use the tourniquet on only one client. This avoids cross-contamination to other clients. Be sure to ask if the client has a latex allergy.

   - For older adults with fragile skin, instead of applying a tourniquet, place the arm in a dependent position to allow the veins to engorge. **Rationale:** *The tourniquet can cause tissue damage and may not be needed to allow the vein to dilate.*

SKILL 7.3   Performing Venipuncture with All Variations (continued)

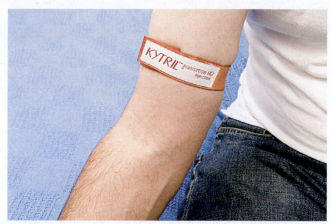

A

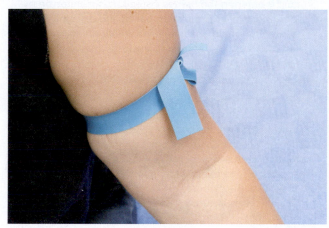

B

⑩ Two types of tourniquets.

- If the vein is not sufficiently dilated:
  a. Massage or stroke the vein distal to the site and in the direction of venous flow toward the heart. **Rationale:** *This action helps fill the vein.*
  b. Encourage the client to clench and unclench the fist. **Rationale:** *Contracting the muscles compresses the distal veins, forcing blood along the veins and distending them.*
  c. Lightly tap the vein with your fingertips. **Rationale:** *Tapping may distend the vein.*
- If the preceding steps fail to distend the vein so that it is palpable, remove the tourniquet and wrap the extremity in a warm, moist towel for 10 to 15 minutes. **Rationale:** *Heat dilates superficial blood vessels, causing them to fill. Then repeat steps to dilate the vein.*

6. Minimize insertion pain as much as possible.
- Although the pain of insertion should be brief, prevention can and should be offered. Simple refrigeration of the skin by placing ice topically for 3 minutes provides enough analgesia to carry out the insertion with minimal pain (Movahedi et al., 2007). Transdermal analgesic creams (e.g., EMLA, Synera) may also be used, depending on policy. Allow at least 30 minutes for the topical analgesic to take effect (Phillips, 2010).

- If desired and permitted by policy, inject 0.03 mL of 1% lidocaine (without epinephrine) or normal saline intradermally over the site where you plan to insert the IV catheter. (Be sure to first apply gloves and clean the skin site as described in step 7 below.) Allow 5 to 10 seconds for the anesthetic to take effect (Phillips, 2010).

7. Apply clean gloves and clean the venipuncture site. **Rationale:** *Gloves protect the nurse from contamination by the client's blood.*
- Clean the skin at the site of entry with a topical antiseptic swab (e.g., 2% CHG or alcohol). Some institutions may use an anti-infective solution such as povidone-iodine (check agency protocol). Check for allergies to iodine or shellfish before cleansing skin with Betadine or other iodine products.
- Use a back-and-forth motion for a minimum of 30 seconds to scrub the insertion site and surrounding area (Phillips, 2010).
- Allow the site to dry completely before insertion of the catheter. Povidone-iodine should be in contact with the skin for 1 minute to be effective. Alcohol should not be applied after the application of the povidone-iodine preparation because it negates the effects of the povidone-iodine (Infusion Nurses Society [INS], 2006).

> **CLINICAL ALERT**
> If using a needleless angiocath system, once the "flash" is noted and the catheter is advanced, the retract button is pushed and the needle automatically shielded.

8. Insert the catheter and initiate the infusion.
- Remove the catheter assembly from its sterile packaging. Review instructions for using the catheter because a variety of needle-safety devices are manufactured. Remove the cover of the needle (stylet).
- Use the nondominant hand to pull the skin taut below the entry site. **Rationale:** *This stabilizes the vein and makes the skin taut for needle (stylet) entry. It can also make initial tissue penetration less painful.*
- Holding the over-the-needle at a 15- to 30-degree angle with the needle (stylet) bevel up, insert the catheter through the skin and into the vein. A sudden lack of resistance is felt as the needle (stylet) enters the vein. Use a slow, steady insertion technique and avoid jabbing or stabbing motions.
- Once blood appears in the lumen or clear "flashback" chamber, lower the angle of the catheter until it is almost parallel with the skin, and advance the needle (stylet) and catheter approximately 0.5 to 1 cm (about 1/4 in.) farther **⑪**. Holding the assembly steady, advance the catheter until the hub is at the venipuncture site. The exact technique depends on the type of device used. **Rationale:** *The catheter is advanced to ensure that it, and not just the needle (stylet), is in the vein.*
- If there is no blood return, try redirecting the catheter assembly again toward the vein. If the needle/stylet has been withdrawn from the catheter even a small distance, or

(continued on next page)

SKILL 7.3   Performing Venipuncture with All Variations (continued)

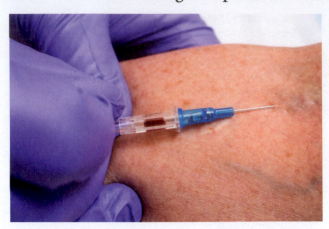

⑪ Blood is noted in the flashback chamber once the stylet has entered the vein.

the catheter tip has been pulled out of the skin, the catheter must be discarded and a new one used. **Rationale:** *Reinserting the needle (stylet) into the catheter can result in damage or slicing of the catheter. A catheter that has been removed from the skin is considered contaminated and cannot be reused.*

CLINICAL ALERT

If no blood is observed and you did not feel the catheter enter the vein, pull back on entire catheter apparatus without exiting skin. Reassess vein position, then reattempt venipuncture. If you are not successful, remove catheter and look for a different site. Remember the catheter is now contaminated and cannot be used again. Most facilities allow the nurse to attempt two venipunctures; if unsuccessful, they must notify another professional to attempt venipuncture.

- If blood begins to flow out of the vein into the tissues as the catheter is inserted, creating a hematoma, the insertion has not been successful. This is sometimes referred to as a "blown vein." Immediately release the tourniquet and remove the catheter, applying pressure over the insertion site with dry gauze. Attempt the venipuncture in another site, in the opposite arm if possible. **Rationale:** *Placing the tourniquet back on the same arm above the unsuccessful site may cause it to bleed. Placing the IV below the unsuccessful site could result in infusing fluid into the already punctured vein, causing it to leak.*
- Release the tourniquet.
- Put pressure on the vein proximal to the catheter to eliminate or reduce blood oozing out of the catheter. Stabilize the hub with thumb and index finger of the nondominant hand.
- Remove the protective cap from the distal end of the tubing and hold it ready to attach to the catheter, maintaining the sterility of the end.

- Stabilize the catheter hub and apply pressure distal to the catheter with your finger. **Rationale:** *This prevents excessive blood flow through the catheter.*
- Carefully remove the needle (stylet), engage the needle-safety device (if it does not engage automatically), and attach the end of the infusion tubing to the catheter hub. Place the needle (stylet) directly into a sharps container. If this is not within reach, place the needle (stylet) into its original package and dispose in a sharps container as soon as possible.
- Initiate the infusion or flush the catheter with sterile normal saline. **Rationale:** *Blood must be removed from the catheter lumen and tubing immediately. Otherwise, the blood will clot inside the lumen.* Watch closely for any signs that the catheter has been infiltrated. Infiltration occurs when the tip of the IV is outside the vein and the fluid is entering the tissues instead. It is manifested by localized swelling, coolness, pallor, and discomfort at the IV site. **Rationale:** *Inflammation or infiltration necessitates removal of the IV catheter to avoid further trauma to the tissues.*

9. Stabilize the catheter and apply a dressing.

- Secure the catheter according to the manufacturer's instructions and agency policy. Several methods are used to stabilize the catheter, including the use of a dressing and securement device. If tape is used, it must be sterile tape or surgical strips and they should be applied only to the catheter adapter and not placed directly on the catheter–skin junction site (INS, 2006). Use of a manufactured stabilization device is preferred (INS, 2006).
- Two methods are used for applying a dressing: a sterile gauze dressing secured with tape and a TSM dressing. Most common is the TSM because it allows for continuous assessment of the site, it is more comfortable than gauze and tape, and the client can bathe or shower without saturating the dressing (Phillips, 2010, p. 337). Do not use ointment of any kind under a TSM dressing. Additional tape may be used to secure the IV catheter below the TSM, if necessary. Do not place tape on the TSM dressing.
- Label the dressing with the date and time of insertion; type, gauge and length of catheter used; and your initials.
- Apply an IV site protector, if available. Protective devices are available that help prevent dislodgment of the IV catheter and still provide easy assessment of the IV site.
- Loop the tubing and secure it with tape. **Rationale:** *Looping and securing the tubing prevent the weight of the tubing or any movement from pulling on the IV catheter.*

10. Discard the tourniquet. Remove and discard gloves. Perform hand hygiene.

11. Discard all used disposable supplies in appropriate receptacles. Cleanse any blood spills according to agency policy. Clean any reusable supplies.

SKILL 7.3   Performing Venipuncture with All Variations (continued)

12. Document relevant data, including assessments.

- Record the venipuncture on the client's chart. Some agencies provide a special form for this purpose. Include the date and time of the venipuncture; type, length, and gauge of the IV catheter; venipuncture site; how many attempts were made and the location of each attempt; and the type of dressing.

Sample Documentation

4/7/2015 0600 Inserted 20-gauge, 1-inch angiocath in the right cephalic vein 4 inches above the (L) wrist on first attempt. Stat-Lock used to stabilize catheter and Tegaderm dressing applied. IV infusing at 125 mL/hr. Explained reason for IV. Verbalized understanding. _____A. Luis, RN

Developmental Considerations

INFANTS/CHILDREN

- Because infants do not have large veins in the antecubital fossa, blood specimens for examination are usually taken from the external jugular and femoral veins.
- Use a doll to demonstrate venipuncture for children and explain the procedure to the parents.
- Explain the procedure to the young client, encourage questions, and be alert for nonverbal cues. Children may not understand things that seem obvious to adults. For example, a child may think the IV therapy is a punishment.
- Venipuncture can be extremely frightening for children. Simply numbing the skin with ice prior to insertion will reduce the discomfort. When prior planning is an option, EMLA cream (lidocaine and prilocaine) topical anesthetic can be applied ahead of time with an occlusive dressing to cover. Remove all of the cream and clean the site prior to insertion.
- Even with analgesia, many children will resist, cry, and even become combative. Parents, in turn, may become upset. Offering distractions and rewards may help. Helping the child to take deep, slow breaths can also trigger some degree of relaxation. Sometimes it is necessary to restrain the child. Most pediatric professionals believe that it is best if a person other than the child's parent holds the child, so the child doesn't associate the parent with the fear and pain. It is important for the parent to remain with the child, soothing the child with voice, closeness, and touch. Some parents are not able to do this, and they need support and understanding from nursing staff. A calm demeanor on the nurse's part (and relaxation breathing) will help ease this potentially upsetting situation for all concerned.
- A 24-gauge catheter or needle is commonly indicated for use with children.
- Apply age-appropriate restraints, arm boards, or other devices to protect the IV site.

OLDER ADULTS

- Skin is often fragile and bruises easily. Select an IV site with adequate healthy tissue to support the IV catheter.
- To distend the vein, tap only lightly to prevent trauma.
- Consider not using a tourniquet. The older adult's superficial veins are often large enough to insert the needle (stylet) without further distention. Using a tourniquet can cause the vein to burst when the needle (stylet) enters.
- Minimize the use of alcohol and tape to avoid irritating sensitive skin.

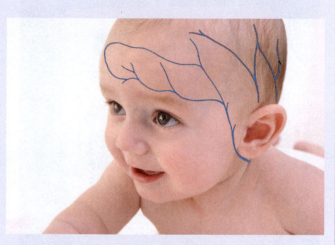

Scalp veins on an infant are frequently used for peripheral IV access. Villareal/Photo Researchers, Inc.

Practice Guidelines

VEIN SELECTION

- Use distal veins of the arm first; subsequent IV starts should be proximal to the previous site.
- Use the client's nondominant arm whenever possible. **Rationale:** *This minimizes the client's restricted mobility and function.*
- Select a vein that is:
  a. Easily palpated and feels soft and full.
  b. Naturally splinted by bone.
  c. Large enough to allow adequate circulation around the catheter.
- Avoid using veins that are:
  a. In areas of flexion (e.g., the antecubital fossa).
  b. Highly visible. **Rationale:** *These veins tend to roll away from the needle (style).*
  c. Damaged by previous use, phlebitis, infiltration, or sclerosis.
  d. Continually distended with blood, knotted, or tortuous.
  e. In a surgically compromised or injured extremity (e.g., following a mastectomy). **Rationale:** *These sites may have impaired circulation and cause discomfort for the client.*
  f. In the foot or legs unless arm veins are inaccessible, and with a primary care provider's order. **Rationale:** *Lower extremity sites are more prone to thrombus formation and subsequent emboli.*

SKILL 7.4 Regulating Infusion Flow Rate

Equipment

- Electronic infusion device (pump) ❶
- Device-compatible IV administration set
- Needless cannula
- Gloves

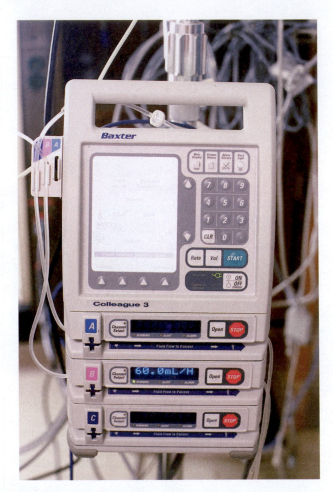

❶ Baxter multiple-channel pump.

Procedure

1. Prior to performing the procedure, check physician's order, introduce self and verify the client's identity using agency protocol. Explain to the client what you are going to do, why it is necessary, and how he or she can participate. Discuss the various sounds that can be heard during the use of the equipment.
2. Perform hand hygiene and observe other appropriate infection control procedures.
3. Close regulating clamp on the set tubing before hanging bag.
4. Spike IV solution bag.
5. Fill drip chamber to minimum one third full. **Rationale:** *This amount allows sufficient air space in drip chamber.*
6. Prime tubing by opening regulating clamp slowly and allowing tubing to fill with IV solution. If using a cassette-type tubing, follow package instructions to correctly prime the cassette portion of the tubing that engages into the control device.

Note: Check if tubing has an anti-free-flow device that must be opened prior to primary tubing.

7. Follow manufacturer's instructions to load administration set into device, taking care to fit tubing and cassette into appropriate receptor sites. (One type of pump is a multiple-channel pump that can infuse three different IV solutions at one time.)
8. Close device door and latch.
9. Perform hand hygiene and don gloves.
10. Check that client's venipuncture site is free from signs of vein irritation or infiltration.
11. Connect administration set tubing to establish infusion site.
12. Open regulating clamp on administration set.
13. Turn device ON.
14. Set device parameters for operation, again following manufacturer's instructions or machine's setup prompts. Parameters may include:
    - Infusion (e.g., primary)
    - Volume to be infused
    - Rate (mL/hr)
    - Pressure (measure can vary; e.g., mmHg, cm H_2O, or psi).
15. START device when parameters are set.
16. Observe that infusion is running properly.
17. Remove and discard gloves. Perform hand hygiene.
18. Check client's infusion site frequently.

VARIATION: MANUALLY SETTING FLOW RATE

- Check manufacturer's drip-rate calibration on administration set package. Macrodrip sets vary from 10 to 15 gtt per 1 mL. Microdrip factor is 60 drops/mL.
- Check physician's order for amount of fluid to be delivered per unit of time (e.g., 1 L every 8 hr, or hourly flow rate such as 100 mL/hr).
- Calculate flow rate.
  - To find the number of milliliters to be given per hour:

    $\dfrac{\text{Total solution}}{\text{No. of hours to run}} = \text{mL/hr}$
  - To find drops per minute:

    $\dfrac{\text{mL/hr}* \text{drop factor}}{60 \text{ minutes}} = \text{gtts/minute}$
- Note drip chamber; count the drops in 1 minute (or in 15 seconds and multiply by 4).
- Adjust tubing clamp until the chamber drips the desired number of drops per minute (or 15-second increment).
- Monitor flow rate frequently—adjustments to maintain desired delivery are often necessary.

Nurses need to check infusions at least every hour to ensure that the indicated milliliters per hour have infused and to assess the IV site. A strip of adhesive marking the exact time and/or amount to be infused should be taped to the solution container. Some agencies make premarked labels available. Do not write directly on the IV bag. Writing directly on the IV bag with a ballpoint pen could damage the bag and contaminate the solution. A felt-tip pen should not be used directly on the bag or on the label because the ink could penetrate the label or bag surface, causing contamination of the solution. Additionally, the writing from felt-tip pens may become illegible with time.

SKILL 7.4   Regulating Infusion Flow Rate *(continued)*

Flow-regulating mechanisms that attach to the primary infusion administration set are called mechanical gravity control devices or mechanical controllers (Phillips, 2010, p. 282). The *Dial-A-Flo* in-line device ❷ is an example of a manual controller that delivers the amount of fluid to be administered. The Dial-A-Flo device may be used in situations where a pump is not available or required, but prevention of fluid overload is important. The nurse presets the volume to be infused by rotating the dial to the desired rate. It is still necessary for the nurse to count the drops to verify that the controller is working accurately. Another variation is a *volume-control set,* or *Volutrol,* which is used if the volume of fluid administered is to be carefully controlled. The set, which holds a maximum of 100 mL of solution, is attached below the solution container, and the drip chamber is placed below the set. Volume control sets are frequently used in pediatric settings, where the volume administered is critical.

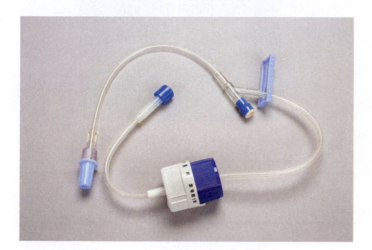

❷ The Dial-A-Flo mechanical gravity control device.

Devices such as battery-operated controllers and infusion pumps with alarm systems facilitate a regulated flow. An infusion pump delivers fluids intravenously by exerting positive pressure on the tubing or on the fluid. In situations where the fluid flow is unrestricted, the pump pressure is comparable to that of gravity flow. However, if restrictions develop (increased venous resistance), the pump can maintain the flow by increasing the pressure applied to the fluid.

Newer systems are programmable and include drug libraries with dose rate calculators, automatic flushing between medications, dual or triple simultaneous line control, memory, multiple alarm settings (air in line, pressure/resistance, battery), schedule

reminders, volume settings down to 0.1 mL, panel locks, and digital displays ❸ ❹. Pumps can exert pressure on the tubing or on the fluid if restrictions develop (increased venous resistance) to maintain the fluid flow.

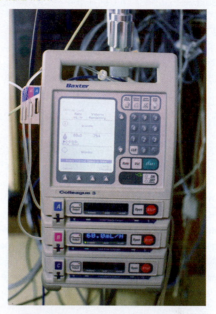

❸ Programmable infusion pump.

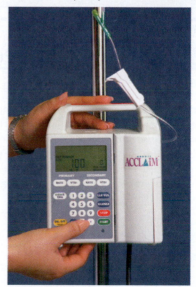

❹ An intravenous infusion pump.

If Alarm Sounds, Check the Following

Most devices have a message system that specifies the exact problem. You should be prepared to troubleshoot various components of the system.

- *Infusion complete:* When the exact volume to be delivered is set and the volume limit has been reached, an alarm sounds and the machine goes to a KVO "keep-vein-open" mode. Establish if the total volume of the container has been delivered; change the solution container if needed, and reset the volume to be infused.

- *Occlusion:* All devices sound an alarm when they cannot maintain delivery in the face of increasing resistance. In this instance, check the insertion site for infiltration, and look for position problems, pinched tubing, closed clamp, turned stopcock, or clogged filter.
- *Other problems:* Other messages may indicate "air in the line," "low battery," "cassette (improperly loaded)," or "free flow."
- *Nursing action:* Check trouble spot carefully, readjust, and restart the infusion.

(continued on next page)

SKILL 7.4 Regulating Infusion Flow Rate *(continued)*

IV Calorie Calculation

- 1,000 mL D_5W provides 50 g of dextrose.
- 50 g of dextrose provides 4 Cal/g; therefore, multiply 50 g × 4 Cal = 200 Cal.
- 1,000 mL D_5W provides 200 Cal.
- Usual IV fluid maintenance is 2,000 to 3,000 mL/day (400 to 600 Cal/day).
- 4 Cal/g is used in calculation; however, it is actually 3.4 Cal/g.

Factors That Influence IV Flow Rates When Using Gravity for Infusion

- Warm fluids drip faster than cold fluids.
- The higher the bag is above the insertion site, the faster the infusion.
- The greater the tilt of the IV administration equipment, the larger each drop from the drip chamber.
- The larger the catheter diameter, the faster the flow rate.
- The longer the catheter, the slower the flow rate because of resistance.
- Increased blood pressure or coughing will slow the flow rate (this is a temporary situation usually).

    Note: Because of these variables, manual control of IVs is not recommended. IV pumps are the most predictable method of infusing fluids.

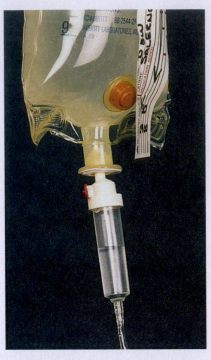

Count drops per minute to check accuracy of drip rate.

SKILL 7.5 Using an Infusion Pump or Controller

Delegation

Due to the need for sterile technique and technical complexity, use of infusion devices is not delegated to UAP. UAP may care for clients with such devices, and the nurse must ensure that the UAP knows how to perform routine tasks such as positioning and changing gowns when a device is in place. The UAP should also know what complications or adverse signs, such as alarms, should be reported to the nurse.

Equipment

- Infusion pump or controller
- IV solution or medication
- IV pole
- IV administration set with compatible IV tubing
- Alcohol swabs and tape
- Label for tubing
- Time strip for container

Preparation

- Review the use of the pump outside of the client's room. Read all appropriate materials and confirm how to set the device.
- Ensure that the tubing is the correct type for the device. Each manufacturer and model may require different tubing.

Procedure

1. Prior to performing the procedure, introduce self and verify the client's identity using agency protocol. Explain to the client what you are going to do, why it is necessary, and how he or she can participate. Explain what the device sounds like during normal use, the various alarms, and to notify the nurse if an alarm sounds.

2. Perform hand hygiene and observe other appropriate infection control procedures.

3. Prepare the client.

    - Check the client's identification band against the IV fluid container. **Rationale:** *This ensures that the correct client receives the infusion.*

    - Assist the client to a comfortable position, either sitting or lying. Expose the limb as needed but provide for client privacy. Make sure that the clothing or gown can be removed over the IV apparatus if necessary. Some agencies provide special gowns that open over the shoulder and down the sleeve for easy removal.

For an Infusion Controller

4. Attach the controller to the IV pole.

    - Attach the controller to the IV pole so that it will be below and in-line with the IV container.

    - Plug the machine into the electric outlet, unless battery power is used.

5. Set up the IV infusion.

    - Open the IV container, maintaining the sterility of the port, and spike the container with the administration set. Place the IV container on the IV pole, and position the drip chamber above the infusion controller.

    - Fill the drip chamber of the IV tubing one third full. **Rationale:** *If the drip chamber is filled more than halfway, the drops may be miscounted.*

SKILL 7.5 Using an Infusion Pump or Controller *(continued)*

- Prime the tubing according to the manufacturer's directions, and close the clamp.
6. Attach the IV drop sensor, and insert the IV tubing into the controller.
   - Attach the IV drop sensor (electronic eye) to the drip chamber so that it is below the drip orifice and above the fluid level in the drip chamber ❶. **Rationale:** *This placement ensures an accurate drop count. If the sensor is placed too high, it can miss drops; if placed too low, it may mistake splashes for drops.*

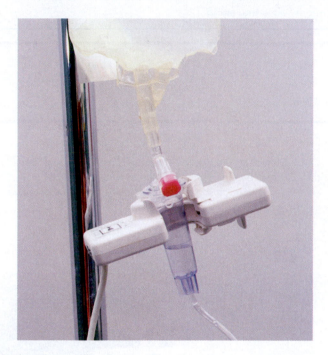

❶ The IV controller drop sensor.

- Make sure the sensor is plugged into the controller.
- Insert the tubing into the controller according to the manufacturer's instructions.
7. Initiate the infusion.
   - Perform a venipuncture or connect the tubing to the existing IV catheter.
8. Set volume control for the appropriate volume per hour.
   - Press the power button.
   - Close the door to the controller, and ensure that all tubing clamps are wide open. **Rationale:** *This enables the controller to regulate the fluid flow.*
   - Set the controls on the front of the controller to the appropriate infusion rate and volume.
   - Press the start button.
   - Count the drops for 15 seconds, and multiply the result by 4. **Rationale:** *This verifies that the rate has been correctly set and the controller is operating accurately.* (*Note:* In some cases the drops may fall at an uneven rate. If so, count the drops for 30 to 60 seconds to verify that the per-minute rate is correct.) Continue with step 9 below.

For an Infusion Pump

4. Attach the pump to the IV pole.
   - Attach the pump at eye level on the IV pole. **Rationale:** *Because the pump does not depend on gravity pressure,*

it can be placed at any level. Eye level is convenient for checking its functioning.
- Plug the machine into an electric outlet, unless battery power is used.
5. Set up the infusion.
   - Check the manufacturer's directions before using an IV filter or before infusing blood. **Rationale:** *Infusion pump pressures may damage filters or cause rate inaccuracies.*
   - Open the IV container, maintaining the sterility of the port, and spike the container with the administration set.
   - Place the IV container on the IV pole above the pump.
   - Fill the drip chamber.
   - Prime the tubing, and close the clamp. Some pumps have a cassette that must also be primed. Manufacturers give instructions for doing this. Often, the cassette must be tilted to be filled with fluid. Some pumps must have the power on and the tubing and cassette in place in order to perform priming.
6. Insert the IV tubing into the pump.
   - Press the power button to the on position.
   - Load the machine according to the manufacturer's instructions.
7. Initiate the infusion.
   - Perform venipuncture or connect the tubing to the IV catheter.
8. Set the controls for the required drops per minute or milliliters per hour.
   - Press the start button.
   - Check the drip chamber to ensure that fluid is flowing from the container.
9. Set the alarms. **Rationale:** *The alarms notify the nurse when a set volume of fluid has been infused or indicate malfunctioning of the equipment.*
10. Monitor the infusion.
   - Check the volume of fluid infused at least every hour, and compare it with the time tape on the IV container. This confirms the actual volume of fluid infused.
   - If the volume infused does not coincide with the time tape or the alarm sounds, begin at the client level and check that:
     a. The IV has not infiltrated or clotted at the insertion site.
     b. The tubing is not pinched, kinked, or disconnected.
     c. The appropriate tubing clamps are fully open.
     d. The sensors are correctly placed.
     e. The rate/volume settings are accurate.
     f. The drip chamber is correctly filled.
     g. The container still has solution.
     h. The time tape is accurate.
     i. The IV container is correctly placed.
11. Document relevant information.
   - Record the date and time of starting the infusion, the type and amount of fluid being infused, the rate at which it is being infused, the infusion device used, the status of the IV insertion site, and any adverse responses of the client.

CLINICAL ALERT
Observe IV site frequently when pumps are used. IV pumps do not normally detect infiltration at the IV site. Infiltration does not produce enough pressure to trigger an alarm. Check for edema, cool skin, discomfort, and tenderness at the IV site.

(continued on next page)

SKILL 7.5 Using an Infusion Pump or Controller *(continued)*

Developmental Considerations

INFANTS/CHILDREN

- Emphasize to children that the IV controller or pump is not a toy and should not be touched unless an adult is present. Children are naturally curious and will want to examine the equipment.
- Use a volume control infusion set (Volutrol, Buretrol, or Soluset) with a pump/controller for pediatric clients.
- Explain the procedure to young clients, encourage questions, and be alert for nonverbal cues. Children may not understand things that seem obvious to adults. For example, a child may think the IV therapy is a punishment.

OLDER ADULTS

- Check the IV flow rate frequently for older adults. Older adults are at increased risk to develop fluid overload if IV fluid is infused too rapidly.
- Check the IV site often for signs of infiltration. Veins become more fragile with aging.

SKILL 7.6 Using a "Smart" Pump

Equipment

- Point-of-care computer specific to nursing unit
- IV tubing
- IV fluids and/or IV medications

Procedure

1. Identify client by checking the client's identity band and asking client to state name and birth date. Explain pump's function.
2. Assemble equipment and bring to client's bedside.
3. Perform hand hygiene and observe other appropriate infection control procedures.
4. Verify IV site is patent and without signs of infiltration.
5. Plug pump into electrical outlet.
6. Insert the pump module into the point-of-care computer ("brain").
7. Spike IV fluid bag.
8. Prime IV tubing with appropriate solution.
9. Insert the IV tubing into the pump module and close the door to the pump ①–④.
10. View screen will ask which client care area is being used. **Rationale:** *The pump automatically configures itself to provide the infusion parameters for that area.*
11. Choose the intended drug and concentration from the list outlined on the screen ⑤ ⑥.
12. Enter the ordered dose and infusion rate; the pump checks this information against the drug library. If what was programmed matches the pump's drug library, the pump allows the infusion to begin. Follow manufacturer's directions on how to program the pump. Each manufacturer's equipment is somewhat different.
13. If an audible and visual alert occurs, the programmed data are outside the specified limits. The alert informs you about which parameter is out of the recommended range.
14. Depending on the medication or client care area, the pump will sound a "soft" alarm or a "hard" alarm. Some facilities allow a "soft" alarm to be overridden. If you override the alarm, the infusion will begin. This alarm is considered a minor error ⑦.

CLINICAL ALERT

Check the facility's policies and procedures to determine whether the pump can be run with the override or whether a verbal verification of the order with a physician or pharmacist must be obtained before proceeding.

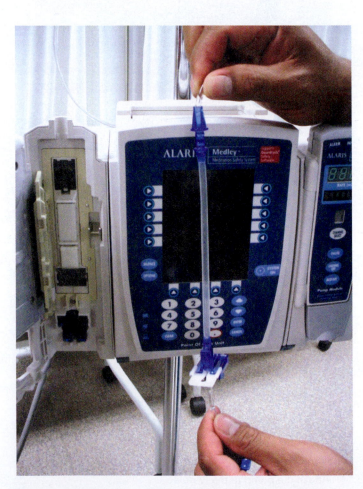

① Hang IV bag on pole. Prime tubing and insert into pump module cassette.

SKILL 7.6 Using a "Smart" Pump *(continued)*

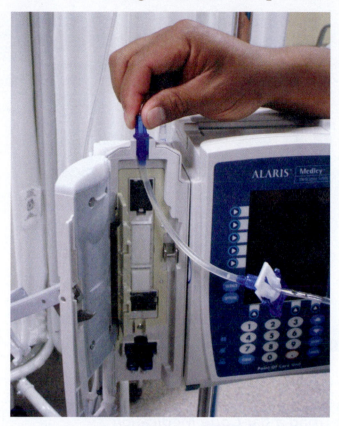

2 Place top of IV tubing into top of cassette; listen for click indicating it is seated.

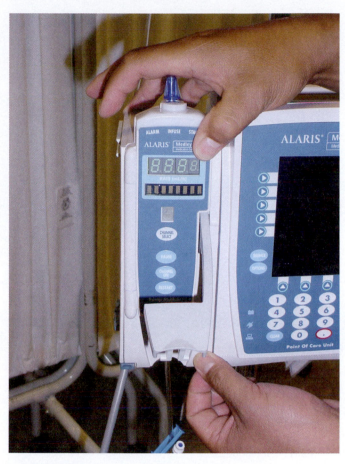

4 Close pump module door and lower locking lever.

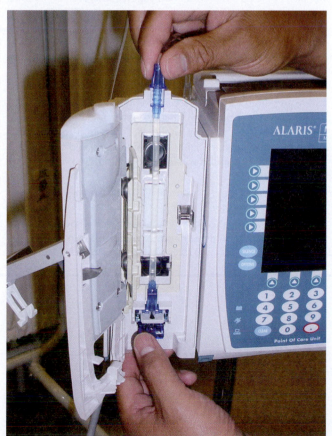

3 Insert white slide clamp into cassette; listen for click.

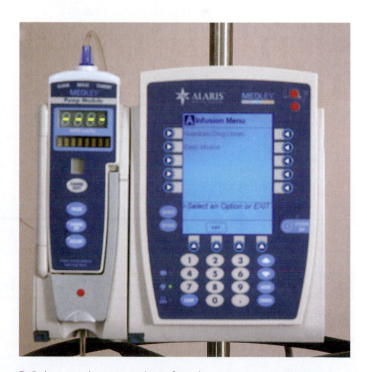

5 Select medication to be infused.

(continued on next page)

SKILL 7.6 Using a "Smart" Pump (continued)

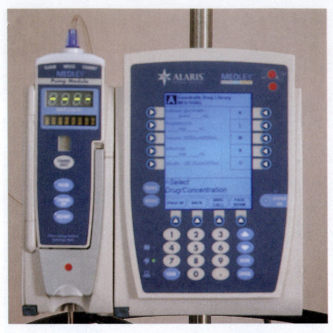

6 Check screen for drug name and infusion rate.

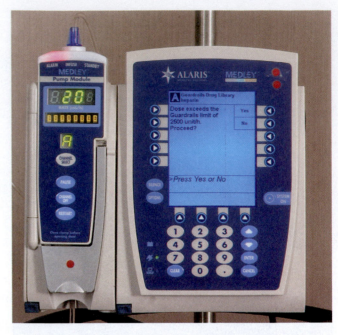

7 Check screen when "soft alert" sounds to determine problem.

15. When a "hard" alarm occurs, the pump shuts down. It cannot be overridden. Reprogram the pump with settings that are within your facility's specified limits to begin infusing when a "hard" alarm sounds.

    Note: The smart pump's software logs and tracks all alerts, recording the time, date, drug, concentration, and infusion rate, as well as any action taken, whether the pump is overridden or not.

16. Observe the screen to ensure medication is infusing at prescribed rate.

LEGAL ALERT

By 2006, the FDA had mandated that all drug manufacturers must label most prescription medications and certain over-the-counter drugs with machine-readable bar codes, using the National Drug Code number that uniquely identifies each drug, its dosage form, and its strength. The FDA predicts that using bar codes will prevent up to 500,000 adverse drug events and transfusion errors during the next 20 years.

Source: U.S. Food and Drug Administration (2005).

Using a Bar-Code Medication Administration System

- If a facility uses a bar-code medication administration (BCMA) system, a computerized prescriber order entry (CPOE) system, automatic medication dispensing, and electronic medication records, smart pumps can provide a very high level of client safety. The system will tell you which IV medications were ordered via a CPOE for your client and when the medication is due.
- When the nurse enters the client's room with the scanning device, she/he scans the bar-code labels on the medication, the client's ID band, and the nurse's ID badge. The information from the bar-code label attached to the medication IV bag will be transmitted wirelessly to and programmed into the infusion pump.
- The pump will begin infusing only when scanning of all pieces of information is completed.
- The pump automatically communicates with a computer in the pharmacy, providing the status of the infusion.

SKILL 7.7 Using a Syringe Pump (Mini-Infuser Pump)

Equipment

- Battery-operated or electronic syringe infusion pump
- Pharmacy-prepared and -labeled syringe with prescribed medication
- Microbore tubing with needleless access device
- Chlorhexidine gluconate

Procedure

1. Check syringe label with physician's order for drug, dosage, and amount of drug to be delivered over specified time.
2. Ensure that medication is compatible with primary infusing solution.

SKILL 7.7 Using a Syringe Pump (Mini-Infuser Pump) (continued)

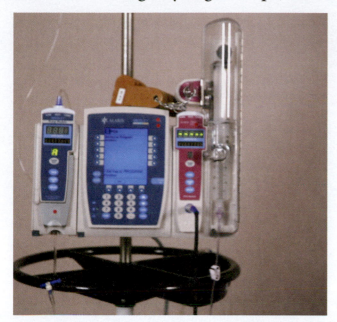

❶ Smart pumps have syringe modules available for attachment to point-of-care computers. To attach such a module, follow manufacturer's directions.

3. Calculate amount of medication to be delivered per minute.
4. Attach microbore tubing to syringe, and holding syringe upright, expel air from medication syringe before priming tubing.
5. Holding syringe downward, carefully prime microbore tubing with medication (about 0.5 mL).
6. Insert syringe into cradle of pump, squeezing clamp around designated parts of syringe; attach pusher to plunger ❶.
7. Verify that IV site is free from infiltration or vein irrigation.
8. Swab primary IV tubing port closest to client.
9. Insert microbore cannula into port.
10. Set rate for drug delivery according to pharmacy specifications on syringe label, or as prescribed. Drug will be infused *independent* of the primary infusion rate.
11. Start syringe pump.
12. Check infusion indicator to verify pump is infusing.
13. Monitor site and pump function frequently.
14. For subsequent doses, the pharmacy dispenses a new syringe but microbore tubing may be reused for 48 to 72 hours (according to agency policy). A sterile cap is used each time a client's primary tubing is accessed.

Note: For other brands of syringe pumps, follow directions for setup and delivery of meds with their product.

SKILL 7.8 Maintaining Infusions

Delegation

Due to the need for sterile technique and technical complexity, inspection of IV sites and regulation of IV rates are not delegated to UAP. UAP may care for clients with such devices, and the nurse must ensure that the UAP knows what complications or adverse signs should be reported to the nurse. In many states, an LPN or LVN with special IV therapy training may manage infusions. Check the state's nurse practice act.

Equipment

None

Procedure

1. Prior to performing the procedure, introduce self and verify the client's identity using agency protocol. Explain to the client what you are going to do, why it is necessary, and how he or she can participate.
2. Perform hand hygiene and observe other appropriate infection control procedures.
3. Position the client appropriately.
   - Assist the client to a comfortable position, either sitting or lying.
   - Expose the IV site but provide for client privacy.
4. Ensure that the correct solution is being infused.
   - Compare the label on the container (including added medications) to the order. If the solution is incorrect, slow the rate of flow to a minimum to maintain the patency of the catheter. If the infusing solution is contraindicated for the client, stop the infusion and saline-lock the catheter. **Rationale:** *Just stopping the infusion may allow a thrombus*

to form in the IV catheter. If this occurs, the catheter must be removed and another venipuncture performed before the infusion can be resumed. Because IV tubing contains approximately 12 to 15 mL, it may be desirable to prevent even this much additional incorrect solution to infuse when the correct IV solution container is hung on existing tubing. In this case, all tubing should be removed until new tubing, primed with the correct solution, can be started.
   - Change the solution to the correct one, using new tubing if indicated.
   - Document and report the error according to agency protocol.
5. Observe the rate of flow every hour.
   - Compare the rate of flow regularly, for example, every hour, against the infusion schedule. **Rationale:** *Infusions that are off schedule can be harmful to a client.* To read the volume in an IV bag, pull the edges of the bag apart at the level of the fluid and read the volume remaining. **Rationale:** *Stretching the bag allows the fluid meniscus to fall to the proper level.*
   - Observe the position of the solution container. If it is less than 1 m (3 ft) above the IV site, readjust it to the correct height of the pole. **Rationale:** *If the container is too low, the solution may not flow into the vein because there is insufficient gravitational pressure to overcome the pressure of the blood within the vein.*
   - If too much fluid has infused in the time interval, check agency policy. The primary care provider may need to be notified.
   - In some agencies, you will slow the infusion to less than the ordered rate so that it will be completed at the planned time. **Rationale:** *Solution administered too quickly may cause a significant increase in circulating blood volume (which is about 6 L in an adult). Hypervolemia may result in*

(continued on next page)

SKILL 7.8   Maintaining Infusions (*continued*)

pulmonary edema and cardiac failure. Assess the client for manifestations of hypervolemia and its complications, including dyspnea; rapid, labored breathing; cough; crackles (rales); tachycardia; and bounding pulses.

- In other agencies, if the order is for a specified amount of fluid per hour, the IV may be adjusted to the correct rate and the client monitored for signs of fluid overload. In this case, make the appropriate revisions on the container time strip.
- If the rate is too slow, check agency policy. Some agencies permit nursing personnel to adjust a rate of flow by a specified amount. Adjustments above this amount may require a primary care provider's order. **Rationale:** *Solution that is administered too slowly can supply insufficient fluid, electrolytes, or medication for a client's needs.*
- If the prescribed rate of flow is 150 mL/hr or more, check the rate of flow more frequently, for example, every 15 to 30 minutes.

6. Inspect the patency of the IV tubing and catheter.
   - Observe the drip chamber. If it is less than half full, squeeze the chamber to allow the correct amount of fluid to flow in.
   - Inspect the tubing for pinches, kinks, or obstructions to flow. Arrange the tubing so that it is lightly coiled and under no pressure. Sometimes the tubing becomes caught under the client's body and the weight blocks the flow.
   - Observe the position of the tubing. If it is dangling below the venipuncture site, coil it carefully on the surface of the bed. **Rationale:** *The solution may not flow upward into the vein against the force of gravity.*
   - Determine catheter position. Some methods include:
     a. Aspirate the catheter for a blood return. Do this slowly and gently.
     b. Apply a tourniquet several inches above the venipuncture site (for a gravity drip). **Rationale:** *Compression from the tourniquet should stop or slow the fluid flow. If it doesn't, the fluid could be leaking into the tissue (Hadaway, 2009).*
     c. Lower the solution container below the level of the infusion site and observe for a return flow of blood from the vein. **Rationale:** *A return flow of blood indicates that the IV catheter is patent and in the vein. Blood returns in this instance because venous pressure is greater than the fluid pressure in the IV tubing. Absence of blood return may indicate that the IV catheter is no longer in the vein or that the tip of the catheter is partially obstructed by a thrombus, the vein wall, or a valve in the vein.* (*Note:* With some catheters, no blood may appear even with patency because the soft catheter walls collapse during siphoning.)
   - If there is leakage, locate the source. If the leak is at the catheter connection, tighten the tubing into the catheter. If the leak is elsewhere in the tubing, slow the infusion and replace the tubing. If leakage is substantial, estimate the amount of solution lost. If the IV insertion site is leaking, the catheter will have to be removed and IV access reestablished at a new site.

CLINICAL ALERT
To check for extravasation, place constrictive band proximal to infusion site tight enough to restrict blood flow through the vein. Set tubing roller clamp to a "keep open" (or slow) rate, and

remove tubing from infusion pump. If the infusion continues to drip, fluid is extravasating into the surrounding tissue.

Clients receiving hypertonic, acidic, or irritating agents, older clients with fragile veins, and pediatric clients who are active are at particular risk for IV site problems.

7. Inspect the insertion site for fluid infiltration.
   - If infiltration is present, stop the infusion and remove the catheter. Restart the infusion at another site.
   - For hypertonic or hyperosmolar fluid infiltration, apply a cold compress to the site of the infiltration. For certain nonvesicant drugs, apply heat to the site; for isotonic or hypotonic fluid infiltration, choose heat or cold based on client comfort (Hadaway, 2009). **Rationale:** *Warmth promotes comfort and vasodilation, facilitating absorption of the fluid from interstitial tissues; cold restricts contact with additional tissue and limits the tissue affected by osmotic fluid shift.*
   - If the infiltration involves a vesicant—"any medication or fluid with the potential for causing blisters, severe tissue injury, or necrosis if it escapes from the vein" (Hadaway, 2007, p. 64)—it is called extravasation and other measures are indicated. The extravasation of a vesicant drug should be considered an emergency. Usually, vesicants are administered only through central venous infusions and by specially certified nurses. An example of a vesicant is the chemotherapy medication paclitaxel.
   - Stop the infusion immediately.
   - Disconnect the tubing from the catheter hub and attach a 3- or 5-mL syringe. Aspirate any fluid remaining in the hub and catheter.
   - Photograph the site if that is agency policy.
   - For a peripheral-short catheter, remove the dressing and withdraw the catheter. Use a dry gauze pad to control bleeding. Apply a new dry dressing. Do not apply excessive pressure to the area.
   - For a central venous catheter, do not remove the catheter. Clamp and cap the catheter hub. Follow agency procedure for flushing when extravasation is suspected.
   - Assess motion, sensation, and capillary refill distal to the injury. Measure the circumference of the extremity and compare it with the opposite extremity.
   - Notify the primary care provider.
   - The affected arm should be elevated and, depending on the drug, heat or cold therapy should be implemented.

8. Inspect the insertion site for phlebitis (inflammation of a vein).
   - Inspect and palpate the site at least every 8 hours. Phlebitis can occur as a result of mechanical trauma or chemical irritation. Chemical injury to a vein can occur from IV electrolytes (especially potassium and magnesium) and medications. The clinical signs are redness, warmth, and swelling at the IV site and burning pain along the course of the vein.
   - If phlebitis is detected, discontinue the infusion, and apply warm or cold compresses to the venipuncture site. Do not use this injured vein for further infusions.

9. Inspect the IV site for bleeding.
   - Oozing or bleeding into the surrounding tissues can occur while the infusion is freely flowing but is more likely to occur after the catheter has been removed from the vein.

SKILL 7.8   Maintaining Infusions (*continued*)

- Observation of the venipuncture site is extremely important for clients who bleed readily, such as those receiving anti-coagulants.
10. Teach the client ways to maintain the infusion system, for example:
    - Inform of any limitations on movement or mobility.
    - Explain alarms if an electronic control device is used.
    - Instruct to notify a nurse if:
      a. The flow rate suddenly changes or the solution stops dripping.
      b. The solution container is nearly empty.
      c. There is blood in the IV tubing.
      d. Discomfort or swelling is experienced at the IV site.
    - Inform that the nurse will be checking the venipuncture site.
11. Document relevant information (often on a specified form).
    - Record the status of the IV insertion site and any adverse responses of the client.
    - Document the client's IV fluid intake at least every 8 hours according to agency policy. Include the date and time; amount and type of solution used; container number; flow rate; and the client's general response. In most agencies, the amount remaining in each IV container is also recorded at the end of the shift.

CLINICAL ALERT

Some facilities use a single secondary tubing for all agents. The tubing is back-flushed with the primary solution prior to administering a new agent, providing the agents are compatible.

Regard IV systems as closed sterile systems and maintain as such. All entries into the tubing should be made through injection ports that are disinfected just before entry.

Client Teaching

Teach the client ways to help maintain the infusion system, for example:

- Avoid sudden twisting or turning movements of the arm with the catheter.
- Avoid stretching or placing tension on the tubing.
- Try to keep the tubing from dangling below the level of the IV catheter.
- Notify a nurse if:
  a. The flow rate suddenly changes or the solution stops dripping.
  b. The client notices the solution container is nearly empty.
  c. There is blood in the IV tubing.
  d. Discomfort or swelling is experienced at the IV site.
  e. The pump or controller alarm sounds.

Setting of Care

- In the home, plant hangers, robe hooks, or over-the-door S hooks may be used to hang an IV container.
- Evaluate the client's or caregiver's ability to operate the infusion device at home.
- Emphasize the need for hand hygiene and clean technique when handling IV equipment. Set aside a clean area in the home to store the IV equipment.

- Demonstrate the device, and ask for a return demonstration from the client or caregiver.
- Discuss complications, such as infiltration, power failure, or equipment problems, and the measures to take when they arise.
- Make certain the client knows how and where to obtain supplies.

SKILL 7.9   Maintaining Intermittent Infusion Devices

Evidence-Based Nursing Practice

Flushing Using Saline or Heparin

The efficacy of peripheral intravenous infusion devices (PIIDs) is extremely important in administering intermittent IV medications, minimizing the number of IV catheter placements, and decreasing the cost of supplies. Heparin has been shown to be effective in maintaining PIIDs, but it is a medication that can cause allergic reactions and pain at the infusion site. It may also be incompatible with some medications, and it costs considerably more than normal saline. The debate over whether heparin or normal saline is better continues.

A group in the Evidence-Based Scholars Program at Children's Hospital of Orange County, California, reviewed 15 studies from 1998 to 2008 that compared heparin versus normal saline for flushing PIIDs (Rodriguez, n.d.). Based on this review, the group determined that saline flush is as efficacious as heparin flush for maintaining patency in PIIDs of young children and adolescents with catheter gauges of 24 and larger. They suggested that saline flushes of 0.6 to 3.0 mL be administered every 6 to 12 hours for optimal catheter maintenance. They also stated that, when saline flush

is used, the technique of positive-pressure displacement is important. This technique involves injecting the last 0.1 mL of saline while simultaneously removing the syringe tip or closing the white side clamp on a T-connector to create positive pressure. Finally, they recommended that policies and procedures be changed to reflect use of saline flush rather than heparin flush to maintain patency of PIIDs.

In contrast, Bertolino and colleagues (2012) performed a randomized study of 214 clients with PIIDs to determine whether flushing PIIDs with 3 mL of a 100 units of heparin/mL solution instead of saline would improve the outcome of infusion devices. This study concluded that heparin 100 units/mL was more effective than saline solution in maintaining PIIDs. They reported reductions both in the number of catheter-related phlebitis/occlusions and in the number of catheters per client. However, they cautioned that since the study excluded clients with platelet or coagulation defects, caution should be used when prescribing heparin flushes for use in such clients.

Source: Data from Rodriguez (n.d.) and Bertolino et al. (2012).

(*continued on next page*)

SKILL 7.9 Maintaining Intermittent Infusion Devices *(continued)*

Delegation

Due to the need for sterile technique and technical complexity, this procedure is not delegated to UAP. UAP may care for clients with such devices, and the nurse must ensure that the UAP knows what complications or adverse signs should be reported to the nurse.

In many states, a licensed practical nurse or licensed vocational nurse with special IV therapy training may manage intermittent infusion devices. Check the state's nurse practice act.

Equipment

- Intermittent infusion cap or device ❶
- Clean gloves
- TSM dressing
- Sterile 2 × 2 or 4 × 4 gauze
- Sterile saline for injection (without preservative) in a prefilled syringe, a 3-mL syringe with a needleless infusion device
- Alcohol wipes
- Tape
- Clean emesis basin

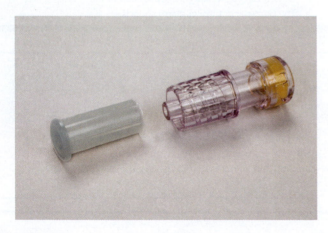

❶ Intermittent infusion device with injection port.

Procedure

1. Prior to performing the procedure, introduce self and verify the client's identity using agency protocol. Explain to the client what you are going to do, why it is necessary, and how he or she can participate. Explain the reason for the intermittent device and that changing an IV to a saline lock should cause no discomfort other than that associated with removing tape from the IV tubing.
2. Perform hand hygiene and observe other appropriate infection control procedures.
3. Assist the client to a comfortable position, either sitting or lying. Expose the IV site but provide for client privacy.
4. Assess the IV site and determine the patency of the catheter. If the catheter is not fully patent or there is evidence of phlebitis or infiltration, discontinue the catheter and establish a new IV site.
   - Expose the IV catheter hub and loosen any tape that is holding the IV tubing in place or that will interfere with insertion of the intermittent infusion plug into the catheter.

- Clamp the IV tubing to stop the flow of IV fluid.
- Open the gauze pad and place it under the IV catheter hub. **Rationale:** *This absorbs any leakage that might occur when the tubing is disconnected.*
- Open the alcohol wipe and intermittent infusion cap, leaving the plug in its sterile package.

5. Remove the IV tubing and insert the intermittent infusion plug into the IV catheter.
   - Apply clean gloves.
   - Stabilize the IV catheter with your nondominant hand and use the little finger to place slight pressure on the vein above the end of the catheter. Twist the IV tubing adapter to loosen it from the IV catheter and remove it, placing the end of the tubing into a clean emesis basin ❷.

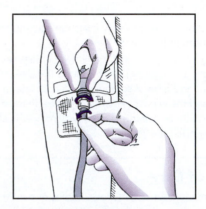

❷ Separating the IV catheter from the infusion tubing.

   - Pick up the intermittent infusion plug from its package and remove the protective sleeve from the male adapter, maintaining its sterility. Insert the plug into the IV catheter, twisting it to seat it firmly or engage the Luer-Lok.
6. Instill saline solution per agency policy. **Rationale:** *Saline is used to maintain patency of the IV catheter when fluids are not infusing through the catheter.*
7. Cover the site with a TSM dressing. **Rationale:** *The TSM dressing provides protection from infection, allows for ease of assessment of the venipuncture site, and also promotes comfort, preventing the plug from catching on clothing or bedding.*
8. Access the device to infuse fluids or medication.
   - Cleanse the cap with povidone-iodine or alcohol according to agency policy.
   - Use a threaded-lock needleless connector for infusions.
9. Flush the device with prescribed solution after each use or every 8 to 12 hours if not in use, according to agency policy. Flush the lock by injecting saline using the push–pause method (a rapid succession of push–pause–push–pause movements exerted on the plunger of the syringe barrel). **Rationale:** *This creates a turbulence within the catheter lumen that causes a swirling effect to remove any debris (e.g., blood or medication) attached to the catheter lumen* (Phillips, 2010, p. 351).
10. Remove and discard gloves. Perform hand hygiene.
11. Teach the client how to maintain the lock.
    - Notify the nurse or primary care provider if the plug or catheter comes out; if the site becomes red, inflamed, or painful; or if any drainage or bleeding occurs at the site.

SKILL 7.9   Maintaining Intermittent Infusion Devices *(continued)*

12. Document relevant information.
    - Record the date and time of converting the infusion device, the status of the IV insertion site, and any adverse responses of the client.

CLINICAL ALERT

If the gauge of the catheter is small (i.e., 22 gauge or smaller), you may not get a blood return. This can be due to the collapse of the tip of the catheter as negative pressure is applied when attempting to aspirate blood. This does not always mean that the catheter is occluded. You may attempt to gently inject the saline while feeling for resistance. If any resistance is felt, it is possible that the catheter is occluded and needs to be removed and a new catheter inserted.

Studies have not definitively shown whether saline or heparin is best to maintain catheter patency, maintain dwell time, and avoid phlebitis. Some hospitals still use a small amount of dilute heparin for flushing peripheral locks; it is usually prepared with 1 mL heparin (1,000 units/mL) added to 9 mL of normal saline to produce 100 units/mL solution. Prefilled syringes of heparin and saline for infusion comes in 10 units of heparin/mL. Caution should be exercised because heparin-induced thrombocytopenia can occur with as little as 500 units of heparin/day.

Client Teaching

Teach the client how to maintain the lock.

- Avoid manipulating the catheter or infusion plug and protect it from catching on clothing or bedding. A gauze bandage such as Kerlix or Kling may be wrapped over the plug to protect it when it is not in use.
- Cover the site with an occlusive dressing when showering; avoid immersing the site.
- Flush the catheter with saline solution as directed.
- Notify the care provider if the plug or catheter comes out, or if the site becomes red, inflamed or painful, or if any drainage or bleeding occurs at the site.

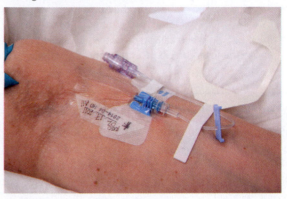

Intermittent infusion device in place.

SKILL 7.10   Discontinuing Infusion Devices

Delegation

In some states and agencies, removal of a peripheral IV catheter may be delegated to UAP. In others, removal of IV infusions or devices is not delegated to UAP. In any case, the nurse must ensure that the UAP knows what complications or adverse signs following removal should be reported to the nurse. In many states, an LPN or LVN with special IV therapy training may discontinue IV infusions. Check the applicable state's nurse practice act.

Equipment

- Clean gloves
- Linen-saver pad
- Small sterile dressing and tape

Procedure

1. Before the procedure, check the physician's order, introduce self and verify the client's identity using agency protocol. Explain to the client what you are going to do, why it is necessary, and how he or she can participate. Explain the reason for discontinuing the IV and that the procedure should cause no discomfort other than that associated with removing the tape.
2. Perform hand hygiene and observe other appropriate infection control procedures.

3. Assist the client to a comfortable position, either sitting or lying. Expose the IV site but provide for client privacy. Place a linen-saver pad under the extremity that has the IV.
4. Prepare the equipment.
    - Clamp the infusion tubing. **Rationale:** *Clamping the tubing prevents the fluid from flowing out of the IV catheter onto the client or bed.*
    - Apply clean gloves.
    - Remove the dressing, stabilization device, and tape at the venipuncture site while holding the IV catheter firmly and applying countertraction to the skin. **Rationale:** *Movement of the IV catheter can injure the vein and cause discomfort to the client. Countertraction prevents pulling the skin and causing discomfort.*
    - Assess the venipuncture site. **Rationale:** *Assess for signs of infection or phlebitis.*
    - Apply the sterile gauze above the venipuncture site. Only touch the upper (top) portion of the gauze pad and maintain sterility of the lower (bottom) portion that is in contact with the venipuncture site.
5. Withdraw the catheter from the vein.
    - Withdraw the catheter by pulling it out along the line of the vein. **Rationale:** *Pulling it out in line with the vein avoids pain and injury to the vein. Do not press down on the sterile gauze pad while removing the catheter.*

(continued on next page)

SKILL 7.10 Discontinuing Infusion Devices (continued)

- Immediately apply firm pressure to the site, using sterile gauze, for 2 to 3 minutes. **Rationale:** *Pressure helps stop the bleeding and prevents hematoma formation.*
- Hold the client's arm or leg above heart level if any bleeding persists. **Rationale:** *Raising the limb decreases blood flow to the area.*
- Teach the client to inform the nurse if the site begins to bleed at any time or the client notes any other abnormalities in the area.

6. Examine the catheter removed from the client.
   - Check the catheter to make sure it is intact. **Rationale:** *If a piece of tubing remains in the client's vein, it could move centrally (toward the heart or lungs).*
   - Report a broken catheter to the nurse in charge or primary care provider immediately.
   - If the broken piece can be palpated, apply a tourniquet above the insertion site. **Rationale:** *Application of a*

tourniquet decreases the possibility of the piece moving until a primary care provider is notified.

7. Cover the venipuncture site.
   - Apply the sterile dressing. **Rationale:** *The dressing continues the pressure and covers the open area in the skin, preventing infection.*
   - Discard used supplies appropriately.
8. Remove and discard gloves. Perform hand hygiene.
9. Read the amount remaining in the IV solution container prior to discarding the IV solution.
10. Document all relevant information.
    - Record the amount of fluid infused on the I&O record and in the record, according to agency policy. Include the container number, type of solution used, time of discontinuing the infusion, and the client's response.

Developmental Considerations

OLDER ADULTS

Older adult clients' veins are fragile and roll easily, and frequently the needle punctures the wall of the vessel.

- Insert small-gauge winged catheter in distal vein first to preserve proximal vessel.
- Tourniquet (constricting band) may not be necessary for venipuncture. If used, it should be applied loosely.
- If used, release tourniquet as soon as venipuncture yields blood return to prevent excessive pressure in vein.
- Maintain close assessment of IV sites to promote long-term use of vessel.

Older adult clients are prone to fluid and electrolyte disorders as a result of the normal aging process.

- Thirst mechanism is decreased.
- Renal threshold is altered.
- Total body fluid is less due to decreased lean muscle mass.
- Fluid replacement therapy requires close monitoring to prevent fluid overload, leading to pulmonary edema and electrolyte imbalance.
- Dehydration is a common reason for IV therapy.
- When infusing IV fluids, monitor closely for signs of fluid volume overload.
- Monitor BUN and electrolytes regularly for signs of overload.

- Use IV pump whenever infusing fluids into older adult clients. If dextrose solution is being infused, IV pumps *must* be used. Dextrose overload can lead to cerebral edema if infused too rapidly.

Stabilizing IV catheter and dressing is problematic due to older clients' fragile skin.

- Avoid excessive use of tape.
- Apply skin protector solution before dressing site.
- Use stretch mesh gauze to cover site and tubing to prevent catching on bed (avoid roll-type gauze).

Protect fragile skin that is susceptible to injury, infiltration, and discomfort from irritating drugs.

- Observe IV site carefully for signs of infiltration. Because of skin's loose folds and decreased tactile sensation, a large amount of fluid can sequester in subcutaneous tissue and go unnoticed before client complains of pain.
- Check IV site frequently when client receives drugs that can cause irritation and even necrosis if they infiltrate.
- At first sign of phlebitis or infiltration, remove IV and restart in a new site.
- If client complains of discomfort during IV therapy, apply a moist and warm pack to site, decrease rate of fluid infusion.

SKILL 7.11 Infusing IV Fluids Through a Central Line

Equipment

- Primed IV fluid administration set with needleless Luer-Lok connector
- Infusion delivery pump
- Antimicrobial swabs
- 10-mL needleless syringe with 5 mL of preservative-free 0.9% normal saline solution

- CLC 2000 positive-pressure cap (or another brand) ❶
- Clean gloves

Preparation

- Check physician's order sheet and client's medication record for IV order.
- Check IV order with IV solution bag.

SKILL 7.11 **Infusing IV Fluids Through a Central Line** (*continued*)

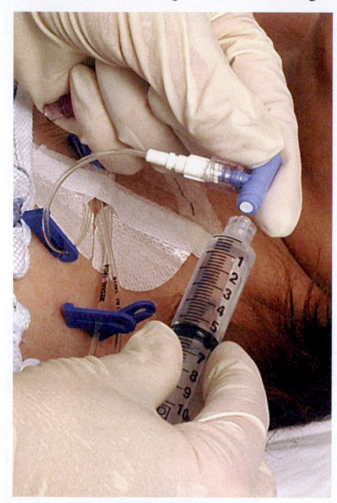

❶ Positive fluid displacement and positive end pressure prevent blood reflux into a catheter lumen. The device provides the saline flush to prevent clotting of the catheter.

- Take equipment to client's room.
- Identify client by checking the client's identity band and asking client to state name and birth date.
- Explain procedure to client and provide privacy.

Procedure

1. Perform hand hygiene and don gloves.
2. Hang IV solution on IV stand ❷ ❸.
3. Wipe access port with antimicrobial swab and allow to dry ❹.
4. Insert needleless cannula from saline flush syringe and unclamp lumen (Clamp is not found on PICC lines or Groshong valve catheter.) ❺ ❻.
5. Aspirate for blood return, using very little force, to check for lumen patency and placement ❼.

> **CLINICAL ALERT**
> To minimize pressure on the catheter during injection, NEVER use less than a 10-mL syringe for central lines. Smaller syringes increase pressure within the catheter.

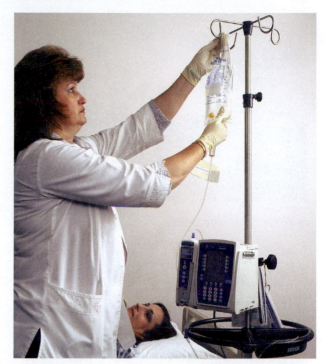

❷ Hang IV solution on IV stand.

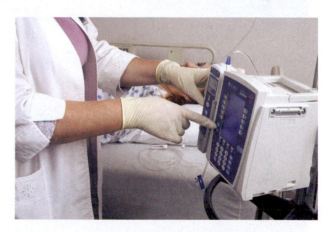

❸ Attach point-of-care module and program.

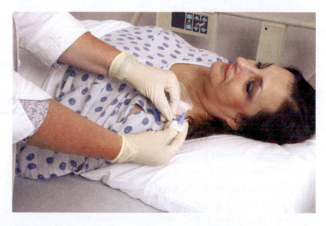

❹ Wipe access cap or positive-pressure clamp with antimicrobial swab and allow to dry.

(*continued on next page*)

SKILL 7.11   Infusing IV Fluids Through a Central Line *(continued)*

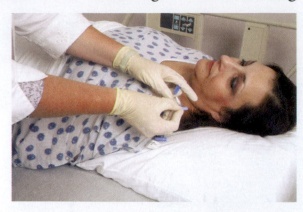

5 Ensure clamp is open before attaching syringe.

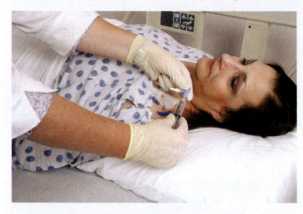

6 Attach 10-mL needleless syringe with saline to pressure valve.

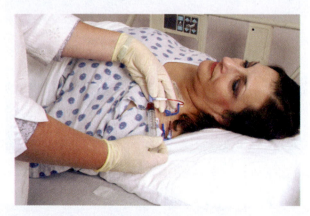

7 Aspirate and check for blood return before infusing saline solution.

6. Instill saline solution slowly. The central venous catheter (CVC) and tubing has a volume of 1–3 mL; therefore, about 5 mL of solution in a 10-mL syringe should be used to flush the catheter thoroughly. **Rationale:** *To clear lumen of in-line dilute heparin.*

7. Maintain positive pressure when withdrawing syringe by clamping catheter before removing syringe or by maintaining pressure on syringe plunger before you clamp or use the CLC 2000 positive-pressure cap. **Rationale:** *This prevents aspiration of blood into lumen and decreases risk of catheter occlusion.*

8. Swab access port again with antimicrobial swabs.

9. Insert IV tubing with Luer-Lok connector into access port. Unclamp lumen.

10. Set electronic device to prescribed rate and begin infusing IV fluids **8**.

11. Ensure central line dressing is clean and intact.

12. Remove gloves and perform hand hygiene.

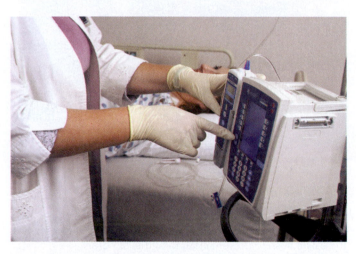

8 After connecting IV tubing to catheter, turn on electric device to prescribed setting.

> **CLINICAL ALERT**
> Nontunneled central vascular access devices (CVADs) have the highest infection rate of all types of CVADs; therefore, it is crucial that aseptic techniques be used in all aspects of catheter care.

SKILL 7.12   Assisting with Percutaneous Central Vascular Catheterization

Equipment

- Specific nontunneled catheter
- Routine IV setup (tubing and solution)
- Through-the-needle radiopaque central catheter
- Local anesthetic, syringes, and needles
- Sterile gloves, gown, masks, drapes, and sutures
- Antimicrobial swabs 2% chlorhexidine gluconate swabs
- Intermittent infusion caps or positive-pressure device
- Prefilled syringes with preservative-free normal saline
- Transparent semipermeable dressing
- Securement device

Procedure

1. Identify client by checking the client's identity band and asking client to state name and birth date. Validate signed consent for catheter insertion.

2. Perform hand hygiene and explain procedure to client, including rationale for mask, positioning, and the Valsalva maneuver.

SKILL 7.12   Assisting with Percutaneous Central Vascular Catheterization (*continued*)

3. Place client in Trendelenburg position. **Rationale:** *This position prevents air embolism and helps distend subclavian and jugular veins.*

4. According to licensed practitioner's preference, extend client's neck and upper chest by placing a rolled pillow or blanket between shoulder blades. **Rationale:** *Usual insertion sites are either the subclavian or right jugular vein.*

5. Place mask on client, and turn client's head away from side of venipuncture. **Rationale:** *This facilitates filling the vessel with blood and prevents contamination.*

6. Maintain sterility while opening glove packet and sterile drape pack.

7. Open antimicrobial prep pads.

   Note: New guidelines to prevent catheter-related bloodstream infection recommend that the licensed provider don a cap and sterile gown in addition to mask and sterile gloves (Institute for Healthcare Improvement, 2012).

8. Don mask and gloves and assist with central catheter insertion.
   - Licensed provider dons mask, gown, and sterile gloves for this procedure.
   - Licensed provider prepares the client's skin, drapes area, and, using a sterile syringe and needle, draws up anesthetic to infiltrate the site.
   - As licensed provider inserts catheter, client is instructed to perform the Valsalva maneuver to prevent air embolism.
     a. Instruct client to exhale against a closed glottis or to hum.
     b. If client is unable to do this, compress client's abdomen. **Rationale:** *Both these procedures help to decrease chances of an air embolism forming.*

   Note: A 14-gauge needle is inserted into the subclavian vein, using the clavicle as a guide ❶. When blood returns in the syringe, the syringe is removed from the needle and a wire is threaded through the needle into the subclavian vein. The needle is removed and the catheter is fed over the wire into the subclavian and brachiocephalic vein. The wire is removed when the tip of the catheter rests in the superior vena cava.

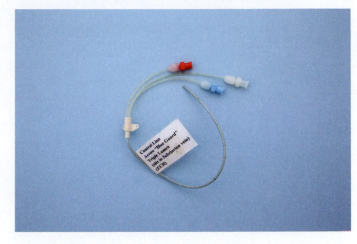

❶ Central line "Blue Guard." Triple-lumen catheter—subclavian vein.

9. When catheterization is complete, insert injection cap, flush with 5 mL of normal saline, and then heparinize with 3 mL dilute heparin (according to agency policy).

10. Apply securement device to skin and place catheter in clamp.

11. Cover securement device and catheter with sterile transparent dressing (according to hospital policy).

12. Label insertion site dressing with date, nurse's initials, and time of insertion.

13. Obtain x-ray for validation of placement into superior vena cava before initiating infusion (unless emergency placement performed).

14. Monitor client's vital signs. **Rationale:** *Bleeding or pneumothorax may occur.*

> **CLINICAL ALERT**
> All continuous IV infusions administered via a central line must have an electric infusion controller device in place.

Evidence-Based Nursing Practice

Antimicrobial Swabs

Studies have shown that 2% chlorhexidine gluconate solution significantly lowers catheter-related bloodstream infection rates when compared with 70% povidone-iodine and 70% isopropyl alcohol. The Centers for Disease Control recommend use of a 2% chlorhexidine wash for daily skin cleansing to reduce CRBSI. It also may be useful with in combination with silver sulfadiazine for its microbactericidal action in clients with placement of long-term catheter (>5 days).

Source: Data from Centers for Disease Control and Prevention (2011).

Role of CHG-Impregnated Sponges in Reducing Infections in ICU

Sponges impregnated with chlorhexidine gluconate (CHG) reduced the rate of catheter-related infections in the ICU. Using CHG-impregnated sponge dressings with intravascular catheters reduced the risk for major catheter-related infections by 60% among clients treated in the ICU. Changing unsoiled, adherent dressings weekly was not inferior to a 3-day changing schedule, according to data from a randomized controlled trial.

A randomly assigned study consisted of 1,636 clients over the age of 18 in an ICU setting. The clients were expected to need an arterial catheter, central vein catheter, or both for 48 hours or longer. Some of the clients received CHG-impregnated sponges and some the standard dressings, scheduled for change either once every 7 days or once every 3 days. The rate for major catheter-related infection decreased from 1.40 per 1,000 catheter days to 0.60 per 1,000 catheter days with the use of the CHG-impregnated sponge. The 3-day group had a 7.8% rate of catheter colonization versus 8.6% for the 7-day group, which proves noninferiority for the 7-day dressing schedule compared with the 3-day dressing schedule. Use of CHG-impregnated dressings decreases the rate of major catheter-related infection when the baseline rate is lower than 2 per 1,000 catheter days.

Source: Timsit (2009).

(*continued on next page*)

SKILL 7.12   Assisting with Percutaneous Central Vascular Catheterization (*continued*)

Practice Guidelines to Prevent Catheter-Related Bloodstream Infections

HAND HYGIENE

- Wash hands or decontaminate hands with alcohol-based waterless hand cleaner to help prevent contamination of central line sites and resulting infection:

  Before and after palpating, caring for catheter insertion sites, or invasive procedures

  Before donning and after removing gloves

  Between clients and after using the bathroom.

BARRIER PRECAUTIONS

- Use maximum barrier precautions when inserting or assisting with insertion of central venous catheters, including PICC lines. Include a cap that covers all hair, mask covering mouth and nose tightly, sterile gown, and sterile gloves.
- Cover client from head to toe with large sterile drape leaving small opening for insertion of catheter.

CHLORHEXIDINE SKIN ASEPSIS

- Prepare site using 2% chlorhexidine gluconate in 70% isopropyl alcohol.
- Pinch wings on chlorhexidine applicator to break open ampule. Hold applicator down to allow solution to saturate pad.
- Press sponge against skin and apply chlorhexidine using a back-and-forth friction rub for at least 30 seconds and then allow to dry thoroughly, approximately 2 minutes. Do not wipe or blot area.

CATHETER SITE SELECTION

- Use central venous catheters (CVCs) impregnated with antimicrobial agents, if available.

- Nontunneled percutaneously inserted CVCs are available with three different agents: chlorhexidine/silver sulfadiazine, rifampin/minocycline, and silver/platinum ionic metals. PICC brand uses rifampin/minocycline agents.
- Catheter should be inserted in the subclavian vein for nontunneled catheter.
- These catheters should be used for clients with a dwell time of more than 5 days and in healthcare facilities where catheter-related bloodstream infection rates are high.
- There is inconclusive evidence that multiple-lumen catheters should not be used; even though they have higher infection rates, they also have fewer mechanical complications than single-lumen catheters.

DAILY ASSESSMENT

Risk for infection increases the longer a line stays in place. However, routine or scheduled replacement does not in itself reduce the risk of infection.

- Include daily review of line necessity as part of rounds and define an appropriate time frame for regular review of necessity for the line when a line is placed for long-term use.
- Record time and date of line placement for documentation and evaluation.
- Name the line day during rounds and in communications (e.g., "Today is line day 6.").

Source: Institute for Healthcare Improvement (2012).

SKILL 7.13   Managing Central Lines

Central venous catheters are available with one, two, three, or four lumens. The triple-lumen catheter is commonly used because it provides multiple venous access. Each lumen has a color-coded port and specific uses. Color coding and port size may vary according to the manufacturer. The distal port is often used for the administration of blood products and for general venous access. The middle port is used for medication administration and provides a general venous access. The proximal port can be used as a general venous access to obtain blood for diagnostic tests or can be dedicated for the administration of total parenteral nutrition.

Delegation

Due to the need for sterile technique and technical complexity, the maintaining and monitoring of central venous lines are not delegated to UAP. UAP may care for clients with central lines, and the nurse must ensure that the UAP knows what complications or adverse signs should be reported to the nurse.

Equipment

- Soft-tipped clamp without teeth
- Alcohol, chlorhexidine gluconate (CHG) wipes

- TSM dressing
- 10-mL syringe
- Sterile normal saline
- Heparin flush solution (e.g., 100 units heparin per milliliter of saline)

Procedure

1. Prior to performing the procedure, introduce self and verify the client's identity using agency protocol. Explain to the client what you are going to do, why it is necessary, and how he or she can participate.
2. Perform hand hygiene and observe other appropriate infection control procedures.
3. Position the client appropriately.
   - Assist the client to a comfortable position, either sitting or lying. Expose the IV site but provide for client privacy.
4. Label each lumen of a multiple-lumen catheter.
   - Mark each lumen or port of the tubing with a description of its purpose (e.g., the distal lumen for CVP monitoring and infusing blood, the middle lumen for parenteral nutrition, and the proximal lumen for other IV solutions or for blood samples).

SKILL 7.13 Managing Central Lines (continued)

or

- Use a color code established by the agency to label the proximal, middle, and distal lumens. **Rationale:** *Labeling prevents mixing of incompatible medications or infusions and reserves each lumen for specific therapies.*

5. Monitor tubing connections.
   - Ensure that all tubing connections are secured according to agency protocol.
   - Check the connections every 2 hours.
   - Tape cap ends if agency protocol indicates.
6. Change tubing according to agency policy.
   - Parenteral nutrition tubing should be changed every 24 hours (Phillips, 2010).
7. Change the catheter site dressing according to agency policy.
   - Use strict aseptic technique (including the use of sterile gloves and mask) when caring for central lines and long-term venous access devices.
   - The frequency of dressing changes is dependent on the dressing material. TSM dressings or tape and gauze are acceptable; however, gauze dressings do not allow for visualization of the insertion site and need to be changed every 48 hours. In contrast, TSM dressings allow for visualization and can be left in place for a maximum of 7 days if they remain clean, dry, and intact **1**. All dressings should be changed when loose or soiled.

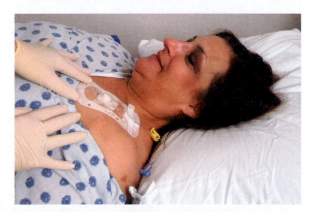

1 TSM dressing. Gauze dressings are used only if the catheter insertion site is oozing. The dressing should be changed every 48 hr or if soiled.

- Assess the site for any redness, swelling, tenderness, or drainage. Compare the length of the external portion of the catheter with its documented length to assess for possible displacement. Report and document any position changes or signs of infection.
- Follow agency protocol for cleaning solutions and types of dressings. CHG is the preferred agent to clean the insertion site.
- Clean the skin around the site with CHG solution, using a back-and-forth or side-to-side motion. Allow the site to air dry. A round dressing impregnated with CHG can also be applied to the insertion site to prevent catheter-related bloodstream infections (CRBSIs) **2**.
- Apply a new stabilization device **3**.
- Apply a sterile dressing.
8. Administer all infusions as ordered.
   - Use a controller or pump for all fluids.

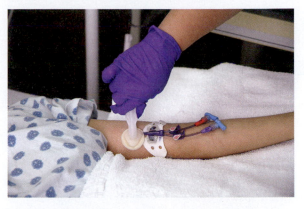

2 Cleanse site with chlorhexidine gluconate swab using back-and-forth motion.

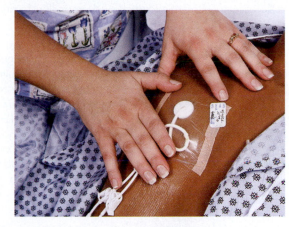

3 BioPatch® with transparent dressing over insertion site.

- Maintain the fluid flow at the prescribed rate.
- Whenever the line is interrupted for any reason, instruct the client to perform the Valsalva maneuver. If the client is unable to perform the Valsalva maneuver, place the client in a supine position, and clamp the lumen of the catheter with a soft-tipped clamp. Place a strip of tape over the catheter (about 3 in. from the end) before applying the clamp. **Rationale:** *The clamp is placed over the taped area to prevent damage to the tubing. A clamp without teeth prevents piercing.*
9. Cap lumens without continuous infusions, and flush them regularly.
   - Change the catheter cap as indicated by agency protocol. The catheter hub can be a source of infection. A 15-second scrub of the connection surface of the needleless connector has been shown to prohibit microorganism entry on the surface (Moureau & Dawson, 2010) **4**. Also available are commercial single-use Luer access valve disinfection caps. This cap contains isopropyl alcohol, which cleans the needleless connector before access and also protects it from contamination between uses. The cap is twisted onto the needleless connector and left in place until the next access to the connector is needed. The nurse removes and discards the old cap, and the connector is ready for use without further wiping.
   - The solution used and frequency of flushing are determined by agency protocol for the specific type of port being used. Heparin-induced thrombocytopenia (HIT) has been reported with the use of heparin flush solutions. If heparin is

(continued on next page)

SKILL 7.13   Managing Central Lines (*continued*)

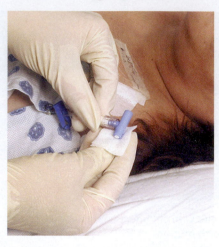

④ Wipe access cap with antimicrobial swab and allow to dry.

used as part of the flushing protocol, the concentration should not be in amounts that cause systemic anticoagulation but in the lowest possible concentration to maintain patency. Many agencies are switching to needleless IV connectors that can be flushed with normal saline solution only.

- Flush the catheter before and after each dose of medication ⑤. **Rationale:** *The initial flush is to assess patency of the catheter, and the flush after administration of the medication is to ensure that the complete dose has entered the bloodstream.*

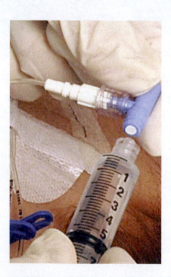

⑤ Flush a lumen regularly to prevent clotting of the catheter.

- Use a 10-mL syringe to flush the catheter. **Rationale:** *Smaller syringes can exert too much pressure, which can damage the catheter.* Create turbulent flow with the flush by pushing, then pausing and then pushing again but do not use excessive force if you feel resistance. **Rationale:** *Turbulent flow may help keep the catheter free of residue but forcing a blocked catheter can cause rupture of the catheter or push a clot free into the bloodstream.*
- Blood reflux into the catheter lumen after flushing increases the risk of infection. This can be avoided by either using prefilled syringes designed specifically for catheter flushing or leaving 0.5 to 1 mL of 0.9% sodium chloride solution in the syringe (Hadaway, 2008, p. 38).

10. Administer medications as ordered.
    - If a capped lumen used for medication has been flushed with heparin solution, aspirate and discard or flush the line with 5 to 10 mL of normal saline according to agency protocol before giving the medication. **Rationale:** *Many medications are incompatible with heparin.*
    - After the medication is instilled through the lumen, inject normal saline first and then the heparin flush solution if indicated by agency protocol. **Rationale:** *The saline solution flushes the line of the medication. The heparin maintains the patency of the catheter by preventing blood clotting.*
11. Monitor the client for complications.
    - Assess the client's vital signs, skin color, mental alertness, appearance of the catheter site, and presence of adverse symptoms at least every 4 hours.
    - If an air embolism is suspected, give the client 100% oxygen by mask, place the client in a left Trendelenburg position, and notify the primary care provider. **Rationale:** *Lowering the head increases intrathoracic pressure, decreasing the flow of air into the vein during inhalation. A left side-lying position helps prevent the air from moving to the pulmonary artery.*
    - If sepsis is suspected, replace a parenteral nutrition, blood, or other infusion with 5% or 10% dextrose solution, change the IV tubing and dressing, save the remaining solution for lab analysis, record the lot number of the solution and any additives, and notify the primary care provider immediately. When changing the dressing, take a culture of the catheter site as ordered by the primary care provider or according to agency protocol.
    - If a lumen appears to be occluded, the cause could be thrombus, precipitate, or mechanical. An x-ray is done to determine if the catheter is properly located. Fluoroscopy can demonstrate the presence of a thrombus by indicating the fluid path through the catheter. If a thrombus is found, thrombolytic therapy using an enzyme such as recombinant tissue plasminogen activator (t-PA) is indicated (Hadaway, 2005). Follow agency guidelines for use of these agents. If drugs infused into the lumen may have created a precipitate, the pharmacist can assist in determining whether an acidic, alkaline, or lipid precipitate is likely and the appropriate solution to dissolve it. If the occlusion is mechanical, consult policy to determine if the nurse may reposition the catheter or if the primary care provider must be notified.
12. Document all relevant information.
    - Record the date and time of any infusion started; type of solution, drip rate, and number of milliliters infusing per hour; dressing or tubing changes; appearance of insertion site; and all other nursing assessments.

SKILL 7.14   Changing a Central Line Dressing

Delegation

Due to the need for sterile technique and technical complexity, changing a central line dressing is not delegated to UAP. UAP may care for clients with central lines, and the nurse must ensure that the UAP knows what complications or adverse signs should be reported to the nurse.

Equipment

- Central line dressing set

  or

- Two face masks (one for the nurse and one for the client)
- 2% chlorhexidine gluconate (CHG) wipes
- Clean gloves
- Sterile gloves
- Catheter securement device (according to agency policy)
- Dressing (e.g., Op-Site, Tegaderm)
- Nonallergenic 2.5-cm (1-in.) tape
- Dressing label
- Sterile drape

Procedure

1. Prior to performing the procedure, introduce self and verify the client's identity using agency protocol. Explain to the client what you are going to do, why it is necessary, and how he or she can participate.
2. Perform hand hygiene and observe other appropriate infection control procedures.
3. Provide for client privacy and position the client.
   - Assist the client to a comfortable position, either sitting or lying. The client should be supine if the tubing or injection cap is also being changed. **Rationale:** *An upright position during these techniques increases the chances of an air embolism forming.* Expose the central line site but provide for client privacy.
4. Prepare the client.
   - Apply a mask, and have the client apply a mask (if tolerated or as agency protocol indicates) and/or ask the client to turn the head away from the insertion site. **Rationale:** *This helps protect the insertion site from the nurse's and client's nasal and oral microorganisms. Turning the client's head also makes the site more accessible.*
5. Prepare the equipment.
   - Establish a sterile field and place the sterile supplies.
6. Remove the old dressing.
   - Apply clean gloves.
   - For a TSM dressing, pull both sides away from the insertion site, stretching it to lift it off the skin. For taped dressings, hold the catheter with one hand and gently pull the tape in the direction of the catheter. **Rationale:** *This prevents catheter displacement and skin irritation.*
   - Inspect the skin for signs of irritation or infection. Inspect the catheter for signs of drainage. If infection is suspected, take a swab of the drainage for culture, label it, send it to the laboratory, and notify the primary care provider. Measure the length of the external portion of the catheter extending from the skin exit site to the injection cap or

infusion tubing. **Rationale:** *This measurement allows comparison with previous measurements to determine if the catheter is migrating in or out.*

7. Remove and discard gloves. Perform hand hygiene.
8. Cleanse the site.
   - Apply sterile gloves.
   - Clean the catheter insertion site with CHG-based skin prep in a back-and-forth motion, with plenty of friction for a minimum of 30 seconds. **Rationale:** *The friction allows the solution to get as far as possible into the skin. The prepped site will be approximately the size of the dressing, 5 to 10 cm (2 to 4 in.)* (Phillips, 2010, p. 528). Let the skin dry.
   - If possible, use one hand to lift the catheter so you can clean under it.
   - For additional protection against CRBSI, some agencies use CHG-impregnated sponges at the catheter exit site.
9. Apply the new dressing.
   - Apply the securement device. **Rationale:** *Standards of practice recommend the use of a manufactured catheter stabilization device to prevent catheter movement (INS, 2006).*
   - Apply a new transparent dressing over the exposed catheter, including the hub. **Rationale:** *This type of dressing allows gas exchange but is impermeable to liquids and microorganisms. It also allows visualization of the site.*

Evidence-Based Nursing Practice

Evaluation of Biopatch® Antimicrobial Dressing

A controlled, randomized study of 687 clients with 1,699 central venous or arterial catheter insertion sites was conducted in two centers. Results indicated as 44% reduction in local infections and a 60% reduction in catheter-related bloodstream infections. There were no serious device-related adverse events during the study. Data regarding use of the patch on children under age 16 is limited. The patch should not be used on premature infants because hypersensitivity reactions and necrosis of the skin have occurred.

Source: Maki et al. (2000).

---

10. Remove and discard gloves. Perform hand hygiene.
11. Label the dressing with catheter information, date and time of the dressing change, and your initials.
12. Document all relevant information.
    - Record the appearance of catheter insertion site: presence of drainage, the type of dressing applied, client complaints or concerns, and patency of tubing (if evaluated).

Sample Documentation

4/13/15 2030 Dressing changed on Broviac catheter. External portion 12.7 cm unchanged from previous. Skin without redness, drainage, or swelling. IV infusing freely. No c/o discomfort. Transparent dressing reapplied using sterile technique. _____ J. Valenzuela, RN

SKILL 7.15 Working with Implanted Vascular Access Devices

Delegation

Due to the need for sterile technique and technical complexity, accessing an implanted vascular access device (IVAD) is not delegated to UAP. UAP may care for clients with such devices, and the nurse must ensure that the UAP knows what complications or adverse signs should be reported to the nurse.

Equipment

- IV solution container and administration set

  or
- Blood or blood product with transfusion set and priming saline

  or
- Blood specimen tubes and syringe and needle
- Sterile gloves
- Clean gloves
- Mask
- 10-mL syringes of normal saline flush and 5-mL syringes of heparinized saline (100 units/mL of heparin) according to agency policy
- 2% lidocaine with subcutaneous syringe and needle (optional)
- Chlorhexidine gluconate (CHG) swabs
- Straight or right-angled Huber needle with attached extension tubing and in-line clamp ❶
- Adhesive or nonallergenic tape
- Dressing materials (e.g., 2 × 2 gauze, TSM dressing)

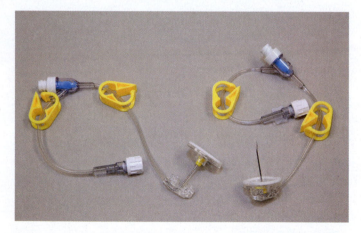

❶ A winged infusion set with right-angled Huber needle.

Preparation

- Assemble the equipment.
- Attach the IV tubing to the infusion or transfusion container.
- Prime the infusion tubing with fluid.
- Prepare and label syringes of normal saline and heparinized saline. Connect the first of these to be used to the Huber needle. Saline followed by heparinized saline is used to flush the device before and after medications or periodically if not in use (check agency policy). **Rationale:** *Heparinized saline may help prevent clotting. There is also some risk of heparin-induced thrombocytopenia so that heparin is not used without clear policy.*

Procedure

1. Prior to performing the procedure, introduce self and verify the client's identity using agency protocol. Explain to the client what you are going to do, why it is necessary, and how he or she can participate.
2. Provide for client privacy and prepare the client.
   - Assist the client to a comfortable position, either sitting or lying. Expose the IVAD site but provide for client privacy.
3. Perform hand hygiene and observe other appropriate infection control procedures.
4. Prepare the site.
   - Locate the IVAD device and its septum, the disk at the center of the port where the needle will be inserted.
   - Prepare the skin in accordance with agency policy and let the area dry after applying solutions.
   - Apply sterile gloves.
   - *Optional:* Inject 2% lidocaine subcutaneously over the needle insertion site. **Rationale:** *This anesthetizes the area for injection.* It may be ordered during the first few weeks after the implant surgery, when the area is tender and swollen and more pain from the needle puncture is felt. Other topical anesthetics may be used.
   - An ice pack may be placed over the site for several minutes to reduce discomfort from the needle puncture.
5. Insert the Huber needle.
   - Grasp the base of the IVAD device between two fingers of your nondominant hand to stabilize it. IVADs may have top entry or side entry ports, depending on the design.
   - Insert the needle at a 90-degree angle to the septum, and push it firmly through the skin and septum until it contacts the base of the IVAD chamber.
   - Avoid tilting or moving the needle when the septum is punctured. **Rationale:** *Needle movement can damage the septum and cause fluid leakage.*
   - When the needle contacts the base of the septum, aspirate for blood to determine correct placement. If no blood is obtained, remove the needle and repeat the procedure after having the client move the arms and change position. **Rationale:** *Movement can free the catheter tip from the vessel wall, where it may be lodged.*
   - Infuse the saline flush. There should be no discomfort or sign of subcutaneous infiltration with infusion of the flush.
6. Prevent manipulation or dislodgement of the needle.
   - If the needle will remain in place for longer than needed to withdraw a blood sample or flush an unused port, secure the needle.
   - Support the Huber needle with 2 × 2 dressings and apply an occlusive transparent dressing to the needle site. Some manufacturer's devices include a safety lock to decrease accidental needlesticks and a client comfort pad that sits between the needle hub and the skin.
   - Loop and tape the tubing. **Rationale:** *Looping prevents tension on the needle.*
7. Attach infusion tubing or an intermittent infusion access cap to the Huber needle.
   - A Huber needle can remain in place for 1 week before it needs to be changed.
8. After use, perform a final flush with heparinized saline.
   - When flushing, maintain positive pressure, and clamp the tubing immediately before the flush is finished. **Rationale:** *These actions avoid reflux of the heparinized saline.*

SKILL 7.15 Working with Implanted Vascular Access Devices *(continued)*

VARIATION: OBTAINING A BLOOD SPECIMEN

To obtain a blood specimen:

- Withdraw 10 mL of blood (or an amount according to agency policy) and discard it. **Rationale:** *This initial specimen may be diluted with saline and heparin from previous flushes.*
- Draw up the required amount of blood and transfer it to the appropriate containers.
- Slowly instill 10 mL of normal saline, according to agency policy. **Rationale:** *This thoroughly flushes the catheter of blood.*
- Inject 5 mL of heparin flush solution to prevent clotting.

9. Remove and discard gloves. Perform hand hygiene.
10. Document all relevant information.
    - Record the appearance of the IVAD site; any difficulty accessing the port and interventions used; presence of drainage; the type of dressing applied; infusions given; and client complaints or concerns. Note any clinical signs indicating venous thrombosis (pain in the neck, arm, and/or shoulder on the side of the insertion site; neck and/or supraclavicular swelling); infection (redness and swelling at the site); and dislodgement of the needle or catheter (shortness of breath, chest pain, coolness in the chest).

Sample Documentation

4/9/15 0900 Implanted port right chest with skin intact and no swelling. Accessed with 20-gauge 1-inch Huber needle. Prompt blood return, flushed without difficulty. IV infusion begun. No c/o of discomfort. _____
G. Young, RN

SKILL 7.16 Changing a PICC Line Dressing

Equipment

- 2% chlorhexidine gluconate (CHG) antimicrobial swabs
- Securement device
- Transparent semipermeable dressing
- BioPatch disc (optional)
- Clean gloves
- Sterile gloves
- Mask

Procedure

1. Identify client by checking the client's identity band and asking client to state name and birth date. Check electronic medical record and client care plan for last dressing change (review facility policy and procedure).
2. Explain procedure to client.
3. Perform hand hygiene and don mask and clean gloves.
4. Remove old transparent dressing by gently pulling in an upward direction ❶. **Rationale:** *Prevents dislodgement of catheter.*

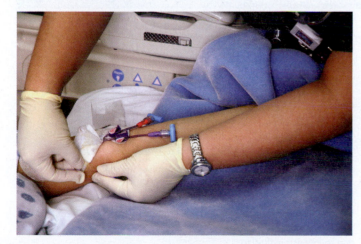

❶ Remove dressing by gently pulling in an upward direction.

5. Check site for bleeding, infection, or signs of phlebitis. **Rationale:** *Bleeding may occur with arm use. Phlebitis is the most common complication.*

6. Discard old dressing and gloves. Perform hand hygiene.

> **CLINICAL ALERT**
> Unless absolutely necessary, avoid blood pressure measurement in the arm with a PICC and avoid venipunctures on the extremity with a PICC line.

7. Prepare sterile supplies.
8. Don sterile gloves.
9. Clean exit site and catheter with antimicrobial swabs using back-and-forth movement ❷.
   Note: The catheter is anchored by a securement device, which does not require suturing of PICC line. Approximately 1 in. of catheter extends from the insertion site.

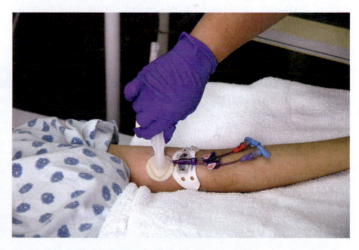

❷ Cleanse site with CHG swab using back-and-forth motion.

10. Allow time for antimicrobial solution to dry. Do not blow on arm or wave hand to hasten drying ❸. **Rationale:** *Waving hand or blowing may contaminate site—antibacterial action does not take effect until solution is dry.*
11. Place securement device over catheter. **Rationale:** *Catheter is not sutured in place, so securement device is used to prevent catheter migration* ❹.

(continued on next page)

SKILL 7.16 **Changing a PICC Line Dressing** (*continued*)

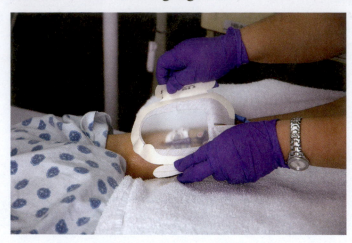

❸ Allow site to dry before applying dressing. Place transparent dressing over site.

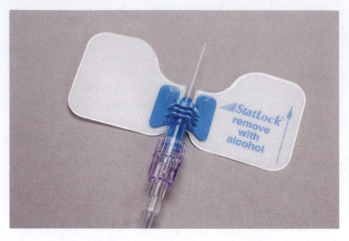

❹ StatLock device, the only evidence-based catheter stabilization device that meets national standards.

12. Cover exit site with transparent semipermeable dressing. Avoid stretching the dressing. Press down on dressing to seal catheter site. No part of actual catheter should be outside transparent dressing.
    Note: Transparent dressings are not occlusive; they allow air to circulate through the semipermeable dressing and thus

prevent perspiration from collecting under the dressing.
13. Remove gloves, mask, and perform hand hygiene.
14. Initial and date dressing.
15. Change initial transparent dressing in 24 hours and then every 7 days or whenever it is soiled or loose. **Rationale:** *First dressing change is done to check insertion site.*

▶ CRITICAL THINKING OPTIONS FOR UNEXPECTED OUTCOMES

Not all unexpected outcomes require further nursing intervention; however, many times they do. When the client demonstrates a change in signs/symptoms indicating an emerging problem, the nurse should immediately assess and troubleshoot what is happening. The assessment data must be processed quickly to formulate a hypothesis so the nurse can make a clinical judgment. The nurse then decides how best to resolve the problem and improve the client's situation for a better appropriate outcome.

EXPECTED OUTCOME	PROBLEM SOLVING	NURSING ACTIONS
Client's intake and output are maintained within expected parameters of 200–300 mL of each other.	Recorded I&O do not balance.	■ Correlate I&O imbalance with weight changes. ■ Emphasize importance of accurate measurements to client and family. ■ Check that entries into computer are accurate (i.e., entering 100 mL instead of 1,000 mL). ■ Identify possible nonmeasurable sources of I or O. ■ Report to charge nurse so she can ensure that all nurses are keeping accurate records. ■ Check if client or family can help with keeping the I&O record. ■ Check the addition on the I&O record to see if an error was made.
	Fluid intake and output do not balance (intake greater than output).	■ Initiate daily weight measurements (weigh before breakfast, after voiding, same scale, same clothing). ■ Compare losses or gains with client's daily weight measurement. ■ Fluid intake and output generally are relatively equal (assuming numbers are accurate). Output should be about 500 mL less per 24 hours due to insensible fluid loss. ■ Determine whether treatment goal is to rehydrate or diurese the client. ■ Use graduated container to accurately measure output in "hat." ■ Search for sources of unmeasured output (fever, wound drainage, diarrhea).

EXPECTED OUTCOME	PROBLEM SOLVING	NURSING ACTIONS
	Fluid output is greater than intake.	■ Analyze whether treatment goal (rehydration, diuresis) has been achieved. ■ Reposition client cautiously, monitoring for possible orthostatic hypotension. ■ Identify when "dry weight" has been achieved (intake balances output after therapy received). ■ Search for sources of unrecorded intake (family offerings, flush solutions, ice chips, full-liquid foods).
Fluid intake is at least 2,600 mL unless contraindicated by diagnosis.	Client unable to maintain an intake of at least 2,600 mL/day.	■ Ensure that fluid restriction is not ordered. ■ Offer fluids in small amounts more frequently. ■ Determine client fluid preferences. ■ Determine client preference for fluid to be hot, cold, or room temperature. ■ Consider "other" fluids such as Jell-O, popsicles. ■ Assess client's ability to use a straw (hemiplegic client is often unable to suck through a straw). ■ Check if client is able to drink fluids independently or if assistance is needed. ■ Ensure that adequate fluids are accessible at the bedside for the client. ■ Do not administer fluids with a bulb syringe. ■ Address client's toileting needs every 2 hours—some clients restrict their fluid intake for fear of incontinence. ■ Use a thickening additive in liquids to facilitate swallowing for the client with aspiration precautions.
IV fluids infuse at prescribed rate without complications.	IV flow not maintained at appropriate rate.	■ Monitor IV fluid intake hourly. ■ Observe IV site for complications. ■ Restart IV immediately when infiltrated to ensure continuous IV fluid intake. ■ Document IV fluid intake every shift. ■ Account for interruption of primary infusion and the delivery of intermittent infusions of medications. ■ Check accuracy of IV administration equipment: electronic device, Dial-A-Flow, etc. ■ Inform physician of alterations in fluid received from what was ordered.
	IV solution does not flow properly.	■ Ensure that the control clamp is open. ■ Check that blood pressure readings are not taken on arm in which IV is running, because flow is impeded and a clot can form on the end of the needle. ■ Ensure that IV administration set is properly loaded. Check pump for flow problem indicator (e.g., cassette seating, air in line). ■ Check IV tubing from insertion site to IV solution for kinks/obstructions. ■ Check for extremity causing positional obstruction to flow (e.g., elbow bent, arm rotated).
IV site remains clean, without signs of infection or infiltration.	Phlebitis is suspected at infusion site (tenderness, warmth, erythema, and pain).	■ Check infusion solution and medications being administered. (Potassium chloride and hypertonic solutions are particularly irritating to veins.) ■ Discontinue IV. ■ Apply warm compress per hospital policy.
	Infiltration occurs.	■ Place warm moist pack, using warm towel, enclose area from fingertips to elbow. Place extremity in plastic bag with open end at elbow. Leave in place no more than 10 minutes.
IV catheter inserted at an appropriate site without difficulty.	Venipuncture is unsuccessful for needle insertion.	■ Remove needle/catheter, apply pressure at insertion site until bleeding stops. (This prevents ecchymosis at site.) Apply bandage. ■ Apply small pressure dressing if client on anticoagulant therapy. ■ Select another site more proximal in vein, or use another extremity. ■ Avoid the one-step entry method since this frequently results in a through-and-through vein puncture. ■ After two failed attempts, seek a more experienced person to perform venipuncture. ■ Place extremity in dependent position before placing tourniquet. Allows vein to fill. ■ Place warm compress on extremity to increase vasodilation, before placing tourniquet.

EXPECTED OUTCOME	PROBLEM SOLVING	NURSING ACTIONS
Infusions of medications or fluids are accomplished without difficulty.	Secondary bag solution does not infuse adequately.	■ Check that primary IV bag is lower than secondary bag (if infusion device requires). ■ Ensure that secondary needleless connector is properly attached in the primary injection port and second bag is sufficiently spiked. ■ Check that the roller clamp of the secondary tubing is open fully.
	Solution in primary IV tubing is incompatible with medication to be administered via secondary "piggyback."	■ Turn primary infusion off. ■ Before administering medication, flush primary tubing with solution compatible with medication (e.g., normal saline, 5% D/W). ■ Hang a separate solution compatible with medication and run through line to flush during drug administration.
	CVP system does not infuse.	■ Check lines for kinks. Change client's position. Check to make sure the manometer stopcock is in the IV→ client position. ■ Obtain order for placing heparin in IV bag to maintain patency. ■ Notify physician and prepare for possible reinsertion.
Blood samples are obtained without difficulty.	Air enters central vein, producing air embolism from system being open at atmosphere.	■ Immediately clamp catheter and place client in Trendelenburg position (turned to the left so right ventricle is uppermost). ■ Immediately inform physician and monitor until physician arrives. Assess vital signs and breath sounds. ■ Administer high-flow O_2 as necessary. ■ Prevent air embolism by having client perform the Valsalva maneuver any time catheter is open to air, or use in-line catheter clamp. ■ Ensure client has a patent peripheral IV line.
Central vascular line remains patent and free of infection.	Infection occurs at insertion site.	■ Prepare for catheter removal and possible reinsertion at another site. ■ If catheter is removed, cut off catheter tip with sterile scissors and place in sterile container. Send tip to laboratory for culture. ■ Administer antibiotics as ordered. ■ Observe client carefully for signs of systemic infection.
IV catheter maintains patency with use of CLC 2000 device.	Catheter appears to be or becomes occluded.	■ Reposition client. ■ Ask client to raise arms over head. ■ Follow facility policy and procedure. ■ Assess mechanical problem: tubing, pumps, catheter, clamps, insertion site, or securement device. ■ Assess nonthrombotic problem: medications infused, fluids or withdrawal of blood. Use of precipitate clearance agent is established by individual facility policies and procedures. ■ Assess thrombotic problem: use of thrombolytic clearance agents is established by individual facility policy and procedures. ■ Perform the Valsalva maneuver. Turn head to one side. ■ Attempt to flush catheter with normal saline, using gentle pressure. ■ Notify physician for order to administer fibrinolytic agent or other agents.
	CVP readings vary greatly.	■ Assess patency of setup. ■ Assess client's level of pain; pain increases the CVP reading. ■ Assess if position of client has been changed; raising the head of the bed alters the reading unless setup is adjusted. ■ Check that the marked area at midaxillary level is at the level of the client's right atrium (fourth ICS). ■ If client has COPD, heart failure, or hypovolemia, expect readings to differ from normal range. However, once baseline is established for individual client, trends should be watched and evaluated against goals of therapy.

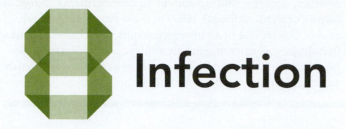

8 Infection

Skills-at-a-Glance

Planned nursing strategies to reduce the risk of transmission of organisms from one person to another include the use of meticulous asepsis. **Asepsis** is the freedom from infection or infectious material. There are two basic types of asepsis: medical and surgical. *Medical asepsis* includes all practices intended to confine a specific microorganism to a specific area, limiting the number, growth, and spread of microorganisms. *Surgical asepsis*, or *sterile technique*, refers to those practices that keep an area or objects free of all microorganisms. It includes practices that destroy all microorganisms and spores (microscopic dormant structures formed by some pathogens that are very hardy and often survive common cleaning techniques).

Evidence-Based Nursing Practice
Intervention Improves Hand Washing Practice

A 6-month program was run at Miami Children's Hospital to test the ability to improve hand washing compliance among healthcare providers. It involved an electronic monitoring system to confirm that providers engage in proper hand hygiene before client contact. After providers apply soap or gel, they place their hands under wall-mounted sensors that verify that hand washing has taken place and send a signal to a specially designed badge worn by all staff and physicians. When the clinician approaches the bedside, a bed monitor causes the badge to vibrate if appropriate hand hygiene has not taken place, thus reminding the provider to wash his or her hands before coming into contact with the client. The system also generates customized reports to inform individualized provider education on hand hygiene as needed.

The program generated high levels of adherence to appropriate hand hygiene (94%). This led to significant reductions in the overall number of healthcare-associated infections (HAIs) (by 61%) and in non–*Clostridium difficile* infections (91%). *C. difficile* HAIs were not meaningfully reduced, likely because these infections live on environmental surfaces for long periods of time; thus, they would have to be targeted by other types of infection prevention initiatives in addition to hand hygiene.

Data from U.S. Department of Health and Human Services, Agency for Healthcare Research and Quality (2013).

▶ BASIC MEDICAL ASEPSIS

Expected Outcomes

1. Care is delivered with pathogen-free hands to clients.
2. The spread of microorganisms from healthcare workers or the environment to clients is prevented.
3. Client-to-client spread of endogenous and exogenous flora is prevented.
4. Hospital personnel are protected from infection.

SKILL 8.1   Hand Hygiene (Medical Asepsis)

Equipment

- Nonantimicrobial soap (according to 1997 Healthcare Infection Control Practices Advisory Committee [HICPAC] recommendations) for routine hand washing
- Orangewood stick for cleaning nails
- Running warm water
- Paper towels
- Trash basket

Procedure

1. Stand in front of but away from sink. **Rationale:** *Uniform should not touch sink to avoid contamination.*
2. Ensure that paper towel is hanging down from dispenser.
3. Turn on water using foot pedal or faucet so that flow is adequate, but not splashing ❶.
4. Adjust temperature to warm. **Rationale:** *Cold water does not facilitate sudsing and cleaning; hot is damaging to skin.*

CLINICAL ALERT
Compliance Studies for Hand Hygiene

- A study of 2,800 opportunities for hand washing showed only a 48% compliance rate.
- Another study showed hands were washed for only 8.5 to 9.5 seconds, although a minimum of 20 seconds is necessary to prevent spread of infection.

- Compliance with hand washing technique is higher among nurses than physicians and other healthcare personnel; however, it is estimated to be only 30% to 50%.

Data from Centers for Disease Control and Prevention (CDC) (2013).

Length of Hand Washing
Nurses must wash hands for 20 seconds before and after each direct contact with a client or each use of client care items to prevent spread of infection (CDC, 2013).

5. Wet hands under running water, keeping hands below elbow level ❷. **Rationale:** *Wet hands facilitate distribution of soap over entire skin surface.*
6. Place 1 to 2 teaspoons (5 to 10 mL) of liquid soap on hands ❸. Thoroughly distribute over hands. Soap should come from a dispenser, not bar soap. **Rationale:** *This prevents spread of microorganisms.*
7. Rub vigorously, using a firm, circular motion, while keeping your fingers pointed down, lower than the wrists ❹. Start with each finger, then between fingers, then palm and back of hand. **Rationale:** *This creates friction on all surfaces.*
8. Wash your hands for least 20 seconds. **Rationale:** *Duration of washing is important to produce mechanical action and to allow antimicrobial products time to achieve desired effect.*
9. Clean under your fingernails with an orangewood stick. (This should be done at least at start of day and if hands are heavily

SKILL 8.1   Hand Hygiene (Medical Asepsis) *(continued)*

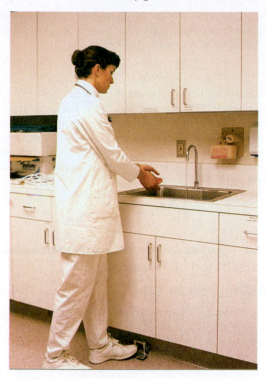

1 Use foot pedals when available to prevent contamination of hands.

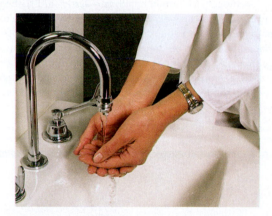

2 Wet hands thoroughly before applying soap to facilitate removal of pathogens.

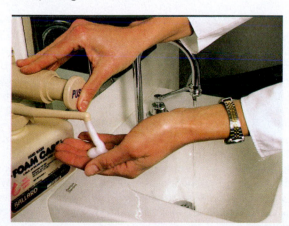

3 Use a generous amount of soap and friction during hand washing procedure.

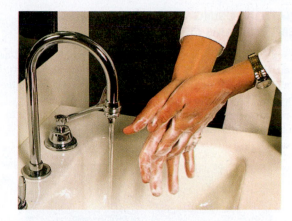

4 Keep fingers pointed down during hand washing to prevent contaminating arms.

        contaminated.) Move rings up and down fingers to clean if rings are left on.

10. Rinse your hands under running water, keeping fingers pointed downward. **Rationale:** *This position prevents contamination of arms.*

11. Resoap your hands, rewash, and rerinse if heavily contaminated.

12. Dry hands thoroughly with a paper towel, while keeping hands positioned with fingers pointing up. **Rationale:** *Moist hands tend to gather more microorganisms from the environment.*

13. Turn off water faucet with dry paper towel, if not using foot pedal **5**. **Rationale:** *To avoid recontaminating the hands.*

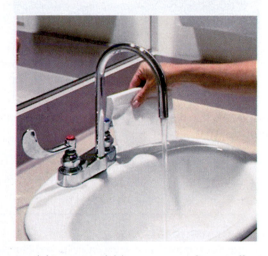

5 If foot pedal is not available, turn water faucet off using paper towel.

14. Restart procedure at step 5 if your hands touch the sink anytime between steps 5 and 13.

CLINICAL ALERT

OSHA requires that hands be washed with soap and water every third time the hands are cleansed.

Antimicrobial soap or waterless agent should be used when identified resistant bacteria, colonization outbreaks, or hyperendemic infections are present with the exception of *C. difficile* and *norovirus*, which are not killed by an alcohol-based gel.

(continued on next page)

SKILL 8.1 Hand Hygiene (Medical Asepsis) *(continued)*

VARIATION: USING WATERLESS ANTISEPTIC AGENTS (FOAMS OR GELS)

- Check dirt on hands and use waterless agent only if hands are clean. **Rationale:** *Hands soiled with dirt or organic matter require soap or detergents that contain antiseptic and water to effectively clean.*
- Apply small amount of alcohol-based rub, foam, or gel (3 to 5 mL) on palm or hand ⑥.

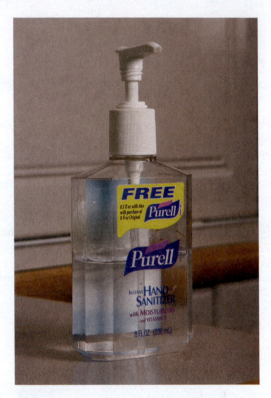

⑥ Waterless hand sanitizer kills 99.9% of the most common germs in 15 seconds.

- Rub hands together vigorously, covering all surfaces, sides of hands and fingers. **Rationale:** *Failure to cover all surfaces can leave contaminated areas on the hands.*
- Rub hands until dry—waterless agent will dry quickly and automatically without using a towel.

Note: Disposable germicidal wipes are now available that are effective at killing 99.99% of harmful bacteria. These wipes are also effective at removing soil from hands because of natural friction when wiping. The wipes are made from cloth saturated with ethyl alcohol gel solution, free of fragrance and dye. These products are approved by the Environmental Protection Agency (EPA) for both hepatitis B and viruses.

For the technique for sterile hand washing, see Skill 15.2.

Evidence-Based Nursing Practice

Nail Polish, Artificial Nails, and Microbial Threat

The World Health Organization (WHO), the American Organization of periOperative Nurses, the Joint Commission, and the CDC recommend that healthcare providers avoid the use of nail polish and artificial nails. Studies have not shown a definitive link between use of nail polish or artificial nails and increased risk of infection. However, the WHO (2009b) states that a growing body of evidence suggests that wearing artificial nails may contribute to the transmission of certain healthcare-associated pathogens. Healthcare workers who wear artificial nails are more likely to harbor gram-negative pathogens on their fingertips than those who have natural nails, both before and after hand washing or use of a an alcohol-based gel. It is not clear if the length of natural or artificial nails is an important risk factor, since most bacterial growth occurs along the proximal 1 mm of the nail, adjacent to subungual skin.

Data from Arrowsmith & Taylor (2012) and World Health Organization (2009b).

Cultural Considerations

It is imperative that nurses remember the unfamiliar and overwhelming nature of healthcare settings. Most clients are uncomfortable in a clinical environment, especially when they are undergoing procedures, hearing unfamiliar terminology, and receiving care from people who may be wearing masks and gloves. Imagine if English is not a client's primary language, or if the client is deaf. Under those circumstances, the challenges to a client's psychoemotional and even physical safety increase. When clarity of communication is compromised, therapeutic efficacy and client safety are compromised. It is essential to clarify all aspects of care with clients, and to provide trained interpreters whenever necessary. It is also necessary for members of the healthcare team to make sure that they themselves understand each other, because English may not be the primary language of every nurse, UAP, physician, or other healthcare provider. Asking for clarification frequently and not making assumptions are two habits that can help prevent clinical care errors. When in doubt, ask.

When it comes to cultural diversity, it is especially important to ask the client about nutritional and exercise patterns, health and healing practices, family organization and roles, social support network, spiritual and religious beliefs and practices, communication styles, gender relation patterns, and attitudes toward individuals in authority. Personal space issues, time orientation, and the client's explanation of his or her health status are also important to explore.

For essential resources regarding cultural considerations in healthcare environments, search the web for Culturally and Linguistically Appropriate Services (CLAS) for healthcare settings. *Holistic Nursing: A Handbook for Clinical Practice* (Dossey & Keegan, 2008) also includes resources and cultural assessments for nurses to incorporate into their admissions and clinical care processes.

▶ PERSONAL PROTECTIVE EQUIPMENT (PPE) AND ISOLATION PRECAUTIONS

Expected Outcomes

1. Appropriate PPE and isolation measures are used for individual clients.
2. The transfer of microorganisms from healthcare workers or the environment to clients is prevented.
3. Cross-contamination among clients is prevented.
4. Hospital personnel and others are protected from contamination.
5. Appropriate equipment is provided and techniques for preventive measures are followed.
6. The incidence of healthcare-associated infections is reduced.
7. Immunosuppressed clients are prevented from acquiring healthcare-associated infections.

SKILL 8.2   Latex Precautions

Equipment

- Latex-free gloves, syringes, and IV ports on IV bags/lines
- Latex-free bellows on ventilator
- Latex-free bags on masks
- Stockinette and latex-free tape
- Medications and equipment for treatment of anaphylactic reaction

Preparation

- Reduce and/or eliminate the amount of latex used in agencies by eliminating use of latex gloves where feasible as well as reducing the amount of other latex products used; when latex gloves are used, they should be nonpowdered. **Rationale:** *The powder in latex gloves contains latex, which is spread into the environment when the gloves are donned.*
- Identify latex-free materials and supplies in the agency.
- Be aware of signs of latex sensitivity.
- Assess all clients for a history of latex allergy or significant risk factors.
- Be prepared for emergency resuscitation if needed.

Procedure

When clients are identified as latex sensitive or allergic, prepare the environment before their entry and continue practices as long as they remain.

1. Remove all latex-containing products (gloves, tourniquets, tape, etc.) from the room. If latex products cannot be removed, the items should be located in a closed storage area, such as cabinets and drawers.
2. After removing latex items, thoroughly clean the room/exam area using latex-free (nitrile or vinyl) gloves to remove contaminated latex-containing dust. Do not wear latex or rubber gloves to clean the room. When an allergic individual has surgery or another procedure, the room should be properly prepared and the case should be the first of the day.
3. Mattresses/exam tables may contain latex and, therefore, should be covered completely with a nonlatex protective cover.
4. Stock rooms with latex-free material and latex-free gloves.
5. Place a latex precaution sign on the client's door/exam area.
6. Place all monitoring devices and cord/tubes (oximeter, blood pressure, electrocardiograph wires, ports on intravenous tubing) in stockinette, and tape with nonlatex tape to prevent direct skin contact. Items sterilized in ethylene oxide must be rinsed before use. Residual ethylene oxide can cause an allergic response in a latex-allergic client.
7. Use stopcocks rather than latex ports to inject drugs.
8. Label the client's medical record, medication form, and identification bands with allergy alerts. Alert other nurses to the allergy during verbal reports between shifts.
9. Document measures taken.
10. Report promptly and document any signs of sensitivity or allergy.
11. Teach clients and families about latex allergy and how to avoid latex products.
12. Instruct the family about foods that commonly cause allergies in those with latex allergy, and avoid feeding them to the client. They include bananas, avocados, kiwis, plums, peaches, cherries, apricots, figs, papayas, tomatoes, potatoes, and chestnuts.

SKILL 8.3   Donning and Removing Clean Gloves

Evidence-Based Nursing Practice

The Importance of Gloves

The World Health Organization (WHO) provides the following recommendations on glove use:

A. Be aware that glove use *does not* modify hand hygiene indications or replace hand hygiene actions (rubbing hands with alcohol-based product or washing hands with soap and water).
B. Wear gloves when anticipating contact with blood or other body fluids, mucous membranes, nonintact skin, or potentially infectious material.
C. Remove gloves after caring for a client. Do not wear the same pair of gloves for the care of more than one client.
D. Change or remove gloves during client care if moving from a contaminated body site to another body site (including a mucous membrane, nonintact skin, or a medical device within the same client or the environment).
E. Do not reuse gloves after reprocessing or decontamination.

ACTION	INDICATION
Gloves on	1) Before a sterile procedure 2) When anticipating contact with blood or another body fluid, regardless of the existence of sterile conditions 3) During contact precautions
Gloves off	1) As soon as gloves are damaged or damage is suspected 2) When contact with body fluid, nonintact skin, and mucous membrane has ended 3) When contact with a single client and his or her surroundings, or a contaminated body site on a client has ended 4) When there is an indication for hand hygiene

(continued on next page)

SKILL 8.3   Donning and Removing Clean Gloves (*continued*)

The WHO states that although gloves have been proven effective in preventing contamination of healthcare workers' hands and in reducing transmission of pathogens in healthcare environments, they do not provide complete protection against hand contamination.

Data from World Health Organization (2009a).

Cross-Contamination

Several studies have shown that hospital surfaces and frequently used medical equipment become contaminated by pathogens and other microorganisms. Items affected include "critical" equipment such as surgical instruments and urinary catheters and "noncritical" equipment such as bedpans and oximetry sensors. There is now increasing evidence that contaminated environmental surfaces such as bedside tables, IV poles, and walls may be implicated in transmission of pathogens.

Organisms that can persist on dry inanimate surfaces include *Escherichia coli* (up to 16 months), norovirus (up to 7 days), *Staphylococcus aureus* including MRSA (up to 7 months), and *Clostridium difficile* spores (5 months). In one study 14 of 26 clients in an ICU acquired MRSA when no other client with that type of MRSA was present. Therefore, infection prevention measures must include inanimate environmental equipment as well as "critical" equipment. Disposable (single-client-use) items such as pulse oximetry sensors may be useful in reducing spread of transmission and cross-contamination. Strict adherence to infection prevention practices is essential.

Data from Arias (2010).

Equipment

- Clean gloves
- Trash receptacle

Procedure

1. Complete hand hygiene ❶. **Rationale:** *Donning gloves with unclean hands can transfer microorganisms outside gloves.*
2. Remove glove from glove receptacle ❷.
3. Hold glove at wrist edge and slip fingers into openings. Pull glove up to wrist.
4. Place gloved hand under wrist edge of second glove and slip fingers into opening.
5. Remove glove by pulling off, touching only outside of glove at cuff, so that glove turns inside out.
6. Place rolled-up glove in palm of second hand.
7. Remove second glove by slipping one finger under glove edge and pulling down and off so that glove turns inside out. Both gloves are removed as a unit.
8. Dispose of gloves in proper container, not at bedside ❸.
9. Complete hand hygiene.

CLINICAL ALERT

Ungloved hands should not touch anything that is moist coming from a body surface. The moisture coming from a body surface should be considered potentially contaminated.

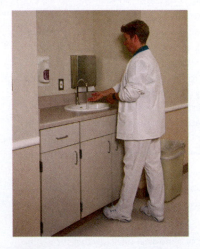

❶ Wash your hands or complete hand hygiene before donning gloves.

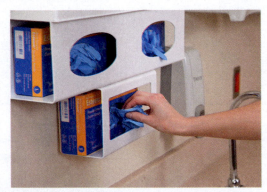

❷ Remove glove from dispenser.

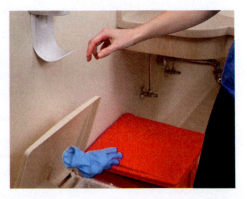

❸ Dispose of gloves in proper container, not at bedside. Complete hand hygiene.

SKILL 8.4   Donning and Removing Isolation Attire

Equipment

- Gown
- Clean gloves

Procedure (for Donning Attire)

1. Complete hand hygiene.
2. Take gown from isolation cart or cupboard. Put on a new gown each time you enter an isolation room.

SKILL 8.4   Donning and Removing Isolation Attire *(continued)*

3. Hold gown so that opening is in back when you are wearing the gown.
4. Put gown on by placing one arm at a time through sleeves. Pull gown up and over your shoulders.
5. Wrap gown around your back, tying strings at your neck.
6. Wrap gown around your waist, making sure your back is completely covered. Tie strings around your waist.
7. Don eye shield and/or mask, if indicated ❶. **Rationale:** *Mask is required if there is a risk of splashing fluids.*
8. Don clean gloves and pull gloves over gown wristlets ❷. **Rationale:** *To prevent contamination of exposed skin.*

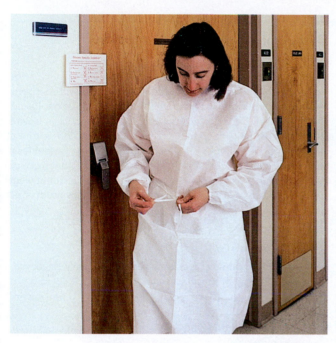

❶ Isolation gown is put on before mask, eye shield, or gloves.

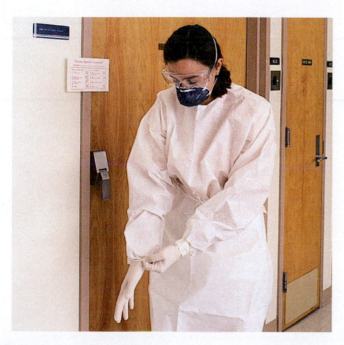

❷ Cover wristlets completely to prevent contamination of exposed skin.

Procedure (For Removing Attire)

1. Untie gown waist strings.
2. Remove gloves and dispose of them in garbage bag ❸ ❹.

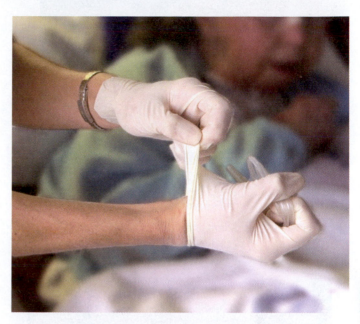

❸ Remove gloves before gown, mask, or eye shield.

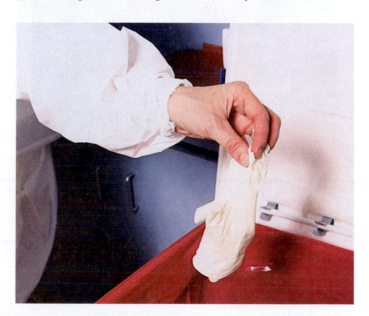

❹ Dispose of gloves in an appropriate receptacle.

3. Next, untie neck strings, bringing them around your shoulders so that gown is partially off your shoulders.
4. Using your dominant hand and grasping clean part of wristlet, pull sleeve wristlet over your nondominant hand. Use your nondominant hand to pull sleeve wristlet over your dominant hand.
5. Grasp outside of gown through the sleeves at shoulders. Pull gown down over your arms ❺.
6. Hold both gown shoulders in one hand. Carefully draw your other hand out of gown, turning arm of gown inside out. Repeat this procedure with your other arm.

(continued on next page)

SKILL 8.4   Donning and Removing Isolation Attire *(continued)*

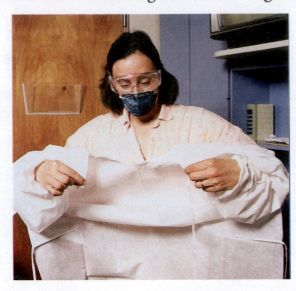

⑤ Pull gown off shoulders, then down over arms.

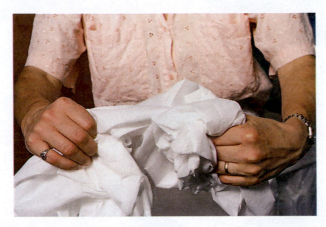

⑥ Hold gown away from body when rolling inside out.

7. Hold gown away from your body. Fold gown up, inside out ⑥.
8. Discard gown in appropriate place.
9. Remove eye shield and/or mask and place in receptacle.
10. Complete hand hygiene. **Rationale:** *This prevents cross-infection to other clients.*

CLINICAL ALERT
Some isolation gowns do not tie at the neck; they slip over the head. When removing these gowns, pull shoulders forward to loosen the Velcro at the neck area. Remove gown in the same manner as you would if tied at the neck.

Developmental Considerations

CHILDREN
Isolation precautions can increase an already stressful situation for a hospitalized child. Younger children have limited cognitive abilities to understand the implications of isolation. Particularly frightening for them is the presence of people in gowns and masks. To help decrease their fears, preparation is important. Letting the children see and play with the equipment lessens some of the anxiety. Healthcare workers should introduce themselves to the child before donning a mask. Frequent visits to the child can also lessen the fear and loneliness associated with isolation.

Setting of Care
- All aspects of standard precautions and PPE apply equally in the clinic, home, or long-term care setting.
- Ensure that the supply of gloves, gowns, masks, and eyewear is adequate.
- Ensure that procedures are in place for removal and disposal of used materials.
- Teach the client and family appropriate aspects of standard precautions.

SKILL 8.5   Using a Mask

Equipment
- Clean mask

Procedure

1. Obtain mask from box ❶.
2. Position mask to cover your nose and mouth.
3. Bend nose bar so that it conforms over bridge of your nose.
4. If you are using a mask with string ties, tie top strings on top of your head to prevent slipping. If you are using a cone-shaped mask, tie top strings over your ears ❷.

CLINICAL ALERT
Respiratory N95 or HEPA (high-efficiency particulate air) respirator masks are recommended for infectious diseases transmitted by the airborne mode, for example, influenza or suspected or confirmed multidrug-resistant tuberculosis.

- Masks are fitted to worker. Mask should have a good sealing surface with no leakage around the edge, providing a tight seal over the nose and mouth.
- Wear mask until it becomes difficult to breathe. This indicates mask is clogged.
- When not in use, store mask in zip-lock bag in safe area.
- Masks are expensive and can be used repeatedly until it is difficult to breathe through them.

Protective eyewear such as goggles and face shield are worn when there is a risk of splashes or sprays from blood, secretions, excretions, or body fluids. Eyewear is removed before taking off mask.

5. Tie bottom strings around your neck to secure mask over your mouth. There should be no gaps between the mask and your face.

SKILL 8.5   Using a Mask (*continued*)

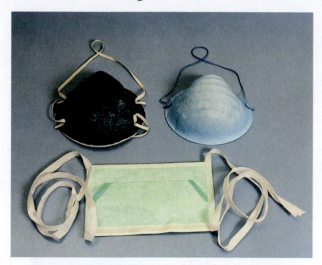

❶ Sample masks used for isolation protocol.

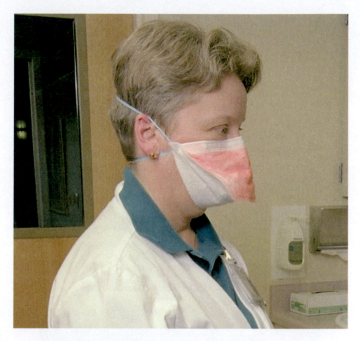

❷ Particulate filter respirator mask must be airtight.

6. *Important*: Change mask every 30 minutes or sooner if it become damp. **Rationale:** *Effectiveness is greatly reduced after 30 minutes or if mask is moist.*
7. Complete hand hygiene before removing mask.
8. To remove mask, untie lower strings first, or slip elastic band off without touching mask. **Rationale:** *Only strings are considered clean.*

9. Discard mask in a trash container.
10. Complete hand hygiene.

SKILL 8.6   Assessing Vital Signs of Infectious Client

Equipment

- Thermometer
- Stethoscope
- Blood pressure cuff and sphygmomanometer
- Thermometer stand
- Watch with sweep second hand
- Isolation clothing

Procedure

1. Complete hand hygiene and identify client by checking the client's identity band and asking client to state name and birth date.

2. Don isolation clothing as required by type of isolation.
3. Proceed to take and to document vital signs as you would for any client.
4. Place equipment in appropriate area if it is to be left in room. Follow appropriate protocol to remove equipment from isolation room (see Skill 8.7).
5. Remove isolation clothing according to protocol.
6. Complete hand hygiene.
7. Wipe watch if accidentally contaminated. Use appropriate solution.

SKILL 8.7   Removing Items from Isolation Room

Equipment

- Large red isolation bags
- Specimen container
- Plastic bag with biohazard label
- Laundry bag
- Red plastic container for sharps
- Cleaning articles

Procedure

1. Place laboratory specimen in biohazard plastic bag.
2. Dispose of all sharps in appropriate red plastic container in room.

3. Place all linen in linen bag.
4. Place reusable equipment such as procedure trays in plastic bags. **Rationale:** *Appropriate separation of equipment from isolation room alerts central supply staff that it is contaminated and special handling needs to be carried out.*
5. Dispose of all garbage in plastic bags. Close bag tightly ❶.
6. Double bag all material from isolation room in anteroom (if available) ❷. **Rationale:** *All material removed from an isolation room is potentially contaminated. This will prevent spread of microorganisms.*

(continued on next page)

SKILL 8.7   Removing Items from Isolation Room (*continued*)

7. Replace all bags, such as linen bag and garbage bag, in appropriate container in room ❸.
8. Clean client's room as necessary, using germicidal solution, according to facility protocol.
9. Prepare to leave the client's room.

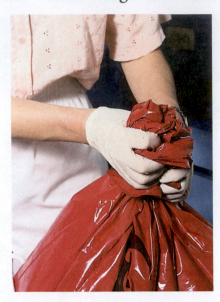

❶ Close bag securely and label contents, if necessary.

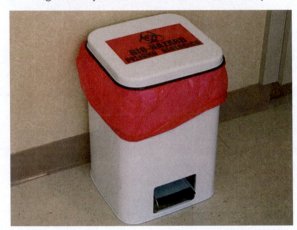

❷ Place red biohazard bag in specified area for disposal.

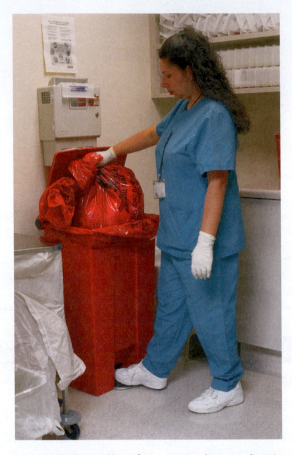

❸ Set up new biohazard bag for continued use in client's room.

SKILL 8.8   Removing Specimen from Isolation Room

Equipment

- Specimen container
- Clean biohazard bag ❶

Procedure

1. Follow dress protocol for entering isolation room, or, if you are already in the isolation room, continue with step 2.
2. Mark a specimen container with the client's name, type of specimen, and the word "isolation" before entering an isolation room.
3. Collect specimen, and place container in a clean plastic biohazard bag outside the room. **Rationale:** *Use clear bags so that laboratory personnel can see the specimen easily.*
4. Complete hand hygiene.
5. Send specimen to laboratory with appropriate laboratory request form.

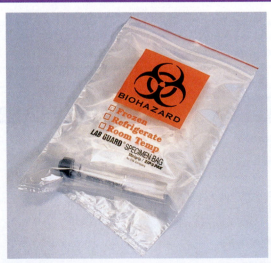

❶ Biohazard bag for transportation of specimens from isolation room.

SKILL 8.9 Transporting Isolation Client Outside Room

Equipment

- Transport vehicle
- Bath blanket
- Mask for client if needed

Procedure

1. Explain procedure to client.
2. If client is being transported from a respiratory isolation room, instruct him or her to wear a mask for the entire time out of isolation ❶. **Rationale:** *This prevents the spread of airborne microbes.*
3. Cover the transport vehicle with a bath blanket if there is a chance of soiling when transporting a client who has a draining wound or diarrhea.
4. Help client into transport vehicle. Cover client with a bath blanket.
5. Tell receiving department what type of isolation client needs and what precautions hospital personnel should follow.
6. Remove bath blanket, and handle as contaminated linen when client returns to room.
7. Instruct all hospital personnel to complete hand hygiene before they leave the area.
8. Wipe down transportation vehicle with an antimicrobial solution if soiled.

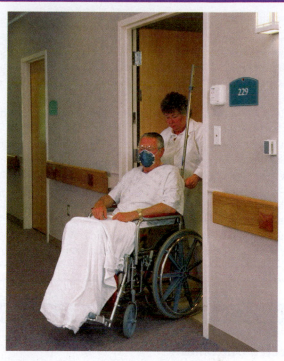

❶ Place surgical mask on client if he or she needs to be transported outside room.

SKILL 8.10 Removing Soiled Large Equipment from Isolation Room

Equipment

- Antimicrobial agent and articles needed to wash equipment
- Plastic bag

Procedure

1. Don isolation garb as recommended.
2. Wash equipment with an antimicrobial agent ❶. **Rationale:** *Washing is preferred to spraying in order to ensure all surfaces are cleaned.*
3. Cover equipment with a plastic bag.
4. Remove garb, and complete hand hygiene outside the room. Take equipment to the decontamination area of central supply room.

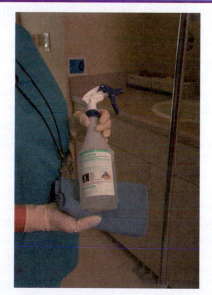

❶ Wash isolation equipment with antimicrobial agent.

Practice Guidelines

PROTOCOL FOR LEAVING ISOLATION ROOM

- Untie gown at waist.
- Take off gloves.
- Untie gown at neck.

- Pull gown off and place in laundry hamper.
- Take off goggles or face shield.
- Take off mask.
- Complete hand hygiene.

(continued on next page)

SKILL 8.10 Removing Soiled Large Equipment from Isolation Room (continued)

DISPOSING OF CONTAMINATED EQUIPMENT

- **Disposable glass:** Place in isolation bag separate from burnable trash and direct to appropriate hospital area for disposal.
- **Glass equipment:** Bag separately from metal equipment and return to CSR.
- **Metal equipment:** Bag all equipment together, label, and return to central supply room (CSR).
- **Rubber and plastic items:** Bag items separately and return to CSR for gas sterilization.
- **Dishes:** Require no special precautions unless contaminated with infected material; then bag, label, and return to kitchen.
- **Plastic or paper dishes:** Dispose of these items in burnable trash bins.
- **Soiled linens:** Place in laundry bag, and send to separate area of laundry room for special care. If possible, place linens in

hot-water–soluble bag. This method is safer for handling, because bag may be placed directly into washing machine. (Double-bagging is usually required because these bags are easily punctured or torn. They also dissolve when wet.)

- **Food and liquids:** Dispose of these items by putting them in the toilet—flush thoroughly.
- **Needles and syringes:** Do not recap needles; place in puncture-resistant container.
- **Sphygmomanometer and stethoscope:** Require no special precautions unless they are contaminated. If contaminated, disinfect using the appropriate cleaning protocol based on the infective agent.
- **Thermometers:** Dispose of electronic probe cover with burnable trash. If probe or machine is contaminated, clean with appropriate disinfectant for infective agent. If reusable thermometers are used, disinfect with appropriate solution.

▶ PERSONAL PROTECTIVE EQUIPMENT IN THE HOME SETTING

Expected Outcomes

1. Equipment is cleaned appropriately.
2. Waste is disposed of in proper manner.
3. Clients do not acquire infections during home care visits.
4. Infections are treated appropriately and not transmitted to other home care clients or the nurse because effective preventive measures are utilized.

In the home setting, medical asepsis, or clean technique, is often used instead of sterile technique. The major reasons for this protocol change are the nature of the setting and the personnel providing care.

The greatest infection control problem in hospitals is healthcare-associated infections due to the large numbers of antibiotic-resistant organisms present in a hospital setting. When clients are in their own environment, however, they tend to develop fewer infections because they are subjected to fewer organisms. In the home setting, focus is on protecting home care staff and family, not other clients. While there may be transmission of organisms between individuals in the home, there are minimal data on the incidence of home care–acquired infections. Infection preventing strategies in the home should focus on IV therapy and urinary tract, respiratory, and wound care.

Sterile equipment, such as prepackaged catheter and irrigation kits, parenteral fluid equipment, and dressings, are often purchased for home care. When sterile technique is required, it is the responsibility of the nurse to provide the instruction and evaluate the family's ability to perform the skill accurately. Hospital techniques may need to be modified for the home setting, and ideal environmental working conditions may not be present. Unfortunately, the Division of Healthcare Quality Promotion of the CDC has not developed guidelines for infection control in home care settings at this time. Therefore, adaptations must be made, and essential infection control measures must be maintained.

Just as in the hospital, effective hand hygiene is the most effective means of infection control in the home setting. There is one major difference between hospital and home. Equip-

ment (soap, running water, and paper towels) that is readily available to the nurse in the hospital may not be available in the home. Even if running water is available, there may not be soap or clean towels. Nurses must bring their own hand washing supplies.

A decrease in the duration of hospital stays has dramatically increased the expanded scope of the home care nurse. Unfortunately, infection surveillance, prevention, and control efforts have not kept up. Many of the home care infection control practices have been based on ritual and acute care practice, rather than scientific principles. Changes in infection control procedures in the home are currently occurring based on a scientific approach.

Home care assessment for potential infections relies on clinical signs and symptoms and tests, such as the urine dipstick, that can be performed in the home. Routine tests used in hospitals to diagnose infections of the urinary tract, respiratory tract, and wound or skin sites are not routinely done, as the current reimbursement system does not support cultures and laboratory tests. Only cultures that confirm and treat bloodstream infections for clients requiring home infusion therapy are obtained.

If the home care client is suspected of or diagnosed as having an infectious disease or the client is infected or colonized with VRE or MSRA, the nurse should use the same PPE and protocol used in the hospital setting. The equipment includes gloves, disposable gown or apron, mask, cap, and goggles. Reusable equipment, such as stethoscopes and blood pressure cuffs, should stay in the home and not be used on other home care clients. If possible, these clients should be seen at the end of the day.

SKILL 8.11 Preparing for Client Care

Equipment

- Community health nursing bag
- Liquid soap
- Antibacterial gel for hand hygiene
- Disposable gloves
- Disposable apron or gown
- Goggles
- Masks, air-purifying mask
- Thermometers (oral and rectal)
- Thermometer sheaths
- Nex Temp (disposable thermometer)
- Petroleum jelly or other lubricant
- Cotton balls
- Alcohol, one small bottle
- Antimicrobial wipes
- Cotton-tipped applicators
- Tongue depressors
- Sterile 4 × 4s
- Band-Aids
- Bandage scissors
- Nonallergic tape
- Plastic bags with ties
- Keto-Diastix and Chemstrips
- Sphygmomanometer
- Stethoscope
- Paper cups
- Bleach, one small bottle

Procedure

1. Arrange equipment in bag before making home visit so that hand hygiene equipment is accessible. Bring only the supplies needed. **Rationale:** *This procedure decreases the possibility of cross-contamination.*
2. Place bag on flat, dry surface to establish a clean work area during visit. Use of disposable barrier under bag is recommended. **Rationale:** *To prevent potential spread of infection between clients' homes. The risk can be high for transmitting undiagnosed infections between home clients.*
3. Perform hand hygiene.
   - Use liquid soap and paper towels from bag and client's water supply. Wash hands with clean running water and apply soap. Rub hands together to make a lather and scrub all surfaces. Rub hands for 10 to 15 seconds. Rinse hands well under running water. Dry hands using paper towel from nurse's bag. Turn off faucet using paper towel.
   - Use antimicrobial gel as alternative to hand washing when soap and water are not available. Squeeze small amount of germicide onto palm of hand and rub all surfaces of hands, fingers, and nails. Germicide evaporates into air, making towels unnecessary.
4. Don disposable gloves when appropriate for infection control, especially when handling blood and body fluids.
5. Take other equipment that will be needed during the visit out of the bag and place on clean work surface.
6. Keep bag closed when not in use to promote cleanliness, safety, and security. Care should be taken not to reenter bag wearing soiled gloves. Washing hands between reentering bag is not necessary unless soiled.
7. Wear disposable apron or gown, goggles, or masks if necessary. **Rationale:** *This protects the caregiver from blood or body fluid exposure.*
8. Cleanse thoroughly any equipment that left clean area and is to be returned to the bag on completing care.
   - Rinse equipment (such as bandage scissors, forceps) under *cold* water, wash with soap and water. Use client's personal equipment or disposable equipment whenever possible.
   - Return stethoscope and blood pressure cuff to nursing bag. **Rationale:** *Clean items can be returned to nursing bag if no visible soiling.*
9. Ensure nursing bag is monitored regularly for safety.
   - Keep bag out of reach of children.
   - Keep bag in trunk of car or keep in your home overnight. **Rationale:** *Unattended bags in cars are more often stolen.*
   - Clean bag monthly and PRN.

> **CLINICAL ALERT**
> If item is soiled and cannot be returned to the bag, place in separate container for transport to agency. Clean item when it is returned to agency. Most items for home care are disposable.

Client Teaching

Infection Control

- Describe ways to manipulate the bed, the room, and other household facilities to prevent injury or to contain possible cross-contamination.
- Instruct to clean obviously soiled linen separately from other laundry. Wash in hot water if possible, adding a cup of bleach or phenol-based disinfectant such as Lysol concentrate to the wash, and rinse in cold water.
- Based on assessment of client and family knowledge, teach proper hand hygiene (e.g., before handling foods, before eating, after toileting, before and after any required home care treatment, and after touching any body substances such as wound drainage) and related hygienic measures to all family members.
- Promote nail care. Keep fingernails short, clean, and well manicured to eliminate rough edges or hangnails, which can harbor microorganisms.
- Instruct not to share personal care items such as toothbrushes, washcloths, and towels. Describe how infections can be transmitted from shared personal items.
- Discuss antimicrobial soaps and effective disinfectants.
- Discuss the relationship between hygiene, rest, activity, and nutrition in the chain of infection.
- Instruct about cleaning reusable equipment and supplies. Use soap and water, and disinfect with a chlorine bleach solution.
- Teach the client and family members the signs and symptoms of infection, and when to contact a healthcare provider. Determine by verbal questions the level of understanding of the topic after each teaching session.

(continued on next page)

SKILL 8.11 Preparing for Client Care *(continued)*

- Teach the client and family members how to avoid infections.
- Suggest techniques for safe food preservation and preparation (e.g., wash raw fruits and vegetables before eating them, refrigerate all opened and unpackaged foods).
- Remind to avoid coughing, sneezing, or breathing directly on others. Cover the mouth and nose to prevent the transmission of airborne microorganisms.

- Inform of the importance of maintaining sufficient fluid intake to promote urine production and output. This helps flush the bladder and urethra of microorganisms.
- Emphasize the need for proper immunizations of all family members.

Developmental Considerations

CHILDREN

Infections are an expected part of childhood. The majority of these infections are caused by viruses. In some cases, severe, even life-threatening infections occur. Considerations related to children include the following:

- Newborns may not be able to respond to infections due to an underdeveloped immune system. As a result, in the first few months of life, infections may not be associated with typical signs and symptoms (e.g., an infant with an infection may not have a fever).
- Newborns are born with some naturally acquired immunity transferred from the mother across the placenta.
- Breastfed infants enjoy higher levels of immunity against infections than formula-fed infants.
- Children who are immune compromised (e.g., leukemia, HIV) or have a chronic health condition (e.g., cystic fibrosis, sickle cell disease, congenital heart disease) need extra precautions to prevent exposure to infectious agents.

OLDER ADULTS

Normal aging may predispose older adults to increased risk of infection and delayed healing. Anatomical and physiological agents that are protective when an individual is younger often change in structure and function with increasing age and then provide a decrease in their protective ability. Changes take place in the skin, respiratory tract, gastrointestinal system, kidneys, and immune system. Special considerations for older adults include the following:

- Nutrition may be poor in older adults. Certain components, especially adequate protein, are necessary to build up and maintain the immune system.
- Diabetes mellitus, which occurs more frequently in older adults, increases the risk of infection and delayed healing by causing an alteration in nutrition and impaired peripheral circulation, which decrease the oxygen transport to the tissues.
- The normal inflammatory response is delayed. This often causes atypical responses to infections with unusual presentations. Instead of displaying the redness, swelling, and fever usually associated with infections, atypical symptoms such as confusion and disorientation, agitation, incontinence, falls, lethargy, and general fatigue are often seen first.

Recognizing these changes in older adults is important in the early detection and treatment of the related potential for infections and delayed healing. Nursing interventions to promote prevention include the following:

- Provide and teach ways to improve nutritional status.
- Use strict aseptic technique (especially in healthcare facilities).
- Encourage older adults to have regular immunizations for flu and pneumonia.
- Be alert to subtle atypical signs of infection and act quickly to diagnose and treat.

Setting of Care

INFECTION CONTROL

- Assist with injury-proofing the home to prevent the possibility of tissue injury (e.g., use of padding, installation of handrails, removal of hazards).
- Explore ways to control the environmental temperature and airflow (especially if client has an airborne pathogen).
- Determine the advisability of visitors and family members in proximity to an infected client.
- Ensure access to and proper use of hand-cleansing supplies, gloves, and other barriers as indicated by the type of infection or risk.

SKILL 8.12 Disposing of Waste Material

Equipment

- Plastic bags, heavy-duty
- Disposable gloves
- Receptacle, rigid and puncture-proof
- Bleach
- Germicide

Procedure

1. Dispose of wastes contaminated with blood or body fluids.
   - Place waste products in impenetrable, heavy-duty plastic bag.
   - Remove plastic gloves by rolling inside out (so contaminated side is on inside) and drop into plastic bag.
   - Seal plastic bag with tie.
   - Discard in client's trash.
   - Perform hand hygiene with soap and water or germicide.
2. Dispose of body wastes, such as urine, feces, respiratory secretions, vomitus, and blood, by flushing them down the toilet. (This is true whether the toilet empties into a septic tank or a sewage system.)

SKILL 8.12   Disposing of Waste Material (*continued*)

3. Dispose of needles and sharp objects.
   - Do *not* remove needle from syringe or bend, break, clip, or recap after use.
   - Drop entire disposable safety syringe intact into rigid, puncture-proof receptacle provided by agency.
   - Complete hand hygiene.
4. Discard other trash.
   - Place in plastic bag.
   - Discard in client's trash.

Note: Clothes and bedding do not need to be destroyed. They are laundered separately in hot water with a 10% bleach solution added to the detergent in the washer.

CLINICAL ALERT

All items contaminated with blood, exudates, or other body fluids should be considered to present a risk of transmission of HIV or hepatitis B. These items should be disposed of by incineration if possible. Use mechanisms for disposal of waste into normal trash only when incineration is not available.

Do not use glass bottles or plastic bottles that can be returned to store. Bleach bottle with screw lid can be left in home for use as a sharps container. Tape closed before disposing of bottle. Small biohazard containers can be obtained from drugstores.

SKILL 8.13   Caring for a Client with HIV or AIDS

Equipment

- Gloves
- Disposable mask, gown, or apron
- Protective eyewear
- Specimen container if needed
- Plastic bag for transport of specimen
- Chlorine bleach solution (Clorox)

Procedure

1. Perform hand hygiene before and after client care and after disposing of soiled materials.
2. Don disposable gloves for any procedure.
   - Don double gloves if tearing is likely during the procedure.
   - If staff member has any type of open wound or weeping dermatitis, she or he should not administer care (even with gloves) until condition is resolved.
3. Don disposable gown or apron to protect clothing from soilage.
4. Put on mask and protective eyewear if splattering is anticipated during the procedure (e.g., suctioning, wound irrigations).
5. Collect specimens in appropriate containers. Place in plastic sealable biohazard bags.
6. Use extraordinary care to avoid puncture wounds with needles and other sharp objects.
   - If puncture occurs, bleed wound and wash with soap and water.
   - Notify supervisor immediately, and fill out unusual occurrence report.
7. Transport all specimens in an impermeable container, keeping the container separate from nurse's bag and supplies.
8. Clean spills of blood and body fluids with 10% bleach solution (one part liquid chlorine bleach to nine parts water). Make solution fresh each visit.
9. Wash eating utensils (dishes and silverware) in hot soapy water. Water should be hot enough to need gloves to tolerate the temperature. No other special precautions are required. It is best to use a dishwasher, if available. It is not necessary to wash client's dishes separately.
10. Store linens and laundry soiled with body fluids in a plastic bag and then wash separately with very hot water. Use a detergent and a 10% bleach solution. (Nonchlorine bleaches such as Clorox II are acceptable for colored clothing.)
11. Dispose of gown or apron in plastic bag after completing care.
12. Take off gloves by peeling them down and turning them inside out so that contaminated side is on the inside. Place in plastic bag.
13. Perform hand hygiene.
14. Take off mask and goggles.
15. Perform hand hygiene. Document care and client response.

SKILL 8.14   Teaching Preventive Measures

Procedure

1. Discuss the inadvisability of allowing any person who is ill or who has depressed immune function to come in contact with the client.
2. Teach the client these appropriate hygiene principles:
   - Wash hands after use of toilet or contact with any body fluids.
   - Do not share thermometers, razors, razor blades, toothbrushes, douche, or enema equipment.
   - Do not cough without covering mouth.
   - Be careful to dispose of nasal secretions in tissue, then in plastic bags.
3. Teach these guidelines for sharing kitchens and bathrooms:
   - Good household cleaning practices prevent spread of infection.
   - Don't share eating and drinking utensils. After use, they must be cleaned with hot water (hot enough to necessitate use of gloves) and soap. Use of a dishwasher and soap is appropriate.
   - Kitchen and bathroom surfaces should be cleaned every day with scouring powder or with chlorine bleach solution (10%—one part bleach to nine parts water). Use disposable bathroom cups. Use covered individual toothbrush holders.

(continued on next page)

SKILL 8.14   Teaching Preventive Measures (*continued*)

- Clean refrigerators regularly with soap and water; remove old food to prevent mold.
- Mop floors in bathroom and kitchen weekly. Pour dirty water down the toilet and disinfect with bleach solution.
- Clean toilet, tub, and shower weekly or as often as necessary with 10% bleach solution. If urine or diarrhea spills on toilet or floor, wipe immediately with the 10% bleach solution.
- Sponges used to clean floors or body fluid spills should be soaked for 5 minutes in a 10% bleach solution.

4. Teach the following principles of food preparation:
- Discuss the fact that people infected with HIV may prepare food for others. They should follow usual practices for safe food preparation and be especially diligent about hand washing.
- Wash hands thoroughly before any food preparation.
- Do not lick fingers or taste from the mixing spoon while cooking.
- Avoid unpasteurized milk (danger of contact with *Salmonella*); do not eat old or moldy food (danger of food poisoning); and carefully wash and thoroughly cook chicken.
- Wash all fresh (raw) fruits and vegetables before eating.

5. Teach how to care for linens and laundry.
- When clothing or linen is soiled with blood or body fluids, it should be stored separately in a plastic bag. Wash separately with very hot water, detergent, and bleach. Use Clorox II for colored clothing.
- Wear disposable gloves when touching soiled clothes or linen.
- Do not share used towels or washcloths, and wash separately. (Towels and washcloths are, however, safe to use after washing.)
- Change towels and washcloths daily.

6. Inform client and family of measures for disposing of trash.
- Flush body wastes down the toilet.
- Discard dressings, diapers, Chux, or any materials soiled with secretions in a plastic bag. Discard into the regular trash.

- Sharp items (e.g., razors, needles) should be placed in a rigid, puncture-proof container with a solution of 10% bleach. Incinerate when container is full. Pharmacies collect the used containers in some areas.

7. Discuss procedures for caring for pets.
- Clean birdcages wearing gloves. Birds can spread psittacosis (*Chlamydia psittaci*) or *Cryptococcus*.
- Clean cat litter boxes wearing gloves to prevent spread of toxoplasmosis.
- Tropical fish tanks should not be cleaned by an individual with AIDS to prevent spread of *Mycobacterium*.

8. Teach general principles of preventing cross-infection.
- Wear gloves when handling body fluids, linens, or other objects contaminated with body fluids.
- Disposable gowns or aprons protect clothing from becoming soiled.
- Caregivers should not provide care when ill themselves. If this is not possible. they should wear a mask when in close contact with an individual with AIDS. Clients with AIDS are very susceptible to infections.
- Maintain adequate ventilation in the living quarters.

9. Discuss steps to prevent spread of contagious disease; cold, flu, strep throat.
- Clean hands thoroughly before eating or touching food, after using the bathroom, taking out trash, playing with a pet, or being in contact with someone who is ill.
- Use tissues when sneezing or coughing, cover mouth and nose, and discard tissue immediately. If tissue is not available, cover mouth and nose with bend in your elbow or your hands. Clean hands immediately.
- Avoid contact with others if you are ill.
- Maintain up-to-date vaccinations.

10. Medical supplies should be kept in a clean, dry location. If refrigeration is required, place medications in sealed plastic storage bag.

SKILL 8.15   Teaching Safer Practices to Clients Who Abuse IV Drugs

Procedure

1. Inform individuals of risk behaviors and factors associated with IV drug use.
- Direct transmission occurs with shared needles and syringes; permits blood-to-blood contact, the most direct method of transmitting the AIDS virus and hepatitis B.
- Transmission to sexual partners; permits contact of body fluids.
- Transmission to fetus during pregnancy.
- Suppression of the immune system caused by alcohol or drug use.
- Impaired judgment while under the influence of drugs.

2. Teach IV drug users how to reduce the risk.
- Do not share needles or syringes with others.
- Clean needles and other equipment vigorously. Wash twice with full-strength bleach or alcohol; rinse twice with water.

- Boil needles and other equipment for 15 minutes.
- Do not borrow or use needles or equipment from others, even if they appear healthy or say that they do not have AIDS.

3. Teach basic health maintenance measures.
- Decrease use of all immunosuppressive drugs (marijuana, speed, cocaine, alcohol).
- Maintain an adequate, nutritionally sound diet.
- Reduce stress on self by practicing stress-reduction practices or removing self from a stressful situation (living with others who routinely use drugs).
- Obtain regular medical and dental care.
- Follow lifestyle that provides adequate rest and exercise.
- Obtain counseling to assist in living life without dependence on drugs.

4. Document teaching and client response.

▶ CRITICAL THINKING OPTIONS FOR UNEXPECTED OUTCOMES

Not all unexpected outcomes require further nursing intervention; however, many times they do. When the client demonstrates a change in signs/symptoms indicating an emerging problem, the nurse should immediately assess and troubleshoot what is happening. The assessment data must be processed quickly to formulate a hypothesis so the nurse can make a clinical judgment. The nurse then decides how best to resolve the problem and improve the client's situation for a better appropriate outcome.

EXPECTED OUTCOME	PROBLEM SOLVING	NURSING ACTIONS
PPE and Isolation Precautions The transfer of microorganisms from healthcare workers or environment to clients is prevented.	Infection occurs in client.	▪ Assess mode of transmission of microorganism. ▪ Administer antibiotics specific to microorganism as ordered. ▪ Review hand washing technique. ▪ Attend in-service program on infection control procedures. ▪ Notify nurse manager of allergy.
Appropriate PPE and isolation measures are used for individual clients.	Latex allergy identified in healthcare worker or client.	▪ Institute latex safety procedures for staff and client (if identified). ▪ Educate staff about latex allergy. ▪ Replace latex-containing objects (particularly gloves) with nonlatex alternatives. ▪ Create a latex-free environment in which those who are allergic can work safely.
Hospital personnel and others are protected from contamination.	Contaminated blood or body fluid comes in contact with skin or mucous membranes.	▪ Report incident, and complete unusual occurrence report (very important for follow-up legal and medical implications). ▪ Follow hospital guidelines for postexposure prophylaxis (PEP). ▪ HIV exposure should be immediately reported, because most hospitals offer AZT preventive therapy. This therapy should be administered within 1 hr and not more than 24 hr after exposure. ▪ Obtain AIDS antibody test in ensuring months. ▪ Continue to monitor own health status and carry out specific activities to build immune system. Maintain wellness activities to build immune system.
Hospital personnel are protected from infection.	Hospital personnel become infected.	▪ Request consultation therapy to handle feelings and learn new methods of coping with stress. ▪ Leave this type of work temporarily. ▪ Change other aspects of your life to reduce stress. ▪ Take measures to enhance immune system.
The incidence of healthcare-associated infections is reduced.	Healthcare-associated infection occurs in isolation environment.	▪ Identify source of infection and contact the infection control practitioner for consultation. ▪ Examine isolation precautions and hand washing practices among staff. ▪ Provide educational activity on isolation precautions and hand washing to refresh awareness of appropriate guidelines.
PPE in the Home Setting Infections are treated appropriately and not transmitted to other home care clients or the nurse because effective preventive measures are utilized.	The home environment has potential infection sources.	▪ Explain the necessity of keeping the environment free of potential organisms and of keeping it clean and uncluttered. ▪ Instruct the client and family members on proper hand hygiene technique. ▪ Explain and develop a plan for family members to discard soiled dressings, diapers, etc., to prevent potentially infecting other household members.

9 Intracranial Regulation

RELATED CONCEPTS

The Concept of Intracranial Regulation

Exemplar 11.1
Increased Intracranial Pressure

Exemplar 11.2
Seizure Disorders

Skills-at-a-Glance

Intracranial regulation focuses on the processes that affect intracranial compensation and adaptive neurological function. All body functions, muscle movements, senses, mental process-ing, and emotions are regulated by the neurological system. It takes in intrinsic and extrinsic information, processes it, interprets it, and causes motor or sensory responses.

Expected Outcomes

1. Lumbar puncture is performed with minimal discomfort and no untoward effects.
2. Appropriate tools are used to evaluate a neurological client's level of consciousness.
3. Ongoing assessment of a client's brainstem reflects and vital signs are used to determine compensating versus decompensating neurological status.
4. Signs and symptoms of increased intracranial pressure are recognized.
5. Factors that increase intracranial hypertension are identified.
6. Measures to prevent/manage intracranial hypertension are initiated.
7. Client responses to pain management and sedation are evaluated.

SKILL 9.1   Glasgow Coma Scale

The Glasgow Coma Scale (GCS) has been used for several decades to evaluate level of consciousness (LOC) by requiring the client to hear the examiner and respond with (1) eye opening, (2) oral responses, and (3) motor responses. If the client is unresponsive to these, then abnormal posturing response (decortication, decerebration) to shaking or noxious stimuli is assessed. Clients with a score of 8 or less are considered to be comatose and are typically intubated to protect the airway and facilitate mechanical ventilation if required. A "T" is added to their GCS score to indicate this functional limitation. Using this scale, a client with spinal cord injury who is paralyzed may receive a coma score of 8, be intubated, but not be comatose. It follows that the GCS cannot be used to assess neurological signs in clients who are unable to respond orally (e.g., clients who are intubated, sedated, aphasic, have impaired hearing or altered level of consciousness).

Procedure

1. Prior to performing the procedure, introduce self and verify the client's identity using agency protocol. As appropriate, explain what you are going to do and why. Perform hand hygiene and observe other appropriate infection control procedures. Provide for client privacy.
2. When the client has an injury to the head or altered consciousness, assess each of the three categories of the Glasgow Coma Scale according to the criteria in the table. In some cases the client will need stimulation to obtain a response that can be scored. Initially, observe the client to see if all categories can be assessed (e.g., the client who is intubated cannot be assessed for verbal response).
3. Note the score for each category. Document the total score and time performed. Total the scores for all three categories to get the Glasgow Coma Score. See **Table 9–1** ● for score interpretation.
4. Repeat the test at regular intervals for clients defined in step 1. **Rationale:** *Because the test provides a numeric score for altered consciousness, regular measurements help detect subtle changes in the client's condition.*

Note: Because the Glasgow Coma Scale has limitations, the Full Outline of Un-Responsiveness (FOUR Score) Coma Scale is sometimes used for assessing the comatose client, especially one with an acute metabolic or other nonstructural brain injury/disorder. FOUR Score detects early changes in consciousness such as inability to follow the examiner's commands, altered brainstem reflexes, and Cheyne-Stokes breathing. It is also used to differentiate vegetative from minimally conscious states, locked-in syndrome, uncal herniation, and brain death.

TABLE 9–1   Glasgow Coma Scale for Assessment of Coma

CATEGORY	SCORE*	INFANT OR YOUNG CHILD CRITERIA	OLDER CHILD AND ADULT CRITERIA
Eye opening	4	Spontaneous; opens with blinking	Spontaneous
	3	To voice or shout	To voice
	2	To pain	To pain
	1	No response	No response
Verbal response	5	Smiles, coos; uses appropriate words for age	Oriented to time, place, person, and situation
	4	Irritable but consolable; disoriented	Confused
	3	Persistent cries or inappropriate words	Inappropriate
	2	Moans, grunts, is restless	Incomprehensible sounds
	1	No response	No response
Motor response	6	Spontaneous for infant; young child obeys commands	Obeys commands
	5	Localizes pain	Localizes pain
	4	Flexion/withdrawal	Withdraws
	3	Flexion/decorticate posturing	Abnormal flexion (decorticate)
	2	Extension/decerebrate	Abnormal extension (decerebrate)
	1	No response	No response

*Add the score from each category to get the total. The maximum score is 15, indicating the best level of neurological functioning. The minimum is 3, indicating total neurological unresponsiveness.
Data from Comprehensive Advanced Life Support (2011) and Rainbow Rehabilitation Centers (2009).

SKILL 9.2   Assisting with Lumbar Puncture

In a lumbar puncture (LP, or spinal tap), cerebrospinal fluid (CSF) is withdrawn through a needle ❶ inserted into the subarachnoid space of the spinal canal between the third and fourth lumbar vertebrae or between the fourth and fifth lumbar vertebrae ❷. At this level the needle avoids damaging the spinal cord and major nerve roots.

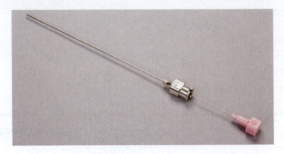

❶ A spinal needle with the stylet protruding from the hub.

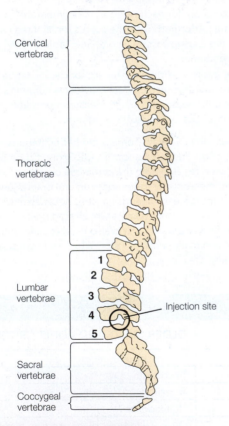

Cervical vertebrae

Thoracic vertebrae

Lumbar vertebrae
1
2
3
4
5
Injection site

Sacral vertebrae

Coccygeal vertebrae

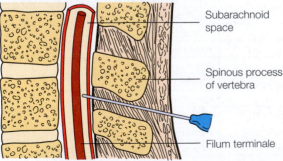

Subarachnoid space

Spinous process of vertebra

Filum terminale

❷ A diagram of the vertebral column, indicating a site for insertion of the lumbar puncture needle into the subarachnoid space of the spinal canal.

Equipment

- Supplies for procedure to be performed
- Infection control/protective gear as needed, generally clean gloves, gown, and mask

Procedure

1. Prior to performing the procedure:
   a. Introduce self and verify the client's identity using agency protocol. Explain what you are going to do and why. Ask client to void and clear bowels just prior to procedure.
   b. Perform hand hygiene and observe other appropriate infection control procedures. Provide for client privacy.
2. Assist the client to a lateral position with the head bent toward the chest, the knees flexed onto the abdomen, and the back at the edge of the bed or examining table; explain the importance of remaining still during procedure. ❸. **Rationale:** *In this position the back is arched, increasing the spaces between the vertebrae so that the spinal needle can be inserted readily.*

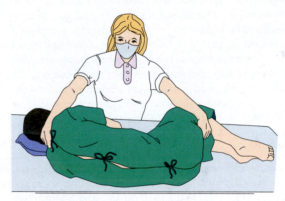

❸ Supporting the client for a lumbar puncture.

3. The nurse helps the client maintain the lumbar puncture position, monitors client, and provides encouragement as needed. **Rationale:** *Holding the position helps prevent accidental needle displacement. Monitoring and reassuring client maintain safety.*
4. Ask client to report headache or persistent pain at insertion site. **Rationale:** *This provides information about potential complications.*
5. During a lumbar puncture, the primary care provider frequently takes CSF pressure readings using a manometer, a glass or plastic tube calibrated in millimeters ❹. The primary care provider collects samples of CSF.

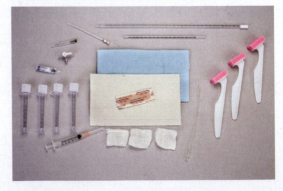

❹ A preassembled lumbar puncture set. Note the manometer at the top of the set.

SKILL 9.2   Assisting with Lumbar Puncture *(continued)*

6. After the procedure, apply a small sterile dressing over the puncture site. **Rationale:** *This protects the site from infection.*
7. Assist client to dorsal recumbent position with one pillow. Monitor often.
8. Document relevant information.

VARIATION: POSITIONING A CHILD FOR LUMBAR PUNCTURE

Preparation

- Determine if the parent wants to be present during an uncomfortable procedure or to be available after the procedure to comfort the child.
- When the parent wishes to be present, discuss the parent's role (e.g., providing distraction or comfort during the procedure).
- Make sure the individual positioning and holding the child clearly understands what body parts must be held still and how to do this safely.

Equipment

- Supplies for procedure to be performed
- Infection control/protective gear as needed, generally clean gloves, gown, and mask

Procedure

1. Don protective gear. Place the child in the side-lying or sitting position that is preferred by the practitioner. The assistant can hold the child in position by wrapping one arm behind the knees and the other behind the neck, keeping the back curved. **Rationale:** *This position ensures the best possible access to spinal processes and disc spaces.*
2. The infant can be held in the desired position by holding the neck and thighs in your hands ❺.
3. The older child can be quite strong, and someone with enough strength will be needed to hold him or her in the side-lying position. Lean over the child with your entire body, using your forearms against the thighs and around the shoulders and head ❻. Alternatively, the older child may be in a seated position, bending forward and supported by the assistant.

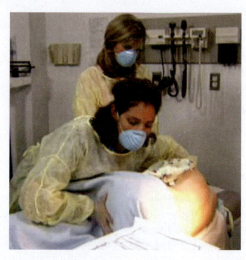

❻ Child in side-lying and flexed position for a lumbar puncture.

4. Be certain that the child has free air exchange. Another assistant may be assigned to monitor respirations and perform other assessments during the procedure.

CLINICAL ALERT

Lumbar puncture requires that the child be held still to prevent injury and to ensure success in obtaining fluid. It is advisable to have an experienced staff member hold the child in position for the procedure. Ensure that the child has free air exchange and receives no injuries. The practitioner performing the procedure may choose a variety of positions: side lying with or without flexion of the knees and hips or sitting upright (Abo et al., 2010).

Developmental Considerations

CHILDREN

- Briefly demonstrate the procedure on a doll or stuffed animal. Allow time to answer questions.
- One member of the child healthcare team should stay in close physical contact with the child, maintain eye contact, and talk to and reassure the child during the procedure.

OLDER ADULTS

- Some clients need help maintaining the flexed position due to arthritis, weakness, or tremors.
- Provide an extra blanket to keep the client warm during the procedure. Older adults have a decreased metabolism and less subcutaneous fat.
- If the client has a hearing loss, speak slowly, distinctly, and loud enough, especially when unable to make eye contact.

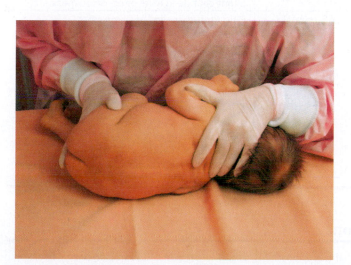

❺ Infant in side-lying and flexed position for a lumbar puncture.

SKILL 9.3 — Intracranial Pressure Monitoring and Daily Care

Preparation

- Review the client's chart related to indications for intracranial pressure monitoring.
- Review the physician's orders for monitoring and drainage parameters.
- Verify the identity of the client by checking the client's identity band and asking client to state name and birth date.
- Provide explanations to the client and family or significant other about the need for intracranial pressure (ICP) monitoring.
- Perform hand hygiene.

Equipment

- ICP transducer system and monitor
- Sterile gloves, mask, and gown

Procedure

1. Ensure that the fluid-filled transducer system is placed and maintained at the level of the foramen of Monro, the line between the top of the ear and the outer canthus of the eye. Balance the ICP transducer to zero for calibration according to hospital guidelines and when the client's position changes. **Rationale:** *This ensures the accuracy of pressure readings and waveforms by the transducer system.*
2. ICP monitoring is usually continuous. When an external ventricular drain is present, document ICP and CPP at the frequency ordered by the physician or by hospital protocol. Monitor and print ICP waveforms. See **Table 9–2** ●.
3. Assess the client's responsiveness, vital signs, and neurological status. Assess for signs of increased ICP. See **Table 9–3** ●. **Rationale:** *Clients with brain injuries are at risk for seizures and cerebral edema, which further compromise CPP.*

> ### CLINICAL ALERT
> Cerebral perfusion pressure (CPP) is calculated by subtracting the ICP from the mean arterial pressure. Normal CPP is 60 to 150 mmHg. Normal ICP is 5 to 15 mmHg.

4. Assess pain and comfort level. Administer sedation and pain medication as prescribed. **Rationale:** *Clients may experience pain at the catheter insertion site and pain from increased ICP. Medications promote the client's comfort and help reduce elevations in ICP.*
5. Maintain the client's position with the head at midline with the remainder of the body and the head of the bed elevated 15 to 30 degrees or according to physician order. **Rationale:** *This position prevents compression of blood vessels in the neck and obstruction of venous blood flows.*
6. Monitor client's neurological status during nursing care and continue or stop nursing interventions depending on client's response. Document care and client's response.

TABLE 9–2 ICP Waveforms and Implications

WAVEFORM	PRESSURE (mmHg)	IMPLICATIONS
A	50–100	Symptoms related to cerebral dysfunction; changes in vital signs, respiratory pattern, and motor function; headache; and emesis
B	20–50	Decreasing level of consciousness, agitation, varying respiratory pattern
C	4–20	No clinical significance
Normal	4–15	Normal

Rationale: *Anxiety, agitation, pain, hypoxia, hypertension, head position out of neutral alignment, some environmental stimuli, and nursing care procedures may elevate the ICP (Rangel-Castillo, Gopinath, & Robertson, 2008). Signs indicating poor client response to interventions include deterioration in clinical signs, increase in ICP greater than 10 mmHg above baseline longer than 3 minutes, and wide-amplitude waveform and/or the appearance of plateau waves.*

7. Document the ICP reading, CPP, waveforms, and the client's neurological status at intervals specified by hospital guidelines or physician order.

TABLE 9–3 Signs of Increased Intracranial Pressure

TIMING OF SIGNS	SIGNS
Early signs	Headache Visual disturbances, diplopia Nausea and vomiting Dizziness or vertigo Slight change in vital signs Pupils not as reactive or equal Sunsetting eyes Seizures Slight change in level of consciousness
Additional signs in infants	Bulging fontanelle Wide sutures, increased head circumference Dilated scalp veins High-pitched, catlike cry
Late signs	Significant decrease in level of consciousness Cushing triad: ■ Increased systolic blood pressure and widened pulse pressure ■ Bradycardia ■ Irregular respirations Fixed and dilated pupils

SKILL 9.4 — Implementing Seizure Precautions

Delegation

UAP should be familiar with establishing and implementing seizure precautions and methods of obtaining assistance during a client's seizure. Care of the client during a seizure, however, is the responsibility of the nurse due to the importance of careful assessment of respiratory status and the potential need for intervention.

SKILL 9.4   Implementing Seizure Precautions (continued)

Equipment

- Blankets or other linens to pad side rails
- Oral suction equipment and clean gloves
- Oxygen equipment

Procedure

1. Prior to performing the procedure, gather equipment. Introduce self and verify the client's identity using agency protocol. Explain to the client what you are going to do, why it is necessary, and how he or she can participate.
2. Perform hand hygiene and observe appropriate infection control procedures. If the client is actively seizing, apply clean gloves in preparation for performing respiratory care measures.
3. Provide for client privacy. Position the bed at an appropriate height.
4. Pad the bed of any client who might have a seizure. Secure blankets or other linens around the head, foot, and side rails of the bed ①.

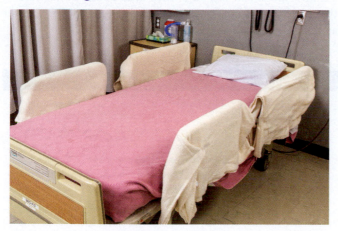

① Padding a bed for seizure precautions.

5. Put oral suction equipment in place and test to ensure that it is functional. **Rationale:** *Suctioning may be needed to prevent aspiration of oral secretions.*

VARIATION: MANAGING SEIZURE ACTIVITY

If a seizure occurs:

- Remain with the client and call for assistance. Do not restrain the client.

- If the client is not in bed, assist client to the floor and protect the client's head by holding it in your lap or on a pillow. Loosen any clothing around the neck and chest.
- Turn the client to a lateral position if possible. **Rationale:** *Turning to the side allows secretions to drain out of the mouth, decreasing the risk of aspiration, and helps keep the tongue from occluding the airway.*
- Move items in the environment to ensure the client does not experience an injury.
- Do not insert anything into the client's mouth.
- Time the seizure duration.
- Observe the progression of the seizure, noting the sequence and type of limb involvement. Observe skin color. When the seizure allows, check pulse and respirations.
- Apply gloves and use equipment to suction the mouth if the client vomits or has excessive oral secretions.
- Apply oxygen via mask or nasal cannula
- Administer anticonvulsant medications, as ordered.
- When the seizure has subsided, assist client to a comfortable position. Reorient. Explain what happened. Reassure the client. Provide hygiene as necessary. Allow the client to verbalize feelings about the seizure.
- If applied, remove and discard gloves. Perform hand hygiene.

6. Document the event in the client record using forms or checklists supplemented by narrative notes when appropriate. Notify the physician of the seizure.

Sample Documentation

7/8/15 1815 Upon entering room, observed generalized muscle spasms/contractions of arms and legs lasting 25 seconds. Seizure padding previously placed on bed. Incontinent of urine. Cyanotic. Placed on left side. Suctioned. Airway clear. Respirations 14/min with irregular pattern. Oxygen applied at 4 L/min via mask. Oxygen sat. 90% on O_2. Not currently responding to verbal stimuli. Dr. Smith notified. Diazepam 10 mg given IV per order. VS taken every 15 min. See neuro flow sheet. _____ M. Faustino, RN

1835 Respirations 15/min, regular. Responding to verbal stimuli, oriented to person, place, and time. Oxygen sat. 95% on O_2. O_2 discontinued per physician's order. VS taken every 15 min. See neuro flow sheet.

_____ M. Faustino, RN

Developmental Considerations

INFANTS

- The most common cause of seizures in young infants is birth injury (e.g., intracranial trauma, hemorrhage, anoxia) or congenital brain defects. Onset of epilepsy is highest in the first few months of life (Hockenberry & Wilson, 2012).

CHILDREN

- In children over 3 years of age, the most common cause of seizures is idiopathic epilepsy.
- Febrile seizures associated with acute infections occur more commonly in children than in adults and are usually preventable through the use of antipyretics and tepid baths.

- Determine oxygenation. Apply oxygen if pulse oximetry reading is less than 95%. Oxygen can be applied via head hood, tent, nasal cannula, or mask, depending on the age and response of the child. Oxygen is drying and must be humidified. Tents are cooling, and the child's thermal balance must be monitored. The concentration of oxygen in tents is more difficult to regulate.
- Children who have frequent seizures may need to wear helmets for protection.
- Children on anticonvulsant medications should wear a medical identification tag (bracelet or necklace).

(continued on next page)

SKILL 9.4 Implementing Seizure Precautions (*continued*)

Setting of Care

- Discuss with the client and family the factors that may precipitate a seizure.
- If clients have frequent or recurrent seizures or take anticonvulsant medications, they should wear a medical identification tag (bracelet or necklace) and carry a card delineating any medications they take.
- When making home visits, inspect anticonvulsant medications and confirm that clients are taking them correctly. Blood level measurements may be required periodically.

- Discuss safety precautions for inside and out of the home. If seizures are not well controlled, activities that may require restriction or direct supervision by others include tub bathing, swimming, cooking, using electric equipment or machinery, and driving.
- Assist clients in determining which individuals in the community should or must be informed of their seizure disorder (e.g., employers, healthcare providers such as dentists, motor vehicle department if driving, and companions).

▶ CRITICAL THINKING OPTIONS FOR UNEXPECTED OUTCOMES

Not all unexpected outcomes require further nursing intervention; however, many times they do. When the client demonstrates a change in signs/symptoms indicating an emerging problem, the nurse should immediately assess and troubleshoot what is happening. The assessment data must be processed quickly to formulate a hypothesis so the nurse can make a clinical judgment. The nurse then decides how best to resolve the problem and improve the client's situation for a better appropriate outcome.

EXPECTED OUTCOME	PROBLEM SOLVING	NURSING ACTIONS
Lumbar puncture is performed with minimal discomfort and no untoward effects.	Client has spinal fluid leak after lumbar puncture.	■ Keep client in supine position. ■ Notify physician. ■ Keep sterile dressing over puncture site. Do not allow dressing to become wet. ■ If leak persists, physician may place client in the Trendelenburg position to prevent headache. This position is contraindicated in clients with increased intracranial pressure or after a craniotomy.
Appropriate tools are used to evaluate a neurological client's level of consciousness.	Neurological client's comatose state cannot be determined using Glasgow Coma Scale due to inability to respond verbally.	■ Recognize that a nonverbal client cannot respond to parameters assessed using the Glasgow Coma Scale. ■ Utilize the FOUR Score Coma Scale to assess separate components of eye response, motor response, brainstem reflexes, and respiration for the nonverbal client.
Ongoing assessment of a client's brainstem reflects and vital signs are used to determine compensating versus decompensating neurological status.	Client shows signs of decreasing level of consciousness.	■ Reassess to validate findings. ■ Notify physician of findings immediately.
Client responses to pain management and sedation are evaluated.	Client is very agitated with frequent nonpurposeful movements, despite increased frequency of sedative administration.	■ Try to find a cause for the client's change in behavior. ■ Attempt an analgesic trial to determine whether the client's pain is managed. This trial may be therapeutic as well as diagnostic.

10 Metabolism

The primary function of the endocrine system is to regulate the body's internal environment. Hormones secreted by endocrine glands regulate growth, reproduction and sex differentiation, metabolism, and fluid and electrolyte balance. The endocrine system helps the body adapt to constant changes in the internal and external environment.

Hormones are chemical messengers of the body. They act on specific target cells, causing either an increase or decrease in body function. Hormone levels are regulated by a process called *negative feedback*. Negative feedback acts similar to the way the thermostat in a house regulates temperature. When too much hormone is released, the target cell sends back a message to reduce its hormone release. If too little hormone is released, the target cell sends back a message to increase the hormone to the normal level. **Figures 10–1 ●** and **10–2 ●** show selected endocrine glands and effects of their hormones on the body.

Expected Outcomes

1. Assessment data supports differential endocrine disorder diagnoses.
2. Lifestyle changes assist in management of client's altered health status.
3. Client demonstrates understanding (verbalized knowledge) of behavioral modification strategies provided.
4. Paracentesis is completed without complications.

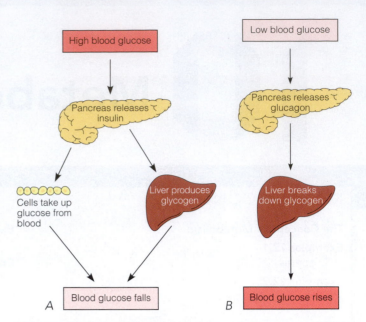

Figure 10–2 ● Action of insulin and glucagon on blood glucose levels. *A,* High blood glucose is lowered by insulin release. *B,* Low blood glucose is raised by glucagon release.

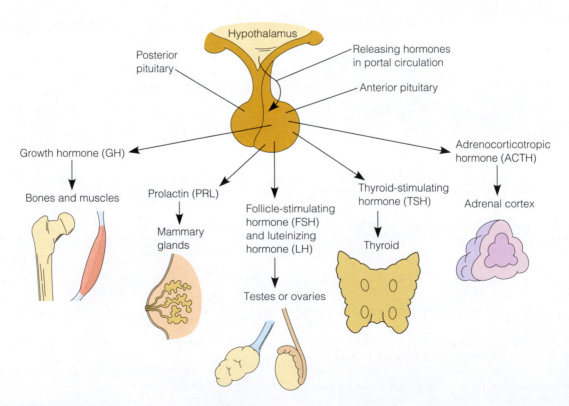

Figure 10–1 ● Actions of the major hormones of the anterior pituitary.

SKILL 10.1   Assessing for Endocrine Disorders

Because hormones affect all body systems, manifestations of endocrine dysfunction are often nonspecific. This makes assessment of endocrine function more difficult. Subjective and objective data can be collected, however, that support assessment of endocrine disorders.

Procedure

1. Before entering client's room, check physician's order and gather equipment and supplies needed to take into client's room. After entering, introduce self and explain what procedure will be done and why. Perform hand hygiene, follow infection control measures, and verify client's identity. Provide privacy. Provide comfort and safety for client and yourself including raising bed to appropriate height for procedure.

2. Ask specific questions to obtain subjective data from the client:
   - Changes in energy level and fatigue and how activities of daily living are affected
   - Increased sensitivity to heat or cold, weight loss or gain, diarrhea or constipation
   - Increased appetite, urination, or thirst; salt cravings
   - History of hypertension, abnormally fast or slow heart rate, palpitations, or shortness of breath
   - Changes in vision, excessive tearing, or swelling around the eyes
   - History of numbness or tingling in lips or extremities, nervousness, hand tremors, change in memory, mood, or sleep patterns
   - Thinning or loss of hair, dry or moist skin, brittle nails, easy bruising, or slow wound healing
   - History of taking any hormone replacements such as thyroid, steroids, or insulin
   - History of previous surgery, chemotherapy, or radiation, especially of the neck area, as well as brain surgery or a head injury
   - Any family history of diabetes mellitus, diabetes insipidus, goiter, obesity, Addison disease, or infertility
   - Changes in sexual function or secondary sex characteristics. Ask women about changes in menstruation or menopause.

3. Focus assessment to obtain objective data about the client:
   - General appearance, vital signs, height, and weight. Note extremely short height.
   - Skin color, temperature, texture, and moisture. Observe for rough, dry or smooth, flushed skin. Note bronze color over knuckles, purple striae over the abdomen, and bruising.
   - Inspect the lower extremities for lesions and any signs of healing.
   - Assess the texture and condition of hair and nails. Observe for thinning and loss of hair, as well as thick or thin brittle nails. Look for excessive hair growth on face, chest, or abdomen.
   - Inspect the face for shape and symmetry. Inspect the eyes for the presence of exophthalmos (forward protrusion of the eyeballs). Determine visual acuity.
   - Inspect the neck for visible signs of masses. Gently palpate the thyroid gland from behind the client ❶. Palpate only one side of the neck at a time.

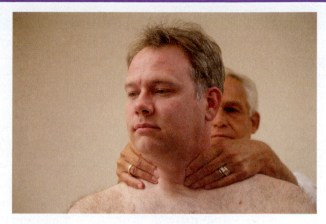

❶ Palpating the thyroid gland from behind the client.

   - Assess for increased size of hands and feet, trunk obesity, and thin extremities.
   - Inspect men for gynecomastia, enlargement of the breasts.
   - Evaluate muscle strength and deep tendon reflexes. Assess for the Chvostek sign (facial grimacing in response to tapping your finger at jaw) and Trousseau sign (carpal spasm when blood pressure cuff inflated higher than systolic pressure for 2 to 4 minutes).
   - Assess ability to sense touch, hot/cold, and vibration in the extremities.
   - Auscultate lungs for adventitious sounds and heart for extra heart sounds.
   - Palpate hands and feet for edema.
   - Perform hand hygiene and return bed to lowest height.

4. Review results of diagnostic tests.
   - To diagnose an endocrine disorder, several laboratory tests are used. **Table 10–1** ● lists these tests, their normal values, what the test measures and its significance, and any nursing implications for the test.
   - Other nonspecific laboratory tests are done to give clues about endocrine disorders. A chemistry panel, which includes serum electrolytes such as sodium, potassium, calcium, and phosphate, and blood glucose levels are used to monitor disease progression. For instance, serum sodium and blood glucose levels increase in Cushing syndrome but decrease in Addison disease. In people with diabetes, serum cholesterol and triglyceride levels help to evaluate the risk of developing atherosclerosis.

5. Review results of imaging studies. Imaging techniques used to diagnose endocrine disorders are noninvasive.

Magnetic Resonance Imaging (MRI)
   - Used to identify tumors of the pituitary gland and hypothalamus.
   - Clients with metallic implants cannot have an MRI due to its magnetic field.

(continued on next page)

SKILL 10.1 Assessing for Endocrine Disorders (continued)

TABLE 10–1 Common Laboratory Tests for Endocrine Disorders

TEST	NORMAL ADULT VALUES	EXPLANATION	NURSING IMPLICATIONS
Pituitary			
Growth hormone (GH)	Less than 5 ng/mL for men Less than 10 ng/mL for women	Used to evaluate growth hormone excess or deficiency. Increased values indicate acromegaly.	The client must be fasting, well rested, and not physically or emotionally stressed.
Water deprivation test	1–5 pg/mL	Increased level indicates SIADH, decreased level means diabetes insipidus.	Tell client to fast for 12 hours and to withhold fluids and smoking at midnight.
Thyroid			
Thyroid-stimulating hormone (TSH)	0.35–5.5 mcg/mL	This is the most sensitive test to evaluate thyroid function by measuring pituitary TSH secretion.	No fluid restriction is required. Avoid shellfish several days before test.
T_3	80–200 ng/dL	Measures triiodothyronine (T_3) and thyroxine (T_4) to evaluate thyroid function. Increased level indicates hyperthyroidism and decreased reflects hypothyroidism.	No fluid restriction is required. Avoid shellfish several days before test.
T_4	4.5–11.5 mcg/dL		
Parathyroid			
Serum calcium	9–11 mg/dL	This test evaluates parathyroid function and calcium metabolism.	Fasting not required; however, it is part of a chemistry panel in which fasting is required.
Serum phosphate	2.5–4.5 mg/dL	It measures serum phosphate. Increased levels in both tests indicate hyperparathyroidism; decreased levels indicate hypoparathyroidism.	Fasting not required; however, it is part of a chemistry panel in which fasting is required.
Adrenal			
Cortisol	8 to 10 am 5–23 mcg/dL 4 to 6 pm 3–13 mcg/dL	This test measures total serum cortisol, which evaluates adrenal cortex function. Levels are increased in Cushing's syndrome and decreased in Addison's disease.	Advise client to rest in bed 2 hours before blood is drawn. Explain that two blood samples are drawn—one at 8:00 to 10 am, the other at 4 to 6:00 pm.
Aldosterone	4–30 ng/dL sitting position Less than 16 ng/dL supine position	Levels are drawn to diagnose hyperaldosteronism.	Ask client to be in supine position for 1 hour before test is drawn.
Urinary 17-ketosteroids	5–15 mg/24 hours men 5–25 mg/24 hours women	17-KS are metabolites of testosterone, which are released from adrenal cortex. Levels increase with Cushing's syndrome and decrease in Addison's disease.	Teach client about 24-hour urine collection, which must be iced or refrigerated during collection.
Pancreas			
Fasting blood glucose	70–110 mg/dL	This test measures circulating blood glucose level. Increases are seen in diabetes mellitus, acute pancreatitis; decreased level is seen in Addison's disease.	This test is done fasting.
Glycosylated hemoglobin (Hb A1c)	5.5%–7%	Test used to measure glucose control during the previous 3 months. Levels are increased in newly diagnosed or poorly controlled diabetic. It is not used to diagnose diabetes mellitus.	No fasting is required.
Two-hour oral glucose tolerance test (OGTT)	Less than 125 mg/dL	Determines the level of glucose 2 hours after drinking 75 g of glucose. Glucose level should return to premeal levels, but in diabetics, the level is higher than 200 mg/dL.	Client is NPO for 12 hours before test. Then client must drink entire 100 g of glucose and not eat anything else until blood is drawn.
Urine glucose	Negative	Estimates the amount of glucose in urine, which should be negative.	Collect a fresh urine sample; stagnant urine may alter test results.
Urine ketones	Negative	Measures ketones excreted in urine from incomplete fat metabolism. Positive result means lack of insulin or diabetic ketoacidosis.	Some drugs may interfere with both test results.
Urine test for microalbumin	0.2–1.9 mg/dL	Microalbumin is the earliest indicator for development of diabetic nephropathy. Elevated microalbumin levels increase the risk for end-stage renal disease.	Collect a fresh urine sample and send to laboratory for analysis.

SKILL 10.1   Assessing for Endocrine Disorders (continued)

Computed Tomography (CT) Scan

- In a thyroid scan iodine-125 is injected IV.
  - Abdominal CT is used to detect tumors of the adrenal gland and pancreas. "Cold spots," which do not take up the I-125, indicate malignancy.
  - Ask about allergies to iodine and seafood.
- For the radioactive iodine (RAI) uptake test, iodine-131 or I-125 (capsule or liquid form) is given.
  - Increased uptake indicates Graves disease; decreased uptake means hypothyroidism.
  - Ask about allergies to iodine and seafood. Thyroid drugs or medications containing iodine are withheld for weeks before the study.
6. Document assessment findings.

Sample Documentation

Case Example: A 48-year-old female has an appointment with her family physician to rule out a diagnosis of hyperthyroidism. She states that she eats all the time but has lost 10 lb in the past 2 months. She has a family history of Graves disease.

12/11/15 BP 168/90 mmHg, P 110 bpm, R 26/min. Alert and oriented but cannot sit still, keeps fidgeting with purse. Hands visibly shake. Has difficulty focusing on interview questions. Appears exhausted. Eyeballs protrude and cannot close eyelids completely. Denies blurry vision. Patchy hair loss with thin, brittle nails noted. Skin warm, smooth, and moist. C/O heart palpitations, denies chest pain. Bowel tones hyperactive.

SKILL 10.2   Teaching the Client Lifestyle and Behavioral Modification Strategies for Endocrine Disorders

Clients with endocrine disorders require care for multiple problems. They often face changes in physical appearance and emotional responses, and permanent alterations in lifestyle.

1. Before entering client's room, check physician's order and gather equipment and supplies needed to take into client's room. After entering, introduce self and explain what procedure will be done and why. Perform hand hygiene, follow infection control measures, and verify client's identity.

Provide privacy. Provide comfort and safety for client and yourself.

2. Focus on teaching clients how to meet physical and emotional needs for themselves and their families.
3. Depending on the endocrine disorder, discuss necessary lifestyle and behavioral modifications. **Table 10–2** ● lists selected strategies that apply.
4. Document teaching and client response.

TABLE 10–2   Select Endocrine Disorders and Common Strategies

ENDOCRINE DISORDERS	LIFESTYLE/BEHAVIORAL MODIFICATION STRATEGY
Anterior Pituitary Gland	
Gigantism Dwarfism	■ Coping with body image changes ■ Coping with possible surgery ■ Adapt environment to meet size needs ■ Need for lifetime hormone replacement therapy
Posterior Pituitary Gland	
Diabetes insipidus	■ Recognize excess fluid and electrolyte imbalance problems ■ Monitor weight daily ■ Maintain low-sodium diet ■ Need for periodic healthcare visits ■ Need for lifetime medication therapy
Hyperthyroidism	
Graves disease	■ Coping with body image changes of goiter and exophthalmos ■ Schedule rest times for fatigue ■ Maintain balanced diet and weight ■ Maintain cool environment ■ Wear tinted eyeglasses or eye shields to protect the cornea ■ Apply artificial tears as needed ■ Coping with possible surgery ■ Coping strategies for emotional control ■ Need for lifetime medications ■ Need for periodic healthcare visits

(continued on next page)

SKILL 10.2   Teaching Modification Strategies for Endocrine Disorders (*continued*)

TABLE 10–2   Select Endocrine Disorders and Common Strategies (*continued*)

ENDOCRINE DISORDERS	LIFESTYLE/BEHAVIORAL MODIFICATION STRATEGY
Hypothyroidism	
Hashimoto thyroiditis	▪ Coping with body image of goiter ▪ Slow movements, need for rest periods ▪ Maintain warm environment ▪ Maintain appropriate diet and weight ▪ Monitor weight weekly ▪ Periodic healthcare visits ▪ Utilize preventive infection practices ▪ Use stool softeners or laxatives as prescribed ▪ Need for lifetime medications
Myxedema coma	▪ Have a plan to get immediate medical help with seizures or extreme lethargy ▪ Need for lifetime medications
Adrenal Gland	
Cushing syndrome	▪ Coping with body image of buffalo hump over upper back, thinning of hair, moon face, and increased body hair ▪ Safety measures to prevent injuries, especially bone injuries and bruising ▪ Utilize preventive infection practices ▪ Maintain appropriate weight through fluid intake and meals ▪ Need for lifetime medications ▪ Coping with possible surgery ▪ Periodic healthcare visits ▪ Seek counseling for depression
Addison disease	▪ Monitor for hypotension, rapid pulse ▪ Monitor serum electrolytes, mainly potassium ▪ Monitor daily fluid intake and output ▪ Need to carry emergency kit containing parenteral cortisone and a syringe ▪ Assess for signs of dehydration ▪ Need for lifetime medications ▪ Periodic healthcare visits

SKILL 10.3   Assisting with Paracentesis

Normally the body creates just enough peritoneal fluid for lubrication. The fluid is continuously formed and absorbed into the lymphatic system. However, in some disease processes, a large amount of fluid accumulates in the abdominal cavity; this condition is called **ascites**. Normal ascitic fluid is serous, clear, and light yellow in color. An abdominal paracentesis is carried out to obtain a fluid specimen for laboratory study and to relieve pressure on the abdominal organs due to the presence of excess fluid ❶.

1. Before entering client's room, check physician's order and gather equipment and supplies. Introduce self and explain what procedure will be done and why. Perform hand hygiene, follow infection control measures, and verify client's identity. Provide privacy. Provide comfort and safety for client and yourself, including positioning in bed or chair at appropriate height for procedure.

2. Have client void just before the procedure. **Rationale:** *This reduces bladder size to minimize risk of puncturing the bladder.*

3. Help client assume correct position for procedure. Explain importance of remaining still during the procedure.

4. Provide verbal support; monitor for signs of distress during the procedure.
   - Using strict sterile technique, the primary care provider makes a small incision midway between the umbilicus and the symphysis pubis on the midline. A trocar (a sharp, pointed instrument) and cannula (tube) are inserted. The trocar, which is inside the cannula, is then withdrawn ❷.

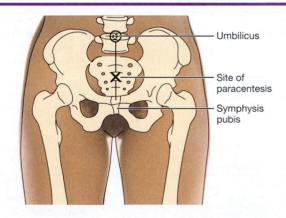

❶ A common site for an abdominal paracentesis.

- Tubing is attached to the cannula and the fluid flows through the tubing into a receptacle. If the purpose of the paracentesis is to obtain a specimen, the primary care provider may use a long aspirating needle attached to a syringe rather than making an incision and using a trocar and cannula. Normally about 1,500 mL is the maximum amount of fluid drained at one time and it is drained very **slowly**. **Rationale:** *Limiting the amount and speed of fluid withdrawal prevents hypovolemic shock.* Some fluid is placed in the specimen container before the cannula is withdrawn.

SKILL 10.3   Assisting with Paracentesis (*continued*)

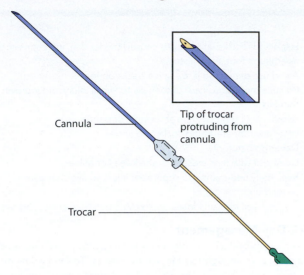

Cannula

Tip of trocar protruding from cannula

Trocar

2 A trocar and cannula may be used for an abdominal paracentesis.

5. The small incision may or may not be sutured; it is covered with a small sterile bandage. **Rationale:** *This helps prevent infection at the site.* Perform hand hygiene and put bed in lowest position.
6. Label and transport specimens to the laboratory as ordered.
7. Monitor client after the procedure.
8. Document relevant information.

Developmental Considerations

OLDER ADULTS

- Provide pillows and blankets to help older adults remain comfortable during the procedure.
- Ask the client to empty the bladder just before the procedure. Older adults may need to void more frequently and in smaller amounts.
- Remove ascitic fluid slowly and monitor the client for signs of hypovolemia. Older adults have less tolerance for fluid loss and may develop hypovolemia if a large volume of fluid is drained rapidly.

▶ DIABETES

Expected Outcomes

1. Accurate blood glucose level is obtained.
2. Insulin injection is administered without complications.
3. Medication therapeutic effect is achieved.
4. Client's diabetic teaching is completed before discharge.

SKILL 10.4   Nursing Management of the Client with Diabetes

Diabetes mellitus is a common chronic disease of adults. It is not a single disorder but a group of metabolic disorders characterized by hyperglycemia (too much glucose in the blood). This condition is due to an insufficient supply of insulin, ineffective insulin action, or both. Blood glucose control is essential to reduce complications that most often affect the cardiovascular system, kidneys, eyes, and nerves.

The nurse monitors for complications and teaches clients to be aware of potential complications associated with diabetes (**Table 10–3 ●**). The longer the client has been diagnosed with diabetes, the greater the risk for complications. Frequent blood glucose monitoring with insulin injections, exercise, and a healthy diet help to reduce these risks.

TABLE 10–3	Potential Complications Associated with Diabetes Mellitus		
BODY FOCUS	INITIAL COMPLICATION	FURTHER COMPLICATION	LATE DEVELOPMENT
Cardiovascular system	■ Atherosclerosis ■ Hypertension ■ Impaired peripheral circulation	■ Coronary artery disease ■ Stroke ■ Peripheral vascular disease	■ Myocardial infarction with heart failure ■ Lower leg ulcers ■ Gangrene tissue and amputations of lower leg
Eyes	Diabetic retinopathy	■ Progressive blindness ■ Cataracts	■ Blurry vision ■ Loss of vision
Kidneys	Diabetic nephropathy	■ Albumin in urine ■ Hypertension, edema ■ Progressive renal insufficiency	■ End-stage renal disease ■ Renal failure
Nerves	Diabetic autonomic neuropathy	■ Sensory and motor impairment ■ Postural hypotension ■ Delayed gastric emptying, diarrhea ■ Impaired genitourinary function	■ Peripheral neuropathies begin in toes and progress upward; distal paresthesia, pain, cold sensation ■ Urinary retention ■ Frequent urinary tract infections ■ Sexual dysfunction ■ Increased risk for infection

(continued on next page)

SKILL 10.4 Nursing Management of the Client with Diabetes (continued)

Client Teaching

Management of Potential Complications

- Maintain balance of nutrition, activity, and blood glucose levels.
- Monitor blood glucose levels regularly and give insulin and/or oral antidiabetic agents as prescribed.
- Rotate insulin injection sites.
- Eat appropriate meals and snacks at given times.
- Maintain skin integrity, especially feet.
- Have an adequate fluid intake appropriate for chronic conditions.
- Do not smoke.
- Assess for signs/symptoms of infection: fever, chills; cloudy, foul-smelling urine; tachycardia; red, swelling, or pain at skin breakdown site.
- Maintain good oral hygiene with a soft toothbrush.
- Be aware of environmental hazards to avoid injury.
- Develop an adequate support system with family and friends, or join a support group.
- Utilize community resources as needed.
- Have periodic medical assessment of general condition and any potential risk factors.
- Take all medications as prescribed.
- Report any change in chronic conditions to physician.
- Maintain self-care as able and secure assistance as needed.

The Diabetic Foot

People with diabetes mellitus have high incidence of problems with their feet and subsequent amputations. Guidelines for management of the diabetic foot include the following:

- Inspect daily for injury, cuts, bruises, red areas, or burns, from foot trauma occurring without knowing it happened.

- Inspect for cracks and fissures caused by dry skin, infections such as athlete's foot, and blisters.
- Avoid use of heating pads or ice packs on feet.
- Practice meticulous care of toenails to avoid injury and ingrown toenails.
- Avoid use of garters, knee stockings, or pantyhose.
- Wear appropriate-fitting socks and shoes.
- Never go barefoot.
- Do not sit with legs crossed at the knees or ankles.
- Seek early treatment of a superficial injury to avoid deeper progression.
- Get bed rest, take antibiotics, and provide debridement wound care.

Sick-Day Management

When an individual with diabetes is sick, blood glucose levels increase, even though food intake decreases. The individual may mistakenly alter or omits the insulin dose or oral antidiabetic agent, causing further problems. Dietary guidelines during illness focus on preventing dehydration and providing nutrition for promoting recovery. The nurse teaches the following sick-day management:

- Monitor blood glucose at least four times a day throughout the illness.
- Test urine for ketones if the blood glucose level is greater than 250 mg/dL.
- Continue to take the usual insulin dose or oral antidiabetic agent.
- Drink 8 to 12 oz of fluid each waking hour.
- Eat a small amount of carbohydrate every 1 to 2 hours, such as Jell-O, fruit juice, or a popsicle.
- Call the healthcare provider if unable to eat for >24 hours or if vomiting and diarrhea last for >6 hours.

SKILL 10.5 Obtaining a Capillary Blood Specimen and Measuring Blood Glucose

Equipment

- Blood glucose meter (glucometer)
- Blood glucose reagent strip compatible with the meter
- 2 × 2 gauze
- Antiseptic swab
- Clean gloves
- Sterile lancet (a sharp device to puncture the skin)
- Lancet injector (a spring-loaded mechanism that holds the lancet)
- Warm cloth or other warming device (optional)

Preparation

- Review the type of meter and the manufacturer's instructions. Assemble the equipment at the bedside.

Procedure

1. Prior to performing the procedure, introduce self and verify the client's identity using agency protocol. Explain to the client what you are going to do, why it is necessary, and how he

or she can participate. Discuss how the results will be used in planning further care or treatments.
2. Perform hand hygiene and observe other appropriate infection control procedures (e.g., gloves).
3. Provide for client privacy.
4. Prepare the equipment.
   - Some meters turn on by inserting the test strip into the meter.
   - Calibrate the meter and run a control sample according to the manufacturer's instructions and/or confirm the code number.
5. Select and prepare the vascular puncture site.
   - Choose a vascular puncture site (e.g., the side of an adult's finger). Avoid sites beside bone. Wrap the finger first in a warm cloth, or hold a finger in a dependent (below heart level) position. If the earlobe is used, rub it gently with a small piece of gauze. **Rationale:** *These actions increase the blood flow to the area, ensure an adequate specimen, and reduce the need for a repeat puncture.*
   - Clean the site with an antiseptic swab or soap and water and allow it to dry completely. **Rationale:** *Alcohol can*

SKILL 10.5   Obtaining a Capillary Blood Specimen *(continued)*

affect accuracy, and the site burns when punctured if wet with alcohol.

6. Obtain the blood specimen.
   - Apply clean gloves.
   - Place the injector, if used, against the site, and release the needle, thus permitting it to pierce the skin ❶. Make sure the lancet is perpendicular to the site. **Rationale:** *The lancet is designed to pierce the skin at a specific depth when it is in a perpendicular position relative to the skin.*

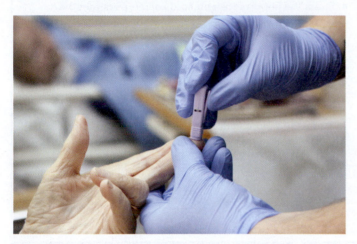

❶ Place the injector against the site. Life-in-View/Science Source

or

   - Prick the site with a lancet or needle, using a darting motion.
   - Gently squeeze (but do not touch) the puncture site until a large drop of blood forms. The size of the drop of blood can vary depending on the meter. Some meters require as little as 0.3 mL of blood to accurately test blood sugar.
   - Hold the reagent strip under the puncture site until adequate blood covers the indicator square ❷. The pad will

absorb the blood and a chemical reaction will occur. Do not smear the blood. **Rationale:** *Smearing the blood will cause an inaccurate reading. Some meters wick the blood by just touching the puncture site with the strip.*
   - Ask the client to apply pressure to the skin puncture site with a 2 × 2 gauze. **Rationale:** *Pressure will assist hemostasis.*

7. Expose the blood to the test strip for the period and the manner specified by the manufacturer. As soon as the blood is placed on the test strip:
   - Follow the manufacturer's recommendations on the glucose meter for the amount of time indicated by the manufacturer. **Rationale:** *The blood must remain in contact with the test pad for a prescribed time to obtain accurate results.*
   - Some glucometers have the test strip placed in the machine before the specimen is obtained.

8. Measure the blood glucose.
   - Place the strip into the meter according to the manufacturer's instructions. Refer to the specific manufacturer's recommendations for the specific procedure.
   - After the designated time, most glucose meters will display the glucose reading automatically. Correct timing ensures accurate results ❸.

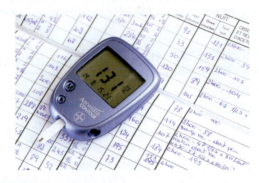

❸ Read the results. John Thys/Reporters/Science Source

   - Turn off the meter and discard the test strip and 2 × 2 gauze in a biohazard container. Discard the lancet into a sharps container.

9. Remove and discard gloves. Perform hand hygiene.

10. Document the method of testing and results on appropriate documents in the client's record. If appropriate, record the client's understanding and ability to demonstrate the skill. The client's record may also include a flow sheet on which capillary blood glucose results and the amount, type, route, and time of insulin administration are recorded. Always check if a diabetic flow sheet is being used for the client.

11. Check for orders for sliding-scale insulin based on capillary blood glucose results. Administer insulin as prescribed.

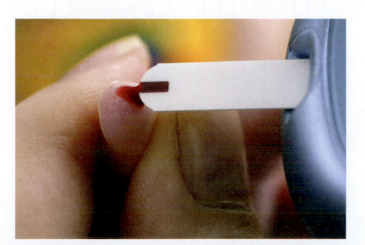

❷ Apply the blood to the test strip. John Thys/Reporters/Science Source

(continued on next page)

SKILL 10.5   Obtaining a Capillary Blood Specimen *(continued)*

Developmental Considerations

INFANTS

The outer aspect of the heel is the most common site on neonates and infants for obtaining a capillary blood specimen. Placing a warm cloth on the infant's heel often increases the blood flow to the area.

CHILDREN

- Use the side of a fingertip for a young client older than age 2, unless contraindicated.
- When possible, allow the child to choose the puncture site.
- Praise the young client for cooperating and assure the child that the procedure is not a punishment.

OLDER ADULTS

- Older adults may have arthritic joint changes, poor vision, or hand tremors and may need assistance using the glucose meter or obtaining a meter that accommodates their limitations.
- Older adults may have difficulty obtaining diabetic supplies due to financial concerns or homebound status.
- Older adults often have poor circulation. Warming the hands by wrapping with a warm washcloth for 3 to 5 minutes or placing the hand dependent for a few moments may help in obtaining a blood sample.

Setting of Care

- Assess the client or caregiver's ability and willingness to perform blood glucose monitoring at home.
- Teach the proper use of the lancet and glucose meter, and provide written guidelines. Allow time for a return demonstration. The client may need several visits to completely learn the procedure.
- Ensure the client's ability to obtain supplies and purchase reagent strips. The strips are relatively expensive and may not be covered by the client's insurance.
- Stress the importance of record keeping. Instruct the client on when to do glucose monitoring, how to record the blood glucose levels, and when to notify the primary care provider.
- Children with diabetes who need to perform fingersticks should be taught about safe practices for cleaning blood from surfaces (household bleach is best) and about safe storage of equipment to prevent young children from having access to it. Identify a place in the school where the child can store glucose-monitoring equipment and perform the procedure in private.

SKILL 10.6   Preparing Insulin Injections

Equipment

Insulin Vials

- Unopened vials of insulin should be stored in a refrigerator.
- An opened vial of insulin may be refrigerated or kept at room temperature; recommend discard after 28 days.
- Insulin should not be exposed to light, or to temperatures over 27°C (80°F).
- Do not use insulin that exhibits clumping, frosting, or precipitation.
- Insulin vials
- Insulin syringe, available in 3/10-, 1/2-, and 1-mL sizes (*Note:* Syringes are no longer called U40, U100, etc.)
- Needles, 29- to 31-gauge short needles
- Antimicrobial swab
- Dry gauze sponge
- Clean gloves if indicated

Preparation

- Check physician's order. Follow steps for preparing injections ❶.
- Obtain client's blood glucose level before preparation to determine appropriate administration of insulin.

For Newly Diagnosed Diabetic Client

- Explain to client that the dose of short-acting insulin must be adjusted according to blood glucose test results.
- Explain that there is a variation in levels—the lowest blood glucose level is before meals and the highest 1 to 2 hours after meals.
- Goal of treatment is to eliminate wide swings in glucose levels.

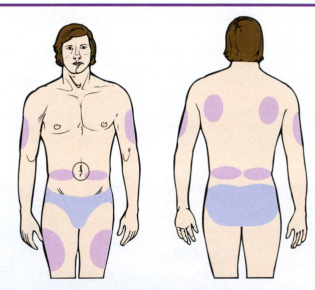

❶ Sites for subcutaneous injections given routinely. (Avoid umbilicus area.) Abdomen site preferred for insulin injection as absorption is more predictable.

Procedure

Procedure for One-Insulin Solution

1. Perform hand hygiene.
2. Turn intermediate or long-acting (cloudy) insulin vial top-to-bottom 10 times. **Rationale:** *This brings cloudy insulin solution into suspension. Clear insulins do not require this.*

SKILL 10.6   Preparing Insulin Injections (*continued*)

3. Wipe top of insulin bottle with antimicrobial swab.
4. Remove needle guard and place on tray.
5. Pull plunger of syringe down to desired amount of medication (e.g., 12 units). Inject amount of air into air space, not into insulin solution. **Rationale:** *Injecting air directly into insulin solution causes bubbles*.
6. Withdraw ordered amount of insulin into syringe.
7. Validate medication record, insulin bottle, and prepared syringe with an RN for accuracy. **Rationale:** *Double checking insulin helps safeguard against errors*.
8. Remove needle from vial and expel air from syringe.
9. Replace needle guard.
10. Take medication to client's room.
11. Follow steps for administration of medications by subcutaneous injection.

Procedure for Two-Insulin Solutions

1. Check medication orders (**Table 10–4 ●**).
2. Perform hand hygiene.
3. Follow steps for combining medications in one syringe using two vials.

4. Turn cloudy intermediate insulin bottle (Bottle A) top to bottom 8 to 10 times. **Rationale:** *This brings cloudy solution into suspension*.
5. Wipe top of both insulin bottles with alcohol.
6. Take needle guard off and place on tray.
7. Pull plunger of syringe down to desired total units of insulin.
8. Insert needle and inject prescribed amount of air into Bottle A (cloudy) insulin ❷.

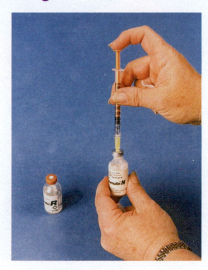

❷ Step 1: Inject prescribed amount of air into intermediate-acting (cloudy) insulin vial—withdraw needle without needle touching solution.

TABLE 10–4   Insulin Types and Therapeutic Action (in min/hr*)

TYPES	INJECT**	ONSET	PEAK	DURATION
Very Rapid Acting (clear solution)				
Humalog® (lispro)	Within 15 min AC or immediately PC	5–15 min	30–90 min	3–5 hr
NovoLog® (aspart)	Within 5–10 min AC			
Apidra® (glulisine)	15 min AC or within 20 min after *starting* a meal			
Short Acting (clear solution)				
Novolin R	Per order	0.5–1 hr	2–4 hr	5–7 hr
Humulin R	Within 30–60 min AC			
Intermediate Acting (cloudy solution)				
Humulin N (NPH)	Per order	1–2 hr	6–10 hr	16–24 hr
Novolin N (NPH)	Per order	1–3 hr	8 hr	12–16 hr
Mixtures (cloudy solution)				
Novolin 70/30 (70% NPH, 30% Regular)	Per order	30 min	Varies	10–16 hr
Humulin 70/30 (70% NPH, 30% Regular)	Within 30–60 min AC	30 min		
Humulin 50/50 (50% NPH, 50% Regular)				
Humalog 75/25 (75% lispro protamine suspension, 25% lispro)	Within 15 min AC	10–15 min		
Humalog 50/50 (50% lispro protamine suspension, 50% lispro)	Within 15 min AC			
NovoLog 70/30 (70% aspart protamine suspension, 30% aspart)	Within 15 min AC	5–15 min		
Long Acting				
Lantus (glargine) (*clear solution*)	Daily	4–6 hr	No peak	24 hr
Levemir (detemir) (*clear solution*)				

*The time of insulin action may vary significantly in different clients and in the same client at different times.
**AC = before meals; PC = after meals.

(*continued on next page*)

SKILL 10.6   Preparing Insulin Injections (*continued*)

9. Withdraw needle.
10. Pull plunger of syringe down to prescribed units of clear insulin.
11. Insert needle and inject air into clear insulin bottle (Bottle B) **3**.

12. Invert and withdraw medication **4**. **Rationale:** *Withdrawing clear insulin first prevents inadvertent injection of intermediate-acting insulin into rapid- or short-acting insulin bottle, which would slow its rapid action.*
13. Double check your preparations with another nurse.

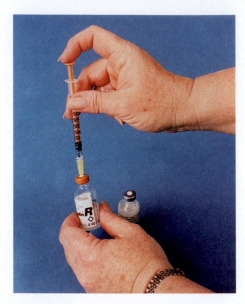

3 Step 2: Inject prescribed amount of air into rapid- or short-acting (clear) insulin vial. Do not withdraw needle.

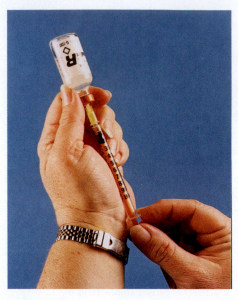

4 Step 3: Invert vial of rapid or short-acting insulin; withdraw prescribed amount of medication and withdraw needle from vial.

Evidence-Based Nursing Practice
Double Checking Drug Doses

Double checks of medications have sometimes been considered a "weak" intervention because even when done, many medication errors still occur. Vague reminders to use critical thinking when double checking medications have little positive impact on reducing errors. A new systematic review showed there is not enough evidence to draw conclusions about double checking medication administration. Certain factors have been linked to ongoing medication errors:

- The expectation that someone else will make sure a mistake is not made
- The lack of focus that comes of attempting to do math while the "double checking" nurse is watching (This produces ambiguity about who is doing the calculation and who is approving it.)

- Lack of time
- The tendency not to check the order again after a distraction has occurred.

Further research into the value of double checks is advised. Current recommendations for the double-checking process include the following:

- Eliminate language such as "That's right, isn't it?" and substitute language that suggests independent calculation, such as "What dose did you get?"
- Perform an audit for processes that require double checks and determine how often they are being done correctly.
- Learn from errors discovered after a double check process.
- Limit double checks to high alert medications, such as insulin.

Data from Alsulami, Conroy, & Choonara (2012) and Intermountain University (n.d.)

14. Withdraw needle from bottle and expel all air bubbles from syringe.
15. Invert Bottle A and insert needle. Take care not to inject any rapid or short-acting (clear) insulin into intermediate-acting (cloudy) insulin bottle. This can be avoided by holding steady pressure on plunger when inserting needle into bottle.
16. Pull back on plunger to obtain exact prescribed amount of intermediate or long-acting insulin **5**. The total insulin dose now includes both the clear insulin, previously drawn up into syringe, and the intermediate cloudy insulin you have just drawn up.

17. Withdraw needle from bottle and replace needle guard.
18. Follow protocol for administration of medications by subcutaneous injections **6**–**8**. Document actions.

CLINICAL ALERT
Do not massage site following injection of certain drugs such as insulin or heparin because this hastens absorption and drug action and may cause tissue irritation.

SKILL 10.6　Preparing Insulin Injections *(continued)*

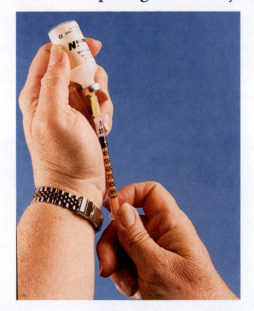

5 Step 4: Invert intermediate-acting insulin vial and withdraw exact amount without injecting insulin into bottle.

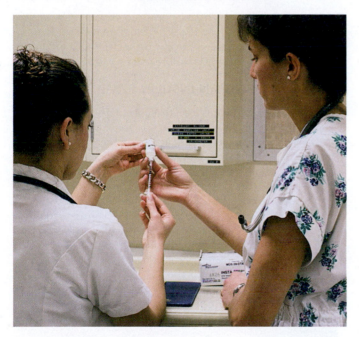

6 Double check insulin dose with a second nurse to help prevent errors in preparation.

Hypoglycemia (blood sugar < 60 mg/dL) is the most common adverse effect of insulins. Client should wear a medical alert bracelet/ID to alert others. The client should be instructed to carry at least 15 g of fast-acting sugar (e.g., glucose tablet, 1 Tbsp sugar, jelly, honey, or tube of cake frosting) to be taken in the event of a hypoglycemic reaction.

The IV route is superior for administering sliding-scale insulin to a client who is obese. Adipose tissue slows onset of insulin action.

Long-acting insulin, Lantus (glargine), is a clear solution. It is not to be mixed with any other type of insulin or solution. It is given subcutaneously and is not intended for IV use.

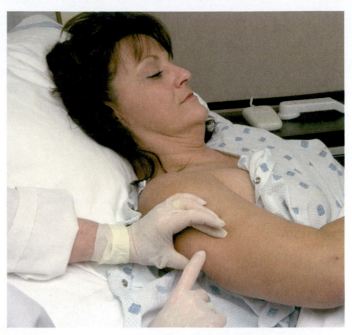

7 Select site on lateral aspect of mid-upper arm for subcutaneous injection.

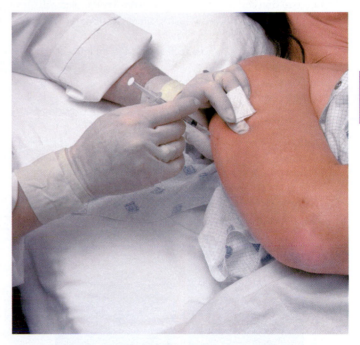

8 Insert needle at a 45- or 90-degree angle, using a short needle for a subcutaneous injection.

VARIATION: USING AN INSULIN PEN

Equipment

- Insulin delivery device labeled with client's name
- Prefilled pen or cartridge with correct insulin type with instructions for use
- Device-compatible needle
- Antimicrobial swab

(continued on next page)

SKILL 10.6 Preparing Insulin Injections (*continued*)

Preparation

- Check physician's order. Perform hand hygiene.
- Identify client by checking the client's identity band and asking client to state name and birth date.
- Review device instructions with the client.
- Have client perform hand hygiene.
- Instruct client to perform steps below.

Procedure

1. Remove pen cap and insert insulin cartridge if indicated.
2. Turn pen up and down at least 10 times. **Rationale:** *This creates suspension of cloudy insulin.*
3. Remove needle cap and attach sterile needle immediately before injecting.
4. Prime insulin pen by pulling dose knob out in direction of arrow until a "0" appears in the dose window. **Rationale:** *A dose cannot be dialed until the dose knob is pulled out.*
5. Dial 2 units, then push plunger and repeat until drop of insulin appears at tip of needle ❾. **Rationale:** *This removes air and ensures proper dosing. This may require six "air shots" for the InnoLet (an easy-to-use doser that has a large, easy-to-read dial).*
6. Dial required number of insulin units to be injected.
7. Swab injection site.

8. Pinch up skin, insert needle, and release skin before injection.
9. Press pen/device "push button" completely and keep depressed for 10 seconds before removing needle from skin ❿.
10. Do not massage the area.
11. Remove needle from pen/device and dispose in sharps container.
12. Replace pen/device cap and store according to directions.
13. Document relevant information.

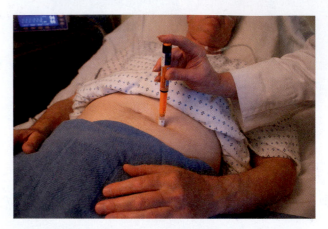

❿ Press pen firmly on client's abdomen to engage needle; inject dialed units and hold 10 seconds before releasing. Remove needle, dispose in sharps receptacle. Recap and return pen to storage area for future use.

VARIATION: USING AN INSULIN PUMP

- Continuous subcutaneous insulin infusion (CSII) is a form of intensive insulin therapy utilized as an alternative to multiple daily injections in an attempt to achieve optimal glycemic control and decrease risk of long-term complications of diabetes. Insulin pumps are manufactured by a number of companies that provide 24-hr emergency and clinical specialists to assist clients with start-up of their pump. All models consist of a battery-powered pump with insulin reservoir, an infusion catheter, and microcomputer that allows programming to deliver basal and bolus doses according to the physician orders ⓫. Only rapid-acting or short-acting insulin is used.
- CSII more closely mimics release of insulin by the pancreas with continuous-delivery basal and bolus insulin infusion.

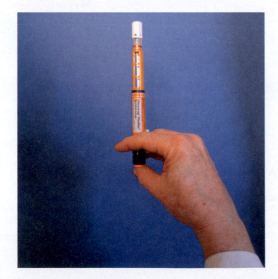

❾ Air shot clears cartridge and needle of air and primes needle for injection.

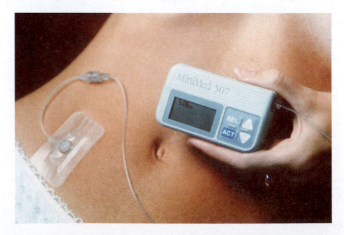

⓫ MiniMed 507 insulin pump attached to infusion set. Abdominal site is preferred because insulin absorption is faster and most predictable.

SKILL 10.6 Preparing Insulin Injections *(continued)*

- Basal rate(s): amount of insulin delivered (units per hour) to keep blood glucose levels in target range between meals and overnight.
- Bolus: additional amount of insulin delivered immediately before meals or for episodes of hyperglycemia, the greatest risk associated with insulin pump therapy.
- The client should be referred to a certified diabetes educator before the start of pump use. Insulin boluses will be based on blood glucose readings and carbohydrate grams intake.
- The client performs frequent fingerstick blood glucose checks: before adjusting any insulin dose, fasting, before meals, 2 hours after eating, at bedtime, and at 3 a.m. weekly.
- Lifestyle advantages: flexibility; insulin needs can be tailored to changes in schedule (mealtime, exercise, or sleep).

CLINICAL ALERT

Insulin pump management and education should be done by a certified diabetes educator who is also a certified insulin pump trainer.

If insulin must be discontinued (e.g., for MRI, CT scan), the pump should be disconnected. Blood glucose level should be checked before disconnecting and upon reconnecting. Ketoacidosis can occur within 2 hours if insulin delivery is interrupted.

Practice Guidelines

Premixing Types of Insulin

- Mixtures of rapid-acting (Humalog) and intermediate or long-acting insulin should be administered within 10 minutes before a meal.
- Mixtures of NPH and regular (short-acting) insulin should be administered 20 to 30 minutes prior to a meal.

- Mixtures may be stored in refrigerator for up to 30 days and should be gently resuspended prior to injection.
- Insulin type and brand should remain consistent for an individual client.

▶ CRITICAL THINKING OPTIONS FOR UNEXPECTED OUTCOMES

Not all unexpected outcomes require further nursing intervention; however, many times they do. When the client demonstrates a change in signs/symptoms indicating an emerging problem, the nurse should immediately assess and troubleshoot what is happening. The assessment data must be processed quickly to formulate a hypothesis so the nurse can make a clinical judgment. The nurse then decides how best to resolve the problem and improve the client's situation for a better appropriate outcome.

EXPECTED OUTCOME	PROBLEM SOLVING	NURSING ACTIONS
Lifestyle changes assist in management of client's altered health status.	Client does not adhere to diet.	■ Elicit client's feelings to determine reason for nonadherence. ■ Check method of diet preparation and administration to see if it is attractive and appealing. ■ Ensure that environment is conducive to eating. ■ Collaborate with dietitian to discuss diet with client.
Paracentesis is completed without complications.	Urine output is blood tinged after paracentesis.	■ Notify physician at once; bladder may have been punctured during procedure. ■ Monitor vital signs for shock. ■ Maintain client on bed rest. ■ Observe for urine output.
Diabetes Insulin injection is administered without complications.	Medication is administered using wrong parenteral route.	■ Notify physician; medications may need to be administered to reverse the action of the medication. ■ Monitor client's response closely and report adverse findings immediately. ■ Medication administered IM or IV rather than subcutaneously leads to faster absorption rates; therefore, ongoing assessment must be done to determine effects. (IV administration has immediate action.) ■ Complete unusual occurrence report according to agency policy.
Client's diabetic teaching is completed before discharge.	Client is to be discharged before diabetic teaching is completed.	■ Collaborate with agency's diabetic nurse. ■ Continue to complete discharge teaching, and send to referral agency. ■ Notify physician of the situation (may need to schedule office visits to complete teaching). ■ Verbally communicate to referral agency and discuss discharge needs of client (i.e. this may include home care nurse visits to ensure a client with diabetes does appropriate diabetic checks and insulin is administered as needed).

11 Mobility

In this chapter, readers will be given essential safe and efficient strategies for assisting clients to move and change positions. The use of assistive equipment, adequate numbers of staff, and proper body alignment of nurse and client are discussed. Skills for assisting clients into various positions, turning clients in bed, and transferring clients from a bed to a chair or stretcher are included. During all positional changes, the comfort and dignity of clients must be protected. Ensure modesty by preventing improper exposure throughout all positional changes. Protect dignity by giving careful and complete instructions, by not rushing, by encouraging clients to help themselves as much as possible, and by using a caring tone of voice and eye contact.

Expected Outcomes

1. Correct body mechanics are utilized by caregiver.
2. Injuries are prevented to both the nurse and the client.
3. Proper body mechanics facilitate client care.
4. Client improves range of motion and muscle tone after performing range-of-motion exercises.
5. Client is able to progress through range of motion with minimal to no pain.
6. Joint movement is maintained.

SKILL 11.1 Applying Body Mechanics

Equipment

None

Procedure

1. Determine need for assistance in moving or turning a client following OSHA lifting guidelines. **Rationale:** *Half of all back pain is associated with lifting or turning clients. The most common back injury is strain on the lumbar muscle group.*

2. Introduce self, explain what procedure is to be done and why. Perform hand hygiene, follow infection control measures, and verify client's identity. Provide privacy. Provide comfort and safety for client and self, including raising bed to appropriate height for procedure.

3. Establish a firm base of support by placing both feet flat on the floor, with one foot slightly in front of the other.

4. Distribute weight evenly on both feet.

5. Slightly bend both knees. **Rationale:** *Allows strong muscles of legs to do the lifting.*

6. Hold abdomen firm and tuck buttocks in so that spine is in alignment. **Rationale:** *This position protects the back.*

7. Hold head erect, and secure firm stance.

8. Use this stance as the basis for all actions in moving, turning, and lifting clients.

9. Maintain weight to be lifted as close to your body as possible. **Rationale:** *This position maintains the center of gravity and provides leverage that reduces lower back strain.*

10. Align the three natural curves in your back (cervical, thoracic, and lumbar). **Rationale:** *Weight of client is evenly distributed throughout spine, lowering risk of back injury.*

11. Prevent twisting your body when moving the client. Use a gait belt if needed ❶. **Rationale:** *This prevents injury to the back.*

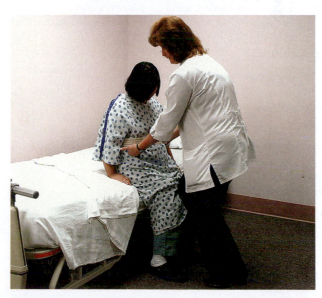

❶ Gait belts are routinely used to assist in manual transfer in most facilities.

(continued on next page)

SKILL 11.1 Applying Body Mechanics (*continued*)

Evidence-Based Nursing Practice
Preventing Back Injury

According to OSHA (2011), in 2011 the Bureau of Labor Statistics reported that hospital workers suffered injuries and illnesses at nearly twice the national average and that close to 50% of reported injuries and illnesses among nurses and nursing support staff were musculoskeletal disorders. Client handling injuries accounted for 25% of all workers' compensation claims for the healthcare industry. More than 30 years of evidence have demonstrated that manual client handling and relying on body mechanics are unsafe (Waters et al., 2009).

Data from the BLS show that in 2011, the overexertion injury rate for hospital workers was 76 per 10,000—twice the average over all occupations; the rate for nursing home workers was over three times the average (132 per 10,000). The single greatest risk factor for overexertion injuries in healthcare workers is the manual lifting, moving, and repositioning of residents or clients, that is, manual client handling.

Rising obesity rates in the United States have increased the physical demands on caregivers. Also, the aging of the healthcare workforce likely contributes to the problem; recent data indicate that the average registered nurse in the United States is in his or her mid-40s. Nursing work demands have been strained by an ongoing shortage of nurses, projected to reach 260,000 unfilled nursing positions by the year 2025 in the United States.

Safe client handling has been associated not only with fewer injuries but also with a decrease in severity of injuries. The use of back braces, a subject of debate in the past, is no longer promoted, because newer devices and methods have shown substantial results. Mechanical lifts and lift teams have dramatically reduced the incidence of injury. For example, 23 high-risk hospital units across seven Southeast Veterans Health Administration facilities were able to reduce their injury rate from 24.0 to 16.9 per 100 workers per year (a 30% drop).

The benefits of safer client handling for nurses is obvious, but the quality of client care also improves when safe handling programs are implemented. Use of mechanical lifts and lift teams leads to fewer falls, skin tears, and pressure ulcers for clients. Safe lift equipment increases client mobility, which can reduce length of hospital stay. Mechanical transfer devices can increase a feeling of safety, a sense of dignity, and client satisfaction.

Evidence-based research has shown that safe client handling interventions can significantly reduce overexertion injuries by replacing manual client handling with safer methods.

Data from Waters et al. (2009), National Institute for Occupational Safety and Health (2013), and Occupational Safety and Health Administration (2011).

SKILL 11.2 Performing Passive Range-of-Motion Exercises

Delegation

Performing passive range-of-motion (ROM) exercises can be delegated to unlicensed assistive personnel (UAP). Some agencies may have specially trained nursing assistants who perform restorative activities, such as ROM, for clients. For UAP who do not have this special training, however, it is important for the nurse to review the general guidelines for performing passive ROM exercises to avoid injury to the UAP or client. Encourage the UAP to perform ROM during the bath. Emphasize the importance of reporting anything unusual to the nurse. If a client has a recent spinal cord injury or some form of orthopedic trauma, the nurse or a physical therapist should do the ROM.

Equipment

No special equipment is needed other than a bed.

Preparation

- Prior to initiating the exercises, review any possible restrictions with the primary care provider or physical therapist. Also refer to the agency's protocol.

Procedure

1. Prior to performing the skill, introduce self and verify the client's identity using agency protocol. Explain to the client what you are going to do, why it is necessary, and how he or she can participate. Listen to any suggestions made by the client or support people. Discuss the importance of ROM exercises in the plan of care. Provide comfort and safety for client and self, including raising bed to appropriate height for procedure. **Rationale:** *The more a client can assist, the better. Whenever possible, progress should be made toward active ROM exercises.*

2. Perform hand hygiene and observe other appropriate infection control procedures.

3. Provide for client privacy, and use client-selected music when possible. **Rationale:** *The ROM session is an opportunity to use touch with the client in a relaxing and therapeutic manner. Any measures that will enhance relaxation are warranted, such as privacy, scent, and sound.*

4. Assist the client to a supine position near you and expose only the body parts requiring exercise. **Rationale:** *This ensures thermal comfort and protects modesty.*

5. Place the client's feet together, place the arms at the sides, and leave space around the head and the feet. **Rationale:** *Positioning the client close to you prevents excessive reaching.*

6. Perform exercises in a head-to-toe format. Follow a repetitive pattern and return to the starting position after each motion. Repeat each motion three to five times on the appropriate limb. **Rationale:** *This ensures thoroughness in the movement and reduces chances of forgetting any part of the body.*

7. Support the limb being ranged above and below the joint. **Rationale:** *This facilitates support and comfort. It also allows the nurse to detect ease/resistance to movement.*

8. Assess for pain by eliciting client self-report before, throughout, and after the session. Observe the client for nonverbal/behavioral cues of discomfort or pain, as well as verbal. Accept the client's self-report or behavioral cues and address pain fully in a timely manner. **Rationale:** *Monitoring for pain is an essential nursing responsibility. Using verbal self-report and observing behavior will enable the nurse to respond therapeutically to any clients who experience pain, whether or not they are able to verbalize for themselves.*

9. Assess the client for changes in cardiopulmonary status (e.g., dyspnea, fatigue, change in vital signs). **Rationale:** *Weak or*

SKILL 11.2 Performing Passive Range-of-Motion Exercises (*continued*)

debilitated clients may have decreased tolerance for activity when beginning the ROM exercises. If a change occurs, stop and note the length of the recovery time for the client. **Rationale:** *A decrease in recovery time can indicate improved activity tolerance.*

10. Perform ROM slowly, gently, and smoothly. **Rationale:** *This will encourage relaxation and lengthening of muscles so they can be ranged further.*

11. Neck (pivot joint):
    - Remove the client's pillow.
    - Flex and extend the neck (ROM: 45 degrees from midline):
        - Place the palm of one hand under the client's head and the palm of the other hand on the client's chin.
        - Move the head from the upright midline position forward until the chin rests on the chest ❶.
        - Move the head from the flexed position back to the resting supine position without the head pillow ❷.
    - Lateral flexion of the neck (ROM: 40 degrees from midline):
        - Place the heels of the hands on each side of the client's cheeks.
        - Move the head laterally toward the right and left shoulders ❸.

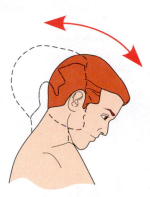

❶ Flexion/extension of neck.

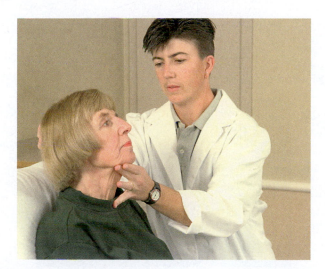

❷ Extension of neck; move head up from chest 90 degrees.

- Rotation (ROM: 70 degrees from midline):
    - Place the heels of the hands on each side of the client's cheeks.
    - Turn the face as far as possible to the right and left.

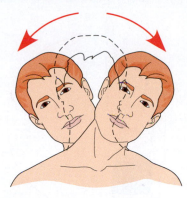

❸ Lateral flexion of neck.

12. Shoulder (ball-and-socket joint):
    - Flexion (ROM: 180 degrees from the side):
        - Begin with the client's arm at the side. Grasp the arm beneath the elbow with one hand and beneath the wrist with the other hand unless otherwise indicated.
        - Raise the arm from a position by the side forward and upward to a position beside the head. The elbow may need to be flexed if the headboard is in the way.
    - Extension (ROM: 180 degrees from vertical position beside the head):
        - Move the arm from a vertical position beside the head forward and down to a resting position at the side of the body ❹.

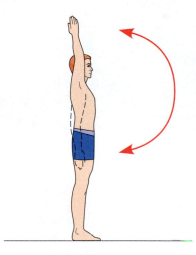

❹ Flexion/extension of shoulder.

- Abduction (ROM: 180 degrees):
    - Move the arm laterally from the resting position at the side to a side position above the head, palm of the hand away from the head ❺.
- Adduction (ROM: 230 degrees):
    - Move the arm laterally from the position beside the head downward laterally and across the front of the body as far as possible. The elbow may be straight or bent ❻.
- External rotation (ROM: 90 degrees):
    - With arm held out to the side at shoulder level and the elbow bent to a right angle, fingers pointing down, move the arm upward so that the fingers point up and the back of the hand touches the mattress ❼.

(*continued on next page*)

SKILL 11.2   Performing Passive Range-of-Motion Exercises (*continued*)

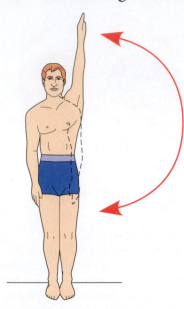

5 Abducting the shoulder.

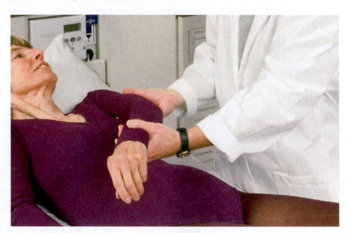

6 Adducting the shoulder.

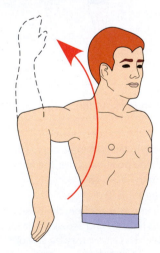

7 External/internal rotation of shoulder.

- Internal rotation (ROM: 90 degrees):
  - With the arm held out to the side at shoulder level and the elbow bent to a right angle, fingers pointing up, bring the arm forward and down so that the palm touches the mattress.

- Circumduction (ROM: 360 degrees):
  - Move the arm forward, up, back, and down in a full circle **8**.

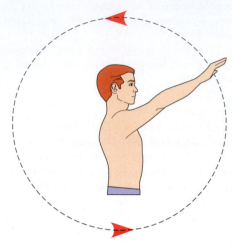

8 Circumduction of shoulder.

13. Elbow (hinge joint):
    - Flexion (ROM: 150 degrees):
      - Bring the lower arm forward and upward so that the hand is level with the shoulder.
    - Extension (ROM: 150 degrees):
      - Bring the lower arm forward and downward, straightening the arm **9** **10**.

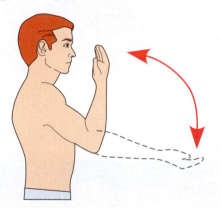

9 Flexion/extension of elbow.

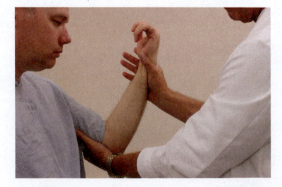

10 Elbow flexion with supination of the forearm.

- Rotation for supination (ROM: 70 to 90 degrees):
  - Grasp the client's hand as for a handshake and turn the palm upward. Make sure that only the forearm (not the shoulder) moves.

SKILL 11.2 Performing Passive Range-of-Motion Exercises (*continued*)

- Rotation for pronation (ROM: 70 to 90 degrees):
  - Grasp the client's hand as for a handshake and turn the palm downward ⓫. Make sure that only the forearm (not the shoulder) moves.

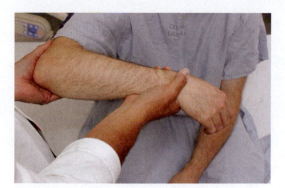

⓫ Pronating the forearm.

14. Wrist (condyloid joint):
    - Flexion (ROM: 80 to 90 degrees):
      - Flex the client's arm at the elbow until the forearm is at a right angle to the mattress. Support the wrist joint with one hand while your other hand manipulates the joint.
      - Bring the fingers of the hand toward the inner aspect of the forearm ⓬.

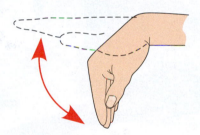

⓬ Flexion/extension of wrist.

- Extension (ROM: 80 to 90 degrees):
  - Straighten the hand to the same plane as the arm.
- Hyperextension (ROM 70 to 90 degrees):
  - Bend the fingers of the hand back as far as possible ⓭.

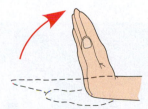

⓭ Hyperextension of wrist.

- Radial flexion (abduction) (ROM: 0 to 20 degrees):
  - Bend the wrist laterally toward the thumb side ⓮.
- Ulnar flexion (adduction) (ROM: 30 to 50 degrees):
  - Bend the wrist laterally toward the fifth finger.

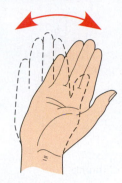

⓮ Radial and ulnar flexion.

15. Hand and fingers (metacarpophalangeal joints—condyloid; interphalangeal joints—hinge):
    - Flexion (ROM: 90 degrees):
      - Make a fist ⓯.

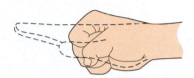

⓯ Flexion/extension of fingers.

- Extension (ROM: 90 degrees):
  - Straighten the fingers.
- Hyperextension (ROM: 30 degrees):
  - Gently bend fingers back.
- Abduction (ROM: 20 degrees):
  - Spread the fingers of the hand apart ⓰.

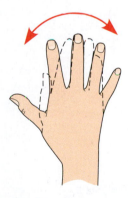

⓰ Abduction/adduction of fingers.

- Adduction (ROM: 20 degrees):
  - Bring fingers together.
16. Thumb (saddle joint):
    - Flexion (ROM: 90 degrees):
      - Move the thumb across the palmar surface of the hand toward the fifth finger ⓱.
    - Extension (ROM: 90 degrees):
      - Move the thumb away from the hand.

(*continued on next page*)

SKILL 11.2 **Performing Passive Range-of-Motion Exercises** (*continued*)

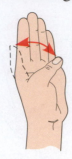

17 Flexion/extension of thumb.

- Abduction (ROM: 30 degrees):
  - Extend the thumb laterally (can be done when placing fingers in abduction and adduction) 18.

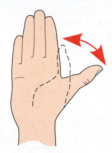

18 Abduction/adduction of thumb.

- Adduction (ROM: 30 degrees):
  - Move the thumb back to the hand.
- Opposition:
  - Touch thumb to the top of each finger of the same hand. The thumb joint movements involved are abduction, rotation, and flexion 19.

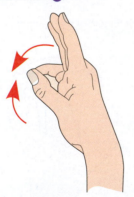

19 Opposition.

17. Hip (ball-and-socket joint):
  - To carry out hip and leg exercises, place one hand under the client's knee and the other under the ankle 20.

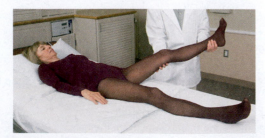

20 Position for knee and hip movements.

- Flexion (ROM: knee extended, 90 degrees; knee flexed, 120 degrees):
  - Lift the leg and bend the knee, moving the knee up toward the chest as far as possible 21.

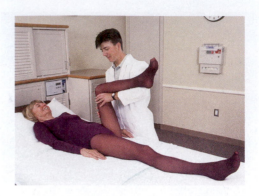

21 Flexing the knee and the hip.

- Extension (ROM: 90 to 120 degrees):
  - Bring the leg down, straighten the knee, and lower the leg to the bed.
- Abduction (ROM: 45 to 50 degrees):
  - Move the leg to the side away from the client 22.

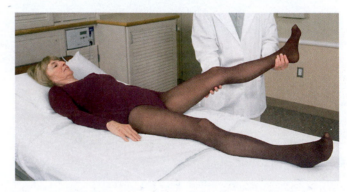

22 Abducting the leg.

- Adduction (ROM: 20 to 30 degrees beyond other leg):
  - Move the leg back across and in front of the other leg 23.

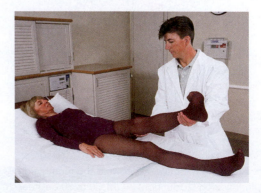

23 Adducting the leg.

SKILL 11.2   Performing Passive Range-of-Motion Exercises (*continued*)

- Circumduction (ROM: 360 degrees):
  - Move the leg in a circle ㉔.

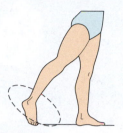

㉔ Circumduction of hip.

- Internal rotation (ROM: 90 degrees):
  - Roll the foot and leg inward ㉕.

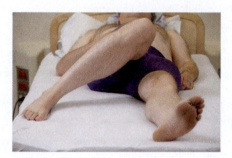

㉕ Internal rotation of hip.

- External rotation (ROM: 90 degrees):
  - Roll the foot and leg outward. *Note:* An alternative method is to flex the knee and hip to 90 degrees. Place the foot away from the midline. Move the thigh and knee toward the midline for internal rotation (ROM: 40 degrees). Place the foot toward the midline and move the thigh and knee away from the midline for external rotation (ROM 45 degrees) ㉖.

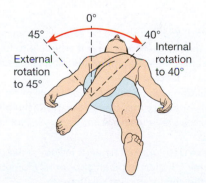

㉖ Internal and external hip rotation.

18. Knee (hinge joint):
    - Flexion (ROM: 120 to 130 degrees):
      - Bend the leg, bringing the heel toward the back of the thigh (done with hip flexion) ㉗.

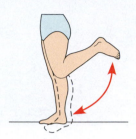

㉗ Flexion/extension of knee.

- Extension (ROM: 120 to 130 degrees):
  - Straighten the leg, returning the foot to the bed.
19. Ankle (hinge joint):
    - Extension (plantar flexion) (ROM: 45 to 50 degrees):
      - Move the foot so the toes are pointed downward ㉘.

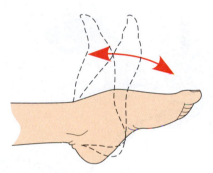

㉘ Extension/flexion of ankle.

- Flexion (dorsiflexion) (ROM: 20 degrees):
  - Move foot so toes are pointed upward.
20. Foot (gliding):
    - Eversion (ROM: 5 degrees):
      - Place one hand under the client's ankle and the other over the arch of the foot.
    - Turn the whole foot outward ㉙.

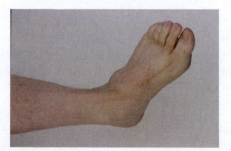

㉙ Everting the foot.

(*continued on next page*)

SKILL 11.2   Performing Passive Range-of-Motion Exercises (continued)

- Inversion (ROM: 5 degrees):
  - Using the same hand placement as above, turn the whole foot inward **30**.

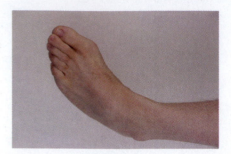

30 Inverting the foot.

21. Toes (interphalangeal joints—hinge; metatarsophalangeal joints—hinge; intertarsal joints—gliding):
    - Flexion (ROM: 35 to 60 degrees):
      - Place one hand over the arch of the foot.
      - Place the fingers of the other hand over the toes to curl the toes downward **31**.

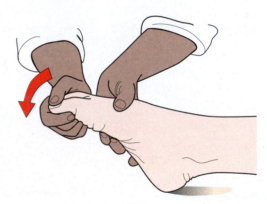

31 Flexing the toes.

- Extension (ROM: 35 to 60 degrees):
  - Place one hand over the arch of the foot.
  - Place the fingers of the other hand under the toes to bend the toes upward **32**.

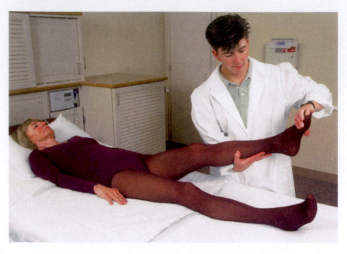

32 Extending the toes against resistance.

- Abduction (ROM: 0 to 15 degrees):
  - Spread the toes apart.
- Adduction (ROM: 0 to 15 degrees):
  - Bring the toes together.
22. Move to the other side of the bed and repeat exercises for other arm and leg.
23. Return bed to lowest position.
24. Document the following:

- Type of ROM exercise (e.g., active, passive, active-assistive)
- Joints exercised and their degree of joint motion
- Length of exercise
- Client's tolerance level to the activity
- Any abnormalities.

Sample Documentation

8/16/15 1000 Passive ROM performed with bath. All joints ranged fully with 4 reps each. Resistance in shoulders resolved when pace slowed. Tolerated well, no c/o pain. _____ M. Foti, RN

Developmental Considerations

CHILDREN

- Perform exercises gently and with full range of motion, avoiding hyperextension of joints. **Rationale:** *Some children may have lax ligaments, and overstretching can cause injury and pain.*
- A small roll can be made of soft cloth to place in the palms. **Rationale:** *The roll is used to prevent contractures of the fingers. Ensure that the thumb is adducted with finger opposition.* Consult an occupational therapist for a well-fitting splint if needed.
- Special boots (ankle-foot orthotics, often ordered by a physical therapist) or high-top sneakers can be used. These should be

properly fitted, and skin should be carefully examined for pressure areas. Usually, there is an on/off schedule to follow. Footboards can also be placed. **Rationale:** *This helps prevent footdrop (plantar flexion of the foot).*
- In some children with impaired mobility, splinting of the wrist, knees, or ankles may be necessary. **Rationale:** *Splinting helps prevent severe contractures* (Hockenberry & Wilson, 2012).
- Children have developmental needs including the need to play. Performing ROM can be an opportunity for fun and for enhancing the child–caregiver relationship.

SKILL 11.2   Performing Passive Range-of-Motion Exercises *(continued)*

OLDER ADULTS
Changes in the Musculoskeletal System that Affect Nursing Care

■ Contractures—muscles atrophy, regenerate slowly; tendons shrink and sclerose.

■ Range of motion of joints decreases—lack of adequate joint motion, ankylosis.

■ Avoid hyperextending the joints of older adults. **Rationale:** *Such movements can cause pain or nerve damage because joints become less flexible with age.*

■ Work slowly and assess for pain when working with older adults, especially those who have arthritis. **Rationale:** *Arthritis changes can cause contractures and enlarged, painful joints.*

■ Assess for skin breakdown or reddened areas during the range-of-motion procedure. **Rationale:** *Older adults are at risk for skin breakdown due to decreased subcutaneous fat and increased thinning of the skin.*

■ Mobility level is limited—muscle strength lessens and gait may be unsteady.

■ Kyphosis occurs—cervical vertebrae may be flexed; intervertebral discs narrow.

■ Bodies of thoracic vertebrae compress slowly with aging leading to the hunchback appearance—loss of overall height results from disc shrinkage and kyphosis.

■ Bone changes—loss of trabecular bones and bones become brittle.

■ Osteoporosis occurs as a result of calcium loss from the bone and insufficient replacement.

■ Osteoarthritis increases with age, equally affecting men and women. This condition results in physical stress on joints as a result of long-term mechanical, horizontal, chemical, and genetic factors.

■ Nursing care for older adult clients includes the following:

 • Ambulate within limitations of age.

 • Alter position every 2 hours; align correctly.

 • Prevent osteoporosis of long bones by providing exercises against resistance as ordered.

 • Provide active and passive exercises—rest periods necessary and exercise paced throughout the day for older adults.

 • Provide ROM exercises to all joints three times a day.

 • Educate family that allowing the client to be sedentary is not helpful.

 • Encourage walking, which is the best single exercise for older adults.

Changes in Immobilized Older Adults

■ At risk for confusion, depression and disorientation—keep clock and calendar in room to help reorient to time and place.

■ More susceptible to hazards of immobility—maintain own ADLs as much as possible and change position every 2 hours.

Changes in Ability to Maintain Activity Levels

■ As aging occurs, there is a decrease in the rate or speed of activity.

■ Loss of muscle mass interferes with activities that require strength such as bending down, dressing, and reaching for objects.

■ Dexterity decreases, leading to a change in performing manipulative skills.

Impaired Mobility and Disability

■ Nearly 23% of older people living in the community have some degree of disability.

■ Individuals 85 years and older constitute 27% of those who have impaired mobility.

■ Impaired mobility can lead to many subsequent problems, including depression, negative self-image, dependent behavior, and loss of independence.

■ Effects of disability can influence the individual's body image, physical appearance, and bodily sensations.

■ Posture becomes more flexed and center of gravity shifts.

Special Assessment Parameters for Older Adults

■ Consider the following assessment parameters for older adults.

 • Specific source of disability or impaired mobility

 • Presence of accompanying disease state: arthritis, stroke, dementia, diabetes, heart failure, COPD

 • Presence of pain

 • Condition of skin

 • Drug effects: sedation, incontinence, orthostatic hypotension

 • Motivation for rehabilitation

 • Nutritional status

 • Best assistive aid for client

■ Be aware of any vision problems your client may have, especially cataracts, glaucoma, or macular degeneration. Note poorly lighted areas in the home or dark areas in the corridors, throw rugs, uneven or uncarpeted areas adjoining carpeted areas, etc., that may cause the client to stumble or fall.

■ Check your client's ability to be mobile—gait, balance, posture, and whether the client shuffles or is able to pick up his or her feet. Check if the client leans forward and is therefore off balance. Poor or unsteady mobility is often a direct cause of falling.

■ Assess the client's degree of muscle strength on both sides of body and/or loss of flexibility because as age increases, strength declines, resulting in a fall. Check the degree of range of motion to all joints before ambulating. Even a poor handgrip can be dangerous if the client is walking downstairs. If leg muscles are weak, it may be difficult to get off a bed or up from a chair and the client may lose his or her balance.

■ Assess for certain medications the client is taking that can cause vertigo, poor balance, blurred vision, weakness, or even drowsiness. Review the medications of older adult clients, keeping in mind the fact that they may require only half the normal dose due to their age and inability to metabolize drugs. The use of alcohol may contribute to falls in the home environment, so if the client uses alcohol there should be client teaching that focuses on the potential danger.

■ Chronic diseases such as osteoarthritis, Parkinson's, Alzheimer's, and diabetes with peripheral neuropathy can all contribute to falls. Clients who have these diseases may require special assessment and interventions to prevent falls.

■ Most older adult clients are aware of the danger of falling and breaking a hip or a leg, so fear is usually present when they are moving or walking. Proper intervention and instructions with an assistive device (canes, walkers, wheelchairs, etc.) will help to allay these fears, which may become so overpowering that

(continued on next page)

SKILL 11.2   Performing Passive Range-of-Motion Exercises (*continued*)

they cause immobilization and depression. Even fear itself, with its concomitant caution, may result in a fall; if the nurse can work with the client to discuss fears about falling and specific behaviors to prevent falling, it would be very therapeutic.

Nursing Care Plan to Meet Older Adult Clients' Needs

- Focus on disability or impaired mobility.
- Establish supportive relationship.
- Teach activities of daily living. Determine activities that must be accomplished each day for individual to care for own needs and be as independent as possible.
- Use assistive devices until client is stable and able to ambulate independently.

- Increase activities as individual progresses and is able to assume activity.
- Give positive reinforcement for all effort expended.

Setting of Care

Teach the client's caregiver:

- The purpose and importance of performing ROM exercises at home.
- To move gently and slowly through each exercise.
- To perform the exercises at least twice daily and to do five repetitions of each exercise.
- How to use correct body mechanics to prevent muscle strain while performing the exercises.

▶ POSITIONING A CLIENT

Expected Outcomes

1. Client's comfort is increased.
2. Skin remains intact without evidence of breakdown as a result of moving and turning.
3. Footdrop is prevented.

4. Body alignment is maintained.
5. Mechanical equipment and devices are used in client transfers and repositioning as needed.
6. Client is moved safely using appropriate device.

SKILL 11.3   Supporting a Client's Position in Bed

Delegation

Positioning clients in bed can be delegated to unlicensed assistive personnel (UAP). The nurse must give specific directions to UAP about the appropriate positions for the client and the reporting of any changes in skin integrity. The UAP should be encouraged to have the client participate as much as possible in the position change. The nurse is responsible for evaluating the client's comfort and alignment after the repositioning and for assessing skin integrity, particularly at pressure points.

Equipment

The following equipment can be used when positioning clients:
- Pillows—one to six depending on client need
- Trochanter rolls
- Footboard or suspension boots
- Hand rolls or wrist splints, if needed
- Folded towel
- Sandbag or rolled towel

Preparation

- Check the position-change schedule for the next time and type of position change.
- Administer an analgesic, if appropriate, before changing the client's position.
- Obtain required assistance, as needed.

Procedure

1. Prior to performing the procedure, introduce self and verify the client's identity using agency protocol. Explain to the

client what you are going to do, why it is necessary, and how he or she can participate.
2. Perform hand hygiene and observe other appropriate infection control procedures.
3. Provide for client privacy.
4. Raise the height of the bed to bring the client close to your center of gravity to avoid back strain.

VARIATION: SUPPORTING A CLIENT IN THE FOWLER POSITION

- Position the client.
  - Have the client flex the knees slightly before raising the head of the bed. **Rationale:** *Slight knee flexion prevents the person from sliding toward the foot of the bed as the bed is raised.* Be certain the client's hips are positioned directly over the point where the bed will bend when the head is raised. **Rationale:** *An appropriate hip position ensures that the client will be sitting upright when the head of the bed is raised.*
  - Raise the head of the bed to 45 degrees or the angle required by or ordered for the client ❶. See **Table 11–1** ● for commonly used client positions.
- Provide supportive devices to align the client appropriately.
  - Place a small pillow or roll under the lumbar region of the back if you feel a space in the lumbar curvature. **Rationale:** *The pillow supports the natural lumbar curvature and prevents flexion of the lumbar spine.*
  - Place a small pillow under the client's head. **Rationale:** *The pillow supports the cervical curvature of the vertebral column. Alternatively, have the client rest the head against*

SKILL 11.3   Supporting a Client's Position in Bed *(continued)*

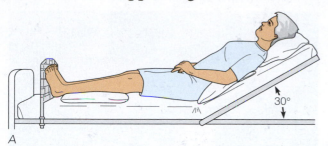
A

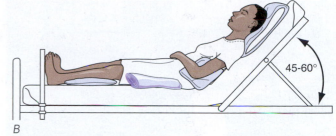
B

1 *A,* Low Fowler (semi-Fowler) position (supported); *B* Fowler position (supported). The amount of support depends on the needs of the individual client.

TABLE 11–1	Bed Positions for Client Care	
POSITIONS	PLACEMENT	USE
High-Fowler **2**	Head of bed 60° angle	Thoracic surgery, severe respiratory conditions
Orthopneic **3**	Head of bed at 90° or client on side of bed leaning over bed table	Difficulty breathing, especially difficulty exhaling (COPD); can press the lower part of the chest against the table to aid exhalation
Fowler **4**	Head of bed 45°–60° angle; hips may or may not be flexed	Postoperative, gastrointestinal conditions; promotes lung expansion
Semi-Fowler **5**	Head of bed 30° angle	Cardiac, respiratory, neurosurgical conditions
Low-Fowler **6**	Head of bed 15° angle	Necessary degree elevation for ease of breathing; promotes skin integrity, client comfort
Knee-gatch **7**	Lower section of bed (under knees) slightly bent	For client comfort; contraindicated for vascular disorders
Trendelenburg's **8**	Head of bed lowered and foot raised	Percussion, vibration, and drainage (PVD) procedure; promotes venous return
Reverse Trendelenburg's **9**	Bed frame is tilted up with foot of bed down	Gastric conditions; prevents esophageal reflux

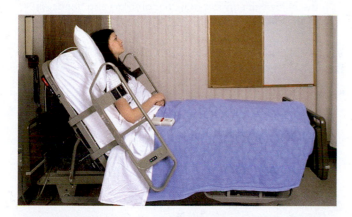

2 High-Fowler position at 60-degree angle.

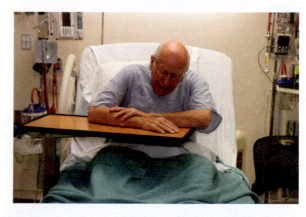

3 Orthopneic position.

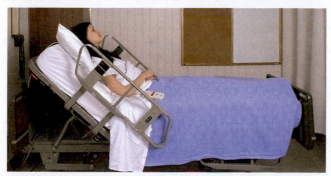

4 Fowler position at 45° to 60° angle.

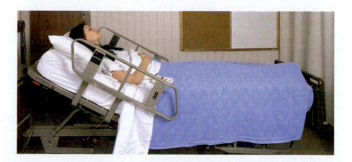

5 Semi-Fowler position at 30° angle.

(continued on next page)

SKILL 11.3   Supporting a Client's Position in Bed (*continued*)

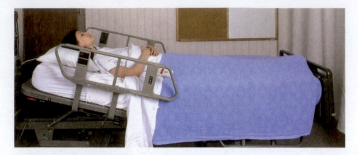

6 Low-Fowler position at 15° angle.

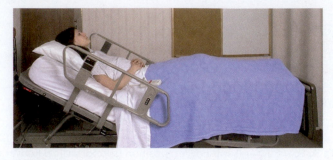

7 Elevate knee-gatch position.

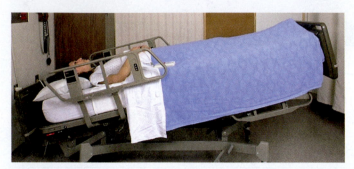

8 Trendelenburg's position.

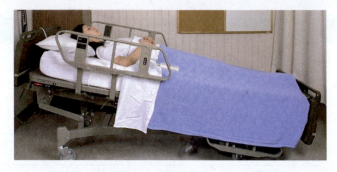

9 Reverse Trendelenburg's position.

the mattress. **Rationale:** *Too many pillows beneath the head can cause neck flexion contracture and respiratory issues in obese clients.* Clients with a cervical collar should not use a pillow. **Rationale:** *This can lead to increased risk of pressure ulcers under the collar.*

- Place one or two pillows under the lower legs from below the knees to the ankles. **Rationale:** *The pillows provide a broad base of support that is soft and flexible, prevent uncomfortable hyperextension of the knees, and reduce pressure on the heels.* Make sure that no pressure is exerted on the popliteal space and that the knees are flexed. **Rationale:** *Pressure against the popliteal space can damage nerves and vein walls, predisposing the client to thrombus formation. Keeping the knees slightly flexed also prevents the person from sliding down in the bed.*

- Avoid using the knee-gatch of a hospital bed to flex the client's knees. **Rationale:** *The position of the knee-gatch rarely coincides with the position of the client's knees. Even when the knee-gatch does bend at the client's knees, considerable pressure (due to the narrow base of support beneath the knees and the firm, unyielding mattress) can be exerted against the popliteal space and beneath the client's calves.*

- Put a trochanter roll lateral to each femur (optional). **Rationale:** *This prevents external rotation of the hips.*

- Support the client's feet with heel boots, high-top tennis shoes, or a footboard. **Rationale:** *This prevents plantar flexion.* The footboard should protrude several inches above the toes. **Rationale:** *This protects the toes from pressure exerted by the top bedding.* The footboard should be placed 1 inch away from the heels. **Rationale:** *This prevents undue pull on the Achilles tendon and discomfort.*

- Place pillows to support both arms and hands if the client does not have normal use of them. **Rationale:** *These*

pillows prevent shoulder and muscle strain from the effects of downward gravitational pull, dislocation of the shoulder in paralyzed individuals, edema of the hands and arms, and flexion contracture of the wrist. Arrange the pillows to support only the forearms and hands, up to the elbow.*

VARIATION: SUPPORTING A CLIENT IN THE DORSAL RECUMBENT POSITION

- Assist the client to the supine position **10**.

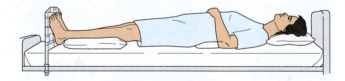

10 Dorsal recumbent position (supported).

- Provide supportive devices to align the client appropriately.
  - Place a pillow of suitable thickness under the client's head and shoulders as needed. **Rationale:** *This prevents hyperextension of the neck. Too many pillows beneath the head may cause or worsen neck flexion contracture.*
  - Place a pillow under the lower legs from below the knees to the ankles. **Rationale:** *This prevents hyperextension of the knees, keeps the heels off the bed, and reduces lumbar lordosis.*
  - *Optional:* Place trochanter rolls or sandbag laterally against the femurs. **Rationale:** *These prevent external rotation of the hips and legs.*
  - Place a rolled towel or small pillow under the lumbar curvature if you feel a space between the lumbar area and the bed. **Rationale:** *This pillow supports the lumbar curvature and prevents flexion of the lumbar spine.*

SKILL 11.3 Supporting a Client's Position in Bed (continued)

- Place a small pillow under thigh to flex knee slightly. **Rationale:** *This prevents hyperextension of knees.*
- Put heel boots or high-top tennis shoes on the client or a footboard on the bed to support the feet. **Rationale:** *This prevents plantar flexion (footdrop).*
- If the client is unconscious or has paralysis of the upper extremities, elevate the forearms and hands (*not the upper arm*) on pillows. **Rationale:** *This position promotes comfort and prevents edema. Pillows are not placed under the upper arms because they can cause shoulder flexion.*
- If the client has actual or potential finger and wrist flexion deformities, use hand rolls or wrist/hand splints. **Rationale:** *This prevents flexion contractures of the fingers.* Hand rolls, having a circumference of 13 to 15 cm (5 to 6 in.), exert even pressure over the entire flexor surface of the palm and fingers ⓫.

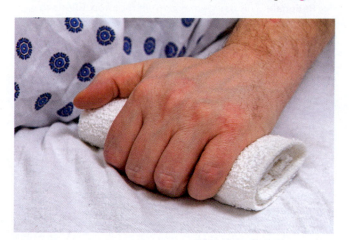

⓫ A hand roll may be made from a folded and rolled washcloth. It is used to maintain functional position of the wrist and fingers and to prevent contractures.

VARIATION: SUPPORTING A CLIENT IN THE PRONE POSITION

- Assist the client to a prone position ⓬.

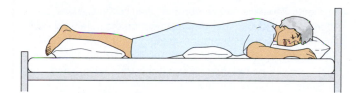

⓬ Prone position (supported).

- Provide supportive devices to position the client appropriately.
  - Turn the client's head to one side, and either omit the pillow entirely if drainage from the mouth is being encouraged, or place a small pillow under the head to align the head with the trunk. **Rationale:** *This prevents flexion of the neck laterally.* Avoid placing the pillow under the shoulders. **Rationale:** *A pillow placed under the shoulders increases lumbar lordosis.*
  - Place a small pillow or roll under the abdomen in the space between the diaphragm (or the breasts of a woman) and the iliac crests. **Rationale:** *The pillow prevents hyperextension of the lumbar curvature, difficulty breathing, and, for some women, pressure on the breasts. Supports placed too low can increase lumbar lordosis and pressure on bony prominences.*

- Place a pillow under the lower legs from below the knees to just above the ankles. **Rationale:** *This raises the toes off the bed surface and reduces plantar flexion. This pillow also flexes the knees slightly for comfort and prevents excessive pressure on the patellae.* Or, position the client on the bed so that the feet are extended in a normal anatomical position over the lower edge of the mattress. **Rationale:** *There should be no pressure on the toes.*

VARIATION: SUPPORTING A CLIENT IN THE LATERAL POSITION

- Assist the client to a lateral position ⓭.

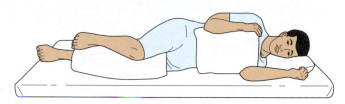

⓭ Lateral position (supported).

- Provide supportive devices to align the client appropriately.
  - Place a pillow under the client's head so that the head and neck are aligned with the trunk. **Rationale:** *The pillow prevents lateral flexion and discomfort of the major neck muscles (e.g., the sternocleidomastoid muscles).*
  - Have the client flex the lower shoulder and position it forward so that the body does not rest on it. Rotate it into any position of comfort. **Rationale:** *In this way, circulation is not disrupted.*
  - Place a pillow under the upper arm. **Rationale:** *This prevents internal rotation and adduction of the shoulder and downward pressure on the chest that could interfere with chest expansion during respiration.* If the client has respiratory difficulty, increase the shoulder flexion and position the upper arm in front of the body off the chest.
  - Place two or more pillows under the upper leg and thigh so that the extremity lies in a plane parallel to the surface of the bed. **Rationale:** *A position parallel to the bed most closely approximates correct standing alignment and prevents internal rotation of the thigh and adduction of the leg. The pillow also prevents pressure caused by the weight of the top leg resting on the lower leg. Such pressure can damage the vein walls in the lower leg and predispose the client to thrombus formation.*
  - Ensure that the two shoulders are aligned in the same plane as the two hips. If they are not, pull one shoulder or hip forward or backward until all four joints are aligned in the same plane. **Rationale:** *Proper alignment prevents twisting of the spine.*
  - *Optional:* Place a folded towel under the natural hollow at the waistline. **Rationale:** *This prevents postural scoliosis of the lumbar spine.* Take care to fill in only the space at the waistline. **Rationale:** *A towel support that extends too high or too low creates undue pressure against the rib cage or iliac crests.*
  - Place a rolled pillow (fold pillow lengthwise) alongside the client's back to stabilize the position. This pillow may not be needed when the client's upper hip and knee are appropriately flexed.

(continued on next page)

SKILL 11.3   Supporting a Client's Position in Bed (continued)

VARIATION: SUPPORTING A CLIENT IN THE SIMS POSITION

Procedure

- Turn the client as for the prone position ⑭.

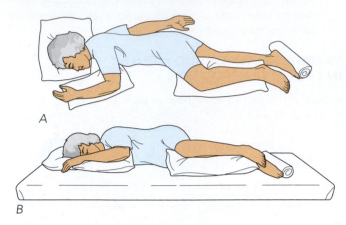

A

B

⑭ The Sims position (supported).

- Provide supportive devices to align the client appropriately.
  - Place a small pillow under the client's head, unless drainage from the mouth is being encouraged. **Rationale:** *The pillow prevents lateral flexion of the neck and cushions the cranial and facial bones and the ear. It is contraindicated if drainage of mucus is required. Too large a pillow produces an uncomfortable lateral flexion of the neck.*
  - Place the lower arm behind and away from the client's body in a position that is comfortable and does not disrupt circulation. **Rationale:** *This position prevents damage to the nerves and blood vessels in the axillae.*
  - Position the upper shoulder so that it is abducted slightly from the body and so the shoulder and elbow are flexed.

Place a pillow in the space between the chest and abdomen and the upper arm and bed. **Rationale:** *This position and support prevent internal shoulder rotation and adduction and maintain alignment of the upper trunk.*

- Place a pillow in the space between the abdomen and pelvis and the upper thigh and bed. **Rationale:** *This position prevents internal rotation and adduction of the hip and also reduces lumbar lordosis.*
- Ensure that the two shoulders are aligned in the same plane as the two hips. If they are not, pull one shoulder or hip forward or backward until all four joints are aligned in the same plane. **Rationale:** *This prevents twisting of the spine.*
- Place a support device (e.g., foot boot on the client or a sandbag or rolled towel against the lower foot of the client). **Rationale:** *This device may prevent footdrop. Efforts to correct plantar flexion in this position, however, are usually unsuccessful.*

- Document all position changes carefully, recording:
  - Time and change of position moved from and position moved to (according to agency protocol).
  - Number of personnel required for turning and positioning.
  - Safety precautions and the use of any premedications.
  - Ways client is able to assist with positioning.
  - Any signs of pressure areas or contractures.
  - Any difficulty client has with breathing (the Fowler, prone, and Sims positions).
  - Use of support/assistive devices and any special requirements.

Sample Documentation

10/15/15 1030 Turned to (L) side by 2 staff. Pillows under head, upper arm & upper leg. Skin intact without redness over bony prominences.

_____M. Foti, RN

Developmental Considerations

INFANTS
- Position infants on their back for sleep, even after feeding. There is little risk of regurgitation and choking, and the rate of sudden infant death syndrome (SIDS) is significantly lower in infants who sleep on their back.
- The skin of newborns can be fragile and may be abraded or torn (sheared) if the infant is pulled across a bed.

CHILDREN
- Carefully inspect the dependent skin surfaces of all infants and children confined to bed at least three times in each 24-hour period.

OLDER ADULTS
- In clients who have had cerebrovascular accidents (strokes), there is a risk of shoulder displacement on the paralyzed side from improper moving or repositioning techniques. Use care when moving, positioning in bed, and transferring. Pillows or foam devices are helpful to support the affected arm and shoulder and prevent injury.
- Decreased subcutaneous fat and thinning of the skin place older adults at risk for skin breakdown. Repositioning approximately every 2 hours (more or less, depending on the unique needs of the individual client) helps reduce pressure on bony prominences and avoid tissue trauma.

▶ MOVING AND TRANSFERRING A CLIENT

Expected Outcomes

1. Appropriate assistive devices are utilized to transfer client.
2. Caregiver is able to manage turning, repositioning, and assistive devices.

SKILL 11.4 Moving a Client Up in Bed

Evidence-Based Nursing

Use of Drawsheet for Moving Clients

Evidence-based studies agree that the critical task of repositioning a client in bed places caregivers at an increased risk of back injury due to high spinal loads. In spite of equipment options such as ceiling track lifts and repositioning slings to minimize the risks, staff continue to reposition clients manually on a regular basis. This study focused on use of slider sheet units (a bottom slider sheet and a slider drawsheet) versus "soaker pads" on jersey sheets for shifting client position. Analysis showed that any combination of slider sheets is a safer option than the traditional lift-and-shift maneuver with soaker pads. Interestingly, many nurses chose a combination of items, most commonly the slider bottom sheet coupled with the "soaker" pad. Use of the slider bottom sheet/soaker pad combination results in significantly less friction than the slider drawsheet/jersey bottom sheet combination that has recently become an acceptable combination within health care.

The study identified an area of caution. It determined that slider sheet components must be standard and readily available in order to be successful. Facilities that did not have items directly on hand for caregivers did not experience success in implementing their use.

Negative feedback for slider sheet use included concerns about excess material, a tendency to wrinkle under clients, and being "too slippery" for some clients.

An unforeseen benefit of slider sheets was their use by clients. Many clients were able to turn and/or boost themselves or assist with bed mobility because of the slider sheets. This had several benefits:

- Increased client independence and self-esteem
- Maintained or increased client strength
- Decreased assistance required from staff.

Source: Filek et al. (2010).

Delegation

The skills of moving and turning clients in bed can be delegated to UAP. The nurse should make sure that any needed equipment and additional personnel are available to reduce risk of injury to the healthcare personnel. Emphasize the need for the UAP to report changes in the client's condition that require assessment and intervention by the nurse.

Equipment

- Assistive devices such as pull and/or turn sheet, friction-reducing device, or a mechanical lift

Preparation

- Determine if assistive devices will be required.
- Determine if any encumbrances to movement, such as an IV or an indwelling urinary catheter, are present.
- Be aware of medications the client is receiving, because certain medications may hamper movement or alertness of the client.
- Decide if assistance will be required from other healthcare personnel.

Procedure

1. Prior to performing the procedure, introduce self and verify the client's identity using agency protocol. Explain to the client what you are going to do, why it is necessary, and how he or she can participate. Listen to any suggestions made by the client or support people.
2. Perform hand hygiene and observe other appropriate infection control procedures.
3. Provide for client privacy.
4. Adjust the bed height and the client's position.
   - Adjust the head of the bed to a flat position or as low as the client can tolerate. **Rationale:** *Moving the client upward against gravity requires more force and can cause back strain.*
   - Raise the height of the bed as appropriate to enhance personnel safety (at the elbows).
   - Lock the wheels on the bed and raise the rail on the side of the bed opposite you.
   - Remove all pillows, then place one against the head of the bed. **Rationale:** *This pillow protects the client's head from inadvertent injury against the top of the bed during the upward move.*
5. For the client who is able to reposition without assistance:
   - Place the bed in flat or reverse Trendelenburg's position (as tolerated by the client). Stand by and instruct the client to move self. Encourage the client to reach up and grasp the upper side rails with both hands, bend knees, and push off with the feet and pull up with the arms simultaneously. Assess if the client is able to move without causing friction to skin.
   - Ask if a positioning device is needed (e.g., pillow).
6. For the client who is partially able to assist:
   - For a client who weighs less than 200 pounds: Use a friction-reducing device and two to three assistants. **Rationale:** *Moving a client up in bed is not a one-person task. During any client handling, if the caregiver is required to lift more than 35 lb of a client's weight, then the client should be considered fully dependent and assistive devices should be used (Waters, 2007).*
   - For a client who weighs more than 200 pounds: Use a friction-reducing device and three assistants. **Rationale:** *Moving a client up in bed is not a one-person task. During any client handling, if the caregiver is required to lift more than 35 lb of a client's weight, then the client should be considered fully dependent and assistive devices should be used (Waters, 2007).*
   - Ask the client to flex the hips and knees and position the feet so that they can be used effectively for pushing. **Rationale:** *Flexing the hips and knees keeps the entire lower leg off the bed surface, preventing friction during movement, and ensures use of the large muscle groups in the client's legs when pushing, thus increasing the force of movement.*
   - Place the client's arms across the chest. Ask the client to flex the neck during the move and keep the head off the

(continued on next page)

SKILL 11.4   Moving a Client Up in Bed (continued)

bed surface. **Rationale:** *This keeps the arms off the bed surface and minimizes friction during movement.*

- Use a friction-reducing device and assistants to move the client up in bed. Ask the client to push on the count of three.

7. Position yourself appropriately, and move the client **1**.
   - Face the direction of the movement, and then assume a broad stance with the foot nearest the bed behind the forward foot and weight on the forward foot. Lean your trunk forward from the hips. Flex hips, knees, and ankles.

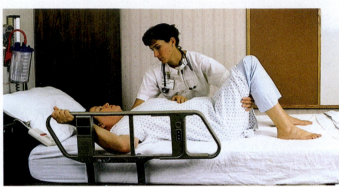

A

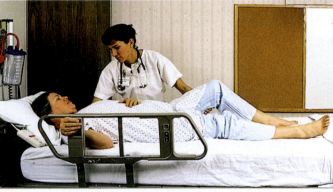

B

1 A, Place one arm under shoulders and other under thighs. B, Maintain proper body alignment when moving client up in bed.

- Tighten your gluteal, abdominal, leg, and arm muscles and rock from the back leg to the front leg and back again. Then, shift your weight to the front leg as the client pushes with the heels and pulls with the arms so that the client moves toward the head of the bed.

8. For the client who is unable to assist:
   - Use a ceiling lift with supine sling or floor-based lift and two or more caregivers. Follow the manufacturer's guidelines for using the lift. **Rationale:** *Moving a client up in bed is not a*

one-person task. During any client handling, if the caregiver is required to lift more than 35 lb of a client's weight, then the client should be considered fully dependent and assistive devices should be used (Waters, 2007). This reduces risk of injury to the caregiver.

9. Ensure client comfort.
   - Elevate the head of the bed and provide appropriate support devices for the client's new position.
   - See the sections on positioning clients earlier in this chapter.

VARIATION: TWO NURSES USING A TURN SHEET

Two nurses can use a turn sheet to move a client up in bed. **Rationale:** *A turn sheet distributes the client's weight more evenly, decreases friction, and exerts a more even force on the client during the move. In addition, it prevents injury of the client's skin, because the friction created between two sheets when one is moved is less than that created by the client's body moving over the sheet.*

- Place a drawsheet or a full sheet folded in half under the client, extending from the shoulders to the thighs. Each person rolls up or fanfolds the turn sheet close to the client's body on either side.
- Both individuals grasp the sheet close to the shoulders and buttocks of the client. **Rationale:** *This draws the weight closer to the nurse's center of gravity and increases the nurse's balance and stability, permitting a smoother movement.*
- Assist the client to flex the hips and knees. Place the client's arms across the chest. **Rationale:** *This keeps them off the bed surface and minimizes friction during movement.* Ask the client to flex the neck during the move and keep the head off the bed surface.
- Position yourself appropriately, and move the client.
  - Face the direction of the movement, and then assume a broad stance with the foot nearest the bed behind the forward foot and weight on the forward foot. Lean your trunk forward from the hips. Flex hips, knees, and ankles.
  - Tighten your gluteal, abdominal, leg, and arm muscles and rock from the back leg to the front leg and back again. Then, shift your weight to the front leg as the client pushes with the heels so that the client moves toward the head of the bed.
- Ensure client comfort.
  - Elevate the head of the bed and provide appropriate support devices for the client's new position.
- Document all relevant information. Record:
  - Time and change of position moved from and position moved to.
  - Any signs of pressure areas.
  - Use of support devices.
  - Ability of client to assist in moving and turning.
  - Response of client to moving and turning (e.g., anxiety, discomfort, dizziness).

Cultural Considerations

Different cultures have cultural variances regarding distance and personal space, which refers to the physical distance between two people. Providing nursing care often means interacting with clients in their personal space, such as moving a client up in the bed or transferring to a bed or gurney, resulting in the client being brought close to the nurse's body. Nurses can show respect to clients by giving them explanations about what they are doing to help clients understand their actions instead of feeling threatened by invasion of their personal space.

SKILL 11.5   Turning a Client to the Lateral or Prone Position in Bed

Preparation

- Determine if any assistive devices will be required (e.g., friction-reducing device or mechanical lift).
- Determine if any encumbrances to movement, such as an IV or an indwelling urinary catheter, are present.
- Be aware of medications the client is receiving, because certain medications may hamper movement or alertness of the client.
- Decide if assistance will be required from other healthcare personnel. **Rationale:** *Moving a client is not a one-person task. During any client handling, if the caregiver is required to lift more than 35 lb of client's weight, then the client should be considered fully dependent and assistive devices should be used (Waters, 2007). This reduces risk of injury to the caregiver.*

Procedure

1. Prior to performing the procedure, introduce self and verify the client's identity using agency protocol. Explain to the client what you are going to do, why it is necessary, and how he or she can participate.
2. Perform hand hygiene and observe other appropriate infection control procedures.
3. Provide for client privacy.
4. Position yourself and the client appropriately before performing the move. Other person(s) stand on the opposite side of the bed.
   - Adjust the head of the bed to a flat position or as low as the client can tolerate. **Rationale:** *This provides a position of comfort for the client.*
   - Raise the height of the bed appropriate to personnel safety (i.e., at the elbows).
   - Lock the wheels on the bed.
   - Move the client closer to the side of the bed opposite the side the client will face when turned. **Rationale:** *This ensures that the client will be positioned safely in the center of the bed after turning.* Use a friction-reducing device or mechanical lift (depending on level of client assistance required) to pull the client to the side of the bed. Adjust the client's head and reposition the legs appropriately.
   - While standing on the side of the bed nearest the client, place the client's near arm across the chest. Abduct the client's far shoulder slightly from the side of the body and externally rotate the shoulder ❶. **Rationale:** *Pulling the*

one arm forward facilitates the turning motion. Pulling the other arm away from the body and externally rotating the shoulder prevents that arm from being caught beneath the client's body during the roll.*

   - Place the client's near ankle and foot across the far ankle and foot. **Rationale:** *This facilitates the turning motion. Making these preparations on the side of the bed closest to the client helps prevent unnecessary reaching.*
   - The person on the side of the bed toward which the client will turn should be positioned directly in line with the client's waistline and as close to the bed as possible.
5. Roll the client to the lateral position. The second person standing on the opposite side of the bed helps roll the client from the other side.
   - Place one hand on the client's far hip and the other hand on the client's far shoulder. **Rationale:** *This position of the hands supports the client at the two heaviest parts of the body, providing greater control in movement during the roll.*
   - Position the client on his or her side with arms and legs positioned and supported properly ❷.

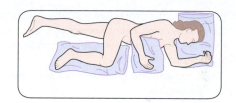
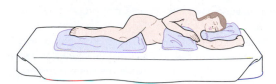

❷ Lateral position with pillows in place.

VARIATION: TURNING A CLIENT TO A PRONE POSITION

To turn a client to the prone position, follow the preceding steps, with two exceptions:

- Instead of abducting the far arm, keep the client's arm alongside the body for the client to roll over. **Rationale:** *Keeping the arm alongside the body prevents it from being pinned under the client when the client is rolled.*
- Roll the client completely onto the abdomen. **Rationale:** *It is essential to move the client as close as possible to the edge of the bed before the turn so that the client will be lying on the center of the bed after rolling. Never pull a client across the bed while the client is in the prone position.* **Rationale:** *Doing so can injure a woman's breasts or a man's genitals.*

6. Document all relevant information. Record:
   - Time and change of position moved from and position moved to
   - Any signs of pressure areas
   - Use of support devices
   - Ability of client to assist in moving and turning
   - Response of client to moving and turning (e.g., anxiety, discomfort, dizziness).

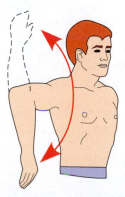

❶ External rotation of the shoulder prevents the arm from being caught beneath the client's body when the client is turned.

SKILL 11.6 Logrolling a Client

Logrolling is a technique used to turn a client whose body must at all times be kept in straight alignment (like a log). An example is the client with a spinal injury. Considerable care must be taken to prevent additional injury. This technique requires a minimum of two nurses or four to five staff, depending on agency policy. For the client who has a cervical injury, one nurse must maintain the client's head and neck alignment.

Preparation

- Determine if assistive devices will be required.
- Determine if any encumbrances to movement, such as an IV or an indwelling catheter, are present.
- Be aware of medications the client is receiving, because certain medications may hamper movement or alertness of the client.
- Obtain assistance from other healthcare personnel. At least two or three additional people are needed to perform this skill safely.

Procedure

1. Prior to performing the procedure, introduce self and verify the client's identity using agency protocol. Explain to the client what you are going to do, why it is necessary, and how he or she can participate.
2. Perform hand hygiene and observe other appropriate infection control procedures.
3. Provide for client privacy.
4. Position yourselves and the client appropriately before the move.
   - Place the client's arms across the chest. **Rationale:** *Doing so ensures that the arms will not be injured or become trapped under the body when the client is turned.*
5. Pull the client to the side of the bed.
   - Use a turn sheet or friction-reducing device to facilitate logrolling. First, stand with another nurse on the same side of the bed. Assume a broad stance with one foot forward, and grasp half of the fanfolded or rolled edge of the turn sheet or friction-reducing device. On a signal, pull the client toward both of you ❶.

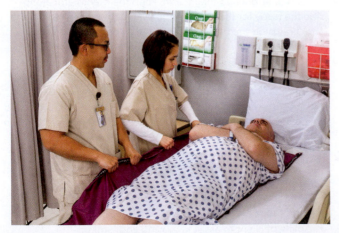

❶ Using a friction-reducing slide sheet, the nurses pull the sheet with the client on it to the edge of the bed.

- One nurse counts: "One, two, three, go." Then, at the same time, all staff members pull the client to the side of the bed by shifting their weight to the back foot. **Rationale:** *Moving the client in unison maintains the client's body alignment.*
6. One person moves to the other side of the bed, and places supportive devices for the client when turned.
   - Place a pillow where it will support the client's head after the turn. **Rationale:** *The pillow prevents lateral flexion of the neck and ensures alignment of the cervical spine.*
   - Place one or two pillows between the client's legs to support the upper leg when the client is turned. **Rationale:** *This pillow prevents adduction of the upper leg and keeps the legs parallel and aligned.*
7. Roll and position the client in proper alignment.
   - The person farthest from the client assumes a stable stance.
   - This person reaches over the client and grasps the far edges of the turn sheet or friction-reducing device ❷.

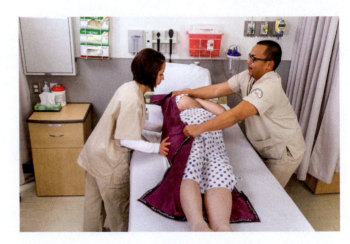

❷ The nurse on the right uses the far edge of the friction-reducing slide sheet to roll the client toward him; the nurse on the left remains behind the client and assists with turning.

- One nurse counts: "One, two, three, go." Then, at the same time, all nurses roll the client to a lateral position.
- The nurse behind the client helps turn the client and provides pillow supports to ensure good alignment in the lateral position.
- Support the client's head, back, and upper and lower extremities with pillows.
- Raise the side rails and place the call bell within the client's reach.
8. Document all relevant information. Record:
   - Time and change of position moved from and position moved to
   - Any signs of pressure areas
   - Use of support devices
   - Ability of client to assist in moving and turning
   - Response of client to moving and turning (e.g., anxiety, discomfort, dizziness).

SKILL 11.7   Assisting a Client to Sit on Side of Bed (Dangling)

The client assumes a sitting position on the edge of the bed to allow neurovascular equilibration before walking, moving to a chair or wheelchair, eating, or performing other activities.

Preparation

- Determine if assistive devices will be required.
- Determine if any encumbrances to movement, such as an IV or an indwelling catheter, are present.
- Be aware of medications the client is receiving, because certain medications may hamper movement or alertness of the client.
- Decide if assistance will be required from other healthcare personnel. At least two or three additional people are needed to perform this skill safely.

Procedure

1. Prior to performing the procedure, introduce self and verify the client's identity using agency protocol. Explain to the client what you are going to do, why it is necessary, and how he or she can participate.
2. Perform hand hygiene and observe other appropriate infection control procedures.
3. Provide for client privacy.
4. Position yourself and the client appropriately before performing the move.
   - Assist the client to a lateral position facing you.
   - Raise the head of the bed slowly to its highest position. **Rationale:** *This decreases the distance that the client needs to move to sit up on the side of the bed.*
   - Position the client's feet and lower legs at the edge of the bed. **Rationale:** *This enables the client's feet to move easily off the bed during the movement, and the client is aided by gravity into a sitting position.*
   - Stand beside the client's hips and face the far corner of the bottom of the bed (the angle in which movement will occur). Assume a broad stance, placing the foot nearest the client forward. Lean your trunk forward from the hips.
5. Move the client to a sitting position ❶.
   - Place one arm around the client's shoulders and the other arm beneath both of the client's thighs near the knees. **Rationale:** *Supporting the client's shoulders prevents the client from falling backward during the movement. Supporting the client's thighs reduces friction of the thighs against the bed surface during the move and increases the force of the movement.*
   - Tighten your gluteal, abdominal, leg, and arm muscles.

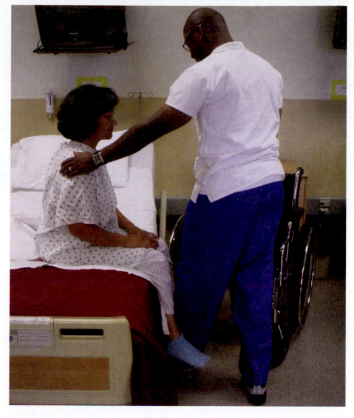

❶ Pivot client to dangling position before placing feet on floor.

- Pivot on the balls of your feet in the desired direction facing the foot of the bed while pulling the client's feet and legs off the bed. **Rationale:** *Pivoting prevents twisting of the nurse's spine. The weight of the client's legs swinging downward increases downward movement of the lower body and helps move the client's upper body into a vertical position.*
- Keep supporting the client until the client is well balanced and comfortable. **Rationale:** *This movement may cause some clients to become light-headed or dizzy.*
- Assess vital signs (e.g., pulse, respirations, and blood pressure) as indicated by the client's health status.
6. Document all relevant information. Record:
   - Ability of client to assist in moving and turning
   - Response of client to moving and turning (e.g., anxiety, discomfort, dizziness).

Setting of Care

- Assess the height of the bed and the person's leg length to ensure that self-movements in and out of the bed are smooth.
- When making a home visit, it is particularly important to inspect the mattress for support. A sagging mattress, a mattress that is too soft, or an underfilled waterbed used over a prolonged period can contribute to the development of hip flexion contractures and low back strain and pain. Bed boards made of plywood and placed beneath a sagging mattress are increasingly recommended for clients who have back problems or are prone to them.
- Assess the caregivers' knowledge and application of body mechanics to prevent injury.
- Demonstrate how to turn and position the client in bed.
- Observe the caregiver performing a return demonstration. Reevaluate this technique periodically to reinforce correct application of body mechanics.

(continued on next page)

SKILL 11.7 Assisting a Client to Sit on Side of Bed (Dangling) *(continued)*

- Teach caregivers the basic principles of body alignment and how to check for proper alignment after the client has been changed to a new position.
- Warn caregivers of the dangers of lifting and repositioning and encourage the use of assistive devices and a "no solo lift" policy.
- Teach the caregiver to check the client's skin for redness and integrity after repositioning the client. Stress the importance of informing the nurse about the length of time skin redness remains over pressure areas after the person has been repositioned. Emphasize that reddened areas should not be massaged because it may lead to tissue trauma. Teach the caregiver that open areas must be inspected and treated by a healthcare professional.

SKILL 11.8 Transferring a Client Between Bed and Chair

Delegation

The skill of transferring a client can be delegated to UAP who have demonstrated safe transfer technique for the involved client. It is important for the nurse to assess the client's capabilities and communicate specific information about what the UAP should report back to the nurse.

Equipment

- Robe or appropriate clothing
- Slippers or shoes with nonskid soles
- Gait/transfer belt
- Chair, commode, wheelchair, or stretcher as appropriate to client need
- Sliding board, if appropriate
- Lift, if appropriate

Preparation

- Plan what to do and how to do it.
- Obtain essential equipment before starting (e.g., gait/transfer belt, wheelchair) and check that all equipment is functioning correctly.
- Remove obstacles from the area so clients do not trip, and make sure there are no spills or liquids on the floor on which clients could slip.

Procedure

1. Prior to performing the procedure, introduce self and verify the client's identity using agency protocol. Explain the transfer process to the client. During the transfer, explain step by step what the client should do, for example, "Move your right foot forward."
2. Perform hand hygiene and observe other appropriate infection control procedures.
3. Provide for client privacy.
4. Position the equipment appropriately.
   - Lower the bed to its lowest position so that the client's feet will rest flat on the floor. Lock the wheels of the bed.
   - Place the wheelchair parallel to the bed as close to the bed as possible ❶. Put the wheelchair on the side of the bed that allows the client to move toward his or her stronger side. Lock the wheels of the wheelchair and raise the footplate.
5. Prepare and assess the client.
   - Assist the client to a sitting position on the side of the bed.
   - Assess the client for orthostatic hypotension before moving the client from the bed.
   - Assist the client in putting on a bathrobe and nonskid slippers or shoes.

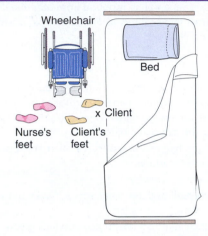

❶ The wheelchair is placed parallel to and as close to the bed as possible. Note that placement of the nurse's feet mirrors that of the client's feet.

   - Place a gait/transfer belt snugly around the client's waist. Check to be certain that the belt is securely fastened.
6. Give explicit instructions to the client. Ask the client to:
   - Move forward and sit on the edge of the bed (or surface on which the client is sitting) with feet placed flat on the floor. **Rationale:** *This brings the client's center of gravity closer to the nurse's.*
   - Lean forward slightly from the hips. **Rationale:** *This brings the client's center of gravity more directly over the base of support and positions the head and trunk in the direction of the movement.*
   - Place the foot of the stronger leg beneath the edge of the bed (or sitting surface) and put the other foot forward. **Rationale:** *In this way, the client can use the stronger leg muscles to stand and power the movement. A broader base of support makes the client more stable during the transfer.*
   - Place the client's hands on the bed surface (or available stable area) so that the client can push while standing. **Rationale:** *This provides additional force for the movement and reduces the potential for strain on the nurse's back.* The client should **not** grasp your neck for support. **Rationale:** *Doing so can injure the nurse.*
7. Position yourself correctly.
   - Stand directly in front of the client. Lean the trunk forward from the hips. Hold the gait/transfer belt with the nearest hand; the other hand supports the back of the client's shoulder ❷. Lean the trunk forward from the hips. Flex the hips, knees, and ankles. Assume a broad stance, placing one foot forward and one back. Mirror the placement of

SKILL 11.8   Transferring a Client Between Bed and Chair *(continued)*

the client's feet, if possible. **Rationale:** *This helps prevent loss of balance during the transfer.*

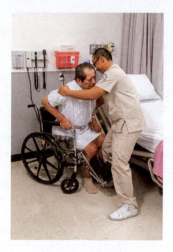

2 Using a gait/transfer belt to assist in transfer to a wheelchair.

8. Assist the client to stand, and then move together toward the wheelchair or sitting area to which you wish to transfer the client. Count to three or give the verbal instructions of "Ready—Steady—Stand." On the count of three or the word "Stand," ask the client to push down against the mattress/side of the bed while you transfer your weight from one foot to the other (while keeping your back straight) and stand upright, moving the client forward (directly toward your center of gravity) into a standing position. (If the client requires more than a very small degree of pulling, even with the assistance of two nurses, a mechanical device should be obtained and used.)

    *   Support the client in an upright standing position for a few moments. **Rationale:** *This allows the nurse and the client to extend the joints and provides the nurse with an opportunity to ensure that the client is stable before moving away from the bed.*
    *   Together, pivot or take a few steps toward the wheelchair, bed, chair, commode, or car seat.

9. Assist the client to sit.

    *   Move the wheelchair forward or have the client back up to the wheelchair (or desired seating area) and place the legs against the seat. **Rationale:** *Having the client place the legs against the wheelchair seat minimizes the risk of the client falling when sitting down.*
    *   Make sure the wheelchair brakes are on.
    *   Have the client reach back and feel/hold the arms of the wheelchair.
    *   Stand directly in front of the client. Place one foot forward and one back.
    *   Tighten your grasp on the transfer belt, and tighten your gluteal, abdominal, leg, and arm muscles.
    *   Have the client sit down while you bend your knees/hips and lower the client onto the wheelchair seat.

10. Ensure client safety.

    *   Ask the client to push back into the wheelchair seat. **Rationale:** *Sitting well back on the seat provides a broader base of support and greater stability and minimizes the risk of falling from the wheelchair. A wheelchair or bedside commode can topple forward when the client sits on the edge of the seat and leans far forward.*

*   Remove the gait/transfer belt.
*   Lower the footplates, and place the client's feet on them, if applicable.

VARIATION: ANGLING A WHEELCHAIR

For clients who have difficulty walking, place the wheelchair at a 45-degree angle to the bed. **Rationale:** *This enables the client to pivot into the chair and lessens the amount of body rotation required.*

VARIATION: TRANSFERRING A CLIENT WITH A BELT AND TWO NURSES

*   Even if a client is able to partially bear weight and is cooperative, it still may be safer to transfer a client with the assistance of two nurses. If so, you should position yourselves on both sides of the client, facing the same direction as the client. Flex your hips, knees, and ankles. Grasp the client's transfer belt with the hand closest to the client, and with the other hand support the client's elbows.
*   Coordinating your efforts, all three of you stand simultaneously, pivot, and move to the wheelchair. Reverse the process to lower the client onto the wheelchair seat.

VARIATION: TRANSFERRING A CLIENT WITH AN INJURED LOWER EXTREMITY

When a client has an injured lower extremity, movement should always occur toward the client's unaffected (strong) side. For example, if the client's right leg is injured and the client is sitting on the edge of the bed preparing to transfer to a wheelchair, position the wheelchair on the client's left side. **Rationale:** *In this way, the client can use the unaffected leg most effectively and safely.*

VARIATION: USING A SLIDING BOARD

*   For clients who cannot stand but are able to cooperate and possess sufficient upper body strength, use a sliding board to help them move without nursing assistance **3**. **Rationale:** *This method not only promotes the client's sense of independence but also preserves your energy.*

11. Document relevant information:

    *   Client's ability to bear weight and pivot
    *   Number of staff needed for transfer and safety measures/precautions used
    *   Length of time up in chair
    *   Client response to transfer and being up in chair or wheelchair.

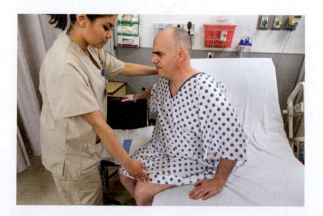

3 Using a sliding board.

SKILL 11.9   Transferring a Client Between Bed and Stretcher

Delegation

The skill of transferring a client can be delegated to UAP who have demonstrated safe transfer technique for the involved client. It is important for the nurse to assess the number of staff needed, assistive devices needed, client's ability to assist, and to communicate specific information about what the UAP should report to the nurse.

Equipment

- Stretcher
- Transfer assistive devices (e.g., rolling transfer board, friction-reducing device, lift) ❶ ❷

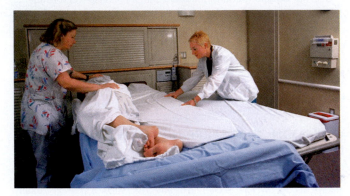

❶ Positioning a rolling transfer board.

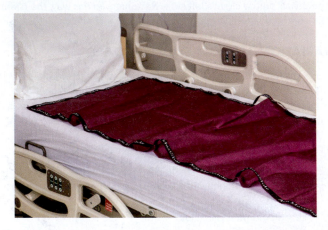

❷ Friction-reducing device with handles.

Preparation

- Obtain the necessary equipment and nursing personnel to assist in the transfer.

Procedure

1. Prior to performing the procedure, introduce self and verify the client's identity using agency protocol. Explain to the client what you are going to do, why it is necessary, and how he or she can participate. Explain the transfer to the nursing personnel who are helping and specify who will give directions (one person needs to be in charge).

2. Perform hand hygiene and observe other appropriate infection control procedures.
3. Provide for client privacy.
4. Adjust the client's bed in preparation for the transfer.
   - Lower the head of the bed until it is flat or as low as the client can tolerate.
   - Place the friction-reducing device under the client.
   - Raise the bed so that it is slightly higher (i.e., ½ in.) than the surface of the stretcher. **Rationale:** *It is easier for the client to move down a slant.*
   - Ensure that the wheels on the bed are locked.
   - Place the stretcher parallel to the bed next to the client and lock the stretcher wheels.
   - *Optional:* Fill the gap that exists between the bed and the stretcher loosely with the bath blankets.
5. Transfer the client securely to the stretcher.
   - If the client can transfer independently, encourage him or her to do so and stand by for safety.
   - If the client is partially able or not able to transfer:
     a. One caregiver needs to be at the side of the client's bed, between the client's shoulder and hip.
     b. The second and third caregivers should be at the side of the stretcher: one positioned between the client's shoulder and hip and the other between the client's hip and lower legs.
     c. All caregivers should position feet in a walking stance.
     d. On a planned command, the caregivers at the stretcher's side pull (shifting weight to the rear foot) and the caregiver at the bedside pushes the client toward the stretcher (shifting weight to the front foot).

VARIATION: USING A TRANSFER BOARD

The transfer board is a lacquered or smooth polyethylene board ❸ measuring 45 to 55 cm (18 to 22 in.) by 182 cm (73 in.) with handholds along its edges. Transfer mattresses are also available, as are mechanical assistive devices. It is imperative to have enough people assisting with the transfer to prevent injury to staff as well as clients. Turn the client to a lateral position away from you, position the board close to the client's back, and roll the client onto the board. Pull the client and board across the bed to the stretcher. Safety belts may be placed over the chest, abdomen, and legs.

6. Document relevant information:
   - Equipment used
   - Number of people needed for transfer
   - Destination if reason for transfer is transport from one location to another.

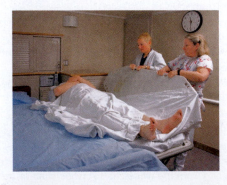

❸ A smooth polyethylene transfer board for transferring clients.

SKILL 11.10   Using a Hydraulic Lift

Delegation

The skill of using a hydraulic lift can be delegated to UAP who have demonstrated competent use of the equipment for the involved client.

Equipment

- Hydraulic lift (such as a mobile floor or ceiling-mounted lift) with any necessary accessories

Preparation

- Obtain the lift and put in the client's room. Arrange for assistance from others at a designated time.

Procedure

1. Prior to performing the procedure, introduce self and verify the client's identity using agency protocol. Explain to client what you are going to do, why it is necessary, and how he or she can participate. Explain the procedure and demonstrate the lift. **Rationale:** *Some clients are afraid of being lifted and will be reassured by a demonstration.*
2. Wash hands and observe other appropriate infection control procedures.
3. Provide for client privacy.
4. Prepare the equipment.
   - Lock the wheels of the client's bed and raise the bed to the high position.
   - Put up the side rail on the opposite side of the bed and lower the side rail near you.
   - Position the lift so that it is close to the client.
   - Place the chair that is to receive the client beside the bed. Allow adequate space to maneuver the lift.
   - Lock the wheels if a chair with wheels is used.
5. Position the client on the sling.

   Note: The remaining steps of this procedure need to be performed by at least two healthcare personnel working together with the client.

   - Roll the client away from you.
   - Place the canvas seat or sling under the client with the wide lower edge under the client's thighs to the knees and the more narrow upper edge up under the client's shoulders. **Rationale:** *This places the sling under the client's center of gravity and greatest part of body weight. Correct placement permits the client to be lifted evenly, with minimal shifting.*
   - With the help of your assistant, roll the client to the opposite side, and pull the canvas sling through.
   - Roll the client to the supine position and center the client on top of the canvas sling.
6. Attach the sling to the swivel bar.
   - Wheel the lift into position, with the footbars under the bed on the side where the chair is positioned. Set the adjustable base at the widest position to ensure stability. Lock the wheels of the lifter.
   - Lower the side rail.
   - Move the lift arms directly over the client and lower the horizontal bar by releasing the hydraulic valve. Lock the valve.
   - Attach the lifter straps or hooks to the corresponding openings in the canvas seat. Check that the hooks are correctly placed and that matching straps or chains are of equal length. Face the hooks away from the client. **Rationale:** *This prevents the hooks from injuring the client.*
7. Lift the client gradually.
   - Elevate the head of the bed to place the client in a sitting position.
   - Ask the client to remove eyeglasses and put them in a safe place. **Rationale:** *The swivel bar may come close to the face and cause breakage of eyeglasses.*
   - *Nurse 1:* Close the pressure valve, and gradually pump the jack handle until the client is above the bed surface. **Rationale:** *Gradual elevation of the lift is less frightening to the client than a rapid rise.*
   - *Nurse 2:* Assume a broad stance, and guide the client with your hands as the client is lifted. **Rationale:** *This prepares the nurse to hold the client and provide control during the movement.*
   - Check the placement of the sling before moving the client away from the bed.
8. Move the client over the chair.
   - *Nurse 1:* With the pressure valve securely closed, slowly roll the lift until the client is over the chair. Use the steering handle to maneuver the lift.
   - *Nurse 2:* Guide movement by hand until the client is directly over the chair. **Rationale:** *Slow movement decreases swaying and is less frightening. Guidance also decreases swaying and gives a sense of security.*
9. Lower the client into the chair.
   - *Nurse 1:* Release the pressure valve very gradually. **Rationale:** *Gradual release is less frightening than a quick descent.*
   - *Nurse 2:* Guide the client into the chair. ❶

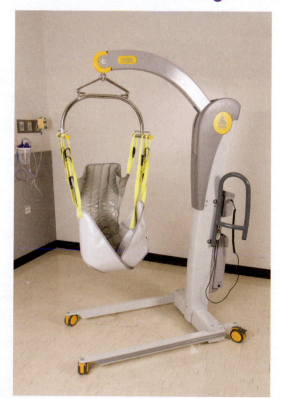

❶ A mobile floor-based hydraulic lift.

(continued on next page)

SKILL 11.10 Using a Hydraulic Lift *(continued)*

10. Ensure client comfort and safety.
    - Remove the hooks from the canvas seat. Leave the seat in place. **Rationale:** *The seat is left in place in preparation for the lift back to bed.*
    - Align the client appropriately in a sitting position and return the client's eyeglasses, if appropriate.

    - Apply a seat belt as needed.
    - Place the call bell within reach.

11. Document the type of equipment, number of assistants needed, safety precautions taken, and the client's physiological and psychological response.

SKILL 11.11   Assisting a Client to Ambulate

Delegation

Ambulation of clients is frequently delegated to UAP. However, the nurse should conduct an initial assessment of the client's abilities in order to direct other personnel in providing appropriate assistance. Any unusual events that arise from assisting the client in ambulation must be validated and interpreted by the nurse.

Equipment

- Gait/transfer belt whether or not the client is known to be unsteady
- Wheelchair for following client, or chairs along the route if the client needs to rest
- Portable oxygen tank, if needed

Preparation

- Be certain that others are available to assist you if needed. Also, plan the route of ambulation that has the fewest hazards and a clear path for ambulation.

Performance

1. Prior to performing the procedure, introduce self and verify the client's identity using agency protocol. Explain to the client what you are going to do, why ambulation is necessary, and how he or she can participate. Discuss how this activity relates to the overall plan of care.
2. Perform hand hygiene and observe other appropriate infection control procedures.
3. Ensure that the client is appropriately dressed to walk and has shoes or slippers with nonskid soles.
4. Prepare the client for ambulation.
    - Have client sit up in bed for at least 1 minute prior to preparing to dangle legs.
    - Assist the client to sit on the edge of the bed and allow dangling for at least 1 minute (see Skill 11.7).
    - Assess the client carefully for signs and symptoms of orthostatic hypotension (dizziness, light-headedness, or a sudden increase in heart rate) prior to leaving the bedside. **Rationale:** *Allowing for gradual adjustment can minimize drops in blood pressure (and fainting) that occur with shifts in position from lying to sitting, and sitting to standing.*
    - Assist the client to stand by the side of the bed for at least 1 minute until he or she feels secure.
    - Carefully attend to any IV tubing, catheters, or drainage bags. Keep urinary drainage bags below level of the client's bladder. **Rationale:** *To prevent backflow of urine into bladder and risk of infection.*

- Use a gait/transfer (walking) belt if the client is slightly weak and unstable. Make sure the belt is pulled snugly around the client's waist and fastened securely. Grasp the belt at the client's back, and walk behind and slightly to one side of the client ❶.

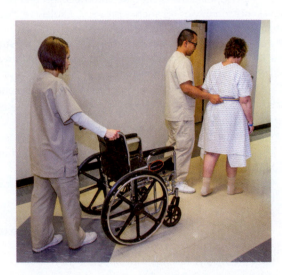

❶ Using a gait/transfer (walking) belt to support the client.

5. Ensure client safety while assisting the client to ambulate.
    - Encourage the client to ambulate independently if he or she is able, but walk beside the client's weak side, if appropriate. If the client has a lightweight IV pole because of infusing fluids, he or she may find that holding on to the pole while ambulating helps with balance. If the pole or other equipment is cumbersome in any way, the nurse must push it to match the client's pace, securing any assistance necessary in order to move smoothly with the client.
    - Remain physically close to the client in case assistance is needed at any point.
    - If it is the client's first time out of bed following surgery, injury, or an extended period of immobility, or if the client is quite weak or unstable, have an assistant follow you and the client with a wheelchair in the event that it is needed quickly.
    - If the client is moderately weak and unstable, walk on the client's weaker side and interlock your forearm with the client's closest forearm. Encourage the client to press the forearm against your hip or waist for stability if desired. This client should definitely wear a gait/transfer belt, and the nurse should maintain a secure grasp of the belt.
    - If the client is very weak and unstable, place your near arm around the client's waist, and with your other arm support

SKILL 11.11   Assisting a Client to Ambulate (continued)

the client's near arm at the elbow. Walk on the client's stronger side. Again, the client should definitely wear a gait/transfer belt in case of an emergency.

- Encourage the client to assume a normal walking stance and gait as much as possible. Ask the client to straighten the back and raise the head so that the eyes are looking forward in a normal horizontal plane. **Rationale:** *Clients who are unsure of their ability to ambulate tend to look down at their feet, which makes them more likely to fall.*

6. Protect the client who begins to fall while ambulating.
   - If a client begins to experience the signs and symptoms of orthostatic hypotension or extreme weakness, quickly assist the client into a nearby wheelchair or other chair, and help the client to lower the head between the knees.
   - Stay with the client. **Rationale:** *A client who faints while in this position could fall head first out of the chair.*
   - When the weakness subsides, assist the client back to bed.
   - If a chair is not close by, assist the client to a horizontal position on the floor before fainting occurs.
     a. Assume a broad stance with one foot in front of the other. **Rationale:** *A broad stance widens your base of support. Placing one foot behind the other allows you to rock backward and use the femoral muscles when supporting the client's weight and lowering the center of gravity (see the next step), thus preventing back strain.*
     b. Bring the client backward so that your body supports the person. **Rationale:** *Clients who faint or start to fall usually pitch slightly forward because of the momentum of ambulating. Bringing the client's weight backward against your body allows gradual movement to the floor without injury to the client.*
     c. Allow the client to slide down your leg, and lower the person gently to the floor, making sure the client's head does not hit any objects.

VARIATION: TWO NURSES

If the client is very weak and unstable, two nurses or a nurse and a UAP should support the client, using a gait belt, during ambulation. Apply a gait belt before the client gets out of bed. Each nurse should have one hand on the gait belt, at the back of the client, and support the client by holding on to his or her forearm or the lower upper arm with the other hand. **Rationale:** *This provides a secure grip for each nurse.*

- Walk in unison with the client, using a smooth, even gait, at the same speed and with steps the same size as the client's. **Rationale:** *This gives the client a greater feeling of security.*
- If the client starts to fall and cannot regain strength or balance, each nurse should place one hand under the client's nearer axilla and continue to grasp the gait/transfer belt and lower the person gently to the floor or to a nearby chair. **Rationale:** *Placing the nurse's arms under the client's axillae evenly balances the client's weight between the two nurses, preventing injury to both the nurses and the client. Keeping hold of the gait belt allows for more control and direction of the client who can no longer effectively protect himself or herself.*

7. Document distance and duration of ambulation in the client record using forms or checklists supplemented by narrative notes when appropriate. Include description of the client's gait (including body alignment) when walking, pace, activity tolerance when walking (e.g., pulse rate, facial color, any shortness of breath, feelings of dizziness, or weakness), degree of support required, and respiratory rate and blood pressure after initial ambulation to compare with baseline data.

Sample Documentation

8/22/15 1030 Ambulated length of hall (120 ft) and returned with minimal assistance of 2 staff. Steady gait, tolerated well. VS remain at baseline after walking. _____ B. Snyder, RN

Developmental Considerations

CHILDREN

- Children and adolescents who have suffered a sports injury (e.g., sprained ankle) may want to be more active than they should be. A cast, splint, or boot may be put in place to limit activity and assist in healing. Teach children the importance of appropriate activity and the use of assistive devices (e.g., crutches) if necessary. Help them focus on what they can do rather than what they cannot do (e.g., "You can stand at the free-throw line and shoot baskets").

OLDER ADULTS

- Inquire how the client has ambulated previously and/or check any available chart notes regarding the client's abilities and modify assistance accordingly.
- Take into account a decrease in speed, strength, resistance to fatigue, reaction time, and coordination due to a decrease in nerve conduction, muscle strength, and the effects of aging on baroreceptors and proprioceptors.
- Be cautious when using a transfer belt with a client with osteoporosis. Too much pressure from the belt can increase the risk of vertebral compression fractures. If a client has had abdominal surgery, it may be necessary to use a gait vest instead of a gait belt.

- If assistive devices such as a walker or cane are used, make sure clients are supervised in the beginning to learn the proper method of using them. Crutches may be much more difficult for older adults due to decreased upper body strength. In general, older individuals do much better with walkers than with crutches.
- Be alert to signs of activity intolerance, especially in older adults with cardiac and lung problems.
- Break up the eventual desired client mobility goal into shorter, more easily attained but progressively more ambitious client goals. Increase slowly to build endurance, strength, and flexibility.
- Be aware of any fall risks the older adult may have, such as the following:
  - The normal effects of aging on the body's mobility abilities
  - Effects of medications
  - Neurological disorders
  - Orthopedic problems
  - Presence of equipment that must accompany the client when ambulating
  - Environmental hazards
  - Orthostatic hypotension.

(continued on next page)

SKILL 11.11 Assisting a Client to Ambulate (*continued*)

- In older adults, the body's responses return to normal more slowly. For instance, an increase in heart rate from exercise may stay elevated for hours before returning to normal.

Setting of Care
- When making a home visit, assess carefully for safety issues for ambulation. Counsel the client and family about unfastened rugs, slippery floors, and loose objects on the floors.

- Check the surroundings for adequate supports such as railings and grab bars.
- Recommend that nonskid strips be placed on outside steps and inside stairs that are not carpeted.
- Ask to see the shoes the person intends to wear while ambulating. They should be in good repair and supportive of the foot.

SKILL 11.12 Transporting an Infant or Toddler

Equipment

- Transporting vehicle (e.g., stretcher, crib, wheelchair)
- Wheeled poles for any necessary equipment
- Necessary supportive equipment such as oxygen tank or ventilation bags/masks
- Blankets

Preparation

- Obtain necessary transporting equipment.
- Securely fasten intravenous lines, feeding lines, ECG leads, and other equipment. **Rationale:** *Lines that are securely fastened are less likely to be dislodged during transport.*
- Explain the transport to the family. **Rationale:** *Adequate explanation helps to decrease anxiety.*

Procedure

1. Perform an assessment of the child. **Rationale:** *A baseline assessment provides comparison with later findings. At times, transport may adversely affect the child's condition. Initial assessment data provide necessary baseline information.*

2. The infant is placed in a bassinet or crib for transport. If the bassinet has a bottom shelf, it is used for carrying the IV pump or monitor.
3. Attach intravenous poles and other equipment to the crib. When this is not possible, adequate personnel are needed to push all of the equipment. **Rationale:** *Lines can be more easily kept intact if they are on one transport vehicle.*
4. Keep the infant covered with blankets. **Rationale:** *Adequate covers help to prevent hypothermia resulting from a cool environment.*
5. Allow parents to accompany the child on the transport when possible. **Rationale:** *The parent's presence can provide a sense of security for the young child.*

VARIATION: TRANSPORTING A TODDLER

Preparation

- Explain the transport plan to the family and child. **Rationale:** *Adequate explanation helps to decrease anxiety.*

Procedure

- Transport the toddler in a high-top crib (also used for infants), with the side rails up and the protective top in place ❶. The

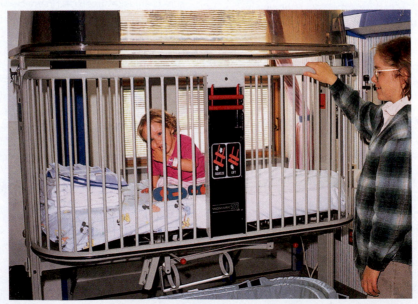

❶ High-top crib for infant or toddler transport.

SKILL 11.12   Transporting an Infant or Toddler (*continued*)

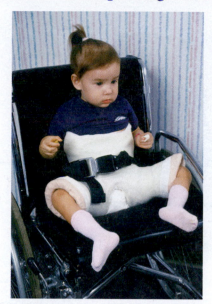

2 Toddler in a wheelchair with a safety strap.

child may be sitting or lying down. Alternatively, secure the child in a stroller or wheelchair of the proper size for the child's age **2**. **Rationale:** *Stretchers should not be used because the mobile toddler may roll or fall off.*

- Be sure to secure the child in the device with the seat safety strap. **Rationale:** *The child is secured to avoid falls and injury during transport.*

> **CLINICAL ALERT**
> Specialized wheelchairs and other equipment are available to carry enteral feeding solutions, motors necessary for equipment, and other supplies. These transporters are helpful for families when the child has a long-term disability, enabling them to take the child and equipment to school, stores, and other settings.

6. Document the time the client leaves the unit and where client is going, how client is traveling (i.e., via crib, wheelchair, or ambulation), who accompanies the client, and how client responds.

▶ CLIENT USING ASSISTIVE DEVICES

Expected Outcomes

1. Feelings of physical and mental well-being increase.
2. Balance and muscle tone improve.
3. Client progresses from being dependent to becoming independent in ambulation.
4. Complications of immobility are prevented with ambulation.
5. Client correctly uses assistive devices without assistance.
6. Client appropriately uses crutches to ambulate.
7. Crutches are measured correctly to prevent numbness or tingling in fingers.
8. Client is able to resume routines of daily living.

SKILL 11.13   Assisting a Client to Use a Cane

Delegation

Due to the extent of knowledge required, teaching the client to use assistive devices is not delegated to UAP. The nurse or the physical therapist does the teaching. However, once the client has demonstrated adequate skill, UAP may assist the client in ambulating with this equipment.

Equipment

- Appropriately sized cane with rubber tip(s)

Preparation

- Ensure that the client's path is free from clutter and hazards.

Procedure

1. Prior to performing the procedure, introduce self and verify the client's identity using agency protocol. Explain to the client what you are going to do, why it is necessary, and how he or she can participate. Discuss how this activity will be used in planning further care.
2. Perform hand hygiene and observe appropriate infection control procedures.

3. Ensure that client is appropriately dressed for walking, especially in regards to stability of footwear.
4. Prepare the client for walking.
   - Ask the client to hold the cane on the stronger side of the body. **Rationale:** *This provides support and body alignment when walking. The arm opposite the advancing foot normally swings forward when walking, so the hand holding the cane will come forward and the cane will support the weaker leg.*
   - Position the tip of a standard cane (and the nearest tip of other canes) about 15 cm (6 in.) to the side and 15 cm (6 in.) in front of the near foot, so that the elbow is slightly flexed. **Rationale:** *This provides the best balance and prevents the person from leaning on the cane. In this position, the client stands erect, with the center of gravity within the base of support.*
5. When maximum support is required, instruct the client to move as follows:
   - Move the cane forward about 30 cm (1 ft), or a distance that is comfortable while the body weight is borne by both legs **1**.
   - Then, move the affected (weak) leg forward to the cane while the weight is borne by the cane and stronger leg.

(*continued on next page*)

SKILL 11.13 Assisting a Client to Use a Cane *(continued)*

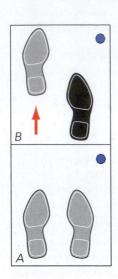

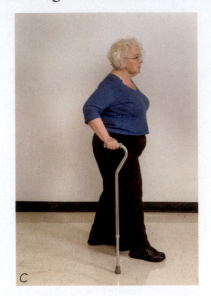

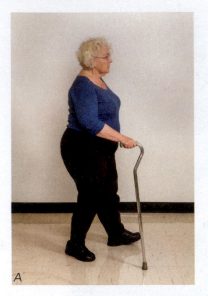

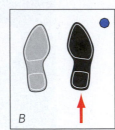

1 Steps involved in using a cane to provide maximum support.

2 Steps involved in using a cane when less than maximum support is required.

- Next, move the unaffected (stronger) leg forward ahead of the cane and weak leg while the weight is borne by the cane and weak leg.
- Repeat the above three steps. **Rationale:** *This pattern of moving provides at least two points of support on the floor at all times.*

6. If the client requires minimal support from the cane, for instance, just a little assist with balance, instruct the client to follow these steps:
   - Move the cane and weak leg forward at the same time, while the weight is borne by the stronger leg **2**.
   - Move the stronger leg forward while the weight is borne by the cane and the weak leg.

7. Ensure client safety.
   - Walk beside the client on the affected side. **Rationale:** *The client is most likely to fall toward the affected side.*
   - Walk the client for the time or distance indicated in the plan of care, being prepared to revise this plan if the client's condition warrants it.
   - If the client loses balance or strength and is unable to regain it, slide your hand up to the client's axilla, and take a

broad stance to provide a base of support. If there was any indication that this situation might occur, the client should have had a gait belt placed before ambulation began. Have the client rest against your hip until assistance arrives, or gently lower yourself and the client to the floor.

- For stair climbing, the phrase "up with the good, down with the bad" can help clients remember which pattern of movement to use. This means that when climbing stairs the client should ascend first with the good leg, bringing the weaker leg up to that level afterward. The pattern is reversed when descending stairs. This is also the pattern used with crutches on stairs.

8. Document the client's progress in the client record using forms or checklists supplemented by narrative notes when appropriate. Describe the distance ambulated and any difficulties the client experienced.

CLINICAL ALERT
Instruct clients to use the cane opposite the side of pain or weakness to facilitate balance and decrease weight on painful extremities.

SKILL 11.14 Assisting a Client to Use Crutches

Equipment

- Appropriately sized crutches

Preparation

- Ensure that the crutches are the proper length.

Procedure

1. Assist the client to assume the tripod (triangle) position, the basic crutch stance used before crutch walking.
   - Ask the client to stand and place the tips of the crutches 15 cm (6 in.) in front of the feet and out laterally about 15 cm (6 in.). This is the starting position for all the different variations of ambulation with crutches **1**. **Rationale:** *The tripod*

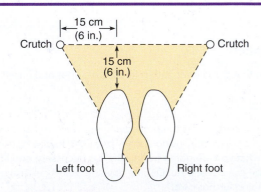

1 The tripod position.

SKILL 11.14 Assisting a Client to Use Crutches (*continued*)

position provides a wide base of support and enhances both stability and balance.

- Make sure the feet are slightly apart. A tall person requires a wider base than a short person.
- Ensure that posture is erect; that is, the hips and knees should be extended, the back straight, and the head held straight and high. There should be no hunch to the shoulders and thus no weight borne by the axillae. The elbows should be extended sufficiently to allow weight bearing on the hands.
- Stand slightly behind and on the client's affected side. **Rationale:** *By standing behind the client and toward the affected side, the nurse can provide support if the client loses balance.*
- If the client is unsteady, place a walking belt around the client's waist, and grasp the belt from above, not from below. **Rationale:** *A fall can be prevented more effectively if the belt is held from above. In addition, this manner of holding the belt is less likely to result in a twisting injury to the nurse's hands.*

2. Teach the client the appropriate crutch gait. Specific gaits are chosen based on client capabilities and ability to bear weight. This varies from client to client.

VARIATION: FOUR-POINT ALTERNATE GAIT

- This is the most elementary and safest gait, providing at least three points of support at all times, but it requires coordination. It can be used when walking in crowds because it does not require much space. It is a slow gait because it requires the client to move crutches and legs and shift weight constantly. To use this gait, the client has to be able to bear some weight on both legs (❷, reading from bottom to top).
- Ask the client to:
  - Move the right crutch ahead a suitable distance (e.g., 10 to 15 cm [4 to 6 in.]).
  - Move the left foot forward, preferably to the level of the crutch.
  - Move the left crutch forward.
  - Move the right foot forward.

VARIATION: THREE-POINT GAIT

- To use this gait, the person must be able to bear entire body weight on the unaffected leg. It is a fast gait that requires strength in the three unaffected extremities. The two crutches and the unaffected leg bear weight alternately (❸, reading from bottom to top).
- Ask the client to:
  - Move both crutches and the weaker leg forward.
  - Move the stronger leg forward.

VARIATION: TWO-POINT ALTERNATE GAIT

- This gait is intermediate in pace and in required strength between the four-point gait and the three-point gait. It requires more balance than the four-point gait, because only two points support the body at one time; it also requires at least partial weight bearing on each foot. In this gait, arm movements with the crutches are similar to the arm movements during normal walking (❹, reading from bottom to top).

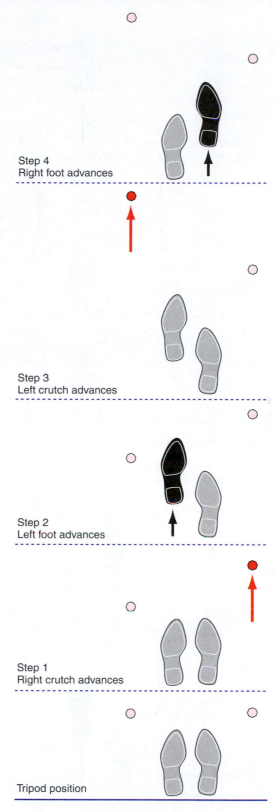

Step 4
Right foot advances

Step 3
Left crutch advances

Step 2
Left foot advances

Step 1
Right crutch advances

Tripod position

❷ The four-point alternate crutch gait.

- Ask the client to:
  - Move the left crutch and the right foot forward together.
  - Move the right crutch and the left foot ahead together.

(*continued on next page*)

SKILL 11.14 Assisting a Client to Use Crutches (*continued*)

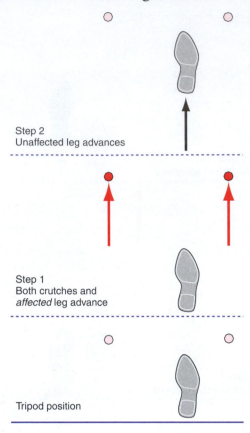

Step 2
Unaffected leg advances

Step 1
Both crutches and
affected leg advance

Tripod position

❸ The three-point crutch gait.

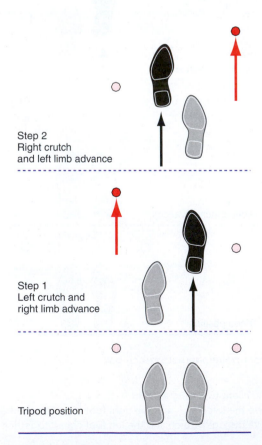

Step 2
Right crutch
and left limb advance

Step 1
Left crutch and
right limb advance

Tripod position

❹ The two-point alternate crutch gait.

VARIATION: SWING-TO GAIT

- People with paralysis of the legs and hips use the swing-to or swing-through gait. Prolonged use of these gaits results in atrophy of the unused muscles. The swing-to gait is the easier of these two gaits ❺.

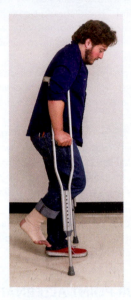

❺ The swing-to-crutch gait.

- Ask the client to:
  - Move both crutches ahead together.
  - Lift body weight by the arms and swing *to* the crutches.

VARIATION: SWING-THROUGH GAIT

- This gait requires considerable client skill, strength, and coordination ❻.

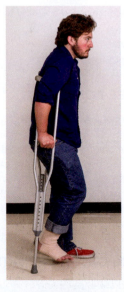

❻ The swing-through crutch gait.

- Ask the client to:
  - Move both crutches forward together.
  - Lift body weight by the arms and swing through and beyond the crutches.

SKILL 11.14   Assisting a Client to Use Crutches (continued)

3. Teach the client to get into and out of a chair. Teach the client to always leave the crutches within arms' reach when sitting or reclining, as they are needed for safe ambulation.

VARIATION: GETTING INTO A CHAIR

- Ensure that the chair has armrests and is secure or braced against a wall.
- Instruct the client to:
  - Stand with the back of the unaffected leg centered against the chair.
  - Transfer the crutches to the hand on the affected side, hold the crutches by the hand bars, and then grasp the arm of the chair with the hand on the unaffected side ❼. **Rationale:** *This allows the client to support the body weight on the arms and the unaffected leg.*
  - Lean forward, flex the knees and hips, and lower into the chair.

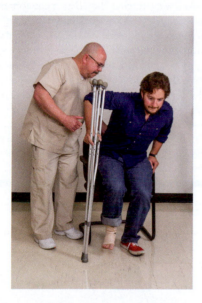

❼ A client using crutches getting into a chair.

VARIATION: GETTING OUT OF A CHAIR

- Instruct the client to:
  - Move forward to the edge of the chair and place the unaffected leg slightly under or at the edge of the chair. **Rationale:** *This position helps the client stand up from the chair and achieve balance, because the unaffected leg is supported against the edge of the chair.*
  - Grasp the crutches by the hand bars in the hand on the affected side, and grasp the arm of the chair with the hand on the unaffected side. **Rationale:** *The body weight is placed on the crutches and the hand on the armrest to support the unaffected leg when the client rises to stand.*
  - Push down on the crutches and the chair armrest while elevating the body out of the chair.
  - Assume the tripod position before moving.
4. Teach the client to go up and down stairs.

VARIATION: GOING UP STAIRS

- Stand behind the client and slightly to the affected side.
- Ask the client to:
  - Assume the tripod position at the bottom of the stairs.
  - Transfer the body weight to the crutches and move the unaffected leg onto the step ❽.

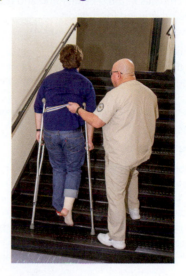

❽ Climbing stairs: Place weight on the crutches while first moving the unaffected leg onto a step.

- Transfer the body weight to the unaffected leg on the step and move the crutches and affected leg up to the step. The crutches always support the affected leg.
- Repeat steps b and c until the top of the stairs is reached.

VARIATION: GOING DOWN STAIRS

- Stand one step below the person on the affected side.
- Ask the client to:
  - Assume the tripod position at the top of the stairs.
  - Shift the body weight to the unaffected leg, and move the crutches and affected leg down onto the next step ❾.

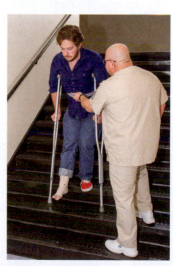

❾ Descending stairs: Move the crutches and affected leg to the next step.

(continued on next page)

SKILL 11.14 Assisting a Client to Use Crutches (continued)

- Transfer the body weight to the crutches, and move the unaffected leg to that step. The crutches always support the affected leg.
- Repeat steps b and c until the bottom of the stairs is reached.

or

- Ask the client to:
  - Hold both crutches in the outside hand and grasp the handrail with the other hand for support.
  - Move as in steps b and c, above.

5. Reinforce client teaching.
6. Document the client's progress in the client record using forms or checklists supplemented by narrative notes when appropriate. Describe the distance ambulated and any difficulties the client experienced, including changes in vital signs as compared to baseline.

Sample Documentation

8/22/15 1500 Attempted crutch walking up steps. Unable to lift affected leg to next step, balance remained stable. Became dyspneic and upset. Vital signs (when seated) at baseline after activity. Reassured that this skill takes time. Encouraged to continue seated leg exercises and frequent ambulation. Will try again tomorrow. _____ B. Schneider, RN

Client Teaching

Teaching the Client to Use Crutches

- If you have been given a plan of exercises developed for you to strengthen your arm muscles, follow this plan. It is necessary for a healthcare professional to establish the correct length for your crutches and the correct placement of the hand pieces. Crutches that are too long force your shoulders upward and make it difficult for you to push your body off the ground. Crutches that are too short will make you hunch over and develop an improper body stance.
- The weight of your body should be borne by the arms rather than the axillae (armpits). Continual pressure on the axillae can injure the radial nerve and eventually cause crutch palsy, a weakness of the muscles of the forearm, wrist, and hand. Injuries to the radial nerve may cause pain, numbness and tingling, and muscle atrophy, but these problems are reversible by using crutches correctly so weight is not borne by the axillae (Hoch & Zieve, 2008).
- Maintain an erect posture as much as possible to prevent strain on muscles and joints and to maintain balance.
- Each step taken with crutches should be a comfortable distance for you. It is wise to start with a small rather than large step.
- Inspect the crutch tips regularly, and replace them if worn.
- Keep the crutch tips dry and clean to maintain their surface friction. If the tips become wet, dry them well before use.
- Wear a shoe with a low heel that grips the floor. Rubber soles decrease the chances of slipping. Adjust shoelaces so they cannot come untied or reach the floor where they might catch on the crutches. Consider shoes with alternative forms of closure (e.g., Velcro), especially if you cannot easily bend to tie laces. Slip-on shoes are acceptable only if they are snug and the heel does not come loose when the foot is bent.

Measuring Clients for Crutches

When nurses measure clients for axillary crutches, it is most important to determine the correct length for the crutches and the correct placement of the hand piece. Two methods are used to measure crutch length:

1. The client lies in the supine position, and the nurse measures from the anterior fold of the axilla to a point 2.5 cm (1 in.) lateral from the heel of the foot.
2. The client stands erect and positions the crutch tips 5 cm (2 in.) in front of and 15 cm (6 in.) to the side of the feet. The nurse makes sure the shoulder rest of the crutch is at least three fingerwidths, that is, 2.5 to 5 cm (1 to 2 in.), below the axilla. *Note:* Alternatively, for a quick and easy estimate, 40 cm (16 in.) can be subtracted from the client's height for the length of the crutches (Kunkler, 2007).

To determine the correct placement of the hand bar:

1. The client stands upright and supports the body weight by the hand grips of the crutches.
2. The nurse measures the angle of elbow flexion. It should be about 30 degrees. A goniometer (a handheld instrument used to measure joint angles) may be used to verify the correct angle.

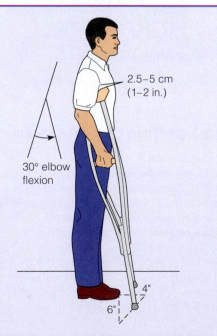

2.5–5 cm (1–2 in.)

30° elbow flexion

4"

6"

The standing position for measuring the correct length for crutches.

SKILL 11.14   **Assisting a Client to Use Crutches** (*continued*)

Setting Crutch Height for Children

- While the child is standing, the child's elbows should be slightly and comfortably flexed.
- Place the tip of the crutches about 8 to 15 cm (3 to 6 in.) to the upper, outer border of the toes on each foot.
- The upper pad on the crutches should now be lightly placed in the child's axilla. **Rationale:** *Crutches that are too high*

can put pressure on the brachial plexus, causing pain and injury. Crutches that are too low require that the child bend over to walk, and can cause injury or discomfort of the back and neck.

- The child should be taught safe crutch walking, a procedure generally taught by a physical therapist or other specialist.

SKILL 11.15   **Assisting a Client to Use a Walker**

Equipment

- Walker of appropriate size

Preparation

- Ensure client has adequate arm strength to use walker.
- Ensure walker is at correct height. The walker should reach to the level of the client's hip joint, and the elbows should be bent at about a 30-degree angle while using it.
- Ensure client has a clear path free from obstacles.
- Use shoes that support the feet and are resistant to skidding and slipping.

Procedure

1. Give the client these instructions when maximum support is required:
   - Move the walker ahead about 15 cm (6 in.) while your body weight is borne by both legs.
   - Then move the right foot up to the walker while your body weight is borne by the left leg and both arms.
   - Next, move the left foot up to the right foot while your body weight is borne by the right leg and both arms.
2. Give the client these instructions if one leg is weaker than the other:
   - Move the walker and the weak leg ahead together about 15 cm (6 in.) while your weight is borne by the stronger leg.
   - Then move the stronger leg ahead while your weight is borne by the affected leg and both arms.
3. Document the client's progress in the client record using forms or checklists supplemented by narrative notes when appropriate. Describe the distance ambulated, any difficulties the client experienced, and changes in vital signs in relation to baseline.

Developmental Considerations

CHILDREN

- Children learn and adapt quickly to the use of assistive devices.
- Care should be taken to check regularly that they are using proper technique.
- Children may reach the point where they prematurely believe they no longer need them.

OLDER ADULTS

- Older adults' conditions can change rapidly. Check regularly to see that the current assistive device is the most appropriate one and that it fits the client properly.
- Reinforce teaching regarding proper use of mechanical aids. Clients can easily fall into bad habits such as leaning the axillae on the crutches.
- Be aware that there may be a social stigma attached to the use of walkers in the minds of older adults. They may avoid using needed devices because of a need to perceive themselves as other than "old."

Setting of Care

- When making a home visit, assess carefully for safety issues for ambulation with mechanical devices. Counsel the client and family about poor lighting, unfastened rugs, slippery floors, and loose objects on the floors.
- Recommend nonskid strips be placed on outside steps and inside stairs that are not carpeted.
- Check that appropriate chairs are available. Such chairs should be high enough to sit on and rise from comfortably, with sturdy arms from which to push oneself up.
- Reinforce client teaching about proper gaits with canes, crutches, and walkers. Ask the client to demonstrate how the appliance is normally used, because inappropriate gaits and transferring techniques can develop.
- Ensure that the equipment is properly maintained and stored out of the way when not in use.
- Tennis balls with a cross cut in them may be applied over walker tips to make sliding easier.

▶ TRACTION AND CAST CARE

Expected Outcomes

1. Extremity is maintained in correct alignment.
2. Pin site remains free of infection.
3. Cast integrity is maintained to provide adequate site immobilization.
4. Client experiences minimal swelling.
5. Neurovascular complications do not occur.

SKILL 11.16   Caring for a Client in Traction

Evidence-Based Nursing Practice

Traction vs. No Traction for Hip Fracture

A review of the literature related to traction for hip fractures was done to evaluate the effects of traction applied to an injured limb prior to surgery for a fractured hip. Eleven trials, involving a total of 1,654 predominantly older adult clients with hip fractures, were included in the review.

Ten of the 11 trials compared skin traction with no traction and found no evidence of benefit from traction in relief of pain soon after immobilization, in ease of fracture reduction, or in quality of fracture reduction at surgery. Although data for pressure sores and other complications were inconclusive, minor adverse effects related to skin traction (skin blisters and sensory disturbance) were reported. Two trials compared skeletal traction with skin traction. No important differences between the two methods were noted, except that the initial skeletal traction application was more painful and costly.

The evidence suggests that the routine use of any type of traction prior to surgery had no particular benefit. More controlled studies are needed to confirm the value of this intervention.

Source: Handoll et al. (2011).

Equipment

- Orthopedic traction apparatus including traction straps, ropes, pulleys, and weights
- Trapeze bar

Preparation

- Determine the following: bruises and abrasions in the area where the traction is to be applied, any history of circulatory problems and skin allergies, mental and emotional status and ability to understand activity restrictions.
- Check physician's order for type of traction, and inspect the traction apparatus regularly, that is, whenever you are at the bedside or at prescribed intervals, such as every 2 hours.

Procedure

VARIATION: CARING FOR A CLIENT IN SKIN TRACTION

1. Maintain the client in the appropriate traction position.
   - Maintain the client in the supine position unless there are other orders. **Rationale:** *Changing position can change the body alignment and the amount of force supplied by the traction.*
   - Maintain body alignment when turning the client. In some cases, the person can turn to a lateral position if a pillow placed between the legs maintains body alignment. Refer to the client's record for information about permitted movement.
   - Provide a trapeze to assist the client to move and lift the body for back care if he or she is unable to turn.
   - Provide a fracture or slipper bedpan as required to minimize the client's movement during elimination.
2. Assess the neurovascular status of the affected extremity.
   - Conduct a neurovascular assessment 30 minutes following reapplication of the bandage, then every 2 hours for the first 24 hours. If the client's status is stable, then assess every 4 hours during the traction. If the client's status is not normal, continue assessments hourly.
3. Provide protective devices and measures to safeguard the skin.
   - Place heel protectors or sheepskins under the heels, sacrum, shoulders, and other pressure areas.
   - Change or clean the sheepskin lining at least weekly.
   - Massage the skin with rubbing alcohol or lotion every 4 hours, or if redness and signs of pressure appear, every 2 hours. **Rationale:** *Alcohol tends to toughen the skin and leave it less vulnerable to breakdown. Because alcohol is drying to the skin, however, lotion may be preferred for those who have dry skin (e.g., older adults).*
   - Make sure the spreader bar is wide enough to prevent the traction tape from rubbing on the client's bony prominences.
4. Remove only intermittent nonadhesive skin traction in accordance with agency protocol or orders.
   - To remove a nonadhesive skin traction:
     - Remove the weights first.
     - Unwrap the bandage and provide skin care.
     - Rewrap the limb and slowly reattach the weights.
5. Teach the client ways to prevent problems associated with immobility.
   - Teach the client deep-breathing and coughing exercises to prevent hypostatic pneumonia.
   - Teach the client appropriate exercises to maintain and develop muscle tone, prevent muscle contracture and atrophy, and promote blood circulation:
     - Range-of-motion exercises (discussed earlier in this chapter).
     - Teach isometric exercises, like tightening the knees, to strengthen the quadriceps. Pushing the knees down without moving them also strengthens the hamstring muscles. Tensing the buttocks and the inner thighs promotes

SKILL 11.16   Caring for a Client in Traction *(continued)*

stabilization of the hips. Tensing the inner thighs also helps stabilize the knees.

- Circulation to the extremities can be promoted by encouraging the client to flex and extend the feet and to perform the isometric exercises.
- Specific exercises to strengthen the biceps and triceps in preparation for using crutches can be taught as indicated. For example, raising the buttocks off the bed by pushing down with the arms develops the triceps, and pulling the body up with a trapeze develops the biceps.

6. Document findings in the client record using forms or checklists supplemented by narrative notes when appropriate.
7. Perform a detailed follow-up examination based on findings that deviated from expected or normal for the client. The client should be able to demonstrate usual ROM in all unaffected body joints, move all fingers or toes of the affected extremity, feel normal sensation and have normal skin color and temperature in all fingers or toes of the affected extremity, and be free of pressure signs (pallor, redness, increased warmth or tenderness) over pressure areas. Relate findings to previous assessment data if available. Report significant deviations from normal to the primary care provider.

> ### CLINICAL ALERT
> Do not apply Buck's traction over or under a calf compression device. Foot pumps (only around the foot) are acceptable for deep venous thrombosis prophylaxis.

VARIATION: APPLYING AND MONITORING SKIN TRACTION FOR A CHILD

Equipment

- Poles, pulleys, rope, weight, pads
- Elastic wrap for skin traction

Preparation

- Verify the identity of the child. Explain to the child and family the type of traction and what it involves.
- Gather equipment needed and review proper setup.
- Check the weights to be certain they are the same as those ordered by the physician.

Procedure

1. Set up the prescribed type of traction with proper weights.
2. Apply skin traction as ordered to the particular extremity. Wrap the extremity and apply straps to freely movable prescribed weights.
3. Perform assessments every 30 minutes initially, and then advance to every 1 to 2 hours when stable. Include the following areas:
   - Proper position of traction
   - Proper body alignment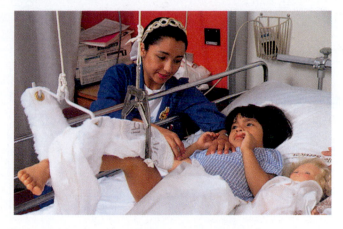
   - Neurovascular status of the extremity
   - Skin condition under and around the traction application
   - Skin on prominences exposed to the surface of the bed
   - Vital signs
   - Pain and psychological status. **Rationale:** *Traction can lead to skin breakdown or neurovascular impairment. Infections can result, especially with internal traction. Regular assessments help to identify problems early. Children may be*

❶ The child in traction needs close monitoring for alignment and proper traction application. Parents can often provide distraction and activities to help the child pass the time during his or her immobility.

pulled out of correct alignment by traction and movement in bed and may require frequent repositioning.

4. Check the child's alignment in bed and reposition as needed.
5. Remove traction according to agency policy, performing assessments and skin care. Reapply as directed in the medical orders.
6. Provide teaching and evaluation of technique if the family will maintain traction at home.

VARIATION: SKELETAL TRACTION

Delegation

Care of clients in traction may be delegated to trained UAP. However, assessment and pin site care must be performed by the nurse.

Equipment

- Supplies for providing pin site care according to agency policy (e.g., normal saline, cotton-tipped swabs, gauze dressings, clean or sterile gloves)

Preparation

- Verify the primary care provider's orders. Determine the degree of movement permitted and any special precautions (e.g., bed positions permitted).

Procedure

1. Prior to performing the procedure, introduce self to the client and verify the client's identity using agency protocol. Explain to client what you are going to do, why it is necessary, and how he or she can participate. Discuss how the results will be used in planning further care of treatments.
2. Perform hand hygiene and observe other appropriate infection control procedures.
3. Provide for client privacy.
4. Inspect the traction apparatus ❷ *A* and *B*:
   - Is the appropriate countertraction provided? For example, is the foot of the bed elevated 2.5 cm (1 in.) for every pound of traction or is the knee of the bed flexed 20 to 30 degrees?

(continued on next page)

SKILL 11.16   Caring for a Client in Traction (continued)

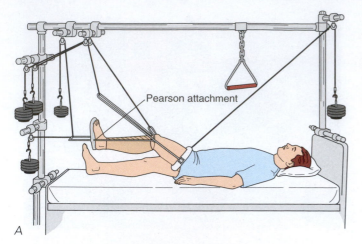

Pearson attachment

A

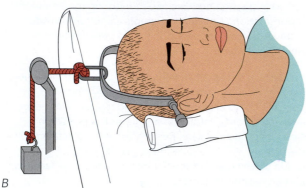

B

❷ A, Thomas splint with Pearson attachment for fracture of the femur for balanced suspension skeletal traction. B, Gardner-Wells skull tongs for skeletal traction immobilize fractures of cervical and upper thoracic vertebrae.

- Are the correct weights applied? For example, Buck's traction should have no more than 5 pounds.
- Is there free play of the ropes on the pulleys; that is, does the groove of the pulley support the rope? Are the knots positioned no closer than 30 cm (12 in.) to the nearest pulley?
- Do all weights hang freely and not rest against or on the bed or floor when the bed is in the lowest position?
- Are the ropes intact, that is, not frayed, knotted, or kinked between their points of attachment?
- Are the ropes securely attached with slipknots and the short ends of ropes attached with tape?
- Is the line of the traction straight and in the same plane as the long axis of the bone?
- Are bedclothes and other objects free from the traction?
- Is the spreader bar wide enough to prevent the traction tape from rubbing on bony prominences?

5. Maintain the client in the appropriate traction position. Check that the head, knee, and foot of the bed are properly elevated.
   - For clients with skull tongs or a halo ring, turn the client as a unit. Do not allow the neck to twist. A special bed may be required.
   - If skull tongs or pins become dislodged, support the head, remove the weights, place sandbags or liter fluid bags on

either side of the head to maintain alignment, and notify the primary care provider immediately.

CLINICAL ALERT

Skeletal traction is never released without a physician's order.

6. Assess the neurovascular status of the affected extremity.
   - Conduct a neurovascular assessment every hour for the first 24 hours. If the client's status is "normal," then assess every 4 hours during the traction. If the client's status is not normal, continue assessments hourly.
7. Provide pin site care daily if indicated by the primary care provider's orders and agency protocol. Analysis of randomized clinical trials of pin site care concluded that there was insufficient evidence to determine the best management of pin sites (Lethaby, Temple, & Santy, 2008). Thus, all agency protocols should emphasize reduction of the potential for infection.
   - Carefully inspect the site. Regular inspection of the pin site ensures early detection of minor infections, as manifested by signs of serosanguineous drainage, crusting, swelling, and erythema.
   - Use clean or sterile technique as agency protocol dictates. **Rationale:** *Sterile technique is most often used in the hospital setting, clean technique in the ambulatory setting.*
   - According to agency policy, remove crusts using normal saline or other agent such as diluted alcohol, povidone-iodine, or hydrogen peroxide recommended by the agency. Use a cotton-tipped swab with a gentle, rolling technique to reduce irritation to the tissue. **Rationale:** *Removing crusted secretions permits the pin site to drain freely. Initial crusts around pins do not create a problem and can serve as a barrier to infection, but accumulated crusts around external fixator pins may cause secondary infection.*
   - If purulent (containing pus) drainage is present, notify the primary care provider and obtain specimens for culture and sensitivity.
   - Apply sterile ointment if ordered. Determine agency practices regarding pin site care; ointment could interfere with proper drainage.
   - Loosely apply gauze dressing around pin site.
   - Adjust frequency of care according to the amount of drainage. If no drainage is present, daily site care is adequate. If drainage is present, perform site care every 8 hours.
   - Dispose of soiled equipment according to agency protocol.
   - Remove and discard gloves. Perform hand hygiene.
8. Teach the client ways to prevent problems associated with immobility.
9. Document findings in the client record using forms or checklists supplemented by narrative notes when appropriate.

Sample Documentation

9/17/15 1230 Traction maintained at 20 pounds with FOB↑ 50 cm. Skin intact and pink, sensation present, no pain. Pin sites clean and dry without sign of infection. _____ G. Merritt, RN

SKILL 11.16   Caring for a Client in Traction (continued)

Developmental Considerations

INFANTS/CHILDREN

- Bryant's traction is an adaptation of a bilateral Buck's extension. It is used to stabilize fractured femurs or correct congenital hip dislocations in young children under 17.5 kg (35 lb). The skin traction is applied to both the affected and the unaffected leg to maintain the position of the affected leg. A spreader bar attached to the strips or positioning of the pulleys maintains leg alignment. Unless otherwise ordered, the hips are flexed at right angles (90 degrees) to the body with the knees extended, and the buttocks raised about 2.5 cm (1 in.). Pressure areas include skin over the tibia, malleoli, hamstring tendon, soles of feet, and upper back.

OLDER ADULTS

- Adhesive skin traction should not be used due to the fragility of older adults' skin.
- Skin breakdown can occur more easily with any form of traction in older adults than in younger clients.

Setting of Care

TRACTION IN THE HOME SETTING

- Cervical traction may be done in the home setting using electrical systems or over-the-door mechanical systems. Clients may be instructed to use the system several times a day for up to 30 minutes at a time. A physical therapist should establish the system and conduct initial client and family teaching. The nurse should reinforce proper technique and assess effectiveness during home or clinic visits.
- Clients in halo-thoracic vest traction are ambulatory and need not be hospitalized. Client and family teaching regarding

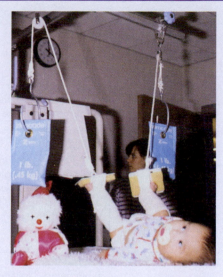

Bryant's traction. Ensure that the sacrum is elevated sufficiently to allow the nurse to slip a hand between the child's buttocks and the bed.

hygiene, care of the device, and when to contact healthcare providers must be reinforced.

- Children are increasingly being treated with traction at home. Be certain that the family understands how to set up and maintain the traction. Teach the observations to be made on the extremity involved. Siblings may change the weights or ropes, so close supervision may be needed by parents in some families. A home visit soon after traction begins is often made to evaluate the family's understanding and ability to carry out the regimen.

SKILL 11.17   Performing Initial Cast Care

Delegation

The nurse should perform baseline assessment of all new casts (Table 11–2 ●). Care of clients with stable casts may be delegated to unlicensed assistive personnel (UAP). The status of the cast is observed during usual care and may be recorded by individuals other than the nurse. However, assessment of complications from the cast requires the expertise of a nurse. Abnormal findings detected by UAP must be validated and interpreted by the nurse.

Equipment

- Pillows to support the casted areas
- Ice packs
- Pen

Preparation

- Review the client record to determine the reason for the cast and the initial status of the client's extremity. Examine the record regarding pain assessment findings and interventions.

Procedure

1. Prior to performing the procedure, introduce self to the client and verify the client's identity using agency protocol. Explain to the client what you are going to do, why it is necessary, and how he or she can participate. Discuss how the results will be used in planning further care or treatments.
2. Perform hand hygiene and observe other appropriate infection control procedures.
3. Provide for client privacy as indicated.
4. Assess the neurovascular status of the affected limbs.
   - Assess the toes or fingers for nerve and circulatory impairments every 30 minutes for 4 hours following cast application, and then every 3 hours for the first 24 to 48 hours or until all signs and symptoms of impairment are negative. Increase the frequency of neurovascular assessments in accordance with the client's condition (e.g., presence of circulatory impairment). **Rationale:** *Rapid swelling under a cast can cause neurovascular problems, so frequent neurovascular assessments by the nurse are a priority.*

(continued on next page)

SKILL 11.17   Performing Initial Cast Care (continued)

TABLE 11–2   Cast Materials

TYPE OF MATERIAL	DESCRIPTION	APPLICATION	SETTING TIME AND WEIGHT-BEARING RESTRICTIONS
Plaster (e.g., Gypsona)	Open-weave cotton rolls or strips saturated with powdered calcium sulfate crystals (gypsum)	Applied after being soaked in tepid water for a few seconds until bubbling stops	Dries in 48 hr, no weight bearing allowed until dry
Synthetics; polyester and cotton (e.g., Hygia Cast, Nemoa)	Open-weave polyester and cotton tape permeated with water-activated polyurethane resin	Applied after being soaked in cool water, 26°C (80°F); used within 2–3 min of soaking	Sets in 7 min, weight bearing allowed in 15 min
Fiberglass; water-activated (e.g., Scotchcast, Delta-Lite) or light-cured (e.g., Lightcast II); fiberglass-free/latex-free (e.g., Delta-Cast Elite, FlashCast Elite)	Open-weave fiberglass tape impregnated with water-activated polyurethane resin or photosensitive polyurethane resin	Applied after being immersed in tepid water for 10–15 sec or applied with gloves or silicone-type hand cream to keep it from sticking	Sets in 7–15 min, weight bearing allowed in 20–30 min; light-cured version sets after being exposed for 3 min to a special ultraviolet lamp (curing), weight bearing allowed immediately
Thermoplastic (e.g., Hexcelite)	Knitted thermoplastic polyester fabric in rigid rolls	Applied after being heated in water at 76°–82°C (170°–180°F) for 3–4 min to make the rolls soft and pliable	Remove excess water by squeezing between towels before applying

CLINICAL ALERT

When casting material inhibits palpation of peripheral pulses, assess capillary refill and for edema, comfort level, and other parameters of circulation-motor-sensory status as an indication of neurovascular status.

5. Support and handle the cast appropriately.
   • Immediately after the cast is applied, place it on pillows. Avoid using plastic or rubber pillows. **Rationale:** *The pillows provide even pressure and support the curves of the cast and promote venous blood return, thereby decreasing the possibility of swelling. Plastic or rubber pillows do not allow the heat of a drying cast to dissipate and so cause discomfort.*
   • Until a cast has set or hardened (10 to 20 minutes), support the cast in the palms of your hands rather than with the fingertips, and extend your fingers so that your fingertips do not touch the plaster. **Rationale:** *Fingertip pressure can cause dents in unset plaster and subsequent skin pressure areas.*
   • When the cast is set, continue to handle the cast in your palms, but you may then wrap your fingers around the contour of the cast.
6. Implement measures to reduce swelling.
   • Control swelling by elevating arms or legs on pillows or, for a leg fracture, by elevating the foot of the bed. Immediately after injury and surgery, elevate the limb to 45 degrees (Bakody, 2009). Generally, three pillows are needed to achieve high elevation of a leg. As circulation improves and healing progresses, the elevation can be gradually reduced to two pillows (moderate elevation) and then to one pillow (low elevation). **Rationale:** *Swelling can cause neurovascular impairment.*
   • Apply ice packs to control perineal edema associated with a hip spica cast. Although ice packs are a less effective method of control than elevation, elevation of the area is obviously difficult.
   • Report excessive swelling and indications of neurovascular impairment to the primary care provider or nurse in charge. The primary care provider may bivalve a cast if it appears to

be too tight. Bivalving a cast is cutting the cast partially or completely and wrapping it with bandage material to hold it together ❶. **Rationale:** *This relieves the pressure of the cast but still provides support.*

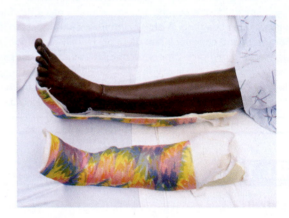

❶ Bivalved cast.

CLINICAL ALERT

Casted extremity should be assessed every half hour for 4 hours and then every 4 hours.

7. Use appropriate means to dry the plaster cast thoroughly.
   • Extremity plaster casts usually take 24 to 48 hours to dry completely; spica or body casts require 48 to 72 hours. Drying time depends on the temperature, humidity, size of the cast, and method used for drying. The cast is dry when it no longer feels damp. A dry cast feels dry, looks white and shiny, and is odorless, hard, and resonant when tapped. Synthetic casts take only 10 to 15 minutes to harden completely.
   • Expose the cast to the circulating air. Place sheets and blankets only over areas that do not have the cast.
   • Check agency policy about the recommended turning frequency for clients with different kinds of casts. **Rationale:** *Frequent turning promotes even drying of the cast.*

SKILL 11.17 Performing Initial Cast Care *(continued)*

- Turn the client with an extremity cast or body spica every 2 to 4 hours.

CLINICAL ALERT

Do not use abductor bars (incorporated into cast) for moving the client. Move the client as a unit instead.

- Use regular pillows. **Rationale:** *Plastic or rubber pillows hinder drying and do not allow the heat of a drying cast to dissipate.*
- Do not facilitate drying by artificial means (e.g., by using a fan, hair dryer, infrared lamp, or electric heater). **Rationale:** *Artificial methods dry the outer surface of the cast while the inner portion remains soft and spongy. Such a cast cracks readily at points of strain. Natural methods dry the cast evenly.*

8. Monitor bleeding if an open reduction was done or if the injury was a compound fracture.
   - Monitor bloodstains or other drainage on the cast for 24 to 72 hours after surgery or injury or longer if necessary.
   - Outline the stained area with a pen at least every 8 hours if it is changing, and note the time and date, so that any further bleeding can be determined.

CLINICAL ALERT

If the client has had an open reduction, wound drainage will be absorbed and spread rapidly, or seep down the back of cast. The visible drainage does not necessarily indicate the amount of actual drainage.

Inspect all cast surfaces and mark drainage regularly if it is increasing. Bleeding should not persist after 24 hours.

9. Assess pain and pressure areas.
   - Never ignore any complaints of pain, burning, swelling or pressure. If a client is unable to communicate, be alert to changes in temperament, restlessness, or fussiness that may indicate a problem. **Rationale:** *Compartment syndrome is a serious complication that can result when swelling and pressure within the closed fascial compartment build to dangerous levels, preventing nourishment from reaching nerve and muscle cells. The skin overlying the area may be red and hard. Apply ice, elevate, and notify primary care provider immediately. An absent or diminished distal pulse necessitates immediate surgical action to allow expansion and blood flow and prevent nerve damage.*

CLINICAL ALERT

Always assess active extension, flexion, adduction, and abduction of the fingers, flexion and extension of the toes, and inversion and dorsiflexion of the foot. Pain on passive stretching of the muscle or distal digits is an *early* indicator of circulatory compromise. Diminished or absent pulses, coolness, and pallor are *late* signs and unreliable indicators of acute compartment syndrome.

Neurovascular impairment under a cast is an emergency. If assessments indicate impaired circulation or neurological status, notify the physician immediately. Have a cast cutter at the bedside so the cast can be removed if needed and the pressure relieved.

- Determine particularly whether the pain is persistent and if it occurs over a bony prominence or joint.
- Do not disregard a cessation of persistent pain or discomfort complaints from the client. **Rationale:** *Cessation of complaints can indicate a skin slough. When a skin slough occurs, superficial skin sensation is lost and the client no longer feels pain.*
- When a pressure area under the cast is suspected, the primary care provider may either bivalve the cast so that all of the skin beneath the cast can be inspected or cut a window in the cast over only the area of concern. When a cast is windowed:
  a. Retain the piece (cast and padding) that was cut out. Some primary care providers order that it be taped back if no skin problem is present, but left out if a pressure area is present. **Rationale:** *Putting back the piece prevents window edema, which occurs when skin pressure at the window is not equal to that from the remainder of the cast.*
  b. Inspect the skin under the window at scheduled time intervals.

10. Document findings in the client record using forms or checklists supplemented by narrative notes when appropriate. Record each assessment (whether or not there are problems).

Sample Documentation

9/18/15 1100 Cast still damp, elevated on one pillow. Fingers warm to touch, color pink, full ROM of fingers, no numbness or tingling. Arm pain at 2/10. Declined pain med. Will reassess in 30 minutes. _____ E. Mitchell, RN

Client Teaching

- For itching, suggest that the client use a hair dryer on cool, a vacuum cleaner on reverse, or an ice bag over the outside of the itching area. Emphasize the importance of not putting anything inside the cast, because serious infections and tissue damage can occur. **Rationale:** *These are safer ways to resolve itching and less irritating to the skin than inserting an object into the cast.*
- Before discharge from the hospital, instruct the client to:
  a. Observe for indications of nerve or circulatory impairment, such as extreme coldness or blueness of toes or fingers; extreme continuous swelling of casted toes or fingers; numbness or tingling ("pins and needles" sensation) in casted toes or fingers; continuous complaints of pain; or inability to move the toes or fingers.
  b. Keep the plaster cast dry.
  c. Avoid strenuous activity and follow medical advice about exercise.
  d. Elevate the arm or leg frequently to prevent dependent edema.
  e. Move the toes or fingers frequently.
  f. Observe the skin around the cast edges frequently, and keep it clean and dry.
  g. Report any increase in pain; unexplained fever; foul odor from within the cast; decreased circulation; numbness; inability to move the fingers or toes; or a weakened, cracked, loose, or tight cast.
- Review modifications that may be necessary in clothing, toileting, sleeping, and other ADLs.
- When it is time for cast removal, reassure clients that the saw, though loud, oscillates rather than rotates, and is not dangerous. Skin under the cast will look macerated and pale and hair growth can be increased. Muscle atrophy usually occurs, leading to asymmetry of limbs. Muscles may regain strength through substantial physical effort although this is more likely in younger clients than in older adults (Carlson et al., 2009).

(continued on next page)

SKILL 11.17 Performing Initial Cast Care (continued)

Developmental Considerations

CHILDREN

- Teach parents of young children ways to prevent the child from placing small items inside the cast. Serious infections and damage to tissues can occur as a result of sticking anything inside the cast. Parents also need to ensure that the top of a body cast is covered during meals so that food does not fall inside the cast.
- If possible, allow the child to choose the color of the synthetic cast. Wearing a cast can cause disturbances in body image and self-concept. Education regarding cast care, how to adapt activities of daily living (ADLs), efficient ambulation, and what to expect as far as cast removal will help the child cope effectively.
- Reassure the child that the saw used for windowing, bivalving, and removing the cast is not painful. It rapidly vibrates back and forth rather than rotates, so injury from the blade is

unlikely. The saw is rather loud and can scare children, so have an adult present to support the child during these procedures. Let the child keep the cast pieces when removed if desired and they are not needed.

OLDER ADULTS

- Older adults who are immobilized are at increased risk for skin breakdown and pressure ulcers.
- Wound healing may be slower in older adults than in younger clients.
- Older adults may be less able to manage the additional weight and imbalance caused by a cast.
- Take appropriate steps in planning for use of crutches or other mobility aids to keep older adults moving safely.

SKILL 11.18 Performing Ongoing Cast Care

Delegation

Care of clients with stable casts may be delegated to UAP. The status of the cast is observed during usual care and may be recorded by individuals other than the nurse. However, assessment of complications from the cast requires the expertise of a nurse. Abnormal findings detected by UAP must be validated and interpreted by the nurse.

Equipment

Assemble any of the following equipment items necessary to complete client care:

- Pillows to support the casted areas
- Damp cloth
- Swab
- Alcohol
- Acetone or nail polish remover
- Waterproof tape or adhesive strips
- Bib or towels
- Slipper (fracture) bedpan
- Plastic covering
- Soap and water
- Handheld blow dryer
- Mineral, olive, or baby oil

Preparation

- Review the client record to determine previous status of the cast and the client's extremities. Examine the record regarding pain assessment findings and interventions.

Procedure

1. Prior to performing the procedure, introduce self to the client and verify the client's identity using agency protocol. Explain to the client what you are going to do, why it is necessary, and how he or she can participate. Discuss how the results will be used in planning further care or treatments.

2. Perform hand hygiene and observe other appropriate infection control procedures.

3. Provide for client privacy as indicated.

4. Continue to assess the client for problems.
   - Assess the neurovascular status of the affected limb at regular intervals in accordance with agency protocol.
   - Inspect the skin near and under the cast edges whenever neurovascular assessments are made and/or whenever the client is turned.
   - Check the cast daily for a foul odor. **Rationale:** *This kind of odor may indicate skin excoriation from pressure or an infected area beneath the cast.*

5. Implement measures to prevent skin irritation at the edges of the cast.
   - Wash crumbs of plaster from the skin with a damp cloth and feel along the cast edges to check for rough edges or areas that press into the client's skin. **Rationale:** *As a plaster cast dries, small bits of plaster frequently break off from its rough edges. If they fall inside the cast, they can cause discomfort and irritation.*
   - Remove the resin of synthetic casting materials with a swab moistened with alcohol, acetone, or nail polish remover. Check the manufacturer's directions.
   - When it is dry, cover any rough edges and protect areas of the cast that may come in contact with urine. "Petal" the edges with small strips of waterproof tape or moleskin as follows:
     a. Cut several strips of 2.5-cm (1-in.) adhesive, 5 to 7.5 cm (2 to 3 in.) long. Then curve all corners of each strip. **Rationale:** *Square or pointed ends tend to curl.*
     b. Insert one end of each strip as far as possible inside the cast, and bring the other end out over the cast edge ❶.
     c. Press the petals firmly against the plaster.
     d. Overlap successive petals slightly ❷.

6. Provide skin care to all areas vulnerable to pressure.
   - Examine all areas vulnerable to pressure and breakdown at least every 4 hours. For clients with sensitive skin or potential

SKILL 11.17   Performing Initial Cast Care *(continued)*

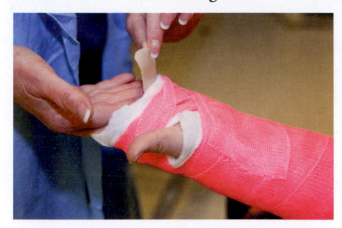

① Gently insert the strip under the cast and fold over the exposed edge.

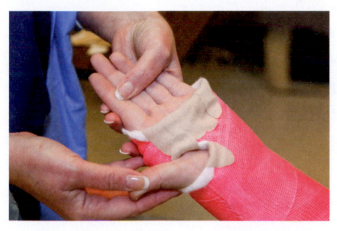

② Overlapping the strips ensures that there are no remaining exposed cast edges.

skin problems, provide care every 2 hours during the day and every 3 hours at night.
  a. Reach under the cast edges as far as possible and massage the area.
  b. Also provide skin care over all bony prominences not under the cast (e.g., the sacrum, heels, ankles, wrists, elbows, and feet). **Rationale:** *These are potential pressure areas if the client is confined to bed.*
7. Keep the cast clean and dry.

VARIATION: PLASTER CAST

- Place a bib or towel over a body cast to catch spills. If a spill does wet the cast, allow the area to air-dry.
- Use a slipper (fracture) bedpan for people with long leg, hip spica, or body casts. **Rationale:** *The flat end placed correctly under the client's buttocks lessens the chance of spillage and minimizes the amount of lifting required by the client and/or nurse.*
- Before placing the client on the bedpan, tuck plastic or other waterproof material around the top of a long leg cast or around the perineal cutout. For a perineal cutout, funnel one end of the plastic into the bedpan.
- Remove the plastic when elimination is completed. **Rationale:** *If left in place, waterproof material makes the cast edge airtight and prevents evaporation of perspiration, which is irritating to the skin.*

- For people with long leg casts, keep the cast supported on pillows while the client is on the bedpan. **Rationale:** *If the cast dangles, urine may run down the cast.*
- For clients with hip spica casts, support both extremities and the back on pillows so that they are as high as the buttocks. **Rationale:** *This prevents urine from running back into the cast.*
- When removing the bedpan, hold it securely while the client is turning or lifting the buttocks. **Rationale:** *This prevents dripping and spilling.*
- After removing the bedpan, thoroughly clean and dry the perineal area.

VARIATION: SYNTHETIC CAST

- Wash the soiled area with warm water and a mild soap.
- Thoroughly rinse the soap from the cast.
- Dry thoroughly to prevent skin maceration and ulceration under the cast.
- If the cast is immersed in water, dry the cast and underlying padding and stockinette thoroughly. First, blot excess water from the cast with a towel. Then, use a handheld blow dryer on the cool or warm setting, directing the air stream in a sweeping motion over the exterior of the cast for about 1 hour or until the client no longer feels a cold clammy sensation like that produced by a wet bathing suit. **Rationale:** *This drying procedure is essential to prevent skin maceration and ulceration.*

8. Turn and position the client in correct alignment to prevent the formation of pressure areas.

  • Place pillows in such a way that:
    a. Body parts press against the edges of the cast as little as possible.
    b. Toes, heels, elbows, and so on, are protected from pressure against the bed surface.
    c. Body alignment is maintained.
  • Plan and implement a turning schedule that will incorporate all of the possible positions. Generally, clients can be placed in lateral, prone, and supine positions unless surgical procedures or any other factors contraindicate them. Attach a trapeze to the overhead frame to enable the client to assist with moving. **Rationale:** *Repositioning prevents pressure areas.*
  • Turn people with large casts or those unable to turn themselves at least once every 4 hours. If the person is at risk for skin breakdown, turn every 1 to 3 hours as needed.
  • When turning the client in a long leg cast to the unaffected side, place a pillow between the legs to support the cast.
  • Use at least three individuals to turn a person in a *damp* hip spica cast. When the cast is dry, the individual can usually turn with the assistance of one nurse. To turn a client from the supine to prone position, follow these steps:
    a. Remove the support pillows only when an assistant is supporting the cast.
    b. Move the client to one side of the bed.
    c. Ask the client to place the arms above the head or along the sides.
    d. Have two assistants go to the other side of the bed while you remain to provide security for the person who is at the edge of the bed.
    e. Place pillows along the bed surface to receive the cast when the client turns.

(continued on next page)

SKILL 11.17 Performing Initial Cast Care (continued)

f. Roll the client toward the two assistants onto the pillows.

g. Adjust the pillows as needed so that they provide proper support and comfort, and prevent pressure areas.

9. Encourage range-of-motion (ROM) and isometric exercises.

- Unless contraindicated, encourage active ROM exercises for all joints on the unaffected extremities, as well as on the joints proximal and distal to the cast. If active exercises are contraindicated, implement active–assistive or passive exercises, depending on the client's abilities and disabilities. **Rationale:** *Exercise helps prevent joint stiffness, muscle atrophy, and venous stasis.*

- Encourage the client to move toes and/or fingers of the casted extremity as frequently as possible. **Rationale:** *Moving these extremities enhances peripheral circulation and decreases swelling and pain.*

- Teach isometric (muscle-setting) exercises for extremities in a cast. **Rationale:** *Isometric exercise will minimize muscle atrophy in the affected limb.*

  a. Teach the isometric exercises on the client's unaffected limb before the person applies it to the affected limb.

  b. Demonstrate muscle palpation while the client is carrying out the exercise. **Rationale:** *Palpation enables the person to feel the changes that occur with muscle contraction and relaxation.*

- Determine if the client can be safely assisted out of bed. To protect both the nurse and the client, ensure that sufficient caregivers and equipment are available and properly used (Patterson et al., 2009). Hospitals should have a designated process for the use of "lift teams." Zero-lift legislation is under consideration at both the federal and state levels that would mandate hospitals to provide both lift equipment and trained lift teams (Kutash et al., 2009). Some facilities have Safe Patient Handling programs, and others support the program but have not yet initiated it.

10. Provide client teaching to promote self-care, comfort, and safety.

- Teach people immobilized in bed with large body casts ways to turn and to move safely by using a trapeze, the side rails, and other such devices.

- Instruct clients with leg casts about ways to walk effectively with crutches.

- Instruct people with arm casts how to apply slings.

- Teach clients how to resolve itching under the cast safely. Discourage the person from using long sharp objects to scratch under the cast. **Rationale:** *These objects can break the skin and cause an infection, because bacteria flourish in the warm, dark, moist environment under the cast. Sticking objects under a cast can also cause folding or bunching of padding material and subsequent pressure and discomfort.*

- When healing is complete and the cast is removed, the underlying skin is usually macerated, pale, flaky, and encrusted, since layers of dead skin have accumulated. Instruct clients to remove this debris gently and gradually:

  a. Apply oil (e.g., mineral, olive, or baby oil).

  b. Soak the skin in warm water and dry it.

  c. Caution the client not to rub the area too vigorously. **Rationale:** *Vigorous rubbing can cause bleeding or excoriation of fragile skin.*

  d. Repeat steps a and b for several days. **Rationale:** *Gradual removal of skin exudates reduces skin irritation.*

11. Document findings in the client record using forms or checklists supplemented by narrative notes when appropriate. Record each assessment (whether or not there are problems).

Sample Documentation

9/15/15 1000 Cast intact, leg elevated on 2 pillows. Toes warm to touch, pink, capillary refill 2 seconds. Moves toes readily and fully; states no numbness or tingling. Pain 0/10. _____ B. Snyder, RN

VARIATION: CARING FOR A CHILD WITH A CAST

Equipment

- Cast material (if assisting in application)
- Large basin with water (if assisting in application)
- Pillows with waterproof covering
- Absorbent pads and protectors
- Clean gloves

Preparation

- Consult the child's chart for description of the injury or surgery.

Procedure

Following cast application:

1. Perform hand hygiene and don clean gloves.

2. Elevate a wet cast on pillows covered in plastic. **Rationale:** *Elevation decreases edema under the cast, which can restrict circulation.*

3. Use the palm of the hands when lifting a wet or damp cast. **Rationale:** *Fingertips can indent plaster and create pressure points.*

4. Circle and note the date and time of any drainage on the cast. **Rationale:** *Some drainage is common after surgery. Monitoring its presence provides clues to the amount and type of fluid lost.*

5. Assess circulation and neurological status every 15 minutes after surgery or cast placement and then progress to every 30 minutes, 60 minutes, and 2 hours. Report abnormal findings or changes in condition. Include the following observations on the involved extremities:

   - Distal pulses
   - Color
   - Warmth
   - Sensation
   - Capillary refill
   - Edema
   - Movement
   - Pain, tingling
     Rationale: *Circulation and nerves under the cast can be injured if it is too tight.*

6. Use pain-control measures as needed and reassess pain. Report immediately worsening pain or pain that is not controlled by prescribed medication.

7. Check the edges of the cast for roughness or crumbling. Pull the inner stockinette over the edge of the cast and tape once the cast has dried. **Rationale:** *These actions can prevent discomfort and skin breakdown.*

8. Keep the cast clean and dry. Cover it with a plastic bag during bathing or toileting.

SKILL 11.17 Performing Initial Cast Care *(continued)*

9. Avoid use of lotions and powders under the cast. **Rationale:** *These products can cause skin irritation.*
10. Keep shirts or other clothing over the top edges of casts on young children. **Rationale:** *This action helps to prevent the child from placing objects down into the cast, which can result in areas of discomfort or skin damage.*
11. Instruct the family about care of the cast at home and when to return for checks and removal of the cast.
12. Document the cast application, how the child tolerated the procedure, cast care provided, and assessment of vascular and neurological status.

▶ CRITICAL THINKING OPTIONS FOR UNEXPECTED OUTCOMES

Not all unexpected outcomes require further nursing intervention; however, many times they do. When the client demonstrates a change in signs/symptoms indicating an emerging problem, the nurse should immediately assess and troubleshoot what is happening. The assessment data must be processed quickly to formulate a hypothesis so the nurse can make a clinical judgment. The nurse then decides how best to resolve the problem and improve the client's situation for a better appropriate outcome.

EXPECTED OUTCOME	PROBLEM SOLVING	NURSING ACTIONS
Correct body mechanics are utilized by caregiver.	Incorrect body mechanics are used while giving client care.	▪ Identify areas of your body where you feel stress and strain. ▪ Evaluate the way you use body mechanics. ▪ Attend an in-service program on using body mechanics appropriately. ▪ Concentrate on how you are using your body when moving and turning clients. ▪ Position bed and equipment at a comfortable height and proximity to working area. ▪ Use your longest and strongest muscles to prevent injury.
Injuries are prevented to both the nurse and the client.	Nurse injures self while giving client care.	▪ Prevent future episodes of injury by increasing physical activity and exercises, changing ergonomics, and evaluating use of orthosis. ▪ Report any back strain immediately to supervisor. ▪ Complete unusual occurrence form. ▪ Go to health service or emergency department for evaluation and immediate care. ▪ Evaluate any activities that led to injury to determine incorrect use of body mechanics. ▪ Prevent additional injury by obtaining assistance when needed. ▪ Use devices such as turning sheets or assistive devices to assist in turning difficult clients.
Positioning a Client Use of proper body mechanics facilitates client care.	Nurse uses poor body mechanics and injures client.	▪ Assess the extent of client's injury. ▪ Notify client's physician. ▪ Complete unusual occurrence form. ▪ Carry out physician's orders for follow-up treatment.
Moving and Transferring Mechanical equipment and devices are used in client transfers and repositioning as needed.	Client unable to assist with movement.	▪ Use a friction-reducing sheet to provide more support for client. ▪ Obtain additional assistance to help with moving "dead" weight.
	Client afraid of using assistive device.	▪ Request physician's order for therapeutic mattress or dressings for pressure ulcer(s) care. ▪ Explain use of equipment (i.e., comfort and safety in transferring). ▪ Demonstrate equipment before using.
Client is moved safely using appropriate device. Body alignment is maintained.	Client unable to maintain any type of position without assistance.	▪ Use trochanter roll to prevent external rotation of client's hip. ▪ Use foam bolsters to maintain side-lying positions. ▪ Use folded towels, blankets, or small pillows to position client's hands and arms to prevent dependent edema.
Appropriate assistive devices are utilized to transfer client.	Unable to transfer client from bed to wheelchair due to excess weight.	▪ Determine if wheelchair without arms or transfer board can aid in transfer. ▪ Contact social services to obtain bariatric assist devices. ▪ Determine if other family members can assist with transfer. ▪ May need home health aide services to assist with transfer.

(continued on next page)

EXPECTED OUTCOME	PROBLEM SOLVING	NURSING ACTIONS
Injuries are prevented to both the nurse and the client.	Injury occurs to client when caregiver attempts transfer to wheelchair.	▪ Do not continue to reposition client, place in bed. ▪ Complete sensory, motor, and pain assessment. ▪ Notify physician. ▪ Document findings.
Client is able to progress through range-of-motion exercises with minimal to no pain.	Client experiences pain and discomfort during range-of-motion exercises.	▪ Assess amount and type of pain and report findings to physician. ▪ Reevaluate your technique to ensure you are performing the exercises correctly. ▪ Start exercises with less stress on joints. Do exercises for a shorter period of time and gradually increase time and range of joint mobility.
Client progresses from being dependent to becoming independent in ambulation.	Client experiences vertigo or feels faint.	▪ If in the client's room, help the client return to the chair or bed. ▪ If in the hall, ease the client down the wall to the floor. Do not attempt to hold the client. ▪ Summon help if possible.
Feelings of physical and mental well-being increase.	Client is too weak to ambulate.	▪ Provide active and passive ROM before attempting ambulation. ▪ Begin ambulation protocol as soon as possible using assistive device.
Balance and muscle tone improve.	Client is heavy or has poor balance.	▪ Ask other nurses or staff to help you ambulate the client until able to walk on his or her own. ▪ If necessary, enlist the aid of a stronger assistant whose presence may give the client additional psychological as well as physical support. ▪ Gradually increase ambulation as muscle tone improves and balance improves. ▪ Request assistance for ambulation from physical therapist. ▪ Obtain walker to assist client with ambulation. The walker will also provide reassurance to client.
Assistive Devices Client appropriately uses crutches to ambulate.	Client fears falling while dependent on crutches.	▪ Place safety or gait belt on client until he/she feels confident. ▪ Observe as the client practices the procedures to make sure that he or she is completing the steps correctly for each gait. ▪ Slow down crutch protocol until client gains confidence at every level of mastery (e.g., four-point gait to two-point gait). ▪ Remain with client and give verbal reassurance and feedback for improvement.
	Client not stable ambulating with crutches or cane.	▪ Place safety belt on client and ambulate with walker. ▪ Increase both upper and lower muscle strength to increase ambulation with cane or crutches.
Client uses assistive devices correctly without assistance.	Slipping occurs with crutch walking.	▪ Check crutch tips to ensure they cover all metal or wood. ▪ Observe the client's stance or gait to determine if it is too broad. ▪ Be sure that floor surface is dry and free of scatter rugs.
Crutches are measured correctly to prevent numbness or tingling in fingers.	Client complains of numbness and tingling in fingers when crutch walking.	▪ Remeasure distance between axilla and crutch bars to determine if two fingerbreadths can be inserted. ▪ Observe client's gait to determine if he or she is leaning on crutch inappropriately.
Caregiver is able to manage turning, repositioning, and assistive devices.	Unable to lift client up in bed with single healthcare worker.	▪ If a second person is available, utilize him/her to assist in moving. ▪ Use sliding board if two healthcare workers are available. ▪ Rent a hydraulic lift or Hoyer lift to assist with moving up in bed or getting out of bed.
Assistive Devices Client progresses from being dependent to becoming independent in ambulation.	Client is not ambulating.	▪ Discuss with caregiver and client reasons why client is not ambulating. ▪ If client is afraid of falling, ensure that a gait belt is worn and the client uses a walker to start with and then moves to a cane, if possible. ▪ Use two individuals to assist with walking, if available.
Traction and Cast Care Extremity is maintained in correct alignment.	Client in skeletal traction keeps migrating to foot of bed.	▪ Without releasing traction, use pull sheet and an assistant to reposition client up in bed. ▪ Elevate lower part of bed to provide countertraction. ▪ Increase weight of countertraction at head of bed.

EXPECTED OUTCOME	PROBLEM SOLVING	NURSING ACTIONS
Neurovascular complications do not occur.	Client experiences "tightness" in thigh after fracture of the femur.	■ Measure thigh circumference and compare with contralateral thigh. ■ Assess for presence of ecchymosis. ■ Monitor vital signs closely for hypovolemia (several units of blood may be sequestered in the thigh after fracture of the femur). ■ Notify physician for significant changes.
	Client in Buck's traction is unable to dorsiflex the foot.	■ Release proximal strap as it may be compressing peroneal nerve over head of fibula. ■ Assess sensation over dorsum of foot and between big and second toes. ■ Notify physician.
	Client develops pain not relieved by analgesics, pain that worsens with extremity elevation and passive stretching of digits.	■ Maintain extremity in dependent position. ■ Notify orthopedic technician immediately: windowing or bivalving of cast may be indicated. ■ Suspect acute compartment syndrome and notify physician immediately to obtain measurement of compartment pressure. ■ Fasciotomy may be indicated if tissue swelling or external device compromises circulation within a muscle compartment.
Pin site remains free of infection.	Halo pin site appears to be infected.	■ Notify physician. ■ Obtain culture of drainage for antibiotic sensitivity studies. ■ Cleanse pin site as prescribed, using aseptic technique and separate applicator for each site. ■ Remove crusts to allow drainage. ■ Monitor for systemic signs of infection.
Cast integrity is maintained to provide adequate site immobilization.	Cast cracks from improper drying or stress.	Notify physician immediately. ■ Reassure client. ■ Do not reposition client until physician assesses.
	Cast edges begin to crumble.	"Petal" edges of cast with 1- to 2-inch strips of tape. ■ Place half of tape inside cast, pull tape over cast, and anchor on outside of cast. ■ Continue to petal cast until all edges are covered.
Client experiences minimal swelling.	Fingers swell after application of arm cast.	■ Assess that there is room for two fingers to be slipped under cast. ■ Apply ice alongside of cast and maintain elevation after cast application. ■ Maintain arm positioning with hand higher than elbow. ■ Encourage client to exercise fingers to help reduce edema. ■ Monitor neurovascular status frequently.

12 Nutrition

Skills-at-a-Glance

Nutrition is the sum of all interactions between an organism and the food it consumes. In other words, nutrition is what an individual eats and how the body uses it. **Nutrients** are organic, inorganic, and energy-producing substances found in foods and required for body functioning. People require the essential nutrients in foods for the growth and maintenance of all body tissues and the normal functioning of all body processes.

Many factors affect the ways that the body uses food. Table 12–1 ● describes factors affecting nutrition.

TABLE 12–1   Factors Affecting Nutrition

FACTOR	COMMENTS
Development	People in rapid periods of growth (i.e., infancy and adolescence) have increased needs for nutrients. Older adults, on the other hand, need fewer calories and often need to make dietary changes in view of the risk of coronary heart disease, osteoporosis, and hypertension.
Gender	Nutrient requirements are different for men and women because of body composition and reproductive functions. The larger muscle mass of men means a greater need for calories and proteins. Because of menstruation, women require more iron than men prior to menopause. Women who are pregnant or lactating have increased caloric and fluid needs.
Ethnicity and culture	Ethnicity often determines food preferences and eating behaviors. Traditional foods may be eaten long after other customs are abandoned. Food preferences, however, probably differ as much among individuals of the same cultural background as they do generally among cultures. See Individual Variations in Nutritional Practices and Preferences section. Between 30 million and 50 million Americans have lactose intolerance (also called lactose maldigestion), a shortage of the enzyme lactase, which is needed to break down the sugar in milk. Certain populations are more widely affected: As many as 80% of African Americans, 80% to 100% of American Indians, and 90% to 100% of Asian Americans are lactose intolerant although they may not always show symptoms (Gaskin & Ilich, 2009).
Beliefs about food	Beliefs about effects of foods on health and well-being can affect food choices. Many people acquire their beliefs about food from television, magazines, and other media.
Personal preferences	Some adults are very adventuresome and eager to try new foods. Others prefer to eat the same foods over and over again. Preferences in the tastes, smells, flavors (blends of taste and smell), temperatures, colors, shapes, and sizes of food influence an individual's food choices.
Religious practices	Some Roman Catholics avoid meat on certain days, and some Protestant faiths prohibit meat, tea, coffee, or alcohol. Both Orthodox Judaism and Islam prohibit pork. Orthodox Jews observe kosher customs, eating certain foods only if they are inspected by a rabbi and prepared according to specific dietary laws.
Lifestyle	Certain lifestyles are linked to food-related behaviors. People who are always in a hurry probably buy convenience grocery items or eat restaurant meals. Individual differences also influence lifestyle patterns (e.g., cooking skills, concern about health). Some people work at different times, such as evening or nightshifts. They might need to adapt their eating habits as a result.
Economics	What, how much, and how often an individual eats are frequently affected by socioeconomic status. People with limited income, including some older adults, may not be able to afford meat and fresh vegetables. In contrast, people with higher incomes may purchase more proteins and fats and fewer complex carbohydrates. Not all individuals have the financial resources for extensive food preparation and storage.
Medications and therapy	The effects of drugs on nutrition vary considerably. Drugs may alter appetite, disturb taste perception, or interfere with nutrient absorption or excretion. Conversely, nutrients can affect drug utilization. Some nutrients can decrease drug absorption; others enhance absorption. Therapies prescribed for certain diseases (e.g., chemotherapy and radiation for cancer) may also adversely affect eating patterns and nutrition. For example, oral ulcers, intestinal bleeding, or diarrhea resulting from the toxicity of antineoplastic agents used in chemotherapy can seriously diminish an individual's nutritional status. The effects of radiotherapy depend on the area that is treated. For example, radiotherapy of the head and neck may cause decreased salivation, taste distortions, and swallowing difficulties.
Health	An individual's health status greatly affects eating habits and nutritional status. The lack of teeth, ill-fitting teeth, or a sore mouth makes chewing food difficult. Difficulty swallowing (dysphagia) due to a painfully inflamed throat or a stricture of the esophagus can prevent an individual from obtaining adequate nourishment. Disease processes and surgery of the gastrointestinal tract can affect digestion, absorption, metabolism, and excretion of essential nutrients.
Alcohol consumption	The calories consumed in alcoholic drinks include both those of the alcohol itself and of the other beverages added to the drink. Drinking alcohol can lead to weight gain through the addition of these calories to the regular diet plus the effect of alcohol on fat metabolism. Excessive alcohol use can contribute to nutritional deficiencies. Alcohol may replace food in an individual's diet, and it can depress the appetite. Excessive alcohol can have a toxic effect on the intestinal mucosa, thereby decreasing the absorption of nutrients.
Advertising	Food producers try to persuade people to change from the product they currently use to the brand of the producer.
Psychological factors	Although some people overeat when stressed, depressed, or lonely, others eat very little under the same conditions. Anorexia and weight loss can indicate severe stress or depression.

▶ INDIVIDUAL VARIATIONS IN NUTRITIONAL PRACTICES AND PREFERENCES

The following are selected variations in nutritional practices and preferences among different individuals.

Availability

- Including geographical location, climate, season, accessibility of foods inside and outside the home
- For example, a drought season, lack of refrigeration, extremes of weather, diseased animal population, lack of food quantity needed, and lack of funds

Body Image

- Self-imposed eating habits that can influence physical body such as, losing weight, gaining weight, or gaining muscle mass
- For example, eating less than or more than the body requires each day, or overtaking dietary supplements

Convenience

- Includes eating in the home or at restaurants, ready-to-cook foods, using eatery take-out services, or buying fast foods
- For example, using packaged and processed foods often, mindless eating, and increased eating outside the home

Financial

- Includes having an income, money to buy food, the cost of food, availability of food and means to acquire food
- For example, not having enough money to buy food or not having access to food products

Eating Habits

- Includes eating patterns such as number of meals per day, grazing or fasting, quantity of food eaten, and snacking
- For example, family recipes and methods of cooking foods, adding excess salt or sugar to foods, and poor meal planning

Emotions

- Emotional eating driven by level of anxiety or stress, depression, guilt, need for comfort, boredom, fatigue, and anger
- For example, salty snacks, warm creamy foods, sugar snacks, and other comfort foods

Food Choices

- Dependent on factors such as, food knowledge, beliefs and culture, familiar foods, favorite foods, peer group, cooking or non-cooking foods, feeling hungry, dietary regimens, chronic diseases, and personal habits
- For example, ease of preparation, adequate money to buy foods, advertisements, hunger level, and health status

Health Benefits

- Provision of energy and nutritional components needed by the body to maintain homeostasis and body functions

- For example, taking adequate amounts of protein, carbohydrates, and fats such as meats, vegetables, and fruits

Taste and Smell

- Includes desire for sweetness, avoidance of bitterness, feelings of satisfaction upon eating certain foods, and feeling of fullness after eating
- For example, use of spices, herbs, and flavors such as garlic, cloves, broth, and salt

▶ NUTRITIONAL VARIATIONS THROUGHOUT THE LIFE CYCLE

Nutritional requirements vary throughout the life cycle. Guidelines follow for the major developmental stages. **Table 12–2** ● describes problems and interventions for older adults.

Neonate to 1 Year

- Fluid and nutritional needs are met by breast milk or formula.
- Fluid needs of infants are proportionally greater than those of adults because of a higher metabolic rate, immature kidneys, and greater water losses through the skin and the lungs. Fluid balance is critical.
- The total daily nutritional requirement is about 80 to 100 mL of breast milk or formula per kilogram of body weight. Stomach capacity is about 90 mL so feedings are required every $2\frac{1}{2}$ to 4 hours.
- During feeding, the infant sucks readily and needs burping every few minutes.
- Infant bottles should never be propped up for feeding to avoid aspiration or choking.
- After feeding, healthy infants can be placed in a supine position for sleep during their first 6 months to reduce the risk of sudden infant death syndrome (SIDS).
- **Regurgitation**, or spitting up, during or after a feeding is a common occurrence during the first year.
- Adequate weight gain demonstrates the infant is receiving adequate nutrition.
- Adding solid food to the diet usually takes place between 4 and 6 months of age.
- Solid foods (strained or pureed) are generally introduced in the following order: cereals (rice), fruits, vegetables (yellow before green), and strained meats. Foods are introduced one at a time every 5 days to ensure that the infant tolerates and demonstrates no allergy to it. This sequence can vary according to cultural preferences.
- With the eruption of teeth at about 7 to 9 months, the infant is ready to chew and experience different textures of food.
- Because honey can contain spores of *Clostridium botulinum* and this has been a source of infection (and death) for infants, children less than 12 months old should not be fed

TABLE 12–2   Problems Associated with Nutrition in Older Adults

PROBLEMS	NURSING INTERVENTIONS
Difficulty chewing	Encourage regular visits to the dentist to have dentures repaired, refitted, or replaced. Chop fruits and vegetables finely; shred green, leafy vegetables; select ground meat, poultry, or fish.
Lowered glucose tolerance	Eat more complex carbohydrates (e.g., breads, cereals, rice, pasta, potatoes, and legumes) rather than sugar-rich foods.
Decreased social interaction, loneliness	Promote appropriate social interaction at meals, when possible. Encourage the client and spouse to take an interest in food preparation and serving, perhaps as an activity they can do together. Encourage family or caregivers to present the food at a dining table with place mats, tablecloths, and napkins to trigger eating associations for the older adult. If food preparation is not possible, suggest community resources, such as Meals-on-Wheels. Suggest picnics in the yard or inviting friends over for meals.
Loss of appetite and senses of smell and taste	Eat essential, nutrient-dense foods first; follow with desserts and low-nutrient-density foods. Review dietary restrictions, and find ways to make meals appealing within these guidelines. Eat small meals frequently instead of three large meals a day.
Limited income	Suggest using generic brands and coupons. Substitute milk, dairy products, and beans for meat. Avoid convenience foods if able to cook. Buy foods that are on sale and freeze for future use. Suggest community resources and nutrition programs.
Difficulty sleeping at night	Have the major meal at noon instead of in the evening. Avoid tea, coffee, or other stimulants in the evening.

honey. According to the Centers for Disease Control and Prevention (CDC) (2011), honey is safe for individuals 1 year of age and older.

- At about 6 months of age, infants require iron supplementation to prevent **iron deficiency anemia**, a decrease in red blood cells needed for synthesis of hemoglobin. Cow's milk is low in iron and, thus, iron-fortified cereals or formulas are recommended until the child reaches 18 months.
- Weaning from the breast or bottle to the cup is usually achieved by 12 to 24 months of age.
- Having the bottle in bed could lead to **bottle mouth syndrome**, decay of the teeth caused by constant contact with sweet liquid from the bottle. Some dentists advocate brushing or cleaning the infant's teeth as prevention. Weaning from the bottle can be facilitated by diluting the formula with water increasingly until the infant is drinking plain water.
- By the age of 1, most infants can be completely fed on table food, and milk intake is about 20 ounces per day.

Toddler

- Can eat most foods and adjust to three meals each day.
- Fine motor skills are sufficiently developed for learning how to feed themselves. Before the age of 20 months, most toddlers require help with glasses and cups because their wrist control is limited.
- By age 3, most of the deciduous teeth have emerged so the toddler is able to bite and chew adult table food.
- Independence may be exhibited through the toddler's refusal of certain foods.
- Meals should be short because of the toddler's brief attention span and environmental distractions.
- Toddlers often eat foods in a certain order, cut foods a specific way, or accompany certain foods with a particular drink.

- The gastrointestinal function is more mature, and the percentage of fluid body weight is lower. A healthy toddler weighing 15 kg (33 lb) needs about 1,250 mL of fluid per 24 hours.
- During the toddler stage, the caloric requirement is 900 to 1,800 kcal/day.
- Table foods offer more variety and are less expensive and more nutritious than prepared toddler foods. Common toddler deficiencies are iron, calcium, and vitamins C and A.
- The following suggestions may help meet the child's nutritional needs and promote effective parent–child interactions:
  a. Make mealtime a pleasant time by avoiding tensions at the table and discussions of bad behavior.
  b. Offer a variety of simple, attractive foods, and avoid one-dish meals, such as a stew.
  c. Do not use food as a reward or punish a child who does not eat.
  d. Schedule meals, sleep, and snack times that will allow for optimum appetite and behavior.
  e. Avoid the routine use of sweet desserts.

Preschooler

- Eats adult foods.
- Very active and may rush through meals to return to playing. May require snacks between meals like cheese, fruit, yogurt, raw vegetables, and milk.
- Requires help in cutting meat and may spill milk when pouring from a large container.
- Need to be taught how to use utensils and have the opportunity to practice (e.g., buttering bread).

- Four- and 5-year-olds often use their fingers to pick up food.
- They may enjoy helping in the kitchen, and both girls and boys should be encouraged to do so.
- Less at risk for fluid imbalances. The average 5-year-old weighing 20 kg (45 lb) requires at least 75 mL of liquid per kilogram of body weight per day, or 1,500 mL every 24 hours.

School-Age Child

- Requires a balanced diet including approximately 2,400 kcal/day in three meals and one to two snacks.
- Needs a protein-rich food at breakfast to sustain the prolonged physical and mental effort required at school. Skipping breakfast results in becoming inattentive and restless by late morning and experiencing decreased problem-solving ability.
- Undernourished children become fatigued easily and face a greater risk of infection.
- The average healthy 8-year-old weighing 30 kg (66 lb) requires about 1,750 mL of fluid per day.
- Many school-age children have only one meal a day with their family, at dinner. Mealtime should be a social time. Eating a balanced diet should be the norm for both parent and child.
- Generally eats lunch brought from home or bought at school. They may trade their food, not eat lunch at all, or buy sweets or junk food with their lunch money.
- Poor eating habits may result in obesity. Childhood obesity is an increasing problem. More than 17% of American children ages 6 to 19 are overweight (Ogden, Carroll, & Flegal, 2008).
- Obesity in school-age children tends to result in adult obesity and all the related health risks. It is both caused by and results in decreased activity as well as psychosocial problems. Children with obesity may be ridiculed and discriminated against by peers, which reinforces low self-esteem. The CDC's Division of Adolescent and School Health has established many programs to address both prevention and treatment of childhood obesity. The goal of treatment is to reduce weight gain, allowing their weight to increase more slowly than their height. Counseling and teaching for parents should include the following:
  a. Review the child's eating habits, including snacks.
  b. Alter meal content.
  c. Use rewards other than food.
  d. Promote regular exercise.

Adolescent

- Need for nutrients and calories increases, particularly during the growth spurt. In particular, the need for protein, calcium, vitamin D, iron, and B vitamins increases.
- An adequate diet is 1 quart of milk per day as well as appropriate amounts of meat, vegetables, fruits, breads, and cereals. Calcium intake (1,200 to 1,500 mg/day) may help decrease osteoporosis (a decrease in bone density) in later life (Rolfes, Pinna, & Whitney, 2009).
- Teenagers, particularly boys, seem to be eating all the time. They have active lifestyles and irregular eating patterns. They tend to diet or snack frequently often eating high-calorie foods such as fast foods.
- Healthy snacks such as fruits and cheese need to be made available in the home. The teenager's food choices relate to physical, social, and emotional factors and impulses.
- Need to take responsibility for decisions they make and to avoid conflicts that relate to food.
- Common problems related to nutrition and self-esteem include obesity, anorexia nervosa, and bulimia.
- Obesity continues to be a problem. Depression is not unusual among adolescents who are obese. Treatment of obesity includes education as well as assessment of psychosocial problems that may produce overeating.
- Under social pressure to be slim, some adolescents severely limit their food intake to a level significantly below that required to meet the demands of normal growth. In some instances, the adolescent may develop an eating disorder, such as anorexia or bulimia. **Anorexia nervosa** is characterized by a prolonged inability or refusal to eat, rapid weight loss, and emaciation in individuals who continue to believe they are fat. People with anorexia may also induce vomiting and use laxatives and diuretics to remain thin. **Bulimia** is an uncontrollable compulsion to consume enormous amounts of food (binge) and then expel it by self-induced vomiting or by taking laxatives (purge).

Young Adult

- Nutritional habits during young adulthood often become patterns maintained throughout an individual's life.
- Many are aware of the food groups but not about how many or size of servings they need.
- Females need to maintain adequate iron intake. To prevent iron deficiency anemia, menstruating females should ingest 18 mg of iron daily by eating iron-rich foods, such as organ meats (liver and kidneys), eggs, fish, poultry, leafy vegetables, and dried fruits.
- The World Health Organization (WHO) recommends folate/folic acid supplements for child-bearing women to prevent neural tube defects in the fetus if taken prior to and during the early portion of the pregnancy (Rolfes et al., 2009).
- Calcium is needed to help decrease development of osteoporosis in later life. Along with calcium, adequate vitamin D is necessary for the calcium to enter the bloodstream.
- Obesity may occur for the sedentary adult who does not decrease caloric intake. Being overweight or obese is a risk factor for hypertension, which is a risk factor in the development of cardiovascular disease. Low-fat and/or low-cholesterol diets play a significant role in the prevention and treatment of these medical problems.

Middle-Aged Adult

- Eats a healthy diet, following the recommended portions of the food groups, with special attention to protein, calcium, and limiting cholesterol and caloric intake.
- Two or three liters of fluid should be included in the daily diet.
- Postmenopausal women need to ingest sufficient calcium and vitamin D to reduce osteoporosis, and antioxidants such as vitamins A, C, and E, which are helpful in reducing the risks of heart disease.

- May gain weight due to decreased metabolic activity and decreased physical activity. Also should be warned that being overweight is a risk factor for many chronic diseases, such as diabetes and hypertension, and for problems of mobility, such as arthritis. Programs are available that use behavior modification techniques and group support to assist clients in reaching weight goals after they have discussed any major changes in their diets with their physician.

- During late middle age, gastric juice secretions and free acid gradually decline. As a result, some individuals may complain of "heartburn" (acid indigestion) or an increase in belching.

- Clients should be advised to develop sensible eating habits and avoid fried or fatty foods.

Older Adult

- Requires the same basic nutrition as the younger adult.
- Fewer calories are needed because of the lower metabolic rate and the decrease in physical activity.

- May need more fiber and bulk, but most nutrient requirements remain relatively unchanged.

- Physical changes like tooth loss and impaired sense of taste and smell may affect eating habits.

- Decreased saliva and gastric juice secretion may also affect an individual's nutrition.

- Psychosocial factors may also contribute to nutritional problems. Those who live alone may not want to cook for themselves or eat alone. As a result, they may adopt poor dietary habits. Other factors, such as lack of transportation, poor access to stores, and inability to prepare food, also affect nutritional status. Loss of spouse, anxiety, depression, dependence on others, and lowered income all affect eating habits. See also Table 12–2.

- Include each group on the federal government's MyPlate program. For example, a 65-year-old female who performs less than 30 minutes of exercise per day requires 1,600 kcal consisting of all food groups.

Expected Outcomes

1. Client's nutritional needs are met with a balanced diet appropriate for developmental age.
2. Client experiences no complications while eating.
3. Client with dysphagia maintains appropriate body weight.
4. Client demonstrates understanding (verbalized knowledge) of dietary information provided.

SKILL 12.1   Taking a Nutritional Assessment

No single parameter is sufficient to determine nutritional status. Initial screening performed on hospital admission includes:
- Changes in body weight of ≤10 pounds in the last 6 months
- Nausea, vomiting, diarrhea lasting >5 days
- Declining food intake, difficulty chewing/swallowing, and time/duration of recent hospitalizations.

See also **Table 12–3** ●.

If results of this initial screening classify the client at "nutrition risk," a dietitian consult is indicated.

1. Take objective measures of nutritional status, to include:
   - Weight in relation to height (body mass index)
   - Monitoring nutrient intake and calorie counts
   - Laboratory tests: serum albumin, transferrin, and prealbumin; tests of cellular immunity; and total lymphocyte count
   - Evaluation of body composition by visual inspection or anthropometric measurements (triceps skinfold, midarm muscle circumference).
2. Document all relevant findings.

TABLE 12–3   Nutritional Assessment Parameters

CLINICAL ASSESSMENT	NORMAL	ABNORMAL
Dietary Data		
Appetite	Remains unchanged	Increased or decreased recently Particular cravings
Nutritional intake	Adequate foods and fluids to supply body nutrients Nonallergic response to major food groups	Elimination of certain food categories that results in limited nutrients Emphasis on some food groups (sugar) to the exclusion of others (vegetables) Allergic response to certain foods
Caloric intake	Average 28 kcal/kg/day	Constant use of fad diets to lose weight Use of drugs or chemicals that interfere with appetite or nutrient assimilation
Meal patterns	3–6 home-prepared meals/day Adequate time and calm atmosphere for meals	Fast-food or packaged foods Missed meals, constant snacking, or overeating Eating "on the run" or hurried
General Appearance		
	Alert, responsive, healthy-appearing eyes and skin	Listless, dull, nonresponsive Skin and eyes appear unhealthy

(continued on next page)

SKILL 12.1   Taking a Nutritional Assessment (continued)

TABLE 12–3   Nutritional Assessment Parameters (continued)

CLINICAL ASSESSMENT	NORMAL	ABNORMAL
Physical factors	Adequate chewing and swallowing capability Mouth and gums healthy so food can be ingested Physical exercise adequate for calorie intake	Teeth or gums in poor condition or ill-fitting dentures Swallowing impairs ingestion Inadequate physical exercise to burn calories
Presence of disease	No disease process that interferes with nutrient assimilation No congenital condition or postsurgery condition that interferes with nutrient assimilation	Disease present that interferes with ingestion, digestion, assimilation, or excretion Congenital condition, rehabilitation phase, or post-surgery that interferes with food assimilation
Elimination schedule	Regular, adequate elimination of foods Absence of constant flatus, discharge, or mucus	Irregular or painful elimination Presence of constant flatus Presence of discharge, blood, or mucus
Anthropometric Measurements		
Height	For bedridden clients, measure arm span—fully extend arms 90° angle to body and measure from tip of one middle finger to the tip of other middle finger for estimated height	Loss of 5 to 8 cm (2–3 in.) in height may indicate osteoporosis
Weight—compared to ideal and usual body weight.	Ideal body weight 100 lb (female); 106 lb (male) for 5 feet height + 5 lb for each 1 in. over 5 feet (female) and 6 lb for each 1 in. over 5 feet (male); small frame minus 10%; large frame plus 10%	Changed—markedly increased or decreased recently: important indicator of changed nutritional status Loss of more than 10% weight for prior 6 months should be clinically evaluated
Body mass index ratio of weight in kilograms and height in meters	18.5–24.9	Less than 18.5—underweight 25–29—overweight 30–39—obese
Triceps skinfold measurement (mm)	Standard values—male to female 12.5–16.5	If values change over months, may indicate a chronic condition
Circumference of upper arm (cm)	29.3–28.5	
Midarm muscle circumference (cm)	25.3–23.2	Hydration status may influence results
Biochemical Assessments*		
Serum albumin	3.5–5.0 g/dL	Examples of possible disease conditions: Decrease signifies lowered nutritional status—protein deficient
Serum transferrin binds iron to plasma and transports to bone marrow	200–430 mg/dL	Reduced levels may indicate chronic diseases and protein deficiency Elevated levels—anemias, liver damage, lead toxicity
Hemoglobin	Male—13.5–17 g/dL Female—12–15 g/dL	Decreased related to iron deficiency (anemias and leukemia)
Prealbumin (PA) serum	20–50 mg/dL	Decreased—protein wasting diseases, malnutrition (10.7 indicates severe nutritional deficiency) Elevated—Hodgkin's disease
Blood urea nitrogen: creatinine	10:1–20:1	Nitrogen imbalance, inadequate renal functioning; ratio increased in heart failure, decreased in renal perfusion
24-hr urinary nitrogen	Positive balance	Inadequate protein intake
Sociocultural Data		
Cultural–religious factors	Ability to afford adequate foods in all food categories Cultural beliefs that do not eliminate whole food groups Religious beliefs that do not eliminate whole food groups	Economic position that precludes purchase of adequate food Religious or cultural beliefs that interfere with receiving balanced diet (macrobiotic diets) Inadequate knowledge, experience, or intelligence to prepare healthy meals
Ethnicity	Traditional foods that do not eliminate whole food groups	Beliefs and ethnic preference that eliminate major nutrients from the diet
Lifestyle	Well-balanced meals that include all nutrients Food does not lose all nutrient value in preparation	Fast-paced stressful lifestyle that incorporates fast food or convenience foods deficient in nutrients or imbalanced (high-fat)

*Laboratory test parameters differ among laboratories. Check the reference range for the specific lab where the client's blood or urine was tested.

SKILL 12.1   Taking a Nutritional Assessment (*continued*)

Evidence-Based Practice

The Mini-Nutritional Assessment (MNA) is an assessment tool that helps identify older adults who are at risk for malnutrition. A PDF is available, and a video demonstration has been posted by the source listed below.

Source: DiMaria-Ghalili & Guenter (2008).

Developmental Considerations

Nutrition Teaching

CHILDREN

- Children learn eating habits from their parents. It is the parents' responsibility to be good nutritional role models, both in terms of what they eat and how they incorporate food into their lifestyle.
- During the preschool and early school-age years, children learn lifelong eating habits. It is the parents' responsibility to provide the child with adequate amounts of nutritious foods in an environment that is relaxed and comfortable for eating.

  It is the child's responsibility to decide what and how much of the nutritious foods to eat. Parents should be counseled that eating can become a source of conflict if the parent tries to tell the child what and how much to eat, or if the child tries to tell the parent what foods should be eaten.
- Children's access to "junk food" should be limited, but completely forbidding a food may also create conflict.
- Although adolescents who are vegetarians are at risk for some nutritional deficits, the diet of adolescents who eat eggs, milk products, and, on occasion, non–red meat is more healthful than that of their red-meat-eating peers (Grant et al., 2008).

ADULTS

- For many years, the WHO has recommended weekly iron folic acid supplementation for sexually active women of fertile age worldwide to prevent fetal birth defects.

OLDER ADULTS

Most older adults take several medications as a result of having an increase in the number of chronic illnesses. Considerations for potential problems include:

- Some foods interact adversely or decrease the effectiveness of certain medications, such as foods high in vitamin K and the

anticoagulant warfarin (Coumadin). Older adults should not change their diet significantly without consulting their healthcare provider because drug dosage may have been based on the older adult's previous dietary intake.
- Some medications increase appetite, such as glucocorticoids.
- Some medications decrease appetite by their actions or by causing an unpleasant taste.
- Certain tablets should not be crushed to be given by mouth or by gastric tubes, such as enteric-coated or slow-release medications.

Conditions such as neuromuscular disorders and dementia can make it difficult for older adults to eat or to be fed. Safety should always be a priority concern with attention paid to prevent aspiration. All healthcare personnel and family caregivers should be taught proper techniques to reduce this risk. Effective techniques include:

- Use the chin-tuck method when feeding clients with dysphagia. Having them flex the head toward the chest when swallowing decreases the risk of aspiration into the lungs.
- Use foods of prescribed consistency. Many older adults can swallow foods with thicker consistency more easily than thin liquids.
- Try to focus on food preferences—the family can help provide this information.
- Try to maintain mealtime as a positive social occasion with conversations and extra attention to having a pleasant environment.

Economic factors may influence older adults' nutritional status if they cannot afford food, especially if a prescribed diet requires expensive supplements. Inexpensive or convenience foods such as canned soups are often high in fat and sodium.

SKILL 12.2   Assisting an Adult to Eat

Clients may need assistance in preparing and consuming foods and liquids on their meal trays. This is an opportunity to observe the client's ability to self-feed and note any difficulties with chewing and swallowing. Further information about assisting the client can be found in Chapter 5, Skill 5.1, Variation: Serving a Food Tray.

Delegation

Assisting or feeding a client is often delegated to UAP. It is, however, the responsibility of the nurse to assess the client's ability to eat and to identify actual or potential risk factors that may affect

the client's nutritional status. The nurse must instruct the UAP about strategies that promote the client's nutritional health as well as the importance of the UAP reporting any unusual or different client behaviors to the nurse.

Equipment

- Meal tray with the correct food and fluids
- Extra napkin or small towel
- Straw, special drinking cup, weighted glass, or other adaptive feeding aid as required

(*continued on next page*)

SKILL 12.2   Assisting an Adult to Eat (*continued*)

Preparation

Prepare the client and overbed table.

- Assist the client to the bathroom or onto a bedpan or commode if the client needs to urinate.
- Offer the client assistance in washing the hands prior to a meal. If the client has problems with oral hygiene, brushing the teeth or using a mouthwash can improve the taste in the mouth and hence the appetite.
- Clear the overbed table so that there is space for the tray. If the client must remain in a lying position in bed, arrange the overbed table close to the bedside so that the client can see the food.

Procedure

1. Prior to feeding the client, introduce self and verify the client's identity using agency protocol. Explain to the client what you are going to do, why it is necessary, and how he or she can participate.
2. Perform hand hygiene and observe other appropriate infection control procedures.
3. Provide for client privacy if appropriate.
4. Position the client and yourself appropriately.
   - Assist the client to a comfortable position for eating. Most people sit during a meal; if it is permitted, assist the client to sit in bed ❶ or in a chair.

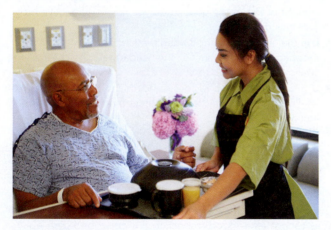

❶ A supported sitting position contributes to a client's comfort while eating. Monkey Business Images/Shutterstock

   - If the client is unable to sit, assist the client to a lateral position. **Rationale:** *It is easier to swallow in a lateral position than in a back-lying position.*
   - If the client requires assistance with feeding, assume a sitting position, if possible, beside the client. **Rationale:** *This conveys a more relaxed presence and encourages the client to eat an adequate meal.*
5. Assist the client as required.
   - Check tray for the client's name, the type of diet, and completeness. If the diet does not seem to be correct, check it against the client's chart. Do *not* leave an incorrect diet for a client to eat.
   - Encourage the client to eat independently, assisting as needed. Do not take over the feeding process. **Rationale:** *Participation by the client enhances feelings of independence.*

- Remove the food covers, butter the bread, pour the drink, and cut the meat, if needed.
- For a client with a visual impairment, identify the placement of the food as you would describe the time on a clock. For instance, say "The potatoes are at 8 o'clock, the chicken at 12 o'clock, and the green beans at 4 o'clock" ❷.

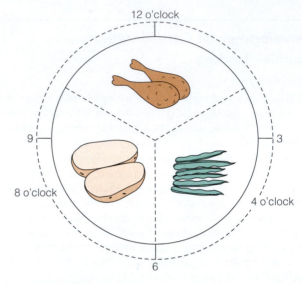

❷ For a client with a visual impairment, the nurse can use the clock system to describe the location of food on the plate.

- If the client needs assistance with feeding:
  a. Ask in which order the client desires to eat the food.
  b. Use normal utensils whenever possible. **Rationale:** *Using ordinary utensils enhances self-esteem.*
  c. If the client has a visual impairment, tell which food you are giving.
  d. Warn the client if the food is hot or cold.
  e. Allow ample time for the client to chew and swallow the food before offering more.
  f. Provide fluids as requested or, if the client is unable to ask, offer fluids after every three or four mouthfuls of solid food.
  g. Use a straw or special drinking cup for fluids that would spill from normal containers.
  h. Make the time a pleasant one, choosing topics of conversation that are of interest to the client, if the individual wants to talk.
6. After the meal, ensure client comfort.
   - Assist the client to clean the mouth and hands.
   - Reposition the client.
   - Replace the food covers and remove the food tray from the bedside.
7. Document all relevant information.
   - Note how much and what the client has eaten and the amount of fluid taken. In many agencies, nurses record the percent of the meal consumed, but describing the amount and size of individual items eaten provides greater accuracy.
   - Record fluid intake and calorie count as required. In a hospital or subacute inpatient setting, a calorie count is usually calculated by the dietary department. It is based on a

SKILL 12.2   Assisting an Adult to Eat (continued)

detailed list of foods and fluids consumed that has been recorded by nursing personnel.

- If the client is on a special diet or is having problems eating, record the amount of food eaten and any pain, fatigue, or nausea experienced.

- If the client is not eating, notify the nurse in charge so that the diet can be changed or other nursing measures can be taken (e.g., rescheduling the meals, providing small, more frequent meals, or obtaining special self-feeding aids).

Developmental Considerations

OLDER ADULTS

- Offer fluids frequently to prevent dry mouth. Initially avoid dry foods such as crackers and sticky foods such as bananas. **Rationale:** *Saliva production decreases with age.*
- Allow the older client time to eat and offer to rewarm the food if needed. **Rationale:** *Hand tremors and arthritic joint changes may slow the eating process for older clients.*
- Observe for dysphagia and adapt the older client's diet accordingly. **Rationale:** *Esophageal nerve degeneration, which often occurs with aging, can affect the ability to swallow.*
- Older clients may need extra seasoning on food. **Rationale:** *Aging decreases the ability to taste, especially sweet and salty foods.*

Setting of Care

- Assess the home for adequate facilities to prepare and store food such as a working refrigerator and stove.
- Assess the client's and caregiver's ability to obtain food and prepare meals.
- Evaluate problems that can interfere with eating such as ill-fitting dentures, sore gums, constipation, diarrhea, or a special diet.
- Instruct the caregiver about the importance of regular, nutritious meals and allowing the client to remain independent when possible.
- Provide written guidelines for the client's diet and any special feeding techniques.

SKILL 12.3   Assisting a Client with Dysphagia to Eat

Equipment

- Provision for oral care and hand hygiene
- Towel
- Penlight to inspect oral cavity
- Oral suction catheter connected to suction source

Preparation

- Note specific instructions for feeding technique (diet and positioning) prescribed by speech or swallowing specialist; for example, use cornstarch, Thickit, or rice cereal to thicken food, as prescribed. **Rationale:** *Clients with swallowing problems find it easier to swallow thickened liquids.*
- Check if client is receiving both oral and enteral feeding; stop the enteral solution about 1 hour before oral feeding.
- Check that client has not recently received sedating medication.
- Eliminate environmental distractors such as television, radio.
- Provide a 30-minute rest period before mealtime.
- Ensure that temperature of food is appropriate.

Procedure

1. Wash your hands.
2. Check client's identification and allergy bracelet and have client state name and birth date.
3. Provide client privacy.
4. Maintain bed in LOW position.
5. Assist client to sit upright (90°) in a chair or in bed with hips flexed, shoulders and face slightly forward, and chin parallel to the floor or slightly tucked. **Rationale:** *Gravity assists proper bolus movement to the stomach.*

Note: Prescribed position is different for specific forms of dysphagia. Some types of dysphagia necessitate client positioning to one side, or with head rotated toward the stronger or weaker side, or even side-lying. Instructions should be placed in client's record and care plan and posted at client's head of bed.

6. Assist client to perform hand hygiene before eating.
7. Place towel over client's chest.
8. Place tray on overbed table and towel under plate. **Rationale:** *This stabilizes plate while feeding.*
9. Suction oral secretions before feeding, if necessary.
10. Sit at client's side, or sit facing client.
11. Encourage self-feeding.
12. Instruct client to take (or offer) small portions of food at first (0.5 to 1 tsp at a time), bites manageable in size but large enough to require chewing.
13. Instruct client to eat food first, without accompanying liquid, reserving all liquid intake until after finishing food. **Rationale:** *Using liquids to wash down boluses of food pushes the food down too rapidly, although some authorities recommend alternating solids with liquids.*
14. Instruct client to perform an exaggerated sucking motion at the beginning of each swallow with chin tucked slightly. **Rationale:** *Decreases risk of aspiration.*
Note: Clients with advanced dementia may not remember how to chew or swallow. Demonstrating chewing and gently stroking the area under the client's chin with a downward motion during swallowing may be helpful cues.
15. Allow client to concentrate on swallowing without distractions such as conversation or television. **Rationale:** *For the client with dysphagia, swallowing takes concentration; talking increases risk for aspiration.*

(continued on next page)

SKILL 12.3   Assisting a Client with Dysphagia to Eat *(continued)*

16. Avoid rushed or forced feeding and make sure client is swallowing every mouthful.
17. Visually inspect oral cavity and under dentures for retained food. **Rationale:** *Buildup may occur on weak side of mouth or pharynx.*
18. Observe client closely for evidence of aspiration (e.g., cough, drooling, voice change such as hoarseness or a gurgling noise after swallowing), and suction oropharynx if indicated.

> **CLINICAL ALERT**
> The use of a straw increases risk of aspiration because the client with dysphagia has less control over the amount of fluid intake. Similarly, the client with dysphagia should not be fed with a syringe.

19. Help with feeding only if client shows signs of weakness, fatigue.
20. Provide positive reinforcement for accomplishment.
21. Assist with oral care and hand hygiene following meal. **Rationale:** *To reduce oral colonization with pathogens and risk of aspiration pneumonia.*
22. Remove food tray and raise side rails as indicated.
23. Place call bell within reach.
24. Document percentage of food eaten and amount of liquid intake (if indicated).
25. Maintain client's sitting position for 30 minutes after eating.
26. Carefully observe client with impaired communication for 30 minutes after the first few servings.

▶ ENTERAL NUTRITION USING A FEEDING TUBE

Alternative feeding methods to ensure adequate nutrition include enteral (through the gastrointestinal system) methods. **Enteral nutrition (EN)**, also referred to as **total enteral nutrition (TEN)**, is provided when the client is unable to ingest foods or the upper gastrointestinal tract is impaired but the remainder of the intestinal tract is functional. Enteral feedings are administered through nasogastric and small-bore feeding tubes, or through gastrostomy or jejunostomy tubes.

Expected Outcomes

1. Client's nutritional needs are met with nasogastric feeding.
2. Client's nutritional needs are met with continuous enteral feeding.
3. Gastrostomy tube site is free of signs of irritation/inflammation.
4. Client experiences no complications with nasogastric feeding.

SKILL 12.4   Inserting a Nasogastric Tube

Delegation

Insertion of a nasogastric tube is an invasive procedure requiring application of knowledge (e.g., anatomy and physiology, risk factors) and problem solving. In some agencies, only healthcare providers with advanced training are permitted to insert nasogastric tubes that require use of a stylet. Delegation of this skill to UAP is not appropriate. The UAP, however, can assist with the oral hygiene needs of a client with a nasogastric tube.

Equipment

- Large- or small-bore tube (nonlatex preferred)
- Nonallergenic adhesive tape, 2.5 cm (1 in.) wide
- Clean gloves
- Water-soluble lubricant
- Facial tissues
- Glass of water and drinking straw
- 20- to 50-mL syringe with an adapter
- Basin
- pH test strip or meter
- Bilirubin dipstick
- Stethoscope
- Disposable pad or towel
- Clamp or plug (optional)
- Antireflux valve for air vent if Salem sump tube is used
- Suction apparatus
- Safety pin and elastic band
- CO_2 detector (optional)

> **CLINICAL ALERT**
> Nurses never insert or withdraw an NG tube for clients recovering from gastric surgery. The suture line could be interrupted, or hemorrhage could occur. The physician should be notified of dislodgement.
>   Never insert an NG tube in a client after nasal, craniofacial, or hypophysectomy surgery.

Preparation

- Check physician's order.
- Assist the client to a high-Fowler position if the client's health condition permits, and support the head on a pillow. **Rationale:** *It is often easier to swallow in this position, and gravity helps the passage of the tube.*
- Place a towel or disposable pad across the chest.

Procedure

1. Prior to performing the insertion, introduce self and verify the client's identity using agency protocol. Explain to the client what you are going to do, why it is necessary, and how he or she can participate. The passage of a gastric tube is unpleasant because the gag reflex is activated during insertion. Establish a method for the client to indicate distress and a

SKILL 12.4   Inserting a Nasogastric Tube (*continued*)

desire for you to pause the insertion. Raising a finger or hand is often used for this.

2. Perform hand hygiene and observe other appropriate infection control procedures (e.g., clean gloves).
3. Provide for client privacy. Raise bed to appropriate height.
4. Assess the client's nares.
   - Apply clean gloves.
   - Ask the client to hyperextend the head and, using a flashlight, observe the intactness of the tissues of the nostrils, including any irritations or abrasions.
   - Examine the nares for any obstructions or deformities by asking the client to breathe through one nostril while occluding the other.
   - Select the nostril that has the greater airflow.
5. Prepare the tube.
   - If a small bowel feeding tube (SBFT) is being used, ensure the stylet or guidewire is secured in position. **Rationale:** *An improperly positioned stylet or guidewire can traumatize the nasopharynx, esophagus, and stomach.*
   - If a large-bore tube (e.g., Salem sump tube) is being used, place the tube in a basin of warm water while preparing the client. **Rationale:** *This allows the tubing to become more pliable and flexible.*
6. Determine how far to insert the tube. (Measure the tube.)
   - Use the tube to mark off the distance from the tip of the client's nose to the tip of the earlobe and then from the tip of the earlobe to the tip of the xiphoid ❶. **Rationale:** *This length approximates the distance from the nares to the stomach. This distance varies among individuals.*
   - Mark this length with adhesive tape if the tube does not have markings.

nose to numb the area (Durai, Venkatraman, & Ng, 2009). **Rationale:** *A water-soluble lubricant dissolves if the tube accidentally enters the lungs. An oil-based lubricant, such as petroleum jelly, will not dissolve and could cause respiratory complications if it enters the lungs.*

- Insert the tube, with its natural curve toward the client, into the selected nostril. Ask the client to hyperextend the neck, and gently advance the tube toward the nasopharynx. **Rationale:** *Hyperextension of the neck reduces the curvature of the nasopharyngeal junction.*
- Direct the tube along the floor of the nostril and toward the ear on that side. **Rationale:** *Directing the tube along the floor avoids the projections (turbinates) along the lateral wall.*
- Slight pressure and a twisting motion are sometimes required to pass the tube into the nasopharynx, and client's eyes may water at this point. **Rationale:** *Tears are a natural body response.* Provide the client with tissues as needed.
- If the tube meets resistance, withdraw it, relubricate it, and insert it in the other nostril. **Rationale:** *The tube should never be forced against resistance because of the danger of injury.*
- Once the tube reaches the oropharynx (throat), the client will feel the tube in the throat and may gag and retch. Ask the client to tilt the head forward, and encourage the client to drink and swallow ❷. **Rationale:** *Tilting the head forward facilitates passage of the tube into the posterior pharynx and esophagus rather than into the larynx; swallowing moves the epiglottis over the opening to the larynx.*

❶ Measuring the appropriate length for a nasogastric tube.

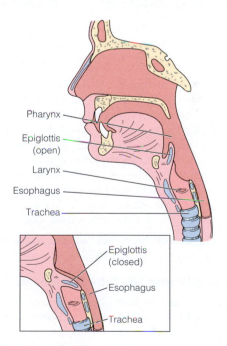

❷ Swallowing closes the epiglottis.

7. Insert the tube.
   - Lubricate the tip of the tube well with water-soluble lubricant or water to ease insertion. In some agencies, topical lidocaine anesthetic is used on the tube or in the client's

- If the client gags, stop passing the tube momentarily. Have the client rest, take a few breaths, and take sips of water to calm the gag reflex.

(*continued on next page*)

SKILL 12.4   Inserting a Nasogastric Tube (*continued*)

- In cooperation with the client, pass the tube 5 to 10 cm (2 to 4 in.) with each swallow, until the indicated length is inserted.
- If the client continues to gag and the tube does not advance with each swallow, withdraw it slightly, and inspect the throat by looking through the mouth. **Rationale:** *The tube may be coiled in the throat. If so, withdraw it until it is straight, and try again to insert it.*
- If a CO_2 detector is used, after the tube has been advanced approximately 30 cm (12 in.), draw air through the detector. Any change in color of the detector indicates placement of the tube in the respiratory tract. Immediately withdraw the tube and reinsert ❸.

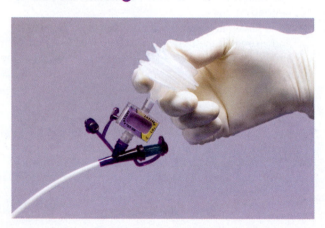

❸ After drawing air into the tube using a syringe or attached bellows, match the sensor color to the legend on the detector. This example shows purple—no CO_2 present.

8. Ascertain correct placement of the tube.
   - Aspirate stomach contents, and check the pH, which should be acidic. **Rationale:** *Testing pH is one way to determine location of a feeding tube. Gastric contents are commonly pH 1 to 5; pH of 6 or greater would indicate the contents are from lower in the intestinal tract or in the respiratory tract. However, pH of esophageal aspirates can also be low (de Aguilar-Nascimento & Kudsk, 2007). Some researchers suggest that a pH of greater than 5 should be followed by further confirmation of tube location (Stock, Gilbertson, & Babl, 2008).*

Evidence-Based Nursing Practice

Determining Proper NG Tube Placement

A number of methods have been proposed to determine whether a tube has been inadvertently placed into the pulmonary tree, including air insufflation, observation of respiratory symptoms, pH testing of aspirated fluid, visual inspection of aspirated fluid, detection of carbon dioxide in the tube, and x-ray tube location verification. The best method of confirming the location of a blindly inserted gastrointestinal tube is by chest/abdominal x-ray.

Source: Rauen et al. (2008).

- Aspirate can also be tested for bilirubin. Bilirubin levels in the lungs should be almost zero, while levels in the stomach will be approximately 1.5 mg/dL and in the intestine over 10 mg/dL.
- Almost all nasogastric tubes are radiopaque, and position can be confirmed by x-ray. Check agency policy. If a SBFT is used, leave the stylet or guidewire in place until correct position is verified by x-ray.

- Place a stethoscope over the client's epigastrium and inject 5 to 20 mL of air into the tube while listening for a whooshing sound. Although still one of the methods used, do not use this method as the *primary* method for determining placement of the feeding tube. **Rationale:** *This method does not guarantee tube position.*
- If the signs indicate placement in the lungs, remove the tube and begin again.
- If the signs do not indicate placement in the lungs or stomach, advance the tube 5 cm (2 in.), and repeat the tests.

9. Secure the tube by taping it to the bridge of the client's nose.
   - If the client has oily skin, wipe the nose first with alcohol to defat the skin.
   - Cut 7.5 cm (3 in.) of tape, and split it lengthwise at one end, leaving a 2.5-cm (1-in.) tab at the end.
   - Place the tape over the bridge of the client's nose, and bring the split ends either under and around the tubing, or under the tubing and back up over the nose ❹. Ensure that the tube is centrally located prior to securing with tape to maximize airflow and prevent irritation to the side of the nares. **Rationale:** *Taping in this manner prevents the tube from pressing against and irritating the edge of the nostril.*

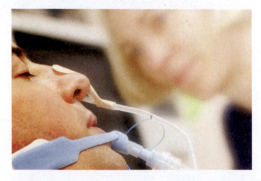

❹ A nasogastric tube taped to the bridge of the nose.
Bodenham, LTH NHS Trust/Science Source

10. Once correct position has been determined, attach the tube to a suction source or feeding apparatus as ordered, or clamp the end of the tubing.
11. Secure the tube to the client's gown.
    - Loop an elastic band around the end of the tubing, and attach the elastic band to the gown with a safety pin.

SKILL 12.4   Inserting a Nasogastric Tube (*continued*)

or

- Attach a piece of adhesive tape to the tube, and pin the tape to the gown. **Rationale:** *The tube is attached to prevent it from dangling and pulling.* If a Salem sump tube is used, attach the antireflux valve to the vent port (if used) and position the port above the client's waist. **Rationale:** *This prevents gastric contents from flowing into the vent lumen.*
- Remove and discard gloves. Perform hand hygiene. Return bed to lowest position.

12. Document relevant information: the insertion of the tube, the means by which correct placement was determined, and client responses (e.g., discomfort or abdominal distention).

13. Establish a plan for providing daily nasogastric tube care.
- Inspect the nostril for discharge and irritation.
- Clean the nostril and tube with moistened, cotton-tipped applicators.
- Apply water-soluble lubricant to the nostril if it appears dry or encrusted.
- Change the adhesive tape as required to secure the tube and prevent skin trauma from either tape or pressure of the tube against the nares.
- Give frequent mouth care. Due to the presence of the tube, the client may breathe through the mouth.

14. If suction is applied, ensure that the patency of both the nasogastric and suction tubes is maintained.
- Irrigations of the tube may be required at regular intervals. In some agencies, irrigations must be ordered by the primary care provider. Prior to irrigation, always recheck placement.
- If a Salem sump tube is used, follow agency policies for irrigating the vent lumen with air to maintain patency of the suctioning lumen. Often, a sucking sound can be heard from the vent port if it is patent.
- Keep accurate records of the client's fluid intake and output, and record the amount and characteristics of the drainage.

15. Document the type of tube inserted, date and time of tube insertion, type of suction used, color and amount of gastric contents, and the client's tolerance of the procedure.

Sample Documentation

11/5/15 1030 Feeding tube (8 Fr) inserted without difficulty through (R) nare with stylet in place. To x-ray to check placement. Radiologist reports tube tip in stomach. Stylet removed. Aspirate pH 4. Tube secured to nose. Verbalizes understanding of need to not pull on tube
_____ L. Traynor, RN

Gastric (Salem) Sump Pump

The gastric Salem tube is a double-lumen radiopaque plastic tube. One lumen is used for decompression. The blue lumen with a blue pigtail provides an air vent to allow atmospheric pressure to enter the stomach to prevent tube adherence to gastric mucosa when the tube is attached to suction. It is NOT used for irrigation, obtaining a specimen, etc. However, if the vent lumen is blocked and requires flushing, after the flush, the pigtail should be cleared with an injection of 20 mL air. The pigtail should be kept above the level of the client's stomach to prevent stomach contents from siphoning into the air vent lumen, making it dysfunctional.

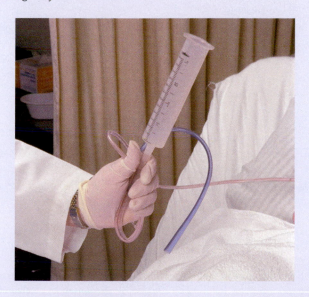

Developmental Considerations

INFANTS AND YOUNG CHILDREN

- Restraints may be necessary during tube insertion and throughout therapy. **Rationale:** *Restraints will prevent accidental dislodging of the tube.*
- Place the infant in an infant seat or position the infant with a rolled towel or pillow under the head and shoulders.
- When assessing the nares, obstruct one of the infant's nares and feel for air passage from the other. If the nasal passageway is very small or is obstructed, an orogastric tube may be more appropriate.
- Measure appropriate nasogastric tube length from the nose to the tip of the earlobe and then to the point midway between the umbilicus and the xiphoid process.
- If an orogastric tube is used, measure from the tip of the earlobe to the corner of the mouth to the xiphoid process.
- Do not hyperextend or hyperflex an infant's neck. **Rationale:** *Hyperextension or hyperflexion of the neck could occlude the airway.*
- Tape the tube to the area between the end of the nares and the upper lip as well as to the cheek.

SKILL 12.5 Flushing/Maintaining a Nasogastric Tube

Equipment

- Disposable irrigation set with 50-mL syringe with catheter tip
- Emesis basin
- Towel
- Normal saline irrigation solution
- I&O record sheet
- Clean gloves

Preparation

- Check physician's orders and client care plan.
- Perform hand hygiene.
- Check client's identification and have client state name and birth date.
- Provide privacy.
- Explain procedure to client.
- Place client in semi-Fowler position. Position bed at an appropriate level.

Procedure

1. Don clean gloves.
2. Disconnect NG tube from suction source if used.
3. Place towel under NG tube to protect sheets and place emesis basin nearby.
4. Check for NG tube placement ❶. **Rationale:** *Solution could be instilled in lungs if NG tube is not in the stomach.*
5. Draw up 20 to 30 mL normal saline into irrigating syringe.
6. Gently instill normal saline (NS) into NG tube or remove syringe plunger, pour NS into syringe barrel, and allow solution to flow in by gravity ❷.

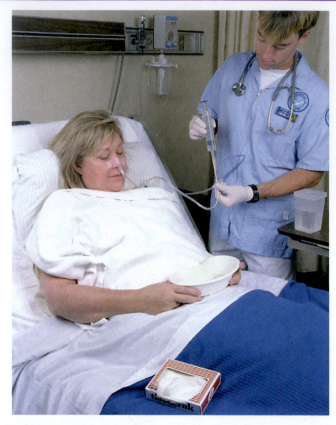

❷ Gently instill normal saline into NG tube by syringe, or allow solution to flow by gravity.

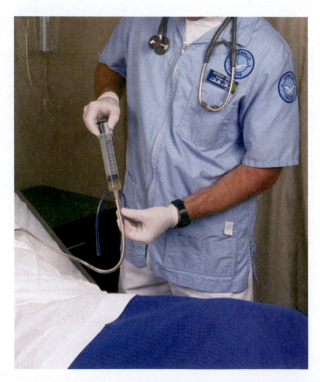

❶ Aspirate secretions to check tube placement before instilling saline solution.

CLINICAL ALERT

- If water rather than normal saline is used to flush enteral decompression tubes, the production of gastric secretions will increase and increasing amounts of electrolytes will be washed out. Similarly, if the client is NPO but ingests ice chips ad lib, electrolyte imbalance due to washout can occur, causing metabolic alkalosis.
- Limit the use of ice chips by substituting chips made from an electrolyte solution, and provide oral hygiene to keep the client's mucous membranes moist for comfort.
- If the client is receiving adequate parenteral hydration (IV fluids), excessive thirst should not be experienced.

7. Repeat procedure if necessary.
8. Reconnect NG tube to suction or plug tube.
9. Document instilled amount on I&O record.
10. Remove and discard gloves. Perform hand hygiene. Place bed in lowest position.
11. Reposition client for comfort.

CLINICAL ALERT

If secretions siphon into blue vent lumen, clear it by instilling 20 mL of normal saline followed by 20 mL of air. Air vent must be cleared of secretions to restore proper functioning.

SKILL 12.6   Performing Gastric Lavage

Equipment

- Large-bore (37- to 40-Fr) soft Ewald or orogastric tube (*Note:* Client must have cuffed endotracheal tube in place if comatose.)
- Large irrigating syringe with adapter
- Container for aspirate
- Lavage fluid, normal saline, or lukewarm water
- Activated charcoal for drug/toxin adsorption
- Container for specimen
- Water-soluble lubricant
- Standby suction available
- Towel
- Pen and tape
- Gloves

Preparation

- Check physician's orders for gastric lavage and solution to be used.
- Determine if client is alert or comatose.
- Gather equipment.

Procedure

1. After entering, introduce self, explain what procedure will be done, and why. Perform hand hygiene and don gloves, follow infection control measures, and verify client's identity. Provide privacy for the client. Provide comfort and safety for client and yourself, including raising bed to appropriate height for procedure.
2. Per agency protocol (physician may insert) measure for tube insertion using the following guidelines.
   - Measure distance from bridge of nose to earlobe to xiphoid process (NEX).
   - Mark with pen or tape.
3. Place client in head-down, left side-lying position. **Rationale:** *This reduces risk of aspiration if client vomits.*

4. Lubricate tube with water-soluble lubricant.
5. Insert tube nasogastrically or orogastrically, about 50 cm (20 in.).
6. Aspirate gastric contents with syringe before instilling solution. Save specimen for analysis.
7. Repeatedly instill 50 to 100 mL normal saline or water and aspirate contents. **Rationale:** *Some authorities recommend water to lavage the stomach of blood since it breaks up clots more easily than saline solution, is less expensive, and is readily available.*

CLINICAL ALERT
Gastric lavage used to remove unabsorbed poison or drug ingestion is generally ineffective if more than 60 minutes have passed, and the procedure may delay administration of activated charcoal or antidotes; therefore, it is not recommended to manage overdose. It is not used for corrosive agents or petroleum distillates due to risk of aspiration, and induced vomiting is no longer considered safe.

8. Carefully monitor volume instilled and character and volume of aspirated contents. **Rationale:** *This will assist in determining net volume if there is blood loss.*
9. Continue repeating process until gastric return is clear, or as ordered.
10. Stomach will be left empty for decontamination. Activated charcoal may be instilled (as ordered) or a saline cathartic may be given. **Rationale:** *Activated charcoal adsorbs drugs in the stomach or intestine.*
11. Pinch tube for removal, wrap in towel, and dispose of equipment.
12. Remove and discard gloves. Perform hand hygiene. Return bed to lowest height.
13. Document procedure and client response. Record vital signs frequently and monitor client's response closely.

SKILL 12.7   Removing a Nasogastric Tube

Delegation

Due to the need for assessment of client status, the skill of removing a nasogastric tube is not delegated to UAP.

Equipment

- Disposable pad or towel
- Tissues
- Clean gloves
- 50-mL syringe (optional)
- Plastic trash bag

Preparation

- Confirm the primary care provider's order to remove the tube.
- Assist the client to a sitting position if health permits.
- Place the disposable pad or towel across the client's chest to collect any spillage of secretions from the tube.

- Provide tissues to the client to wipe the nose and mouth after tube removal.

Procedure

1. Prior to performing the removal, introduce self and verify the client's identity using agency protocol. Explain to the client what you are going to do, why it is necessary, and how he or she can participate.
2. Perform hand hygiene and observe other appropriate infection control procedures (e.g., clean gloves).
3. Provide for client privacy. Position bed at appropriate height for the procedure.
4. Detach the tube.
   - Apply clean gloves.
   - Disconnect the nasogastric tube from the suction apparatus, if present.
   - Unpin the tube from the client's gown.
   - Remove the adhesive tape securing the tube to the nose.

(continued on next page)

SKILL 12.7 Removing a Nasogastric Tube (continued)

5. Remove the nasogastric tube.
   - *Optional:* Instill 50 mL of air into the tube. **Rationale:** *This clears the tube of any contents such as feeding or gastric drainage and decreases the chances of dragging any drainage through the esophagus and nasopharynx.*
   - Ask the client to take a deep breath and to hold it. **Rationale:** *This closes the glottis, thereby preventing accidental aspiration of any gastric contents.*
   - Pinch the tube with the gloved hand. **Rationale:** *Pinching the tube prevents any contents inside the tube from draining into the client's throat.*
   - Smoothly withdraw the tube.
   - Place the tube in the plastic bag. **Rationale:** *Placing the tube immediately into the bag prevents the transference of microorganisms from the tube to other articles or people.*
   - Observe the intactness of the tube.
6. Ensure client comfort.
   - Provide mouth care if desired.
   - Assist the client as required to blow the nose. **Rationale:** *Excessive secretions may have accumulated in the nasal passages.*
7. Dispose of the equipment appropriately.
   - Place the pad, bag with tube, and gloves in the receptacle designated by the agency. **Rationale:** *Correct disposal prevents the transmission of microorganisms.*
   - Place bed in lowest position. Remove and discard gloves. Perform hand hygiene.
8. Document all relevant information.
   - Record the removal of the tube, the amount and appearance of any drainage if connected to suction, and any relevant assessments of the client.

Sample Documentation

11/8/15 1500 NG tube removed intact s̄ difficulty. Oral & nasal care given. No bleeding or excoriation noted. States is hungry & thirsty. 60 mL apple juice given. No c/o nausea. _____ L. Traynor, RN

Evidence-Based Nursing Practice

Postoperative GI Motility

Nurses in a practice project discontinued bowel sound assessment to determine the return of gastrointestinal motility after abdominal surgery, since bowel sounds reflect the normal activity of the small intestine alone but do not represent return of functional GI motility. Primary indicators of the return of GI motility include the return of flatus, bowel movement, client's tolerance of oral intake without nausea or vomiting, return of appetite, and absence of abdominal distention, bloated feeling, and cramps. Recent work on early feeding and reducing the routine use of nasogastric tubes has also contributed to a growing body of evidence on recovery of postoperative GI motility.

Source: Madsen et al. (2005).

SKILL 12.8 Administering a Tube Feeding

Delegation

Administering a tube feeding requires application of knowledge and problem solving and it is not usually delegated to UAP. Some agencies, however, may allow a trained UAP to administer a feeding. In this case, it is the responsibility of the nurse to assess tube placement and determine that the tube is patent. The nurse should reinforce major points, such as making sure the client is sitting upright, and instruct the UAP to report any difficulty administering the feeding or any complaints voiced by the client.

Equipment

- Correct type and amount of feeding solution
- 60-mL catheter-tip syringe
- Emesis basin
- Clean gloves
- pH test strip or meter
- Large syringe or calibrated plastic feeding bag with label and tubing that can be attached to the feeding tube or prefilled bottle with a drip chamber, tubing, and a flow-regulator clamp
- Measuring container from which to pour the feeding (if using open system)
- Water (60 mL unless otherwise specified) at room temperature
- Feeding pump as required

CLINICAL ALERT

Do not add colored food dye to tube feedings. Previously, blue dye was often added to assist in recognition of aspiration. However, the U.S. Food and Drug Administration reports cases of many adverse reactions to the dye, including toxicity and death.

Preparation

- Check physician's order.
- Assist the client to a Fowler position (at least 30 degrees elevation) in bed or a sitting position in a chair, the normal position for eating. If a sitting position is contraindicated, a slightly elevated right side-lying position is acceptable. **Rationale:** *These positions enhance the gravitational flow of the solution and prevent aspiration of fluid into the lungs.*

Procedure

1. Prior to performing the feeding, introduce self and verify the client's identity using agency protocol. Explain to the client what you are going to do, why it is necessary, and how he or she can participate. Inform the client that the feeding should not cause any discomfort but may cause a feeling of fullness.
2. Perform hand hygiene and observe other appropriate infection control procedures.
3. Provide privacy for this procedure if the client desires it. **Rationale:** *Tube feedings are embarrassing to some people.*

SKILL 12.8   Administering a Tube Feeding (*continued*)

4. Assess tube placement prior to initiating a feeding or three times per day for continuous feedings.
   - Apply clean gloves.
   - Examine the placement mark on the tube to determine if it has advanced or slipped out.
   - Attach the syringe to the open end of the tube and aspirate. Check the pH.
   - Allow 1 hour to elapse before testing the pH if the client has received a medication.
   - Use a pH meter rather than pH paper if the client is receiving a continuous feeding. Follow agency policy if the pH is 6 or greater.
5. Assess residual feeding contents.
   - If the tube is placed in the stomach, aspirate all contents and measure the amount before administering the feeding. **Rationale:** *This is done to evaluate absorption of the last feeding; that is, whether undigested formula from a previous feeding remains. If the tube is in the small intestine, residual contents cannot be aspirated.*
   - If 100 mL (or more than half of the last feeding) is withdrawn, check with the nurse in charge or refer to agency policy before proceeding. The precise amount of residual requiring intervention is usually determined by the primary care provider's order or by agency policy. **Rationale:** *At some agencies, a feeding is delayed when the specified amount or more of formula remains in the stomach.*

   or

   - Reinstill the gastric contents into the stomach if this is the agency policy or primary care provider's order. **Rationale:** *Removal of the contents could disturb the client's electrolyte balance.*
   - If the client is on a continuous feeding, check the gastric residual every 4 to 6 hours or according to agency protocol.
6. Administer the feeding.
   - Before administering feeding:
     a. Check the expiration date of the feeding.
     b. Warm the feeding to room temperature. **Rationale:** *An excessively cold feeding may cause abdominal cramps.*
     c. When an open system is used, clean the top of the feeding container with alcohol before opening it. **Rationale:** *This minimizes the risk of contaminants entering the feeding syringe or feeding bag.*

VARIATION: FEEDING BAG (OPEN SYSTEM)

- Hang the labeled bag from an infusion pole about 30 cm (12 in.) above the tube's point of insertion into the client.
- Clamp the tubing and add the formula to the bag.
  - Apply a label that indicates the date, time of starting the feeding, and nurse's initials on the feeding bag.
- Open the clamp, run the formula through the tubing, and reclamp the tube. **Rationale:** *The formula will displace the air in the tubing, thus preventing the instillation of excess air into the client's stomach or intestine.*
- Attach the bag to the feeding tube ❶ and regulate the drip by adjusting the clamp to the drop factor on the bag (e.g., 20 drops/mL) if not placed on a pump.

VARIATION: SYRINGE (OPEN SYSTEM)

- Remove the plunger from the syringe and connect the syringe to a pinched or clamped nasogastric tube. **Rationale:** *Pinching*

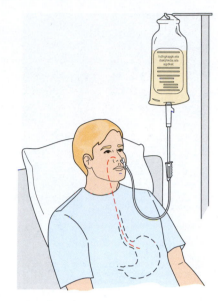

❶ Using a calibrated plastic bag to administer a tube feeding.

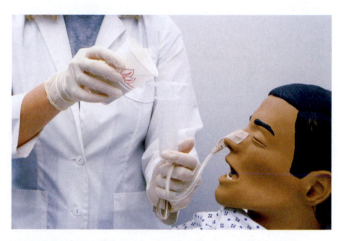

❷ Using the barrel of a syringe to administer a tube feeding.

or clamping the tube prevents excess air from entering the stomach and causing distention.

- Add the feeding to the syringe barrel ❷.
- Permit the feeding to flow in slowly at the prescribed rate. Raise or lower the syringe to adjust the flow as needed. Pinch or clamp the tubing to stop the flow for a minute if the client experiences discomfort. **Rationale:** *Quickly administered feedings can cause flatus, cramps, and/or vomiting.*

VARIATION: PREFILLED BOTTLE WITH DRIP CHAMBER (CLOSED SYSTEM)

- Remove the screw-on cap from the container and attach the administration set with the drip chamber and tubing ❸.
- Close the clamp on the tubing.
- Hang the container on an intravenous pole about 30 cm (12 in.) above the tube's insertion point into the client. **Rationale:** *At this height, the formula should run at a safe rate into the stomach or intestine.*
- Squeeze the drip chamber to fill it to one third to one half of its capacity.

(continued on next page)

SKILL 12.8 Administering a Tube Feeding *(continued)*

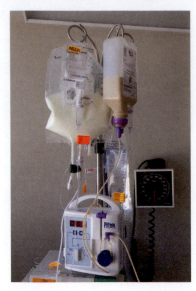

❸ Infusion pumps delivering tube feeding and total parenteral nutrition. Copyright © Slaven MD/Custom Medical Stock Photo—All rights reserved.

■ Open the tubing clamp, run the formula through the tubing, and reclamp the tube. **Rationale:** *The formula will displace the air in the tubing, thus preventing the instillation of excess air.*

■ Attach the feeding set tubing to the feeding tube and regulate the drip rate to deliver the feeding over the desired length of time or attach to a feeding pump.

7. If another bottle is not to be immediately hung, flush the feeding tube before all of the formula has run through the tubing.
   • Instill 50 to 100 mL of water through the feeding tube or medication port. **Rationale:** *Water flushes the lumen of the tube, preventing future blockage by sticky formula.*
   • Be sure to add the water before the feeding solution has drained from the neck of a syringe or from the tubing of an administration set. **Rationale:** *Adding the water before the syringe or tubing is empty prevents the instillation of air into the stomach or intestine and thus prevents unnecessary distention.*

8. Clamp the feeding tube.
   • Clamp the feeding tube before all of the water is instilled. **Rationale:** *Clamping prevents leakage and air from entering the tube if done before water is instilled.*

9. Ensure client comfort and safety.
   • Secure the tubing to the client's gown. **Rationale:** *This minimizes pulling of the tube, thus preventing discomfort and dislodgment.*
   • Ask the client to remain sitting upright in Fowler position or in a slightly elevated right lateral position for at least 30

minutes. **Rationale:** *These positions facilitate digestion and movement of the feeding from the stomach along the alimentary tract, and prevent the potential aspiration of the feeding into the lungs.*
   • Check the agency's policy on the frequency of changing the nasogastric tube and the use of smaller lumen tubes if a large-bore tube is in place. **Rationale:** *These measures prevent irritation and erosion of the pharyngeal and esophageal mucous membranes.*
   • Remove and discard gloves. Perform hand hygiene.

10. Dispose of equipment appropriately.
    • If the equipment is to be reused, wash it thoroughly with soap and water so that it is ready for reuse.
    • Change the equipment every 24 hours or according to agency policy.
    • Remove and discard gloves. Perform hand hygiene.

11. Document all relevant information.
    • Document the feeding, including amount and kind of solution taken, duration of the feeding, and assessments of the client.
    • Record the volume of the feeding and water administered on the client's intake and output record.

12. Monitor the client for possible problems.
    • Carefully assess client receiving tube feedings for problems.
    • To prevent dehydration, give the client supplemental water in addition to the prescribed tube feeding as ordered.

VARIATION: CONTINUOUS-DRIP FEEDING

■ Interrupt the feeding at least every 4 to 6 hours, or as indicated by agency protocol or the manufacturer, and aspirate and measure the gastric contents. **Rationale:** *This determines adequate absorption and verifies correct placement of the tube. If placement of an SBFT is questionable, a repeat x-ray should be done.*

■ Determine agency protocol regarding withholding a feeding. Many agencies withhold the feeding if more than 75 to 100 mL of feeding is aspirated. If the feeding is withheld, flush the tubing with water to prevent formula from clogging the tube.

■ To prevent spoilage or bacterial contamination, do not allow the feeding solution to hang longer than 4 to 8 hours. Check agency policy or manufacturer's recommendations regarding time limits.

■ Follow agency policy regarding how frequently to change the feeding bag and tubing. Changing the feeding bag and tubing every 24 hours reduces the risk of contamination.

Sample Documentation

11/5/15 1330 Aspirated 20 mL pale yellow fluid from NG tube, pH 5. Returned residual. Placed in Fowler position. 1 liter room-temperature ordered formula begun @ 60 mL/hour on pump. No nausea reported.
—————————————————— L. Traynor, RN

Client Teaching

Clients and caregivers need the following instructions to manage these feedings:

■ *Preparation of the formula.* Include name of the formula and how much and how often it is to be given; the need to inspect the formula for expiration date and leaks and cracks in bags or cans; how to mix or prepare the formula, if needed; and aseptic techniques such as swabbing the container's top with alcohol before

opening it, and changing the syringe administration set and reservoir every 24 hours.

■ *Proper storage of the formula.* Include the need to refrigerate diluted or reconstituted formula and formula that contains additives.

■ *Administration of the feeding.* Include proper hand washing technique; how to fill and hang the feeding bag; operation of an

SKILL 12.8 Administering a Tube Feeding *(continued)*

infusion pump, if indicated; the feeding rate; and client positioning during and after the feeding.

- *Management of the enteral access device.* Include site care; aseptic precautions; dressing change, as indicated; how the site should look normally; and flushing protocols (e.g., type of irrigant and schedule).

- *Daily monitoring needs.* Include temperature, weight, and intake and output.

- *Signs and symptoms of complications to report.* Include fever, increased respiratory rate, decrease in urine output, increased stool frequency, and altered level of consciousness.

- *Whom to contact about questions or problems.* Include emergency telephone numbers of home care agency, nursing clinician, and/or primary care provider, or other 24-hour on-call emergency service.

Developmental Considerations

INFANTS

- Feeding tubes may be reinserted at each feeding to prevent irritation of the mucous membrane, nasal airway obstruction, and stomach perforation that may occur if the tube is left in place continuously. Check agency practice.

CHILDREN

- Position a small child or infant in your lap, provide a pacifier, and hold and cuddle the child during feedings. This promotes comfort, supports the normal sucking instinct of the infant, and facilitates digestion.

OLDER ADULTS

- Physiological changes associated with aging may make the older adult more vulnerable to complications associated with enteral feedings. Decreased gastric emptying may necessitate checking frequently for gastric residual. Diarrhea from administering the feeding too fast or at too high a concentration may cause dehydration. If the feeding has a high concentration of glucose, assess for hyperglycemia because with aging, the body has a decreased ability to handle increased glucose levels.

- Conditions such as hiatal hernia and diabetes mellitus may cause the stomach to empty more slowly. This increases the risk of aspiration in a client receiving a tube feeding. Checking for gastric residual more frequently can help document this if it is an ongoing problem. Changing the formula or the rate of administration, repositioning the client, or obtaining a primary care provider's order for a medication to increase stomach emptying may resolve this problem.

Setting of Care

- Teach and provide the client or caregiver the rationale for how to assess for tube placement using pH measurement before administering the feeding. Instruct regarding actions to take if the pH is greater than 5.

- Provide instructions and rationale for care of the tube and insertion site.

- Discuss strategies for hanging formula containers if an IV pole is unavailable or inconvenient.

- Plan for optimal timing of feedings to allow for daily activities. Many clients can tolerate having the majority of their feedings run during sleep so they are free from the equipment during the day.

- Teach signs and symptoms to report to the primary care provider or home health nurse.

SKILL 12.9 Administering a Gastrostomy or Jejunostomy Feeding

Planning

Before commencing a gastrostomy or jejunostomy feeding, determine the type and amount of feeding to be instilled, frequency of feedings, and any pertinent information about previous feedings (e.g., the positioning in which the client best tolerates the feeding).

Equipment

- Correct amount of feeding solution
- Graduated container and tubing with clamp to hold the feeding
- 60-mL catheter-tip syringe

For a Tube That Remains in Place

- Mild soap and water
- Clean gloves
- Petrolatum, zinc oxide ointment, or other skin protectant
- Precut 4 × 4 gauze squares
- Uncut 4 × 4 gauze squares

For Tube Insertion

- Clean gloves
- Moisture-proof bag
- Water-soluble lubricant
- Feeding tube (if needed)

Preparation

- Check physician's order. Review steps in Skill 12.8, Administering a Tube Feeding.

Procedure

1. Prior to performing the feeding, introduce self and verify the client's identity using agency protocol. Explain to the client what you are going to do, why it is necessary, and how he or she can participate ❶.

2. Perform hand hygiene and observe other appropriate infection control procedures.

(continued on next page)

SKILL 12.9 Administering a Gastrostomy or Jejunostomy Feeding (*continued*)

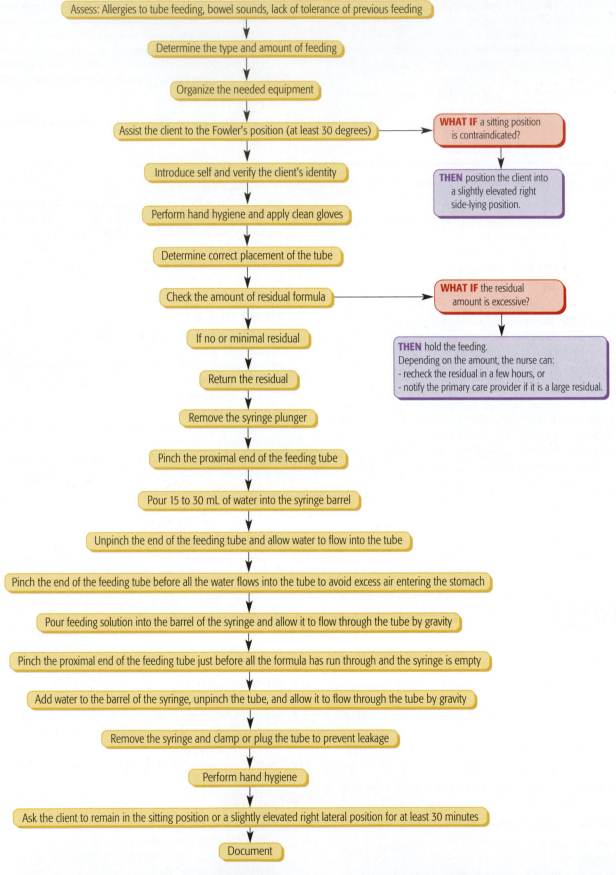

Assess: Allergies to tube feeding, bowel sounds, lack of tolerance of previous feeding

Determine the type and amount of feeding

Organize the needed equipment

Assist the client to the Fowler's position (at least 30 degrees)

WHAT IF a sitting position is contraindicated?

THEN position the client into a slightly elevated right side-lying position.

Introduce self and verify the client's identity

Perform hand hygiene and apply clean gloves

Determine correct placement of the tube

Check the amount of residual formula

WHAT IF the residual amount is excessive?

THEN hold the feeding. Depending on the amount, the nurse can:
- recheck the residual in a few hours, or
- notify the primary care provider if it is a large residual.

If no or minimal residual

Return the residual

Remove the syringe plunger

Pinch the proximal end of the feeding tube

Pour 15 to 30 mL of water into the syringe barrel

Unpinch the end of the feeding tube and allow water to flow into the tube

Pinch the end of the feeding tube before all the water flows into the tube to avoid excess air entering the stomach

Pour feeding solution into the barrel of the syringe and allow it to flow through the tube by gravity

Pinch the proximal end of the feeding tube just before all the formula has run through and the syringe is empty

Add water to the barrel of the syringe, unpinch the tube, and allow it to flow through the tube by gravity

Remove the syringe and clamp or plug the tube to prevent leakage

Perform hand hygiene

Ask the client to remain in the sitting position or a slightly elevated right lateral position for at least 30 minutes

Document

❶ Administering a gastrostomy feeding using an open system.

SKILL 12.9   Administering a Gastrostomy or Jejunostomy Feeding (continued)

3. Provide for client privacy. Raise bed to appropriate height for the procedure.
4. Assess and prepare the client.
   - Apply clean gloves.
5. Insert a feeding tube, if one is not already in place.
   - Remove the dressing. Then discard the dressing and gloves in the moisture-proof bag. Perform hand hygiene.
   - Apply new clean gloves.
   - Lubricate the end of the tube, and insert it into the ostomy opening 10 to 15 cm (4 to 6 in.).
6. Check the location and patency of a tube that is already in place.
   - Determine correct placement of the tube by aspirating secretions and checking the pH of the return.
   - Follow agency policy for amount of residual formula. This may include withholding the feeding, rechecking in 3 to 4 hours, or notifying the primary care provider if a large residual remains.
   - For continuous feedings, check the residual every 4 to 6 hours and hold feedings according to agency policy.
   - Remove the syringe plunger. Pour 15 to 30 mL of water into the syringe, remove the tube clamp, and allow the water to flow into the tube. **Rationale:** *This determines the patency of the tube. If water flows freely, the tube is patent.*
   - If the water does not flow freely, notify the nurse in charge and/or primary care provider.
7. Administer the feeding.
   - Hold the barrel of the syringe 7 to 15 cm (3 to 6 in.) above the ostomy opening.
   - Slowly pour the solution into the syringe and allow it to flow through the tube by gravity.
   - Just before all of the formula has run through and the syringe is empty, add 30 mL of water. **Rationale:** *Water flushes the tube and preserves its patency.*
   - If the tube is to remain in place, hold it upright, remove the syringe, and then clamp or plug the tube to prevent leakage.
   - If a catheter was inserted for the feeding, remove it.

- Remove and discard gloves. Perform hand hygiene. Reposition bed to lowest height.
8. Ensure client comfort and safety.
   - After the feeding, ask the client to remain in the sitting position or a slightly elevated right lateral position for at least 30 minutes. **Rationale:** *This minimizes the risk of aspiration.*
   - Assess status of peristomal skin. **Rationale:** *Gastric or jejunal drainage contains digestive enzymes that can irritate the skin.* Document any redness and broken skin areas.
   - Check orders about cleaning the peristomal skin, applying a skin protectant, and applying appropriate dressings. Generally, the peristomal skin is washed with mild soap and water at least once daily. The tube may be rotated between thumb and forefinger to release any sticking and promote tract formation. Petrolatum, zinc oxide ointment, or other skin protectant may be applied around the stoma, and precut 4 × 4 gauze squares may be placed around the tube. The precut squares are then covered with regular 4 × 4 gauze squares, and the tube is coiled over them.
   - Observe for common complications of enteral feedings: aspiration, hyperglycemia, abdominal distention, diarrhea, and fecal impaction. Report findings to primary care provider. Often, a change in formula or rate of administration can correct problems.
   - When appropriate, teach the client how to administer feedings and when to notify the primary care provider concerning problems.
9. Document all assessments and interventions.

Sample Documentation

1/24/15 2045 No fluid aspirated from gastrostomy tube. Placed in Fowler position. 30 mL water flowed freely by gravity through tube. 250 mL room-temperature Ensure formula given over 20 minutes. No complaints of discomfort. _____L. Traynor, RN

SKILL 12.10   Providing Continuous Feeding via a Small-Bore Nasointestinal/Jejunostomy Tube

Equipment

- Prescribed formula in closed container (ready to infuse system preferred; note expiration date)
- Antimicrobial swabs
- Formula reservoir or bag if necessary for open system (date and replace daily)
- Container of ready-to-use sterile formula (cover, label for client, refrigerate unused portion, and discard in 48 hours) or closed system formula ❶
- Administration tubing compatible with pump (replace daily)
- Infusion pump (not to exceed 40 psi)
- Label or pen
- 60-mL sterile syringe
- Sterile normal saline solution or warm water
- Gloves
- Mask (if caregiver has URI)

Preparation

- Check physician's order for feeding formula type and rate of administration.
- Check x-ray report. **Rationale:** *Validates desired tube placement.*
- Check length of exposed tubing. **Rationale:** *An increase in length may indicate tube tip has dislocated upward, from duodenum to stomach, or from stomach into the esophagus.*
- Perform hand hygiene.
- Gather equipment.
- Don clean gloves and mask if indicated.

Procedure

1. If using reservoir or bag for continuous intestinal feeding, rinse bag with sterile water, and fill with enough formula to limit hang time to 8 hours. *Note:* Bring unused formula to

(continued on next page)

SKILL 12.10 Providing Continuous Feeding via a Small-Bore Nasointestinal *(continued)*

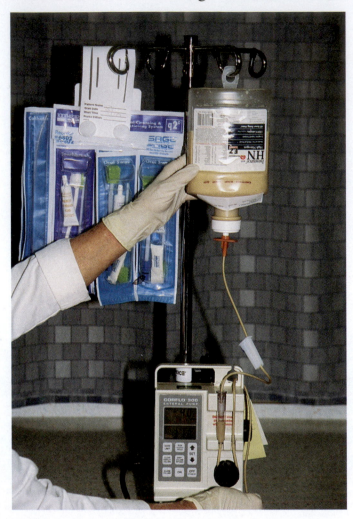

❶ Closed system formula can hang to 48 hours if sterile technique is used.

room temperature before use. **Rationale:** *To reduce risk of infection. Advancement of tube to intestine places it in less protected (alkaline) environment.*

CLINICAL ALERT

If client is receiving continuous feeding, maintain HOB elevation at 30 to 45 degrees at all times. Turn off feeding 1 hour before client must be repositioned at less than 30-degree elevation for any procedure or transport.

Transition from nutrition support to oral feeding requires careful monitoring. Enteral tubes or parenteral access should not be removed until the client has tolerated oral nutrition for 2 to 3 days.

Enteral nutrition via naso/orointestinal infusion should be withheld if the client is hypotensive (mean arterial pressure or MAP < 60 mm Hg), especially if receiving catecholamine agents to maintain hemodynamic stability. Signs of intolerance may indicate gut ischemia.

2. Disinfect ports with antiseptic swab before and after handling.
3. Connect administration tubing to formula reservoir (container or bag) and prime tubing per manufacturer's instructions.
4. Thread tubing through pump per manufacturer's instructions ❷.

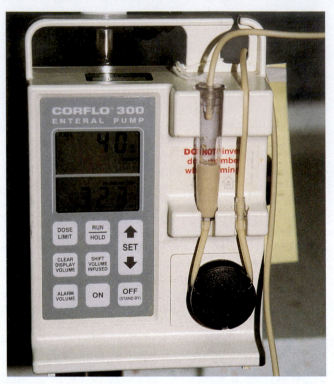

❷ Thread tubing through pump per manufacturer's instructions. Pump must not exceed 40 psi.

5. Note mark on client's feeding tube to determine if migration has occurred.
6. Connect primed formula tubing to client's small-bore feeding tube. Initiate feeding with isotonic (300 mOsm) or slightly hypotonic formula. **Rationale:** *To prevent dumping syndrome (cramping and diarrhea).*

Note: Alternate method is to connect formula tubing to client's surgically established jejunostomy feeding tube ❸.

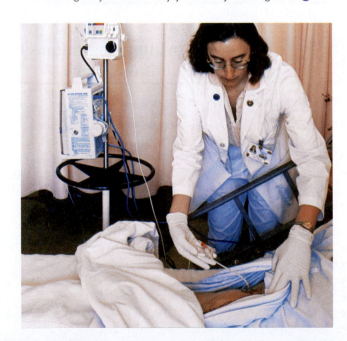

❸ Connect continuous feeding system to client's surgically placed jejunostomy tube.

SKILL 12.10 Providing Continuous Feeding via a Small-Bore Nasointestinal (*continued*)

7. Start feeding at slow constant infusion rate (25 to 50 mL/hr). **Rationale:** *Slow increase in feeding volume is better tolerated. (Maximum rate is 100 to 150 mL/hr.)*
8. If client tolerates feeding, increase rate in 8 to 24 hours (increase by 25 to 50 mL/hr to prescribed rate).
9. Keep client's head of bed elevated at 30 to 45 degrees, or maintain client with obesity in reverse Trendelenburg position ❹. **Rationale:** *To lower intra-abdominal pressure and reduce risk of aspiration.*

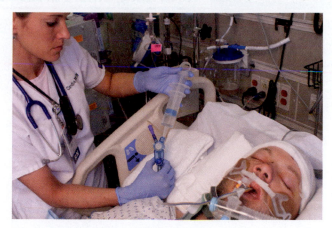

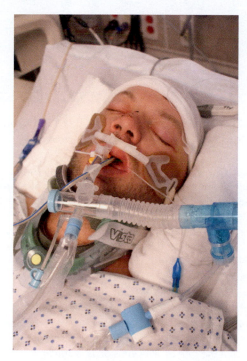

❹ Maintain head-of-bed (HOB) elevation at 30 to 45 degrees to reduce risk of aspiration in clients receiving continuous enteral feeding.

10. Prep side port with antimicrobial swab and, using 60-mL syringe, flush small-bore continuous feeding tube every 4 hours; flush before and after medication administration with 15 mL sterile water or saline ❺. **Rationale:** *To prevent tube clogging.*
11. Check residual volume regularly. **Rationale:** *Small-bore feeding tube residuals are usually less than 10 mL. Residuals as much as 50 mL may indicate upward displacement from the bowel into the stomach.*
12. Document feeding and client response.

Documentation for Enteral Tube Feedings

- Date and time of procedure
- Placement of small-bore enteral tube and x-ray validation of proper placement

❺ Use 60-mL syringe to flush feeding tube with 15 mL sterile water or saline every 4 hours, and before and after medication administration. Do not use tap water.

- External length of exposed tubing
- Methods of validating tube placement
- Quantity and character of aspirated residuals (color, pH, other tests)
- Amount and type of formula administered
- HOB elevation during and following feeding
- Frequency of tube irrigation and irrigant used
- Abdominal assessment findings (distention, nausea, vomiting, flatus, bowel movement)
- Bowel elimination pattern and characteristics
- Daily weight
- Intake and output
- Tube exit site assessment
- Application of dressing to exit site
- Oral hygiene provided

CLINICAL ALERT

Many devices, both enteral and parenteral are the color purple. While enteral connectors have gone to purple in an attempt to have the nurse note that this is not an IV device color, two manufacturers' peripherally inserted central (PIC) catheters use purple and thus the risk for enteral misconnection may be increased

Clients who are obese cannot efficiently mobilize fat stores, but use protein as a primary source of energy, have marked loss of muscle and lean body mass, and become nutrient depleted when critically ill. Nutrient support, however, can cause refeeding syndrome in these as in other protein-deficient clients. This adverse response is characterized by volume overload, heart failure, pulmonary edema, glucose intolerance, excess carbon dioxide production (by-product of glucose metabolism), increased respiratory work, and respiratory failure.

▶ PARENTERAL NUTRITION USING INTRAVENOUS INFUSION

Expected Outcomes

1. Lipids infuse within time frame.
2. Adequate calories and essential fatty acids are provided to clients unable to ingest orally.
3. Parenteral nutrients provided without complications or adverse effects.
4. Normal pancreatic function is maintained.

(*continued on next page*)

SKILL 12.11 Providing Total Parenteral Nutrition (TPN)

Delegation

Due to the need for sterile technique and technical complexity, administration of TPN is not delegated to UAP. UAP may care for clients receiving TPN, and the nurse must ensure that the UAP knows what complications or adverse signs should be reported to the nurse.

Equipment

- TPN solution
- Timing tape
- Infusion pump
- Tubing with filter

Preparation

- Review the client record regarding previous TPN. Note any complications and how they were managed.
- Check physician's order. Inspect and prepare solution.
- Remove the ordered TPN solution from the refrigerator 1 hour before use, and check each ingredient and the proposed rate against the order on the chart. **Rationale:** *Infusion of a cold solution can cause pain, hypothermia, and venous spasm and constriction.*
- Inspect the solution for cloudiness or presence of particles, and ensure that the container is free from cracks. For lipids, examine the bag for separation of emulsion, fat globules, or froth.
- Before administering any TPN solution:
  a. Check its expiration date. Most solutions must be used within 24 hours of preparation, unless they are refrigerated.
  b. Two licensed nurses need to check the nutrients in the bag with the order written by the primary care provider. **Rationale:** *This is another check that ensures the solution was properly prepared by the pharmacist.*
  c. Apply a timing tape on the solution container.

Procedure

1. Prior to performing the procedure, introduce self and verify the client's identity using agency protocol. Explain to the client what you are going to do, why it is necessary, and how he or she can participate.
2. Provide for client privacy and prepare the client.
   - Assist the client to a comfortable position, either sitting or lying. If necessary, expose the central line site but provide for client privacy.
3. Perform hand hygiene and observe other appropriate infection control procedures.
4. Change the solution container to the TPN solution ordered.
   - Ensure that correct placement of the central line catheter has been confirmed by x-ray examination.
   - Ensure that the tubing has an in-line filter connected at the end of the TPN tubing. For plain TPN, use a 0.22-micron filter ❶ A. For TPN with lipids, the filter must be 1.2 microns ❶ B. Plain lipids are infused without a filter. **Rationale:** *The filter traps bacteria and particles that can form in the TPN solution.*
   - Attach and connect the tubing to an infusion pump, if not present. **Rationale:** *A pump eliminates the changes in flow rate that occur with alterations in the client's activity and position.*

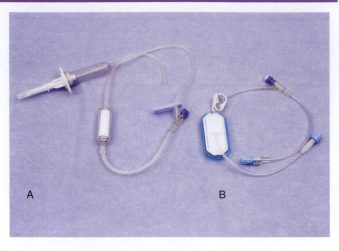

❶ A, A 0.22-micron filter used for TPN; B, a 1.2-micron filter for use with TPN containing lipids.

- Attach the TPN solution to the IV administration tubing. If a multiple-lumen tube is in place, attach the infusion to the appropriate lumen. If possible, a lumen should be dedicated to TPN use only.
- If lipids are being infused separately from the TPN, connect the lipid tubing to the injection port closest to the client (below the TPN filter).

5. Regulate and monitor the flow rate.
   - Establish the prescribed rate of flow and monitor the infusion at least every 30 minutes.
   - Never accelerate an infusion that has fallen behind schedule. **Rationale:** *Wide fluctuations in blood glucose can occur if the rate of TPN infusion is irregular.*
   - Never interrupt or discontinue the infusion abruptly. If TPN solution is temporarily unavailable, infuse a solution containing at least 5% to 10% dextrose. **Rationale:** *This prevents rebound hypoglycemia.*
   - During the initial stage of a lipid infusion (i.e., the first hour), closely monitor vital signs and signs of any side effects (e.g., fever, flushing, diaphoresis, dyspnea, cyanosis, headache, nausea, or vomiting).
   - Start lipid infusions very slowly according to the primary care provider's orders, the manufacturer's directions, and agency policy. For a 10% emulsion, start at 1 mL/min for the first 5 minutes then up to 4 mL/min for the next 25 minutes. If well tolerated, set ordered rate thereafter.

6. Monitor the client for complications.
   - Change the administration set and filter every 24 hours.
   - Monitor the vital signs every 4 hours. If fever or abnormal vital signs occur, notify the primary care provider. **Rationale:** *An elevated temperature is one of the earliest indications of catheter-related sepsis.*
   - Collect double-voided urine specimens in accordance with agency policy, and test the urine for specific gravity. If the specific gravity is abnormal, notify the primary care provider, who may alter the constituents of the TPN solution.
   - Assess capillary (fingerstick) blood glucose levels every 6 hours according to agency protocol. **Rationale:** *Blood glucose is tested to make certain the infusion is not running too rapidly for the body to metabolize glucose*

SKILL 12.11   Providing Total Parenteral Nutrition (TPN) (continued)

or too slowly for caloric needs to be met. Notify the primary care provider of abnormal glucose levels. For hyperglycemia, supplementary insulin may be ordered subcutaneously or added directly to the TPN solution. For hypoglycemia the infusion rate may need to be increased.

- Measure the daily fluid intake and output and calorie intake. **Rationale:** *Precise replacement for fluid and electrolyte deficits can then be more readily determined.*
- Monitor the results of laboratory tests (e.g., serum electrolytes and blood urea nitrogen) and report abnormal findings to the primary care provider.
7. Assess weight and anthropometric measurements.
- Weigh the client daily, at the same time and in the same garments. A gain of more than 0.5 kg (1.1 lb) per day indicates fluid excess and should be reported.
- Measure arm circumference and triceps skinfold thickness weekly or in accordance with agency protocol to assess the physical changes.

8. Document all relevant information.
- Record the type and amount of infusion, rate of infusion, vital signs every 4 hours, fingerstick blood glucose levels as ordered, client's weight daily, and anthropometric measurements.

CLINICAL ALERT
TPN and lipids are frequently infused together in the same bottle to prevent microorganism growth from lipid emulsion.

Do not "catch up" a deficit in infused volume, as doing so could result in complications for the client. To ensure constant flow rate, check rate every 2 hours.

No medication or blood products are to be added or piggybacked into a TPN line.

No blood specimen should be withdrawn from an IV line infusing TPN.

TPN is never stopped abruptly. It should be tapered off.

SKILL 12.12   Infusing IV Lipids

Equipment

- IV lipid solution in container ❶
- Non-phthalate vented IV tubing infusion set (to prevent pooling of fat in IV tubing)
- Needleless cannula

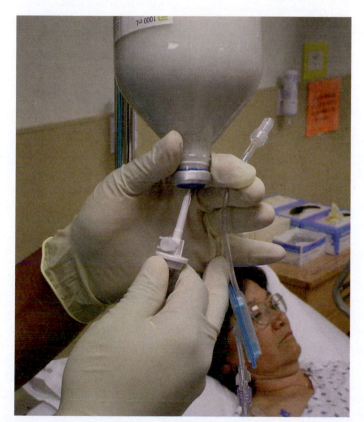

❶ Lipids are administered from glass container or non–polyvinyl chloride (non-PVC) infusion sets.

- 2% chlorhexidine gluconate swabs
- Volume control device

Note: Many facilities do not infuse lipids alone but combine with TPN.

Preparation

- Review physician's orders and medication administration record (MAR).
- Obtain lipid emulsion (refrigerated) from the pharmacy and warm the solution to room temperature (may take 1 to 2 hours).
- Examine solution for separation of emulsion into layers or fat globules or for accumulation of froth. Do not use if any of these appear.
- Label bottle with client name, medical record number, room number, date, time, flow rate, bottle number, and start and stop times.
- Identify client using two forms of identification.
- Explain procedure to client. Follow infection control measures and provide privacy to client. Provide comfort and safety for client and yourself.

Procedure

1. Take vital signs for baseline assessment. **Rationale:** *Baseline information is needed because an immediate reaction can occur.*
2. Perform hand hygiene, and then swab stopper on IV bottle with antimicrobial swab and allow to dry.
3. Attach vented non-PVC infusion set to bottle, twisting the spike to prevent particles from stopper falling into the emulsion, or spike bag with regular IV tubing ❷.
4. Hang IV bottle at least 75 cm (30 in.) above IV site. **Rationale:** *Due to solution viscosity, lipid emulsion needs to be at this height to prevent it from backing up into infusion tubing.*

(continued on next page)

SKILL 12.12 Infusing IV Lipids (*continued*)

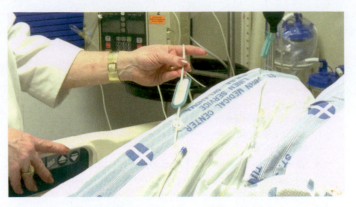

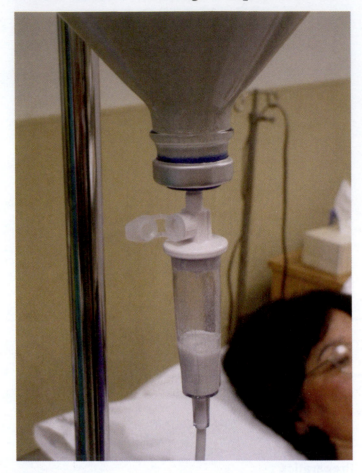

❷ Vented tubing is required for lipid infusion.

5. Fill drip chamber two thirds full, slightly open clamp on the tubing, and prime the tubing slowly. **Rationale:** *Priming more slowly reduces chance of air bubbles with this solution.*
6. Attach the tubing to the IV site.
7. If piggybacking lipids into hyperalimentation, use port closest to client, below tubing filter ❸.

> **CLINICAL ALERT**
>
> Administration sets that contain di-(2-ethylhexyl)phthalate (DEHP) plasticizers extract lipids from the infusion set. Therefore, use of a separate administration set, glass infusate container, or special non-PVC IV bag is recommended.
>
> Lipid emulsions alone promote growth of specific bacteria and yeasts as soon as 6 hours after the infusion. When lipids are combined with a total parenteral nutrition (TPN) solution (amino acids, lipid emulsion, and glucose) in the same bag, it does not appear to support any greater microbial growth than non–lipid-containing TPN fluids. Thus, TPN solution can hang safely for 24 hours.

8. Infuse lipid solutions initially at 1 mL/min for adults and 0.1 mL/min for children for first 15 to 30 minutes. Then increase rate to 2 mL/min for adults and 0.2 mL/min for children.
9. Monitor vital signs according to facility policy and observe for side effects during first 30 minutes of the infusion. If side effects occur, stop the infusion and notify the physician.
10. Adjust flow to prescribed IV rate if no adverse reactions occur.

❸ Check facility policy regarding use of in-line filters for lipid administration. Filters are not recommended by the CDC, but the Infusion Nurses Society favors them.

11. Monitor and maintain the infusion at the ordered rate.
12. Monitor serum lipids 4 hours after discontinuing infusion. **Rationale:** *If you draw blood too soon after infusion is completed, incorrect blood values result.*

> **CLINICAL ALERT**
>
> Observe for IV lipid side effects after starting lipid infusion:
>
> Chills
> Chest and back pain
> Fever
> Nausea and vomiting
> Flushing
> Headache
> Diaphoresis
> Pressure over the eyes
> Dyspnea
> Vertigo
> Cyanosis
> Sleepiness
> Allergic reactions
> Thrombophlebitis.

13. Monitor liver function tests for evidence of impaired liver function. **Rationale:** *These tests indicate the liver's ability to metabolize the lipids.*
14. Discard partially used bottles/bags. **Rationale:** *This action prevents contamination.*
15. Discard administration set after each unit unless additional units are administered consecutively.
16. Continue to monitor vital signs, and observe client for adverse reactions during the entire process of infusion.
17. Answer any questions the client may have about the procedure, and make client comfortable before leaving room.
18. Document nursing actions and client response.

> **CLINICAL ALERT**
>
> In-line filters are not recommended by the CDC as a routine infection control measure; however, the Infusion Nurses Society favors the use of filters. Always check hospital policies and procedures to determine use of filters.

SKILL 12.12   Infusing IV Lipids *(continued)*

Practice Guidelines

IV Lipid Infusion

- IV lipid solutions are isotonic and provide 1.1 kcal/mL of solution in a 10% solution or 2.0 kcal/mL in a 20% solution.
- Do not put additives into IV lipid bottle.
- Do not use an IV filter because the particles are large and cannot pass through.

FOR ADULTS

- Lipid 10%: Up to 500 mL 4–6 hr on first day to maximum of 2.5 g/kg body weight per day. Do not exceed 60% of client's total caloric intake per day.
- Liposyn 10%: No more than 500 mL/day in 4–6 hr.

FOR CHILDREN

- Lipid 10%: Up to 1 g/kg in 4 hr. Do not exceed 60% of total caloric intake.

▶ CRITICAL THINKING OPTIONS FOR UNEXPECTED OUTCOMES

Not all unexpected outcomes require further nursing intervention; however, many times they do. When the client demonstrates a change in signs/symptoms indicating an emerging problem, the nurse should immediately assess and troubleshoot what is happening. The assessment data must be processed quickly to formulate a hypothesis so the nurse can make a clinical judgment. The nurse then decides how best to resolve the problem and improve the client's situation for a better appropriate outcome.

EXPECTED OUTCOME	PROBLEM SOLVING	NURSING ACTIONS
Client's nutritional needs are met with balanced diet appropriate for developmental age.	Client is nauseated and vomits.	• Withhold food if client is nauseated or vomiting. • Provide antiemetic or client's preferred comfort measures (cold cloth to throat, soda drink). • Identify potential source for nausea: specific foods or odors, experience of pain, side effects of medication (e.g., morphine sulfate), or positional changes.
	Older client with visual impairment only eats food on one half of food tray.	• Client may have homonymous hemianopia due to cerebrovascular accident (CVA) and is unable to see the half of the tray on his or her paralyzed side. • Move food tray so that ignored side is within client's restricted range of vision (move tray leftward if client has had a left CVA and right side of tray has been ignored). • Encourage client to turn head so that client's visual field includes the half of tray with food that has not been seen or eaten.
Client experiences no complications while consuming nutrients.	Client has signs of aspirating food (coughing, hoarseness, noisy breathing).	• Request speech pathologist consult for swallow evaluation. • Ensure that assistive personnel are following individualized feeding instructions/precautions (e.g., client positioning, use of thickening agents, and avoiding use of straws). • Remind client not to talk while eating and to concentrate on swallowing.
Enteral Nutrition Client's nutritional needs are met with nasogastric (NG) feeding.	NG tube feedings are delayed/skipped due to large residual volumes.	• Assess for adequate GI function (no abdominal distention; no nausea or vomiting; presence of flatus, bowel movement). If residual is ≤500 mL, continue feeding but closely monitor client's response. • Change to continuous rather than intermittent feeding. • Continue measures to prevent aspiration. • Consider postpyloric feeding.
Client experiences no complications with NG feeding.	Client develops diarrhea with enteral feeding.	• Use closed system if possible to prevent contamination. • Don clean gloves when setting up or opening system; use sterile technique if client is immunocompromised or critically ill. • Flush bag before refilling with formula. • Use prepackaged, ready-to-use sterile feeding formulas. If using open system, cover, label, and refrigerate unused formula and discard in 24 hours. • Disinfect ports before and after any handling. • Consult dietitian about osmolarity of formula (hyperosmolar or high-fiber formula may cause diarrhea).

(continued on next page)

EXPECTED OUTCOME	PROBLEM SOLVING	NURSING ACTIONS
Client's nutritional needs are met with continuous enteral feeding.	Small-bore feeding tube fails to advance into duodenum.	■ Determine if gastric feeding is acceptable (client does not have gastroparesis, reflux esophagitis, high risk for aspiration, absence of gag or cough reflex). ■ Administer prokinetic agent before rather than after tube insertion. ■ Suggest tube be advanced under fluoroscopy.
Gastrostomy tube site is free of signs of irritation/inflammation.	Gastrostomy tube site becomes irritated.	■ Apply plain antacid (e.g., Mylanta) to area if condition is mild. ■ Use skin prep barrier followed by antifungal powder followed by skin prep barrier. ■ Request tube with external bar or disc be replaced with plain tube that is sutured into place (bars and discs may embed into skin).
Parenteral Nutrition Parenteral nutrients provided without complications or adverse effects.	Client develops dyspnea, cyanosis, or allergic reaction, such as nausea, vomiting, increased temperature, or headache.	■ Stop infusion immediately, and notify physician.
	Client develops hyperlipidemia or hypercoagulability.	■ Monitor laboratory results, particularly liver function tests, and notify physician when any abnormality occurs.
Adequate calories and essential fatty acids are provided to clients unable to ingest orally.	Client's serum triglyceride and liver function test results remain elevated.	■ Continue IV lipid infusion. ■ Begin the feeding with a weaker concentration of formula, and increase the concentration slowly as ordered. ■ Repeat lab values.
Lipids infuse within time frame.	Client experiences side effects and cannot continue with lipid infusion.	■ Reassess client's ability to tolerate fat solution. ■ Notify physician for order to discontinue fat solution, and administer hyperalimentation solution. ■ Monitor liver function test results.

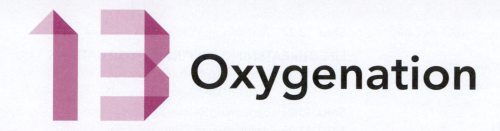

Oxygenation

(continued on next page)

Skills-at-a-Glance (continued)

Living cells require a consistent supply of oxygen. There are three actions necessary to make this process happen. (1) Air needs to be transported to and from the lungs, so there needs to be a patent airway. (2) Oxygen (O_2) exchange and carbon dioxide (CO_2) exchange need to take place in the lungs. An adequate percentage of O_2 must be breathed in and available to diffuse into the blood and CO_2 must be breathed out. (3) The O_2 needs to be transported and made available to all body cells by the cardiovascular system.

Most people in good health give little thought to their respiratory function. Changing position frequently, ambulating, and exercising usually maintain adequate ventilation and gas exchange. Many people tend to breathe in a shallow fashion and do not draw air into the lowest regions of the lungs, thus limiting potential gas exchange.

Mounting evidence supports the use of slow, abdominal breathing to facilitate pain relief (see Chapter 4) and to decrease blood pressure in clients with essential hypertension (Jerath & Barnes, 2009; Jones, Sangthong, & Pachirat, 2010). Deep, slow breathing also facilitates the beneficial "relaxation response" identified by Dr. Herbert Benson in his classic work (1996). This chapter includes interventions to support these mechanics of respiration and ventilation.

▶ ASSESSMENT: OXYGENATION

Expected Outcomes

1. Client receives instructions about all specimen collection procedures before they are begun.

2. Specimens are collected following common guidelines and facility procedures.

SKILL 13.1 Collecting a Sputum Specimen

Delegation

Unlicensed assistive personnel (UAP) can obtain a sputum specimen that is expectorated by a client. It is important to instruct the UAP about when to collect the specimen, how to position the client, and how to correctly collect the specimen. Obtaining a sputum specimen by use of pharyngeal suctioning, however, should be performed by the nurse because it is an invasive, sterile process and requires knowledge application and problem solving.

Equipment

- Sterile specimen container with a cover
- Clean gloves (if assisting the client)
- Disinfectant and swabs, or liquid soap and water
- Paper towels
- Completed label
- Completed laboratory requisition
- Mouthwash

Preparation

Determine the method of collection and gather the appropriate equipment.

Procedure

1. Prior to performing the procedure, introduce self and verify the client's identity using agency protocol. Explain to the client what you are going to do, why it is necessary, and how he or she can participate. Discuss how the results will be used in planning further care or treatments. Give the client the following information and instructions:
   - The purpose of the test, the difference between sputum and saliva, and how to provide the sputum specimen
   - Not to touch the inside of the sputum container or lid
   - To expectorate the sputum directly into the sputum container
   - To keep the outside of the container free of sputum, if possible
   - How to hold a pillow firmly against an abdominal incision if the client finds it painful to cough
   - The amount of sputum required (usually 4–10 mL [1–2 tsp] of sputum is sufficient for analysis)

2. Perform hand hygiene and observe other appropriate infection control procedures.

3. Provide for client privacy.

4. Provide necessary assistance to collect the specimen.
   - Assist the client to a standing or a sitting position (e.g., high-Fowler or semi-Fowler position or on the edge of a bed or in a chair). **Rationale:** *These positions allow maximum lung ventilation and expansion.*
   - Ask the client to hold the sputum cup on the outside, or, for a client who is not able to do so, put on gloves and hold the cup for the client.
   - Ask the client to breathe deeply and then cough up secretions. **Rationale:** *A deep inhalation provides sufficient air to force secretions out of the airways and into the pharynx.*

SKILL 13.1   Collecting a Sputum Specimen (continued)

- Hold the sputum cup so that the client can expectorate into it, making sure that the sputum does not come in contact with the outside of the container. **Rationale:** *Containing the sputum within the cup restricts the spread of microorganisms to others.*
- Assist the client to repeat coughing until a sufficient amount of sputum has been collected.
- Cover the container with the lid immediately after the sputum is in the container. **Rationale:** *Covering the container prevents the inadvertent spread of microorganisms to others.*
- If spillage occurs on the outside of the container, clean the outer surface with a disinfectant. Some agencies recommend washing the outside of all containers with liquid soap and water and then drying with a paper towel.
- Remove and discard the gloves. Perform hand hygiene.
5. Ensure client comfort and safety.
- Assess the client for respiratory difficulty and provide oxygen per the primary care provider's orders.
- Assist the client to rinse his or her mouth with a mouthwash as needed.

- Assist the client to a position of comfort that allows maximum lung expansion as required.
6. Label and transport the specimen to the laboratory.
- Ensure that the specimen label and the laboratory requisition contain the correct information. Attach the label and requisition securely to the specimen. **Rationale:** *Inaccurate identification or information on the specimen container can lead to errors of diagnosis or therapy.*
- Arrange for the specimen to be sent to the laboratory immediately. **Rationale:** *Bacterial cultures must be started immediately before any contaminating organisms can grow, multiply, and produce false results.*
7. Document all relevant information.
- Document the collection of the sputum specimen on the client's chart. Include the amount, color, consistency (e.g., thick, tenacious, watery), evidence of hemoptysis (blood in the sputum), odor of the sputum, any measures needed to obtain the specimen (e.g., postural drainage), the general amount of sputum produced, any discomfort experienced by the client, and any interventions implemented to ensure adequate air exchange postprocedure (such as O_2 saturation monitoring or administration of O_2).

Developmental Considerations

OLDER ADULTS

- Older adults may need encouragement to cough because a decreased cough reflex occurs with aging.

- Allow time for the older adult to rest and recover between coughs when obtaining a sputum specimen.

SKILL 13.2   Obtaining Nose and Throat Specimens

Delegation

Obtaining nose and throat specimens is an invasive skill that requires the application of scientific knowledge and potential problem solving to ensure client safety. Therefore, the nurse needs to perform this skill and does not delegate it to UAP.

Equipment

- Clean gloves
- Two sterile, cotton-tipped swabs in sterile culture tubes with transport medium
- Penlight
- Tongue blade (optional)
- Otoscope with a nasal speculum (optional)
- Container for the used nasal speculum
- Completed labels for each specimen container
- Completed laboratory requisition

Preparation

Prepare the client and the equipment:

- Assist the client to a sitting position. **Rationale:** *This is the most comfortable position for many people and the one in which the pharynx is most readily visible.*
- Don gloves if the client's mucosa will be touched.
- Open the culture tube and place it on the sterile wrapper. **Rationale:** *This prevents microorganisms from entering the tube.*
- Remove one sterile applicator and hold it carefully by the stick

end, keeping the remainder sterile. The swab end is kept from touching any objects that could contaminate it.

Procedure

1. Prior to performing the procedure, introduce self and verify the client's identity using agency protocol. Explain to the client what you are going to do, why it is necessary, and how he or she can participate. Discuss how the results will be used in planning further care or treatments. Inform the client that he may gag while swabbing the throat or feel like sneezing during the swabbing of the nose; however, the procedure will take less than 1 minute.
2. Perform hand hygiene and observe other appropriate infection control procedures.
3. Provide for client privacy.
4. Collect the specimen.

VARIATION: OBTAINING A THROAT SPECIMEN

- Ask the client to tilt the head back, open the mouth, extend the tongue, and say "ah." **Rationale:** *When the tongue is extended, the pharynx is exposed. Saying "ah" relaxes the throat muscles and helps minimize contraction of the constriction muscle of the pharynx (the gag reflex).*
- Use a penlight to illuminate the posterior pharynx while depressing the tongue with a tongue blade. Depress the anterior third of the tongue firmly without touching the throat. ❶ **Rationale:** *Touching the throat stimulates the gag reflex. Check for inflamed areas.*

(continued on next page)

SKILL 13.2 Obtaining Nose and Throat Specimens *(continued)*

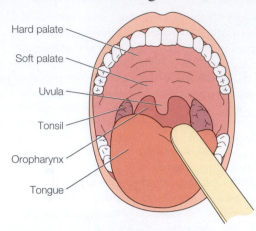

- Hard palate
- Soft palate
- Uvula
- Tonsil
- Oropharynx
- Tongue

❶ Depressing the tongue to view the pharynx.

- Insert a swab into the mouth without touching any part of the mouth or tongue. **Rationale:** *The swab should not pick up microorganisms in the mouth.*
- Gently and quickly, swab along the tonsils, making sure to contact any areas on the pharynx that are particularly erythematous (reddened) or that contain exudates (purulent drainage). **Rationale:** *By moving the swab quickly, you can avoid initiating the gag reflex or causing discomfort. Erythematous areas and areas with exudate will likely have the most microorganisms. Rotating the swab where exudate is present may maximize the amount of specimen collected.*
- Remove the swab without touching the mouth or lips. **Rationale:** *This prevents the swab from transmitting microorganisms to the mouth.*
- Insert the swab into the sterile tube without allowing it to touch the outside of the container. Push the tip of the swab into the liquid medium. Make sure the swab is placed in the correctly labeled tube. **Rationale:** *Touching the outside of the tube could transmit microorganisms to it and then to others.*
- Crush the ampule of culture medium at the bottom of the tube.
- Place the top securely on the tube, taking care not to touch the inside of the cap. **Rationale:** *Touching the inside of the cap could transmit additional microorganisms into the tube.*

- Repeat the above steps with the second swab.
- Discard the tongue blade in the waste container.
- Remove and discard gloves. Perform hand hygiene.

VARIATION: OBTAINING A NASAL SPECIMEN

- Ask the client to blow her nose to clear her nasal passages. Check nostrils with a penlight to check for patency.
- If using a nasal speculum, gently insert the lighted nasal speculum up one nostril.
- Insert the sterile swab carefully through the speculum, without touching the edges. **Rationale:** *This prevents the swab from picking up microorganisms from the speculum.* When working without a speculum, pass the swab along the septum and the floor of the nose.
- When the area of mucosa that is reddened or contains exudate, is reached, rotate the swab quickly.
- Remove the swab without touching the speculum.
- Remove the nasal speculum if used.
- Insert the swab into the culture tube. Crush the ampule at the bottom of the tube and push the tip of the swab into the liquid medium.
- Repeat the above steps for the other nostril.
- Label and transport the specimens to the laboratory.
- Document all relevant information.
  - Record the collection of the nose and/or throat specimens on the client's chart. Include the assessments of the nasal mucosa and pharynx, and any discomfort the client experienced.

VARIATION: OBTAINING A NASOPHARYNGEAL CULTURE

A nasopharyngeal culture uses the same steps as a nasal culture with the following exceptions: A special cotton-tipped swab on a flexible wire is used. While this swab is still in the package, bend the sterile swab in a curve and then open the package without contaminating the swab. Gently pass the swab through the more patent nostril about 8–10 cm (3–4 in.) into the nasopharynx.

Developmental Considerations

Throat Specimens

INFANTS

- When taking a throat swab, avoid occluding an infant's nose because infants normally breathe only through the nose.

CHILDREN

- Have a parent stand the young child between the parent's legs with the child's back to the parent and the parent's arms gently but

firmly around the child. As the parent tips the child's head back, ask the child to open wide and stick the tongue out. Assure the child that the procedure will be over quickly and may "tickle" but should not hurt.

- Cooperative children can be asked to put their hands under their buttocks, open their mouth, and laugh or pant like a dog (Bindler et al., 2014).

SKILL 13.3 Measuring Peak Expiratory Flow Rate

Delegation

PEFR measurement may be delegated to trained UAP. The nurse should double check any values found to be abnormal or significantly different from previous results and must interpret the findings. Modifications in the treatment regimen may not be initiated by UAP.

Equipment

- Peak flow meter

Procedure

1. Prior to performing the procedure, introduce self and verify the client's identity using agency protocol. Explain to the

SKILL 13.3   Measuring Peak Expiratory Flow Rate (*continued*)

client what you are going to do, why it is necessary, and how he or she can participate. Discuss how the results will be used in planning further care or treatments.

2. Perform hand hygiene and observe other appropriate infection control procedures.
3. Provide for client privacy.
4. Position the client.
   * If possible, the client should be sitting with the chest free from contact with the bed or chair. If not possible, place the client in semi-Fowler or high-Fowler position.
5. Reset the marker on the flow meter to the zero position. ❶

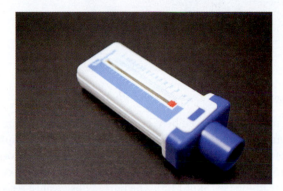

❶ Peak flow meter with marker in the zero position.
(© MediaforMedical/Emmanuel Rogue/Alamy)

6. Assist the client to use the flow meter.
   * Ask the client to take a deep breath in. ❷
   * Client places the mouthpiece in the mouth with the teeth around the opening and the lips forming a tight seal.

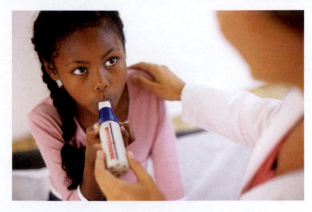

❷ PEFR measurement. (© Science Photo Library/Alamy)

   * Have the client exhale as quickly and forcefully as possible. If you suspect the client is exhaling a significant amount of air through the nose, apply a nose clip.
7. Perform step 6 two more times, allowing the client to rest for 5–10 seconds in between. Record the highest PEFR level achieved.
8. Document findings in the client record using forms or checklists supplemented by narrative notes when appropriate.
9. Normal or expected PEFR is established based on age and size, and a reference chart is included with each peak flow meter. Percentage of predicted PEFR may be calculated by dividing the actual PEFR in milliliters by the predicted PEFR. For example, if the predicted PEFR for a 20-year-old female client 60 inches tall is 554 mL and her actual PEFR is 444 mL, her percentage is approximately 80% of predicted, which is within normal limits. Clients may be taught to use their individual peak flow meter to anticipate early changes in their condition as part of their self-care plan (National Heart, Lung, and Blood Institute, 2007).

▶ INTERVENTIONS: OXYGENATION

Expected Outcomes

1. Promote gas exchange through the use of a sustained maximal inspiration device (incentive spirometer), controlled breathing to sustain maximal expiration (pursed-lip breathing), chest physiotherapy to mobilize secretions, and positioning to support respirations.
2. Encourage breathing exercises to minimize or reverse atelectasis in the lungs.
3. Prevent pulmonary complications for the immediate postoperative client.
4. Maximize COPD client's ability to maintain airway patency, decrease shortness of breath, control breathing rate, and maximize breathing effectiveness.

When people become ill, their respiratory function may be inhibited because of pain and immobility. The result of inadequate chest expansion is pooling of respiratory secretions, which ultimately harbor microorganisms and promote infection. Additionally, shallow respirations may potentiate alveolar collapse, which may cause decreased diffusion of gases and subsequent hypoxemia. This situation is often compounded when opioids are given for pain, because they further depress the rate and depth of respiration.

Interventions by the nurse to maintain the normal respirations of clients include:

■ Positioning the client to allow for maximum chest expansion

■ Encouraging or providing frequent changes in position

■ Encouraging pursed-lip breathing (see Skill 13.5)

■ Encouraging ambulation.

The semi-Fowler or high-Fowler position allows maximum chest expansion and encourages deeper breaths in clients. The nurse should encourage clients to turn from side to side frequently so that each side of the chest experiences maximum expansion. Sitting in a chair and ambulating also increase lung capacity and encourage deeper breaths.

Clients in respiratory distress cannot lie flat in bed. They must sit up to relieve their dyspnea or labored breathing. This is called the **orthopneic position**, which is an adaptation of the high-Fowler position. Some clients also sit upright and lean on their

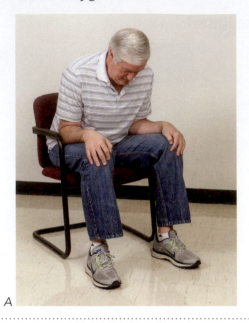

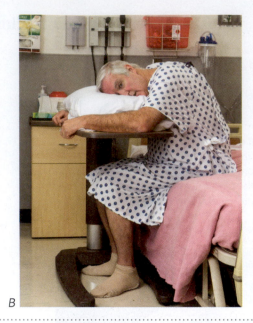

A   *B*

Figure 13–1 ● *A.* Tripod position to assist breathing. *B.* Client using the overbed table to assist with breathing.

arms or elbows. This is called the **tripod position (Figure 13–1 ●)**. Clients with dyspnea often sit in bed and lean over their overbed tables (which are raised to a suitable height), sometimes with a pillow for support. A client in this position can also press the lower part of the chest against the table to help in exhaling.

Breathing exercises are frequently indicated for clients with restricted chest expansion, such as people with **chronic obstructive pulmonary disease (COPD)** or clients recovering from thoracic or abdominal surgery. Instructing and encouraging the client to take deep, sustained breaths is among the safest, most effective, and least expensive strategies for keeping the lungs expanded.

Commonly employed breathing exercises are abdominal (diaphragmatic) and pursed-lip breathing. **Abdominal (diaphragmatic) breathing** permits deep, full breaths with little effort (see Skill 15.1). **Pursed-lip breathing** helps the client develop control over breathing (see Skill 13.5). The pursed lips create a resistance to the air flowing out of the lungs, thereby prolonging exhalation and preventing airway collapse by maintaining positive airway pressure. The client purses the lips as if about to whistle and breathes out slowly and gently, tightening the abdominal muscles to exhale more effectively. The client usually inhales to a count of 3 and exhales to a count of 7 to prolong exhalation.

Client Teaching: Promoting Healthy Breathing

- Sit straight and stand erect to permit full lung expansion.
- Exercise regularly.
- Breathe through the nose.
- Breathe in to expand the chest fully.
- Do not smoke cigarettes, cigars, or pipes.
- Eliminate or reduce the use of household pesticides and irritating chemical substances.
- Do not incinerate garbage in the house.
- Avoid exposure to secondhand smoke.
- Make sure furnaces, ovens, and wood stoves are correctly ventilated.
- Support a pollution-free environment.

SKILL 13.4   Using an Incentive Spirometer

Delegation

The nurse is responsible for teaching clients how to use an incentive spirometer, assessing the client's performance, and evaluating the outcomes of the therapy. UAP, however, can reinforce and assist clients in using the incentive spirometer. The nurse should inform the UAP of the key points to using the incentive spirometer correctly.

Equipment

- Flow-oriented or volume-oriented incentive spirometer (sustained maximal inspiration [SMI] device)
- Mouthpiece or breathing tube
- Label for mouthpiece
- Progress chart
- Nose clip (optional)

Preparation

- Determine if the client has a disposable incentive spirometer at the bedside.
- This skill should not be performed immediately after a meal or other physically stressful activity.

Procedure

1. Prior to performing the skill, introduce self and verify the client's identity using agency protocol. Explain to the client what you are going to do, why it is necessary, and how he or

SKILL 13.4   Using an Incentive Spirometer (continued)

she can participate. Discuss how the results will be used in planning further care or treatments.

2. Perform hand hygiene and observe other appropriate infection control procedures.
3. Provide for client privacy.
4. Prepare the client.
   - Assist the client to an upright position in bed or on a chair. If the person is unable to assume a sitting position for a flow spirometer, have the person assume any position. **Rationale:** *A sitting position facilitates maximum ventilation of the lungs.*

VARIATION: FLOW-ORIENTED INCENTIVE SPIROMETER

Instruct the client to use the spirometer as follows:

- Hold the spirometer in the upright position. **Rationale:** *A tilted spirometer requires less effort to raise the balls or disks; a volume-oriented device will not function correctly unless upright.*
- Exhale normally.
- Seal the lips tightly around the mouthpiece, take in a slow deep breath to elevate the balls, and then hold the breath for 2 seconds initially, increasing to 6 seconds (optimum) to keep the balls elevated if possible. Instruct the client to *avoid* brisk low-volume breaths that snap the balls to the top of the chamber. The client may use a nose clip if the person has difficulty breathing only through the mouth. **Rationale:** *A slow, deep breath ensures maximal ventilation. Greater lung expansion is achieved with a very slow inspiration than with a brisk shallow breath. Sustained elevation of the balls ensures adequate ventilation of the alveoli (lung air sacs).*
- Remove the mouthpiece and exhale normally.
- Cough productively, as needed, after using the spirometer. **Rationale:** *Deep ventilation may loosen secretions and stimulate coughing. Effective coughing can facilitate the removal of the loose secretions.*
- Relax and take several normal breaths before using the spirometer again.
- Repeat the procedure for a total of 10 breaths, encouraging the client to take progressively deeper breaths up to the maximal goal.
- Repeat series of breaths once each hour while awake. **Rationale:** *Practice increases inspiratory volume, maintains alveolar ventilation, and prevents atelectasis (collapse of the air sacs).*

VARIATION: VOLUME-ORIENTED INCENTIVE SPIROMETER

Set the spirometer.

- Set the spirometer to a "target" volume. **Rationale:** *This provides an incentive and motivation for the client. The nurse can start low and increase the "target" after client success.*

Instruct the client to use the spirometer as follows:

- Exhale normally.
- Seal the lips tightly around the mouthpiece and take in a slow, deep breath until the piston is elevated to the predetermined level. The piston level may be visible to the client to identify the volume obtained.
- Hold the breath for 6 seconds to ensure maximal alveolar ventilation.
- Remove the mouthpiece and exhale normally.
- Cough productively, as needed, after using the spirometer. **Rationale:** *Deep ventilation may loosen secretions and stimulate coughing. Effective coughing can facilitate the removal of the loose secretions.*
- Relax and take several normal breaths before using the spirometer again.
- Repeat the procedure for a total of 10 breaths, encouraging the client to take progressively deeper breaths up to the maximal goal.
- Repeat series of breaths once each hour while awake. **Rationale:** *Practice increases inspiratory volume, maintains alveolar ventilation, and prevents atelectasis.*
- Encourage the client to record the top volume achieved at each hour he or she performed the technique. **Rationale:** *This facilitates cooperation of the client and assists in evaluating outcomes of the skill.*

VARIATION: ALL DEVICES

- Clean the equipment.
   - Clean the mouthpiece with water and shake it dry. Label the mouthpiece and a disposable incentive spirometer with the client's name and leave it at the bedside for the client to use as prescribed.
- Document all relevant information.
   - Record the skill, including type of spirometer, number of breaths taken, volume or flow levels achieved, client response, and results of auscultation. Also include, when appropriate, client education and the ability of the client to perform the procedure without prompting.

Sample Documentation

6/12/2015 1030 Coarse rales in RLL. Instructed on use of incentive spirometer (IS). Able to use correctly and raise one ball for 3 seconds. Use of IS stimulated cough, resulting in production of small amount light-colored thick mucus. Encouraged to continue using IS each hour.
_____ *S. Lee, RN*

Developmental Considerations

CHILDREN

- Consider the developmental level of the child when choosing a method to promote breathing exercises. Examples include an incentive spirometer, pinwheels, or other blow toys.
- Use of the incentive spirometer can be presented as a game for young clients. Demonstrate the procedure beforehand and show the child how to take slow, deep breaths.

- Nasal clips may be needed if the younger client does not understand how to refrain from breathing through the nose.

OLDER ADULTS

- Older adults may have trouble sealing their lips around the mouthpiece of a spirometer because of dentures or a dry mouth.

(continued on next page)

SKILL 13.4 Using an Incentive Spirometer (*continued*)

Setting of Care

- Show the client how to use and clean the incentive spirometer.
- Make certain the client understands how often to use the incentive spirometer.

- Ask the client to demonstrate use of the incentive spirometer.
- Evaluate the client's ability to use the incentive spirometer.
- Offer written material to reinforce verbal instructions.

SKILL 13.5 Pursed-Lip Breathing

Delegation

UAP can reinforce and assist clients in performing breathing exercises. However, the nurse is responsible for teaching the client the breathing exercises, evaluating the effectiveness of the teaching, and assessing the outcomes of the breathing exercises (e.g., ease of breathing, effectiveness of cough, breath sounds).

Equipment

None (although a pillow is optional for splinting an abdominal or thoracic incision)

Preparation

- Before starting to teach breathing exercises, determine if a surgical incision prevents deep breathing because of pain. If so, administer analgesic medication 30 minutes prior to implementing deep breathing exercises.

Procedure

1. Prior to performing the procedure, introduce self and verify the client's identity using agency protocol. Explain to the client what you are going to do, why it is necessary, and how he or she can participate. Discuss how pursed-lip breathing will help respirations, thus preventing respiratory complications.
2. Perform hand hygiene and observe other appropriate infection control procedures.
3. Provide for client privacy.
4. Prepare the client.
   - Assist the client to assume a comfortable semi-Fowler or sitting position in bed or on a chair. **Rationale:**

To increase lung capacity and allow for deeper breathing.
5. Teach the client to inhale through the nose and then, pursing lips as if about to whistle, breathe out slowly and gently, making a slow "whooshing" sound without puffing out their cheeks. **Rationale:** *Pursed-lip breathing creates a resistance to air flowing out of the lungs, increases pressure within the bronchi (main air passages), and minimizes collapse of smaller airways, a common problem for people with COPD.*
6. Instruct the client to inhale deeply through the nose and count to 3.
7. Have the client concentrate on tightening the abdominal muscles while breathing out slowly and evenly through pursed lips while counting to 7 or until the client cannot exhale any more. **Rationale:** *Tightening the abdominal muscles and leaning forward helps compress the lungs and enhances effective exhalation.*
8. Teach the client how to perform pursed-lip breathing while walking: Inhale while taking two steps, then exhale through pursed lips while taking the next four steps.
9. Instruct the client to use this exercise whenever feeling short of breath and to increase gradually to 5–10 minutes four times a day. Document teaching. **Rationale:** *Regular practice will help the client do this type of breathing without conscious effort.*

VARIATION: CHILD

- Teach the child to blow through a straw that is in a cup of water and see how long he or she can make a bubbling noise.

SKILL 13.6 Preparing the Client for Chest Physiotherapy (CPT)

Equipment

- Hospital bed or other surface to place client in head-down position
- Gown or towel (optional)
- Tissues
- Container for sputum
- Clean gloves
- Stethoscope
- Pulse oximeter (if indicated)
- Mouthwash/oral hygiene product

Preparation

- Validate physician's order for CPT. **Rationale:** *These procedures are tiring to clients, time consuming, and contraindicated in*

cases of osteoporosis, pulmonary embolism, cardiac conditions, lung cancer, or other conditions not associated with excessive sputum production.
- Administer CPT before or at least 2 hours after meals to prevent vomiting.
- Establish the location of lung segments if the entire lung field is to undergo CPT; the affected segment should be drained first. ❶ **Rationale:** *Usually, the lower areas are the most affected.*

Procedure

1. Prior to performing the procedure, introduce self and verify the client's identity using agency protocol. Explain to the client what you are going to do, why it is necessary, and how

SKILL 13.6 Preparing the Client for Chest Physiotherapy (CPT) *(continued)*

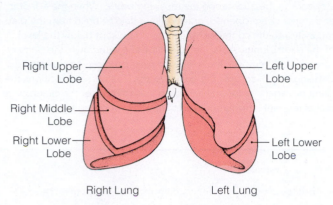

① Lobes of the lungs.

Right Upper Lobe
Right Middle Lobe
Right Lower Lobe
Left Upper Lobe
Left Lower Lobe
Right Lung
Left Lung

he or she can participate. Discuss how the results will be used in planning further care or treatments.

2. Perform hand hygiene and observe other appropriate infection control procedures.
3. Provide for client privacy.
4. Auscultate chest for breath sounds and adventitious sounds prior to therapy.
5. Obtain pulse oximetry (SPO₂) if indicated before therapy.
6. Place towel over skin when performing CPT (optional).
7. Auscultate lungs after therapy. Document procedure and client response.

SKILL 13.7 Assisting with Thoracentesis

Normally, only sufficient fluid to lubricate the pleura is present in the pleural cavity. However, excessive fluid can accumulate as a result of injury, infection, or other pathology. In such a case or in the case of pneumothorax, a primary care provider may perform a thoracentesis to remove the excess fluid or air to ease breathing. Thoracentesis is also performed to introduce chemotherapeutic drugs intrapleurally.

The nurse assists the client to assume a position that allows easy access to the intercostal spaces and explains to client why it is important not to cough during the procedure. This is usually a sitting position with the arms above the head, which spreads the ribs and enlarges the intercostal space. Two commonly used positions are one in which the arm is elevated and stretched forward **①** and

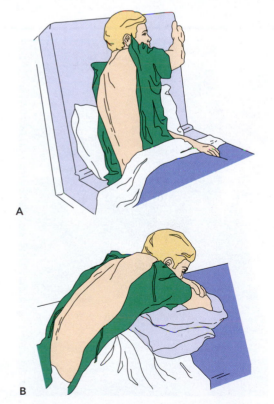

① Two positions commonly used for a thoracentesis: A, Sitting on one side with arm held to the front and up; B, Sitting and leaning forward over a pillow.

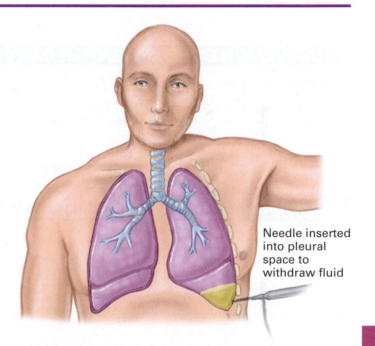

Needle inserted into pleural space to withdraw fluid

② Needle is inserted into the pleural space on the lower posterior chest to withdraw fluid. (*Source:* From *Medical Terminology: A Living Language*, 5th ed. [p. 241, Fig 7.12], by B. Fremgen, and S. Frucht, 2013. Upper Saddle River, NJ: Pearson Education, Inc.)

one in which the client leans forward over a pillow. To make sure that the needle is inserted below the fluid level when fluid is to be removed (or above any fluid if air is to be removed), the primary care provider will palpate and percuss the chest and select the exact site for insertion of the needle. A site on the lower posterior chest is often used to remove fluid, **②** and a site on the upper anterior chest is used to remove air. A chest x-ray prior to the procedure will help pinpoint the best insertion site.

The primary care provider and the assisting nurse follow strict sterile technique. The primary care provider attaches a syringe and/or stopcock to the aspirating needle. The stopcock must be in the closed position so that no air will enter the pleural space.

(continued on next page)

SKILL 13.7   Assisting with Thoracentesis *(continued)*

The primary care provider inserts the needle through the intercostal space to the pleural cavity. In some instances, the primary care provider threads a small plastic tube through the needle and then withdraws the needle. (The tubing is less likely to puncture the pleura.) The nurse monitors the client for signs of distress.

If a syringe is used to collect the fluid, the plunger is pulled out to withdraw the pleural fluid as the stopcock is opened. If a large container is used to receive the fluid, the tubing is attached from the stopcock to the adapter on the receiving bottle. When the adapter and stopcock are opened, gravity allows fluid to drain from the pleural cavity into the container, which should be kept below the level of the client's lungs. After the fluid has been withdrawn, the primary care provider removes the needle or plastic tubing. A small sterile dressing is applied over the puncture site. The nurse repositions the client per agency protocol and continues to monitor the client; documents relevant information; and transports specimen to laboratory.

Developmental Considerations

OLDER ADULTS

- Some older adults will need help maintaining the proper position due to arthritis, tremors, or weakness.
- Provide support with pillows during the procedure.

- Absence of body fat in older adults can help the primary care provider locate the intercostal spaces.
- Provide an extra blanket to keep your client warm during the procedure. Older adults have a decreased metabolism and less subcutaneous fat.

▶ SUPPLEMENTAL OXYGEN THERAPY

Expected Outcomes

1. Supplemental oxygen is delivered] via the most appropriate method to meet individual client's oxygen needs.
2. Respiratory distress will decrease.
3. Oxygen saturation readings will be stable.

4. Client reports improved sleep pattern when using CPAP/BiPAP.
5. The client on a mechanical ventilator will not develop ventilator-associated pneumonia.

SKILL 13.8   Using a Portable Oxygen Cylinder

Equipment

- Steel cylinder portable oxygen tank
- Regulator/flow meter
- Oxygen delivery tubing

Procedure

1. Place oxygen cylinder in carrier in secure upright position. **Rationale:** *If cylinder of compressed air falls accidentally, unit becomes a missile with uncontrollable force and direction.*
2. Using hexagon key, slowly turn cylinder release valve clockwise (left is loose) to crack tank open for a brief period, then close (right to tighten). **Rationale:** *This action removes lint from system.*
3. Check pressure gauge on front of tank to determine amount of oxygen pressure in tank. **Rationale:** *Full status is 2,200 psi.*
4. Attach flow meter regulator unit over neck of cylinder, aligning pins with green "O" ring openings. ❶
5. Use hexagon key to tighten regulator to cylinder neck.
6. Connect delivery tubing to "Christmas tree" adapter on regulator unit.
7. Open cylinder release valve using hexagon key on top of cylinder. **Rationale:** *This allows oxygen flow.*
8. Slowly open regulator/flow meter and adjust to prescribed rate of oxygen delivery in liters per minute.

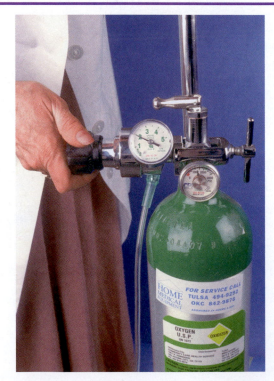

❶ Attach regulator to cylinder neck, attach tubing, open the cylinder release valve, and adjust oxygen flow rate (L/min) as prescribed.

SKILL 13.8   Using a Portable Oxygen Cylinder *(continued)*

Signs and Symptoms of Hypoxia

(SaO_2 < 90% or below desired range for client's situation)

EARLY SYMPTOMS
- Restlessness
- Headache
- Visual disturbances
- Confusion or change in behavior
- Tachypnea
- Tachycardia
- Hypertension
- Dyspnea
- Anxious face

ADVANCED SYMPTOMS
- Hypotension
- Bradycardia
- Metabolic acidosis (production of lactic acid)
- Cyanosis

CHRONIC HYPOXIA
- Polycythemia
- Clubbing of fingers and toes
- Peripheral edema
- Right-sided heart failure
- Chronic PO_2 less than 55 mmHg; O_2 saturation less than 87%
- Elevated PCO_2 (respiratory acidosis)

SKILL 13.9   Administering Oxygen by Nasal Cannula, Face Mask, or Face Tent

Delegation

Initiating the administration of oxygen is considered similar to administering a medication and is not delegated to UAP. However, reapplying the oxygen delivery device may be performed by the UAP and many aspects of the client's response to oxygen therapy are observed during usual care and may be recorded by individuals other than the nurse. Abnormal findings must be validated and interpreted by the nurse. The nurse is also responsible for ensuring that the correct delivery method is being used. The nurse collaborates with the respiratory therapist when a client is receiving oxygen therapy.

Equipment

Cannula

- Oxygen supply with a flow meter and adapter
- Humidifier with distilled water or tap water according to agency protocol
- Nasal cannula and tubing
- Tape (optional)
- Padding for the elastic band (optional)
- Extension tubing and tubing connector (optional)

Face Mask

- Oxygen supply with a flow meter and adapter
- Humidifier with distilled water or tap water according to agency protocol
- Prescribed face mask of the appropriate size
- Padding for the elastic band

Face Tent

- Oxygen supply with a flow meter and adapter
- Humidifier with distilled water or tap water according to agency protocol
- Face tent of the appropriate size

Preparation

- Determine the need for oxygen therapy, and verify the physician's order for the therapy.
- Perform a respiratory assessment to develop baseline data if not already available.
- Prepare the client and support people.

- Assist the client to a semi-Fowler position if possible. **Rationale:** *This position permits easier chest expansion and hence easier breathing.*
- Explain that oxygen is not dangerous when safety precautions are observed. Inform the client and support people about the safety precautions connected with oxygen use.

Procedure

1. Prior to performing the procedure, introduce self and verify the client's identity using agency protocol. Explain to the client what you are going to do, why it is necessary, and how he or she can participate. Discuss how the effects of the oxygen therapy will be used in planning further care or treatments.
2. Perform hand hygiene and observe other appropriate infection control procedures.
3. Provide for client privacy as needed.
4. Set up the oxygen equipment and the humidifier.
   - Attach the flow meter to the wall outlet or tank. ❶ The flow meter should be in the OFF position.

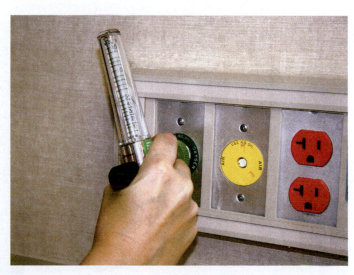

❶ Attach the flow meter to the wall outlet.

(continued on next page)

SKILL 13.9 Administering Oxygen by Nasal Cannula, Face Mask, or Face Tent (continued)

- If needed, fill the humidifier bottle with tap or distilled water, per agency policy. (This can be done before coming to the bedside.)
- Attach the humidifier bottle to the base of the flow meter.
- Attach the prescribed oxygen tubing and delivery device to the humidifier.
5. Turn on the oxygen at the prescribed rate, and ensure proper functioning.
   - Check that the oxygen is flowing freely through the tubing. There should be no kinks in the tubing, and the connections should be airtight. There should be bubbles in the humidifier as the oxygen flows through. You should feel the oxygen at the outlets of the cannula, mask, or tent.
   - Set the oxygen at the flow rate ordered.
6. Apply the appropriate oxygen delivery device.

CLINICAL ALERT
Oxygen is indicated for clients with COPD, but is used conservatively. High levels of oxygen may suppress breathing stimulus, cause hypoventilation and CO_2 retention, and lead to respiratory arrest due to CO_2 narcosis.

VARIATION: USING A NASAL CANNULA

- Put the cannula with the outlet prongs curved downward, fitting into the nares, and the elastic band around the head or the tubing over the ears and under the chin. ❷
- If the cannula will not stay in place, use a short strip of narrow tape to secure it close to the hairline.
- Pad the tubing and elastic band over the ear lobes and cheekbones.

VARIATION: USING A LOW-FLOW OXYGEN NASAL CANNULA ❸

- Assess the client's nares for encrustations and irritation. Apply a water-soluble lubricant as required to soothe the mucous membranes.

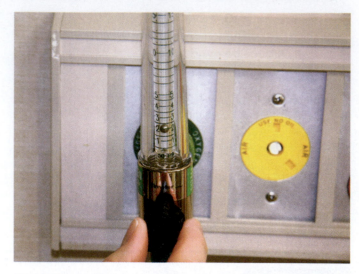

❸ This flow meter is set to deliver 2 L/min.

- Assess the top of the client's ears for any signs of irritation from the cannula strap. If present, padding with a gauze pad may help relieve the discomfort.

CLINICAL ALERT
Humidification of low-flow oxygen through a nasal cannula is contraindicated because it supports bacterial growth.

VARIATION: USING A HIGH-FLOW OXYGEN NASAL CANNULA

- A heated humidification system can be added to the high-flow oxygen nasal cannula to prevent upper airways from drying.
- Assessment of air/oxygen blending in the system ensures that the client who requires a higher percentage of oxygen has a comfortable and more easily tolerated alternative to a face mask.

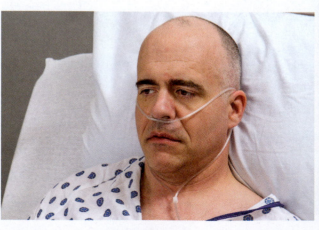
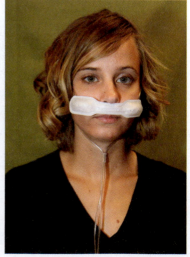
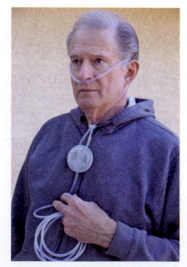

A   B   C

❷ A, Nasal cannula; B, Mustache-style reservoir nasal cannula; C, Pendant-style reservoir nasal cannula.

SKILL 13.9 Administering Oxygen by Nasal Cannula, Face Mask, or Face Tent *(continued)*

VARIATION: USING A FACE MASK

■ Guide the mask toward the client's face, and apply it from the nose downward.

■ Fit the mask and metal nose bracket to the contours of the client's face. ❹ **Rationale:** *The mask should mold to the face, so that very little oxygen escapes into the eyes or around the cheeks and chin.*

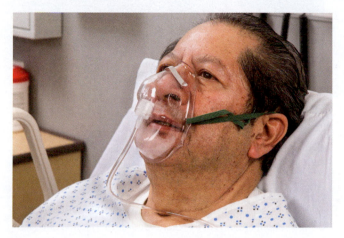

❹ A simple face mask.

■ Secure the elastic band around the client's head so that the mask is comfortable but snug.

■ Pad the band behind the ears and over bony prominences. **Rationale:** *Padding will prevent irritation from the mask.*

VARIATION: SIMPLE FACE MASK

■ A **face mask** that covers the client's nose and mouth may be used for oxygen inhalation. Most masks are made of clear, pliable plastic that can be molded to fit the face. They are held to the client's head with elastic bands. Some have a metal clip that can be bent over the bridge of the nose for a snug fit. There are several holes in the sides of the mask (exhalation ports) to allow the escape of exhaled carbon dioxide and intake of room air. To avoid rebreathing of carbon dioxide by the client while wearing a mask, a minimum 5 L/min oxygen flow rate is required.

■ Some masks have reservoir bags, which provide higher oxygen concentrations to the client. A portion of the client's expired air is directed into the bag. Because this air comes from the upper respiratory passages (e.g., the trachea and bronchi), where it does not take part in gaseous exchange, its oxygen concentration remains the same as that of inspired air.

■ The simple face mask delivers oxygen concentrations from 40% to 60% at liter flows of 5–8 L/min, respectively.

VARIATION: PARTIAL REBREATHER MASK ❺

■ The **partial rebreather mask** delivers oxygen concentrations of from 40% to 60% at liter flows of 6–10 L/min. The oxygen reservoir bag that is attached allows the client to rebreathe about the first third of the exhaled air in conjunction with oxygen.

■ The partial rebreather bag must not totally deflate during inspiration to avoid carbon dioxide buildup. If this problem occurs, the liter flow of oxygen needs to be increased so that the bag remains one third to one half full.

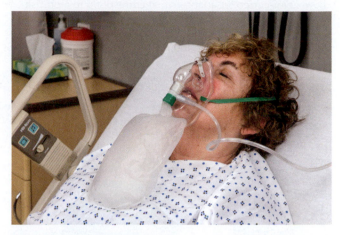

❺ A partial rebreather mask.

VARIATION: NONREBREATHER MASK ❻

■ The **nonrebreather mask** delivers the highest oxygen concentration possible—95%–100%—by means other than intubation or mechanical ventilation, at liter flows of 10–15 L/min. Using a nonrebreather mask, the client breathes only the source gas from the bag.

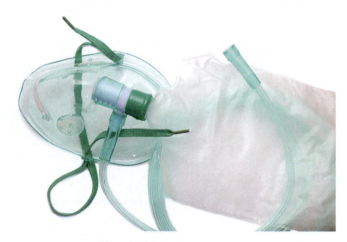

❻ A nonrebreather mask. (Source: © moodboard/fotolia)

■ One-way valves on the mask and between the reservoir bag and the mask prevent the room air and the client's exhaled air from entering the bag. In some cases, one of the side valves is removed so that the client can still inhale room air if the oxygen supply is accidentally cut off.

■ To prevent carbon dioxide buildup, the nonrebreather bag must not totally deflate during inspiration. If it does, the nurse can correct this problem by increasing the liter flow of oxygen.

(continued on next page)

SKILL 13.9 Administering Oxygen by Nasal Cannula, Face Mask, or Face Tent (continued)

VARIATION: VENTURI FACE MASK ⑦

- The **Venturi mask** delivers oxygen concentrations varying from 24% to 50% at liter flows of 4–10 L/min.
- The Venturi mask has a section of wide-bore tubing and can have color-coded jet adapters that correspond to a precise oxygen concentration and liter flow. For example, in some cases, a blue adapter delivers a 24% concentration of oxygen at 4 L/min and a green adapter delivers a 35% concentration of oxygen at 8 L/min. However, colors and concentrations may vary by manufacturers so the equipment must be examined carefully. Other manufacturers use a dial for setting the desired concentration. Turning the oxygen source flow rate higher than specified by the equipment manufacturer will not increase the concentration delivered to the client.

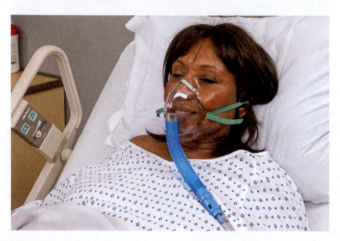

⑦ A Venturi mask.

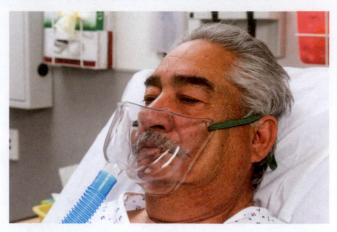

⑧ An oxygen face tent.

9. Inspect the equipment on a regular basis.
   - Check the liter flow and the level of water in the humidifier in 30 minutes and whenever providing care to the client.
   - Make sure that safety precautions are being followed.
10. Document findings in the client record using forms or checklists supplemented by narrative notes when appropriate.

Sample Documentation

9/16/2015 0930 Returned from physical therapy c̄ c/o SOB. R 26/min, shallow. P 92 bpm, BP 160/98 mmHg, SPO₂ 92%. Skin warm, no cyanosis. Lung sounds clear, no retractions. O₂ per nasal cannula applied @ 3 L/min.
_____P. Isola, RN 9/16/2015 1000 No further c/o SOB. R 20/min, P 88 bpm, BP 152/92 mmHg, SPO₂ 96%. O₂ per nasal cannula continues @ 3 L/min._____P. Isola, RN

VARIATION: FACE TENT

- Place the tent over the client's face, and secure the ties around the head. ⑧

For All Face Masks and Tents

7. Inspect the facial skin frequently for dampness or chafing, and dry and treat it as needed.
8. Assess the client regularly.
   - Assess the client's vital signs (including oxygen saturation), level of anxiety, color, and ease of respirations, and provide support while the client adjusts to the device.
   - Assess the client in 15–30 minutes, depending on the client's condition, and regularly thereafter.
   - Assess the client regularly for clinical signs of hypoxia, tachycardia, confusion, dyspnea, restlessness, and cyanosis. Review arterial blood gas results if they are available.

Evidence-Based Practice

Pulse oximetry measures the arterial saturation of available hemoglobin. The client with anemia may have a normal SPO₂ yet not have adequate tissue oxygenation because available hemoglobin is maximally saturated with oxygen. (Bridget, P. [2009]. Pulse points. *Nursing 2009, 39*[2], 8.)

SKILL 13.9   Administering Oxygen by Nasal Cannula, Face Mask, or Face Tent (*continued*)

VARIATION: PROVIDING OXYGEN VIA A TRACHEOSTOMY WITH A T-TUBE OR TRACHEOSTOMY COLLAR

- When a client breathes through a tracheostomy, air is no longer filtered and humidified as it is when passing through the upper airways; therefore, special precautions are necessary.
- Humidity may be provided with a tracheostomy mist collar. ❾ They may also wear a stoma protector such as a 4×4 gauze held in place with a cotton tie over the stoma or a light scarf to filter air as it enters the tracheostomy.

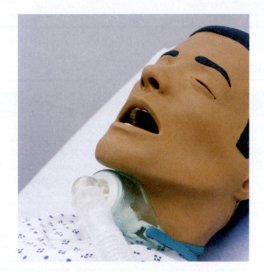

❾ A tracheostomy mist collar.

VARIATION: CONTINUOUS POSITIVE AIRWAY PRESSURE (CPAP) OR BIPHASIC POSITIVE AIRWAY PRESSURE (BiPAP)

- CPAP provides a single positive airway pressure to establish a minimal airway value (e.g., 5 mmHg) at the end of exhalation. ❿
- BiPAP provides two positive airway pressures, one to assist peak pressure on inhalation (e.g., 10 cm H_2O) and a lower one (e.g.,

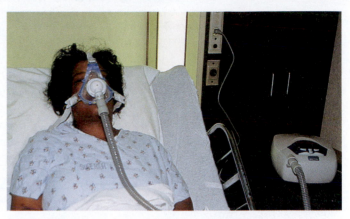

❿ Client receiving CPAP via face mask. Machine is capable of CPAP and BiPAP.

5 cm H_2O) to establish a minimal airway value at the end of exhalation.

- A BiPAP with a rate set feature provides two positive airway pressures and a set respiratory rate to augment breathing for the client with respiratory insufficiency. This capability qualifies this unit as a *noninvasive mechanical ventilator.* The client is spared intubation.
- A BiPAP autotitration device senses and measures the client's airflow and adjusts its pressure setting automatically to maintain airway patency.

CLINICAL ALERT

Clients using CPAP/BiPAP are constantly at risk for aspiration and subsequent respiratory complications. The candidate must be alert and responsive orally, must demonstrate airway protective measures (cough and swallow), and must not be restrained or sedated. Opioids relax the pharynx and contribute further to airway obstruction.

CPAP/BiPAP should never be used on a sedated client. There is great danger of aspiration should the client vomit.

Developmental Considerations

Oxygen Delivery

INFANTS
Oxygen Hood

- An oxygen hood is a rigid plastic dome that encloses an infant's head. It provides precise oxygen levels and high humidity.
- The gas should not be allowed to blow directly into the infant's face, and the hood should not rub against the infant's neck, chin, or shoulder.

CHILDREN
Oxygen Tent

- An oxygen tent consists of a rectangular, clear, plastic canopy with outlets that connect to an oxygen or compressed air source and to a humidifier that moisturizes the air or oxygen.

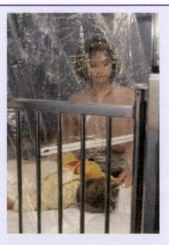

A pediatric tent can be used for oxygen delivery, humidification, temperature control, or a combination of these. (Copyright © B. Kramer/Custom Medical Stock Photo)

(*continued on next page*)

SKILL 13.9 Administering Oxygen by Nasal Cannula, Face Mask, or Face Tent (continued)

- Because the enclosed tent becomes very warm, some type of cooling mechanism such as an ice chamber or a refrigeration unit is provided to maintain the temperature at 20°–21°C (68°–70°F).
- Cover the child with a gown or a cotton blanket. Some agencies provide gowns with hoods, or a small towel may be wrapped around the head. **Rationale:** *The child needs protection from chilling and from the dampness and condensation in the tent.*
- Flood the tent with oxygen by setting the flow meter at 15 L/min for about 5 minutes. Then, adjust the flow meter according to orders (e.g., 10–15 L/min). **Rationale:** *Flooding the tent quickly increases the oxygen to the desired level.*

- The tent can deliver approximately 30% oxygen.
- Children may fight having a mask placed on their faces. They are often fearful when placed in oxygen tents or hoods. These are normal responses that vary based on experience, developmental stage, degree of threat to body image, and attachment/abandonment issues. Providing safe toys and a beloved blanket or pillow to hold can help, as can fostering the parent–child bond even though separated by the plastic. Encourage parents to interact with their child around and through the tubing and tent.

SKILL 13.10 Caring for the Client on a Mechanical Ventilator

Delegation

UAP may provide basic care for clients on mechanical ventilation and collect routine data such as vital signs, but they do not adjust ventilator settings or perform sterile procedures such as suctioning. They report any ventilator alarms, but do not assess the client or troubleshoot the system.

Equipment

- Prescribed type of ventilator
- Oxygen source
- Bag–valve–mask (BVM) ventilator system (Ambu bag)
- Suctioning supplies
- Ventilator setting flow sheet and medical record forms or access to the electronic record system
- Stethoscope
- Pulse oximeter and other vital signs monitors
- End-tidal carbon dioxide (ETCO$_2$) colorimetric measuring device, ❶ or other system for measuring expired carbon dioxide level

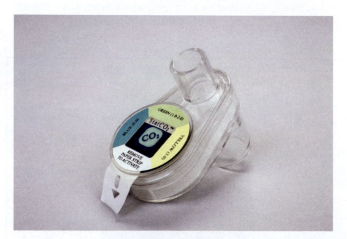

❶ Colorimetric measuring device. (Courtesy of Mercury Medical)

Preparation

- Review information about ventilator modes (**Table 13–1** ●).
- Review physician's order; review the client record for serial ABGs results, data indicating the changes that have been made in the client's ventilator settings over time, and the client's tolerance of mechanical ventilation.

TABLE 13–1 Ventilator Control Modes

MODE	FEATURES
Adaptive support ventilation (ASV)	Inspiratory pressure, inspiratory/expiratory ratio, and mandatory respiratory rate adjusted to maintain target volume and rate
Assist-control (AC)	Set volume with each client-triggered breath and set rate
Pressure control (PC)	Pressure-limited breath delivered at a set rate
Pressure-regulated volume control (PRVC); adaptive pressure ventilation (APV)	Pressure adjusted to deliver a set tidal volume
Pressure support ventilation (PSV)	Set pressure held during the entire inspiration
Synchronized intermittent mandatory ventilation (SIMV)	Set number of breaths and tidal volume while also allowing the client to take spontaneous breaths at a client-determined tidal volume and rate

Procedure

1. Prior to performing ventilator or client care, introduce self and verify the client's identity using agency protocol. Explain to the client what you are going to do and how he or she can participate. Discuss how the results will be used in planning further care or treatments.
2. Perform hand hygiene and observe other appropriate infection control procedures.
3. Provide for client privacy as needed.
4. Measure client temperature, pulse, blood pressure, and oxygen saturation using pulse oximetry. **Rationale:** *Changes in these vital signs may indicate either client improvement or inadequate ventilation requiring adjustments in ventilator settings.*
5. ABGs are ordered routinely or only if the client's condition warrants. Arterial blood may be drawn by the nurse, respiratory therapist, or laboratory technologist, depending on agency policy.
6. Confirm artificial airway tube placement by:
   - Auscultating lungs.
   - Measuring ETCO$_2$ at end expiration.
   - Checking the most recent chest x-ray for tube position.

SKILL 13.10 Caring for the Client on a Mechanical Ventilator (continued)

7. Check the endotracheal tube (ETT) for proper cuff inflation. **Rationale:** *Proper cuff inflation helps prevent ventilator-associated pneumonia (VAP) by ensuring that secretions that collect above the cuff cannot leak down into the lungs.*

8. Suction the client if indicated. Use the BVM device to hyperventilate the client as indicated.

9. Once you have confirmed that the client's status does not require immediate intervention, examine the ventilator equipment and settings.
   - Tubing from the airway to the ventilator should be secured so it does not pull on the client's airway. This includes having adequate slack to allow the client to turn without pulling on the tubing.
   - Verify that ventilator settings are as ordered. ❷
   - Verify that ventilator alarms are set correctly and are active.
   - Check for condensation in the tubing. If condensation is present, empty it appropriately and discard. Never empty fluid back into the humidifier, and use care that the fluid cannot run into the client's airway. **Rationale:** *Liquid in the tubing may be contaminated.* Refill the humidifier if needed.

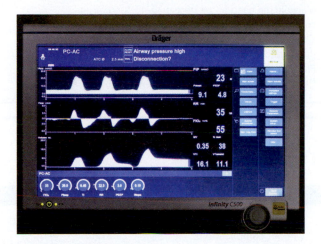

❷ Verify the ventilator settings and client data frequently. (Copyright Zuma Press, Inc./Alamy)

10. Provide oral care every 2 hours. Brush the teeth using a toothbrush and toothpaste at least twice per day. **Rationale:** *VAP can be reduced using this protocol* (Feider, Mitchell, & Bridges, 2010). See the accompanying box about preventing VAP.
    - Use a Yankauer suction tip to suction the mouth.
    - Some ETTs have a lumen above the cuff to allow for continuous suction of secretions that could collect there.
    - If the client has an oral endotracheal airway, it can be moved and resecured to the opposite side of the mouth every 24 hours. **Rationale:** *This minimizes pressure on lips and oral mucosa.* Recheck that the tube is correctly positioned after such a move.

11. Administer medications as ordered to prevent complications of mechanical ventilation. For example, administer histamine receptor inhibitors to prevent gastric ulcers.

12. Administer pain or sedation medications as needed for comfort.

CLINICAL ALERT

Paralytic agents have no effect on wakefulness or sensory perception, including perception of pain. With complete paralysis, pain might be manifested as increased heart rate, increased blood pressure, or sweating. Never assume that a client receiving a paralytic agent is asleep. Continually inform client about care, offer reassurance, and provide pain relief while the paralyzing effect of the drug persists.

The use of sedatives in mechanically ventilated clients prolongs duration of mechanical ventilation as well as length of hospitalization and ICU stay.

13. Institute actions to decrease complications such as deep venous thrombosis that may result from immobility related to the ventilator.
    - Perform range-of-motion exercises.
    - Assist the client to change positions at least every 2 hours, keeping the head of the bed elevated a minimum of 30 degrees.
    - Assist the client to stand or sit in a chair as tolerated.
    - Apply sequential compression devices to lower limbs according to agency policy.
    - If the client has a tracheostomy and is able to eat, encourage adequate intake of fluids and dietary fiber to promote gastrointestinal motility. For clients with an ETT, enteral feedings through a gastric tube are preferred over parenteral nutrition.
    - Administer prophylactic anticoagulant medications according to agency policy.

14. Establish an effective method of communicating with the intubated client.
    - Explain everything you are doing.
    - If the client requires eyeglasses, make them available.
    - If the client does not speak your language, provide a translator.
    - Ask yes/no questions when possible. Ask the client to nod the head if she agrees. Hand signals can also be used. Be sure to allow adequate time for the client to respond.
    - If the client is able to write, provide a writing pad or slate.
    - Be sure that the call light or bell is within reach at all times.
    - Acknowledge signs of frustration and attempt to determine and resolve the cause.

15. Document the ventilator settings and client parameters using checklists, flowcharts, and narrative notes as appropriate. Include results of settings changes, suctioning, activity, physical assessments, and laboratory data.

Sample Documentation

(Note that vital signs and ventilator settings would be recorded on flow sheets.)

10/1/2015 1530 ETT remains in place and secured, ETCO₂ 3%. Lungs clear to auscultation. Oral care provided. No signs of oral trauma or infection. Skin warm, no cyanosis. Active ROM all extremities. Turned to left side, HOB @ 30 degrees. Skin dry & intact. No bowel sounds. Compression devices in place both calves. Indicates pain is 5 on scale of 0 to 10 by holding up fingers. Medicated IV with immediate reduction to pain level of 3. Family in to visit. _____ T. Kourza, RN

(continued on next page)

SKILL 13.10 Caring for the Client on a Mechanical Ventilator *(continued)*

Developmental Considerations

INFANTS AND CHILDREN

- Mechanical ventilation is used for children both in hospitals and in the home. Include the parents and other lay caregivers in all teaching and care instructions.
- When the child's condition is stable, provide age-appropriate activities such as play, art, and educational opportunities.

OLDER ADULTS

- Older clients may be at greater risk for oxygen toxicity, especially if they have chronic lung conditions. As with all clients, the lowest effective oxygen concentration should be used.
- Provide reassurance and emotional support, recognizing that the need for ongoing mechanical ventilation may be viewed by the client or family as a sign of deteriorating health and movement toward death.

Setting of Care

Long-term mechanical ventilation in the home is commonplace in many communities.

- Teach caregivers all of the interventions, emergency, and safety measures needed to provide effective client assistance.
- Assist caregivers in contacting local emergency agencies to inform them that a ventilator-dependent client is in the home.
- Assist the client to determine if a backup power source is needed to run the ventilator should standard power be interrupted.

- Assist the client and family with community resources for obtaining needed equipment and disposal of biohazard waste. Ensure that they have extra supplies that might be needed in an emergency such as a bag and mask system.

Cultural Considerations

Touch-button voice systems are available that allow English or non-English-speaking clients on mechanical ventilation to tap a touch screen that delivers preprogrammed audible words, phrases, or symbols to hold two-way communication with staff.

Practice Guidelines for Preventing Ventilator-Associated Pneumonia (VAP)

Preventing VAP is an important nursing goal. Clients who develop VAP have a significantly greater mortality rate than those clients who do not develop this infection. The Centers for Disease Control and Prevention (2012) describes interventions that can significantly reduce VAP. Interventions to prevent or decrease VAP include the following:

- Maintain rigorous hand hygiene before and after touching the client or the ventilator.
- Maintain the head of the bed at 30–45 degrees unless contraindicated.
- Check the client's ability to breathe on his own every day so that the client can be taken off the ventilator as soon as possible.
- Provide oral care for the client on a regular basis.
- Clean or replace equipment between use on different clients.

▶ MAINTAINING A PATENT AIRWAY

Expected Outcomes

1. As needed, appropriate artificial airway will be used to maintain patency of client's airway.

2. Secretions are removed via appropriate suctioning method without complications.
3. The least invasive method of suctioning will be used to meet individual client's need for a clear airway.

SKILL 13.11 Inserting an Oropharyngeal Airway

Equipment

- Oropharyngeal tube
- Tongue depressor
- Clean gloves
- Suction catheter
- Suction source

Procedure

1. Ensure that client is unresponsive and has NO gag reflex. **Rationale:** *A conscious client may vomit and aspirate or develop laryngospasm during tube insertion.*
2. Select appropriate size airway—length should be from corner of mouth to corner of ear tragus. ❶

3. Perform hand hygiene and observe other appropriate infection control procedures; don gloves.
4. Provide for client privacy.
5. Gently open client's mouth with crossed finger technique, placing your thumb on client's lower teeth and index finger on the upper teeth and gently pushing them apart. You may need to use modified jaw thrust to insert tube.
6. Perform oral suctioning.
7. Hold tongue down with tongue depressor and advance airway to back of tongue **OR** advance airway upside down (curved upward) and, as airway passes uvula, rotate the airway 180 degrees.
8. Check that concave curve fits over tongue. It should extend from the lips to the pharynx, displacing the tongue anteri-

SKILL 13.11   Inserting an Oropharyngeal Airway *(continued)*

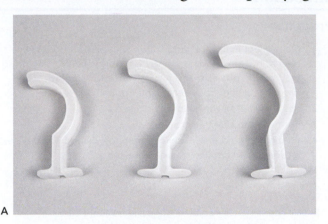

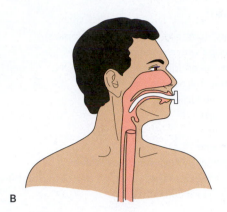

① A, Oropharyngeal airways; B, An oropharyngeal airway in place.

orly. **Rationale:** *Proper positioning helps prevent injury to lips, teeth, tongue, and posterior pharynx.*

9. Tape top and bottom of airway in position. **Rationale:** *Stabilization of the tube prevents injuries.*

10. Position client on side to facilitate drainage of secretions out of the mouth.
11. Remove and discard gloves. Perform hand hygiene.
12. Observe position of airway and evaluate quality of client's spontaneous breathing. Document actions and client response.

SKILL 13.12   Inserting a Nasopharyngeal Airway (Nasal Trumpet)

Equipment

- Flexible nasopharyngeal airway
- Water-soluble lubricant
- Clean gloves

Procedure

1. Prior to performing the procedure, introduce self and verify the client's identity using agency protocol. Explain to the client what you are going to do, why it is necessary, and how he or she can participate. Discuss how the results will be used in planning further care or treatments.
2. Select appropriate size tube (length from tip of nose to earlobe and lumen slightly narrower than client's naris). **①**
3. Perform hand hygiene and observe other appropriate infection control procedures; don gloves.
4. Provide for client privacy.
5. Lubricate entire length of tube.
6. Insert entire tube gently through naris, following anatomical line of nasal passage. If obstructed, try other naris.
7. Validate position **②** by
   - Feeling exhaled air through tube opening
   - Inspecting for tube tip behind uvula.
8. Position client on side to facilitate drainage of secretions.
9. Remove and discard gloves. Perform hand hygiene.
10. Continue to monitor position of airway and client's response.
11. Suction upper airway PRN using clean technique.
12. Document actions and client response.

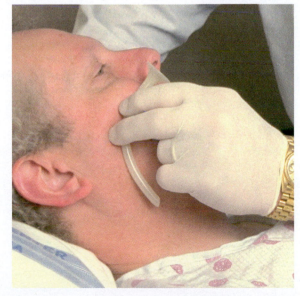

① Nasal trumpet protects airway from repeated trauma with upper airway (nasopharyngeal) suctioning.

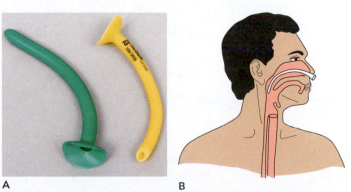

② A, Nasopharyngeal airways; B, A nasopharyngeal airway in place.

SKILL 13.13   Assisting with Endotracheal Intubation

Equipment

- "Crash cart" (contains most needed supplies)
- Laryngoscope with several blade sizes
- Stylet to guide endotracheal tube (ETT) (ONLY for oral intubation)
- Endotracheal tubes
- Water-soluble lubricant
- McGill forceps
- Suction source
- Oxygen source
- Bag–valve–mask (BVM) ventilator system
- Twill tape, adhesive tape, Velcro holder, or Endotube stabilizer
- 10-mL syringe for cuff inflation
- Stethoscope
- CO_2 detector (for airway placement validation)
- Oral airway or bite block
- Clean gloves, personal protective equipment including face shield
- Established pulse oximetry and cardiac monitor if available
- Wrist restraints (if ordered by physician)
- Prepared sedative/neuromuscular blocking agent as ordered
- Labeled container for client's dentures

Note: Noninvasive positive pressure ventilation methods (CPAP, BiPAP) provide an appropriate alternative to intubation for many clients with ventilator insufficiency.

Preparation

- Determine that client has *no protective airway reflexes.*
- Bring crash cart to client's doorway.
- Check that all necessary equipment is functioning: oxygen/ suction source, and delivery systems, laryngoscope batteries.
- Inflate and deflate airway cuff to determine if it is intact.
- Perform hand hygiene and don gloves. Don personal protective equipment.
- Insert stylet into tube (only for oral intubation); ensure that stylus does not extend beyond tube tip.
- Lubricate tube.
- Remove client's dentures/bridgework and place in labeled container.

Procedure

1. Place client in flat supine position with pillow under shoulders to hyperextend neck and help open airway. Position so that mouth, pharynx, and trachea are aligned. **Rationale:** *Proper positioning facilitates intubation.*
2. Restrain client's wrists only if necessary.
3. Premedicate client as ordered.
4. Preoxygenate client for several minutes, using BVM device. **Rationale:** *To create an "oxygen reserve."*

> ### CLINICAL ALERT
>
> Even if spontaneously breathing, the client should be preoxygenated with 100% O_2 for endotracheal tube placement. Ventilation must not be interrupted for over 30 seconds.
>
> Cricoid pressure may be used only if the client:
>
> - Is nonresponsive
> - Is not vomiting
> - Does not have a cuffed tracheal tube in place.
>
> While cuff pressures are typically maintained at 20–25 mmHg, an individual client's tracheal capillary pressure cannot be determined and excessive cuff pressure is the best predictor of tracheolaryngeal injury.

5. Using thumb and index finger, apply cricoid pressure during tube insertion. ❶ **Rationale:** *This facilitates tracheal placement and protects against aspiration of gastric contents.*
6. Maintain cricoid pressure while inflating cuff to "minimal leak" inflation by placing stethoscope at client's suprasternal notch and noting a slight hissing sound at peak of inspiration.
7. Attach BVM device, provide ventilation, and look for chest to rise. **Rationale:** *If chest does not rise, esophageal intubation is likely.*
8. Check tube placement using CO_2 detector. **Rationale:** *Presence of CO_2 indicates tracheal intubation.*
9. Place stethoscope over epigastrium. **Rationale:** *If gurgling is heard, and abdominal distention noted, esophageal placement is likely.*

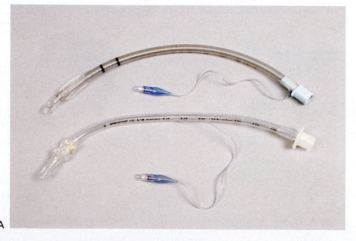

A

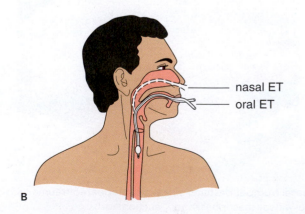

B

❶ A, Endotracheal tubes; B, An endotracheal tube in place.

SKILL 13.13   Assisting with Endotracheal Intubation *(continued)*

10. Auscultate lung fields for bilateral breath sounds. **Rationale:** *This ensures that accidental right main stem intubation has not occurred.*
11. Mark tube at level of client's front teeth and tape securely with twill or adhesive tape, Velcro holder, or Endotube stabilizer. **Rationale:** *Secure taping prevents tube displacement.*
12. Recheck tube placement with the previous measures (steps 8–10).
13. Place bite block or oral airway if ETT has been positioned orally.
14. Attach O_2 source to ETT.
15. Discard disposable equipment, remove protective gear and gloves, and perform hand hygiene.
16. Position client in position as ordered.
17. Obtain chest x-ray to confirm tracheal placement of ETT.
18. Place call bell and writing material within client's reach (as indicated). Document relevant information.
19. Reposition ETT every 4 hours: right, center, left, then repeat (using Velcro or Endotube stabilizer).

> **CLINICAL ALERT**
>
> The presence of an endotracheal tube bypasses defenses that normally protect the lower airways (filtration, humidification, and hydration of inspired air and epiglottal closure). In addition, mucociliary transport of secretions and trapped pathogens is impaired. These alterations place intubated clients at risk for aspiration pneumonia.
>
> Centers for Disease Control and Prevention guidelines recommend orotracheal over nasotracheal intubation to reduce the incidence of sinus infection.

SKILL 13.14   Inflating a Tracheal Tube Cuff

Equipment

- 10-mL syringe
- Suction equipment
- Stethoscope
- Clean gloves

Note: The foam cuff does not require injected air. Air enters the balloon when port is open.

Procedure

1. Don clean gloves.
2. Attach 10-mL syringe to distal end of inflatable cuff port, making sure seal is tight. ❶

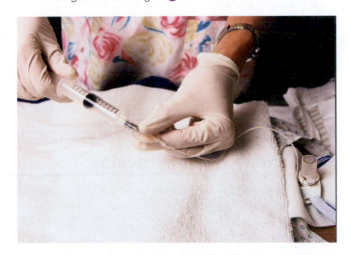

❶ Attach 10-mL syringe to inflate tube cuff.

3. Inflate cuff for a minimal leak or minimal occlusive volume detected by auscultating over the suprasternal notch for a hissing sound at peak of inspiration. **Rationale:** *This provides an adequate seal without risking tracheal pressure necrosis.*

4. Ask client to speak—if voice is heard, inflation is inadequate for mechanical ventilation. ❷

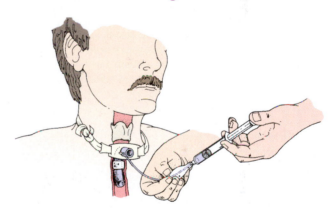

❷ Inflate endotracheal or tracheostomy tube cuff to minimal occlusive volume.

5. Connect ventilator or T-piece to tracheal tube opening if indicated. Document relevant information.
6. Assess breath sounds every 2 hours. **Rationale:** *Presence of bilateral breath sounds indicates proper tube position in trachea.*
7. Monitor cuff pressure regularly. **Rationale:** *This may detect inadvertent cuff overinflation and prevent potential necrosis of tracheal tissue. Pressure is usually maintained at 20–25 mmHg to prevent tracheal necrosis. However, an individual client's tracheal capillary pressure cannot be determined.*

> **CLINICAL ALERT**
>
> Tracheal tube cuff inflation is essential for mechanically ventilated clients. Without cuff inflation, delivered air diverts out through the nose and mouth, and lungs are not ventilated.

SKILL 13.15 Providing Care for the Client with an Endotracheal Tube

Procedure

1. Monitor breath sounds every 4 hours. Breath sounds should be heard equally throughout lung fields bilaterally.
2. Check marked points on tube at insertion level. **Rationale:** *This determines if tube has moved.*
3. Inspect positioning and stabilization of tube. **Rationale:** *A change of position can obstruct airway or cause erosion and necrosis of tissues.*
4. Inspect and clean mouth and nose. Observe for pressure areas or ulceration.
5. Reposition ET tube every 4 hours (right, center, left), noting tube depth each time.
6. Support client's head and tube when turning. **Rationale:** *This prevents tube from becoming dislodged or airway from becoming obstructed.*
7. Place call bell within reach and provide alternative means of communication when cuffed tube is in place. **Rationale:** *No air passes over larynx, so client is not able to summon help or communicate.* Document relevant information.
8. Support client by spending extra time, using touch, and anticipating client's needs.
9. Ensure adequate hydration. **Rationale:** *Artificial airways bypass the humidifying process of normal breathing.*
10. Provide suction toothbrushing every 12 hours, oral swabbing every 2 hours, and oropharyngeal subglottal suctioning every 6 hours. **Rationale:** *This reduces oropharyngeal bacteria and helps prevent pulmonary infection.*

> **CLINICAL ALERT**
> Even with appropriate cuff inflation, intubated clients receiving gastric/enteral tube feedings are at high risk for aspiration.

SKILL 13.16 Extubating the Client with an Endotracheal Tube

Equipment

- Suction source
- Oral suction catheter (or Yankauer)
- Sterile suction catheter set
- Clean gloves
- Sterile gloves
- Personal protective equipment
- Oxygen source
- Postextubation oxygen delivery device
- Syringe for cuff deflation

Preparation

- Check physician's order. Assess client's readiness for extubation.
- Obtain vital signs.
- Explain procedure to client.
- Prepare postextubation oxygen administration device.
- Place client in the Fowler position.

> **CLINICAL ALERT**
> Do not feed client orally immediately after extubation. Seek consult for a feeding trial for clients at risk for aspiration.

Procedure

1. Perform hand hygiene and don clean gloves and personal protective equipment.
2. Perform oral or nasopharyngeal suctioning.
3. Have client take several slow deep breaths. **Rationale:** *This hyperoxygenates client in preparation for extubation.*
4. Deflate tube cuff using syringe or cut pilot tubing.
5. Untie the tracheal tube.
6. Remove gloves, perform hand hygiene, and don sterile gloves.
7. Connect sterile catheter to suction source.
8. Insert sterile suction catheter into airway until resistance is met, then retract slightly.
9. Leave suction catheter in place.
10. Have client take a deep breath. **Rationale:** *This dilates the vocal cords and makes removal easier and less traumatic.*
11. Apply suction while removing catheter and airway at the same time.
12. Immediately apply supplementary oxygen device.
13. Monitor client frequently at first, then regularly.
14. Dispose of equipment, remove gloves and protective gear, and perform hand hygiene. Document action and client response.

SKILL 13.17 Oropharyngeal, Nasopharyngeal and Nasotracheal Suctioning

Delegation

Oral suctioning using a Yankauer suction tube can be delegated to UAP and to the client or family, if appropriate, because this is not a sterile procedure. The nurse needs to review the procedure and important points such as not applying suction during insertion of the tube to avoid trauma to the mucous membrane. Oropharyngeal suctioning uses a suction catheter and, although not a sterile procedure, should be performed by a nurse or respiratory therapist. Suctioning can stimulate the gag reflex, hypoxia, and dysrhythmias that may require problem solving. Nasopharyngeal and nasotracheal suctioning require use of a sterile technique and application of knowledge and problem solving and should be performed by a nurse or respiratory therapist.

Equipment

Oral and Nasopharyngeal/Nasotracheal Suctioning (using sterile technique)

- Towel or moisture-resistant pad
- Portable or wall suction machine with tubing, collection receptacle, and suction pressure gauge
- Sterile disposable container for fluids

SKILL 13.17   Oropharyngeal, Nasopharyngeal and Nasotracheal Suctioning *(continued)*

- Sterile normal saline or water
- Goggles or face shield, if appropriate
- Moisture-resistant disposal bag
- Sputum trap, if specimen is to be collected

Oral and Oropharyngeal Suctioning (using clean technique)

- Yankauer suction catheter or suction catheter kit
- Clean gloves
- Bulb syringe

Nasopharyngeal or Nasotracheal Suctioning (using sterile technique)

- Sterile gloves
- Sterile suction catheter kit (#12 to #18 Fr for adults, #8 to #10 Fr for children, and #5 to #8 Fr for infants)
- Water-soluble lubricant
- Y-connector

Procedure

1. Check physician's order. Prior to performing the procedure, introduce self and verify the client's identity using agency protocol. Explain to the client what you are going to do, why it is necessary, and how he or she can participate. Inform the client that suctioning will relieve breathing difficulty and, although the procedure is painless, it is noisy and can cause discomfort by stimulating the cough, gag, or sneeze reflex. **Rationale:** *Knowing that the procedure will alleviate breathing problems is often reassuring and enlists the client's cooperation.*
2. Perform hand hygiene and observe other appropriate infection control procedures.
3. Provide for client privacy.
4. Prepare the client.
   - Position a conscious person who has a functional gag reflex in the semi-Fowler position with the head turned to one side for oral suctioning or with the neck hyperextended for nasal suctioning. **Rationale:** *These positions facilitate the insertion of the catheter and help prevent aspiration of secretions.*
   - Position an unconscious client in the lateral position, facing you. **Rationale:** *This position allows the tongue to fall forward, so that it will not obstruct the catheter on insertion. The lateral position also facilitates drainage of secretions from the pharynx and prevents the possibility of aspiration.*
   - Place the towel or moisture-resistant pad over the pillow or under the chin.
5. Prepare the equipment.
   - Turn the suction device on and set to appropriate negative pressure on the suction gauge. The amount of negative pressure should be high enough to clear secretions but not too high. **Rationale:** *Too high of a pressure can cause the catheter to adhere to the tracheal wall and cause irritation or trauma.* A rule of thumb is to use the lowest amount of suction pressure needed to clear the secretions. Ireton (2007) suggests suction pressures of 60–80 mmHg for neonates, 80–100 mmHg for children, and 80–120 mmHg for adolescents. LeMone and Burke (2012) recommend suction pressures between 80 and 120 mmHg for adults.

Oral and Oropharyngeal Suction

- Apply clean gloves.

- Moisten the tip of the Yankauer or suction catheter with sterile water or saline. ❶ **Rationale:** *This reduces friction and eases insertion.*

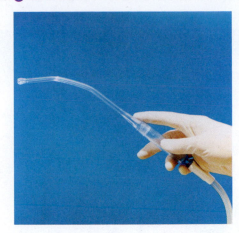

❶ Oral (Yankauer) suction tube.

- Pull the tongue forward, if necessary, using gauze.
- Do not apply suction (that is, leave your finger off the port) during insertion. **Rationale:** *Applying suction during insertion causes trauma to the mucous membrane.*
- Advance the catheter about 10–15 cm (4–6 in.) along one side of the mouth into the oropharynx. **Rationale:** *Directing the catheter along the side avoids stimulating the gag reflex, which can cause vomiting and compromise the airway.*
- It may be necessary during oropharyngeal suctioning to apply suction to secretions that collect in the vestibule of the mouth and beneath the tongue.
- Remove and discard gloves. Perform hand hygiene.

VARIATION: SUCTIONING AN INFANT WITH A BULB SYRINGE

A bulb syringe is used to remove secretions from an infant's nose or mouth.

- An assistant may be needed to gently position and hold the infant or child with the head in midline, and to keep the child's hands out of the way.
- Don gloves and place saline nose drops in a naris. **Rationale:** *The nose drops loosen dried secretions.*
- Deflate the bulb. Insert the tip of the bulb syringe into the infant's naris. ❷ **Rationale:** *Deflating the bulb first prevents pushing the secretions back into the nasopharynx.*

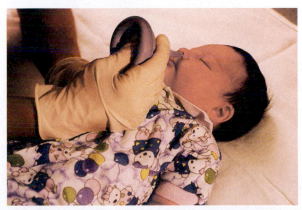

❷ Insertion of a deflated bulb syringe.

(continued on next page)

SKILL 13.17   Oropharyngeal, Nasopharyngeal and Nasotracheal Suctioning (*continued*)

■ Release the bulb and remove the syringe from the naris. ❸
Expel the secretions into the proper receptacle.

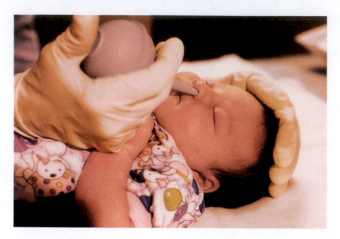

❸ Removal of a reinflated bulb syringe.

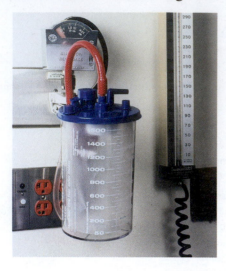

❺ A wall suction unit.

■ Repeat the procedure in the other naris. Assess the child's ability to breathe easily. Repeat the suctioning as necessary.
■ Document the procedure, the character of the secretions, and the infant's response.

Nasopharyngeal and Nasotracheal Suction

■ Open the lubricant if performing nasopharyngeal/nasotracheal suctioning.
■ Open the sterile suction package.
  a. Set up the cup or container, touching only the outside.
  b. Pour sterile water or saline into the container.
  c. Apply the sterile gloves, or apply an unsterile glove on the nondominant hand and then a sterile glove on the dominant hand. **Rationale:** *The sterile gloved hand maintains the sterility of the suction catheter, and the unsterile glove holds the suction connecting tubing and prevents the transmission of microorganisms to the nurse.*
■ With your sterile gloved hand, pick up the sterile suction catheter and attach it to the suction unit. ❹ ❺

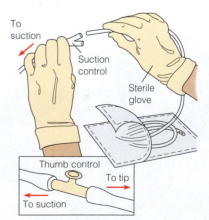

❹ Attaching the catheter to the suction unit.

6. Test the pressure of the suction and the patency of the catheter by applying your sterile gloved finger or thumb to the

port or open branch of the Y-connector (the suction control) to create suction.
  • If needed, apply or increase supplemental oxygen.
7. Lubricate and introduce the catheter.
  • Lubricate the catheter tip with sterile water, saline, or water-soluble lubricant. **Rationale:** *This reduces friction and eases insertion.*
  • Remove oxygen with the nondominant hand, if appropriate.
  • *Without applying suction,* insert the catheter into either naris and advance it along the floor of the nasal cavity. **Rationale:** *This avoids the nasal turbinates.*
  • Never force the catheter against an obstruction. If one nostril is obstructed, try the other.
8. Perform suctioning.
  • Apply your finger to the suction control port to start suction, and gently rotate the catheter. **Rationale:** *Gentle rotation of the catheter ensures that all surfaces are reached and prevents trauma to any one area of the respiratory mucosa due to prolonged suction.*
  • Apply suction for 5–10 seconds while slowly withdrawing the catheter, then remove your finger from the control and remove the catheter.
  • A suction attempt should last only 10–15 seconds. During this time, the catheter is inserted, the suction applied and discontinued, and the catheter removed.
9. Rinse the catheter and repeat suctioning as above.
  • Rinse and flush the catheter and tubing with sterile water or saline.
  • Relubricate the catheter, and repeat suctioning until the air passage is clear.
  • Allow sufficient time between each suction for ventilation and oxygenation. Limit suctioning to 5 minutes total. **Rationale:** *Applying suction for too long may cause secretions to increase or may decrease the client's oxygen supply.*
  • Encourage the client to breathe deeply and to cough between suctions. Use supplemental oxygen, if appropriate. **Rationale:** *Coughing and deep breathing help carry*

SKILL 13.17 Oropharyngeal, Nasopharyngeal and Nasotracheal Suctioning (continued)

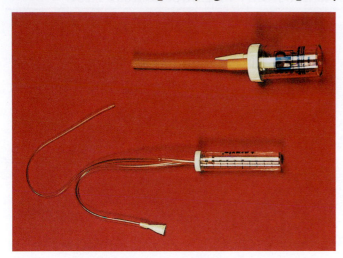

6 Sputum collection traps.

secretions from the trachea and bronchi into the pharynx, where they can be reached with the suction catheter. Deep breathing and supplemental oxygen provide oxygen to the alveoli.

10. Obtain a specimen if required.
    • Use a sputum trap **6** as follows:
    a. Attach the suction catheter to the tubing of the sputum trap.
    b. Attach the suction tubing to the sputum trap air vent.
    c. Suction the client. The sputum trap will collect the mucus during suctioning.
    d. Remove the catheter from the client. Disconnect the sputum trap tubing from the suction catheter. Remove the suction tubing from the trap air vent.
    e. Connect the tubing of the sputum trap to the air vent. **Rationale:** This retains any microorganisms in the sputum trap.
    • Connect the suction catheter to the tubing.
    • Flush the catheter to remove secretions from the tubing.
11. Promote client comfort.
    • Offer to assist the client with oral or nasal hygiene.
    • Assist the client to a position that facilitates breathing.

12. Dispose of equipment and ensure availability for the next suction.
    • Dispose of the catheter, gloves, water, and waste container.
    a. Rinse the suction tubing as needed by inserting the end of the tubing into the used water container.
    b. Wrap the catheter around your sterile gloved hand and hold the catheter as the glove is removed over it for disposal. Perform hand hygiene.
    • Empty and rinse the suction collection container as needed or indicated by protocol. Change the suction tubing and container daily.
    • Ensure that supplies are available for the next suctioning (suction kit, gloves, and water or normal saline).
13. Assess the effectiveness of suctioning.
    • Auscultate the client's breath sounds to ensure they are clear of secretions. Observe skin color, respiratory rate, heart rate, level of anxiety, and oxygen saturation levels.
14. Document relevant data.
    • Record the procedure: the amount, consistency, color, and odor of sputum (e.g., foamy, white mucus; thick, green-tinged mucus; or blood-flecked mucus) and the client's respiratory status before and after the procedure. This may include lung sounds, rate and character of breathing, and oxygen saturation.
    • If the procedure is carried out frequently, it may be appropriate to record only once, at the end of the shift; however, the frequency of the suctioning must be recorded.

Sample Documentation

12/12/2015 0830 Producing large amounts of thick, tenacious white mucus to back of oral pharynx but unable to expectorate into tissue. Uses Yankauer suction tube as needed. O₂ sat increased from 89% before suctioning to 93% after suctioning. RR also decreased from 26 to 18–20 after suctioning. Lungs clear to auscultation. Continuous O₂ at 2 L/min via n/c. Will continue to reassess q hour. _____ L. Webb, RN

Developmental Considerations

INFANTS
■ A bulb syringe is used to remove secretions from an infant's nose and mouth. Care needs to be taken to avoid stimulating the gag reflex.

CHILDREN
■ A catheter is used to remove secretions from an older child's mouth or nose.

OLDER ADULTS
■ Older Adults often have cardiac and/or pulmonary disease, thus increasing their susceptibility to hypoxemia related to suctioning. Watch closely for signs of hypoxemia. If noted, stop suctioning and hyperoxygenate.

Setting of Care

■ Teach clients and families that the most important aspect of infection control is frequent hand washing.
■ Airway suctioning in the home is considered a clean procedure.
■ The catheter or Yankauer should be flushed by suctioning recently boiled or distilled water to rinse away mucus, followed by the suctioning of air through the device to dry the internal surface and, thus, discourage bacterial growth. The outer surface of the device may be wiped with alcohol or hydrogen peroxide. The suction catheter or Yankauer should be allowed to dry and then stored in a clean, dry area.
■ Suction catheters treated in the manner described above may be reused. It is recommended that catheters be discarded after 24 hours. Yankauer suction tubes may be cleaned, boiled, and reused.

SKILL 13.18   Suctioning the Client with a Tracheostomy or Endotracheal Tube

Delegation

Suctioning a tracheostomy or endotracheal tube is a sterile, invasive technique requiring application of scientific knowledge and problem solving. This skill is performed by a nurse or respiratory therapist and is not delegated to UAP.

Equipment

- Bag–valve–mask (BVM) ventilator system connected to 100% oxygen
- Sterile towel (optional)
- Equipment for suctioning (see Skill 13.17)
- Goggles and mask if necessary
- Gown (if necessary)
- Sterile gloves
- Moisture-resistant bag

Preparation

Determine if the client has been suctioned previously and, if so, review the documentation of the procedure. This information can be very helpful in preparing the nurse for both the physiological and psychological impact of suctioning on the client.

Procedure

1. Prior to performing the procedure, introduce self and verify the client's identity using agency protocol. Explain to the client what you are going to do, why it is necessary, and how he or she can participate. Inform the client that suctioning usually stimulates the cough reflex and that this assists in removing the secretions.
2. Perform hand hygiene and observe other appropriate infection control procedures (e.g., gloves, goggles).
3. Provide for client privacy.
4. Prepare the client.
    - If not contraindicated, place the client in the semi-Fowler position to promote deep breathing, maximum lung expansion, and productive coughing. **Rationale:** *Deep breathing oxygenates the lungs, counteracts the hypoxic effects of suctioning, and may induce coughing. Coughing helps to loosen and move secretions.*
5. Prepare the equipment (open suction system). See variation for closed suction system.
    - Attach the resuscitation apparatus to the oxygen source. ❶ Adjust the oxygen flow to 100%.
    - Open the sterile supplies:
       a. Suction kit or catheter
       b. Sterile basin/container.
    - Pour sterile normal saline or water in sterile basin.
    - Place the sterile towel, if used, across the client's chest below the tracheostomy or on a workspace.
    - Turn on the suction, and set the pressure in accordance with agency policy. For a wall unit, a pressure setting between 80 and 120 mmHg is normally used for adults, 60 and 100 mmHg for children.
    - Apply goggles, mask, and gown if necessary.
    - Apply sterile gloves. Some agencies recommend putting a sterile glove on the dominant hand and an unsterile glove on the nondominant hand. **Rationale:** *The sterile gloved hand maintains the sterility of the suction cath-*

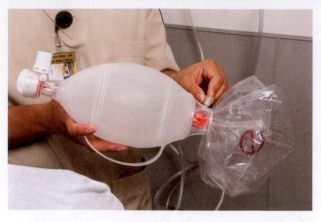

❶ Attaching the resuscitation apparatus to the oxygen source.

eter, and the unsterile glove holds the suction connecting tubing and prevents the transmission of microorganisms to the nurse.
- Holding the catheter in the dominant hand and the connector in the nondominant hand, attach the suction catheter to the suction tubing. ❷

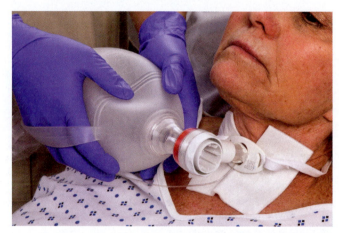

❷ Attaching the resuscitator to the tracheostomy.

6. Flush and lubricate the catheter.
    - Using the dominant hand, place the catheter tip in the sterile saline solution.
    - Using the thumb of the nondominant hand, occlude the thumb control and suction a small amount of the sterile solution through the catheter. **Rationale:** *This determines that the suction equipment is working properly and lubricates the outside and the lumen of the catheter. Lubrication eases insertion and reduces tissue trauma during insertion. Lubricating the lumen also helps prevent secretions from sticking to the inside of the catheter.*

CLINICAL ALERT

Suction client's airway PRN. Secretions are usually more copious following the irritation of intubation.

Suction catheter diameter should be no larger than one half the inner diameter of the artificial airway. To determine catheter diameter size, multiply the artificial airway's diameter times 2 (e.g., for 8-mm tube, use a 16 French suction catheter).

SKILL 13.18 Suctioning the Client with a Tracheostomy or Endotracheal Tube (continued)

Hyperoxygenate the client before and after each time the airway is entered for suctioning, and wait 1 minute before suctioning again to prevent severe hypoxemia.

7. If the client does not have copious secretions, hyperventilate the lungs with a resuscitation bag before suctioning.
   - Summon an assistant, if one is available, for this step.
   - Using your nondominant hand, turn on the oxygen to 12–15 L/min.
   - If the client is receiving oxygen, disconnect the oxygen source from the tracheostomy tube using your nondominant hand.
   - Attach the resuscitator to the tracheostomy or ETT.
   - Compress the BVM device three to five times as the client inhales. This is best done by a second person who can use both hands to compress the bag, thus providing a greater inflation volume.
   - Observe the rise and fall of the client's chest to assess the adequacy of each ventilation.
   - Remove the resuscitation device and place it on the bed or the client's chest with the connector facing up.
8. Document procedure and client response.

VARIATION: CLOSED SUCTION SYSTEM (IN-LINE CATHETER)

- If a catheter is not attached, apply clean gloves, aseptically open a new closed catheter set, and attach the ventilator connection on the T-piece to the ventilator tubing. Attach the client connection to the endotracheal tube or tracheostomy.
- Attach one end of the suction connecting tubing to the suction connection port of the closed system and the other end of the connecting tubing to the suction device.
- Turn suction on, occlude or kink tubing, and depress the suction control valve (on the closed catheter system) to set suction to the appropriate level. Release the suction control valve.
- Use the ventilator to hyperoxygenate and hyperinflate the client's lungs.

- Unlock the suction control mechanism if required by the manufacturer.
- Advance the suction catheter enclosed in its plastic sheath with the dominant hand. Steady the T-piece with the nondominant hand.
- Depress the suction control valve and apply intermittent suction for no more than 10 seconds and gently withdraw the catheter.
- Repeat as needed, remembering to provide hyperoxygenation and hyperinflation as needed.
- When suctioning is complete, withdraw the catheter into its sleeve and close the access valve, if appropriate. **Rationale:** *If the system does not have an access valve on the client connector, the nurse needs to observe for the potential of the catheter migrating into the airway and partially obstructing the artificial airway.*
- Flush the catheter by instilling normal saline into the irrigation port and applying suction. Repeat until the catheter is clear.
- Close the irrigation port and close the suction valve.
- Remove and discard gloves. Perform hand hygiene.

Developmental Considerations

INFANTS AND CHILDREN

- An assistant or parent may be needed to hold the child gently and to keep hands out of the way. The assistant or parent should maintain the child's head in the midline position.

Setting of Care

- Whenever possible, the client should be encouraged to clear the airway by coughing.
- Clients may need to learn to suction their secretions if they cannot cough effectively.
- Clean gloves should be used when endotracheal suctioning is performed in the home environment.
- The nurse needs to instruct the caregiver on how to determine the need for suctioning and the correct process and rationale underlying the practice of suctioning to avoid potential complications of suctioning.
- Stress the importance of adequate hydration: It thins secretions, which can aid in their removal by coughing or suctioning.

SKILL 13.19 Providing Tracheostomy Care

Delegation

Tracheostomy care involves application of scientific knowledge, sterile technique, and problem solving, and therefore needs to be performed by a nurse or respiratory therapist.

Equipment

- Sterile disposable tracheostomy cleaning kit or supplies including sterile containers, sterile nylon brush and/or pipe cleaners, sterile applicators
- Disposable inner cannula if applicable
- Towel or drape to protect bed linens

- Sterile suction catheter kit (suction catheter and sterile container for solution)
- Sterile normal saline (Some agencies may use a mixture of hydrogen peroxide and sterile normal saline. Check agency protocol for soaking solution.)
- Sterile gloves (2 pairs—one pair is for suctioning if needed)
- Clean gloves
- Moisture-proof bag
- Commercially prepared sterile tracheostomy dressing or sterile 4×4 gauze dressing
- Cotton twill ties or Velcro collar
- Clean scissors

(continued on next page)

SKILL 13.19 Providing Tracheostomy Care (*continued*)

Procedure

1. Prior to performing the procedure, introduce self and verify the client's identity using agency protocol. Explain to the client what you are going to do, why it is necessary, and how he or she can participate. Provide for a means of communication, such as eye blinking or raising a finger, to indicate pain or distress. Follow through by carefully observing the client throughout the procedure. Offer periodic eye contact, caring touch, and verbal reassurance. Some clients respond well to a sense of efficiency and gentle humor, and nurses must decide when to use this approach.

2. Perform hand hygiene and observe other appropriate infection control procedures.

3. Provide for client privacy.

4. Prepare the client and the equipment.
   - Assist the client to a semi-Fowler or Fowler position to promote lung expansion.
   - Suction the tracheostomy tube, if needed.
   - If suctioning was required, allow the client to rest and restore oxygenation.
   - Open the tracheostomy kit or sterile basins.
   - Establish a sterile field.
   - Open other sterile supplies as needed including sterile applicators, suction kit, tracheostomy dressing, and, if applicable, the disposable inner cannula.
   - Pour the soaking solution and sterile normal saline into separate containers.
   - Apply clean gloves.
   - Remove oxygen source.
   - Unlock the inner cannula (if present) and remove it by gently pulling it out toward you in line with its curvature. Place the inner cannula in the soaking solution. **Rationale:** *This moistens and loosens dried secretions.*
   - Remove the soiled tracheostomy dressing. Place the soiled dressing in your gloved hand and peel the glove off so that it turns inside out over the dressing. Remove and discard gloves and the dressing. Perform hand hygiene.
   - Apply sterile gloves. Keep your dominant hand sterile during the procedure.

5. Clean the inner cannula. (See the *Variation* section for using a disposable inner cannula.)
   - Remove the inner cannula from the soaking solution.
   - Clean the lumen and entire inner cannula thoroughly using the brush or pipe cleaners moistened with sterile normal saline. ❶ Inspect the cannula for cleanliness by holding it at eye level and looking through it into the light.
   - Rinse the inner cannula thoroughly in the sterile normal saline.
   - After rinsing, gently tap the cannula against the inside edge of the sterile saline container. Use a pipe cleaner folded in half to dry only the inside of the cannula; do not dry the outside. **Rationale:** *This removes excess liquid from the cannula and prevents possible aspiration by the client, while leaving a film of moisture on the outer surface to lubricate the cannula for reinsertion.*

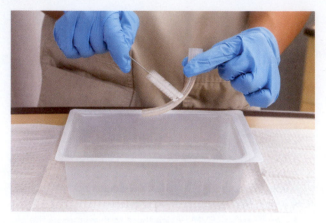

❶ Cleaning the inner cannula with a brush.

6. Replace the inner cannula, securing it in place.
   - Insert the inner cannula by grasping the outer flange and inserting the cannula in the direction of its curvature.
   - Lock the cannula in place by turning the lock (if present) into position to secure the flange of the inner cannula to the outer cannula.

7. Clean the incision site and tube flange.
   - Using sterile applicators or gauze dressings moistened with normal saline, clean the incision site. ❷ Handle the sterile supplies with your dominant hand. Use each applicator or gauze dressing only once and then discard. **Rationale:** *This avoids contaminating a clean area with a soiled gauze dressing or applicator.*

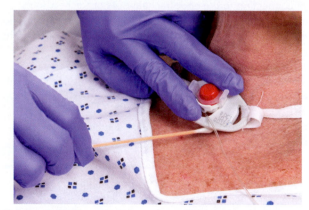

❷ Using an applicator stick to clean the tracheostomy site.

   - Hydrogen peroxide may be used (usually in a half-strength solution mixed with sterile normal saline; use a separate sterile container if this is necessary) to remove crusty secretions around the tracheostomy site. Do not use directly on the site. Check agency policy. Thoroughly rinse the cleaned area using gauze squares moistened with sterile normal saline. **Rationale:** *Hydrogen peroxide can be irritating to the skin and inhibit healing if not thoroughly removed.*
   - Clean the flange of the tube in the same manner.
   - Thoroughly dry the client's skin and tube flanges with dry gauze squares.

8. Apply a sterile dressing.
   - Use a commercially prepared tracheostomy dressing ❸ or open and refold a nonraveling 4×4 gauze dressing into a V shape. Avoid using cotton-filled gauze squares or cutting the

SKILL 13.19   Providing Tracheostomy Care (continued)

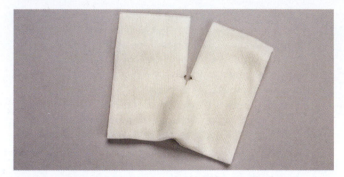

③ A commercially prepared tracheostomy dressing of nonraveling material.

> 4×4 gauze. **Rationale:** *Cotton lint or gauze fibers can be aspirated by the client, potentially creating a tracheal abscess.*
> * Place the dressing under the flange of the tracheostomy tube. **④**
> * While applying the dressing, ensure that the tracheostomy tube is securely supported. **Rationale:** *Excessive movement of the tracheostomy tube irritates the trachea.*

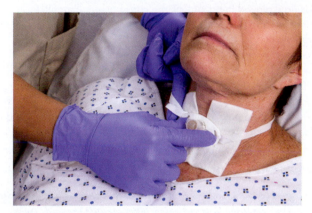

④ *A tracheostomy dressing placed under the flange of the tracheostomy tube.*

9. Change the tracheostomy ties or Velcro collar.
    * Change as needed to keep the skin clean and dry.
    * Twill ties and specially manufactured Velcro collars are available. A twill tie is inexpensive and readily available; however, it is easily soiled and can trap moisture that leads to irritation of the skin of the neck. Velcro collars are becoming more commonly used. **⑤** They are wider, more comfortable, and they cause less skin abrasion (Barnett, 2007).

CLINICAL ALERT

When a child is admitted with a tracheostomy, talk with the parents about the method used for tracheostomy management at home. Develop a nursing care plan for tracheostomy management that integrates home management as well as teaching to enhance home management techniques.

Remember that the child with an endotracheal tube or tracheostomy tube is unable to talk or cry. Implement other ways of communication. Picture boards that illustrate common activities or requests work for younger children. An electronic tablet or a pad and pencil can be used by older children with normal motor skills.

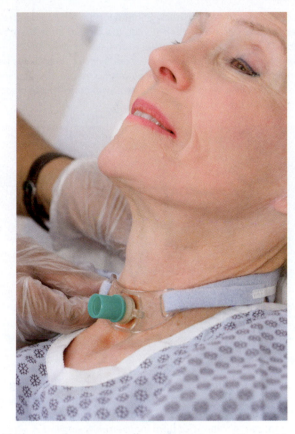

⑤ A Velcro tracheostomy collar.

Two-Strip Method (Twill Ties)

* Cut two unequal strips of twill ties, one approximately 25 cm (10 in.) long and the other about 50 cm (20 in.) long. **Rationale:** *Cutting one tape longer than the other allows them to be fastened at the side of the neck for easy access and to avoid the pressure of a knot on the skin at the back of the neck.*
* Cut a 1-cm (0.5-in.) lengthwise slit approximately 2.5 cm (1 in.) from one end of each tie. To do this, fold the end of the tie back onto itself about 2.5 cm (1 in.), then cut a slit in the middle of the tie from its folded edge.
* Leaving the old ties in place, thread the slit end of one clean tie through the eye of the tracheostomy flange from the bottom side; then thread the long end of the tie through the slit, pulling it tight until it is securely fastened to the flange. **Rationale:** *Leaving the old ties in place while securing the clean ties prevents inadvertent dislodging of the tracheostomy tube. Securing ties in this manner avoids the use of knots in the flange area, which can come untied or cause pressure and irritation.*
* If old ties are very soiled or it is difficult to thread new ties onto the tracheostomy flange with old ties in place, have an assistant don a sterile glove and hold the tracheostomy in place while you replace the ties. **Rationale:** *This is very important because movement of the tube during this procedure may cause irritation and stimulate coughing. Coughing can dislodge the tube if the ties are undone.*
* Repeat the process for the second tie.

(continued on next page)

SKILL 13.19 Providing Tracheostomy Care (continued)

■ Ask the client to flex the neck. Slip the longer tape under the client's neck, place a finger between the tape and the client's neck, ❻ and tie the ties together at the side of the neck. **Rationale:** *Flexing the neck increases its circumference the way coughing does. Placing a finger under the tie prevents making the tie too tight, which could interfere with coughing or place pressure on the jugular veins.*

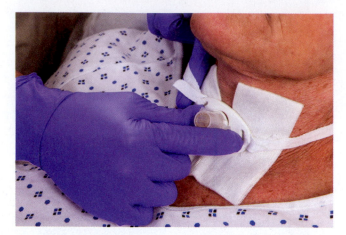

❻ Placing a finger underneath the tie tape before tying it.

■ Tie the ends of the ties using square knots. Cut off any long ends, leaving approximately 1–2 cm (0.5 in.). **Rationale:** *Square knots prevent slippage and loosening. Adequate ends beyond the knot prevent the knot from inadvertently untying.*

■ Once the clean ties are secured, remove the soiled ties and discard.

One-Strip Method (Twill Tie)

■ Cut a length of twill tie 2.5 times the length needed to go around the client's neck from one tube flange to the other.

■ Thread one end of the tie into the slot on one side of the flange.

■ Bring both ends of the tie together. Take them around the client's neck, keeping them flat and untwisted.

■ Thread the end of the tie next to the client's neck through the slot from the back to the front.

■ Have the client flex the neck. Tie the loose ends with a square knot at the side of the client's neck, allowing for slack by placing two fingers under the ties as with the two-strip method. Cut off long ends.

10. Tape and pad the tie knot.
   • Place a folded 4×4 gauze square under the tie knot, and apply tape over the knot. **Rationale:** *This reduces skin irritation from the knot and prevents confusing the knot with the client's gown ties.*

11. Check the tightness of the ties.
   • Frequently check the tightness of the tracheostomy ties and position of the tracheostomy tube. **Rationale:** *Swelling of the neck may cause the ties to become too tight, interfering with coughing and circulation. Ties can loosen in restless clients, allowing the tracheostomy tube to extrude from the stoma.*

12. Remove and discard sterile gloves. Perform hand hygiene.

13. Document all relevant information.
   • Record suctioning, tracheostomy care, and the dressing change, noting your assessments.

VARIATION: USING A DISPOSABLE INNER CANNULA

■ Check policy for frequency of changing the inner cannula because standards vary among institutions.

■ Open a new cannula package.

■ Using a gloved hand, unlock the current inner cannula (if present) and remove it by gently pulling it out toward you in line with its curvature.

■ Check the cannula for amount and type of secretions and discard properly.

■ Pick up the new inner cannula touching only the outer locking portion.

■ Insert new cannula and lock the cannula in place by turning the lock (if present).

Sample Documentation

12/11/2015 0900 Respirations 18–20/min. Lung sounds clear. Able to cough up secretions requiring little suctioning. Inner cannula changed. Trach dressing changed. Minimal amount of serosanguineous drainage present. Trach incision area pink to reddish in color 0.2 cm around entire opening. No broken skin noted in the reddened area. _____ J. Garcia, RN

Developmental Considerations

INFANTS AND CHILDREN

■ An assistant should always be present while tracheostomy care is performed. (See figures top of next page.)

■ Always keep a sterile, packaged tracheostomy tube taped to the child's bed so that if the tube dislodges, a new one is available for immediate reintubation.

OLDER ADULTS

■ Older adult skin is fragile and prone to breakdown. Care of the skin at the tracheostomy stoma is very important.

Setting of Care

■ For tracheostomies older than 1 month, clean technique (rather than sterile technique) is used for tracheostomy care.

■ Stress the importance of good hand hygiene to the caregiver.

■ Tap water may be used for rinsing the inner cannula.

■ Teach the caregiver the tracheostomy care procedure and observe a return demonstration. Periodically reassess caregiver knowledge and/or tracheostomy care technique.

■ Inform the caregiver of the signs and symptoms that may indicate an infection of the stoma site or lower airway.

■ Names and telephone numbers of healthcare personnel who can be reached for emergencies or advice must be available to the client and/or caregiver.

■ If the tracheostomy is permanent, provide contact information for available support groups.

SKILL 13.19 Providing Tracheostomy Care *(continued)*

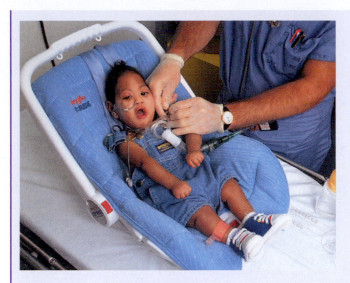

Infant with a tracheostomy collar.

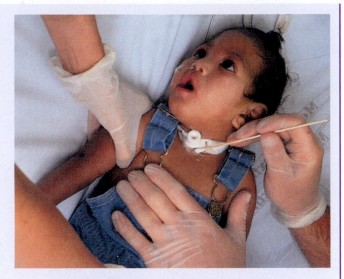

Cleaning the tracheostomy tube.

▶ MAINTAINING LUNG EXPANSION

Expected Outcomes

1. Chest drainage system remains a closed system.

2. Chest tubes remain patent and secured in place.

SKILL 13.20   Assisting with Chest Tube Insertion

Delegation

Assisting the primary care provider with insertion of a chest tube is not delegated to UAP.

Equipment

- Sterile chest tube tray that includes:
  - Drapes
  - 10-mL syringe
  - Gauze sponges
  - #22-gauge needle
  - #25-gauge needle
  - #11 blade scalpel
  - Forceps
- Extra 4×4 gauze sponges or other occlusive bandage material
- Split drain sponges
- Chest tube and Kelly clamps
- Suture materials
- Closed drainage system (water or dry seal)
- Suction source, if indicated
- Sterile gloves
- Local anesthetic vial
- Skin cleansing solution (e.g., povidone-iodine)
- Adhesive or foam tape
- Petrolatum gauze (optional)

Preparation

- Whenever possible, informed consent should be obtained.
- Remove the cap on the water-seal chamber. ❶

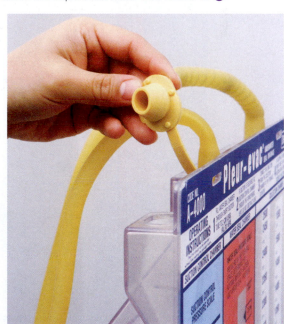

❶ Opening the water-seal filling port.

(continued on next page)

SKILL 13.20 Assisting with Chest Tube Insertion (*continued*)

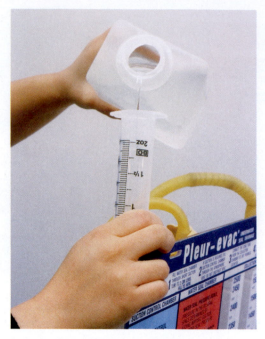

❷ Filling the water-seal chamber with sterile water.

- Fill the water-seal chamber with sterile water or as specified. ❷
- Inject the required amount of water into the self-sealing port of the water-seal chamber using a syringe and needle. ❸
- Although the primary care provider will have already done initial client and family teaching, the nurse reinforces key elements.

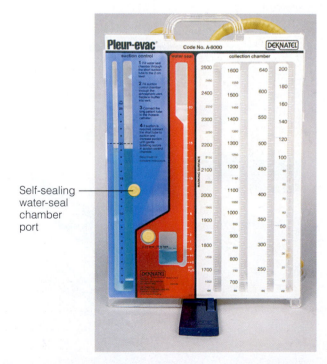

Self-sealing water-seal chamber port

❸ A three-chamber wet-suction/wet-seal disposable chest drainage system.

Rationale: *This reduces client anxiety and assists in efficiency of the procedure.*

- Confirm with the primary care provider the desired types and numbers of equipment needed. Primary care providers have personal preferences for styles and sizes of chest tubes, and needs vary with the purpose of the tube.
- Premedicate the client for pain. Incorporate nonpharmacologic pain and stress-reducing strategies as much as possible.
- Monitor the client closely to ensure that the respiratory status has not worsened from the analgesics.

Procedure

1. Prior to performing the procedure, introduce self and verify the client's identity using agency protocol. Explain to the client what your role will be, why it is necessary, and how he or she can participate. Discuss how the results will be used in planning further care or treatments.
2. Perform hand hygiene and observe appropriate infection control procedures.
3. Provide for client privacy.
4. Position the client as directed by the primary care provider.
   - The client may be placed flat or in semi-Fowler position. **Rationale:** *The flat position is preferred for best access to the second or third intercostal space; a semi-Fowler position is preferred for access into the sixth to eighth intercostal space.*
   - Turn the client laterally so that the area receiving the tube is facing upward.
5. Prepare for the insertion.
   - Open the chest tube tray and sterile gloves on the over-bed table.
   - Assist the primary care provider to clean the insertion site.
   - Assist the primary care provider to draw up the local anesthetic by holding the anesthetic bottle upside down with the label facing the primary care provider. The primary care provider will withdraw the solution.
   - Participate in the Joint Commission's (2011) National Patient Safety Goal—Universal Protocol for Preventing Wrong Site, Wrong Procedure, Wrong Person Surgery, which requires preprocedure verification and a "time-out" to ensure that all members of the team agree about what is to be done and to whom.
6. Provide emotional support to the client during insertion as the primary care provider makes a small incision through the skin and muscle. Often, the practitioner will probe through the incision with a finger to ensure there are no underlying structures that may be damaged during insertion of the tube. The practitioner will use a Kelly clamp to broaden and deepen the insertion site and then pass the tube into the chest. Monitor the client's condition and reaction to the procedure.
7. Dress the site.
   - Apply sterile gloves and wrap the petrolatum gauze (if prescribed) around the chest tube at the insertion site.
   - Place split drain gauze around the chest tube, one from the top and one from the bottom.

SKILL 13.20 Assisting with Chest Tube Insertion (continued)

- Place several additional gauze squares and tape or occlusive bandage materials over the drain gauze. These form an airtight seal at the insertion site.
8. Secure the tube.
    - Assist with connecting the chest tube to the valve or drainage system.
    - Attach the longer tube from the collection chamber to the client's chest tube.
    - Remove and discard gloves. Perform hand hygiene.
    - Tape the chest tube to the client's skin so that any pull on the tubing creates traction on the skin and not on the insertion site.
    - Tape all connections using spiral turns, but do not completely cover the collection tubing with tape. ➍ **Rationale:** *Taping prevents inadvertent separation. Not covering all of the collection tubing allows drainage to be seen.*

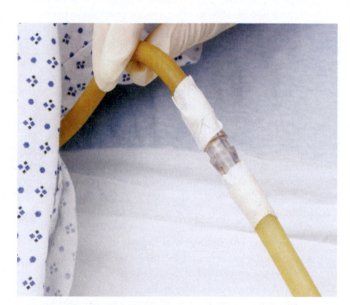

➍ Taped tubing connection with the connector exposed for observation of drainage.

- Coil the drainage tubing and secure it to the linen, ensuring slack for the client to turn and move. **Rationale:** *This prevents kinking of the tubing and impairment of drainage.*
- If suction is ordered, attach the remaining shorter tube from the suction chamber to the suction source and turn it on. If wet suction is used, inspect the suction chamber for bubbling. Gentle bubbling indicates an appropriate suction level.
- If suction has not been ordered, keep the shorter rubber tube unclamped. This maintains negative or equal pressure in the system.
9. When all drainage connections are complete, ask the client to take a deep breath and hold it for a few seconds, then slowly exhale. These actions facilitate drainage from the pleural space and lung reexpansion.

10. Prepare the client for a chest x-ray to check for placement of the tube and lung expansion.
11. Ensure client safety.
    - Monitor intactness of closed chest drainage system. Keep a 250-mL pour bottle of sterile water (or normal saline) and a sterile occlusive dressing (like a petroleum dressing) at the bedside in case of a breech in this system. (See Skill 13.21 for information about maintaining chest tube drainage.) **Rationale:** *The bottle of sterile water (or normal saline) would be used as a water seal if the chest tube becomes disconnected from the drainage system or the system breaks or cracks. The sterile occlusive dressing taped down at the chest tube insertion site would prevent sucking air into the chest and also inhibit air from escaping from the chest (which could result in a tension pneumothorax).*
    - Assess the client for signs of a new or worsening pneumothorax.
    - Assess the client for signs of subcutaneous emphysema (collection of gas under the skin). Palpate around the dressing site for crackling indicative of subcutaneous emphysema. **Rationale:** *Subcutaneous emphysema can result from a poor seal at the chest tube insertion site. This is not an emergency but should be reported, documented, and monitored. It should reabsorb in a few days.*

> **CLINICAL ALERT**
> Subcutaneous emphysema (air in tissue) may be felt around the chest tube insertion site, but should be reported if it extends beyond this.

   - Assess drainage and vital signs every 15 minutes for the first hour and then as ordered. Mark the collection chamber with a line and the date and time. Report bleeding or drainage greater than 100 mL/hr.
12. Document the insertion in the client record using forms or checklists supplemented by narrative notes when appropriate. Include the name of the primary care provider, site of placement, type of tube, type of drainage system, characteristics of the immediate drainage (**Table 13–2 ●**), and other assessment findings.

TABLE 13–2	Characteristics of Chest Tube Drainage
DESCRIPTION OF FLUID	**INDICATION**
Blood tinged or bloody	Anticoagulant use
	Pulmonary infarct
	Trauma
	Malignancy
	Inflammation
Cloudy	Infection or inflammation
Purulent (pus)	Empyema
Food particles	Esophageal rupture
Black	*Aspergillus* (fungal) infection
Low pH	Tuberculosis, malignancy

(continued on next page)

SKILL 13.20   Assisting with Chest Tube Insertion (continued)

Sample Documentation

5/12/15 0130 32-Fr chest tube inserted into l chest by Dr. Novarty & connected to water-seal drainage unit. Suction at 20 cm H₂O. Immediately
drained 120 mL straw-colored fluid. Moderate coughing after insertion,
eased in 10 minutes. All connections taped, tubing taped to chest wall &
attached to draw sheet. Tidaling c̄ respirations. Client instructed re:
positioning & care of tube & collection device. Expresses understanding.
VS 101°F, P 100 bpm, R 26/min, BP 170/94 mmHg.

_____ J. Lygas, RN

SKILL 13.21   Maintaining Chest Tube Drainage

Delegation

Care of chest tubes is not delegated to UAP. However, aspects of the client's condition are observed during usual care and may be recorded by individuals other than the nurse. Abnormal findings must be validated and interpreted by the nurse.

Equipment

- Sterile gloves
- Petrolatum gauze (optional)
- 4×4 gauze sponges
- Split drain sponges
- Drainage system
- Skin cleansing solutions (e.g., povidone-iodine)
- Adhesive or foam tape

Preparation

- Determine when the last dressing change was performed.

Procedure

1. Prior to performing the procedure, introduce self and verify the client's identity using agency protocol. Explain to the client what you are going to do, why it is necessary, and how he or she can participate. Discuss how the results will be used in planning further care or treatments.
2. Perform hand hygiene and observe other appropriate infection control procedures.
3. Provide for client privacy.
4. Assess the client.
   - Determine ease of respirations, breath sounds, respiratory rate and depth, oxygen saturation, and chest movements every 2 hours.
   - Observe the dressing site. Inspect the dressing for excessive and abnormal drainage, such as bleeding or foul-smelling discharge. Palpate around the dressing site for crackling indicative of subcutaneous emphysema. **Rationale:** *Subcutaneous emphysema can result from an inadequate seal (air leak) at the chest tube insertion site.*
   - Determine level of discomfort with and without activity. **Rationale:** *Analgesics may need to be administered before the client moves or does deep breathing and coughing exercises.*
   - Evaluate the impact of possible changes to the client's body image that occur when an individual has tubes extending out from the body. It can be a frightening and disorienting experience for the client and family. They may be afraid of pulling them out, pulling on them and causing pain, or having someone else accidentally pull on them. A nurse who is sensitive to this will be able to offer a more comforting presence to the client.
5. Implement all necessary safety precautions.
   - Monitor intactness of closed chest drainage system. Keep a 250-mL pour bottle of sterile water (or normal saline) and a sterile occlusive dressing (like a petroleum dressing) at bedside in case of a breech in this system (see step 9 for further information).
   - Keep the drainage system below chest level and upright at all times. **Rationale:** *Keeping the unit below chest level prevents backflow of fluid from the drainage chamber into the pleural space (Briggs, 2010). Keeping the unit upright maintains the water seal.*
6. Maintain the patency of the drainage system.
   - Check that all connections are secured with tape. **Rationale:** *This ensures that the system is airtight.*
   - Inspect the drainage tubing for kinks or loops dangling below the entry level of the drainage system.
   - Coil the drainage tubing and secure it to the bed linen, ensuring enough slack for the client to turn and move. **Rationale:** *This prevents kinking of the tubing and impairment of the drainage system.* Be sure that there are no dependent loops of tubing between the bed surface and the collection device. **Rationale:** *This decreases the chances of clots forming in the tubing that can obstruct drainage.*
   - Inspect the air vent in the system periodically to make sure it is not occluded. **Rationale:** *A vent must be present to allow air to escape. Obstruction of the air vent causes an increased pressure in the system that could result in pneumothorax.*
   - Avoid any forceful manipulation of the tube. In some agencies, this includes milking (stripping) the chest tubing. Stripping refers to compressing the chest tube between fingers and thumb, using a pulling motion down the rest of the tubing away from the chest wall. Milking involves squeezing, kneading, or twisting the tubing to create bursts of suction to move any clots. Stripping chest tubes may significantly increase negative pressure that could damage the pleural membranes and/or surround-

SKILL 13.21 Maintaining Chest Tube Drainage (continued)

ing tissues, causing pain and impairing the client's recovery. If clots are present in the tubing, expert opinion recommends gentle squeezing and releasing of small segments of the tubing between the fingers instead of stripping (Halm, 2007). Some providers fear the stripping maneuver may cause more bleeding by generating negative pressure within the pleural cavity (Briggs, 2010; Shalli et al., 2009).

CLINICAL ALERT
Strip and milk chest tubes only with physician's orders. Excessive negative pressure created by stripping and milking increases negative pressure in the intrapleural space.

7. Assess fluid level fluctuations and bubbling in the drainage system.
   • Check for fluctuation (tidaling) of the fluid level in the water-seal chamber as the client breathes. **Rationale:** *Tidaling reflects the pressure changes in the pleural space during inhalation and exhalation. The fluid level rises when the client inhales and falls when the client exhales. The absence of tidaling may indicate tubing obstruction from a kink, dependent loop, blood clot, or outside pressure (e.g., because the client is lying on the tubing), or may indicate that full lung reexpansion has occurred.*
   • Check for intermittent bubbling in the water of the water-seal chamber. **Rationale:** *Intermittent bubbling normally occurs when the system removes air from the pleural space, especially when the client takes a deep breath or coughs. Absence of bubbling may indicate that the drainage system is blocked or that the pleural space has healed and is sealed but this must be verified by x-ray. Continuous bubbling or a sudden change from an established pattern can indicate a break in the system (i.e., an air leak) and should be reported immediately.*
   • Check for gentle bubbling in the suction control chamber in wet systems. **Rationale:** *Gentle bubbling indicates proper suction pressure.*
8. Assess the drainage.
   • Inspect the drainage in the collection container at least every 15 minutes during the first 2 hours after chest tube insertion and every 2 hours thereafter.
   • Every 4–8 hours, mark the time, date, and drainage level on a piece of adhesive tape affixed to the container, or mark it directly on a disposable container. ❶
   • Note any sudden change in the amount or color of the drainage.
   • If drainage exceeds 100 mL/hr or if a color change indicates hemorrhage, notify the primary care provider immediately.
9. Watch for dislodgement of the tubes, and remedy the problem promptly.
   • Keep a 250-mL pour bottle of sterile water (or normal saline) and a sterile occlusive dressing (like a petroleum dressing) at the bedside.

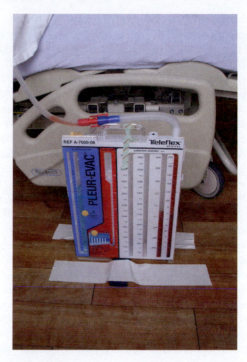

❶ Marking the date, time, and drainage level.

   • If the chest tube becomes disconnected from the drainage system or the system breaks or cracks, the end of the chest tube is immediately inserted 2.5–5 cm (1–2 in.) into the sterile pour bottle of water to create a water seal.
   • Another closed drainage system can then be set up and connected to the chest tube.
   • If the chest tube becomes dislodged from the client, the sterile occlusive dressing would immediately be applied to the insertion site and taped down on three sides.
   • The fourth side is periodically lifted open when the client exhales to allow air trapped in the pleural space to be expelled.
   • The physician is called to insert another chest tube. **Rationale:** *These actions will prevent the client from sucking air into the chest on inspiration and allow air trapped in the pleural space to be expelled on expiration. They are important interventions to prevent a tension pneumothorax, which can develop into an emergency situation for the client.*
   • Assess the client closely for respiratory distress (dyspnea, pallor, diaphoresis, blood-tinged sputum, or chest pain).
   • Check vital signs every 10 minutes until stable.
   • Document the incident in the client's medical record or other appropriate records according to the facility's protocol.
10. If bubbling persists in the water-seal collection chamber or air leak chamber, determine its source. Continuous bubbling in the water-seal collection chamber normally occurs for only a few minutes after a chest tube is attached to drainage.

(continued on next page)

SKILL 13.21 Maintaining Chest Tube Drainage (continued)

11. Take a specimen of the chest drainage as required.
    - Specimens of chest drainage may be taken from a disposable chest drainage system through the resealable connecting tubing. If a specimen is required:
    a. Use a povidone-iodine swab to wipe the self-sealing tubing below the connection to the chest tube. Allow it to dry.
    b. Attach a sterile 18- or 20-gauge needle to a syringe, and insert the needle into the tubing, being careful not to pass all the way through the opposite side of the tubing.
    c. Aspirate the specimen, discard the needle in the appropriate container, and securely cap the syringe, or transfer the specimen to an appropriate collection tube. Label the syringe or tube while still at the client's side, matching it to the requisition slip and the client identification.
12. Ensure essential client care.
    - Encourage deep breathing and coughing exercises every 2 hours, if indicated (this may be contraindicated in clients with a lobectomy). Premedicate the client for pain as needed. Have the client sit upright to perform the exercises, and splint the tube insertion site with a pillow or with a hand to minimize discomfort. **Rationale:** *Deep breathing and coughing help remove accumulations from the pleural space, facilitate drainage, and help the lung to reexpand.*
    - While the client takes deep breaths, palpate the chest for thoracic excursion. Normal thoracic excursion will result in thumbs separating at least 2.5–5.0 cm (1–2 in.) as the client inhales.
    - Auscultate the client's chest every 4 hours. Breath sounds should be symmetric. **Rationale**: *Decreased breath sounds on the side of the chest tube could indicate that air or fluid has reaccumulated in the pleural space. Breath sounds that are louder on the affected side could indicate that fluid has accumulated on the other side of the chest.*
    - Percuss the client's chest. A normal lung should have a resonant (hollow) sound. **Rationale**: *A dull or flat sound indicates fluid or solid tissue. Report any abnormal findings to the primary care provider.*
    - Check that the chest tube site dressing is dry and occlusive. The dressing does not need to be changed unless it is loose or wet. In some agencies, chest tube dressings are changed daily. **Rationale:** *A wet dressing could indicate a fluid leak around the tube.*

- Examine the chest tube insertion site for signs of healing, skin irritation, or infection.
- Reposition the client every 2 hours. When the client is lying on the affected side, place rolled towels on either side of the tubing. **Rationale:** *Frequent position changes promote drainage, prevent complications, and provide comfort. Rolled towels prevent occlusion of the chest tube by the client's weight.*
- Assist the client with range-of-motion exercises of the affected shoulder three times per day to maintain joint mobility.
- Conduct regular pain assessments using a simple scoring system. If necessary, ask the primary care provider for more aggressive pain management (possibly patient-controlled analgesia). **Rationale:** *Pain will limit the client's mobility and will result in shallow breaths and incomplete lung expansion.*
- When transporting and ambulating the client:
  a. Keep the water-seal unit below chest level and upright.
  b. Disconnect the drainage system from the suction apparatus before moving the client, and make sure the air vent is open. Or, if ordered, obtain a portable suction device.

13. Document findings in the client record using forms or checklists supplemented by narrative notes when appropriate. Record patency of chest tubes; type, amount, and color of drainage; presence of fluctuations; appearance of insertion site; laboratory specimens, if any were taken; respiratory assessments; client's vital signs and level of comfort; and all other nursing care provided to the client.

Developmental Considerations

OLDER ADULTS

- Coughing and deep breathing exercises are particularly important because shallow breathing and decreased ability to cough may occur with aging.
- Encourage the client to take pain medication when needed. Older adults may be reluctant to take pain medication.
- Take special care of the client's skin due to the possibility of skin tears from tape and increased risk of skin breakdown over bony prominences as skin becomes thinner and less elastic.
- The older client is at increased risk for respiratory distress due to increased lung stiffness.

SKILL 13.22 Assisting with Chest Tube Removal

Delegation

Assisting with the removal of a chest tube is not delegated to UAP. However, many effects of the removal may be observed during usual care and may be recorded by persons other than the nurse. Abnormal findings must be validated and interpreted by the nurse.

Equipment

- Clean gloves
- Sterile gloves
- Suture removal set with forceps and scissors
- Sterile petrolatum gauze

- 4×4 gauze sponges
- Adhesive or foam tape
- Moisture-proof medical waste bag
- Linen-saver pad
- Sharps container
- Safety goggles

Preparation

Ensure that the client has been informed that the chest tube will be removed and when. Clamp the tube, if ordered. The client should be given the opportunity to discuss and express any concerns. Administer analgesics as ordered.

SKILL 13.22   Assisting with Chest Tube Removal (continued)

Procedure

1. Prior to performing the procedure, introduce self and verify the client's identity using agency protocol. Explain the procedure to the client and how he or she can participate. Discuss how the results will be used in planning further care or treatments.
2. Perform hand hygiene and observe other appropriate infection control procedures.
3. Provide for client privacy.
4. Prepare the client:
   - Assist the client to a side-lying or semi-Fowler position with the chest tube site exposed.
   - Place the linen-saver pad under the client, beneath the chest tube. **Rationale:** *This protects the bed linens and provides a place for the chest tube after removal.*
   - Instruct the client on how to hold the breath during removal. Some experts recommend holding a full inhalation, others recommend holding a full exhalation, and still others recommend the Valsalva maneuver—exhaling against the closed glottis (Briggs, 2010; Hunter, 2008). **Rationale:** *These techniques increase the intrathoracic pressure and prevent air from entering the pleural space.* Verify the preferred method with the provider who will be removing the chest tube and then instruct the client on how to hold the breath during removal.
5. Prepare the sterile field and supplies. Have the petrolatum gauze opened and ready for quick application.
6. Remove the dressing around the chest tube.
   - Apply clean gloves and dispose of the dressing in the moisture-proof bag.
   - Remove and discard gloves. Perform hand hygiene.
7. Assist with removal of the tube.
   - Apply sterile gloves.
   - Assist the client with the breathing technique and provide emotional support during the primary care provider's removal of the sutures and tube.
   - As the primary care provider removes the chest tube, either the provider or the nurse immediately applies the petrolatum gauze, and covers it with dry gauze and adhesive tape. **Rationale:** *This forms an airtight bandage.*
   - Remove all used equipment and place in appropriate medical waste containers.
   - Remove and discard gloves. Perform hand hygiene.
8. Assess and monitor the client's response to tube removal.
   - Obtain vital signs every 15 minutes for the first hour and, if stable, then as indicated.
   - Auscultate lung sounds every hour for the first 4 hours to determine that the lung is remaining inflated.
   - Observe for signs of pneumothorax.
9. Document the date and time of removal, any drainage noted, and the client's response to the procedure in the client record using forms or checklists supplemented by narrative notes when appropriate.
10. Prepare the client for a chest x-ray 1–2 hours after chest tube removal and possibly again in 12–24 hours.

> **CLINICAL ALERT**
> The chest tube can be removed when drainage is less than 50–100 mL in 24 hours, or, if inserted for blood removal, drainage has become serous or serosanguineous and has been less than 100 mL in the past 8 hours.

▶ LIFE-THREATENING RESPIRATORY SITUATIONS

Expected Outcomes

1. Obstructed airway is cleared of foreign body.
2. Rescue breathing or CPR is begun within five minutes after assessment has determined that the client has a life-threatening need for these actions.
3. Client's heart rhythm is restored to normal after defibrillation with an AED or manual defibrillator.
4. Rescue breathing or CPR is continued until rapid-response team arrives.

SKILL 13.23   Clearing an Obstructed Airway

Delegation

Although UAP cannot perform all aspects of a hospital code situation, they are trained in CPR and can perform foreign body airway obstruction (FBAO) techniques. If they are the first responders, UAP should call for help and initiate the intervention without waiting for a nurse.

Equipment

- Standard precautions supplies should always be easily accessible: gloves, CPR mask or manual resuscitator (bag–valve–mask [BVM] device), gowns, and protective eyewear.

Procedure

Conscious Individual

1. State your name and explain to the client that you are trained to help, what you are going to do, and how he or she can cooperate. Speak slowly, clearly, and with confidence.
2. Observe appropriate infection control procedures as much as possible.
3. Provide for as much privacy as possible without interfering with the necessary individuals and activities. If another individual is present and can participate, have that person get help. If family members are present, the nurse may request

(continued on next page)

SKILL 13.23 Clearing an Obstructed Airway (continued)

they leave for the moment. However, research also supports allowing family members to remain during emergencies (Howlett, Alexander, & Tsuchiya, 2010).

4. Give abdominal thrusts (Heimlich maneuver).
   - Stand or kneel behind the individual, and wrap your arms around her waist.
   - Make a fist with one hand, tuck the thumb inside the fist, and place the flexed thumb just above the individual's navel and below the xiphoid process. **Rationale:** *A protruding thumb could inflict injury.*
   - With the other hand, grasp the fist ❶ and press it into the individual's abdomen with a firm, quick upward thrust. ❷ Avoid tightening the arms around the rib cage.

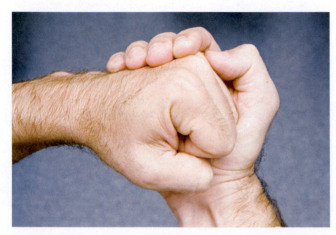

❶ The hand and first position used for abdominal thrusts in a conscious individual.

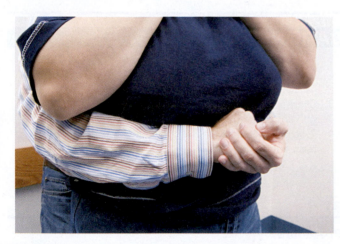

❷ The position for providing abdominal thrusts to a conscious individual.

- Deliver successive thrusts as separate and complete movements until the individual's airway clears or she becomes unconscious.
- If the individual becomes unconscious, lower her carefully to the floor, supporting the head and neck to prevent injury.

Unconscious Individual

5. Activate the emergency response system using "911" or the agency arrest code.

6. Apply clean gloves and other personal protective equipment as soon as possible.

7. Open the airway.
   - Tilt the individual's head back, lift the chin. **Rationale:** *This pulls the tongue away from the back of the throat.*
   - Remove an object only if you see it:
   a. If foreign material is visible in the mouth, it must be expediently removed. The finger sweep maneuver should be used only on unconscious individuals and with extreme caution. **Rationale:** *Foreign material can accidentally be pushed back into the airway, causing increased obstruction.*
   b. To remove solid material, insert the index finger of your free hand along the inside of the person's cheek and deep into the throat. With your finger hooked, use a sweeping motion to try to dislodge and lift out the foreign object. ❸
   c. After removing the foreign object, clear out liquid material, such as mucus, blood, or emesis.

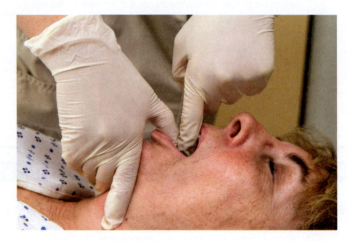

❸ The finger sweep maneuver.

8. Provide ventilations.
   - Apply a CPR resuscitation mask to the individual's face (❹, A–B). If a mask is not available, insert the airway portion of a face shield into his mouth.
   - Give one 1-second breath and check for a visible chest rise.
   - If unable to ventilate, retilt the head and repeat breath.
   - If successful, give an additional 1-second breath.

9. If unsuccessful, proceed with full CPR, repeating ventilation attempts, chest compressions, and foreign object checks until the airway clears or the individual breathes.
   - In the hospital setting, an individual trained in airway interventions will take over responsibility for clearing the airway.

SKILL 13.23 Clearing an Obstructed Airway (*continued*)

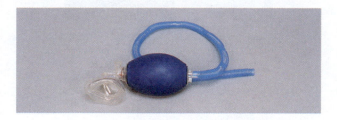

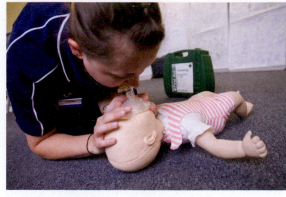

A | B

❹ Face masks: A, Bag–valve–mask (Ambu bag with face mask); B, Face shield. (B: Copyright by Ian Miles—Flashpoint Pictures/Alamy)

- When the emergency care is completed, remove and discard gloves and other personal protective equipment. Perform hand hygiene.

VARIATION: CHEST THRUSTS

Chest thrusts are to be administered only to women in advanced stages of pregnancy and markedly obese persons who cannot receive abdominal thrusts. See all steps above except substitute chest thrusts for the abdominal thrusts.

To administer chest thrusts:

- Place the thumb side of the fist on the middle of the breastbone, not on the xiphoid process.
- Grab the fist with the other hand and deliver a quick backward thrust.
- Repeat thrusts until the obstruction is relieved or the victim becomes unconscious.

To administer chest thrusts to unconscious individuals lying on the ground:

- Position the individual supine and kneel close to the side of her trunk.
- Position the hands as for cardiac compression with the heel of the hand on the lower half of the sternum.
- Deliver five thrusts.

10. Document the date and time of the procedure, including the precipitating events and the client's response to the intervention.
    - Describe the type of procedure, the duration of breathlessness, and the type and size of any foreign object.
    - Note vital signs, any complications, and type of follow-up care.

Developmental Considerations

INFANTS

To administer a combination of back slaps and chest thrusts to infants:

1. Deliver back slaps.
   - Straddle the infant over your forearm with his or her head lower than the trunk.
   - Support the infant's head by firmly holding the jaw in the hand.
   - Rest your forearm on your thigh.
   - With the heel of the free hand, deliver five sharp slaps to the infant's back over the spine between the shoulder blades. (See figure.)
2. Deliver chest thrusts.
   - Turn the infant as a unit to the supine position:
     a. Place the free hand on the infant's back.
     b. While continuing to support the jaw, neck, and chest with the other hand, turn and place the infant on the thigh with the baby's head lower than the trunk.

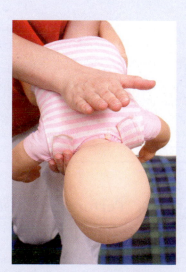

Infant back slaps. (© Roman Milert/Alamy)

(*continued on next page*)

SKILL 13.23   Clearing an Obstructed Airway (*continued*)

- Using two fingers, administer five chest thrusts over the sternum in the same location as external chest compression for cardiac massage, one finger-width below the nipple line, 1 second each. (See figure.)

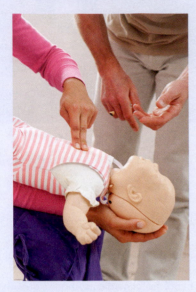

Infant chest thrusts. (Credit: Burger/Phanie/Science Source)

- For a conscious infant, continue chest thrusts and back slaps until the airway is cleared or the infant becomes unconscious.
- If the infant is unconscious, begin CPR.
  a. Assess the airway and give two breaths. As with adults, a mask or barrier should be used whenever possible. If unable to ventilate, retilt the infant's head and try to give two breaths.
  b. If the air does not go in, then give chest compressions. Following the chest compressions, lift the jaw and tongue and check for a foreign object. If an object is noted, sweep it out with finger.
  c. Repeat this sequence of breaths, foreign object checks, and chest compressions until the airway clears or the infant begins to breathe.

CHILDREN
- For conscious children over age 1 who are choking, perform the Heimlich maneuver as for adults. (See figure.)

OLDER ADULTS
- Older clients have a decreased gag reflex and, thus, may be more prone to choking. Preventive measures, such as adjusting the consistency of food, and close surveillance of clients with a history of choking may prevent an obstructed airway.

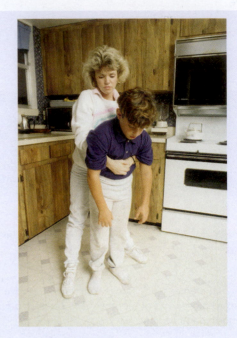

Conscious child abdominal thrusts. (Copyright © Martin/Custom Medical Stock Photo)

- Older clients can be injured by incorrect placement of the rescuer's hands. The sternum becomes more brittle with aging, and fracture of the sternum or ribs is more common.

Setting of Care
- Stay with the individual and call the EMS.
- Any individual who receives intervention to treat an obstructed airway should seek immediate follow-up medical evaluation, even if the person remains conscious and the airway is cleared with abdominal thrusts.
- After removal of an airway obstruction at home, the client should receive a medical evaluation. The client may have aspirated foreign material, which can cause airway edema and infection.
- If the individual becomes unconscious, activate the EMS.

FAMILY ROLE
- If a client has difficulty swallowing, teach the caregiver how to clear an obstructed airway.
- Young children are most likely to choke on objects such as small toys. Children do not understand the danger of placing objects in the mouth. Teach parents how to clear an obstructed airway and emphasize the importance of keeping small objects away from a young child.

SKILL 13.24   Performing Rescue Breathing

Delegation

Although UAP cannot perform all aspects of a hospital code situation, they are trained in CPR and can perform rescue breathing techniques. If they are the first responders, UAP should initiate the intervention and not wait for a nurse.

Equipment

- Standard precautions supplies should always be easily accessible: gloves, CPR mask or manual resuscitator (bag–valve–mask [BVM] device), gowns, and protective eyewear.

SKILL 13.24   Performing Rescue Breathing *(continued)*

- Emergency equipment such as intubation supplies should be centrally located.
- Pocket face mask with one-way valve or mouth shields, or BVM device (often referred to as an Ambu bag)

Procedure

1. Recognize the presence of an emergency.
   - Determine that the individual is unresponsive.
   - Determine the absence of normal breathing (i.e., no breathing or only gasping).
2. Call a "code" or follow agency protocol to call for assistance. If another individual is present and can participate, have that individual go get help. Tell the individual to return and report that help has been called.
3. Take no more than 10 seconds to check for a pulse. To palpate the carotid artery, first locate the larynx, and then slide your fingers alongside it into the groove between the larynx and the neck muscles on the same side you are. Use gentle pressure. **Rationale:** *This avoids compressing the artery. The carotid pulse site is used because it is easy to reach and can often be palpated when more peripheral pulses, such as the radial, are imperceptible.*
   - If there is no pulse, begin CPR with compressions.
   - If only a respiratory arrest exists, proceed with the steps below.
4. Observe appropriate infection control procedures including applying clean gloves as much as possible.
5. Provide for as much privacy as possible without interfering with the necessary individuals and activities. If family members are present, the nurse may request that they leave for the moment.
6. Position the client appropriately.
   - If the individual is lying on one side or face down, turn him onto his back as a unit, while supporting the head and neck. Kneel beside the head.
7. Open the airway.
   - Use the head tilt–chin lift maneuver or the jaw-thrust maneuver. A modified jaw thrust is used for individuals with suspected neck injury. In unconscious individuals, the tongue lacks sufficient muscle tone, falls to the back of the throat, and obstructs the pharynx. ❶ **Rationale:** *Because the tongue is attached to the lower jaw, moving the lower jaw forward and tilting the head backward lifts the tongue away from the pharynx and opens the airway.*
   - If possible, insert an oropharyngeal (oral) airway. **Rationale:** *This prevents the tongue from occluding the oropharynx.* Hold the airway with the curved end upward and insert as far as possible into the mouth to the end of the soft palate. Rotate the airway 180 degrees so the end is directed down the pharynx, gliding it over the tongue. The outer flange remains just outside the client's lips.

Head Tilt–Chin Lift Maneuver

- Place one hand palm downward on the forehead.
- Place the fingers of the other hand under the bony part of the lower jaw near the chin. The teeth should then be almost closed. The mouth should not be closed completely.
- Simultaneously press down on the forehead with one hand, and lift the individual's chin upward with the other. ❷ Avoid press-

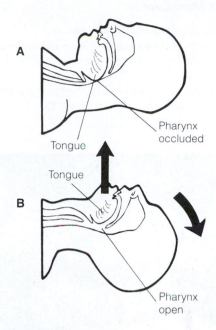

❶ The position of an unconscious individual's tongue: A, Airway occluded; B, Airway open.

ing the fingers deeply into the soft tissues under the chin or hyperextending the neck because too much pressure can obstruct the airway.
- Open the individual's mouth by pressing the jaw downward with the thumb after tilting the head.
- Remove dentures if they cannot be maintained in place. Note, however, that dentures that can be maintained in place make a mouth-to-mouth seal tighter should rescue breathing be required.

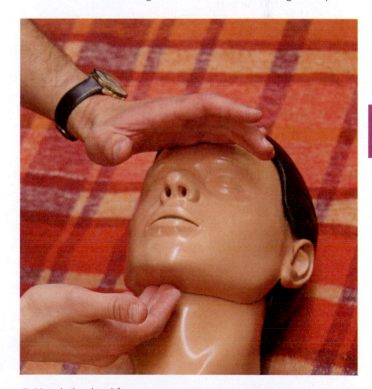

❷ Head tilt–chin lift maneuver. (© Roman Milert/Fotolia)

(continued on next page)

SKILL 13.24   Performing Rescue Breathing (continued)

Jaw-Thrust Maneuver

■ Kneel at the top of the individual's head.

■ Grasp the angle of the mandible directly below the earlobe between your thumb and forefinger on each side of the individual's head.

■ While tilting the head backward, lift the lower jaw until it juts forward and is higher than the upper jaw. **③**

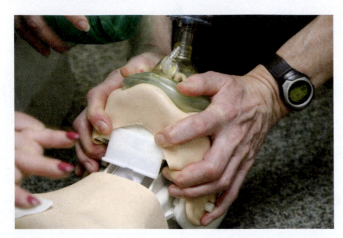

③ Jaw-thrust maneuver. (Credit: Dr. P. Marazzi/Science Source)

■ Rest your elbows on the surface on which the individual is lying.

■ Retract the lower lip with the thumbs prior to giving artificial respiration.

■ If the individual is suspected of having a spinal neck injury, do not hyperextend the neck.

8. Determine if the individual has resumed breathing as a result of the opened airway. This takes 5–10 seconds.

   • Place your ear and cheek close to the individual's mouth and nose.

   • Look at the chest and abdomen for rising and falling movement.

   • Listen for air escaping during exhalation.

   • Feel for air escaping against your cheek.

9. If no breathing is evident, provide rescue breathing.

   • Give two full breaths (1 second per breath). Pause and take a breath after the first ventilation. **Rationale:** *The 1-second time span allows adequate time to provide good chest expansion and decreases the possibility of gastric distention. Excessive air volumes and rapid inspiratory flow rates can cause pharyngeal pressures that are great enough to open the esophagus, thus allowing air to enter the stomach.*

   • Ensure adequate ventilation by observing the individual's chest rise and fall and by assessing his breathing as outlined in step 8.

   • If the initial ventilation attempt is unsuccessful, reposition the individual's head and repeat the rescue breathing as above.

   • If the individual still cannot be ventilated, proceed to clear the airway of any foreign bodies using the finger sweep technique if the foreign object is visible, abdominal thrusts, or chest thrusts.

Mouth-to-Mask Method

■ If not already at hand, remove the mask from its case and push out the dome.

■ Connect the one-way valve to the mask port.

■ Position yourself at the top of the individual's head, and open the airway using the jaw-thrust maneuver.

■ Place the wider rim of the mask between the individual's lower lip and chin. Place the rest of the mask over the face using your thumbs on each side of the mask to hold it in place. **④** **Rationale:** *This keeps the mouth open under the mask.*

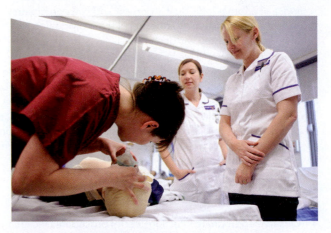

④ Mouth-to-mask rescue breathing. (© wunkley/Alamy)

Bag–Valve–Mask Method

■ Use one hand to secure the mask at the top and bottom and to hold the individual's jaw forward. Use the other hand to squeeze and release the bag every 6–8 seconds (8–10 breaths per minute). **⑤** If two rescuers are available, one holds the head and mask in place while the second compresses the bag.

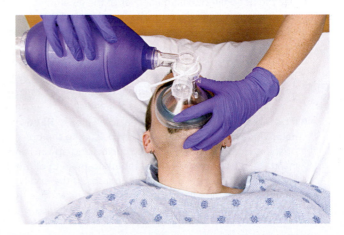

⑤ Bag-to-mask breathing.

Mouth-to-Mouth Method

■ Perform mouth-to-mouth breathing only if a mask is not available. Use a face shield and insert the airway portion of the shield into the individual's mouth.

SKILL 13.24   Performing Rescue Breathing (continued)

- Maintain the open airway by using the head tilt–chin lift maneuver.
- Pinch the individual's nostrils with the index finger and thumb of the hand on the individual's forehead. **Rationale:** *Pinching closes the nostrils and prevents resuscitation air from escaping through them.* Take one normal (not a deep breath).
- Give each ventilation using 1 second per breath. ❻ **Rationale:** *The 1-second time span allows adequate time to provide good chest expansion, and decreases the possibility of gastric distention. Excessive air volumes and rapid inspiratory flow rates can cause pharyngeal pressures that are great enough to open the esophagus, thus allowing air to enter the stomach.*
- Remove your mouth and allow the individual to exhale passively.

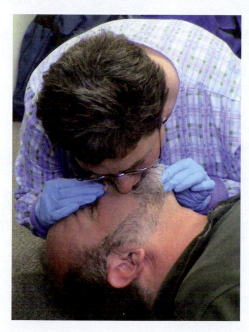

❻ Mouth-to-mouth rescue breathing.

Mouth-to-Nose Method

This method can be used when there is an injury to the mouth or jaw or when the client is edentulous (toothless), making it difficult to achieve a tight seal over the mouth.

- Use a barrier device if a resuscitation mask is not available. Some face shields used for mouth-to-mouth breathing also are effective for mouth-to-nose breathing.

- Maintain the head tilt–chin lift position.
- Close the individual's mouth by pressing the palm of your hand against the individual's chin. The thumb of the same hand may be used to hold the bottom lip closed.
- Take a normal breath and deliver two full breaths of 1 second each.
- Remove your mouth and allow the individual to exhale passively. It may be necessary to separate the individual's lips or to open the mouth for exhaling, since the nasal passages may be obstructed during exhalation.

10. After 2 minutes, recheck for the presence of a carotid pulse ❼ (Berg et al., 2010).

11. If the carotid pulse is palpable, but breathing is not restored, repeat rescue breathing.
    - Inflate at the rate of 8–10 breaths per minute (1 breath every 6–8 seconds).
    - Deliver rescue breaths slowly but with enough force to make the individual's chest rise.
    - If chest expansion fails to occur, ensure that the neck is not hyperextended and the jaw lifted upward, or check again for the presence of obstructive material, fluid, or vomitus.
    - Reassess the carotid pulse every 2 minutes thereafter.

12. When the emergency care is completed, remove and discard gloves and other standard precautions equipment. Perform hand hygiene.

13. Document the date and time of the arrest, including the precipitating events, the duration of breathlessness, and the individual's response to the breathing.
    - Notify the primary care provider of the relevant events if not already notified.

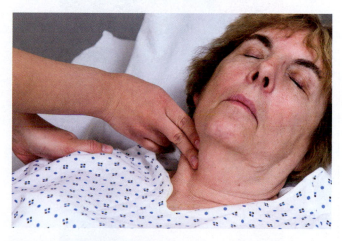

❼ Checking the carotid pulse.

Developmental Considerations

INFANTS AND CHILDREN

- Airway obstruction by a foreign body is the most common cause of respiratory arrest in children. Other common causes include suffocation, poisoning, or trauma.

- Acute epiglottitis can lead to upper airway obstruction in children. Symptoms usually occur suddenly and include drooling, difficulty swallowing, and a croaking sound with inspiration.

(continued on next page)

SKILL 13.24 Performing Rescue Breathing (continued)

RESCUE BREATHING FOR INFANTS

- If the child is not breathing or only gasping, check for a brachial pulse. If the child is unresponsive and not breathing normally and there are no signs of life, the nurse should begin CPR unless a pulse can definitely be felt within 10 seconds (Kleinman et al., 2010).
- If there is a pulse but no breathing, begin ventilations. For infants, place one hand on the forehead and tilt the head back gently. Do not hyperextend the neck because this can cause the soft trachea to collapse.

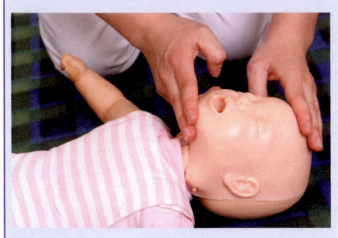

Infant head tilt–chin lift maneuver. (© Roman Milert/Alamy)

- The jaw-thrust maneuver can also be used if a neck injury is suspected.
- When performing mouth-to-mouth breathing, cover both the mouth and nose of an infant.

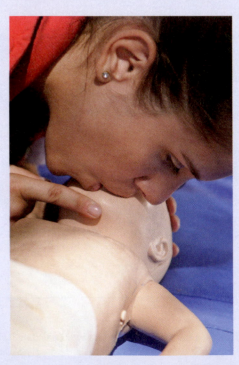

Infant mouth-to-mouth rescue breathing. (Photographer: microgen)

- If an appropriate size mask and bag are available, they should always be used. The mask should reach from the bridge of the nose to the chin but not cover the eyes.

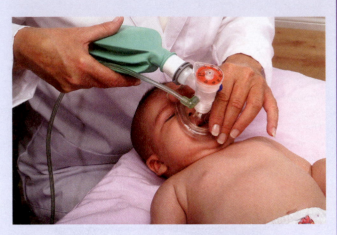

Infant bag-to-mask breathing. (Photo Researchers)

- Deliver 8–10 breaths per minute (1 breath every 6–8 seconds).

Setting of Care

- If an individual has cardiac or breathing problems, encourage the caregiver to learn CPR.
- Carry a pocket mask in the home care nursing bag at all times.
- Know how to activate the EMS. In most cases of respiratory arrest, the individual will need oxygen, respiratory support, and ambulance transport to the emergency department.
- Assist the ambulance crew as needed and provide information about the individual's history.
- Once the individual is en route to the hospital, call the emergency department and give the report to the nurse in charge, including:
  a. A brief health history
  b. Medications the individual takes at home
  c. Findings prior to the respiratory arrest
  d. Duration of respiratory arrest and the individual's response to resuscitation
  e. Vital signs.
- Provide emotional support to family members. If the individual lives alone, contact family members, as needed.
- Notify the primary care provider.

SKILL 13.25   Administering External Cardiac Compressions

Evidence-Based Practice

Chest Compressions for CPR

An observational study concluded that chest compressions are the most important aspect of CPR. The chest is able to fully recoil during each compression, thereby lowering intrathoracic pressures, which promotes improved cardiac preload and improved filling of the coronary arteries. Interruptions in chest compressions, even if brief, produce a dramatic decline in coronary perfusion pressures and worsen outcomes. For a single rescuer, it is believed that continuous cardiac compression will improve outcomes. The use of chest compressions first has now been approved by the American Heart Association and released October 2010.

Source: SOS-KANTO Study Group (2007). Cardiopulmonary resuscitation by bystanders with chest compression only (SOS-KANTO): An observational study. *The Lancet, 369*(9565), 920–926.

Delegation

Although UAP cannot perform all aspects of a hospital code situation, they are trained in CPR and can perform external cardiac compression techniques. If they are the first responders, UAP should initiate the intervention and not wait for a nurse.

Equipment

- Standard precautions supplies should always be easily accessible: gloves, CPR mask or manual resuscitator (bag–valve–mask [BVM] device), gowns, and protective eyewear.
- Emergency equipment such as defibrillation and intubation equipment should be centrally located.
- Face mask with one-way valve or mouth shields or a BVM device
- A hard surface, such as a cardiac board or the floor, on which to place the individual.

Procedure

1. Determine that the individual is unresponsive.
2. If the individual does not respond, call a "code" or follow agency protocol to call for assistance. If another individual is present and can participate, have that individual go get help. Tell the individual to return and report that help has been called.
3. Observe appropriate infection control procedures including applying clean gloves as much as possible.
4. Provide for as much privacy as possible without interfering with the necessary individuals and activities. If family members are present, the nurse may request they leave for the moment. Family members should be allowed the option of remaining in the room (Howlett et al., 2010). This option requires policies and procedures to be in place for a facilitator who can:
   - Explain the options to the family.
   - Support the family before, during, and after the event.
   - Support any family decisions not to be present.
   - Enforce contraindications for family presence such as extreme emotional behavior or interference with medical procedures.
5. Position the individual appropriately if not already done.
   - Place the individual supine on a firm surface. **Rationale:** *Blood flow to the brain will be inadequate during CPR if the individual's head is positioned higher than the thorax. A hard surface facilitates compression of the heart between the sternum and the hard surface.*
   - If the individual is in bed, place a cardiac board—preferably the full width of the bed—under the back. If necessary, place the individual on the floor.
   - If the individual must be turned, turn the body as a unit while firmly supporting the head and neck so that the head does not roll, twist, or tilt backward or forward. **Rationale:** *Turning the individual as a unit prevents further injury (if present) to the neck or spine.*
6. Position the hands on the sternum. Proper hand placement is essential for effective cardiac compression. Position the hands as follows:
   - With the hand nearest the individual's legs, use your middle and index fingers to locate the lower margin of the rib cage.
   - Move the fingers up the rib cage to the notch where the lower ribs meet the sternum. ❶

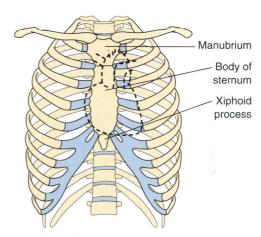

Manubrium
Body of sternum
Xiphoid process

❶ The sternum and ribs.

   - Place the heel of the other hand (nearest the individual's head) along the lower half of the individual's sternum, close to the index finger that is next to the middle finger in the costal-sternal notch. **Rationale:** *Proper positioning of the hands during cardiac compression helps prevent injury to underlying organs and the ribs. Compression directly over the xiphoid process can lacerate the individual's liver.*
   - Then place the heel of the first hand on top of the second hand. The fingers may be extended or interlaced (preferred). Compression occurs only on the sternum and through the heels of the hands.
7. Administer cardiac compression.
   - Lock your elbows into position, straighten your arms, and position your shoulders directly over your hands. ❷

(continued on next page)

SKILL 13.25   Administering External Cardiac Compressions (*continued*)

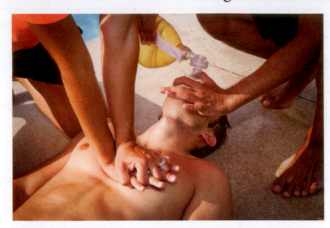

❷ Arm and hand position for external cardiac compression.
(Copyright daviles/Fotolia)

- For each compression, using the weight of your upper body, forcefully push straight down on the sternum. For an adult of normal size, depress the sternum at least 5 cm (2 in.). **Rationale:** *The muscle force of both arms is needed for adequate cardiac compression of an adult. The weight of your shoulders and trunk supplies power for compression. Extension of the elbows ensures an adequate and even force throughout compression.*
- Between compressions, completely release the compression pressure. However, do not lift your hands from the chest or change their position. **Rationale:** *Releasing the pressure allows the sternum to return to its normal position and allows the heart chambers to fill with blood. Leaving the hands on the chest prevents taking a malposition between compressions and possibly injuring the individual.*
- Provide external cardiac compressions at the rate of 100 per minute. Push fast and maintain the rhythm by counting "one, two, three," and so on. **Rationale:** *The specified compression rate and rhythm simulate normal heart contractions.*
- Administer 30 external compressions followed by two rescue breaths.
- After five cycles (approximately 2 minutes) of compressions and breaths (ratio 30:2), reassess the individual's carotid pulse. If there is no pulse, continue with CPR and check for the return of the pulse every few minutes.

VARIATION: CPR PERFORMED BY TWO RESCUERS

- One rescuer provides external cardiac compressions and the other provides rescue breathing, inflating the lungs once after every 30 compressions.
- Pause chest compressions for no longer than 10 seconds for the two breaths unless an advanced airway (e.g., endotracheal tube) is in place. If an advanced airway is in place, the compressing rescuer should deliver at least 100 compressions per minute continuously, without pauses for ventilation. The rescuer delivering the rescue breaths should give 8–10 breaths per minute.
- Providers should switch positions after every five cycles, about 2 minutes. **Rationale:** *Changing positions should help prevent rescuers from becoming fatigued.*
- When relieved from CPR:
  - Stand by to inform the team what has occurred and to assist as needed.
  - Provide emotional support to the individual's family members and any others who may have witnessed the cardiac arrest. This is often a frightening experience for others because it is so sudden and life threatening.
- When the emergency care is completed, remove and discard gloves and other standard precautions equipment. Perform hand hygiene.
- CPR is terminated only when one of the following events occurs:
  - Another trained individual takes over.
  - The individual's heartbeat and breathing are reestablished.
  - Adjunctive life support measures are initiated.
  - A physician states that the individual has died and that CPR is to be discontinued.
  - The rescuer becomes exhausted, and there is no one to take over (this may occur when an arrest occurs outside the healthcare setting).
- Document the date and time of the arrest, including the precipitating events, the duration of respiratory and cardiac arrest and resuscitation efforts, and the individual's response.
  - Record any advanced cardiac life support interventions such as defibrillation or initiation of intravenous therapy.
  - Document vital signs, cardiac rhythm recordings, any complications, and type of follow-up care. Notify the primary care provider of the relevant events.

Developmental Considerations

INFANTS

- Place the infant on a firm, flat surface if possible. If none is available or the infant is being carried, hold the infant's head in your nondominant hand and rest the thorax along your forearm.
- Check carefully for airway obstruction in children with cardiac arrest. Cardiac arrest in children most often occurs after an initial respiratory arrest.
- To find the position for compressions, place two fingers in the center of the infant's chest just below the nipple line. Do not press on the bottom of the breastbone.

- Compress the chest at least one third the depth of the chest (about 4 cm [1.5 in.]) straight down using the pads of two fingers. (See figure.) Release the compression completely, keeping your fingers in the compression position while the other hand remains on the forehead, maintaining the open airway.
- Give compressions at a rate of 100 compressions per minute with cycles of 30 compressions and two breaths if you are alone.
- If two rescuers are present, instead of the two-finger technique described above, encircle the infant's chest with both hands, fingers behind the thorax and the thumbs over the lower half of the

SKILL 13.25   **Administering External Cardiac Compressions** (*continued*)

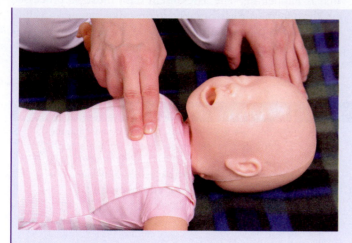

CPR on an infantwith one healthcare provider.
Roman Milert/123RF

sternum for compression. In this fashion, the heart is compressed from both front and back, resulting in more effective CPR (Mutchner, 2007). With two healthcare provider rescuers, the compression-ventilation ratio for infants becomes 15 compressions to two breaths.

CHILDREN (AGES 1 YEAR TO PUBERTY)

- Check carefully for airway obstruction in children with cardiac arrest. Cardiac arrest in children most often occurs after an initial respiratory arrest.
- In children, to find the hand position for compressions, run your index and middle fingers up the ribs until you locate the sternal notch. With those two fingers on the lower end of the sternum, put the heel of the other hand on the sternum just above the location of the index finger. (See figure.)
- Use one or two hands for compressions, keeping the fingers off the chest. Compression depth is at least one third the depth of the chest (5 cm [2 in.]). Never lift the hand(s) off the chest.

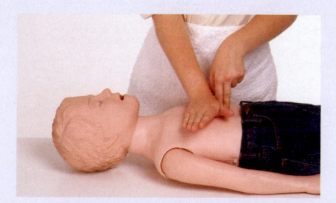

Locating the site for chest compressions on a child.
(Dorling Kindersley—Jules Selmes)

- CPR for a child is given at the following rate: 100 compressions per minute with cycles of 30 compressions and two breaths for single rescuers and 15 compressions to two breaths for two-rescuer CPR (Hazinski, 2010).

OLDER ADULTS

- Older clients are most likely to be injured by incorrect placement of the rescuer's hands. The sternum becomes more brittle with aging and fracture of the sternum or ribs is more common.
- The older client may have an advance directive, or living will, expressing his or her wishes about life support.

Setting of Care

- Always carry a pocket mask in the home care nursing bag.
- Survey the scene for safety hazards, presence of bystanders, and other individuals needing assistance.
- Call for help or have another individual call for EMS or 911.
- The individual who calls the local EMS must be able to impart all of the following information:
  - Location of the emergency
  - Telephone number from which the call is being made
  - What happened
  - Number of people needing assistance
  - Condition of the individuals needing assistance
  - What aid is being given.

The EMS dispatcher may ask for additional information. Dispatchers will also give rescue skills instructions to the caller.

- If the rescuer is alone, summon help and then perform CPR.
- Have a bystander elevate the lower extremities (optional). This may promote venous return and augment circulation during external cardiac compressions.
- If a second individual identifies himself or herself as a trained rescuer, have that individual verify that EMS has been notified. If EMS has been notified, the second rescuer offers to help with CPR.
- After activating the emergency response system, continue resuscitation until the first responder vehicle arrives. This may be a fire truck or an ambulance. Be prepared to give a report to the crew and assist them as needed.
- While the individual is en route to the hospital, contact the emergency department and report the following to the nurse in charge:
  - A brief health history
  - Medications the individual takes at home
  - Findings prior to the cardiopulmonary arrest
  - Duration of the cardiopulmonary arrest and the individual's response to resuscitation
- Provide emotional support to family members. If the individual is alone, contact family members or neighbors, as needed.
- Advise older adults to talk with the primary care provider about preparing an advance directive for life support measures.
- Encourage caregivers or family members to learn CPR.

▶ CRITICAL THINKING OPTIONS FOR UNEXPECTED OUTCOMES

Not all unexpected outcomes require further nursing intervention; however, many times they do. When the client demonstrates a change in signs/symptoms indicating an emerging problem, the nurse should immediately assess and troubleshoot what is happening. The assessment data must be processed quickly to formulate a hypothesis so the nurse can make a clinical judgment. The nurse then decides how best to resolve the problem and improve the client's situation for a better appropriate outcome.

EXPECTED OUTCOMES	PROBLEM SOLVING	NURSING ACTIONS
Introduction 1. Client maintains breathing rate and pattern to support his or her needs adequately. 2. Client maintains patent airway by using preventative actions, effective coughing and expectoration of secretions, frequent repositioning, periodic deep breathing, maintaining hydration, and ambulating as able. 3. Encourage deep breathing to minimize or reverse atelectasis in the lungs. 4. Prevent pulmonary complications for the immediate postoperative client.	■ Client develops atelectasis.	■ Encourage client to change position frequently, cough, take deep breaths, and ambulate as physician orders. ■ Encourage client to use an incentive spirometer. ■ Chest physical therapy may be ordered. ■ Monitor breath sounds.
Supplemental Oxygen Therapy 1. Supplemental oxygen is delivered via the most appropriate method to meet individual client's oxygen needs. 2. Respiratory distress will decrease. 3. Oxygen saturation readings will be stable. 4. Client reports improved sleep pattern when using CPAP/BiPAP. 5. The client on a mechanical ventilator will not develop ventilator-associated pneumonia. 6. Promote gas exchange through the use of a sustained maximal inspiration device (incentive spirometer), controlled breathing to sustain maximal expiration (pursed lips breathing), positioning to support respirations, or chest physiotherapy to mobilize secretions. 7. Maximize COPD client's ability to maintain airway patency, decrease shortness of breath, control breathing rate, and maximize breathing effectiveness.	■ Client remains having difficulty breathing after supplemental oxygen is begun.	■ Place client in high Fowler's position. ■ Check supplemental oxygen set-up and oxygen flow rate is correct. ■ Assess oxygen saturation and lung sounds and compare to previous findings. ■ Ask client to describe what he or she is experiencing. ■ Conduct actions to increase comfort and decrease anxiety.
Maintaining a Patent Airway 1. Secretions are removed via appropriate suctioning method without complications. 2. The least invasive method of suctioning will be used to meet individual client's need for a clear airway.	■ Client's oxygen saturation decreases and tachycardia develops while suctioning.	■ Suction only as needed. ■ Oxygenate client before and after suctioning. ■ Limit suctioning time to <10 seconds. ■ Use correct catheter diameter (less than half the inner diameter of the airway it enters)
	■ Frequent suctioning is required due to the amount of secretions.	■ Suction as needed but pre- and post-oxygenate with 100% oxygen. ■ Allow rest period before suctioning again. ■ Maintain adequate hydration. ■ Reposition client frequently to keep secretions mobile.
As needed, appropriate artificial airway will be used to maintain patency of client's airway.	■ Tracheostomy tube becomes dislodged.	■ Quickly use new obturator to insert new tracheostomy tube (both items should be kept at the bedside). ■ Encourage client to remain calm and take slow deep breaths. ■ Retie tracheostomy ties or secure Velcro tracheostomy collar to secure correct tracheostomy tube position.

EXPECTED OUTCOMES	PROBLEM SOLVING	NURSING ACTIONS
Maintaining Lung Expansion Chest drainage system remains a closed system.	▪ Chest tube becomes disconnected from the drainage system or the system breaks or cracks.	▪ Immediately insert the end of the chest tube one to two inches into a sterile pour bottle of water to create a water seal (a small pour bottle of sterile water should be kept at the bedside). ▪ Then set-up another closed drainage system and connect it to the chest tube.
Chest tubes remain patent and secured in place.	▪ Chest tube becomes dislodged from the client.	▪ Immediately apply a sterile occlusive dressing to the insertion site and tape it down on three sides (a sterile occlusive dressing should be kept at the bedside). ▪ Periodically lift open the fourth side when the client exhales to allow air trapped in the pleural space to be expelled. ▪ Call the physician to insert another chest tube.
Life-Threatening Respiratory Situations Obstructed airway is cleared of foreign body.	▪ Client's airway becomes obstructed during a meal.	▪ Assess and then follow emergency maneuvers to clear the airway. ▪ Call for help. ▪ If unable to clear the airway, call for rapid-response team. ▪ Begin rescue breathing or CPR as client needs. ▪ Use AED with client as appropriate. ▪ Have emergency cart brought to bedside.
1. Rescue breathing or CPR is begun within five minutes after assessment has determined that the client has a life-threatening need for these actions. 2. Client's heart rhythm is restored to normal after defibrillation with an AED or manual defibrillator. 3. Rescue breathing or CPR is continued until rapid-response team arrives.	▪ Client suddenly has a condition change that becomes life-threatening.	▪ Call for help. ▪ Call for rapid-response team. ▪ Assess and begin rescue breathing or CPR as client needs. ▪ Use AED with client as appropriate. ▪ Have emergency cart brought to bedside.

14 Perfusion

Skills-at-a-Glance

Most people in good health give little thought to their cardio-vascular function. Changing position frequently, ambulating, and exercising usually maintain adequate cardiovascular functioning. Immobility is detrimental to cardiovascular function.

Preventing venous stasis is an important intervention to reduce the risk of complications following surgery, trauma, or major medical problems. The use of antiembolism stockings and sequential compression devices is an additional measure that can help prevent venous stasis.

Expected Outcomes

1. Early detection of bleeding occurs and loss of blood is minimized.
2. Pressure dressing is applied, and bleeding is controlled.
3. Vital signs remain stable.

SKILL 14.1   Using Digital Pressure

Equipment

- Towels or gauze dressing if available
- Gloves

Procedure

1. Observe/assess site with active bleeding. Initiate standard precautions immediately and follow infection control measures.
2. Don gloves, sterile preferred.
3. Identify the closest artery proximal to the bleeding site ❶. **Rationale:** *The rapid loss of more than 40% of the total blood volume leads to death if rapid aggressive intervention is not implemented.*
4. Apply direct pressure to artery, using your gloved finger.
5. If towels or 4 × 4 gauze pads are available, apply direct pressure to site if wound does not contain glass particles. **Rationale:** *If pressure is placed on wound when glass is present, additional tissue damage can occur.*
6. Raise the affected limb above the level of the heart about 30 degrees. **Rationale:** *This decreases arterial blood flow to area and promotes venous return.*
7. Maintain direct pressure for 5 minutes. **Rationale:** *This action promotes clot formation.*

> **CLINICAL ALERT**
> Determine if individual is receiving medications or herbal therapies, which affect blood coagulation (e.g., warfarin [Coumadin]). If so, increase time of applied pressure.

8. When bleeding has subsided, proceed to clean and address the wound gently.
9. To control nose bleeds (epistaxis), place client in sitting position, with head tilted forward. Pinch nose for 5 minutes. Apply ice pack to neck. **Rationale:** *This assists in vasoconstriction.*
10. Remove and discard gloves when bleeding subsides.
11. Perform hand hygiene immediately. **Rationale:** *This protects you from possible contamination should any leakage have occurred through the gloves.*
12. Document procedure and client response.

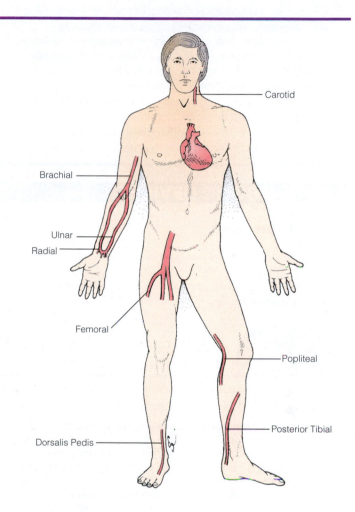

❶ Pulse sites that may be used to control bleeding.

SKILL 14.2   Using a Pressure Dressing

Equipment

- 4 × 4 gauze pad
- Sterile dressings—number and size depends on wound
- Sterile gloves
- Cleansing solution
- Tape

(continued on next page)

SKILL 14.2 Using a Pressure Dressing (*continued*)

Preparation

- Check physician's orders.
- Assemble necessary supplies according to extent of wound
- If time permits, explain procedure to client and provide light and privacy.
- Perform hand hygiene thoroughly if time permits.
- Set up sterile field and prepare cleansing solution if time permits.

Procedure

1. Put on sterile gloves.
2. Cleanse wound and apply dressing. Use several layers of 4 × 4 gauze pads.
3. Place tape tightly over entire dressing to provide an occlusive dressing. Do not completely circle an extremity or the body. **Rationale:** *Encircling an extremity with a bandage acts like a tourniquet and may prevent blood flow.*
4. Check for pulses distal to pressure site. **Rationale:** *This ensures that collateral blood flow is maintained.*
5. Place all soiled material in biohazard bag. **Rationale:** *This prevents cross-contamination and ensures proper disposal.*

6. Remove gloves and perform hand hygiene.
7. Monitor vital signs, and observe for signs of shock.
8. Continue to monitor extremity distal to pressure dressing for adequate circulation. **Rationale:** *This ensures circulation.*
9. Position client for comfort.
10. Elevate extremity to prevent bleeding. **Rationale:** *This minimizes bleeding.*
11. Monitor frequently for signs of bleeding and hematoma. *Note:* Hematomas feel spongy even under bandages.
12. Document care and client response.

Documentation

- Size (in centimeters), location based on anatomical landmark, condition of wound
- Color, odor, consistency, amount of drainage
- Type and number of dressings used
- Approximate amount of blood loss
- Condition of dressing when removed (e.g., saturated with drainage)

▶ ANTIEMBOLIC DEVICES

Expected Outcomes

1. Compression stockings remain wrinkle free and pressure is evenly distributed.
2. Peripheral pulses are present during use of sequential stockings and elastic hosiery.

3. Client's skin remains intact while using compression stockings.

SKILL 14.3 Applying Antiembolism Stockings (Graduated Compression Stockings and Elastic Stockings)

Evidence-Based Nursing Practice

Compression Stockings—Safe Practice Issues

Compression stockings are generally prescribed as a means of preventing deep venous thrombosis (DVT)—blood clots in the legs. Clots from DVT may travel to the lungs, producing a potentially fatal condition called pulmonary embolism (PE). The current recommendation of the American College of Chest Physicians is ambulation with compression as tolerated, after starting anticoagulation, in clients with acute DVT. However, there are several roadblocks to correct and consistent use of compression stockings.

Common issues with compression stockings are proper fit, proper use, and client compliance. Some manufacturers' stockings do not fit client measurements or are too loose or tight. Effectiveness depends on the appropriate amount of compression for the particular client's condition, so it is essential to measure the legs and to obtain properly fitting stockings. Also, regular review measure-

ments should be taken to check for changes in leg size and to correct excessive pressure.

Improper use, such as allowing compression stockings to roll down, increases pressure at the ankle and decreases it in the calf or thigh. Improper application or use can create a tourniquet effect.

Client teaching is important to encourage compliance. Clients should be taught the importance of removing stockings at least once a day and assessing the skin. Nurses should monitor stockings with the client in a seated, not supine, position, to determine whether the stockings are obstructing blood flow. Nurses may need to encourage clients to start or continue to wear compression stockings and explain their purpose, because some clients find compression uncomfortable and simply stop wearing them.

Data from Christakou & Zakynthinos (2014), *Johns Hopkins Medical Letter: Health After 50* (2013a, 2013b), and Pal (2011).

Delegation

Unlicensed assistive personnel (UAP) frequently remove and apply antiembolism stockings as part of hygiene care. The nurse should stress the importance of removing and reapplying the stockings and reporting any changes in the client's skin to the nurse. The nurse is responsible for assessment of the skin.

Equipment

- Single-use tape measure (to prevent cross-infection)
- Clean knee or thigh antiembolism stockings of appropriate size

SKILL 14.3   Applying Antiembolism Stockings *(continued)*

TABLE 14–1   Measuring for Graduated Compression Stockings (Elastic Hosiery)

THIGH-HIGH MEASURING		KNEE-HIGH MEASURING	
Circumference	**Length**	**Circumference**	**Length**
Measure mid-thigh circumference.	Measure leg from bottom of heel to fold of buttocks.	Measure calf at largest circumference.	Measure leg from Achilles tendon to popliteal fold.

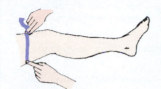 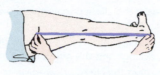 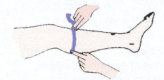 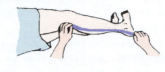

Preparation

- Check physician's order and gather supplies.
- Take measurements as needed to obtain the appropriate size stockings.
  - Measure the length of both legs from the heel to the gluteal fold (for thigh-length stockings) or from the heel to the popliteal space or bend of the knee (for knee-length stockings).
  - Measure the circumferences of each calf and each thigh at the widest point.
  - Compare measurements to the size chart on the back of the manufacturer's package to obtain stockings of correct size (**Table 14–1** ●). Obtain two sizes if there is a significant difference. **Rationale:** *Stockings that are too large for the client do not place adequate pressure on the legs to facilitate venous return, and may bunch, increasing the risk of pressure and skin irritation. Stockings that are too small may impede blood flow to the feet and cause skin breakdown.*

Procedure

1. Prior to performing the procedure, introduce self and verify the client's identity using agency protocol. Explain to the client what you are going to do, why it is necessary, and how he or she can participate.
2. Perform hand hygiene and observe other appropriate infection control procedures.
3. Provide for client privacy.
4. Select an appropriate time to apply the stockings.
   - Apply stockings in the morning, if possible, before the client gets out of bed. **Rationale:** *In sitting and standing positions, the veins can become distended so that edema occurs; the stockings should be applied before this occurs.*
   - Assist the client who has been ambulating to lie down and elevate legs for 15 to 30 minutes before applying the stockings. **Rationale:** *This facilitates venous return, reduces swelling, and facilitates application of the stockings.*
5. Prepare the client.
   - Assist the client to a lying position in bed. Raise bed to appropriate height.
   - Wash and dry the legs as needed.
6. Apply the stockings.
   - Reach inside the stocking from the top, and grasping the heel, turn the upper portion of the stocking inside out so the foot portion is inside the stocking leg. **Rationale:**

Firm elastic stockings are easier to fit over the foot and calf when inverted in this manner rather than bunching up the stocking.

- Ask the client to point the toes, and then position the stocking on the client's foot. With the heel of the stocking down and stretching each side of the stocking, ease the stocking over the toes taking care to place the toe and heel portions of the stocking appropriately ●. **Rationale:** *Pointing the toes makes application easier.*

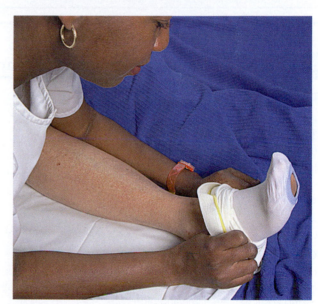

❶ Applying the stocking over the toes.

- Grasp the loose portion of the stocking at the ankle and gently pull the stocking over the leg, turning it right side out in the process. If applying the thigh-length stockings, stretch them over the knee until the top is below the gluteal fold.
7. Return bed to lowest height. Provide comfort and safety for the client.
8. Document procedure, including size and length of stockings used.

CLINICAL ALERT
Postoperative DVT of the lower extremity is often asymptomatic and in many, fatal pulmonary embolism is the first clinical sign of postoperative venous thromboembolism.

(continued on next page)

SKILL 14.3 Applying Antiembolism Stockings *(continued)*

Developmental Considerations

CHILDREN

- Antiembolism stockings are infrequently used on children.

OLDER ADULTS

- Because the elastic is quite strong in antiembolism stockings, older adults may need assistance with putting on the stockings. Clients with arthritis may need to have another person put the stockings on for them.
- Many older adults have circulation problems and wear antiembolism stockings. It is important to check for wrinkles in the stockings and to see if the stocking has rolled down or twisted. If so, correct immediately. **Rationale:** *The stockings must be evenly distributed over the limb to promote rather than hinder circulation.*
- Stockings should be removed at least once a day (check agency policy) so that a thorough assessment can be made of the legs and feet. **Rationale:** *Redness and skin breakdown on the heels can occur quickly and go undetected if not thoroughly assessed on a regular basis.*

- Provide information about the importance of wearing the elastic stockings, how to wear them correctly, and how to take care of them.

Setting of Care

- Teach the client or caregiver how to apply the antiembolism stockings.
- Stress the importance of no wrinkles or rolling down of the stockings and the rationale.
- Instruct the client or caregiver to remove the stockings daily and inspect the skin on the legs.
- Provide instructions about the following:
  - Laundering the stockings (They should be air dried because putting them in a dryer can affect the elasticity of the stockings.)
  - The need for two pairs of stockings to allow for one pair to be worn while the other is being laundered
  - Replacing the stockings when they lose their elasticity
- The slipperiness of stockings if worn without slippers or shoes.
  - If the client is ambulatory, emphasize the need for footwear to prevent falling.

SKILL 14.4   Applying Pneumatic Compression Devices

Equipment

- Disposable leg sleeve(s), knee-length or thigh-length
- Tubing assembly
- Compression controller (motor)
- Measuring tape

Preparation

- Review physician's orders for type of disposable leg sleeve needed.
- Gather equipment and supplies.
- Introduce self, identify client, and perform hand hygiene. Provide privacy by checking the client's identity band and asking client to state name and birth date.
- Explain that this device decreases the risk of developing deep venous thrombosis (DVT) for clients following surgery or those on long-term bed rest. **Rationale:** *This device counteracts blood stasis by increasing peak blood flow velocity. It helps to carry pooled blood from vein.*
- Assess client for potential problems and contraindications for use of these devices. **Rationale:** *Clients on long-term bed rest and clients with ischemic conditions, massive edema of the leg, dermatitis, gangrene, or preexisting DVT within past 6 months are not candidates for these devices.*
- Complete a neurovascular assessment. Include an evaluation of skin color, temperature, sensation, capillary refill, and presence and quality of pedal pulses. Document findings. **Rationale:** *This assessment provides baseline data for evaluating neurovascular changes while devices are used.*
- Assemble equipment. Read manufacturer's directions for connecting and operating compression controller.

- Read directions for setting sleeve pressure (between 35 and 45 mmHg). Maximum pressure should not exceed client's diastolic pressure.
- Locate and identify the indicator lights on the controller for the ankle, calf, and thigh pressure. **Rationale:** *Light is on when the pressure is applied to the three leg sleeves.*

Procedure

1. Provide comfort and safety for client and self, including raising bed to appropriate height.
2. Remove sleeve from plastic bag.
3. Unfold sleeve and follow directions to fit sleeve to client's leg. Leg is placed on white side (lining) of sleeve. Markings on the lining indicate the ankle and popliteal area.
4. Place client's leg on sleeve. Position back of knee over popliteal opening.
5. Starting at the side, wrap sleeve securely around client's leg.
6. Attach Velcro straps securely.
7. Check the fit by placing two fingers between client's leg and sleeve to determine if sleeve fits properly. Readjust Velcro as needed. **Rationale:** *To ensure sleeve does not constrict circulation.*
8. Attach tubing and connect to plugs on leg sleeve by pushing ends firmly together.
9. Connect tubing assembly plug to controller at the tubing assembly connector site.
10. Ensure tubing is free of kinks or twists. **Rationale:** *Kinks and twists can restrict airflow through system.*
11. Plug controller power cable into grounded electric outlet and attach unit to bed frame.

SKILL 14.4   Applying Pneumatic Compression Devices (*continued*)

12. Turn controller power switch to ON. Confirm that alarms are audible.
13. Check that pressure indicator lights are functioning properly. Lower bed to lowest height.
14. Monitor that compression cycles are correct.
15. Conduct neurovascular checks every 2 to 4 hours. Turn machine off immediately if the client complains of numbness or other signs of DVT.
16. Monitor client's tolerance of device.
17. Turn off machine at prescribed time intervals to assess skin and to provide skin care.

> **CLINICAL ALERT**
> Follow hospital policy for amount of time alternating pneumatic compression devices are removed during the day. It is important to keep stockings on most of the day to prevent clot formation.

18. To remove sleeve, turn power switch OFF, disconnect tubing assembly from sleeve at connection site. Unwrap sleeve from leg.
19. Document procedure, care, assessment, and client response.

SKILL 14.5   Applying Sequential Compression Device (SCDs)

Delegation

UAP often remove and reapply SCDs when performing hygiene care. The nurse should check that the UAP knows the correct application process for SCDs. Remind the UAP that the client should not have SCDs removed for long periods of time because the purpose of the SCDs is to promote circulation.

Equipment

- Measuring tape
- SCDs, including disposable sleeves, air pump, and tubing

Procedure

1. Check physician order and gather equipment and supplies.
2. Prior to performing the procedure, introduce self and verify the client's identity using agency protocol. Explain to the client what you are going to do, why it is necessary, and the procedure for applying the sequential compression device. **Rationale:** *The client's participation and comfort will be increased by understanding the reasons for applying the SCD.*
3. Perform hand hygiene and observe other appropriate infection control procedures.
4. Provide for client privacy and drape the client appropriately.
5. Prepare the client. Position bed at correct height for procedure.
   - Place the client in a dorsal recumbent or semi-Fowler position.
   - Measure the client's legs as recommended by the manufacturer if a thigh-length sleeve is required. **Rationale:** *Foot and knee-length sleeves come in just one size; the thigh circumference determines the size needed for a thigh-length sleeve.*
6. Apply the sequential compression sleeves.
   - Place a sleeve under each leg with the opening at the knee ❶.
   - Wrap the sleeve securely around the leg, securing the Velcro tabs. Allow two fingers to fit between the leg and sleeve ❷. **Rationale:** *This amount of space ensures that the sleeve does not impair circulation when inflated.* Ensure that there is no overlapping or increases in the SCD. **Rationale:** *This prevents skin breakdown.*

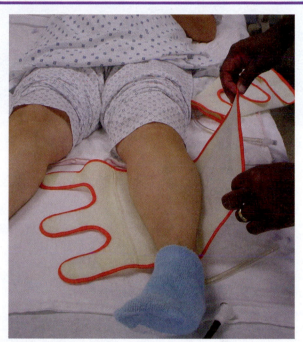

❶ Place inflatable bladder directly behind client's calf.

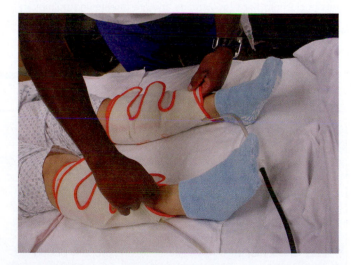

❷ Slip two fingers under wrap to ensure that it is not too tight.

(*continued on next page*)

SKILL 14.5 Applying Sequential Compression Device (SCDs) *(continued)*

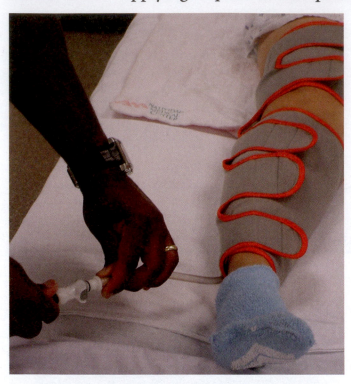

❸ Attach tubing from wrap to tubing connected to pump.

7. Connect the sleeves to the control unit and adjust the pressure as needed ❸. Reposition bed to lowest height.
   - Connect the tubing to the sleeves and control unit ensuring that arrows on the plug and the connector are in alignment and that the tubing is not kinked or twisted.

Rationale: *Improper alignment or obstruction of the tubing by kinks or twists will interfere with operation of the SCD.*

- Turn on the control unit and adjust the alarms and pressures as needed. The sleeve cooling control and alarm should be on; ankle pressure is usually set at 35 to 55 mmHg. **Rationale:** *It is important to have the sleeve cooling control on for comfort and to reduce the risk of skin irritation from moisture under the sleeve. Proper pressure settings prevent injury to the client. Alarms warn of possible control unit malfunctions.*

8. Document the procedure.
   - Record baseline assessment data and application of the SCD. Note control unit settings.

Assess and document skin integrity and neurovascular and peripheral vascular status per agency policy while the SCD is in place. Remove the unit and notify the primary care provider if the client complains of numbness and tingling or leg pain. These may be symptoms of nerve compression.

CLINICAL ALERT
Contraindications to Use of SCDs

- Known or suspected acute DVT, phlebitis, severe atherosclerosis, or ischemic peripheral vascular disease
- DVT within the past 6 months
- Pulmonary embolism
- Any condition where an increase in venous return to the heart might be detrimental
- Local conditions such as dermatitis, gangrene, recent skin graft, infected leg wound, or ulcer.

Evidence-Based Nursing Practice

Recommend Bed Rest for DVT?

Prolonged immobilization has been associated with deep venous thrombosis (DVT) in critically ill clients. However, the value and safety of mobilizing clients with acute DVT has been a concern, largely because of the potential for venous thromboembolism (dislodging of the clot into the bloodstream) and life-threatening pulmonary embolism (PE).

A number of studies have shown that clients with acute DVT who use compression stockings and who begin ambulating early after initiation of anticoagulant therapy experience several benefits from

this approach. Benefits include reduced pain level, more rapid reduction in edema, increased strength maintenance, and improved flexibility. Early ambulation in these clients, with careful monitoring for any evidence of PE, resulted in no increase in incidence of PE. Conversely, bed rest and immobilization did not result in any reduction in incidence of PE. Therefore, the current recommendation of the American College of Chest Physicians is ambulation with compression as tolerated, after starting anticoagulation, in clients with acute DVT.

Source: Christakou & Zakynthinos (2014).

Developmental Considerations

CHILDREN

- Because young children tend to be more active, SCD use is rarely necessary unless the child is immobile (e.g., comatose or in critical care setting).

OLDER ADULTS

- The SCD sleeves may become loose as clients move around in bed. Check that the sleeves are secure and properly positioned.

Setting of Care

- A sequential compression device may be used in the home. Inform the client or caregiver how to apply the device correctly and how to operate the system, including how to respond to the alarm.

▶ ELECTRICAL CONDUCTION IN THE HEART

Any disturbance in the rate or rhythm of the heartbeat is termed *dysrhythmia*. Historically, the term *arrhythmia* has been used in the literature. Although the terms are often used interchangeably, dysrhythmia, which means a disturbance in cardiac rhythm, is more accurate. Dysrhythmias are classified according to their site of origin. The sites include sinus, atrial, junctional, ventricular, and atrioventricular (AV) nodal tissue. A sinus dysrhythmia usually reflects a change in rate or rhythm. An atrial dysrhythmia results from a disturbance with the sinoatrial (SA) node or atria indicated by an abnormality in the P-wave configuration.

A junctional dysrhythmia occurs when there is a problem associated with the AV node as indicated by a change in the PR interval. A ventricular dysrhythmia results from a problem with the ventricle and is indicated by an abnormality in the configuration of the QRS complex. Although many dysrhythmias have no clinical manifestations, many others have serious consequences. A ventricular dysrhythmia is the most life threatening because it compromises cardiac output.

Expected Outcomes

1. ECG leads are applied appropriately and without difficulty.
2. Abnormal ECG findings are interpreted accurately.
3. Monitor wave forms are distinct and readable.
4. Client's cardiac rate is maintained through use of a pacemaker.
5. Client is prepared psychologically and physically for insertion of the pacemaker.
6. Pacemaker is inserted without complications.

SKILL 14.6   Monitoring Clients on Telemetry (Applying ECG Leads)

Equipment

- Telemetry transmitter box with 9-volt battery
- Electrode pouch or gown with transmitter pocket
- 5-lead electrode cable and wires
- Electrodes
- Skin prep pad or alcohol swab

Preparation

- Check physician order and gather equipment.
- Review the client's cardiac assessment. **Rationale:** *The choice of monitoring lead is based on the client's assessment and potential arrhythmias that could occur.*
- Introduce self, identify client, and perform hand hygiene. Provide privacy. Provide comfort and safety for client and self, including raising bed to appropriate height.
- Place a fresh 9-volt battery in the telemetry transmitter box, if needed.
- Attach lead wire securely into transmitter box, ensuring colors match.
- Explain procedure to client. Radio waves transmit the heart's electrical activity to a central monitoring station. This system allows the client to move around while his or her heart is constantly being monitored. Explain that the telemetry range is limited; therefore, client cannot wander out of the range, which is usually the nursing unit. If client goes off the unit, the nurse must be notified.
- Instruct the client to notify the nurse if the electrode falls off.

Procedure

1. Check the expiration date on the electrode packet. **Rationale:** *To ensure electrode gel is moist.*
2. Select electrode sites according to leads to be used for monitoring. Ensure they are not over bony prominences, muscular areas, joints, breasts, or skin creases. **Rationale:** *Placing electrodes on these areas can lead to artifact on the monitor screen.* *Note:* If client is overly obese, electrodes may have to be placed on the bones, since a large amount of adipose tissue results in a poor image on the oscilloscope.

3. Assess skin site before placing electrode. Wipe skin areas using alcohol swab. Allow site to dry thoroughly before affixing electrode. **Rationale:** *This removes oily substances and dead skin for better adherence of electrodes.* Rub skin until slightly red. If client's chest is hairy, then clip hair. **Rationale:** *This enables electrodes to adhere well to skin and minimizes artifact.*
4. Attach lead wires to chest electrodes ❶.

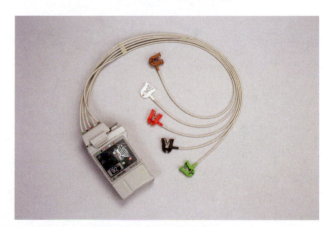

❶ Transmitter box, cable, and lead wires for telemetry.

5. Apply electrodes to client's chest: peel off paper backing on electrode disc ❷. Check that sponge pad in center of electrode is moist with conductive jelly. Place electrode on skin with adhesive side down. Press edges down to secure.
6. Attach wire to transmitter box, matching the color codes of the wires to the telemetry box ❸. **Rationale:** *Mismatch of the colors will cause the client's rhythm pattern to appear inverted.*
7. Have base station run an ECG strip to check clarity of transmission.
8. Reposition bed to lowest height. Perform hand hygiene.
9. Set HIGH and LOW alarm limits on the monitor. Turn alarm buttons to ON per agency/unit protocol (e.g., 50 low, 100 high).
10. Assess skin surrounding the electrode for signs of irritation regularly. Document findings.

(continued on next page)

SKILL 14.6 Monitoring Clients on Telemetry (Applying ECG Leads) *(continued)*

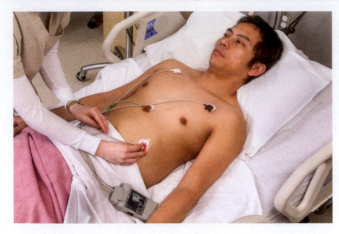

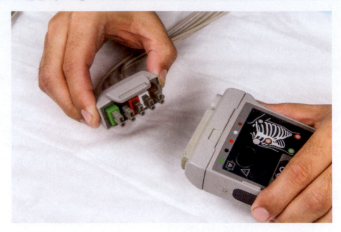

❷ Color-coded lead wires and placement of electrodes for ECG monitoring.

❸ Insert electrode cable into transmitter box.

11. Check lead placement at least once a shift unless notified by client or monitoring station that electrodes are not functioning properly.

12. Change electrodes at least every 3 days or if ECG strip indicates poor conduction of waveform. See **Table 14–2** ● for telemetry electrode placement.

TABLE 14–2   Telemetry Electrode Placement

• **Lead I:** Records activity between a negative electrode (below right clavicle) and a positive electrode (below left clavicle). This lead looks at the heart's left lateral wall. Atrial arrhythmic activity is poorly identified.

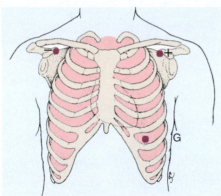

• **Lead II*:** Records activity between a negative electrode (below right clavicle) and a positive electrode (midclavicular line on left flank). This lead looks at left inferior wall. It is used to diagnose supraventricular rhythms, which arise from the atrial and junctional nodes. It best detects atrial activity.

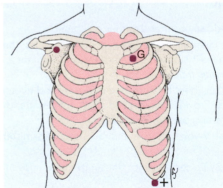

• **Lead III:** Records activity between a negative electrode (below left clavicle) and a positive electrode (lowest rib, left midclavicular line). It looks at left inferior wall.

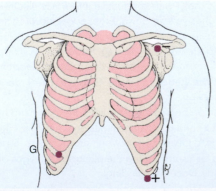

• **Lead MCL₁*:** Records activity between a negative electrode (below left clavicle) and a positive electrode (fourth intercostal space, right of sternum). It is used to analyze ventricular activity so it is beneficial for clients at risk for developing ventricular tachycardia or those with bundle branch block.

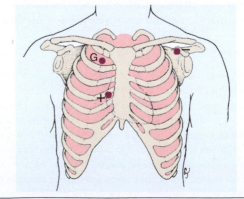

SKILL 14.6 Monitoring Clients on Telemetry (Applying ECG Leads) *(continued)*

TABLE 14–2 Telemetry Electrode Placement *(continued)*

- **Lead MCL$_6$:** Records activity between a negative electrode (below left clavicle) and a positive electrode (fifth intercostal space, left midaxillary line). It monitors ventricular conduction changes much like MCL$_1$. Not as frequently used.

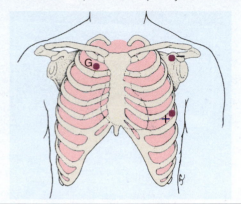

* Most popular leads for telemetry.

Electrode Placement

White to right shoulder

Black to left shoulder

Red to left midclavicular upper abdominal area (lead II positive electrode)

Brown to fourth intercostal space, right sternal border (MCL$_1$, positive chest electrode), or left sternal border, or alternatively at left fifth intercostal space, midaxillary line (V$_6$ position)

Green to right abdomen or other convenient area (ground electrode)

Note: Limb leads and any one chest lead can be monitored using these electrode positions.

SKILL 14.7 Interpreting an ECG Strip

Equipment

- Calipers (optional)
- ECG rhythm strip

Procedure

1. Assess ECG grid ❶ ❷.
   - Each small square represents 0.04 second (horizontal measurement).
   - Each large block (5 small squares) represents 0.20 second.
   - 15 large blocks represent 3 seconds.

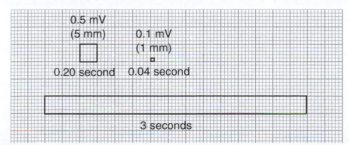

❶ ECG grid.

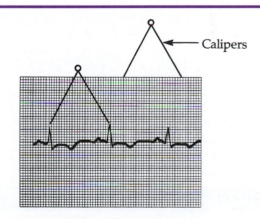

❷ Use calipers to measure heart rate.

2. Determine heart rate by calculating ventricular rate; normal is 60 to 100 per minute.
   - Count the number of R waves in a 6-second period (30 large blocks) and multiply this by 10 to obtain the heart rate.
   - For true accuracy, count client's apical heart rate for 1 full minute.

(continued on next page)

SKILL 14.7 Interpreting an ECG Strip (*continued*)

3. Determine the regularity of ventricular rhythm (R waves should be equally spaced.)

4. Determine the P-wave rate (atrial depolarizations).
   • There should be one P wave in front of each QRS complex.
   • Note if there are more P waves or fewer P waves than QRS complexes.

5. Determine the regularity of the P waves; are they all equally spaced?

6. Measure the PR interval (beginning of the P wave to the beginning of the QRS complex); represents conduction time through the electrical tissue to the ventricles (from the SA node, through the AV node, bundle of His, bundle branches, and Purkinje fibers); normal is 0.12 to 0.20 second.

7. Measure the QRS duration from beginning of the Q wave, if present, to end of the S wave; normal is less than 0.12 second ❸ ❹.

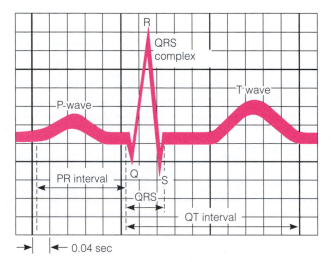

❸ It is important to determine configuration and location of wave pattern to interpret an ECG accurately.

8. Interpret the client's cardiac rhythm (**Tables 14–3** ● and **14–4** ●) and place ECG rhythm sample strip in client's chart, according to hospital policy.

9. Documented information.

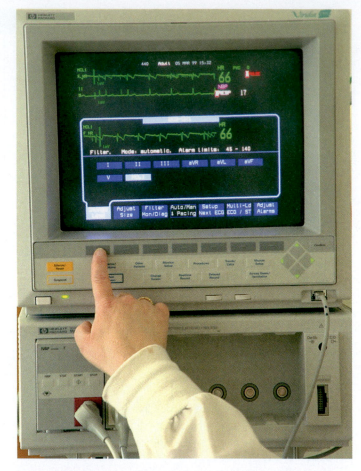

❹ ECG pattern and lead placement are depicted on oscilloscope.

CLINICAL ALERT

Always assess client to determine whether the abnormal rhythm is potentially life threatening and emergency measures should be taken. Signs of hemodynamic instability include:

■ Ongoing chest pain

■ Shortness of breath

■ Change in mental status

■ Systolic blood pressure (SBP) <90 mmHg

■ Heart rate >150 bpm.

TABLE 14–3 Normal Sinus Rhythm

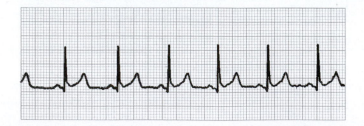

Regular configuration, uniform P wave precedes each QRS
Atrial rate: 60–100
PR interval: 0.12–0.2 second
QRS width: <0.12 second
Ventricular rate: 60–100

SKILL 14.7 Interpreting an ECG Strip *(continued)*

TABLE 14–4   Selected Cardiac Rhythms and Dysrhythmias

Sinus Tachycardia	Sinus Bradycardia
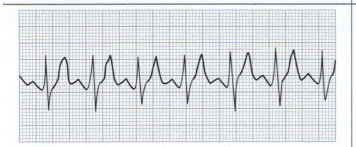	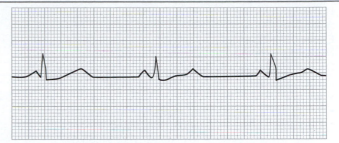
Regular rhythm: >100 beats per min (bpm) P waves: normal Atrial rate: >100 bpm PR interval: 0.12–2.0 second QRS complex width: 0.06–0.08 second usually normal *Note:* A moderately faster heart rate can be a physiological normal variant.	Regular rhythm: <60 bpm P waves: normal Atrial rate: <60 bpm PR interval: 0.20 second QRS complex width: 0.08 second usually normal *Note:* A slow heart rate can be physiologically normal for some clients.
Etiology Underlying causes such as anxiety, fever, shock, drugs, exercise, electrolyte disturbances	**Etiology** Drugs Hypoxia Altered metabolic states (hypothyroidism) Cardiac diseases Athleticism
Initial Treatment Immediately initiate cardioversion if unstable Treatment dependent on elimination of cause Decreasing anxiety Pain relief Antipyretics O_2 Medications (sedatives, tranquilizers, antianxiety, etc.) Calcium channel blockers and beta-blockers	**Initial Treatment** Maintain patent airway; assist breathing as needed Oxygen IV Atropine 0.5–1 mg bolus IV while awaiting pacemaker May repeat to a total dose of 3 mg Then, epinephrine (2–10 mg/min) or dopamine (2–10 mg/kg/min) infusion while awaiting pacemaker Transcutaneous pacing
Multifocal Premature Ventricular Contraction (PVCs)	**Ventricular Tachycardia**
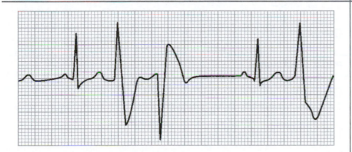	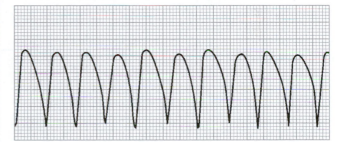
Irregular rhythm P waves: none with premature beat, impulse originates in ventricle Atrial rate: undetermined PR interval: none with premature beat QRS width: greater than 0.12 second for premature beat Ventricular rate: varies *Note:* Each PVC has different configuration as foci are from different areas of heart. PVCs may be the result of imbalance between oxygen demand versus supply, thereby making the myocardium irritable.	Regular rhythm Atrial rate: cannot differentiate PR interval: none QRS width: greater than 0.12 second Ventricular rate: 130–250 bpm *Note:* Ventricular tachycardia is a result of myocardial irritability and is life threatening.

(continued on next page)

SKILL 14.7   Interpreting an ECG Strip (continued)

TABLE 14–4   Selected Cardiac Rhythms and Dysrhythmias (*Continued*)

Etiology Heart disease (myocardial infarction [MI]) Hypoxia Acidosis Electrolyte imbalances Myocardial ischemia Drug toxicity (especially digitalis)	**Etiology** Acute MI Coronary artery disease, cardiomyopathy Electrolyte imbalance Drug intoxication (digitalis)
Initial Treatment • Oxygen • Potassium or magnesium if electrolytes dictate • Lidocaine bolus—1–1.5 mg/kg; may repeat doses of 0.5–0.75 mg/kg every 5–10 minutes up to 3 mg/kg • Refractory to lidocaine: amiodarone or procainamide • Continuous IV drip may be started • Correct underlying cause	**Initial Treatment** Lidocaine 1.5 mg/kg bolus; may repeat in 3–5 minutes to maximum dose of 3 mg/kg Amiodarone 300 mg IV/IO can be followed by 150 mg IV/IO Cardioversion if cardiac output is compromised Pulseless ventricular tachycardia—follow treatment for ventricular fibrillation (epinephrine)

Atrial Fibrillation	Atrial Flutter
Irregularly irregular rhythm Disorganized atrial activity: greater than 350 bpm P waves: none identifiable PR interval: not measured QRS: variable QRS complex: irregular	Regular or irregular rhythm (depending on block) Atrial rate: >250 bpm P wave: usually sawtooth pattern; PR interval cannot be calculated PR interval: regular Ventricular rate can be irregular QRS complex: 0.6–0.10 second
Etiology Heart failure Rheumatoid heart disease Coronary heart disease Hypertension Hyperthyroidism	**Etiology** Sympathetic nervous system stimulation (i.e., anxiety), caffeine, and alcohol intake Thyrotoxins Coronary heart disease, MI, pulmonary embolism
Initial Treatment Cardioversion Diltiazem Beta-blocker: carvedilol (Coreg) or metoprolol (Toprol XL) Digoxin Quinidine Procainamide Amiodarone or dronedarone ibutilide Anticoagulant to reduce risk of clot formation and stroke, if atrial fibrillation duration new in onset but older than 48 hours.	**Initial Treatment** Cardioversion—if symptomatic Diltiazem Calcium channel blocker (Cardizem) or beta-blocking agents to slow ventricular response Followed by ibutilide, quinidine, procainamide

Ventricular Fibrillation	Third-Degree Heart Block

SKILL 14.7   Interpreting an ECG Strip (continued)

SKILL 14.7   **Interpreting an ECG Strip** (continued)

Ventricular Fibrillation (*Continued*)	Third-Degree Heart Block (*Continued*)
Irregular, totally chaotic rhythm Atrial rate: cannot differentiate PR interval: none QRS width: fibrillating waves only Ventricular rate: cannot differentiate *Note:* Ineffective quivering of ventricles with no audible heartbeat, pulse, or respiration.	Regular atrial and ventricular rhythm Atrial rate: greater than ventricular rate PR interval: varies QRS width: less than 0.12 second if pacemaker cell in junction; greater than 0.12 second if cell in ventricle Ventricular rate: 40–60 bpm if pacemaker is from bundle of His; <40 bpm if from Purkinje fibers in ventricle *Note:* Electrical impulse originates in SA node but is blocked in either the AV node, the bundle of His, or the Purkinje fibers. There is no correlation between the atrial rate and the ventricular rate.
Etiology Myocardial ischemia, acute MI Coronary artery disease Cardiomyopathy Acid–base imbalance Severe hypothermia Electrolyte imbalance	**Etiology** Digitalis toxicity Myocardial infarction, inferior or anterior wall Organic heart disease
Initial Treatment Immediately defibrillate, shock CPR—100 chest compressions/minute—no cycles Ventricular fibrillation continues—give a vasopressor (epinephrine 1 mg IV push), repeat 3–5 minutes Defibrillate again and continue CPR Second-line drugs may be used, such as amiodarone (300 mg IV), lidocaine	**Initial Treatment** Atropine bolus Transcutaneous pacing Dopamine or epinephrine Prepare for pacemaker insertion

SKILL 14.8   Recording a 12-Lead ECG

Equipment

- Electrodes
- Skin prep pad or alcohol swab
- ECG machine
- Cable

Preparation

- Review physician's order for ECG and gather ECG machine. Introduce self and perform hand hygiene.
- Identify client by checking the client's identity band and asking client to state name and birth date. Provide for client privacy. Provide comfort and safety for client and self, including raising bed to appropriate height. Reassure client that machine will not cause discomfort or electrocution.
- Assess chest for placement of electrodes.
- Determine if skin site care is necessary. If so, cleanse areas with skin prep pad or alcohol swab, or clip hair if needed. Allow area to dry thoroughly before placing electrodes. **Rationale:** *This will ensure a more secure fit for the electrodes and provide a better ECG tracing.*
- Attach wires to electrodes before pressing onto client's chest. **Rationale:** *This prevents pressure being applied to chest area. This is particularly necessary following open heart surgery or chest trauma.*
- Check the color coding on the manufacturer's directions before placing electrodes to ensure they are correct.

Procedure

1. When placing electrodes, ensure lead wires are all going in the same direction.
2. Place electrodes on fleshy areas, avoiding bone and muscle. **Rationale:** *To ensure good electrical conduction and clear ECG tracings.*
3. Place the four-limb leads, one on each limb, according to the color coding. Three standard leads will be recorded on the 12-lead ECG:
   Lead I: Right arm wrist (negative electrode) white; and left arm (positive electrode) black. Records activity between the two arms.
   Lead II: Right arm (negative electrode) and left leg ankle (positive electrode) red. Records activity between arm and leg.
   Lead III: Left arm (negative electrode) black and left leg (positive electrode) green. Records activity between arm and leg.
4. Three augmented limb lead tracings are obtained on the ECG as follows:
   aVR: Records activity between the center of the heart and right arm.
   aVL: Records activity between the center of the heart and left arm.
   aVF: Records activity between the center of the heart and the left leg or foot.
5. Place the chest leads as follows ❶.
   V_1: Fourth intercostal space, right sternal border. Records activity between the center of the heart and the fourth intercostal space; P wave is shown best here.

(continued on next page)

SKILL 14.8   Recording a 12-Lead ECG (*continued*)

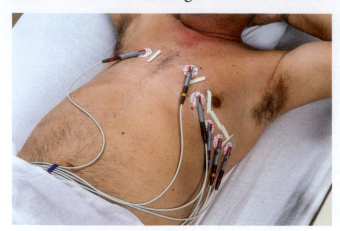

❶ Electrode placement for chest leads V_1 through V_6.

- Palpate the jugular notch above sternum (feels like a depression).
- Move finger down and palpate the manubrium of sternum (feels solid).
- Continue to move finger down to the angle of Louis, which is at the top of the sternal body.
- Move finger to the right of the angle of Louis to the second right rib.
- Below the rib is the second intercostal space.
- Move fingers down, palpating the next two ribs. Below the fourth rib and to the right of the sternal body is the fourth intercostal space. Place electrode in this area.

V_2: Fourth intercostal space, left sternal border.

V_3: Midway between V_2 and V, between fourth and fifth intercostal space.

V_4: Fifth intercostal space, left midclavicular line.

V_5: Fifth intercostal space, anterior axillary line.

V_6: Fifth intercostal space, left midaxillary line.

6. Begin taking the ECG according to manufacturer's directions on machine ❷.
7. Remove electrodes. Reposition bed to lowest height and perform hand hygiene.
8. Place tracing copy in client's chart ❸.

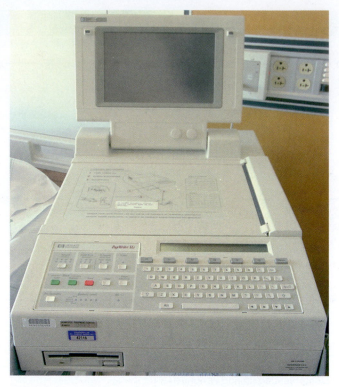

❷ Portable ECG machine for taking 12-lead tracing.

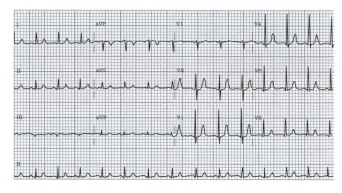

❸ Normal 12-lead ECG.

SKILL 14.9   Monitoring Temporary Cardiac Pacing (Transvenous, Epicardial)

Equipment

- Cardiac monitor
- Transcutaneous: pacing generator, pacing electrodes
- Appropriate temporary pulse generator (select for single- or dual-chamber pacing)
- 9-volt battery for pulse generator (single- or dual-chamber version)
- Bridging cable for epicardial wires
- Clean gloves
- Established continuous cardiac monitoring (see Skill 14.6)

Preparation

- Check physician's order. Validate that informed consent has been obtained for temporary pacing.

- Introduce self and identify client by checking the client's identity band and asking client to state name and birth date. Provide for client privacy. Provide comfort and safety for client. Raise bed to appropriate height for procedure.
- Explain rationale for temporary pacing and necessary restrictions/precautions, and provide reassurance of close continuous monitoring.
- Perform a baseline assessment: vital signs, urinary output, level of consciousness (LOC), heart rate, rhythm, and skin color. If life-threatening dysrhythmia is assessed, assist physician for pacemaker insertion. **Rationale:** *Transcutaneous pacemakers are used for symptomatic bradycardia unresponsive to atropine or high-degree atrioventricular block causing hemodynamic compromise. If transcutaneous pacing is ineffective, then prepare for transvenous pacemaker insertion.*

SKILL 14.9 Monitoring Temporary Cardiac Pacing (Transvenous, Epicardial) *(continued)*

- Assess IV site for patency; if no IV, obtain physician order for one. **Rationale:** *IV access is needed for drug administration.*
- Document client's cardiac rhythm.
- Perform hand hygiene.

Procedure

For Transcutaneous Pacing (TCP)

1. Provide sedation as ordered. **Rationale:** *TCP causes discomfort.*
2. Clip hair, if necessary. Do not shave under electrode placement. Do not use alcohol or tincture of benzoin because they can cause burns to occur. **Rationale:** *Improve conduction between electrode and skin. Shaving may cause nicks in skin, which may increase discomfort with pacing.*
3. Ensure client is on cardiac monitoring with either lead I, II, or III. Lead II is customary as it assesses atrial activity.
4. Provide physician with clean gloves. **Rationale:** *Gloves are worn to prevent microshock to client.*
5. Assist physician performing the following actions as needed.
   - Connect ECG cable to input connection on pacing generator.
   - Turn switch selector to MONITOR ON. ECG waveform will appear.
   - Set alarm, press ALARM ON. Ensure alarm parameters are set 20 beats higher and lower than client's desired rate.
   - Record waveform by pressing START/STOP button.
   - Apply pacing pads as marked, first removing posterior pad covering, then placing posterior (back) pad left of spine between the scapulas. Place anterior "front" pad to left side of lower sternum.
   - Press firmly on and around pacing electrodes. **Rationale:** *This ensures good skin contact.*
   - Attach pacing cable to pace connector on defibrillator/monitor.
   - Select PACER button and green light will appear.
   - Set pacing rate to 60 to 80 bpm.
   - Assess cardiac rhythm on oscilloscope and observe the QRS for sensing marker.
   - Set milliamperes (mA) threshold initially at 0. **Rationale:** *This prevents pacemaker discharge while setting adjustment.*
   - Activate pacing by depressing START/STOP button.
   - Increase mA slowly, increasing it until capture appears.
6. Assess pulse and blood pressure. **Rationale:** *These parameters assess for perfusion.*
7. Return bed to lowest position.
8. Record ECG strip and document pacing parameters, significant events during the procedure, and client's response to the procedure.
9. Monitor for perfusion.
10. Continually assess client's need for sedation. **Rationale:** *Pacing causes discomfort.*

For Epicardial Pacing

1. Provide physician with clean gloves. **Rationale:** *Gloves are worn to prevent microshock to client.*
2. Assist physician performing the following actions as needed:
   - Locate epicardial pacing wires on client's chest wall.

- Securely connect pacing wires to external generator. **Rationale:** *This promotes pacemaker impulse reception from and transmission to the myocardium.*
- Connect cable to pulse generator (positive to positive, negative to negative). **Rationale:** *Pacing stimulus goes from pulse generator to the negative terminal and back to pulse generator by the positive terminal.*
- Remove protective cover to dial settings.
- Select pacing mode (e.g., atrial, ventricular, AV synchronous, or demand).
3. Return bed to lowest position.
4. Record ECG strip and document pacing parameters, significant events during the procedure, and client's response to the procedure.

For Transvenous or Epicardial Pacing

1. Assist physician performing the following actions as needed:
   - Set dial at prescribed pacing rate (atrial and/or ventricular).
   - Set energy output (mA) on pulse generator to prescribed level (set for both atrial and ventricular pacing). **Rationale:** *Energy output setting ensures that pacemaker stimulates the client's myocardium.*
   - Return plastic cover to protect generator dial settings and hang generator from pole at client's bedside.
   - Monitor pacemaker function for sensing (light indicates client's QRS complexes), capture (pacemaker spike is followed by QRS complex), and pacemaker rate.
2. Monitor client's heart rhythm, vital signs, and other responses to pacing, including femoral pulsation palpable with captured beats. **Rationale:** *These demonstrate effectiveness of pacemaker support.*
3. Lower bed to lowest height. Remove and discard gloves. Perform hand hygiene.
4. Evaluate electrode insertion/exit sites and dress according to agency protocol.
5. Record ECG strip and document significant events during the procedure, pacemaker settings, sterile dressing applied, and client's response to the procedure.

CLINICAL ALERT

Transvenous single-chamber (ventricular) pacing is most commonly used as an emergency measure to support ventricular contraction and cardiac output. Epicardial pacing occurs when pacing electrodes are inserted into the epicardium of the right ventricle during cardiac surgery. If the physician wants to initiate atrioventricular sequential pacing, then the surgeon places an additional electrode in the right atrium. The pacing wires are then pierced through the chest wall and may be attached to the external pulse generator, which is placed on standby mode should pacing become necessary. If no pacing is indicated at this time, insert the pacing wires in either a sterile rubber glove or finger cot. Place sterile gauze and occlusive dressing over pacing wires and insertion site to prevent microshock and/or infection. Epicardial pacing electrodes provide either single-chamber atrial pacing, single-chamber ventricular pacing, or dual-chamber pacing, known as A-V sequential pacing, which is used to simulate normal pump function (atrial followed by ventricular stimulation/contraction).

SKILL 14.10 Assisting with Pacemaker Insertion

Equipment

- Emergency cart with defibrillator
- External pacemaker pulse generator ❶ ❷
- Pacing catheter electrodes
- ECG monitor
- Client cable
- Rubber glove
- Sterile antiseptic solution
- Sterile gloves, gown, and mask
- Sterile towels
- Lidocaine, 1%–2%
- Alcohol wipes
- Syringe
- Needles
- Suture with attached needle
- Sterile 4 × 4 gauze pads
- Tape
- Cutdown tray
- Gloves

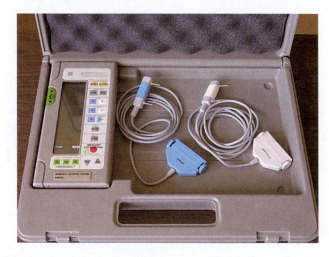

❶ Type of external pacemaker.

Preparation

- Validate that informed consent has been obtained for pacemaker insertion.
- Introduce self, perform hand hygiene, follow infection control measures, and verify client's identity by checking the client's identity band and asking client to state name and birth date.
- Provide for client privacy. Provide comfort and safety for client. Raise bed to appropriate height for procedure.
- Perform a baseline assessment, including vital signs, sensorium, and heart rhythm.
- Provide sedation as ordered. Diazepam (Valium) or Versed is frequently used. Conscious sedation may be used.
- Connect client to a continuous ECG monitor.
- Place the client in a supine position with head flat or slightly lower than body.
- If either the subclavian or external jugular vein is to be used, place a towel roll under the client's shoulders to provide better exposure of the insertion site.

Procedure

1. Assist physician as needed.
   - Physician dons mask, sterile gown, and gloves.
   - Insertion site is cleansed with sterile antiseptic solution.
   - Drape area with sterile towels.
   - Break single-dose vial of lidocaine and hold at angle for physician withdrawal.
   - Physician withdraws lidocaine, using filtered needle, then changes to 25-gauge needle and injects skin.
   - Insertion is accomplished (transvenous method via cutdown or percutaneously). Catheter electrode wires are positioned, and skin sutures are applied.
2. Continuously monitor the ECG and client status during the insertion.
3. Don gloves to prevent microshock to client.
4. Assist in the connection of the pacing electrode to the appropriate outlet terminal (unipolar to negative and bipolar to both the positive and negative terminals).
5. Physician turns on power switch on external pacemaker and sets the rate. The milliamperes (mA) are set by determining

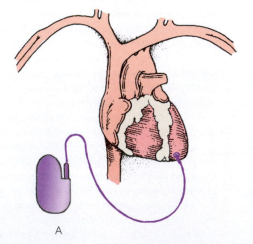
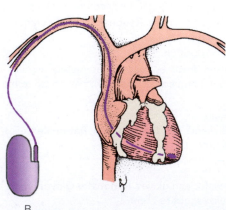

A   B

❷ Temporary pacemakers have two parts, the pulse generator and the electrode. The pulse generator is external to the body. *A,* Epicardial ventricular pacemaker; *B,* transvenous ventricular pacemaker.

SKILL 14.10 Assisting with Pacemaker Insertion *(continued)*

threshold. To do this, the ECG is observed while the physician slowly increases the number of milliamperes from its lowest setting to a point where a QRS complex is captured and preceded by a pacing spike.

6. Physician sets sensitivity mode (usually 1.5 mV).
7. Secure all connections. The plastic cover is put back over pacemaker controls if required.
8. The external pacemaker and exposed wires are placed in a rubber glove to ensure insulation against electric shock to client.

SAFETY ALERT

Electrical

- Use only grounded equipment; use common ground.
- Remove and tag any defective equipment.
- Maintain environmental humidity at 50% to 60%.
- Do not roll equipment over electrical cords.
- Avoid placing wet articles on electrical equipment.
- Insulate exposed pacing electrodes at all times.
- Wear rubber gloves when handling pacing electrodes or terminals.
- Do not touch any electric equipment while handling wire or terminals.
- Discharge static electricity by touching faucets or other metal that communicates with ground.

CLINICAL ALERT

When temporary transvenous pacemakers are used, the balloon air port is not to be used for IV access.

9. Sterile dressings are applied to insertion site and taped securely.
10. Lower bed to lowest height.
11. Record ECG strip and document significant events during the procedure, pacemaker settings, sterile dressing applied, and client's response to the procedure.
12. Chest x-ray is obtained following insertion to validate lead placement if pacemaker not inserted using fluoroscopy.
13. Obtain 12-lead ECG.

Note: A generic code for antibradycardia pacing was developed jointly by the North American Society of Pacing and Electrophysiology and the British Pacing and Electrophysiology Group and can be found at the National Institutes of Health Web site.

SKILL 14.11 Maintaining Temporary Pacemaker Function

Equipment

- Battery
- Oscilloscope

Procedure

1. Check physician's order and gather equipment and supplies. Introduce self, explain to the client what procedure is to be done and why. Perform hand hygiene, follow infection control measures, and verify client's identity by checking the client's identity band and asking client to state name and birth date. Provide for client privacy. Provided comfort and safety for client and self, including raising bed to appropriate height for procedure.
2. Observe for failure to sense.
   - Observe the oscilloscope for presence of pacemaker artifact (spikes); artifact before QRS complex in ventricular paced or preceding the P waves and QRS waves in AV sequential pacing ❶.
   - Check connections for secure, tight fit.
   - Observe that pace–sense needle deflects to right, indicating pacing is occurring.
   - Check sensitivity dial to determine if sensitivity threshold is set correctly.
3. Observe for failure to pace.
   - Check that external generator is ON.
   - Check battery to ensure it is functioning.

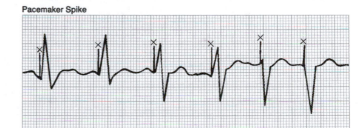

Pacemaker Spike

❶ ECG tracing showing pacemaker spike triggering ventricular depolarization (QRS).

   - Check lead connector sites.
   - Check pace–sense indicator. (Absence of or slight deflection of the pace–sense indicator reveals battery failure.)
4. Observe for failure to capture.
   - Observe for pacing artifact not followed by QRS complex ❷. **Rationale:** *This indicates a failure of the stimulus to trigger a ventricular response.*
   - Check the setting of the mA, or output dial, to determine if setting should be increased. **Rationale:** *The myocardial threshold may be altered as a result of disease or drugs.*
   - Check all connector sites for secure, tight fit.
5. Observe that sutures are intact.
6. Assess insertion site for bleeding, hematoma formation, or infection.

(continued on next page)

SKILL 14.11 Maintaining Temporary Pacemaker Function (*continued*)

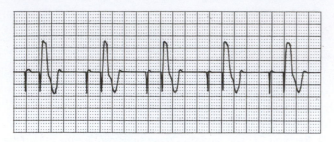

❷ ECG tracing showing pacing spikes not followed by QRS complex.

7. Obtain chest x-ray postinsertion.
8. Monitor client's response to therapy.
   - Assess urine output. **Rationale:** *Decreased urine output indicates poor cardiac output.*
   - Observe for dyspnea, crackles, heart rate, decreased blood pressure.
   - Monitor temperature.
   - Observe client for signs of anxiety. Complete pacemaker teaching as necessary.

9. Obtain and analyze a strip for functioning of pacemaker.
10. Observe for battery failure.
11. Observe for electrical interference and development of microshocks.
    - Ground all electrical equipment in proximity to client.
    - Cover exposed wires with nonconductive material.
    - Wear gloves when handling generator/lead wires.
12. Complete pacemaker teaching as necessary.
13. Document procedure, teaching, and client response.

> **CLINICAL ALERT**
> Observe for the following signs of pacemaker failure:
> - Decreased urine output
> - ECG pattern change
> - Decreased blood pressure
> - Bradycardia
> - Shortness of breath.

SKILL 14.12 Providing Permanent Pacemaker Client Teaching

Equipment

- Audiovisual aids
- Written material

Procedure

1. Ascertain what client already knows and understands.
2. Determine client's ability and level of interest in learning about pacemaker.
3. Recognize client's fears, and provide opportunity to talk about them.
4. Review facts: heart anatomy and physiology and pacemaker information. Use illustrations and audiovisual aids.
5. Clarify misconceptions and allay fears.
6. Provide rationale for any mobility restrictions.
7. Answer questions, and provide additional opportunities to discuss procedure.
8. Check pacemaker function regularly per instructions. With new pacemakers, physicians check them on routine visits.
9. Instruct client in clinical manifestations related to pacemaker failure and when to contact physician or pacemaker clinic.
10. Provide client with pacemaker information ID card (provided by manufacturer) and instruct to carry in wallet.
11. Suggest a medical alert band be worn at all times.
    Note: Inform client of electromagnetic interference restrictions:
    - No MRI; do not place cell phone or cardiovert over generator.
    - Avoid airport hand wand, high-voltage areas, and diathermy.
    - If dizziness experienced, move away from area.
12. Document client teaching and response to it.

Pacemaker Clinics

Many clients use telephone transmission of the generator's pulse rate to determine status of pacemaker function. Special equipment is used to transmit information concerning function of the pacemaker over the telephone to a receiving system in a pacemaker clinic. The equipment converts information to electronic signals that are permanently recorded on an ECG strip. Physicians monitor client's records and can intervene quickly when abnormalities appear on an ECG strip. This type of clinic is very common in outlying areas where clients are unable to go to a clinic easily.

SKILL 14.13 Administering Automated External Defibrillation (AED) to an Adult Client

Delegation

Any person who has been trained in its use can apply and activate the AED.

Equipment

- AED with all components including the automatic override key, event documentation module or tape, electrodes and cables,

SKILL 14.13 Administering Automated External Defibrillation (AED) (*continued*)

and charged battery pack. Brands and models differ in their features.

Procedure

1. Follow steps for CPR. Traditional CPR must be performed until the AED can be attached.
2. Attach the AED.
   - Turn on the power of the AED (usually a green ON/OFF button).
   - Apply the electrode pads to dry skin: one in the upper right chest near the clavicle, and the other in the lower left chest below the nipple.
   - If the person has heavy chest hair, it may be necessary to quickly shave the hair. **Rationale:** *Heavy chest hair may prevent the pads from sticking to the chest and may also catch fire during defibrillation.*
   - Attach the cables to the box if necessary.
3. Initiate rhythm analysis. Be sure no one is touching the person. **Rationale:** *This ensures that the AED is reading only the*

person's cardiac electrical activity. The analysis may take 5 to 15 seconds. In most models, this also charges the AED.
4. Defibrillate as indicated.
   - Before delivering the shock, state loudly "Clear" and check visually to ensure that no one is touching the person or anything that is touching the person (e.g., the bed). **Rationale:** *If a shock is delivered while someone is in contact with the person, that person will also receive the shock.*
   - Press the shock button and observe for the brief contraction of the person's muscles that indicates the shock has been delivered.
5. Resume CPR. The AED will automatically prompt to reanalyze the person in 2 to 3 minutes. Continue the sequence of CPR and defibrillation until the AED specifies that no shock is indicated, the person converts to a functional rhythm (pulse is felt or movement observed), or the code team takes over.
6. Document the events above including data provided by the AED. Attach electrocardiogram strips or other records made by the AED.

Developmental Considerations

Automated External Defibrillation

INFANTS

- Use child-sized pads if available.
- A manual defibrillator is preferred. If a manual defibrillator is not available, an AED with pediatric dose attenuation is desirable. If neither is available, an AED without a dose attenuator may be used.

CHILDREN

- Use child-sized pads if available.
- Select a child shock dose (pediatric dose attenuator) on the AED if available. This may require turning a key or switch. If a child dose is not available, an AED without a dose attenuator may be used.

▶ ARTERIAL LINE CARE

Expected Outcomes

1. Peripheral perfusion distal to arterial catheter placement site remains adequate.
2. Arterial cannulation is accomplished without complication.
3. Arterial blood pressure monitoring system functions reliably and accurately.
4. Arterial blood samples are obtained.

SKILL 14.14 Performing the Allen Test

Procedure

1. Introduce self, explain what procedure is to be done and why. Perform hand hygiene and verify client's identity. Provide comfort and safety for client.
2. Perform the modified Allen Test to determine distal peripheral perfusion. **Rationale:** *This procedure assesses blood supply to client's hand to determine that the radial and ulnar arteries are functioning before an arterial line is inserted.*
   - Compress both arteries at client's wrist for about 1 minute.
   - Instruct client to clench and unclench fist several times. **Rationale:** *This causes blanching in the hand and palm.*

   - With client's hand in open, relaxed position, release pressure on ulnar artery.
   - Observe how quickly (7 seconds) the palm color flushes. **Rationale:** *If color returns quickly, good collateral blood supply to the hand exists. If normal color does not return, there is insufficient collateral circulation to the hand should radial artery occlusion occur.*
3. Repeat procedure with release of the radial artery.
4. Report to physician if collateral blood flow is insufficient. **Rationale:** *A Doppler flow study may be used to help determine collateral blood flow.*
5. Document care and assessments.

SKILL 14.15 Assisting with Arterial Line Insertion

Equipment

- 20-gauge Teflon catheter with introducer and flexible guidewire
- 500 mL of normal saline for flush
- Heparin, 1,000 units/mL
- One-mL unit-dose syringe
- Pressure bag for flush infusion
- IV tubing
- Short wide-bore, high-pressure tubing
- Three-way stopcocks with nonvented caps
- Established pressure monitor system
- Clean gloves, sterile gloves
- Personal protective equipment (PPE)
- Sterile towels and drape
- Skin prep solution (2% chlorhexidine)
- Sterile 4 × 4 gauze sponges
- Lidocaine 1% (without epinephrine)
- 3-mL syringe with 18- and 25-gauge needles for topical anesthetic
- Alcohol wipes
- Silk suture, size 000 (if used)
- Sterile transparent dressing
- Atropine for reversal of bradycardia

Preparation

- Validate that informed consent has been obtained.
- Determine whether client has received anticoagulant therapy. **Rationale:** *Coagulation studies may be indicated.*
- Identify client by checking the client's identity band and asking client to state name and birth date.
- Explain rationale for procedure.
- Check physician's orders and gather equipment and supplies.
- Introduce self and perform hand hygiene. Provide for client privacy. Provide comfort and safety for client. Raise bed to appropriate height.
- Add heparin to normal saline solution and label bag with additive and date (commonly 2 units of heparin/mL fluid). Follow hospital protocols.
- Connect IV tubing to solution bag.
- Remove all air from flush solution bag.
- Insert flush infusion bag into pressure bag and hang bag on IV pole.

CLINICAL ALERT

Arterial catheter alarms should always be enabled to detect disconnection, alterations in blood pressure, or pulseless electrical activity.

- Prepare and assemble pressurized monitoring system (transducer, continuous flush device, and stopcocks) following manufacturer's instructions.
- Level stopcock above transducer to client's phlebostatic axis (see Skill 14.16).
- Inflate pressure bag to 300 mm Hg using hand pump on bag.

Procedure

1. Don gloves and PPE and prepare to assist the physician as needed.
   - Skin is prepped briskly with 2% chlorhexidine for 3 seconds.
   - Lidocaine vial is cleansed with alcohol wipe.
   - Physician dons sterile gloves.
   - Sterile drape is placed over arterial insertion site.
   - Physician aspirates lidocaine with 18-gauge needle, changes needle, and injects client's skin with 25-gauge needle. **Rationale:** *For local anesthesia.*
   - Percutaneous insertion is made at arterial insertion site, and arterial catheter is inserted.
   - Physician advances catheter in artery.
   - Arterial catheter is sutured in place with 000 silk suture secured with transparent dressing.
2. Assist physician performing the following actions as needed:
   - Observe for pulsating bright-red blood spurting retrograde into catheter. **Rationale:** *This evidence ensures arterial catheter position.*
   - Attach catheter to primed pressure-monitoring system tubing. Make sure all connections are secure.
   - Press fast flush valve to clear system.
   - Observe oscilloscope for arterial waveform.
   - Apply sterile transparent dressing (with date and initials) to site after catheter is sutured into place.
3. Remove and discard gloves. Perform hand hygiene.
4. Set monitor alarms for both HIGH and LOW parameters.
5. Document arterial monitor strip, significant events during the procedure, arterial monitor settings, sterile dressing applied, and client's response to the procedure.

CLINICAL ALERT

Mean Arterial Blood Pressure

In general, the mean arterial pressure (MAP) provides a more accurate interpretation of a client's hemodynamic status than a single blood pressure reading. The MAP is the averaging of blood pressure readings over a single cardiac cycle. The MAP reflects perfusion pressure and is notated on a monitor screen in parentheses by the blood pressure reading; 154/86 (108).

SKILL 14.16 Monitoring Arterial Blood Pressure

Equipment

- Disposable pressure transducer, dome, and amplifier
- Flush valve with flush system
- Display monitor (oscilloscope)
- Sterile stopcock cap
- Sterile transparent dressing
- Gloves
- Carpenter's level
- Marker

SKILL 14.16   Monitoring Arterial Blood Pressure (continued)

Procedure

1. Check physician's order and gather equipment and supplies. Introduce self, explain what procedure is to be done and why. Perform hand hygiene, follow infection control measures, and verify client's identity by checking the client's identity band and asking client to state name and birth date. Provide for client privacy. Provide comfort and safety for client and self, including raising bed to appropriate height for procedure.

2. Level and calibrate (zero out) the system.
   - Calibrate system at beginning of each shift. **Rationale:** *Monitor readings are altered by changes in atmospheric pressure.*
   - Position client with head of bed flat or at up to a 45-degree elevation.
   - Using a carpenter's level, align stopcock above transducer level with client's left atrium (phlebostatic axis) and mark client's chest for future readings. **Rationale:** *Readings will be inaccurately high or low if stopcock above transducer is not level with client's phlebostatic axis.*
   - To zero ("calibrate") the system, turn stopcock near transducer off to client. Remove cap from stopcock, opening it to air.
   - Depress ZERO button on monitor, release button, and note monitor reading is zero. **Rationale:** *Zero reading indicates monitor is calibrated to atmospheric pressure.*
   - Replace cap or place new sterile cap on stopcock.
   - Turn stopcock so transducer is open to client.

3. Observe waveform at eye level for the sharp systolic upstroke, peak, dicrotic notch, and end diastole ❶ ❷.

4. Fast flush the continuous flush system and quickly release. A sharp upstroke followed by a horizontal line, then a brisk downstroke descending below, then returning to baseline indicates that the system requires no adjustment ❸.

5. Ensure pressure bag is maintained at 300 mmHg.

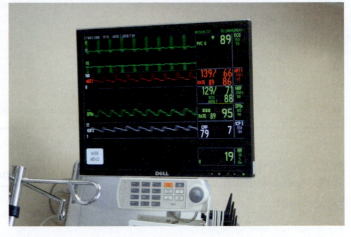

❷ Arterial line allows direct measurement of blood pressure—monitor displays digital and waveform.

Square wave test configuration

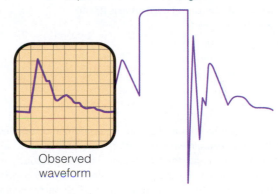

Observed
waveform

❸ Fast flush the continuous flush system and quickly release. A sharp upstroke, followed by a horizontal line, then a brisk downstroke descending below and then returning to baseline indicates the system requires no adjustment (squarewave test).

6. Leave cannulated extremity uncovered for easy observation. Assess site for signs of infection every shift.

7. Assess circulation, motion, and sensation of extremity distal to cannulation site every 2 hours initially, then every 8 hours.

8. Immobilize extremity if necessary.

9. Change flush solution and tubing every 96 hours (according to agency policy).

10. Change dressing weekly or if it becomes wet, loose, or soiled. **Rationale:** *Loose or soiled dressings increase risk of infection at site.*
    - Put on gloves.
    - Remove dressing and discard in biohazard container.
    - Apply transparent dressing, date, and initials.

11. Remove gloves and PPE and perform hand hygiene.

12. Document arterial monitor strip, arterial monitor settings, assessment data, and client's response to the procedure.

13. Monitor site to ensure hemostasis occurs.

14. Monitor extremity distally for adequacy of perfusion.

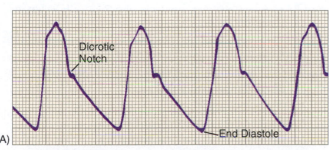

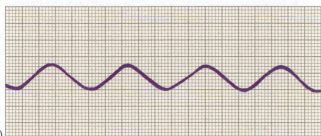

(A) Dicrotic Notch — End Diastole

(B)

❶ A, Arterial line—normal waveform; B, arterial line—flattened waveform. Flattened arterial waveform indicates damping. Damping results from obstruction in arterial line or imbalance of transducer.

(continued on next page)

SKILL 14.16   Monitoring Arterial Blood Pressure (*continued*)

Evidence-Based Practice

Monitoring Arterial Blood Pressure

The use of an indirect brachial blood pressure measurement to determine whether an arterial pressure monitoring system is accurate is not evidence based. It is more important to determine that technical aspects of the method are optimized and the blood pressure is adequate. In addition to obtaining an absolute measure, monitoring for trends or changes in blood pressure over time is equally important for guiding clinical decisions.

Source: Rauen et al. (2008).

SKILL 14.17   Withdrawing Arterial Blood Samples

Equipment

- One 6-mL sterile syringe
- ABG kit with one 3-mL syringe with dry lithium heparin and an air filter device *or* Vacutainer with Luer-Lok adapter cannula and blood specimen tubes
- Gloves
- Face shield
- Container with ice (paper cup, emesis basin)
- Two specimen labels
- Bubble packaging
- Biohazard specimen bag
- Gauze sponges/pads

Preparation

- Check physician's order and gather equipment and supplies. Introduce self, explain what procedure is to be done and why. Perform hand hygiene, follow infection control measures, and verify client's identity by checking the client's identity band and asking client to state name and birth date. Provide for client privacy. Provide comfort and safety for client and self, including raising bed to appropriate height for procedure.
- Attach label to specimen syringe with client's name, hospital number, room number, time, and date. Also add client's current temperature and FIO_2.
- For arterial blood gas (ABG) specimen, maintain client's current oxygen delivery setting for 20 minutes before obtaining specimen.
- Fill paper cup or emesis basin with ice.

Procedure

1. Momentarily disengage arterial alarms.
2. Turn stopcock off to client.
3. Remove protective cap from open blood sampling port on three-way stopcock closest to arterial line insertion site.
4. Attach syringe or Vacutainer with Luer-Lok adapter cannula to open port of three-way stopcock.
5. Turn stopcock off to flush solution.
6. Attach syringe or blood specimen tube into Vacutainer to establish blood draw ❶.
7. Discard obtained sample. **Rationale:** *This discard ensures that the specimen will be free of heparin or flush solution.*

Note: For an ABG sample, discard volume should be twice the dead space volume of the catheter and tubing up to the sampling site. For coagulation studies, discard volume should be six times the dead space volume.

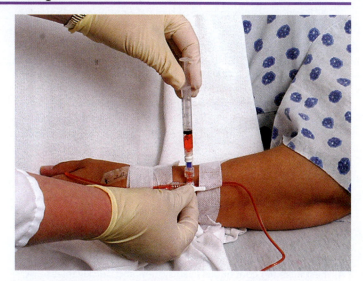

❶ Engage syringe or Vacutainer to sample port to obtain arterial blood.

8. Engage ABG specimen tube in Vacutainer.
9. Obtain ABG specimen. See **Table 14–5** ● for ABG values in acid–base imbalances.
10. Turn stopcock off to open port. **Rationale:** *This reestablishes flow between flush solution and client.*
11. Remove Vacutainers for blood conservatory process.

    For Blood Conservatory Process
    - Don clean gloves.
    - Aspirate blood into reservoir tubing.
    - Close stopcock to reservoir tubing.
    - Access sampling port (closest to client) using blunt cannula with tube holder (Vacutainer).
    - Engage blood collection tubes in tube holder and allow to fill. **Rationale:** *Obtaining specimens using a blood conservatory system helps to prevent nosocomial anemia.*
    - When sampling is complete, remove blunt cannula and tube holder.
    - Open stopcock to reservoir tubing and return contents to client ❷.
12. Place ABG specimen tubes in container filled with ice.
13. Fast flush remaining blood onto gauze pad.
14. Reattach protective cap on open port.
15. Validate good arterial waveform on monitor.
16. Reactivate monitor alarms.

SKILL 14.17 Withdrawing Arterial Blood Samples *(continued)*

TABLE 14–5 Arterial Blood Gas Values in Acid–Base Imbalances

Normal ABG Values		
pH	7.35–7.45	
PCO_2	35–45 mmHg	
HCO_3^-	22–26 mEq	
Respiratory Acidosis		**Compensation**
pH: decreased	<7.35	7.35
PCO_2: increased	>45 mmHg	
HCO_3^-: normal	24	>26 mEq
Respiratory Alkalosis		**Compensation**
pH: increased	>7.45	7.45
PCO_2: decreased	<35 mmHg	
HCO_3^-: normal	24	<22 mEq
Metabolic Acidosis		**Compensation**
pH: decreased	<7.35	7.35
PCO_2: normal	40	<35 mmHg
HCO_3^-: decreased	<22 mEq	
Metabolic Alkalosis		**Compensation**
pH: increased	>7.45	7.45
PCO_2: normal	40	>45 mmHg
HCO_3^-: increased	>26 mEq	

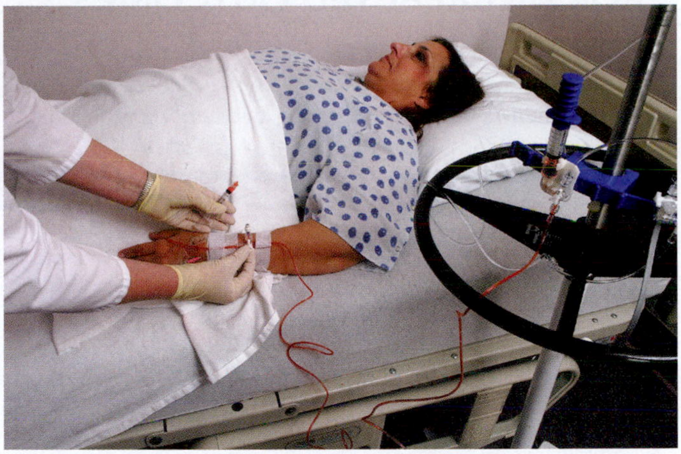

❷ When sampling is complete, open stopcock to reservoir tubing and return contents of blood conservatory system to client.

17. Wrap syringe/specimen in bubble packaging and place in biohazard bag with ice.
18. Remove and discard gloves. Perform hand hygiene.
19. Send specimens to laboratory immediately and notify lab that tubes are being sent.
20. Document output of blood.

SKILL 14.18 Removing an Arterial Catheter

Equipment

- Gloves
- Personal protective equipment (PPE)
- Two 4 ×4 gauze pads
- Suture removal set
- Tape

Preparation

- Check physician's orders.
- Check client's coagulation lab results (values).
- Gather equipment.
- Perform hand hygiene
- Identify client by checking the client's identity band and asking client to state name and birth date, and explain procedure to client.
- Provide for client privacy. Provide comfort and safety for client and self, including raising bed to appropriate height for procedure.
- Disarm monitor alarms.

Procedure

1. Don gloves and PPE.
2. Remove dressing, and discard in appropriate container.
3. Clip retaining sutures if present.
4. Apply finger pressure approximately 2 cm above skin puncture site. **Rationale:** *The artery puncture site is proximal to the skin puncture site.*
5. Place folded 4 × 4 gauze pad over cannula site with nondominant hand, and apply gentle pressure.
6. Pull arterial cannula straight out of artery with quick, even pressure.
7. Apply firm pressure over and just above cannula site for at least 5 to 10 minutes. **Rationale:** *This action achieves hemostasis and prevents formation of a hematoma.*

CLINICAL ALERT

Apply pressure to puncture site for at least 10 minutes if client is on anticoagulation or antithrombotic therapy.

8. Place folded 4 × 4 gauze pad over puncture site, and tape tightly. **Rationale:** *This provides additional pressure to site to prevent bleeding.*
9. Lower bed to lowest height. Discard supplies, remove and discard gloves and PPE, and perform hand hygiene.
10. Check cannulation site frequently. **Rationale:** *To observe for bleeding or thrombosis.*
11. Check distal extremity for temperature, circulation, motion, and sensation intermittently for several hours, then routinely after catheter removal. **Rationale:** *Delayed complications (thrombosis) may occur.*
12. Document care and assessment.

► CRITICAL THINKING OPTIONS FOR UNEXPECTED OUTCOMES

Not all unexpected outcomes require further nursing intervention; however, many times they do. When the client demonstrates a change in signs/symptoms indicating an emerging problem, the nurse should immediately assess and troubleshoot what is happening. The assessment data must be processed quickly to formulate a hypothesis so the nurse can make a clinical judgment. The nurse then decides how best to resolve the problem and improve the client's situation for a better appropriate outcome.

EXPECTED OUTCOMES	PROBLEM SOLVING	NURSING ACTIONS
Pressure dressing is applied, and bleeding is controlled.	Even with direct pressure and application of pressure dressing, bleeding continues.	■ Reinforce pressure dressing. ■ Maintain IV infusion. ■ Notify physician, and be prepared to send client to surgery for wound closure. ■ Monitor closely for signs of shock (LOC, vital signs, oliguria or anuria, tachycardia, narrow pulse pressure, hypotension). ■ Apply pressure directly or proximal to wound. ■ Place tourniquets proximal to site of hemorrhage to control bleeding if all other actions are unsuccessful.
Antiembolic Devices Compression stockings remain wrinkle free and pressure is evenly distributed.	Graduated compression stockings are loose and do not provide support.	■ Remeasure legs and compare to chart to determine correct size. ■ Hosiery may be old with no elasticity and should be discarded; ensure line drying rather than with electric dryer. ■ Need to order different knit design and elastomeric yarn denier that will increase pressure.
Peripheral pulses are present during use of sequential stockings and elastic hosiery.	While compression device is being used, client complains of numbness or tingling in leg.	■ Remove devices immediately. ■ Suggest use of foot pulse device as alternate. ■ Complete neurovascular assessment. ■ Notify physician of assessment findings.
Electrical Conduction in the Heart Monitor waveforms are distinct and readable.	ECG is not clearly displayed on monitor.	■ Ensure that electrodes are applied in correct position and are securely attached. ■ Observe for electrical interference resulting in a 60-cycle interference on oscilloscope. ■ Observe for excessive client activity resulting in artifact display on oscilloscope.
	Electrical interference appears on monitor.	■ Check all other electric equipment in the immediate environment. ■ Check for proper grounding of monitor. ■ Change electrodes and cable; poor conduction may cause 60-cycle interference. ■ Check that monitor is calibrated.
	Telemetry signal not picked up at base station.	■ Check that client hasn't wandered to an area where transmission is not available. ■ Check that transmitter battery is functioning. ■ Check that transmitter is ON. ■ Change wires. ■ Usual cause is a dry electrode. Replace electrodes.
ECG leads applied appropriately and without difficulty.	Electrodes do not adhere to skin, and interference appears on oscilloscope.	■ Change placement of electrodes to another area. Clip hair if needed to improve skin contact. ■ Recleanse skin thoroughly using skin prep or alcohol and allow to dry.
Abnormal ECG findings interpreted accurately.	ECG pattern is abnormal.	■ If client is asymptomatic, recheck lead placement and ensure cables are attached properly. ■ Check if pattern is a life-threatening arrhythmia (for ventricular tachycardia, call rapid response team; for ventricular fibrillation, call code). ■ Increasing PVCs—notify rapid response team. ■ Notify physician immediately.
	Asystole displays on monitor.	■ Check client's LOC and electrodes, wires, and cable connection. ■ If the client has an arterial line, check for an arterial waveform in the absence of an ECG waveform.
Client's cardiac rate is maintained through use of a pacemaker.	Temporary pacing is ineffective.	■ Check for battery depletion and change if necessary (9-V batteries). ■ Record rhythm strip and correlate to client's signs and symptoms. ■ Monitor vital signs, mental status. ■ Check sensitivity setting. (If too high, P or T wave may be sensed; if too low, fixed-rate pacing occurs.) ■ Check milliampere setting (may be too high). ■ Check pace indicator for movement. ■ Check rate setting. ■ Check all connections. ■ Check catheter insertion site for swelling, hematoma.

EXPECTED OUTCOMES	PROBLEM SOLVING	NURSING ACTIONS
Client is prepared psychologically and physically for insertion of the pacemaker.	Client does not understand function of pacemaker.	■ If client is frightened, reassure him or her that a pacemaker is not dangerous. ■ If client does not understand pacemaker or procedure, use illustrated learning aids. ■ Allow time for questions and further explanations. ■ Orient your teaching to the client's intellectual and interest level.
Pacemaker is inserted without complications.	Inflammation occurs at insertion site.	■ Provide daily care using strict aseptic technique. ■ Keep dressing dry at all times. ■ Monitor vital signs. ■ Instruct client to limit extremity movement.
Client's cardiac rate is maintained through use of a pacemaker	Failure to capture is suspected.	■ Check client's heart rate. If heart rate less than the rate set on generator, and if pace indicator shows firing, suspect failure to capture. ■ Check all connections. ■ Anticipate that pacer wires are dislodged. ■ Check battery. ■ Change position of extremity. ■ Turn client on left side; catheter may float back to epicardial wall. ■ Increase amperage (mA) after checking threshold. ■ Obtain chest x-ray and 12-lead ECG. ■ Anticipate change of batteries, electrode terminals, or generator.
	Battery depletion occurs.	■ Have atropine and isoproterenol available. ■ Anticipate possible CPR. ■ Turn on power switch, and observe pace indicator. If there is little or no movement, replace battery immediately. ■ Record clock hours of battery usage. (Record should be taped to back of generator.) ■ Determine rate fluctuations. ■ Label each pacemaker with the date battery is inserted. ■ Store extra batteries in refrigerator and put new battery in pacemaker before use. ■ Disconnect catheter from pacemaker before replacing battery. ■ Contact with battery terminal may be dangerous to the client.
Peripheral perfusion distal to arterial catheter placement site remains adequate.	Cannulated extremity develops diminished distal perfusion.	■ Check periphery for changes in color, temperature, motion, and sensation resulting from possible thrombus occlusion or circulatory "steal." ■ Notify physician immediately. ■ Prepare for catheter removal.
Arterial Line Care Arterial cannulation is accomplished without complication.	Hematoma or bleeding occurs at arterial insertion site.	■ Apply direct pressure over artery while you check for leaks in the system. ■ Check all stopcocks: check if catheter is inserted in artery as it should be. ■ Keep cannulated extremity exposed for observation. ■ Remove catheter if oozing continues.
	Signs of infection or inflammation appear at insertion site.	■ Use sterile transparent dressings exclusively. ■ Always use aseptic technique with dressing changes; change dressing weekly. ■ Cap open port on stopcock to maintain asepsis. ■ Do not apply ointment to insertion site. ■ Change tubing, flush solution, and transducer every 96 hr or with catheter change using sterile technique. ■ Flush open port after obtaining blood specimens. ■ Prepare for catheter removal if infection suspected.
Arterial blood pressure monitoring system functions reliably and accurately.	Arterial waveform loses definition and digital pressures drop.	■ Reverse response with atropine administration. ■ Use low-compliance (rigid), short (<90–120 cm [<3–4 ft]) monitor tubing. ■ Check for thrombus formation by aspirating blood through stopcock and then flushing system. ■ Be sure to fast-flush arterial line thoroughly after arterial blood samples are obtained or system is zeroed. ■ Make sure all stopcocks are closed to air. ■ Maintain 300 mmHg of pressure in pressure bag. ■ Ensure secure fit of all stopcocks and connections. Avoid adding stopcocks and line extensions. ■ Change position of extremity in which catheter is placed.

(continued on next page)

EXPECTED OUTCOMES	PROBLEM SOLVING	NURSING ACTIONS
Arterial blood pressure monitoring system functions reliably and accurately.	Direct blood pressure readings vary significantly.	■ Flick tubing system to remove tiny air bubbles escaping the flush solution. ■ Recheck transducer and client position to ensure accurate data. ■ Recalibrate transducer. ■ Flush system after sampling and zeroing. ■ Keep flush bag adequately filled and cleared of air. ■ Maintain bag external pressure at 300 mmHg. ■ Check that connections are tightly secured.
	Client has decreased urinary output or develops signs of radial artery occlusion.	■ Suspect balloon migration. ■ Maintain head-of-bed elevation at less than 45 degrees to prevent kinking and migration of catheter. ■ Immobilize cannulated extremity to prevent catheter migration.
Arterial blood samples are obtained.	Arterial blood sample is unobtainable.	■ Suspect arterial spasm; allow spasm of artery to stop, then attempt to aspirate blood with gentle pressure using a 6-mL syringe rather than Vacutainer. ■ Reposition client's arm, making sure there is no pressure at catheter insertion site. ■ Check that catheter is in artery (note waveform on oscilloscope), flush catheter, then attempt to obtain sample.

15 Perioperative Care

RELATED CONCEPTS

The Concept of Perioperative Care

Skills-at-a-Glance

The three phases of perioperative care (preoperative, intraoperative, and postoperative) have distinct nursing activities to support best client outcomes when a surgical procedure is done. These phases of care may take place in a variety of settings: a physicians' office, a clinic, a day-surgery unit, an emergency department, or a hospital surgery department. Nursing actions not only provide support to the client and family, but also focus on safety throughout the time before, during, and after the client's surgical experience.

Expected Outcomes

1. Client's physical or emotional deviations from normal are identified preoperatively.
2. Preoperative baseline data are obtained.
3. Surgical site is marked and prepared correctly.
4. Client states expectations regarding intraoperative and post-operative course.

SKILL 15.1   Conducting Preoperative Teaching

Delegation

Assessment of the learning needs of the client and his or her support people and determining the teaching content and appropriate strategies for teaching require application of professional knowledge and critical thinking. Preoperative teaching is conducted by the nurse and is not delegated to unlicensed assistive personnel (UAP). The UAP, however, can reinforce teaching, assist the client with the exercises, and report to the nurse if the client is unable to perform the exercises.

Equipment

- Pillow
- Teaching materials (e.g., videotape, written materials) if available at the agency

Preparation

- Ensure that potential distracters (e.g., pain, TV, visitors) to teaching are not present. Family and significant others should be included in the teaching plan, if appropriate.

Procedure

1. Prior to performing the procedure, introduce self and verify the client's identity using agency protocol. Explain to the client what you are going to teach and the importance of the client's participation in the exercises he or she is going to be taught.
2. Perform hand hygiene and observe other appropriate infection control procedures.
3. Provide for client privacy.
4. Show the client ways to turn in bed and to get out of bed.
   - Instruct a client who will have a right abdominal incision or a right-sided chest incision to turn to the left side of the bed and sit up as follows:
     a. Flex the knees.
     b. Splint the wound by holding the left arm and hand or a small pillow against the incision.
     c. Turn to the left while pushing with the right foot and grasping a partial side rail on the left side of the bed with the right hand.
     d. Come to a sitting position on the side of the bed by using the right arm and hand to push down against the mattress and swinging the feet over the edge of the bed.
   - Teach a client with a left abdominal or left-sided chest incision to perform the same procedure but splint with the right arm and turn to the right.

- For clients with orthopedic surgery (e.g., hip surgery), use special aids, such as a trapeze, to assist with movement.
5. Teach the client the following three leg exercises:
   - Alternate dorsiflexion and plantar flexion of the feet. **Rationale:** *This exercise is sometimes referred to as calf pumping, because it alternately contracts and relaxes the calf muscles, including the gastrocnemius muscles.*
   - Flex and extend the knees, and press the backs of the knees into the bed while dorsiflexing the feet ❶. Instruct clients who cannot raise their legs to do isometric exercises that contract and relax the muscles.

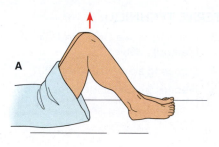

A

B

C

❶ Flexing and extending the knees.

- Raise and lower the legs alternately from the surface of the bed. Flex the knee of the stable leg and extend the knee of the moving leg ❷. **Rationale:** *This exercise contracts and relaxes the quadriceps muscles.*

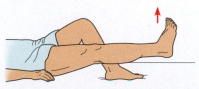

❷ Raising and lowering the legs.

SKILL 15.1   Conducting Preoperative Teaching *(continued)*

6. Demonstrate deep breathing (diaphragmatic) exercises as follows:
   - Place your hands palms down on the border of your rib cage, and inhale slowly and evenly through the nose until the greatest chest expansion is achieved ❸.
   - Hold your breath for 2 to 3 seconds.
   - Then exhale slowly through the mouth.
   - Continue exhalation until maximum chest contraction has been achieved.

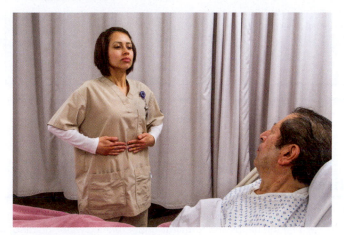

❸ Demonstrating deep breathing.

7. Help the client perform deep breathing exercises.
   - Ask the client to assume a sitting position.
   - Place the palms of your hands on the border of the client's rib cage to assess respiratory depth.
   - Ask the client to perform deep breathing, as described in step 6.
8. Instruct the client to cough voluntarily after five deep inhalations.
   - Ask the client to inhale deeply, hold the breath for a few seconds, and then cough once or twice.
   - Ensure that the client coughs deeply and does not just clear the throat.
9. If the incision will be painful when the client coughs, demonstrate techniques to splint the abdomen.
   - Show the client how to support the incision by placing the palms of the hands on either side of the incision site or directly over the incision site, holding the palm of one hand over the other. **Rationale:** *Coughing uses the abdominal*

and other accessory respiratory muscles. Splinting the incision may reduce pain while coughing if the incision is near any of these muscles.
   - Show the client how to splint the abdomen with clasped hands and a firmly rolled pillow held against the client's abdomen ❹.

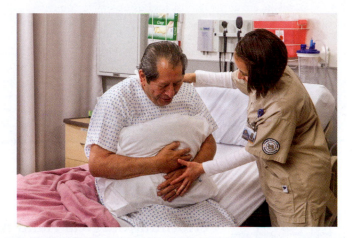

❹ Splinting an incision with a pillow while coughing.

10. Inform the client about the expected frequency of these exercises.
    - Instruct the client to start the exercises as soon after surgery as possible.
    - Encourage clients to carry out deep breathing and coughing at least every 2 hours, taking a minimum of five breaths at each session. Note, however, that the number of breaths and frequency of deep breathing vary with the client's condition. People who are susceptible to pulmonary problems may need deep breathing exercises every hour. People with chronic respiratory disease may need special breathing exercises (e.g., pursed-lip breathing, abdominal breathing, or exercises using various kinds of incentive spirometers).
11. Document the teaching and all assessments. Some agencies may have a preoperative teaching flow sheet. Check agency policy.

Sample Documentation

3/19/15 0900 Instructed how to splint abdomen while deep breathing and coughing. Able to perform correctly. Stated that he will use this technique after surgery. _____ A. Moore, RN

Evaluation

Document the outcome of the teaching plan such as:
- Client's demonstrated ability to perform moving, leg exercises, deep breathing, and coughing exercises.
- Client's verbalization of key information presented.

Developmental Considerations

Preoperative Teaching

CHILDREN
- Parents need to know what to expect and to be able to express their concerns.

- Separation from parents often is the child's greatest fear; the time of separation should be minimized and parents allowed to interact with the child both immediately preceding and following the surgery.
- Teaching and communicating with children (both timing and content) should be geared to the child's developmental level and cognitive abilities (e.g., "You will have a sore tummy").
- Play is an effective teaching tool with children (e.g., the child can put a bandage on an incision on a doll).

(continued on next page)

SKILL 15.1 Conducting Preoperative Teaching (continued)

OLDER ADULTS

- Assess hearing ability to ensure the older client hears the necessary information.
- Assess short-term memory. Presenting one focused idea at a time and repeating or reinforcing information may be necessary.
- Older adults are at greater risk for postoperative complications, such as pneumonia. Reinforce moving and deep breathing and coughing exercises.
- Assess potential postoperative needs at this time. Arrangements can be made preoperatively to obtain necessary items. Examples are medical equipment, such as walkers, raised toilet seats, and bed trapezes; Meals-on-Wheels; and help with transportation.

- If the older adult client will need to be in extended care for a period of time after surgery, this is the time to initiate these plans.
- Assess the client for risk of pressure ulcer development postoperatively, and be extra attentive to use of proper padding and support devices to prevent injury during positioning and transfers in the operating room. Risks include:
  - Older age.
  - Poor nutritional status
  - History of diabetes or cardiovascular problems
  - History of taking steroids, which cause increased bruising and skin breakdown.

SKILL 15.2 Performing Surgical Hand Antisepsis/Scrubs

Delegation

Surgical hand antisepsis/scrub is performed by a perioperative nurse or RNFA. It can, be, however, delegated to a UAP or LVN/LPN in some agencies. The Association of periOperative Nurses (AORN) believes that individuals who are not licensed to practice professional nursing and who perform in the role of scrub person are performing a delegated technical function under the supervision of a perioperative registered nurse (AORN, 2007, p. 407).

Equipment

- Deep sink with foot, knee, or elbow controls
- Antimicrobial solution
- Nail-cleaning tool, such as a file or orange stick
- Surgical scrub brush
- Sterile towels for drying the hands

Preparation

- Ensure that all of the surgical garb is in place (i.e., shoe covers; cap, which should completely cover all the hair; face mask; and protective eyewear).

Procedure

1. Prepare for the surgical hand antisepsis/scrub.
   - Remove wristwatch, bracelets, and all rings. Ensure that fingernails are trimmed. **Rationale:** *Jewelry and long fingernails harbor microorganisms. Removal of jewelry permits full skin contact with the antimicrobial agent.*
   - Turn on the water, using either the foot, knee, or elbow control, and adjust the temperature to lukewarm. **Rationale:** *Warm water removes less protective oil from the skin than hot water. Soap irritates the skin more when hot water is used.*

2. Wash hands.
   - Wet the hands and forearms under running water, holding the hands above the level of the elbows so that the water runs from the fingertips to the elbows. **Rationale:** *The hands will become cleaner than the elbows. The water should run from the least contaminated to the most contaminated area.*
   - Apply 2 to 4 mL (1 tsp) antimicrobial solution to the hands.
   - Use firm, rubbing, and circular movements to wash the palms and backs of the hands, the wrists, and the forearms.
   - Interlace the fingers and thumbs, and move the hands back and forth ❶. Continue washing for 20 to 25 seconds. **Rationale:** *Circular strokes clean most effectively, and rubbing ensures a thorough and mechanical cleaning action. (Other areas of the hands still need to be cleaned, however.)*
   - Hold the hands and arms under the running water to rinse thoroughly, keeping the hands higher than the elbows.

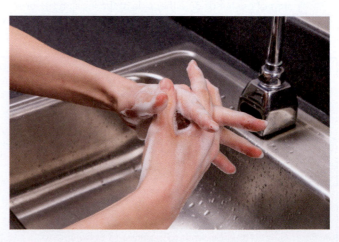

❶ Interlacing the fingers during hand washing.

SKILL 15.2 Performing Surgical Hand Antisepsis/Scrubs (*continued*)

Rationale: *The nurse rinses from the cleanest to the least clean area.*

- Check the nails, and clean them with a file or orange stick if necessary ❷. Rinse the nail tool after each nail is cleaned. **Rationale:** *Sediment under the nails is removed more readily when the hands are moist. Rinsing the nail tool after cleaning each nail prevents the transmission of sediment from one nail to another.*

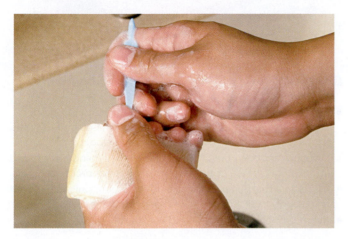

❷ Cleaning the fingernails.

3. Perform surgical hand antisepsis/scrub (with brush/sponge).
   - Apply antimicrobial agent to wet hands and forearms and lather hands again. Using a scrub brush or sponge, scrub each hand. Visualize each finger and hand as having four sides. Wash all four sides effectively ❸. Repeat this process for opposite fingers and hand. **Rationale:** *Scrubbing loosens bacteria, including those in the creases of the hands.*

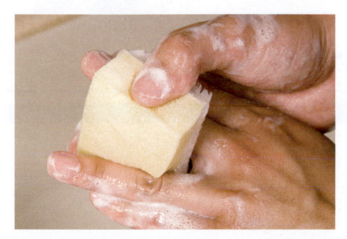

❸ Scrubbing side of finger.

   - Using the scrub brush or sponge, scrub from the wrists to 5 cm (2 in.) above each elbow. Visualize each arm as having four sides. Using agency protocol (e.g., scrubbing by number of strokes or length of time), wash all parts of the arms: lower forearm, upper forearm, and antecubital space to marginal area above elbows. Continue to hold the hands higher

than the elbows. **Rationale:** *Scrubbing thus proceeds from the cleanest area (hands) to the least clean area (upper arm).*
- Discard the scrub brush or sponge.
- Rinse hands and arms thoroughly so that the water flows from the hands to the elbows. **Rationale:** *Rinsing removes resident and transient bacteria and sediment.*
- Avoid splashing water onto surgical attire. **Rationale:** *A sterile gown put over wet or damp surgical attire would be considered contaminated.*
- If a longer scrub is required, use a second brush and scrub each hand and arm with the antimicrobial agent for the recommended time.
- Discard second brush, and rinse hands and arms thoroughly.
- Turn off the water with the foot or knee pedal.
- Keeping hands elevated and away from the body, enter the operating room by backing into the room. **Rationale:** *This position of the hands maintains the cleanliness of the hands and backing into the room prevents accidental contamination.*

4. Dry the hands and arms.
   - Use a sterile towel to dry one hand thoroughly from the fingers to the elbow ❹. Use a rotating motion. Use a second sterile towel to dry the second hand in the same manner. In some agencies, towels are of a sufficient size that one half can be used to dry one hand and arm and the second half for the second hand and arm. **Rationale:** *The nurse dries the hands (the cleanest area) to the least clean area. Using a new towel or the opposite end of a towel prevents the transfer of microorganisms from one elbow (least clean area) to the other hand (cleanest area).*
   - Discard the towel(s).
   - Keep the hands in front and above the waist. **Rationale:** *This position maintains the cleanliness of the hands and prevents accidental contamination.*

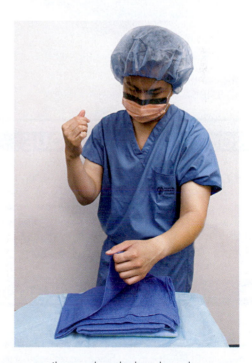

❹ Picking up sterile towel to dry hands and arms.

(*continued on next page*)

SKILL 15.2 *Performing Surgical Hand Antisepsis/Scrubs* (*continued*)

VARIATION: SURGICAL HAND ANTISEPSIS/HAND SCRUB USING ALCOHOL-BASED SURGICAL HAND RUB

- Prepare for the surgical hand antisepsis/scrub and wash hands (see steps 1 and 2 above).
- Dry hands and forearms thoroughly with a paper towel.
- Follow the manufacturer's directions for use of the brushless surgical hand antisepsis product. Following is an example of how to use one brushless product. Note, however, that many products are available and it is imperative to use a product according to the manufacturer's guidelines. **Rationale:** *Following the manufacturer's guidelines helps ensure effective surgical hand antisepsis, which is needed to prevent surgical site infections.*
- Using a foot pump, dispense one pump (2 mL) of the surgical hand rub product into the palm of one hand ❺. **Rationale:** *A foot pump avoids contamination of the hands.*

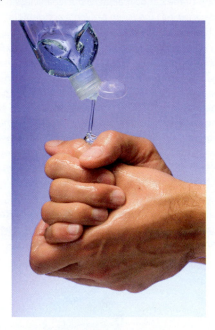

❺ Dispensing hand rub.
(*Source:* © BSIP SA/Alamy.)

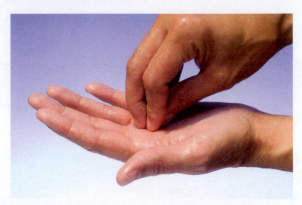

❻ Dip fingers into hand prep. (*Source:* © BSIP SA/Alamy)

- Dip fingertips of the opposite hand into the hand-rub product and work under fingernails ❻. Spread remaining hand-rub product over the hand and up to just above the elbow.
- Dispense another pump (2 mL) of the surgical hand-rub product into the palm of the opposite hand and repeat procedure.
- Dispense a final pump (2 mL) of hand-rub product into either hand and reapply to all aspects of both hands up to the wrists ❼.
- Rub thoroughly until dry. Do not use towels.

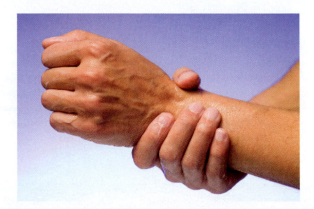

❼ Reapply hand rub to both hands up to wrists.
(*Source:* © BSIP SA/Alamy.)

▶ USING STERILE TECHNIQUE

Expected Outcomes

1. Infection is prevented in clients during surgical procedures.
2. Surgical asepsis is maintained during surgical procedure.
3. Sterile field is maintained on instrument tray during surgical procedure.

SKILL 15.3 Donning Sterile Gown and Gloves (Closed Method)

Delegation

Applying a sterile gown and sterile gloves is performed by a perioperative nurse or RNFA. It can be, however, delegated to a UAP or LVN/LPN in some agencies. A UAP often assists the RN or RNFA or scrub person by preparing the sterile pack containing the sterile gown and gloves.

Equipment

- Sterile pack containing a sterile gown and sterile gloves

Preparation

- Gather sterile pack and ensure its sterility.

SKILL 15.3 Donning Sterile Gown and Gloves (Closed Method) *(continued)*

Procedure

1. Perform surgical hand antisepsis/scrub (see Skill 15.2).

Applying a Sterile Gown

1. Apply the sterile gown.
   - Grasp the sterile gown at the crease near the neck, hold it away from you, and permit it to unfold freely without touching anything, including the uniform. **Rationale:** *The gown will not be sterile if its outer surface touches any unsterile objects.*
   - Put the hands inside the shoulders of the gown without touching the outside of the gown.
   - Work the hands down the sleeves only to the beginning of the cuffs ❶.

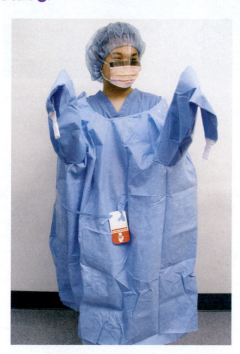

❶ Working the hands down the sleeves of a sterile gown.

   - Have a coworker wearing a hair cover and mask reach inside arm seams and pull gown over shoulders.
   - The coworker grasps the neck ties without touching the outside of the gown and pulls the gown upward to cover the neckline of the scrub person's uniform in front and back ❷.

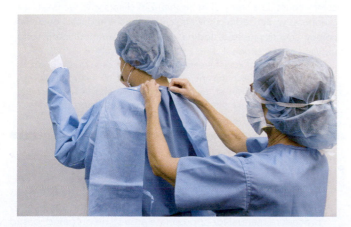

❷ Coworker ties the neck ties of the sterile gown.

Apply Sterile Gloves (Closed Method)

1. Open the sterile glove wrapper ❸.

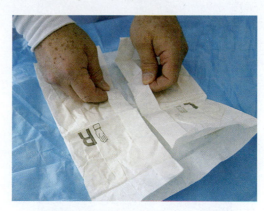

❸ Opening the sterile glove wrapper. If no assistant is present, keep hands inside sleeves of gown to open wrapper.

2. Put the glove on the nondominant hand.
   - With the dominant hand, pick up the opposite glove with the thumb and index finger, handling it through the sleeve.
   - Position the dominant hand palm upward inside the sleeve. Lay the glove on the opposite gown cuff, thumb side down, with the glove opening pointed toward the fingers.
   - Use the nondominant hand to grasp the cuff of the glove through the gown cuff, and firmly anchor it.
   - With the dominant hand working through its sleeve, grasp the upper side of the glove's cuff, and stretch it over the cuff of the gown while extending the fingers of the nondominant hand into the glove's fingers. ❹

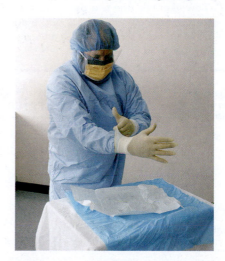

❹ Pulling on the first sterile glove and letting wrist portion snap into place.

3. Put the glove on the dominant hand.
   - Place the fingers of the gloved hand under the cuff of the remaining glove.
   - Place the glove over the cuff of the second sleeve.
   - Extend the fingers into the glove as you anchor the cuff with the nondominant hand. ❺
   - Unfold the second cuff and adjust as for the first hand. Keep gloved hands above the sterile field. ❻

(continued on next page)

SKILL 15.3 Donning Sterile Gown and Gloves (Closed Method) *(continued)*

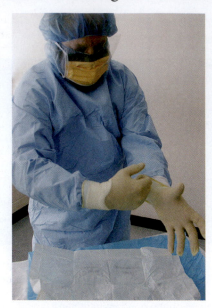

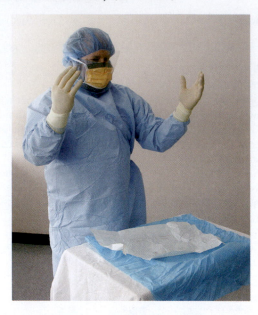

⑤ Extending the fingers into the second glove of the dominant hand.

⑥ Sterile gloved hands must remain above waist level or the level that defines the sterile field.

Completion of Gowning

1. Complete gowning as follows.
   - Have a coworker hold the waist tie of your gown, using sterile gloves or a sterile forceps or drape. **Rationale:** *This approach keeps the ties sterile.*
   - Make a three-quarter turn, then take the tie and secure it in front of the gown.
   or
   - Have a coworker take the two ties at each side of the gown and tie them at the back of the gown, making sure that the scrub person's uniform is completely covered.

- When worn, sterile gowns should be considered *sterile* in front from the waist to the shoulder. Once the nurse approaches a table, the gown is considered contaminated from the waist or table down, whichever is higher. The sleeves should be considered sterile from the cuff to 5 cm (2 in.) above the elbow, since the arms of a scrubbed person must move across a sterile field. Moisture collection and friction areas such as the neckline, shoulders, underarms, back, and sleeve cuffs should be considered unsterile.

SKILL 15.4 Preparing a Surgical Site

Equipment

- Absorbent pad
- Bath blanket or drape
- Scissors or electric clippers (optional)
- Disposable prep kit (for shaving)

If kit not available:

- Disposable razor (number according to area to be shaved)
- 2 sterile bowls
- 4 × 4 gauze pads
- Emesis basin
- Applicator sticks
- Cleansing solution
- Sterile water
- Clean gloves
- Depilatory
- Antiseptic solution
- Tongue blade
- 4 × 4 gauze pad

Evidence-Based Nursing Practice

Surgical Site Infection (SSI)

A preoperative antiseptic shower or bath decreases skin microbial colony count. In a study of more than 700 clients who received two preoperative antiseptic showers, chlorhexidine reduced bacterial colony counts ninefold. Iodine or triclocarban-medicated soap reduced colony counts 1.3- to 1.9-fold, respectively.

Chlorhexidine gluconate–containing products require several applications to obtain maximum antimicrobial benefit, so repeated antiseptic showers are indicated. Even though these showers reduce the colony count, they have not definitively shown a reduction in SSI rate.

Source: Centers for Disease Control and Prevention (2011).

Procedure

1. Refer to physician's orders for specific operative site or area to be prepared. If orders do not state preference for site, refer to procedure manual for appropriate area to be prepared, based on surgical procedure.

SKILL 15.4 Preparing a Surgical Site *(continued)*

Note: Many surgeons do not require hair to be shaved for a surgical site unless it interferes with the surgical procedure or wound closure. Based on clinical research, it has been found that shaving the hair does not prevent surgical site infections, but it does interfere with the client's psychological status. Client's body image can be impaired and he or she senses a loss of control with shaving of the hair, particularly of the head or pubic area.

2. Determine type of preparation to be done: clipping of hair, shaving site, or hair removal using depilatory. Gather equipment.
3. Introduce yourself and identify client by checking the client's identity band and asking client to state name and birth date.
4. Explain procedure to client, and provide privacy.
5. Adjust light to ensure good visualization.
6. Perform hand hygiene.
7. Position client for maximum comfort and site exposure and have bed positioned at correct height.
8. Drape client for comfort and to prevent undue exposure.
9. Protect bed with absorbent pad.
10. Arrange equipment for your convenience.
11. Put on clean gloves.
12. Assess surgical site before skin preparation for moles, warts, rash, and other skin conditions. **Rationale:** *Inadvertent removal of lesions traumatizes skin and may contribute to infection.*
   Note: Centers for Disease Control and Prevention (CDC) standards indicate that clients are to shower or bathe with an antiseptic agent at least the night before surgery. The U.S. Food and Drug Administration (FDA) has also shown that antimicrobial activity of the antiseptic agent prevents skin infections.
13. Prepare site using scissors or clippers according to facility policy/procedures.
   - Use scissors or electric clippers and cut hair 1 cm above surgical site or according to facility policies.
   - Clip small amount of hair each time.
   - Cut in direction hair grows.
   - Remove all hair from site, and discard.
14. Prepare site using depilatory.
   - Clip hair before applying cream.
   - Apply cream to designated area using tongue blade or gloved hand.
   - Leave on skin for designated time, according to directions on package, usually 10 minutes.
   - Remove cream by rubbing off with tongue blade or moistened 4 × 4 gauze pads.
   - Wash skin with antiseptic soap; dry area thoroughly.
   - Remove all hair with washing. **Rationale:** *This provides clean, smooth skin, free of abrasions and cuts.*
15. Prepare site using razor.
   - Lather skin with antiseptic soap and 4 × 4 gauze pads. **Rationale:** *Wet shave results in fewer microabrasions to the skin. Shaving should be done in direction of hair growth.*
   - Discard soiled sponges frequently.
   - Using sharp razor, shave hair moving away from incision site. With free hand, stretch skin taut and shave, following the hair growth pattern and using firm, steady strokes. Shave small area at one time. **Rationale:** *Shave is closer and nicks are prevented.*

- Change razor as often as necessary. Avoid nicking the skin. Report if skin is nicked. **Rationale:** *Nicks, if severe, can cause infection by bacteria normally found on the skin.*
- Wash all hair off site with 4 × 4 gauze pads or use sticky mitt or tape to remove hair.
- The shave should be completed close to the time of surgery. The shave prep is completed before the client enters the operating room. **Rationale:** *Shaving and clipping hair immediately before surgery are associated with a lower risk of infection than if done the night before.*

CLINICAL ALERT

If hair must be removed, scissors or clippers should be used and procedure completed before the client reaches the operating room suite. Many hospitals use the minimal shave and scrub preparation approach. The shaved area may be as small as 2 cm surrounding the surgical incision site. Refer to the policy and procedure manual and physician's orders before beginning the surgical prep.

Electric or battery-powered clippers are preferred to razors to prevent skin irritation and microscopic cuts to the skin. Clippers must have a disposable head that is changed between clients. Handles should be disinfected.

16. After removing hair, apply antiseptic solution with 4 × 4 pads or use disposable prep kit.
17. Begin at incision site and, with light friction, make ever-widening circles, moving outward from the center to the most distant line of area. **Rationale:** *Working from most clean to least clean area prevents contamination.* Scrub area for 2 to 3 minutes.
18. Rinse area with warm water and blot dry with 4 × 4 gauze pads.
19. Remove and dispose of equipment; scissors and razors are disposed of in sharps container. Return bed to lowest height.
20. Remove gloves and discard. Perform hand hygiene.
21. Assist client to put on clean gown.
22. Position the client for comfort. Document care provided.

Evidence-Based Nursing Practice

Skin Preparation and Surgical Site Infections

Hair removal prior to surgery is sometimes necessary, but it can be associated with a high incidence of SSIs. The healthcare costs for clients with SSIs are about double the costs for clients without. Various means of hair removal have been studied, including shaving, clipping, and use of depilatory creams.

Shaving has been associated with a greater number of SSIs than clipping. Depilatory creams have a very low incidence of SSIs; however, they cause hypersensitivity skin reactions in some clients. Clipping hair immediately before an operation results in a lower risk of SSIs (1.8%) than shaving or clipping the night before (4.0%).

The CDC recommends removal of hair only if hair will interfere with surgery. CDC guidelines suggests removing hair immediately prior to surgery to reduce the incidence of SSIs.

Data from Broex et al. (2009), Reichman & Greenberg (2009), and CDC (2011).

SKILL 15.5 Preparing a Client for Surgery

CLINICAL ALERT

The AORN recommends that the preop skin preparation should be an antimicrobial agent that has a broad germicidal range and is non toxic. The most common antiseptic agents used for preoperative skin preparation and surgical scrubs include alcohol, chlorhexidine, iodine/iodophors, and Triclosan.

Alcohol has the most rapid microbial action, which denatures proteins and is effective against both gram-positive and gram-negative bacteria, viruses, and fungi. However, it is not often used as a surgical skin prep because it does not stay on the skin.

Chlorhexidine has an intermediate rapidity of action, disrupting the cell membrane. It should not be used on mucous membranes, eyes, or brain tissue (neurotoxic). It works well against gram-positive bacteria, and less well against gram-negative bacteria.

Iodine/iodophors has an intermediate action and is acceptable for use against a wide range of bacteria, fungi, and viruses.

Triclosan disrupts the cell wall and has an acceptable kill rate against bacteria.

Equipment

- Preoperative checklist
- Operative permit
- Specific equipment needed to provide physical care as ordered, such as enema equipment, nasogastric tube, Foley catheter
- Antiseptic agent for shower

Procedure

1. Check physician's order, introduce self, and explain why you are there. Identify client by checking the client's identity band and asking client to state name and birth date. Provide for client privacy.
2. Obtain client's signature on surgical consent form and check agency policy. Ensure all preoperative forms are complete, with no blank areas ❶–❸.
3. Assist client to complete anesthesia questionnaire if required.
4. Assess if bowel prep was completed at home. **Rationale:** *Most clients complete bowel prep before admission to facility. Administer an enema if ordered.*
5. Assist client to shower if not completed at home. Instruct on how to shower and specific time guidelines according to facility guidelines.
6. Complete skin prep, if ordered. Follow facility guidelines for skin prep.
7. Assess for latex allergy. If present, ensure allergy band is applied, physician is notified, and OR staff personnel are notified. **Rationale:** *All latex products must be removed from OR and client must be scheduled for first case in morning.*
8. Enquire for symptoms and observe for signs of cold or upper respiratory infection.
9. Explain need for client to be NPO for 8 to 10 hours preoperatively.
10. Remove lipstick and nail polish if required by hospital policy.
11. Insert Foley catheter if ordered.
12. Take and record vital signs.
13. Remove earrings, necklaces, medals, watch, rings (ring may be taped to finger or toe in some facilities). If possible, remove body piercing jewelry. Cover with tape if not possible

❶ Sample surgical consent form.

❷ Sample surgical preoperative checklist.

SKILL 15.5   Preparing a Client for Surgery (continued)

3 Sample preanesthesia evaluation form.

to remove. **Rationale:** *Protect skin from possible burns from electrical arcing generated by electrical cautery machines.*

14. Remove contact lenses, glasses, hairpieces, and dentures. Some hospitals/anesthesiologists allow full dentures to remain if using a mask.
15. Assist client to void if catheter not inserted, and record time and amount.
16. Check client's identity, blood band, and allergy bracelet. During this stage the client must be identified by at least two identifiers (i.e., medical record number, birth date, name, charge number).
17. Put antiembolism stockings on client as ordered.
18. Administer preoperative medications.
19. Observe that the operative site is verified and marked, both site and side, by the physician while the client is awake.
20. Place side rails in UP position and bed in LOW position following administration of medications.
21. Darken room, and provide quiet environment following administration of medications. Document care provided.
22. Check client 15 minutes after medication administered to observe for possible side effects.

CLINICAL ALERT

Universal Protocol for Preventing Wrong Site, Wrong Procedure, and Wrong Person Surgery

The Joint Commission (2010) has issued guidelines for preventing wrong site, wrong procedure, and wrong person surgery as discussed here.

Preoperative validation of the right client, procedure, and site should occur while the client is awake, aware, and before he or she leaves the preoperative area or enters the surgical suite.

- The marking should be made by an individual who is familiar with the client and is involved with the client's procedure. This individual is encouraged to be the surgeon or (1) individuals permitted through a residency program to participate in the procedure or (2) a licensed individual who performs duties in collaboration with the surgeon (i.e., nurse practitioners and physician assistants).
- Incision site must be marked, using a marker that is not easily removed, at or near the incision site.
- DO NOT MARK any nonoperative site(s) unless necessary for some other aspect of care.
- Use initials, word "yes," or a line indicating proposed incision site to prevent ambiguous marks.
- Mark must be visible after client is prepped and draped.
- Final verification of site mark must take place in the location where the procedure will take place. This time is identified as the "time-out" period. Nothing happens until this final check has occurred. The entire team must be present during this check.
- Verification must include
  a. Correct client identity.
  b. Correct site and side.
  c. Agreement on procedure to be done.
  d. Correct client position.
  e. Availability of any special equipment or implants needed for procedure.

Exemptions from Marking Procedure

- Single-organ cases (e.g., C-section, cardiac surgery).
- Interventional cases: insertion site of instrument/catheter not predetermined.
- Premature infants: for whom the mark may become a permanent mark.
- Teeth—BUT indicate operative tooth name(s) on documentation OR mark the operative tooth (teeth) on the dental radiographs or dental diagram.

Data from American Academy of Orthopaedic Surgeons (2014) and Joint Commission (2010, 2014).

Evidence-Based Practice

Preventing Wrong Site, Wrong Procedure, Wrong Person Surgeries

Following a 2001 report that surgical mistakes were on the rise, the Joint Commission approved a universal protocol for preventing wrong site, wrong procedure, wrong person surgery. This protocol became effective in 2004. Despite its existence, these "never" events do still occur. Compliance with the protocol continues to be a challenge given the nature of the surgical environment.

Studies show that adjuncts to the protocol may be helpful. Anatomical marking has been used by one facility in addition to the protocol and has had significant success. In four and a half years and

(continued on next page)

SKILL 15.5   Preparing a Client for Surgery *(continued)*

more than 100,000 clients, there was one implementation error, and it led to minimal client harm. Another facility instituted a 2-minute briefing—done after induction of anesthesia and before incision—in which every OR team member states his or her name and role, and the lead surgeon identifies critical aspects of the operation such as the client's identity, the surgical site, and other client safety con-

cerns. This approach has resulted in greatly increased communication among team members. The benefits of a "time-out" prior to surgery seem clear. The Joint Commission names communication as the greatest single factor in preventing wrong site/wrong client/ wrong procedure errors.

Data from Stahel et al. (2010). Knight & Aucar (2010), and Neily et al. (2009).

SKILL 15.6   Pouring from a Sterile Container

Equipment

- Sterile container
- Nonsterile container
- Sterile solution

Procedure

1. Perform hand hygiene.
2. Gather equipment.
3. Open sterile container according to procedure.
4. Place container on firm surface.
5. Take cap off the bottle and invert the cap before placing it on a firm surface. **Rationale:** *This keeps the cap sterile.*
6. Hold the bottle with the label facing up.
7. Pour a small amount of liquid into the nonsterile container ❶. **Rationale:** *This action cleans the lip of the bottle.*

8. Pour the liquid into the sterile container while keeping the label facing up and not touching the container with the bottle ❷. Do not reach over a sterile field if the container has been placed on one. **Rationale:** *Crossing over a sterile field can lead to contamination of the field.*
9. Replace the cap if liquid remains in the bottle. If total contents have been used, dispose of bottle in trash.
10. Date and initial bottle if reusing.
11. Return partially filled bottle to storage area if it is to be reused.

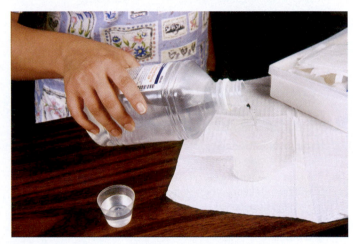

❷ Pour liquid by placing container close to edge of sterile area.

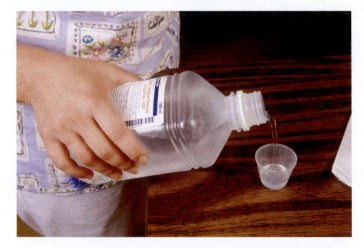

❶ First pour a small amount of liquid into a nonsterile container.

SKILL 15.7   Preparing a Sterile Field Using Prepackaged Supplies

Equipment

- Packaged supplies

Procedure

1. Gather equipment and supplies. Perform hand hygiene, following infection control measures.

2. Ensure working surface is clean and dry. Client's overbed table is frequently used as preparation area. **Rationale:** *This prevents contamination of sterile package.*
3. Remove outer plastic wrap.
4. Place package in center of work area and position so that you first open package flap away from you. **Rationale:** *This prevents reaching across the sterile field as you continue to open package.*

SKILL 15.7   Preparing a Sterile Field Using Prepackaged Supplies (*continued*)

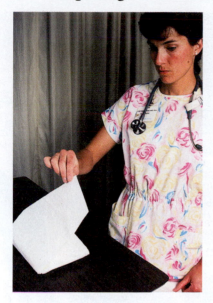

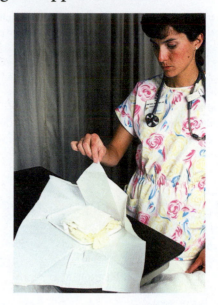

1 Grasp edge of top flap of wrapper and lift it away from you.

2 Open last flap toward you—do not cross over sterile field.

5. Grasp edge of the first flap of the wrapper, move it away from you, and place it on the working surface **1**.

6. Grasp the first side flap, lift it up; grasp the second side flap and together move both hands out toward the sides. Place the flaps down on the working surface.

7. Grasp the last flap of the wrapper and open it toward you, taking care not to touch the inside of the flap or any of the contents of the package **2**. **Rationale:** *This prevents contamination of the supplies.*

Setting of Care

- Clean and wipe dry a flat surface for the sterile field.
- Keep pets and noninvolved small children out of the area when setting up for and performing sterile procedures.
- Dispose of all soiled materials in a waterproof bag. Check with the agency as to how to dispose of medical refuse.
- Remove all instruments from the home or other setting where others might accidentally find them. **Rationale:** *New or used*

instruments can be sharp or capable of causing injury. Used instruments may transmit infection. Check with the agency for instructions on cleansing of reusable supplies and disposal of single-use instruments.

- If appropriate, teach the client and family members the principles and rationale underlying the use of a sterile field.

SKILL 15.8   Preparing for a Dressing Change Using Individual Supplies

Equipment

- Antiseptic cleaner or cleaning solution
- Number and type of dressings needed (i.e., 4 × 4 gauze pads, abdominal pads, application sticks, transparent dressings)
- Tape
- Clean gloves
- Sterile gloves
- Disposal bag
- Mask, if needed

Procedure

1. Gather equipment and supplies. Perform hand hygiene.
2. Clean off bedside stand and wash thoroughly with antiseptic solution. Dry thoroughly.
3. Place supply packages on table in configuration that allows you to open packages without reaching over sterile field. **Rationale:** *Reaching over sterile field will contaminate supplies.*

(*continued on next page*)

SKILL 15.8 **Preparing for a Dressing Change Using Individual Supplies** (*continued*)

4. Grasp cover of 4 × 4 pad plastic container and pull flap back and away from sterile area ❶. Place cover in disposal bag.
5. Grasp edge of transparent dressings package, peel back top covering ❷. Place open package on work surface. Do not cross over any open supply packages.
6. Continue to open all supplies using above steps.
7. Pour solution over pads in plastic container, if ordered ❸.
8. Open sterile gloves ❹. Place in position on table where you do not pass over a sterile field.

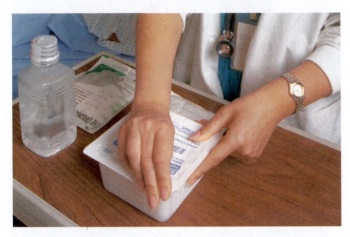

❶ Open sterile 4 ×4 pads container by pulling back on flap.

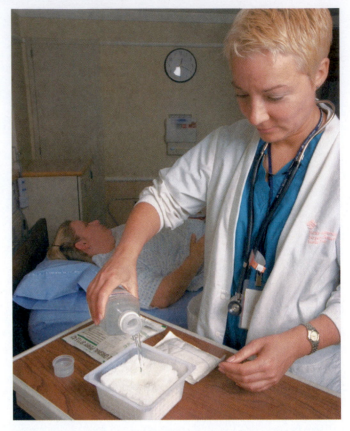

❸ Pour cleaning solution over 4 × 4 pad.

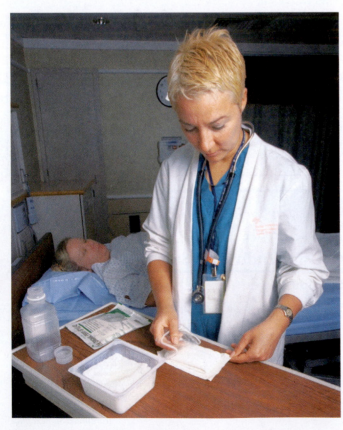

❷ Open transparent dressing packet.

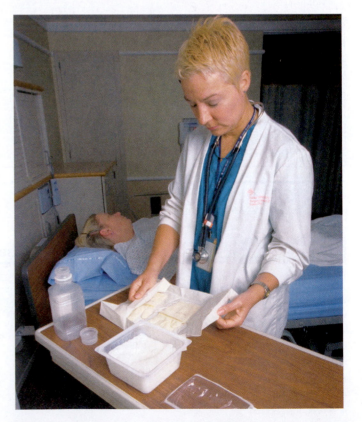

❹ Open sterile glove packet on overbed table.

SKILL 15.9 Changing a Dry Sterile Dressing

Equipment

- Sterile gloves
- Clean gloves
- Mask
- Gown
- Disposal bag for used dressings
- Dressing supplies, as needed
- Micropore tape
- Sterile normal saline (optional)
- Package sterile cotton swabs, or 4 × 4 pads
- Bath blanket or sheet

Preparation

- Check physician's orders and client care plan.
- Perform hand hygiene.
- Gather equipment.
- Introduce self to client. Identify the client by checking the client's identity band and asking client to state name and birth date, and explain procedure.
- Provide privacy.
- Clean off overbed table.
- Place sterile supplies on overbed table.
- Provide comfort and safety for client and self, including raising bed to appropriate height.
- Place bag for soiled dressings near incision site.
- Fanfold linen to expose incision area.
- Cover client with bath blanket or sheet, leaving incision area exposed.
- Open sterile packages, and place on overbed table. Arrange packages to ensure you don't cross over the sterile field when reaching for dressings. **Rationale:** *Commercially prepared sterile packages can be opened and used for the sterile field because the inside of the package is sterile.*
- Cut tape into appropriate length strips.

Procedure

1. Remove tape slowly by pulling tape toward the wound **❶**. **Rationale:** *Pulling toward the wound decreases the pain of tape removal by not putting pressure on the incision line.*

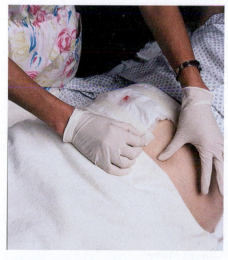

❶ Remove tape by gently lifting toward wound.

2. Don clean gloves.
3. Remove soiled dressing **❷** and dispose of in the proper bag **❸**. Wet dressing with sterile normal saline if it adheres to the suture line.

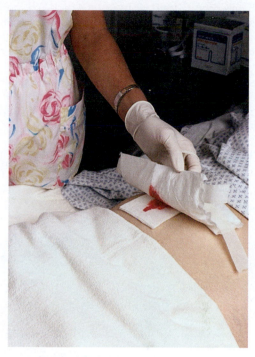

❷ Remove soiled dressing carefully.

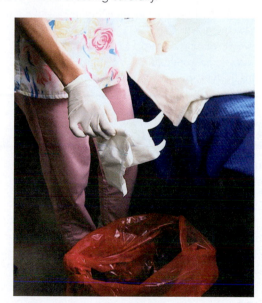

❸ Dispose of dressing in appropriate container.

4. Assess incision area for erythema, edema, or drainage. **Rationale:** *Persistent drainage, edema, or temperature above 38°C (100.4°F) 2 days postop indicates a complication is occurring.*
5. Assess color of incision. (A healing incision looks pink or red.) **Rationale:** *Redness that does not fade 48 hours after surgery may indicate impaired healing.*
6. Remove clean gloves, and discard.

(continued on next page)

SKILL 15.9 Changing a Dry Sterile Dressing *(continued)*

7. Move overbed table next to working area.
8. Don sterile gloves.
9. Cleanse incision area with sterile swabs or 4 × 4 pads soaked in normal saline, according to hospital policy. Cleanse from incision line outward, cleaning from top to bottom, using the swab only once. Discard swabs or 4 × 4 pads in disposal bag. **Rationale:** *Cleaning outward from incision cleans from least to most contaminated area. Cleaning from top to bottom prevents contamination from secretions that accumulate at the bottom of the wound.*
10. Place 4 × 4 gauze pads over incision area, being careful not to touch incision or client with your gloves ❹. **Rationale:** *Touching the incision or client contaminates the gloves.* You need to reglove if this occurs.

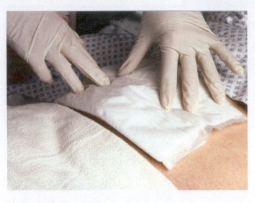

❺ Place abdominal pad over center of incision.

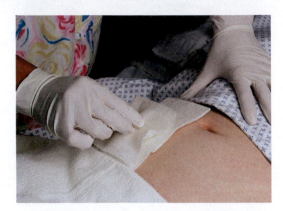

❹ Do not touch incision when applying dressing.

11. Place abdominal pad over incision, being careful not to contaminate the gloves ❺.
12. Remove gloves and discard.
13. Tape dressing securely ❻.
14. Discard trash in appropriate receptacle.

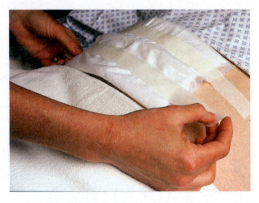

❻ Tape dressing securely to prevent slipping.

15. Return bed to lowest height. Position client for comfort.
16. Perform hand hygiene.
17. Document sterile dressing change done: assessment of wound, incision area cleaned with saline, dry sterile dressing applied, and client tolerance of procedure.

SKILL 15.10 Removing Sutures

Equipment

- Sterile suture removal set
- Antiseptic solution
- Tape
- Butterfly tape
- Paper bag for disposal of dressings
- Two pair clean gloves (1 pair optional)

Procedure

1. Check physician's order and gather equipment and supplies. Introduce self, explain what procedure is to be done and why. Perform hand hygiene, follow infection control measures, and verify client's identity by checking the client's identity band and asking client to state name and birth date. Provide for client privacy. Provide comfort and safety for client and self, including raising bed to appropriate height for procedure.
2. Don clean gloves.
3. Remove dressing and discard in disposal bag. (Discard gloves only if soiled.)
4. Open suture removal set, and don gloves if second pair needed.
5. Pick up forceps with nondominant hand.
6. Grasp suture at the knot with forceps and lift away from skin ❶.
7. Pick up suture scissors with dominant hand.
8. Place curved tip of suture scissors under suture, next to knot.
9. Cut suture and, with forceps, pull suture through skin with one movement ❷.
10. Discard suture into disposal bag.
11. Check that entire suture is removed.
12. Continue to remove remaining sutures according to hospital policy. Some policies state that every other suture is removed and then remaining sutures are removed at a later time. **Rationale:** *To prevent wound dehiscence.*
13. Cleanse suture site with antiseptic solution.
14. Remove gloves, and place in disposal bag.
15. Place dressing or butterfly tape over incision area, if ordered.
16. Discard disposal bag into contaminated waste container.
17. Perform hand hygiene.
18. Document care, assessments, and client response.

SKILL 15.10   Removing Sutures (continued)

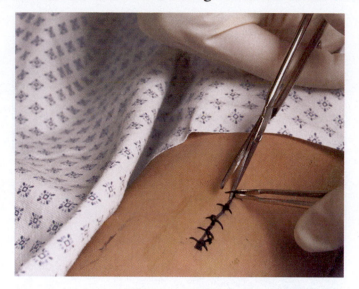

❶ Grasp suture at the knot with forceps and lift away from skin.

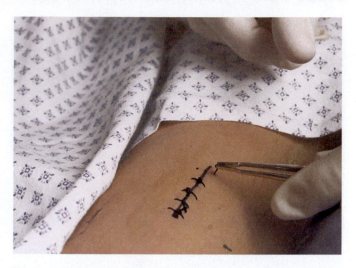

❷ After cutting suture, grasp suture at knot and pull through skin.

Topical Glue for Wound Closure

A product to replace sutures and staples (used in an estimated 80 to 90 million procedures annually) was approved by the FDA after proving itself in clinical trials. This superglue is called Dermabond. It is a synthetic, noninvasive glue that mitigates trauma and post-procedure inflammation, while providing a waterproof seal and protecting underlying tissue without the need for bandages. Dermabond is painless, fast and simple to apply, and naturally sloughs off in 7 to 10 days.

SKILL 15.11   Removing Staples

Equipment

- Sterile staple remover
- Disposal bag
- Clean gloves, 2 pairs (1 pair optional)
- Dressings
- Tape or butterfly tape
- Antiseptic solution

Procedure

1. Check physician's order and gather equipment and supplies. Introduce self, explain what procedure is to be done and why. Perform hand hygiene, follow infection control measures, and verify client's identity by checking the client's identity band and asking client to state name and birth date. Provide for client privacy. Provide comfort and safety for client and self, including raising bed to appropriate height for procedure. Open sterile staple remover.
2. Don clean gloves.
3. Remove dressing, and discard in disposal bag ❶. (Discard gloves only if soiled.)
4. Don gloves if necessary.
5. Place lower tip of staple remover under staple.

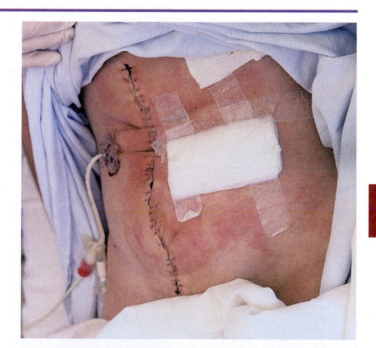

❶ Large abdominal wound with staples closing incision.

(continued on next page)

SKILL 15.11 Removing Staples (continued)

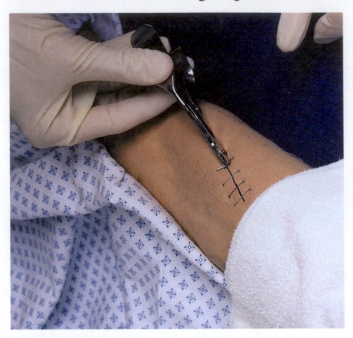

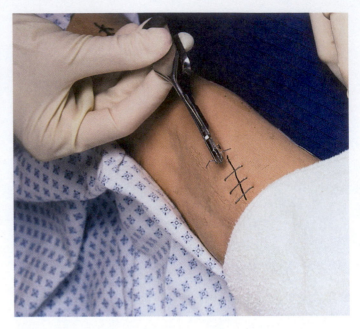

❸ Lift staple remover device upward and away from incision.

❷ With lower tip of staple removal device under staple, press handle together to depress center of staple.

6. Press handles together to depress center of staple ❷.
7. Lift staple remover upward, away from incision site when both ends of staple are visible ❸.
8. Place staple removal device over disposal bag and release handles to release staple.
9. Remove all staples or as directed by hospital policy. Some policies indicate every other staple is removed with remaining staples done at a later time. **Rationale:** *To prevent wound dehiscence.*
10. Cleanse incision area with antiseptic solution if ordered.
11. Remove gloves, and place in disposal bag.
12. Place dressing over incision and secure with tape, or place butterfly tape over incision.

13. Discard disposal bag in contaminated waste container.
14. Perform hand hygiene. Document care and client response.

Client Teaching

Upon discharge:

- Instruct client to eat foods high in protein, carbohydrates, vitamins, and minerals to promote wound healing.
- Splint wound when coughing or moving from chair or bed to prevent separation of wound edges.
- Provide list of signs and symptoms of wound infection or delayed healing. Include when to notify physician.
- Encourage use of daily showers; water may run over wound.
- Instruct not to use soap, lotions, or vitamin creams on incision.
- Instruct in dressing change procedure.
- Instruct to not lift heavy objects (anything over 10 pounds).
- Instruct in measures to promote elimination.

CLINICAL ALERT

Steri-Strips may be applied over incision to protect incision after staples have been removed.

Setting of Care

In the home setting, medical asepsis, or clean technique, is often used instead of sterile technique. The major reasons for this protocol change are the nature of the setting and the personnel providing care.

The greatest infection control problem in hospitals is healthcare-associated infections due to the large numbers of antibiotic-resistant organisms present in a hospital setting. When clients are in their own environment, however, they tend to develop fewer infections because they are subjected to fewer organisms. In the home setting, the focus is on protecting home care staff and family, not other clients. Although organisms may be transmitted among individuals in the home, there are minimal data on the incidence of home care–acquired infections. Infection-preventing strategies in the home should focus on IV therapy and urinary tract, respiratory, and wound care.

Nevertheless, sterile technique and equipment, such as prepackaged catheter and irrigation kits, parenteral fluid equipment, and dressings, are often purchased for home care. When sterile technique is required, it is the responsibility of the nurse to provide the instruction and evaluate the family's ability to perform the skill accurately. Hospital techniques may need to be modified for the home setting, and ideal environmental working conditions may not be present. Unfortunately, the Division of Healthcare Quality Promotion of the CDC has not developed guidelines for infection control in home care settings at this time. Therefore, adaptations must be made, and the essential infection control measures must be maintained.

SKILL 15.11 Removing Staples (continued)

Just as in the hospital, effective hand hygiene is the most effective means of infection control in the home setting. There is one major difference between hospital and home. Equipment (soap, running water, and paper towels) that is readily available to the nurse in the hospital may not be available in the home. Even if running water is available, there may be no soap or clean towels. Nurses must bring their own hand washing supplies.

A decrease in the duration of hospital stays has dramatically increased the expanded scope of the home care nurse. Unfortunately, infection surveillance, prevention, and control efforts have not kept up. Many home care infection control practices have been based on ritual and acute care practice, rather than scientific principles. Changes in infection control procedures in the home are currently occurring based on a scientific approach.

Home care assessment for potential infections relies on clinical signs and symptoms and tests, such as the urine dipstick, that can

be performed in the home. Routine tests used in hospitals to diagnose infections of the urinary tract, respiratory tract, and wound or skin sites are not routinely done, because the current reimbursement system does not support cultures and laboratory tests. Only cultures that confirm and treat bloodstream infections for clients requiring home infusion therapy are obtained.

If the home care client is suspected of or diagnosed as having an infectious disease or the client is infected or colonized with VRE or MRSA, the nurse should use the same personal protective equipment and protocol used in the hospital setting. The equipment includes gloves, disposable gown or apron, mask, cap, and goggles. Reusable equipment, such as stethoscopes and blood pressure cuffs, should stay in the home and not be used on other home care clients. If possible, these clients should be seen at the end of the day.

▶ CRITICAL THINKING OPTIONS FOR UNEXPECTED OUTCOMES

Not all unexpected outcomes require further nursing intervention; however, many times they do. When the client demonstrates a change in signs/symptoms indicating an emerging problem, the nurse should immediately assess and troubleshoot what is happening. The assessment data must be processed quickly to formulate a hypothesis so the nurse can make a clinical judgment. The nurse then decides how best to resolve the problem and improve the client's situation for a better appropriate outcome.

EXPECTED OUTCOME	PROBLEM SOLVING	NURSING ACTIONS
Preoperative baseline data are obtained.	Factors that can affect the postoperative course are identified during the preoperative care (i.e., arthritic changes in client's back, history of thrombophlebitis).	■ Place information in client's care plan and inform charge nurse and surgeon about findings. ■ Write a note in client's chart and alert the operating room and PACU staff of the findings so that they can assess for the problems.
Client's physical or emotional deviations from normal are identified preoperatively.	Client refuses to go to operating room without dentures.	■ Explain to client that dentures are likely to be lost, broken, or inadvertently pushed to back of mouth if not removed. ■ If client refuses to remove dentures, alert anesthesiologist that dentures are in place.
	Client is abnormally stressed.	■ Explore feelings and reasons for client's or family's stressed behaviors. ■ Explore more effective methods to reduce stress for client and family. ■ Clarify misconceptions and inappropriate perceptions. ■ Have physician speak to client and answer questions.
Surgical site is marked and prepared correctly.	Client refuses surgery site marking.	■ Client has right to refuse; document client refusal on appropriate forms. ■ Procedure may be performed without marking. ■ Provide client with information regarding safety aspects for marking procedure. ■ Discuss rationale for client's refusal to determine whether insufficient information was provided regarding marking procedure.
Using Sterile Technique Infection is prevented in clients during surgical procedures.	Client's skin is cut during shave.	■ Notify physician and OR staff of client's condition. ■ Follow specific directions; surgery may be canceled as infection could occur as a result of break in skin integrity.
Surgical asepsis is maintained during surgical procedure.	A hole develops in a glove while performing sterile technique.	■ Discard gloves and replace with sterile gloves. ■ Examine hands for cuts if the hole was caused by sharp object. ■ If hands are cut, scrub hands and replace sterile gloves.
Sterile field is maintained on instrument tray during surgical procedure.	Sterile field becomes wet or damp.	■ Discard supplies on sterile field. ■ Set up new sterile field.

RELATED CONCEPTS

Skills-at-a-Glance

Nursing assessment of the obstetrical client is a major responsibility for any nurse whether she or he works in an office setting or in an acute care facility. The nurse midwife and nurse practitioners have become integral members of the interdisciplinary team that provides care for the family during the birthing process. More advanced practice nurses such as certified nurse midwives and nurse practitioners, have in-depth education and skill in performing assessment responsibilities with the physician. While performing the antepartum physical assessment (see **Table 16–1** ● in Skill 16.1), the nurse should establish an environment in which the woman feels comfortable and free to discuss any concerns. This is also an opportunity to establish rapport with the client to support her during the intrapartum assessment (see **Table 16–2** ● in Skill 16.1) and care. The last phase of the client relationship includes the postpartum maternal assessment (see **Table 16–3** ● in Skill 16.1) and care in addition to the newborn assessment (see **Table 16–4** ● in Skill 16.1) and care. The information collected during the antepartum (prenatal), intrapartum, postpartum, and newborn assessments can be used to identify needed areas for teaching and counseling (Davidson, London, & Ladewig, 2012).

▶ ANTEPARTUM CARE

Expected Outcomes

1. Client is psychologically prepared for a pelvic examination.
2. Client experiences no discomfort throughout assessment of fetal well-being nonstress testing.
3. Client exhibits no signs of side effects or allergic responses at the injection site of administered Rh Immune Globulin.
4. An amniocentesis is completed without complication.
5. Client experiences no physical problems during pregnancy.

SKILL 16.1 Maternal and Newborn Assessments

Procedure

1. Gather equipment and supplies. Introduce self and explain what procedure is to be done and why. Perform hand hygiene, following infection control measures, and verify client's identity. Provide privacy. Provide comfort and safety for client and self, including raising bed to appropriate height for procedure.
2. Perform a systematic assessment (see Tables 16–1 to 16–4).
3. Document all pertinent information.

TABLE 16–1 Antepartum Assessment

ASSESSMENT	NORMAL FINDINGS DURING PREGNANCY	ABNORMAL FINDINGS DURING PREGNANCY
Take vital signs, blood pressure (BP), temperature, pulse, and respiration (TPR)	Temperature: 98°–99°F Pulse: 80–90 bpm (pulse rates can increase 10 beats during pregnancy) Respirations: 16–24 breaths/min (pregnancy may induce a mild form of hyperventilation and thoracic breathing) Blood pressure (BP): 120/80 mmHg	Elevated temperature (infection) Increased pulse rate—anxiety or excitement; cardiac disorder Marked tachypnea—assess for respiratory distress Increased: possible anxiety (client should rest 20–30 minutes before you take BP again) Rise of 30/15 above baseline data: sign of preeclampsia Decreased: sign of supine hypotensive syndrome. If lying on back, turn client on left side and take BP again
Evaluate weight to assess maternal health and nutritional status and growth of fetus	Minimum weight gain during pregnancy: 24 lb If underweight: 28–42 lb If obese: 15 lb or more Normal weight gain: 25–35 to 40 lb	Inadequate weight gain; possible maternal malnutrition Excessive weight gain: if sudden at onset, may indicate preeclampsia; if gradual and continual, may indicate overeating
Skin ■ Color	Nail beds are pink; color of skin is consistent with racial background *Striae* (reddish-purple lines) on breasts, hips, and thighs; after pregnancy, faint silvery-gray *Spider nevi* common in pregnancy	Pallor—anemia; yellowish—liver disease or some form of jaundice Dark-skinned individuals with anemia may have bluish, reddish, mottled skin; dusty or pale appearance of the palms and nails beds Petechiae, multiple bruises, ecchymosis (hemorrhage; abuse)

(continued on next page)

SKILL 16.1   Maternal and Newborn Assessments (continued)

TABLE 16–1   Antepartum Assessment (continued)

ASSESSMENT	NORMAL FINDINGS DURING PREGNANCY	ABNORMAL FINDINGS DURING PREGNANCY
Skin (continued) ■ Condition	Absence of edema (slight edema in lower extremities normal); usually no rashes	Edema could be suggestive of pregnancy-induced hypertension. Presence of rash could indicate dermatitis; allergic reaction Ulcerations could indicate varicose veins or decreased circulation
■ Edema	In lower extremities	In upper extremities and face may indicate pregnancy-induced hypertension
Nose, mouth, and neck	Nasal mucosa redder than oral; nasal mucosa edematous due to increased estrogen resulting in nasal stuffiness and nosebleeds; gingival tissue hypertrophy related to increase in estrogen	Pallor in mucosa may be anemia; edema in mucosa tissue may be inflammation or infection
Chest and lungs Breasts and nipples ■ Contour and size ■ Presence of lumps ■ Secretions	Should be no difference during pregnancy Size increases are noticeable during first 20 weeks; become nodular; tingling sensation may be felt during first and third trimester; breasts feel heavy; darker pigmentation of nipple and areola Colostrum in late first trimester or early second trimester Secondary areola appears at 20 weeks, characterized by series of washed-out spots surrounding primary areola Old striae marks may be present in multiparas	Redness, heat, tenderness, cracked or fissured nipples (infection); "pigskin" or orange peel appearance, nipple retraction, swelling, hardness (carcinoma) Secretions, other than colostrum
Heart	Palpitations during pregnancy may occur due to sympathetic nervous system disturbance Short systolic murmurs that increase in held expiration are normal due to increased volume	Enlargement, thrills, thrusts, gross irregularity or skipped beats, gallop rhythm or extra sounds could indicate cardiac disease
Abdomen	Flat, rounded abdomen; progressive enlargement due to pregnancy Primiparas: coincidentally with growth Linea nigra (black line of pregnancy along midline of abdomen) Primiparas: coincidentally with growth of fundus Multiparas: after 13–15 weeks' gestation	
Fundal height in centimeters (finger-breadths less accurate): measure from symphysis pubis to top of fundus	Fundus palpable just above symphysis at 8–10 weeks Halfway between symphysis and umbilicus at 16 weeks Umbilicus at 20–22 weeks	Large measurements: Expected date of confinement or delivery (EDC) is incorrect; tumor; ascites; multiple pregnancy; polyhydramnios, hydatidiform mole Less than normal enlargement: fetal abnormality, oligohydramnios, placental dysmaturity, missed abortion, fetal death
Fetal heart rate by quadrant, location, and rate	120–160 bpm 110–160 bpm May be heard with Doppler at 10–12 weeks' gestation; with fetoscope at 17–20 weeks	Decreased: indicates fetal distress with possible cord prolapse or cord compression Accelerated: initial sign of fetal hypoxia Absent: may indicate fetal demise
Fetal movement	Trained examiner should be able to feel fetal movement after 18th week	
Ballottement	Tapping the uterus sharply during the 4th or 5th month results in the fetus rising and then returning to the original position	

SKILL 16.1   Maternal and Newborn Assessments *(continued)*

TABLE 16–1   Antepartum Assessment *(continued)*

ASSESSMENT	NORMAL FINDINGS DURING PREGNANCY	ABNORMAL FINDINGS DURING PREGNANCY
Determine fetal position, using Leopold maneuvers: Complete external palpations of the abdomen to determine fetal position, lie, presentation, and engagement		
First maneuver: to determine part of fetus presenting into pelvis	Vertex presentation	Breech presentation or transverse lie
Second maneuver: to locate the back, arms, and legs: fetal heart heard best over fetal back		
Third maneuver: to determine part of fetus in fundus		
Fourth maneuver: to determine degree of cephalic flexion and engagement		

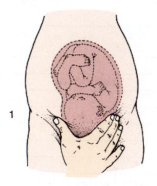 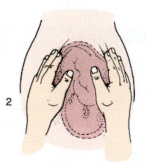 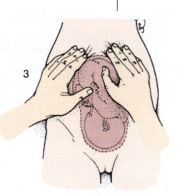 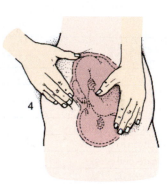

Steps of Leopold maneuvers

Pelvis and perineum	1–4 weeks' gestation: enlargement in anteroposterior diameter	Absence of Goodell sign: inflammatory condition, carcinoma
	4–8 weeks: softening of cervix (Goodell sign); softening of isthmus of uterus (Hegar sign); cervix takes on bluish color (Chadwick sign)	
	8–12 weeks: vagina and cervix appear bluish-violet in color (Chadwick sign)	
	External genital: in multiparas labia majora loose and pigmented; urinary and vaginal orifices visible and appropriately located	
	Vagina: in multiparas, vaginal folds smooth and flattened; may have episiotomy scar	
	Cervix: in multiparas, cervical os allows insertion of one fingertip	
	Pelvic Measurements:	
	Internal measurements:	
	Diagonal conjugate at least 11.5 cm	Deviations in pelvic measurements may indicate that vaginal birth may not be possible
	Obstetric conjugate estimated by subtracting 1.5–2 cm from diagonal conjugate	Disproportion of pubic arch
	Mobility of coccyx: external intertuberosity diameter > 9 cm	Fixed or malposition of coccyx
Reflexes	Normal and symmetrical	Hyperactivity, clonus would be present in pregnancy-induced hypertension

(continued on next page)

SKILL 16.1 Maternal and Newborn Assessments (continued)

TABLE 16–1 Antepartum Assessment (continued)

ASSESSMENT	NORMAL FINDINGS DURING PREGNANCY	ABNORMAL FINDINGS DURING PREGNANCY
Assessment of Pregnant Woman Evaluate lab findings: Complete blood count (CBC) Hemoglobin (Hgb) Hematocrit (Hct)	12–16 g/dL 38%–47%; physiological anemia (pseudoanemia) may occur	
White blood cell count: 5,000–12,000/µL	Elevations in pregnancy and labor are normal	
Red blood cell count	No alteration	4.0–6.0 million/µL
Urinalysis: sugar, protein, albumin	Normal color and specific gravity Negative for protein, red blood cells, white blood cells, casts	Positive for sugar: may indicate subclinical or gestational diabetes Proteinuria between 300 mg/L and 1 g (1+–2+ dipstick indicates mild pregnancy-induced hypertension)
Glucose	Negative or small amount of glycosuria may occur in pregnancy	
Rubella titer	Hemagglutination: inhibition (HAI) test 1:10 indicates immunity	
Hepatitis B screen	Negative	
HIV	Negative	
Syphilis test	Nonreactive	
Gonorrhea culture	Negative	
Illicit drug screen	Negative	
Sickle cell screen	For those of African descent—negative	
Pap smear	Negative	
Blood type and Rh factor	A variety of blood groupings Rh positive Does not require RhoGAM	If Rh negative, father's blood should be typed If Rh positive, titers should be followed; possible RhoGAM at termination of pregnancy
Group B streptococcus test Either cultured (35–37 weeks' gestation) or new (2013) FDA-approved IDI-Strep B provides results in 1 hr	Strep not present	If strep present, woman is given 4 hr of antibiotic treatment during labor (penicillin or ampicillin)
Assess for Signs of Labor Lightening and dropping (the descent of the presenting part into the pelvis)	Several days to 2 weeks before onset of labor Multipara: may not occur until onset of labor Relief of shortness of breath and increase in frequency	No lightening or dropping: may indicate disproportion between fetal presenting part and maternal pelvis
Check if mucus plug has been expelled from cervix Assess for bloody show	Usually expelled from cervix prior to onset of labor Clear, pinkish, or blood-tinged vaginal discharge that occurs as cervix begins to dilate and efface	
Assess for ruptured membranes ■ Time water breaks	Before, during, or after onset of labor	Breech presentation: frank meconium or meconium staining
■ Color of amniotic fluid	Clear, straw color	Greenish-brown: indicates meconium has passed from fetus, possible fetal distress Yellow-stained: fetal hypoxia 36 hr or more prior to rupture of membrane of hemolytic disease

SKILL 16.1 Maternal and Newborn Assessments (continued)

TABLE 16–1 Antepartum Assessment (continued)

ASSESSMENT	NORMAL FINDINGS DURING PREGNANCY	ABNORMAL FINDINGS DURING PREGNANCY
■ Quantity of amniotic fluid	Normal is 500–1,000 mL of amniotic fluid rarely expelled at one time	Polyhydramnios—excessive amniotic fluid (over 2,000 mL) Observe newborn for congenital anomalies: craniospinal malformation, orogastrointestinal anomalies. Down syndrome, and congenital heart defects Oligohydramnios—minimal amniotic fluid (less than 500 mL) Observe newborn for malformation of ear, genitourinary tract anomalies, and renal agenesis
■ Odor of fluid	No odor	Odor may indicate infection: deliver within 24 hr
Assessment of fetal well-being		Hypertensive disorder, diabetes, renal or heart disease are among conditions that may warrant diagnostic testing for fetal well-being in the third trimester: amniocentesis; nonstress testing (NST), contraction stress test (CST), biophysical profile scoring
Evaluate fundal height	Drop around 38th week: sign of fetus engaging in birth canal Primipara: sudden drop Multipara: slower, sometimes not until onset of labor	Large fundal growth: may indicate wrong dates, multiple pregnancy, hydatidiform mole, polyhydramnios, tumors Small fundal growth: may indicate fetal demise, fetal anomaly, retarded fetal growth, abnormal presentation or lie, decreased amniotic fluid

TABLE 16–2 Intrapartum Assessment

ASSESSMENT	NORMAL INTRAPARTUM FINDINGS	ABNORMAL INTRAPARTUM FINDINGS
Take vital signs (TPR): ■ Temperature	Temperature: 98°–99°F;	Elevated temperature: infection
■ Pulse	Pulse: 80–90 bpm (pulse rates can increase 10 beats)	Increased pulse rates (excitement or anxiety; early shock; cardiac disease; drug use)
■ Respiration	Respirations: 16–24 breaths/min (pregnancy may induce a mild form of hyperventilation and thoracic breathing)	Hyperventilation: anxiety/pain Hyperventilation expected in transition phase Decreased respirations with use of narcotics for pain Marked tachypnea with respiration distress
■ Blood pressure (BP)	BP: 120/80 mmHg	Low BP with supine hypotension, hemorrhage, hypovolemia, shock, or drugs High BP with pregnancy-induced hypertension; pain
Pulse oximeter	95% or greater	<90% hypoxia, hypotension, hemorrhage
Fetal heart rate	120–160 bpm	
Weight	25–35 lb > than prepregnancy weight	>35 lb could be fluid retention, obesity, large infant, diabetes mellitus, pregnancy-induced hypertension <15 lb could be a small- for-gestational-age (SGA) infant, substance abuse, psychosocial problems
Fundus	40 weeks: just below xiphoid process	Uterine size not compatible with estimated date of birth: SGA; large for gestational age (LGA); hydramnios; multiple pregnancy; placental/fetal anomalies; malpresentations
Edema	Slight amount of dependent edema in lower extremities expected	Pitting edema of face, hands, legs, abdomen, sacral area indicative of pregnancy-induced hypertension
Hydration	Normal skin turgor	Poor skin turgor with dehydration

(continued on next page)

SKILL 16.1 Maternal and Newborn Assessments (continued)

TABLE 16–2 Intrapartum Assessment (continued)

ASSESSMENT	NORMAL INTRAPARTUM FINDINGS	ABNORMAL INTRAPARTUM FINDINGS
Perineum	Same as antepartum	Varicosities of vulva, herpes lesions/genital warts
Uterine contractions	Frequency: from start of one contraction to start of next Duration: from beginning of contraction to time uterus begins to relax; 50–90 sec Intensity (strength of contraction): measured with monitoring device; Peak 25 mmHg End of labor may reach 50–75 mmHg	Irregular contractions with long intervals between: indicates false labor >90 sec: uterine tetany; stop oxytocin if running >75 mmHg: uterine tetany or uterine rupture
Cervical dilation (progressive cervical dilation from size of fingertip to 10 cm) **First stage:** Latent phase (0–4 cm dilation) Active phase (4–8 cm)	0–4 cm; average 6.4 hr	Failure to dilate could be cervical rigidity, failure of presenting part to engage; cervical edema (pushing effort by woman before full dilation and effacement of the cervix) Prolonged time in any phase: may indicate poor fetal position, incomplete fetal flexion, cephalopelvic disproportion, or poor uterine contractions
Transitional phase (8–10 cm) Assess for bloody show Observe for presence of nausea or vomiting Evaluate urge to bear down	Length of time varies—may be 1–2 hr Beginning to bulge	Often uncontrolled Multipara: can cause precipitous delivery "Panting" (can be controlled until safe delivery area established)
Cervical effacement (progressive thinning of cervix)	Occurs faster than dilation; 0%–100%	Failure to efface could be indicative of cervical rigidity, infections, scar tissue, failure of presenting part to engage, cephalopelvic disproportion
Fetal descent (progressive descent of fetal presenting part from station −5 to + 4)		
Membranes	Ruptured; if ruptured more than 12–24 hr before onset of labor	If not ruptured, physician may perform amniotomy
Fetal status	Fetal heart rate (FHR) 110–160 bpm Auscultation of fetal heart rate	<110 or >160 bpm may indicate fetal distress with cord compression or prolapse of cord; abnormal fetal patterns on fetal monitor (decreased variability, late decelerations, variable decelerations, absence of accelerations with fetal movement)
Evaluate fetal heart rate tracing	Short-term variability is present Long-term variability ranges from 3–5 cycles/min	Absence of variability (no short term or long term present) Severe variable decelerations (fetal heart rate <70 for longer than 30–45 sec with decreasing variability)
Deceleration	Early deceleration (10–20 beat drop) Recovery when acme contraction passes—often not serious	Monitor closely—distinguish from decrease with hypertonic contraction; leads to fetal distress
Variable deceleration; decrease in FHR, below 120 bpm	Mild; may be within normal parameters—continue to monitor	Cord compression—may result in fetal difficulty
Loss of beat-to-beat variation	If lasts less than 15 min, no problem apparent	Late deceleration pattern occurs—monitor for hypertonic contraction; leads to total distress
Evaluate pain and anxiety	Medication required after dilated 4–5 cm unless using natural childbirth methods	Severe pain early in first stage of labor: inadequate prenatal teaching, backache due to position in bed, uterine tetany
Second stage (10 cm to delivery)	Primipara: up to 2 hr Multipara: several minutes to 2 hr	>2 hr: increased risk of fetal brain damage and maternal exhaustion
Assess for presenting part	Vertex with ROA or LOA presentation	Occiput posterior, breech, face, or transverse lie

SKILL 16.1 Maternal and Newborn Assessments (continued)

TABLE 16–2 Intrapartum Assessment (continued)

ASSESSMENT	NORMAL INTRAPARTUM FINDINGS	ABNORMAL INTRAPARTUM FINDINGS
Assess caput (infant head) Multipara: move to delivery room when caput size of dime Primipara: move to delivery room when caput size of half dollar	Visible when bearing down during contraction	"Crowns" in room other than delivery room: delivery imminent (do not move client)
Assess fetal heart rate Bradycardia, drop of 20 bpm below baseline (↓ less than 120 bpm) Tachycardia, increase in FHR over 160 bpm for 10 min	120—160 bpm	Decreased: may indicate supine hypotensive syndrome (turn client on side and take again) Hemorrhage (check for other signs of bleeding; notify physician) Increased or decreased: may indicate fetal distress secondary to cord compression or prolapsed cord
Third stage (from delivery of baby to delivery of placenta)	Placental separation occurs within 30 min (usually 3–5 min)	Failure of placental separation Abnormality of uterus or cervix, weak, ineffectual uterine contraction, titanic contractions causing closure of cervix >3 hr: indicates retained placenta
Fourth stage (first hour postpartum) Assess vital signs every 15 min for 1 hr, every 30 min for 1 hr, every hour		Mother in unstable condition (hemorrhage usual cause) Highest risk of hemorrhage in first postpartum hour
Temperature	36.5°–37.5°C	>37.5°C: may indicate infection Slight elevation: due to dehydration from mouth breathing and NPO
Pulse	60–100 bpm	Increased may indicate pain or hemorrhage
Respirations	Respirations: 12–20 breaths/min	
Blood pressure	Blood pressure: 120–140/80 mmHg	Increased: may indicate anxiety, pain, or post-eclamptic condition Decreased: hemorrhage
Uterine assessment	Fundus firm, midline	Displaced to right indicates full bladder
Lochia assessment	Large amount, bright red	Excessive amounts may be caused by retained placental fragments
Comfort	Shivering response (tremors)	
Apgar scoring	Newborns who score 7–10 are considered free of immediate danger	Newborns who score 4–6 are moderately depressed Newborns who score 0–3 are severely depressed

TABLE 16–3 Postpartum (PP) Maternal Assessment

Procedure F

ASSESSMENT	NORMAL PP FINDINGS	ABNORMAL PP ASSESSMENT
Assess vital signs every hour for 4 hr, every 8 hr, and as needed	Pulse may be 45–60 bpm in stage 4 Pulse to normal range about third day	Decreased BP and increased pulse: probably postpartum hemorrhage Elevated temperature >38°C indicates possible infection Temperature elevates when lactation occurs
Assess breasts and nipples daily	Days 1–2: soft, intact, secreting colostrum Days 2–3: engorged, tender, full, tight, painful Days 3+: secreting milk Increased pains as baby sucks: common in multiparas	Tenderness, heat, edema indicates engorgement Sore or cracked (clean and dry nipples); decrease breastfeeding time; apply breast shield between feedings Milk does not "let down": help client relax and decrease anxiety; give glass or wine or beer if not culturally, religiously, or otherwise contradicted Reddened area could indicate mastitis Palpable mass indicates mastitis Engorgement indicates venous stasis

(continued on next page)

SKILL 16.1   Maternal and Newborn Assessments (continued)

TABLE 16–3   Postpartum (PP) Maternal Assessment (continued)

ASSESSMENT	NORMAL PP FINDINGS	ABNORMAL PP ASSESSMENT
Nipples	Pigmented, intact, become erect when stimulated	Fissures, cracks, soreness can be caused by poor breast-feeding techniques Inverted nipples will cause nipples not to erect when stimulated
Assess fundus every 15 min for 1 hr, every 8 hr for 48 hr, then daily	Firm (like a grapefruit) in midline and at or slightly above umbilicus Return to prepregnant size in 6 weeks: descending at rate of 1 fingerbreadth/day	Boggy fundus: immediately massage gently until firm; report to physician and observe closely; empty bladder; medicate with oxytocin if ordered Fundus misplaced 1–2 fingerbreadths from midline: indicates full bladder (client must void or be catheterized)
Assess lochia every 15 min for 1 hr, every 8 hr for 48 hr, then daily	Scant to moderate amount, earthy odor, no clots	Clots indicates hemorrhage
■ Color	3 days postpartum: dark red (rubra) 4–10 days postpartum: clear pink (serosa) 10–21 days postpartum: white, yellow brown (alba)	Failure to progress from rubra to serosa to alba indicates subinvolution
■ Quantity	Moderate amount, steadily decreases	No lochia: may indicate clot occluding cervical opening (support fundus; express clot) Heavy, bright red: indicates hemorrhage (massage fundus, give medication on order, notify physician) Spurts: may indicate cervical tear
■ Odor	Minimal	Foul: may indicate infection
Assess perineum daily	May have slight edema and bruising	Swelling or bruising: may indicate hematoma
■ Episiotomy	Episiotomy intact, no swelling, no discoloration	Redness, ecchymosis, discharge, or gaping stitches may indicate infection
■ Hemorrhoids	None present; could have a few small, nontender	Full, tender, red could indicate inflammation
Assess bladder every 4 hr	Voiding regularly with no pain	Not voiding: bladder may be full and displaced to one side, leading to increased lochia (catheterization may be necessary) Symptoms of urgency, frequency, and dysuria could be infection
Assess bowels	Spontaneous bowel movement 2–3 days after delivery	Fear associated with pain from hemorrhoids, episiotomy or perineal trauma; no bowel movement could be constipation
Evaluate Rh-negative status	Clients does not require RhoGAM	RhoGAM administered
Assess mother–infant bonding	Touching infant, talking to infant, talking about infant	Refuses to touch or hold infant
Assess extremities	Negative Homans sign; no pain with palpation	Positive findings indicate thrombophlebitis
Material History: Definition of Terms Abortion: pregnancy loss before fetus is viable (usually <20 weeks or 500 g) Gravida: any pregnancy, including present one Primigravida: refers to first-time pregnancy	Multigravida: refers to second or any subsequent pregnancy Para: past pregnancies that continued to viable age (20 weeks); infants may be alive or dead at birth Primipara: refers to female who has delivered first viable infant; born either alive or dead	Nullipara: refers to female who has never carried pregnancy to viable age for fetus Multipara: refers to female who has given birth to two or more viable infants; either alive or dead

SKILL 16.1   Maternal and Newborn Assessments *(continued)*

TABLE 16–4   Newborn Assessment

ASSESSMENT	NORMAL	ABNORMAL
Vital Signs Temperature	Rectal 36.6°–37.2°C (97.8°–99°F) Axilla 36.4°–37.2°C (97.5°–99°F)	Elevated temperatures may be related to room too hot; too much clothing Subnormal temperatures related to cold, sepsis, brainstem involvement Differences of 2 degrees in either direction could indicate infection
Pulse	120–160 bpm; will go higher if crying	Bradycardia indicative of severe asphyxia or cardiac arrhythmia Weak pulse related to decreased cardiac output Tachycardia (>160 bpm) indicates infection, arrhythmia, central nervous system problems
Respirations	Respiration rate 30–50 breaths/min; transient tachypnea Respiration movement irregular in rate and depth Resonant chest (hollow sound on percussion) Abdominal respirations	Tachypnea indicates pneumonia, respiratory distress syndrome (RDS) Rapid, shallow breathing may occur is mother given large doses of magnesium sulfate during labor for pregnancy-induced hypertension (hypermagnesemia) Respirations below 30 breaths/min indicative of maternal anesthesia or analgesia during labor and delivery Expiratory grunting, subcostal and substernal retractions, flaring of nostrils indicative of respiratory distress, apnea, or respiratory disorder
Blood pressure	At birth: 80–60/45–40 Day 10: 100/50	Low BP indicates hypovolemia or shock
Assess cry (see also **Table 16–5** ● on Apgar scoring)	Lusty cry	Weak, groaning cry: possible neurological abnormality High-pitched cry: newborn drug withdrawal (may occur 6–12 months after birth); hoarse or crowing inspirations; catlike cry: possible neurological or chromosomal abnormality
Assess weight	5.5–8.14 lb Normal weight loss during first 3 days: up to 5%–10%	<8 lb indicates SGA or preterm infant >9 lb indicates LGA infant or infant born to a mother with diabetes Greater loss indicates feeding problems, decreased fluid intake, or losses due to meconium or urine
Skin Assessment Note skin color, pigmentation, turgor, and lesions	Pink Mongolian spots may occur over buttocks in dark-skinned babies Erythema	Cyanosis, pallor, beefy red petechiae, ecchymoses, or purpuric spots: signs of possible hematological disorder or clotting disorders Impetigo (group A beta-hemolytic strep or staph
	Capillary hemangiomas on face or neck	Café au lait spots (patches of brown discoloration): possible sign of congenital neurological disorder Raised capillary hemangiomas on areas other than face or neck
	Localized edema in presenting part	Edema of peritoneal wall Poor skin turgor: indicates dehydration
	Cheesy white vernix Desquamation (peeling off)	Yellow discolored vernix (meconium stained)
	Milia (small white pustules over nose and chin)	Impetigo neonatorum (small pustules with surrounding red areas)

(continued on next page)

SKILL 16.1 Maternal and Newborn Assessments (continued)

TABLE 16–4 Newborn Assessment (continued)

ASSESSMENT	NORMAL	ABNORMAL
	Jaundice after 24 hr; gone by second week	Jaundice at birth or within 12 hr
		Dermal sinuses (opening to brain)
		Holes along spinal column
		Low hairline posteriorly: possible chromosomal abnormality
		Sparse or spotty hair: congenital goiter or chromosomal abnormality
Note color of nails	Pink	Yellowing of nail beds (meconium stained)
Note muscle strength/tone	Strong, tremulous	Flaccid, convulsions
		Muscular twitching, hypertonicity
Head and Neck Assessment Note shape of head	Fontanels: anterior open until 18 months; posterior closed shortly after birth; is 3–4 cm long and 2–3 cm wide; diamond shaped	Depressed fontanels indicate dehydration; closed or bulging indicate congenital anomalies; full or bulging indicate edema or increased ICP
	Posterior fontanel is 1–2 cm at birth and triangle shaped	Cephalohematoma that crosses the midline
		Microcephaly and macrocephaly
	Circumference is ¼ size of body and 2 cm larger than the check circumference	Cephalohematoma trauma from birth lasts up to 3 weeks
	Breech and cesarean newborn's heads are rounded and well shaped	Caput succedaneum occurring from a long labor and birth will disappear in about 1 week
Assess eyes	Slight edema of lids	Purulent discharge indicates infection
		Lateral upward slope of eye with an inner epicanthal fold in infants not of Asian descent
		Exophthalmos (bulging of eyeball): may be congenital anomaly, sign of congenital glaucoma or thyroid abnormality
		Enophthalmos (recession of eyeball): may indicate damage to brain or cervical spine
	Pupils equal and reactive to light by 3 weeks of age	Constricted pupil, unilateral dilated; unequal pupils due to CNS damage
	Intermittent strabismus (occasional crossing of eyes)	Fixed pupil, nystagmus (rhythmic nonpurposeful movement of eyeball): continuous strabismus
	Conjunctival or scleral hemorrhages	
	Symmetrical light reflex (light reflects off each eye in the same quadrant): sign of conjugate gaze	Haziness of cornea
	Blink reflex in response to light stimuli	Absence of red reflex; asymmetrical light reflex
	Corneal reflex present	Blink reflex absent indicates CNS injury
	Vision: tracks objects to midline; fixed focus on objects at a distance; prefers faces and black and white to color	Ulceration indicates herpes infection
		Cataracts from congenital infection
	Cry usually tearless	Excessive tearing from plugged tear ducts; could be narcotic withdrawal
Note placement of ears, shape and position	The top of the ear should be on an imaginary line from the edge of the eye	Low-set ears: may indicate chromosomal or renal system abnormality
Assess nose	Sneezes to clear nasal passageways	Flat or broad bridge of nose seen in Down syndrome
	Nose breathers	Flaring nostrils indicates respiratory distress
		Blockage of nares due to mucus or secretions
		Thick, bloody nasal discharge if infection present
Assess mouth	Gag, swallowing, sucking reflexes present	Absent of reflexes
	Hard and soft palates intact	Cleft lip, palate
		Flat, white nonremovable spots (thrush)
	Esophagus intact; drooling in newborns	Frequent vomiting: may indicate pyloric stenosis; esophageal atresia
		Vomitus with bile: fecal vomiting
		Profuse salivation: may indicate tracheoesophageal fistula

SKILL 16.1   Maternal and Newborn Assessments *(continued)*

TABLE 16–4   Newborn Assessment *(continued)*

ASSESSMENT	NORMAL	ABNORMAL
	Tongue moves freely in all directions; pink color; noncoated	Lack of movement indicates neurological damage
		White cheesy coating indicates thrush
Assess neck	Short, straight, extra skinfolds	Short neck in Turner syndrome
	Tonic neck reflex (Fencer position)	Distended neck veins
		Fractured clavicle
		Unusually short neck
		Excess posterior cervical skin
		Resistance to neck flexion
Chest and Lung Assessment Assess chest	2 cm smaller than head; wider than long; lower end of sternum may protrude	Funnel chest with congenital problems
		Depressed sternum
	Bilateral expansion with no retractions	Retractions, asymmetry of chest movements: indicates respiratory distress and possible pneumothorax
Assess respirations/lungs	Breath sounds louder in infants	Thoracic breathing, unequal motion of chest, rapid grasping or grunting respirations, flaring nares
	Bronchial breath sounds bilaterally	
	Rales may indicate normal newborn atelectasis	Deep sighing respirations
	Cough reflex absent until second day	Grunt on expiration: possible respiratory distress
Breasts	Flat with symmetrical nipples	SGA infants lack breast tissue
	Engorgement occurs third day; may have liquid discharge in full-term newborns	
Heart Assessment Assess the rate, rhythm, and murmurs of the heart	Rate: 100–160 bpm at birth; stabilizes at 120–140 bpm	Heart rate >200 or <100 bpm
	Regular rhythm	Irregular rhythm
	Murmurs: significance cannot usually be determined in newborn	Dextrocardia, enlarged heart
Abdomen and Gastrointestinal Tract Assessment Assess the abdomen	Prominent	Distention of abdominal veins: possible portal vein obstruction
	No protrusion of umbilicus, however, protrusion may be seen in infants of African descent	Umbilical hernia
	Umbilical cord with one vein and two arteries; soft granulation tissue at umbilicus; no bleeding	One artery present in umbilical cord: may indicate other anomalies
		Bleeding, redness or exudate indicates infection
Assess the gastrointestinal tract	Bowel sounds present	Visible peristaltic waves
	Liver 2–3 cm below right costal margin	Increased pitch or frequency: intestinal obstruction
	Spleen tip palpable	Decreased sounds: paralytic ileus
		Distention of abdomen
		Enlarged liver or spleen
		Midline suprapubic mass: may indicate Hirschsprung disease
Femoral pulses	Palpable	Absent or diminished in coarctation of aorta
	No bulges in inguinal area	Inguinal hernia
Genitourinary Tract Assessment Assess kidneys and bladder	May be able to palpate kidneys	Enlarged kidney
	Bladder percussed 1–4 cm above symphysis pubis	Distended bladder; presence of any masses
	Voids at birth or within 3 hr	Failure to void with 24–48 hr
Assess the genitalia	Edema and bruising after delivery	Ambiguous genitalia (chromosomal abnormality)
	Unusually large clitoris in females a short time after birth	Excessive vaginal bleeding indicates coagulation defect
	Vaginal mucoid or bloody discharge may be present in the first week	

(continued on next page)

SKILL 16.1   Maternal and Newborn Assessments (continued)

TABLE 16–4   Newborn Assessment (continued)

ASSESSMENT	NORMAL	ABNORMAL
Urethral orifice	Urethra opens on ventral surface of penile shaft Uncircumcised foreskin tight for 2–3 months	Hypospadias (urethra opens on the inferior surface of the penis) Epispadias (urethra opens on the dorsal surface of the penis) Ulceration of urethral orifice
Testes	Testes in scrotal sac or inguinal canal	Hydroceles in males Phimosis if still tight after 3 months Enlarged testes indicate tumor Small testes indicate Klinefelter syndrome or adrenal hyperplasia
Spine and Extremities Assessment Assess the spine	Straight spine; slight lordosis; full-term infant should hold head at 45-degree angle	Spina bifida, pilonidal sinus; scoliosis Unable to hold head or floppy trunk indicates neurological problems
Assess extremities	Soft click with thigh rotation; should abduct to more than 60 deg Skin creases Feet in straight line; flat feet normal for first 3 months; some infants may have a positional club-foot from position in utero	Asymmetry of movement Sharp click with thigh rotation: indicates possible congenital hip Uneven major gluteal folds: indicates possible congenital hip Polydactyly (extra digits on a hand or foot); syndactyly (webbing or fusion of fingers or toes) Talipes equinovarus (clubfoot)
Assess anus and rectum	Patent anus; passage of meconium within 48 hr after birth	Closed anus: no meconium
Reflexes	Rooting and sucking (turns in direction of stimulus to cheek or mouth—disappears about fourth to seventh month Palmar grasp (fingers grasp adult finger when palm is stimulated); goes away about third to fourth month Moro reflex (an involuntary startle response to stimulation; arms extend with palms up and thumbs flexed; normally disappears after 3–4 months) Stepping (will step alternatively when held upright and one foot is touching a flat surface); disappears about 4–5 months Babinski (fanning and extension of toes when sole of foot is stroked from heel across ball of foot); disappears at about 12 months	Poor sucking or fatigability in preterm Absence of reflex in preterm, neurological involvement or depressed newborns Neurological problems if response is asymmetrical Unilateral indicates fractured clavicle or nerve injury; complete absence suggests damage to the brain or spinal cord Neurological problems if asymmetrical Low spinal cord defects if no response

TABLE 16–5   Apgar Scoring

SIGN	0	1	2
Heart rate	Absent	Slow (<100 bpm)	>100 bpm
Respiratory effort	Absent	Slow, irregular	Good, crying
Muscle tone	Flaccid	Some flexion of extremities	Active motion
Reflex irritability	No response	Cry	Vigorous cry
Color	Blue, pale	Body pink, extremities blue	Completely pink

The Apgar scoring system is a method of evaluating a newborn's condition at 1 and 5 minutes after birth.

• Newborns who score 7–10 are considered free of immediate danger.
• Newborns who score 4–6 are moderately depressed.
• Newborns who score 0–3 are severely depressed.

Scores less than 7 at 5 minutes, repeat every 5 minutes for 20 minutes. Infant may be intubated unless two successive scores of 7 or more occur.

SKILL 16.2 Assisting with a Pelvic Examination

Equipment

- Vaginal specula of various sizes, warmed with water or on a heating pad prior to insertion
- Sterile gloves
- Water-soluble lubricant
- Materials for Pap smear or liquid-based Pap test method and cultures
- Good light source

Note: Lubricant may alter the results of tests and cultures and is not used during the speculum examination. Its use is reserved for the bimanual examination.

Preparation

- Introduce self, provide privacy, and ensure that the room is sufficiently warm by checking the room temperature and adjusting the thermostat if necessary. If overhead heat lamps are available, turn them on. Provide comfort and safety for client.
- Explain the procedure to the woman. If she has never had a pelvic examination, show her the equipment to be used as part of the explanation. **Rationale:** *Explaining the procedure helps reduce anxiety and increase cooperation.*
- Ask the woman to empty her bladder and to remove clothing below the waist. **Rationale:** *An empty bladder promotes comfort during the internal examination.*
- Have padding on the stirrups. If stirrups are not padded, the woman may prefer to leave her shoes on during the procedure. **Rationale:** *Stirrups are usually padded to ease the pressure of the feet against the metal and to decrease the discomfort associated with the touch of the cold stirrups. If they are not padded, however, wearing shoes accomplishes the same purpose.*
- Give the woman a disposable drape or sheet to use during the exam. Ask her to sit at the end of the examining table with the drape opened across her lap.
- Position the woman in the lithotomy position with her thighs flexed and adducted. Place her feet in the stirrups. Her buttocks should extend slightly beyond the edge of the examining table.
- Drape the woman with the sheet, leaving a flap so that the perineum can be exposed. **Rationale:** *This position provides the exposure necessary to conduct the examination effectively. The drape helps preserve the woman's sense of dignity and privacy.*

Procedure

1. The examiner dons gloves for the procedure. Explain each part of the procedure as the certified nurse-midwife, nurse practitioner, or physician performs it.

2. Let the woman know that the examiner begins with an inspection of the external genitalia. The speculum is then inserted to allow visualization of the cervix and vaginal walls and to obtain specimens for testing. After the speculum is withdrawn, the examiner performs a bimanual examination of the internal organs using the fingers of one hand inserted in the woman's vagina while the other hand presses over the woman's uterus and ovaries. The final step of the procedure is generally a rectal examination.

> **CLINICAL ALERT**
> With the examiner's consent (obtained beforehand), offer the woman a hand mirror so that she can watch all or part of the examination. This practice removes the "mystery" from the procedure and enables the woman to become familiar with the appearance of her body.

3. Ask the woman to breathe slowly and regularly and to use any method she finds effective in helping her to remain relaxed.
4. Let her know when the examiner is ready to insert the speculum and ask her to bear down. **Rationale:** *Relaxation helps decrease muscle tension. Bearing down helps open the vaginal orifice and relaxes the perineal muscles.*
5. After the speculum is withdrawn, lubricate the examiner's fingers prior to the bimanual examination. **Rationale:** *Lubrication decreases friction and eases insertion of the examiner's fingers.*
6. After the examiner has completed the examination and moved away from the woman, move to the end of the examination table and face the woman. Cover her with the drape. Apply gentle pressure to her knees and encourage her to move toward the head of the table. Assist her to remove her feet from the stirrups, then offer your hand to her and assist her to sit up. **Rationale:** *Assistance is important because the lithotomy position is an awkward one and many women, but especially those women who are pregnant, obese, or older, may find it difficult to get out of the stirrups.*
7. Provide her with tissues to wipe the lubricant from her perineum. **Rationale:** *Vaginal secretions and lubricant may be discharged from the vagina when the woman sits upright.*
8. Provide the woman with privacy while she dresses. Be sure that she is not dizzy and that she is standing or sitting safely before leaving the room. **Rationale:** *Lying supine may cause postural hypotension.*
9. Document per facility policy.

SKILL 16.3 Assessing Deep Tendon Reflexes and Clonus

Equipment

- Percussion hammer

> **CLINICAL ALERT**
> If a percussion hammer is not available, you may use the side of your hand to elicit deep tendon reflexes (DTRs).

Preparation

- Explain the procedure, the indications for its use, and the information that will be obtained.
- Most nurses check the patellar reflex and one other such as the biceps, triceps, or brachioradialis. **Rationale:** *DTRs are assessed*

(continued on next page)

SKILL 16.3 Assessing Deep Tendon Reflexes and Clonus *(continued)*

to gain information about CNS irritability secondary to preeclampsia and to assess the effects of magnesium sulfate if the woman is receiving it.

Procedure

1. Gather equipment and supplies. Introduce self and explain what procedure is to be done and why. Perform hand hygiene, following infection control measures, and verify client's identity. Provide privacy. Provide comfort and safety for client and self, including raising bed to appropriate height for procedure.
2. Elicit reflexes.
   - Patellar reflex. Position the woman with her legs hanging over the edge of the bed (feet should not be touching the floor) **❶**. Briskly strike the patellar tendon, which is located just below the patella. Normal response is extension or a thrusting forward of the foot. **Rationale:** *In an inpatient setting, the patellar reflex is often assessed while the woman lies supine. Flex her knees slightly and support them.*

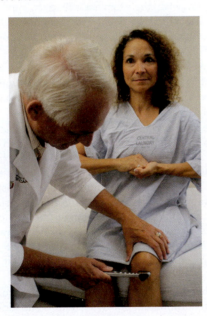

❶ Correct sitting position for eliciting the patellar reflex.

- Biceps reflex. Flex the woman's arm 45 degrees at the elbow and place your thumb on the biceps tendon. Allow your fingers to hold the biceps muscle. Strike your thumb in a slightly downward motion and assess the response. Normal response is flexion of the arm.
- Triceps reflex. Flex the woman's arm up to 90 degrees and allow her hand to hang against the side of her body. Using the percussion hammer, strike the triceps tendon just above the elbow. Normal response is contraction of the muscle, which causes extension of the arm.
- Brachioradialis reflex. Flex the woman's arm slightly and lay it on your forearm with her hand slightly pronated. Using the percussion hammer, strike the brachioradialis tendon, which is found about 2.5 to 5 cm (1 to 2 in.) above the wrist. Normal response is pronation of the forearm and flexion of the elbow. **Rationale:** *The correct position causes the muscle to be slightly stretched. Then when the tendon is stretched, with a tap the muscle should contract. Correct positioning and technique are essential to elicit the reflex.*

3. Grade reflexes. Reflexes are graded on a scale of 0 to 4+, as follows:

   4+ Hyperactive; very brisk, jerky, or clonic response; abnormal

   3+ Brisker than average; may not be abnormal

   2+ Average response; normal

   1+ Diminished response; low normal

   0   No response; abnormal

   Rationale: *Normally reflexes are 1+ or 2+. With CNS irritation, hyperreflexia may be present; with high magnesium levels, reflexes may be diminished or absent.*

4. Assess for clonus. With the woman's knee flexed and the leg supported, vigorously dorsiflex the foot, maintain the dorsiflexion momentarily, and then release. With a normal response, the foot returns to its normal position of plantar flexion. Clonus is present if the foot "jerks" or taps against the examiner's hand. If so, record the number of taps or beats of clonus. **Rationale:** *Clonus occurs with more pronounced hyperreflexia and indicates CNS irritability.*

5. Return bed to lowest height. Perform hand hygiene.
6. Report and document findings. For example: DTRs 2+, no clonus or DTRs 4+, 2 beats clonus.

SKILL 16.4 Assessment of Fetal Well-Being: Nonstress Test (NST)

Equipment

- External fetal heart rate and contraction monitors (ultrasound transducer and tocodynamometer)
- Ultrasonic gel

Preparation

- Identify client by comparing the name and medical record number appearing in the chart against identification arm band information.

- Verify the correct procedure as ordered by the physician/CNM for the correct client.
- Explain the procedure, purpose, and implications of the procedure to the woman and her support person. The purpose of the nonstress test is to assess fetal well-being by monitoring fetal activity and concurrent fetal heart rate (FHR) response to fetal activity.
- Provide for client privacy, comfort, and safety.
- Allow time for and encourage any questions the woman and her support person may have. Reinforce any teaching as necessary.

SKILL 16.4   Assessment of Fetal Well-Being: Nonstress Test (NST) *(continued)*

Procedure

1. Have the woman empty her bladder before the procedure begins.

2. Have the woman lie in a left-tilted semi-Fowler sitting position or in the left lateral position, comfortably, with pillows for support if needed. **Rationale:** *These positions displace the uterus to prevent compression of the vena cava and/or aorta. These positions also promote more fetal movement and are more likely to have a reactive tracing.*

3. Apply fetal heart rate and contraction monitors, applying the ultrasonic gel to the diaphragm of the ultrasound transducer to improve contact.

4. Monitor the fetal heart rate and any contraction activity for at least 20 minutes. Note any fetal movement. **Rationale:** *Accelerations in fetal heart rate should occur spontaneously and in response to fetal movement.*

5. If there are no accelerations in 20 minutes, continue monitoring 20 more minutes. **Rationale:** *The fetus may be in a sleep cycle in which there are usually no heart rate accelerations.*

6. If there are no accelerations or fetal movement during the testing period, stimulation of the fetus may be necessary (acoustic stimulation, maternal intake of cold liquids) ❶.

7. Document the procedure, results, any intervention(s) needed, and any need for further testing in the client's medical record and notify the ordering physician/CNM of the results of the NST per agency policy.

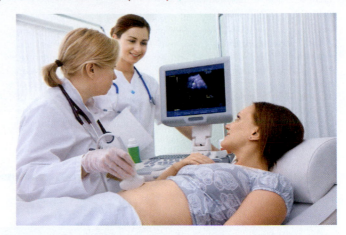

❶ Fetal acoustic stimulation testing. (@Alexander Raths/Fotolia)

TEST INTERPRETATION

Reactive NST (normal): Shows at least two accelerations of FHR with fetal movements of 15 beats per minute, lasting 15 seconds or more, over 20 minutes.

Nonreactive NST: Accelerations are not present or do not meet the reactive criteria. For example, the accelerations do not meet the requirements of 15 beats per minute or do not last 15 minutes. If the test is considered nonreactive (nonreassuring), further testing may be needed.

SKILL 16.5   Assessment of Fetal Well-Being: Biophysical Profile (BPP)

Equipment

- Ultrasound equipment
- Ultrasonic gel

Preparation

- Identify client by comparing the name and medical record number appearing in the chart against identification arm band information.
- Verify the correct procedure as ordered by the physician/CNM for the correct client.
- Introduce self. Explain the procedure, purpose, and implications of the procedure to the woman and her support person.
- Provide for client privacy. Position the client in semi-Fowler or side-lying position.
- Allow time for and encourage any questions the woman and her support person may have. Reinforce any teaching as necessary.

Procedure

This is performed by an ultrasonographer or RN who has had extensive education in ultrasonography for the purpose of obstetrical ultrasound surveillance.

1. Ultrasound scanning is performed to assess for the following:
   - Fetal breathing movement
   - Fetal movement of body or limbs
   - Fetal tone (extension and flexion) of extremities
   - Amniotic fluid volume
   - Reactive nonstress test (reactive FHR with activity).

2. A nonstress test is performed using either an external fetal monitor or ultrasound equipment.

3. A score of 2 is given to each normal finding and a score of 0 is given to each abnormal finding for a maximum total score of 10. Scores of 8 to 10 are considered normal (see **Table 16–6** ●).

4. Document the procedure, results, and any intervention(s) needed in the client's medical record and notify the ordering physician/CNM of the results of the BPP per agency policy.

Evidence-Based Practice

Antepartum Tests for Fetal Well-Being

Numerous tests exist to determine fetal well-being, ranging from maternal reporting of fetal movements ("count to 10" method) to invasive procedures like amniocentesis. However, limited definitive evidence exists regarding the benefit of antenatal testing in decreasing the perinatal mortality rate (PMR). Despite the lack of clear evidence, testing is widely used for various indications during pregnancy.

(continued on next page)

SKILL 16.5   Assessment of Fetal Well-Being: Biophysical Profile (BPP) *(continued)*

For example, the biophysical profile (BPP) is a commonly used set of tests of fetal well-being. BPP includes ultrasound monitoring of fetal movement, fetal tone, and fetal breathing; ultrasound assessment of liquor volume; and assessment of fetal heart rate. Studies of BPP to date have found no significant differences between the BPP and non-BPP groups in perinatal deaths or Apgar scores of less than 7 at 5 minutes, but they do suggest an increased risk of caesarean section. Furthermore, no studies have addressed the impact of BPP on factors like neonatal morbidity, length of hospital stay, or parental satisfaction.

Of all antenatal assessment methods, Doppler ultrasound has been tested most rigorously. Studies indicate that routine umbilical artery Doppler screening has no apparent benefit in low-risk pregnancies (no significant difference in PMR, neonatal morbidity, Apgar scores under 7 at 5 minutes, cesarean section, labor induction, or resuscitation). However, for high-risk pregnancies, use of Doppler ultrasound to evaluate the fetal umbilical artery was associated with a significant reduction in perinatal deaths.

Given that most antenatal tests have not been proven effective in preventing incidence of PMR, obstetricians should be cautious in recommending their use, especially in low-risk clients. Informed consent should always be obtained from the woman before ordering a test.

Data from O'Neill & Thorp (2012), Haws et al. (2009), and Lalor et al. (2008).

TABLE 16–6   Criteria for Biophysical Profile Scoring

COMPONENT	NORMAL (SCORE = 2)	ABNORMAL (SCORE = 0)
Fetal breathing movements	≥1 episode of rhythmic breathing lasting ≥30 sec within 30 min	≤30 sec of breathing in 30 min
Gross body movements	≥3 discrete body or limb movements in 30 min (episodes of active continuous movement considered as single movement)	≤2 movements in 30 min
Fetal tone	≥1 episode of extension of a fetal extremity with return to flexion, or opening or closing of hand	No movements or extension/flexion
Amniotic fluid volume	Single vertical pocket > 2 cm AFI > 5 cm	Largest single vertical pocket ≤ 2 cm AFI < 5 cm
Nonstress test	≥2 accelerations of ≥15 bpm for ≥15 sec in 20–40 min	0 or 1 acceleration in 20–40 min

SKILL 16.6   Performing an Intrapartum Vaginal Examination

Equipment

- Clean, disposable gloves if membranes not ruptured
- Sterile gloves if membranes ruptured
- Lubricant
- Nitrazine test tape
- Slide
- Sterile cotton-tipped swab (Q-tip)

CLINICAL ALERT
Use nonlatex gloves if the woman has a latex allergy.

Preparation

- Check physician's orders, introduce self, identify client, and explain the procedure, the indications for the exam, what the exam may feel like, and that it may cause discomfort.
- Assess for latex allergies. Provide for client privacy, comfort, and safety. Perform hand hygiene.
- Position the woman with her thighs flexed and abducted. Instruct her to put the heels of her feet together. Drape the woman with a sheet, leaving a flap to access the perineum. **Rationale:** *This position provides access to the woman's perineum. The drape ensures privacy.*

- Encourage the woman to relax her muscles and legs. **Rationale:** *Relaxation decreases muscle tension and increases comfort.*
- Inform the woman prior to touching her. Be gentle.

Before the Procedure

Test for Fluid Leakage

- If fluid leakage has been reported or noted, use Nitrazine test tape and a Q-tip with a slide for the fern test before performing the exam.
- The fern test is done by inserting the swab in the pool of fluid in the posterior vagina and then applying the fluid to a slide. **Rationale:** *As long as lubricant has not been used, Nitrazine tape registers a change in pH if amniotic fluid is present.*

Procedure

1. Pull glove on dominant hand. **Rationale:** *A single glove is worn when membranes are intact. If a sterile exam is needed, both hands will be gloved with sterile gloves.*
2. Using your gloved hand, position the hand with the wrist straight and the elbow tilted downward. Insert your well-lubricated second and index fingers of the gloved hand gently into the vagina until they touch the cervix. Use care when

SKILL 16.6   Performing an Intrapartum Vaginal Examination (*continued*)

positioning your hand. **Rationale:** *This position allows the fingertips to point toward the umbilicus and find the cervix.*

3. If the woman expresses discomfort, acknowledge it and apologize. Pause for a moment and allow her to relax before progressing. **Rationale:** *This validates the woman's discomfort and helps her feel more in control.*

4. To determine the status of labor progress, perform the vaginal examination during and between contractions. **Rationale:** *Cervical effacement, dilation, and fetal station are affected by the presence of a contraction.*

5. Palpate for the opening, or a depression, in the cervix. Estimate the diameter of the depression to identify the amount of dilation ❶. **Rationale:** *This allows determination of effacement and dilation.*

6. Determine the status of the fetal membranes by observing for leakage of amniotic fluid. If fluid is expressed, test for amniotic fluid.

7. Palpate the presenting part ❷. **Rationale:** *Determining the presenting part is necessary to assess the position of the fetus and to evaluate fetal descent.*

8. Assess the fetal descent and station by identifying the position of the fetal presenting part in relation to the ischial spines. Station progresses from −5 to +4 ❸.

9. Remove glove and perform hand hygiene.

10. Document findings on the client's chart and on the fetal monitor strip if a fetal monitor is being used.

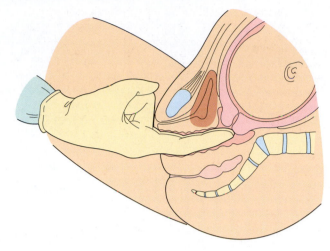

❶ To gauge cervical dilation, place the index and middle fingers against the cervix and determine the size of the opening. Before labor begins, the cervix is long (approximately 2.5 cm [1 in.]), the sides feel thick, and the cervical canal is closed, so an examining finger cannot be inserted. During labor, the cervix begins to dilate, and the size of the opening progresses from 1 to 10 cm (0.4 to 4 in.) in diameter.

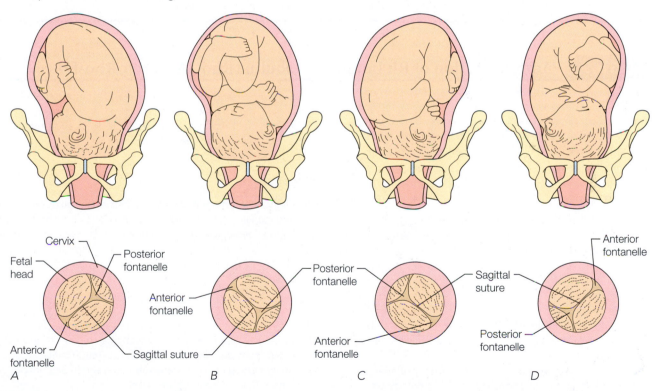

❷ Palpating the presenting part (portion of the fetus that enters the pelvis first). A, Left occiput anterior (LOA). The occiput (area over the occipital bone on the posterior part of the fetal head) is in the left anterior quadrant of the woman's pelvis. When the fetus is LOA, the posterior fontanelle (located just above the occipital bone and triangular in shape) is in the upper left quadrant of the maternal pelvis. B, Left occiput posterior (LOP). The posterior fontanelle is in the lower left quadrant of the maternal pelvis. C, Right occiput anterior (ROA). The posterior fontanelle is in the upper right quadrant of the maternal pelvis. D, Right occiput posterior (ROP). The posterior fontanelle is in the lower right quadrant of the maternal pelvis.

Note: The anterior fontanelle is diamond shaped. Because of the roundness of the fetal head, only a portion of the anterior fontanelle can be seen in each of the views, so it appears to be triangular in shape.

(*continued on next page*)

SKILL 16.6 Performing an Intrapartum Vaginal Examination (continued)

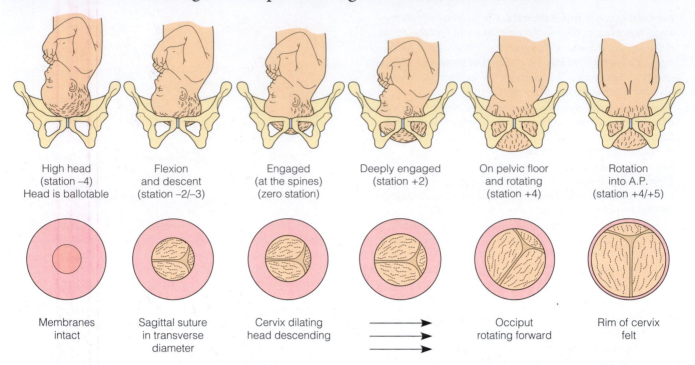

| High head (station –4) Head is ballotable | Flexion and descent (station –2/–3) | Engaged (at the spines) (zero station) | Deeply engaged (station +2) | On pelvic floor and rotating (station +4) | Rotation into A.P. (station +4/+5) |

| Membranes intact | Sagittal suture in transverse diameter | Cervix dilating head descending | | Occiput rotating forward | Rim of cervix felt |

❸ The fetal head progressing through the pelvis. Bottom: The changes that will be detected on palpation of the occiput through the cervix while doing a vaginal examination.

Source: From Myles, M. F. (1975). *Textbook for midwives* (p. 246). Edinburgh, Scotland: Churchill-Livingstone.

SKILL 16.7 Administration of Rh Immune Globulin (RhoGAM, HypRho-D)

Equipment

- Rh immune globulin, which is obtained from the blood bank or pharmacy according to agency protocol (Lot numbers for the drug and the crossmatch should be the same.)
- Syringe and IM needle

Preparation

- Check physician's order. Confirm that Rh immune globulin is indicated by checking the client's prenatal or intrapartum record to verify that she is Rh negative. Then confirm that alloimmunization has not occurred—maternal indirect Coombs' negative. Postpartum, confirm that the baby is Rh positive but not sensitized (direct Coombs' negative) and that the mother's indirect Coombs' is negative. Rh immune globulin is not indicated if the infant is Rh negative. **Rationale:** *Rh immune globulin is only indicated for an Rh-negative, unsensitized woman who gave birth to an Rh-positive infant.*
- Confirm that the woman does not have a history of allergies to immune globulin preparations by checking entries on medication allergies in her chart and by asking her whether she has ever had any allergic reactions to medications, globulins, or blood products. **Rationale:** *Rh immune globulin is made from the plasma portion of blood. Allergic reactions are possible.*
- Explain the purpose and procedure. Have a consent form signed if required by agency policy. **Rationale:** *Many agencies require separate consent for the administration of Rh immune globulin because it is a blood product. The woman should*

clearly understand the purpose of the Rh immune globulin, its rationale, the administration procedure, and any related risks. Generally the primary side effects are redness and tenderness at the injection site and allergic responses.

Procedure

1. Gather equipment and supplies. Introduce self, identify client, and explain what procedure is to be done and why. Perform hand hygiene, following infection control measures, and verify client's identity. Provide privacy. Provide comfort and safety for client and self, including raising bed to appropriate height for procedure.
2. Administer one vial of 300 mg Rh immune globulin IM in the deltoid muscle.
3. An immune globulin microdose is used after miscarriage, elective abortion, ectopic pregnancy, or molar pregnancy occurring within the first 12 weeks' gestation. Antepartum, the Rh immune globulin is generally given within 3 hours but not longer than 72 hours of the event.
4. If a larger bleed is suspected at birth (as in cases of severe abruptio placentae), additional doses may be administered at one time using multiple sites or at regular intervals as long as all doses are given within 72 hours of childbirth. **Rationale:** *The normal 300-mcg dose provides passive immunity following exposure of up to 15 mL of transfused RBCs or 30 mL of fetal blood.*
5. Provide opportunities for the woman to ask questions and express concerns. **Rationale:** *Many women, especially*

SKILL 16.7   Administration of Rh Immune Globulin (RhoGAM, HypRho-D) *(continued)*

primigravidas, are not aware of the risks for an Rh-positive fetus of a sensitized Rh-negative mother. They need to understand the importance of receiving Rh immune globulin for each pregnancy to ensure continued protection.

6. Return bed to lowest height. Perform hand hygiene.
7. Document according to agency policy. Most agencies chart lot number, route, dose, and client education.

SKILL 16.8   Assisting During Amniocentesis

Equipment

- Sterile gloves
- 22-gauge spinal needle with stylet
- 10- and 20-mL syringes
- 1% lidocaine (Xylocaine)
- Povidone-iodine (Betadine)
- Three 10-mL test tubes with tops (amber colored or covered with tape)
  Rationale: *Amniotic fluid must be protected from the light to prevent breakdown of bilirubin.*

Preparation

- Explain the procedure and the indications for it and reassure the woman. **Rationale:** *Explanation of the procedure decreases anxiety.*
- Determine whether an informed consent form has been signed. If not, verify that the woman's physician has explained the procedure and ask her to sign a consent form. **Rationale:** *It is the physician's responsibility to obtain informed consent. The woman's signature indicates her awareness of the risks and gives her consent to the procedure.*
- Provide for client privacy.

Procedure

1. Gather equipment and supplies. Introduce self. Perform hand hygiene, following infection control measures, and verify client's identity. Provide comfort and safety for client and self, including raising bed to appropriate height for procedure.
2. Obtain baseline vital signs, including maternal blood pressure (BP), pulse, respirations, temperature, and fetal heart rate (FHR) before the procedure begins; then monitor BP, pulse, respirations, and FHR every 15 minutes during the procedure.
3. Provide gel for the real-time ultrasound and assist with the procedure to assess needle insertion during the procedure as needed. **Rationale:** *Amniocentesis is usually performed laterally in the area of fetal small parts, where pockets of amniotic fluid are often seen. Real-time ultrasound will identify fetal parts, locate the placenta, and locate pockets of amniotic fluid.*
4. Cleanse the woman's abdomen with Betadine solution. **Rationale:** *Cleansing the abdomen prior to needle insertion helps decrease the risk of infection.*
5. The physician dons gloves, inserts the needle into the identified pocket of fluid, and withdraws a sample ❶.
6. Obtain the test tubes from the physician. Label the tubes with the woman's correct identification and send to the lab with the appropriate lab slips.

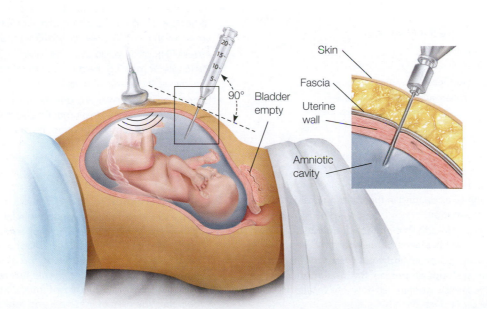

❶ Amniocentesis.

(continued on next page)

SKILL 16.8 Assisting During Amniocentesis (continued)

7. Monitor the woman and reassess her vital signs.
   - Determine the woman's BP, pulse, respirations, and the FHR.
   - Palpate the woman's fundus to assess for uterine contractions.
   - Monitor her using an external fetal monitor for 20 to 30 minutes after the amniocentesis.
   - Assist with treatment course to counteract any supine hypotension and to increase venous return and cardiac output. **Rationale:** *Monitoring maternal and fetal status post-procedure provides information about response to the procedure and helps detect any complications such as inadvertent fetal puncture.*
8. Assess the woman's blood type and determine any need for Rh immune globulin.
9. Administer Rh immune globulin if indicated. **Rationale:** *To prevent Rh sensitization in an Rh-negative woman, Rh immune globulin is administered prophylactically following amniocentesis.*

> **CLINICAL ALERT**
> Have the woman lie on her left side to ensure adequate placental perfusion.

10. Instruct the woman to report any of the following changes or symptoms to her primary caregiver:
    - Unusual fetal hyperactivity or, conversely, any lack of fetal movement
    - Vaginal discharge—either clear drainage or bleeding
    - Uterine contractions or abdominal pain
    - Fever or chills
    Rationale: *The woman needs to know how to recognize changes or symptoms that require further evaluation.*
11. Encourage the woman to engage only in light activities for 24 hours and to increase her fluid intake. **Rationale:** *A decrease in maternal activity will decrease uterine irritability and increase uteroplacental circulation. Increased hydration helps replace amniotic fluid through the uteroplacental circulation.*
12. Return bed to lowest height. Perform hand hygiene.
13. Complete the client record. Document the type of procedure, the date and time, and the name of the physician who performed the procedure. Also record the maternal–fetal response, disposition of the specimen, and discharge teaching.

▶ INTRAPARTUM CARE

Expected Outcomes

1. Ongoing fetal heartbeat documentation occurs with external electronic fetal monitoring.
2. Induction of labor with Pitocin progresses without evidence of fetal distress.
3. The epidural injection is completed as painlessly as possible.

SKILL 16.9 Assisting with Amniotomy (AROM: Artificial Rupture of Membranes)

Equipment

- Sterile vaginal exam glove (for MD/CNM)
- Sterile gloves (for nurse)
- Sterile amnio hook
- Sterile water-soluble lubricant
- Doppler or monitor (external or internal)
- Waterproof linen
- Towels

Preparation

- Introduce self and identify client by comparing the name and medical record number appearing in the chart against identification arm band information.
- Verify the correct procedure for the correct client. Ensure informed signed consent has been obtained from client.
- Explain the procedure, purpose, and implications of the procedure to the woman and support person. **Rationale:** *Anticipatory guidance will decrease the woman's anxiety and facilitate cooperation during the procedure.*
- Provide comfort and safety for client and self, including raising bed to appropriate height for procedure.

- Assist the woman to the lithotomy position, maintaining privacy. **Rationale:** *Proper positioning provides easier access to the cervix and enhances the woman's ability to relax.*
- Assess FHR prior to, during, and following amniotomy. **Rationale:** *Rupturing the amniotic membranes changes the pressure inside the uterus and also causes risk of a prolapsed cord.*
- Encourage and answer any questions the woman or her support person(s) may have at this time. Reassure the woman that amniotic fluid is constantly produced, because she may worry about a "dry birth."

Procedure

1. Don sterile gloves.
2. Using sterile technique, apply sterile lubricant to the MD's/CNM's sterile gloved hand, and open the package containing the amnio hook for the MD/CNM to grasp. **Rationale:** *Lubricant decreases friction between the gloved hand and vaginal wall during the procedure. Sterile technique is essential during amniotomy to prevent potential contamination and decrease the risks of maternal and fetal infection.*
3. Once the membranes are ruptured and fluid is seen, note the color, amount, odor, and presence of meconium or blood.

SKILL 16.9   Assisting with Amniotomy (continued)

Rationale: *Amniotic fluid should be clear or slightly cloudy and without any odor. Meconium-stained or bloody amniotic fluid indicates or places the fetus at risk for complications. Foul-smelling fluid may indicate infection. Absent, decreased, or increased amounts of amniotic fluid may indicate fetal stress.*

4. Assess fetal heart rate immediately before and after the rupture of membranes. **Rationale:** *Fetal well-being must be confirmed prior to and after amniotomy to assess fetal tolerance to the procedure.*

5. Maternal temperature should be assessed every 2 hours or more frequently if febrile and/or MD/CNM ordered. **Rationale:** *A rise in maternal temperature might indicate an intrauterine infection (chorioamnionitis).*

6. While wearing disposable gloves, cleanse the perineum with a warm washcloth, dry the perineal area, and change the waterproof linen pads as needed. **Rationale:** *A dry underpad enhances maternal comfort.*

7. Keep vaginal examinations to a minimum. **Rationale:** *To prevent introducing ascending infections.*

8. Assist the woman to a comfortable position.

9. Return bed to lowest position. Perform hand hygiene.

10. Document date, time of ruptured membranes, color, amount and odor (if applicable), who performed the procedure, cervical exam results, fetal heart rate, and how the client tolerated the procedure.

SKILL 16.10   Auscultating Fetal Heart Rate

Equipment

- Doppler device
- Ultrasonic gel

Preparation

- Explain the procedure, the indications for it, and the information that will be obtained.
- Uncover the woman's abdomen.

Procedure

1. Gather equipment and supplies. Introduce self, identify client, and explain what procedure is to be done and why. Perform hand hygiene, following infection control measures, and verify client's identity. Provide privacy. Provide comfort and safety for client and self, including raising bed to appropriate height for procedure.

2. To use the Doppler:
   - Place ultrasonic gel on the diaphragm of the Doppler. Gel is used to maintain contact with the maternal abdomen and enhances conduction of sound.
   - Place the Doppler diaphragm on the woman's abdomen halfway between the umbilicus and symphysis and in the midline. You are most likely to hear the FHR in this area. Listen carefully for the sound of the fetal heartbeat

3. Check the woman's pulse against the fetal sounds you hear. If the rates are the same, reposition the Doppler and try again. **Rationale:** *If the rates are the same, you are probably hearing the maternal pulse and not the FHR.*

4. If the rates are not similar, count the FHR for 1 full minute. Note that the FHR has a double rhythm and only one sound is counted.

5. If you do not locate the FHR, move the Doppler laterally ❶.

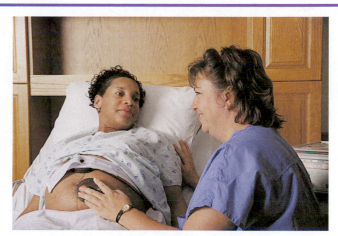

❶ When the fetal heartbeat is picked up by the electronic monitor, the sound can be heard by everyone in the room.

6. Auscultate the FHR between, during, and for 30 seconds following uterine contractions. Frequency recommendations are as follows:
   - *Low-risk women:* Every 30 minutes in the first stage and every 15 minutes in the second stage.
   - *High-risk women:* Every 15 minutes in the first stage and every 5 minutes in the second stage.
   Rationale: *This evaluation provides the opportunity to assess the fetal status and response to labor.*

7. Document FHR data (rate and rhythm), characteristics of uterine activity, and any actions taken as a result of the FHR.

> **CLINICAL ALERT**
> The FHR is heard most clearly through the fetal back. Locate the fetal back using the Leopold maneuvers.

SKILL 16.11   External Electronic Fetal Monitoring

Equipment

- Monitor
- Two elastic monitor belts
- Tocodynamometer ("toco")
- Ultrasound transducer
- Ultrasound gel

(continued on next page)

SKILL 16.11 External Electronic Fetal Monitoring (*continued*)

Preparation

■ Check physician's order. Gather equipment and supplies.

Procedure

1. Introduce self, explain what procedure is to be done, the indications for it, and the information that will be obtained. Perform hand hygiene, following infection control measures, and verify client's identity. Provide privacy. Provide comfort and safety for client and self, including raising bed to appropriate height for procedure.
2. Have the woman empty her bladder.
3. Turn on the monitor and place the two elastic belts around the woman's abdomen.
4. Place the toco over the uterine fundus off the midline on the area palpated to be most firm during contractions. Secure it with one of the elastic belts. **Rationale:** *The uterine fundus is the area of greatest contractility.*
5. Note the UC tracing. The resting tone tracing (that is, without a UC) should be recording on the 10 or 15 mmHg pressure line. Adjust the line to reflect that reading. **Rationale:** *If the resting tone is set on the zero line, there often is a constant grinding noise.*
6. Apply the ultrasonic gel to the diaphragm of the ultrasound transducer. **Rationale:** *Ultrasonic gel is used to maintain contact with the maternal abdomen. The ultrasonic beam is directed toward the fetal heart.*
7. Place the diaphragm on the maternal abdomen in the midline between the umbilicus and the symphysis pubis.

8. Listen for the FHR, which will have a whiplike sound. Move the diaphragm laterally if necessary to obtain a stronger sound ❶.
9. When the FHR is located, attach the second elastic belt snugly to the transducer ❷. **Rationale:** *Firm contact is necessary to maintain a steady tracing.*

CLINICAL ALERT

Evaluating the FHR tracing provides information about fetal status and response to the stress of labor. The presence of reassuring characteristics is associated with good fetal outcomes. Rapid identification of nonreassuring characteristics allows prompt interventions and the opportunity to determine the fetal response to the interventions.

---

10. Place the following information on the beginning of the fetal monitor paper: date, time, woman's name, gravida, para, membrane status, and name of physician or CNM. **Rationale:** *Each birthing unit may have specific guidelines about additional information to include.*
11. Return bed to lowest height. Perform hand hygiene.
12. Ongoing documentation should provide information about FHR, including baseline rate in beats per minute (bpm), presence of variability, response to uterine contractions (accelerations or decelerations), procedures performed, changes in position and the like, as well as any therapy initiated.

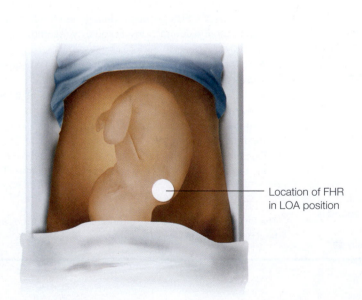

Location of FHR in LOA position

A

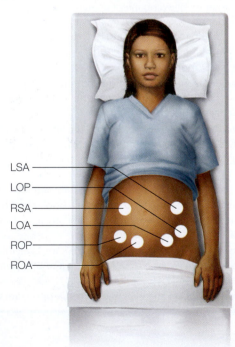

LSA
LOP
RSA
LOA
ROP
ROA

B

❶ Location of the FHR in relation to the more commonly seen fetal positions.

SKILL 16.11   External Electronic Fetal Monitoring *(continued)*

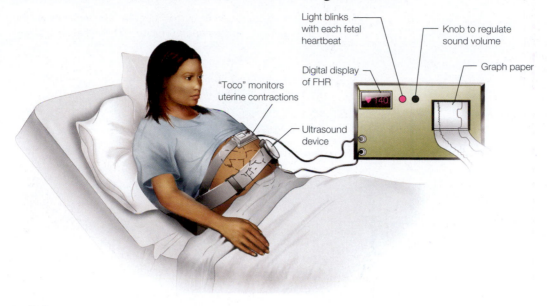

Light blinks with each fetal heartbeat

Knob to regulate sound volume

Digital display of FHR

Graph paper

"Toco" monitors uterine contractions

Ultrasound device

♥140

2 External electronic fetal monitoring.

SKILL 16.12   Internal Electronic Fetal Monitoring: Application of Fetal Scalp Electrode

Equipment

- Sterile exam glove
- Sterile water-soluble lubricant
- Spiral fetal scalp electrode apparatus
- Fetal monitor
- Scalp electrode cable
- Grounding pad (usually found in electrode packaging)

Preparation

- Check physician's orders. Introduce self and identify client by comparing name and medical record number appearing in the chart against identification arm band information.
- Verify correct procedure for correct client.
- Provide for client privacy. Provide comfort and safety for client and self, including raising bed to appropriate height for procedure.
- Explain the procedure, purpose, and implications of using a fetal scalp electrode to client and support person. **Rationale:** *This method of monitoring provides more accurate continuous data than external monitoring because the signal is clearer and movement of the fetus or woman does not interrupt it.*
- Assist the woman into lithotomy position, providing privacy.
- Woman's membranes must have already ruptured spontaneously or been ruptured by the physician or CNM. **Rationale:** *Fetal scalp electrode cannot be applied to the scalp if the membranes are covering the scalp, and RNs are not allowed to rupture membranes.*

Procedure

1. Using sterile technique, open lubricant package, don a sterile glove on the dominant hand, and apply lubricant to the glove with nondominant hand. **Rationale:** *Sterile technique is essential to decrease the risk of intrauterine infection.*
2. Perform vaginal exam to determine dilation and presentation of the fetus. Ensure presenting part is vertex. **Rationale:** *The fetal scalp electrode is placed on the fetal occiput. To do so, the membranes must be ruptured, the cervix must be dilated at least 2 cm, the presenting part must be known, and it must be down against the cervix.*
3. Apply fetal scalp electrode according to package directions on a firm area of the fetal vertex, avoiding fontanelles, face, genitals, etc. This usually involves inserting the electrode within the firm plastic guide. Place end of the guide/electrode against firm area of the scalp, and rotate electrode end clockwise until resistance is met. Release the guide according to package directions and discard. **Rationale:** *Care must be taken to avoid attaching the monitor to soft tissue, which could result in fetal trauma.*
4. Connect spiral electrode wire to a leg plate taped to mother's inner thigh with a grounding pad, following package instructions. This in turn is attached to the electronic fetal monitor **1**.
5. Verify fetal heart rate is tracing before discontinuing the intermittent or continuous external monitor.
6. To remove fetal scalp electrode, disconnect the electrode wire from the cable and rotate the lead counterclockwise. Once removed, visually examine the electrode to ensure it is intact. If unable to remove before going for a cesarean birth, tape electrode wire to the mother's thigh and notify the surgeon.
7. Return bed to lowest height. Perform hand hygiene.
8. Document date and time of application and removal, including the condition of the electrode (intact).

(continued on next page)

SKILL 16.12 **Internal Electronic Fetal Monitoring** (*continued*)

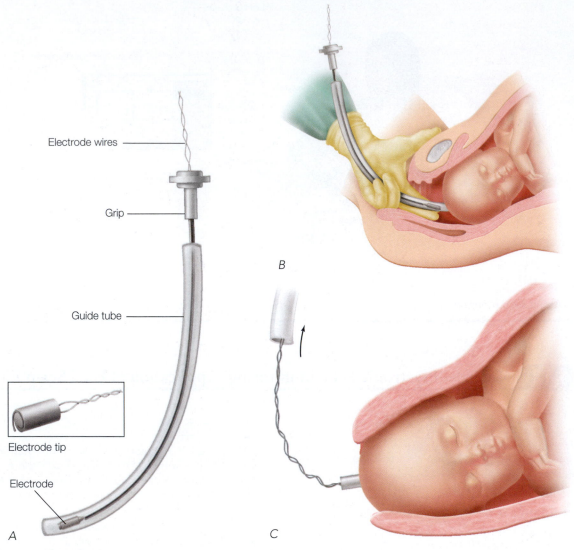

1 Technique for internal, direct fetal monitoring. *A*, Spiral electrode. *B*, Attaching the spiral electrode to the scalp. *C*, Attached spiral electrode with the guide tube removed.

SKILL 16.13 **Assisting with and Monitoring a Client Undergoing Induction of Labor**

Equipment

- Fetal and contraction monitoring equipment (for Pitocin infusion)
- IV fluids (per agency policy, MD/CNM orders)
- IV administration sets (for Pitocin infusion)
- IV infusion pump (two if available) for Pitocin infusion
- Appropriate induction medications
- Sterile exam gloves, sterile lubricant (cervical ripening)

Preparation

- Introduce self and identify client by comparing name and medical record number appearing in the chart against identification arm band information.
- Obtain an order for the procedure, and ensure a written order has been placed in the client's chart.

- Verify correct procedure as ordered by physician/CNM for the correct client.
- Explain the procedure, purpose, and implications of the procedure to the woman and her support person. **Rationale:** *The mother and her family need to be aware that induction of labor may take longer than spontaneous labor. They also need to know there may be limitations on food intake and activity and that continuous fetal monitoring and frequent assessments may be necessary due to the method of induction.*
- Provide for client privacy, comfort, and safety.
- Obtain Pitocin premixed bag from pharmacy or mix 10 units Pitocin per 1,000 mL secondary fluid. Obtain cervical ripening agent.
- Allow time for and encourage any questions the woman and her support person may have. Reinforce any teaching as necessary.

SKILL 16.13   Assisting with and Monitoring a Client Undergoing Induction (*continued*)

Evidence-Based Practice

Possible Side Effects of Oxytocin (Pitocin)

The body of a pregnant woman entering labor typically produces oxytocin, a hormone that increases the intensity and duration of contractions and aids delivery. When this normal process does not occur within 2 weeks of the due date or in the presence of signs like oligohydramnios (insufficient fluid surrounding the baby), synthetic oxytocin (Pitocin) is often administered to initiate the birthing process and provide a more positive outcome for mother and newborn. Side effects of Pitocin for mothers are generally fairly minor and include irritation at the injection site, appetite loss, nausea, vomiting, and cramping. Effects on the newborn have not generally been noted.

A 2013 study, reported at a conference of the American Congress of Obstetricians and Gynecologists (ACOG), examined the effect of Pitocin on 3,000 full-term infants delivered between 2009 and 2011. The study (ACOG, 2013) showed an association between use of Pitocin and Apgar scores lower than 7 at 5 minutes. Pitocin also was an independent risk factor for unexpected admission to the NICU lasting more than 24 hours for full-term infants.

The study concluded that more research is warranted to examine the risk of Pitocin's side effects on newborn babies and to define a systematic process for determining when Pitocin is medically necessary to induce labor.

Data from American Congress of Obstetricians and Gynecologists (2013), Siddique (2013), and Mayo Clinic (2011).

Procedure

Oxytocin (Pitocin)

1. Apply fetal and contraction monitors per unit policy. Assess for reactive or reassuring fetal heart rate tracing. **Rationale:** *A baseline of fetal well-being and uterine activity should be established before induction so that the nurse will recognize complications associated with oxytocin administrations, such as uterine hyperstimulation and fetal distress.*

2. Start IV infusion using aqueous solution at 125 mL/hr. **Rationale:** *This is done to keep the woman hydrated and to have an intravenous line available when the oxytocin infusion is stopped.*

3. Assess maternal vital signs and hydration status. **Rationale:** *Ongoing assessment of the woman's fluid balance (intake and output) is necessary because oxytocin has an antidiuretic effect.*

4. Attach secondary line to an infusion pump. **Rationale:** *An intravenous infusion pump must be used during oxytocin induction to ensure that accurate volume and dosage of oxytocin are administered to the woman.*

5. Start Pitocin infusion per agency policy and increase accordingly. One suggested method is to begin at 1 to 2 milliunits/min and increase by 1 to 2 milliunits/min every 30 to 40 minutes.

6. Evaluate fetal heart rate pattern, contraction pattern, and maternal vital signs before each increase in Pitocin. **Rationale:** *Accurate monitoring of uterine contraction frequency, duration, and intensity and uterine resting tone is essential to evaluate the effect of each oxytocin dosage level and determine the need to increase the infusion rate.*

7. Increase Pitocin rate until adequate labor is established and then maintain at the current rate. Decrease Pitocin if hypersystole occurs, per agency policy. **Rationale:** *Because the half-life of oxytocin is very short (1 to 6 minutes), stopping an oxytocin infusion may quickly reverse the effects of excessive uterine activity and improve fetal oxygenation.*

VARIATION: MISOPROSTOL (CYTOTEC)

- Don sterile glove.
- Monitor fetal heart rate and contractions per agency policy.
- Have IV infusion or IV access established, per agency policy.
- Have the woman empty her bladder prior to insertion of cervical ripening agent.
- Perform sterile vaginal exam, establishing the cervix is "unfavorable" for induction using Pitocin only (1 cm or less, little to no effacement).
- Remove glove, wash hands, don sterile glove, apply minimal lubricant, and insert two fingers (second and third digits) into the vagina with 25 micrograms (1/4 tablet) misoprostol at end of fingers. It is placed in the posterior vaginal fornix.
- Have the woman remain in bed for 30 minutes following insertion and then may allow up to void.
- This process may be repeated every 3 to 6 hours for up to 24 hours. The physician/CNM should be notified if hyperstimulation occurs or if there is no onset of labor.
- Pitocin should not be administered less than 4 hours after the last Cytotec dose.
- The fetal heart rate/contraction pattern should be evaluated for 3 hours following the insertion of misoprostol.
- Monitor closely for uterine hyperstimulation.

VARIATION: DINOPROSTONE (PGE2) (CERVIDIL OR PREPIDIL)

Same procedures as for misoprostol except as follows:

- Cervidil (10 mg): Administer as vaginal insert, × 1 dose. Monitor for 2 hours after insertion.
- Prepidil (0.5 mg): Administer intracervically. Monitor for 1 to 2 hours. May repeat after 6 hours. No more than 3 doses in 24 hours. If hypersystole occurs, remove medication by gently pulling attached string out of vagina.

8. Document the procedures, results, vital signs, fetal heart rate/contraction patterns, and labor progress in the client's medical record, including date and times of administration of medication and any complications.

SKILL 16.14 Assisting With and Caring for a Client with an Epidural

Equipment

- Fetal heart rate and contraction monitoring equipment as ordered
- Intravenous fluid and apparatus as ordered and per hospital policy
- Epidural administration set
- Anesthetic medications per anesthesia department protocol, if certified registered nurse anesthetist (CRNA) or anesthesiologist does not provide it
- High-pressure volumetric pump if epidural will be a continuous infusion
- Ephedrine syringe, dosage according to hospital protocol

Preparation

- Introduce self and identify client by comparing the name and medical record number appearing in the medical record against identification arm band information.
- Verify the correct procedure for the correct client. Document informed consent by the client. Ensure anesthesia personnel and/or the obstetrician explain possible side effects and complications.
- Explain the procedure and interventions that may be required because of the epidural: continuous intravenous infusion, continuous fetal monitoring, complete bed rest, indwelling or intermittent urinary catheterization, frequent blood pressure assessments, and other interventions according to hospital policy. **Rationale:** *The woman may be focused on pain relief and not aware of further interventions that will be required due to epidural infusion.*
- Obtain the physician/CNM order for epidural.
- Notify anesthesia personnel per hospital policy.
- Throughout the procedure and following, allow time to answer any questions the woman or her support person may have. Follow up with further teaching regarding any matter that may have been unforeseen or out of the ordinary.

Procedure

1. Provide for client privacy and perform hand hygiene. Provide comfort and safety for client and self, including raising bed to appropriate height for procedure. Obtain maternal baseline vital signs, fetal heart rate, and variability. The fetal heart rate tracing should show a reassuring tracing before starting the epidural process.
2. Administer an IV fluid bolus per hospital protocol before the epidural is begun (usually 500 to 1,000 mL lactated Ringer solution). **Rationale:** *This is to avoid maternal hypotension associated with the vasodilation common with epidurals.*
3. Assist and support the woman in position per anesthesia personnel request (usually side-lying with knees flexed or sitting up on side of bed with back flexed) ❶. **Rationale:** *This will*

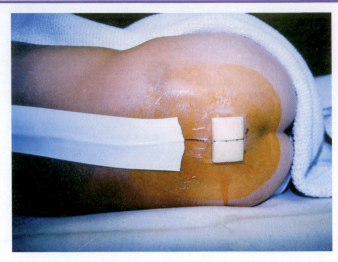

❶ Epidural pain block taped into place and wrapped securely. (Courtesy of Shriners Hospital for Children, Spokane, Washington)

assist the anesthesia personnel in locating the correct vertebrae between which to administer the epidural.

4. Assess BP, heart rate, and fetal heart rate before and after test doses and frequently thereafter according to hospital policy, often every 5 minutes throughout the procedure and immediately following, then regularly according to hospital policy.
5. Return bed to lowest height. Perform hand hygiene.
6. Have ephedrine at bedside in case of hypotensive or fetal bradycardia episode. Administer according to unit protocol and physician orders.
7. Assess the bladder for distention every 30 minutes. Catheterize with intermittent catheter if birth is imminent or indwelling if not. **Rationale:** *A full bladder can slow the descent of the fetus, as well as risk damage to the bladder.*
8. Assess maternal position (from side to side) and body alignment frequently, changing position at least every hour. **Rationale:** *Maximize uteroplacental blood flow, increase circulation, promote comfort, and avoid a one-sided block.*
9. Periodically assess the level of anesthesia and pain control. Notify anesthesia personnel as needed for changes in epidural infusion.
10. Change syringes as needed per hospital policy.
11. After birth, per hospital policy, a qualified RN may remove the epidural catheter.
12. Document the procedure throughout administration of the epidural and removal of the catheter. Document time of removal, condition of epidural puncture site, catheter condition (intact), any dressing applied (if applicable), and how the woman tolerated the procedure.

SKILL 16.15 Care of a Client with a Prolapsed Cord

Equipment

- Sterile exam glove
- Sterile lubricant
- Sterile gauze pad moistened with saline solution, if cord is outside of vagina
- Oxygen and mask
- Fetal monitor/Doppler

Preparation

- A prolapsed cord is an unexpected event and an emergency. Preparation consists of calmly explaining the rationale for interventions, what to expect, and the plan of care to the woman and her support person. Though difficult at times with this particular situation, privacy and safety are priorities.

SKILL 16.15   Care of a Client with a Prolapsed Cord (continued)

■ Allow time for questions from the laboring woman, her support person, and any other family that may be present. Another RN may need to answer questions if the client's RN is busy with the client's care.

Procedure

1. Don sterile gloves.
2. If the cord is visualized extending through the vagina, a sterile gauze moistened with sterile saline must be placed on the cord immediately to prevent the cord from drying. Do not handle the cord. **Rationale:** *Handling the cord may cause it to spasm.*
3. Notify physician/CNM immediately.
4. Place the woman in the knee–chest position ❶. **Rationale:** *This position uses gravity to relieve umbilical cord pressure.*
5. If the cord is palpated during vaginal exam (using sterile glove and lubricant), place two fingers on either side of the cord or both fingers on one side of the cord to avoid compressing it. Exert upward pressure against the presenting part to relieve pressure on the cord.
6. Continue assessing fetal heart rate to determine if interventions and position of fingers are successful in keeping fetal heart rate between 110 and 160 bpm. **Rationale:** *A fetal heart rate in this range indicates that fetal well-being has not been compromised by cord compression.*
7. Start oxygen via face mask at 10 L/min.

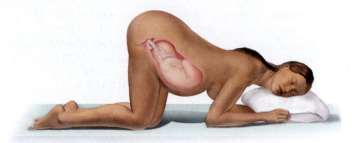

❶ The knee–chest position is used to relieve cord compression during cord prolapse emergency.

8. Examiner must keep fingers on the presenting part until baby is born, usually via cesarean. This may require examiner to travel to the operating room (OR) on the bed with the mother to maintain the position of fingers and presenting part. The woman's position must be maintained until birth or arrival at OR and placement on the OR table. Though difficult, privacy and safety should be maintained during transport to surgery. This may require extra personnel and sheets to cover the woman.
9. Document the course of events, interventions, and maternal and fetal response to interventions in the medical record per agency policy. If there is a poor fetal outcome, further quality assurance documentation may be necessary.

▶ POSTPARTUM CARE

Expected Outcomes

1. Complications are prevented during the postpartum period.
2. Client has progressively less lochia every day.
3. Engorgement of breasts is relieved with breastfeeding.

SKILL 16.16   Assessing the Perineum Postpartum

Equipment

■ Clean perineal pad, clean ice pack if desired/needed
■ Small light source such as a penlight may be necessary
■ Clean gloves

Preparation

■ Gather equipment and supplies. Introduce self, perform hand hygiene, and verify client's identity. Provide privacy. Provide comfort and safety for client and self, including raising bed to appropriate height for procedure. Explain the purpose and the procedure for assessing the perineum during the postpartum period.
■ Complete the assessment of fundal height and lochia. **Rationale:** *Typically, perineal assessment is the final step of the postpartum assessment.*
■ At this point in a postpartum assessment, the woman is lying on her back with her knees flexed. Her perineal pad has already been lifted away from her perineum to permit inspection of the lochia. If an episiotomy was performed or if the birth was diffi-

cult, the woman may be using an ice pack on her perineum to reduce swelling. The ice pack would also have been removed for inspection of the lochia.
■ Ask her to turn onto her side with her upper knee drawn forward and resting on the bed (Sims' position). **Rationale:** *When the woman is supine, even with her knees flexed, it is very difficult to expose the posterior portion of the perineum. Thus, Sims' position makes it easiest to inspect the perineum and anal area.*

Procedure

1. Use a systematic approach to assessment. **Rationale:** *A systematic approach helps ensure that you do not overlook a significant finding.*
2. In evaluating the perineum, begin by asking the woman's perceptions. How does she describe her discomfort? Does it seem excessive to her? Has it become worse since the birth? Does it seem more severe than you would expect? (*Note:* Pain that seems disproportionately severe may indicate that the woman is developing a vulvar hematoma.)

(continued on next page)

SKILL 16.16   Assessing the Perineum Postpartum (*continued*)

Rationale: *Information from the client herself often helps identify developing problems.*

3. After talking with the woman, assess the condition of the tissue. To allow for full visualization, it may be helpful to ask the woman to lift the knee of her upper leg to expose her perineum more fully. In some cases it may help to use the nondominant hand to lift the buttocks and tissue. Note any swelling (edema) or bruising (ecchymosis), and use the REEDA scale to recall what to assess. **Rationale:** *The tissue is often traumatized by the birth, and mild bruising is not unusual. However, excessive bruising may indicate that a hematoma is developing.*

CLINICAL ALERT

In evaluating the perineum, use the REEDA scale as a quick reminder of what to assess.

Specifically:
R = redness
E = edema or swelling
E = ecchymosis or bruising
D = drainage
A = approximation (how well the edges of an incision—the episiotomy—or a repaired laceration seem to be holding together)

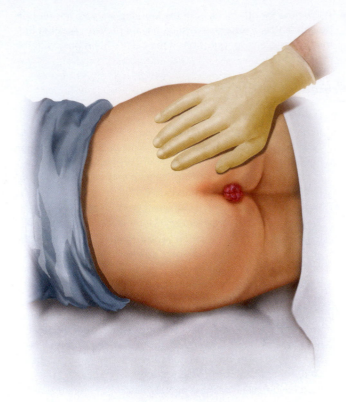

1 Intact perineum with hemorrhoids. Note how the nurse's hand raises the upper buttocks to expose the anal area fully.

4. Evaluate the episiotomy, if there is one, or any repaired laceration for its state of healing. Is it reddened? Note the edges of the incision. Are they well approximated? Tell the woman that you are going to palpate the incision gently, then do so. Note any areas of hardness. Note whether the incision is warmer to the touch than the surrounding tissue. **Rationale:** *Gentle palpation should elicit minimal tenderness and there should be no redness, warmth, or areas of hardness, which suggest infection. Both bruising and infection interfere with normal healing. Typically, within 24 hours the edges of the incision should be "glued" together (well approximated).*

5. During the assessment be alert for odors. Typically the lochia has an earthy, but not unpleasant, smell that is easily identifiable. **Rationale:** *A foul odor associated with drainage often indicates infection.*

6. Finally, assess for hemorrhoids. To visualize the anal area, lift the upper buttocks **1**. If hemorrhoids are present, note the size, number, and pain or tenderness. **Rationale:** *Hemorrhoids often develop during pregnancy or labor and can cause considerable discomfort. If hemorrhoids are present, the woman may benefit from available comfort measures.*

7. During the assessment, talk to the woman about the effectiveness of comfort measures being used. Provide teaching about care of the episiotomy, hemorrhoids, and the like. **Rationale:** *Health teaching is an important part of nursing care. Many women have concerns about the episiotomy and may not know, for example, that the suture used is dissolvable. This is an excellent time to provide information about good healthcare practices in both the short and long term.*

8. Provide the woman with a clean perineal pad. Replenish the ice pack if necessary.

9. Return bed to lowest height and perform hand hygiene.

10. Document findings. For example: "Midline episiotomy; no edema, ecchymosis, or tenderness. Skin edges well approximated. Woman reports pain relief measures are controlling discomfort," or "Perineal repair is approximated, minimal edema, no ecchymosis or tenderness; ice pack to perineum relieves pain."

SKILL 16.17   Assessing the Uterine Fundus Following Vaginal or Cesarean Birth

Equipment

- A clean perineal pad
- Clean gloves

Preparation

- Check physician orders and consider offering to premedicate 30 to 45 minutes before assessing the fundus, especially if the client has had a cesarean section.

- Introduce self and verify client's identity. Provide privacy. Explain the procedure, the information it provides, and what it might feel like.

- Ask the woman when she last voided. Ask her to void if it has been longer than 1 hour. **Rationale:** *A full bladder can cause uterine atony.*

- Perform hand hygiene, following infection control measures. Provide comfort and safety for client and self, including raising bed to appropriate height for procedure.

SKILL 16.17   Assessing the Uterine Fundus Following Vaginal *(continued)*

- Have the woman lie flat in bed with her head on a pillow. If the procedure is uncomfortable, she may find that it helps to flex her legs. Flexing the legs and providing support under them with folded pillows is especially helpful to clients after a cesarean section. **Rationale:** *The supine position prevents falsely high assessment of fundal height. Flexing the legs relaxes the abdominal muscles.*

Procedure

1. Gently place one hand on the lower segment of the uterus for support. Using the side of the other hand, palpate the abdomen until you locate the top of the fundus. **Rationale:** *One hand stabilizes the uterus while the other hand locates the top of the fundus. (Support of the uterus prevents stretching of the ligaments that support the uterus.)*

2. Determine whether the fundus is firm. If it is, it will feel hard and round like a firm grapefruit in the abdomen. If it is not firm, massage the abdomen lightly until it becomes firm, then check for bleeding. **Rationale:** *A firm fundus indicates that the uterine muscles are contracted and bleeding will not occur.*

3. Measure the top of the fundus in fingerbreadths above, below, or at the fundus ❶. **Rationale:** *Fundal height gives information about the progress of involution.*

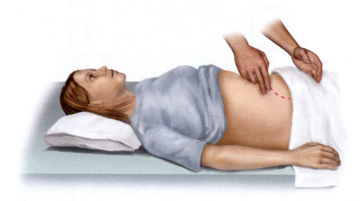

❶ Measuring the descent of the fundus in the woman with a vaginal birth. In this case the fundus is located two fingerbreadths below the umbilicus.

4. Determine the position of the fundus in relation to the midline of the body. If it is not in the midline, locate it and then evaluate the bladder for distention. **Rationale:** *The fundus may* deviate from the midline when the bladder is full because the enlarged bladder pushes the uterus aside.

5. If the bladder is distended, use nursing measures to help the woman void. If she is not able to void after a specified period of time, catheterization may be necessary.

6. Measure urine output for the next few hours until normal elimination is established. **Rationale:** *During the postpartum period, as diuresis occurs, the bladder may fill far more rapidly than normal, putting the woman at risk for uterine atony and hemorrhage. (A diminished tone of the uterus may cause loss of the urge to void.)*

7. Assess the lochia.

> ### CLINICAL ALERT
> Gloves may be put on before assessing the abdomen and fundus or when you are ready to assess the perineum and lochia.

8. During the first few hours postpartum, if the fundus becomes boggy frequently or is located high above the umbilicus and the woman's bladder is empty, the uterine cavity may be filled with clots of blood. In this case, do the following:
   - Release the front of the perineal pad and lay it back so that you can see the perineum and the pad lying between the woman's legs.
   - Massage the uterine fundus until it is firm.
   - Keep one hand in position stabilizing the lower portion of the uterus. With the hand you used to massage the fundus, put steady pressure on the top of the now-firm fundus and see if you are able to express any clots. (Watch the pad between her legs for clots to pass from the vagina.) **Rationale:** *If the woman's uterus is filled with blood, it acts as an irritant and the uterus will not remain contracted. When the muscle fibers relax, bleeding results, further aggravating the problem. Pushing on a uterus that is not firm is dangerous because it is possible to cause the uterus to invert, a true emergency.*

9. Provide the woman with a clean perineal pad.

10. Return bed to lowest height. Perform hand hygiene.

11. Document findings. Fundal height is recorded in fingerbreadths (e.g., "2 FB ↓ U" or "1 FB ↑ U"). If fundal massage was necessary, note that fact: "Uterus boggy → firm with light massage."

12. Communicate bogginess or heavy flow to primary provider.

SKILL 16.18   Evaluating the Lochia

Equipment

- Clean perineal pad
- Clean gloves

Note: Gloves may be put on before assessing the abdomen and fundus or when you are ready to assess the perineum and lochia.

Preparation

- Introduce self, perform hand hygiene, and verify client's identity. Explain why lochia occurs, why it is assessed, how it is assessed, and how it changes during the postpartum. Provide privacy. Provide comfort and safety for client and self, including raising bed to appropriate height for procedure.

- Ask the woman to void. **Rationale:** *A full bladder can cause uterine atony and increase the amount of lochia.*

- Complete the assessment of uterine fundal height and firmness. **Rationale:** *In almost all cases, fundal height and firmness are evaluated with an assessment of lochia. This practice provides a more thorough assessment.*

(continued on next page)

SKILL 16.18   Evaluating the Lochia *(continued)*

■ If she has not already done so for the fundal assessment, ask the woman to flex her legs. Then ask her to spread her legs apart. Use the bed sheet as a drape to preserve her modesty. **Rationale:** *This position allows you to see the perineum and the perineal pad more effectively.*

Procedure

1. Don gloves.

2. Lower the perineal pad and observe the amount of lochia on the pad. Because women's pad-changing practices vary, ask her about the length of time the current pad has been in use, whether the amount of lochia is changed, and whether any clots were passed before this examination, such as during voiding. **Rationale:** *During the first 1 to 3 days, the woman's lochia should be rubra, which is dark red. A few small clots are normal and occur as a result of pooling of blood in the vagina when the woman is lying down. The passage of large clots is abnormal, and the cause should be investigated immediately.*

3. If the woman reports heavy bleeding or clots, ask her to put on a clean perineal pad and then reassess the pad in 1 hour. Also ask her to call you before flushing any clots she passes into the toilet during voiding.

4. When the uterine fundus is firm and stabilized with the non-dominant hand, press down on it with the dominant hand while watching to see if any clots are expelled.

5. Determine the amount of lochia, using the following guide ❶:
   • Heavy amount—Perineal pad has a stain larger than 15 cm (6 in.) in length within 1 hour; 30 to 80 mL lochia.
   • Moderate amount—Perineal pad has a stain less than 15 cm (6 in.) in length within 1 hour; 25 to 50 mL lochia.
   • Small amount—Perineal pad has a stain less than 10 cm (4 in.) in length after 1 hour; 10 to 25 mL lochia.
   • Scant amount—Perineal pad has a stain less than 2.5 cm (1 in.) in length after 1 hour or lochia is only on tissue when the woman wipes.
   Rationale: *Lochia should never exceed a moderate amount such as 4 to 8 partially saturated perineal pads daily. Using a consistent standard for measuring lochia improves the accuracy of the information charted and conveyed to others.*

6. In most cases, a woman is discharged while her lochia is still rubra. Provide her with information about lochia serosa and lochia alba. **Rationale:** *Accurate discharge information enables the woman to assess herself more accurately and enables her to judge better when to contact her caregiver.*

7. Assist client in cleaning peritoneal area and applying clean perineal pad.

8. Return bed to lowest height and perform hand hygiene.

9. Document the findings specifically according to hospital policy. For example, "Uterus firm, 1 FB ↓ U. Lochia moderate rubra, no clots passed."

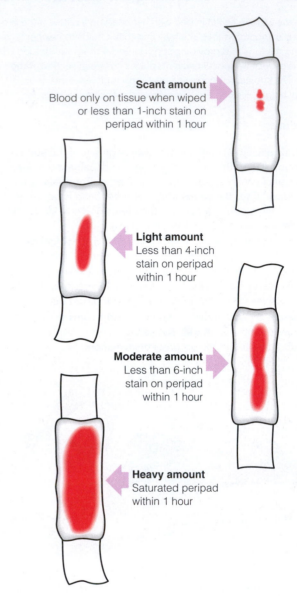

Scant amount
Blood only on tissue when wiped or less than 1-inch stain on peripad within 1 hour

Light amount
Less than 4-inch stain on peripad within 1 hour

Moderate amount
Less than 6-inch stain on peripad within 1 hour

Heavy amount
Saturated peripad within 1 hour

❶ Suggested guidelines for assessing lochia volume.

CLINICAL ALERT

If blood loss exceeds the guidelines given in this chapter, weigh the perineal pads and the chux pads to estimate the blood loss more accurately. Typically, 1 g = 1 mL blood. Because blood can pool below the woman on the chux or peri pad, the pads are included in your assessment.

SKILL 16.19   Assisting with Breastfeeding After Childbirth

Breastfeeding provides newborns and infants with immunological, nutritional, and psychosocial advantages. It also promotes involution in women who have just given birth. Newborns who are put to breast soon after their birth benefit from the physical warmth of their mother's body, from the stimulation of sucking and swallowing, from replenishment of nutrients, and from the opportunity to interact intimately with their mother. As long as the mother is tolerating the birth well and her newborn is adjusting to extrauterine life without complication, breastfeeding can be promoted in the first 1 hour of life when the newborn is usually alert and ready to nurse.

SKILL 16.19   Assisting with Breastfeeding After Childbirth (*continued*)

Equipment

None

Preparation

■ Wash hands.

Procedure

1. Gather supplies. Introduce self and explain what procedure is to be done and why. Perform hand hygiene, following infection control measures, and verify client's identity. Provide for client privacy, comfort, and safety.
2. Assist the mother to a comfortable position. Support her head, shoulders, and arms as necessary for comfort.

Rationale: *A position of comfort allows the new mother to focus on breastfeeding.*

3. Help the mother to wash her hands using a washcloth with soap and water, then rinse well and dry. **Rationale:** *Hands carry a variety of organisms, including* Staphylococcus aureus, Escherichia coli, Streptococcus *species, and* Haemophilus influenzae, *which are all common causes of mastitis, an infection of the breast.*
4. Provide warmed bath blankets to wrap around the mother and newborn together.
5. Help the mother to place the infant skin to skin against her body. Encourage a position that is comfortable for the mother ❶. **Rationale:** *The mother should hold the newborn in a way that feels natural and provides her with a free hand.*

A **Modified cradle.**

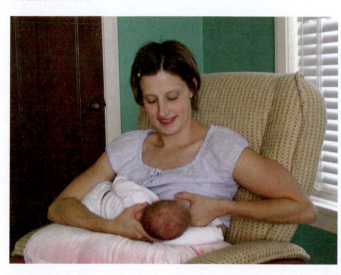

- Have the mother sit comfortably in an upright position using good body alignment. Use pillows for support (may use Boppy, body pillow, or standard bed pillows). Lap pillow should help bring the baby up to breast level so the mother does not lean over baby.
- Place the baby on the mother's lap and turn the baby's entire body toward the mother (the baby is in side-lying position). Position the baby's body so that the baby's nose lines up to the nipple. Maintain the baby's body in a horizontal alignment.
- To feed at left breast, the mother supports the baby's head with her right hand at nape of the baby's neck (allow head to slightly lag back); the mother's right thumb by the baby's left ear, and right forefinger near the baby's right ear.
- With the mother's free left hand, she can offer her left breast.

B **Cradling.**

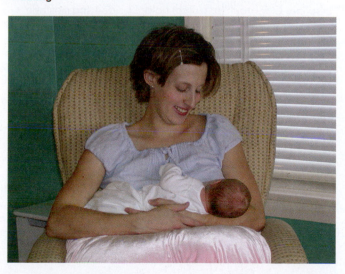

- Position as for modified cradle.
- If feeding from the left breast, have the mother cradle the baby's head near the crook of her left arm while supporting her baby's body with her left forearm.
- With the mother's free right hand, she can offer her left breast.

❶ Four common breastfeeding positions: *A,* Modified cradle; *B,* cradling; *C,* football (or clutch) hold; *D,* side-lying position.
Source: Courtesy of Brigette Hall, MSN, IBLCL.

(*continued on next page*)

SKILL 16.19   Assisting with Breastfeeding After Childbirth (*continued*)

C **Football (or clutch) hold.**

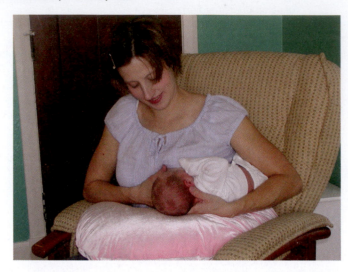

- Have the mother sit comfortably and use pillows to raise the baby's body to breast level. If using a Boppy and the Boppy is in "normal" position on the mother's lap, turn it counterclockwise slightly (if feeding at left breast) to provide extended support for the baby's body resting along the mother's left side and near the back of the mother's chair.
- If feeding at the left breast, place the baby on the left side of the mother's body, heading the baby into position feet first. The baby's bottom should rest on the pillow near the mother's left elbow.
- Turn the baby slightly on her side so that she faces the breast.
- The mother's left arm clutches the baby's body close to the mother's body. The baby's body should feel securely tucked in under the mother's left arm.
- Have the mother support the baby's head with her left hand. With the mother's free right hand, she can offer her breast. (Good position for the mother with a c-section.)

D **Side-lying position.**

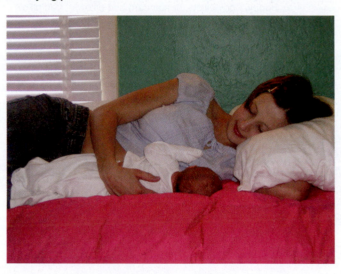

- Have the mother rest comfortably lying on her side (left side for this demonstration). Use pillows to support the mother's head and back, and provide support for the mother's hips by placing a pillow between her bent knees.
- Place the baby in side-lying position next to the mother's body. The baby's body should face the mother's body. The baby's nose should line up to the mother's nipple. Place a roll behind the baby's back, if desired.
- With the mother's free right hand, she can offer her left breast. After the baby is securely attached, mom can rest her right hand anywhere that is comfortable for her.

❶ Four common breastfeeding positions: *A*, Modified cradle; *B*, cradling; *C*, football (or clutch) hold; *D*, side-lying position. (*continued*)

6. Instruct the mother to use the thumb and first two fingers of her dominant hand to make a C-shape around her breast with the nipple in the center of the C-shape and to steadily support her breast ❷. **Rationale:** *This C-hold hand position enables the mother to position the breast correctly in the newborn's mouth.*

7. Help the mother to hold her newborn so that the mouth is in alignment with her breast at the level of the nipple. She then lightly tickles the infant's mouth with the nipple until the baby opens his or her mouth. She then brings the baby closely in to her breast. It is important for the baby to take the whole nipple into the mouth so that the gums are on the areola. Provide firm steady support as the newborn begins to suckle. If sucking does not begin, stroke the cheek gently to elicit the suck–search response and then offer the breast again. Instruct the mother to be sure that the breast tissue does not occlude the newborn's nares. **Rationale:** *The newborn's gums need to be positioned over the areola because this allows the baby's jaws to compress*

the milk ducts located directly beneath the areola as the newborn suckles.

8. If the newborn is sufficiently responsive, have him or her suckle at both breasts. Initially some newborns suck well; others may simply lick or nuzzle the nipple. Reassure the mother that this is a positive interaction. **Rationale:** *Even simple breast stimulation promotes the release of oxytocin, which aids uterine involution and lactation.*

9. Document in the medical record the time and duration of the breastfeeding, the quality of the latch, and interaction between the mother and newborn. Note any difficulties such as flat or inverted nipples, and initiate referral to a lactation consultant.

CLINICAL ALERT
Be patient and allow the newborn and mother to experience breastfeeding in a relaxed way. Your calmness and support can help the mother feel confident and in control.

SKILL 16.19   Assisting with Breastfeeding After Childbirth (*continued*)

C-hold hand position.

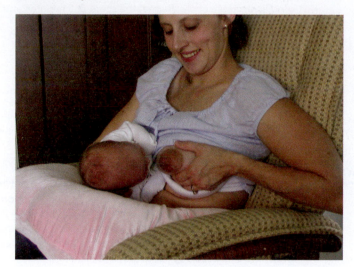

To be ready to draw the baby's mouth onto the mother's breast, as soon as the baby opens the mouth widely enough, the mother needs to have her hand supporting her breast in the ready position. She can use various hand holds, but she needs to keep her fingers well behind the areola. One such hand position is called the "C-hold." In this hold, the thumb is placed on top of the breast near the 12:00 position and the other four fingers are placed on the underside of the breast near the 6:00 position (depends on mother's hand size and length of fingers). The key point is to keep the fingers at least 1½ inches back from the base of the nipple as the fingers support the breast. Mothers are not often aware of where they place their fingers especially on the underside of the breast. If the fingers are too far forward (too close to the nipple), then the infant cannot grasp a large amount of areola in her mouth and this results in a "shallow" latch. A shallow latch is associated with nipple pain and ineffective drainage of the breast. An alternate handhold not shown is a "U-hold" hand position. The thumb and forefinger are near the 3 and 9 position on the breast again with fingers at least 1½ inches back from the base of the nipple; the body of the hand rests on the lower portion of the breast. Using this handhold, the mother's arm position is down at her side rather than sticking outward as it is when supporting the breast using the C-hold position.

❷ C-hold hand position.
Source: Courtesy of Brigette Hall, MSN, IBLCL.

▶ NEWBORN CARE

Expected Outcomes

1. The newborn's Apgar score is 8 to 10 five minutes after birth.
2. The newborn's cord is kept clean and dry.
3. There are no signs of infection at the circumcision site.

SKILL 16.20   Assessing Newborn Apgar Scores

Equipment

- Apgar timer or digital timer that counts seconds or a timepiece with a second hand
- Infant warmer with ISC and probe preheated
- Clean gloves
- Stethoscope
- Sterile baby blanket

Preparation

- Identify the individual responsible for assigning the Apgar score.
- Preheat the radiant warmer to 36.5°C (97.7°F).
- Prewarm blankets under the warmer.

Procedure

1. Perform hand hygiene and don gloves. **Rationale:** *A newborn infant is wet with amniotic fluid, vernix, and secretions. Consequently, universal precautions are indicated when handling the newborn until the initial bath is completed.* Provide comfort and safety during procedure.

2. Using the following five criteria, determine a score for each and assign an Apgar score at 1 minute (see also Table 16–5).
   - Heart rate—Palpate the pulse at the base of the umbilical cord for 6 seconds and multiply by 10, or use the stethoscope to auscultate the heart rate. Score as follows:
     0—no heart rate detected
     1—heart rate below 100 bpm
     2—heart rate greater than 100 bpm.
   - Respiratory effort—Observe respirations and cry. Score as follows:
     0—no respiratory effort or cry
     1—slow to breathe, weak cry
     2—robust cry, good respiratory effort.
   - Muscle tone—Assess flexion of extremities and quality of muscle tone. Score as follows:
     0—flaccid
     1—some flexion of extremities
     2—active motion.
   - Reflex irritability—Assess response to noxious stimuli such as vitamin K injection. Score as follows:
     0—no response

(continued on next page)

SKILL 16.20 Assessing Newborn Apgar Scores *(continued)*

1—grimace
2—cry.
- Color—Assess skin color and score as follows:
0—generally poor color, pale or cyanotic
1—body is pink with some pallor or cyanosis over extremities, around mouth or eyes
2—pink.
  Rationale: *Assessing these five parameters provides a quick indication of the newborn's adaptation to extrauter-*

ine life. With practice, caregivers become skilled at assigning an accurate score. Repeat the score at 5 minutes and again at 10 minutes as indicated.

3. Document appropriately in the medical record.

CLINICAL ALERT
Heart rate and respirations are the two most significant categories to evaluate.

SKILL 16.21 Assisting Thermoregulation of the Newborn

Equipment

- Prewarmed towels or blankets
- Infant stocking cap
- Servocontrol probe
- Infant T-shirt and diaper
- Open crib
- Clean gloves

Preparation

- Check physician's order.
- Prewarm the incubator or radiant warmer. Make sure warm towels and/or lightweight blankets are available.
- Maintain the temperature of the birthing room at 22°C (71°F), with a relative humidity of 60% to 65%. **Rationale:** *The change from a warm, moist intrauterine environment to a cool, dry drafty environment stresses the newborn's immature thermoregulation system.*

Procedure

1. Perform hand hygiene and don gloves. **Rationale:** *Gloves are worn whenever there is the possibility of contact with body fluids—in this case, a newborn wet with amniotic fluid, vernix, and maternal blood. Provide comfort and safety for newborn.*

2. Place the newborn under the radiant warmer. Wipe the newborn free of blood, fluid, and excess vernix, especially from the head, using prewarmed towels. **Rationale:** *The radiant warmer creates a heat-gaining environment. Drying is important to prevent the loss of body heat through evaporation.* Discard gloves and perform hand hygiene.

3. If the newborn is stable, wrap him or her in a prewarmed blanket, apply a stocking cap, and carry the newborn to the mother. The mother and her support person can hold and enjoy the newborn together.

   Alternatively, carry the newborn wrapped to the mother, loosen the blanket, and place the infant skin to skin on the mother's chest under a warmed blanket. **Rationale:** *Use of a prewarmed blanket reduces convection heat loss and facilitates maternal–newborn contact without compromising the newborn's thermoregulation. Skin-to-skin contact with the mother or father helps maintain the newborn's temperature.*

4. After the newborn has spent time with the parents, return him or her to the radiant warmer. Leave the newborn uncovered (except for the cap and diaper) under the radiant warmer. **Rationale:** *Radiant heat warms the outer skin surface, so the skin needs to be exposed.*

5. Tape a servocontrol probe on the newborn's anterior abdominal wall, with the metal side next to the skin. Do not place it over the ribs. Secure the probe with porous tape or a foil-covered aluminum heat deflector patch. The figure shows a newborn with a skin probe ❶. Note that in this picture the newborn is no longer wearing a stocking cap.

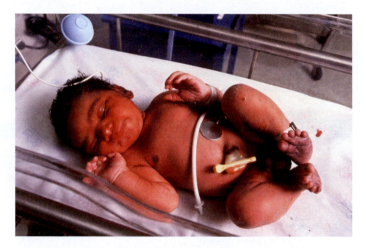

❶ Temperature monitoring for the newborn. A skin thermal sensor is placed on the newborn's abdomen, upper thigh, or arm and secured with porous tape or a foil-covered foam pad.
Source: © Tom McCarthy/Photoedit.

6. Turn the heater to servocontrol mode so that the abdominal skin is maintained at 36.0° to 36.5°C (96.8° to 97.7°F).

CLINICAL ALERT
Take action to help the newborn maintain a stable temperature:

- Keep the newborn's clothing and bedding dry.
- Double-wrap the newborn and put a stocking cap on him or her.
- Use the radiant warmer during procedures.
- Reduce the newborn's exposure to drafts.
- Warm objects that will be in contact with the newborn (e.g., stethoscopes).
- Encourage the mother to snuggle with the newborn under blankets or to breastfeed the newborn with hat and light cover on.

7. Monitor the newborn's axillary and skin probe temperatures per agency protocol. **Rationale:** *The temperature indicator on the radiant warmer continually displays the newborn's probe*

SKILL 16.21   Assisting Thermoregulation of the Newborn *(continued)*

temperature. The axillary temperature is checked to ensure that the machine is accurately recording the newborn's temperature.

8. When the newborn's temperature reaches 37°C (98.6°F), add a T-shirt, double-wrap the infant (two blankets), and place the newborn in an open crib.

9. Recheck the newborn's temperature in 1 hour and regularly thereafter according to agency policy. **Rationale:** *It is important to monitor the newborn's ability to maintain his or her own thermoregulation.*

10. If the newborn's temperature drops below 36.1°C (97°F), rewarm the infant gradually. Place the infant (unclothed except for a diaper) under the radiant warmer with a servocontrol probe on the anterior abdominal wall. **Rationale:** *Rapid heat-*

ing can lead to hyperthermia, which is associated with apnea, insensible water loss, and increased metabolic rate.

11. Recheck the newborn's temperature in 30 minutes, then hourly.

12. When the temperature reaches 37°C (98.6°F), dress the newborn, remove him or her from the radiant warmer, double-wrap, and place in an open crib. Check the temperature hourly until stable, then regularly according to agency policy.

Note: An infant who repeatedly requires rewarming should be observed for other signs and symptoms of illness, and a physician should be notified because it may warrant screening for infection.

13. Document care provided and all relevant information.

SKILL 16.22   Applying, Caring for, and Removing an Umbilical Cord Clamp

Equipment

- Cord clamp
- Prescribed preparations: triple dye, bacitracin ointment, or isopropyl alcohol for initial cord care
- Cord clamp remover or scissors
- Gloves

Preparation

- Check physician's orders and obtain necessary supplies. Confirm that consent has been obtained and documented properly.

Procedure

Assisting with Cord Clamp Application

The goal of applying the cord clamp is to prevent bleeding and promote adaptation to the extrauterine circulation pattern.

1. Assist physician as needed while he or she does the following actions:
   - Places a disposable clamp at the base of the cord about 2.5 cm (1 in.) distal to the skin demarcation line.
   - Secures the clamp by pressing until it clicks and locks.
   - Cuts away excess cord distal to the disposable clamp.
   - Examines the cord and count the vessels.
   - Applies antimicrobial agent over the base of the cord and on 2.5 cm (1 in.) of surrounding skin. **Rationale:** *Antimicrobial ointments may be used for initial cord care in an attempt to minimize microorganisms and promote drying.*

2. Document status of the clamp and cord in the medical record.

Routine Cord Care

The goal of routine cord care is to promote drying and sloughing of the cord and to prevent infection.

1. Apply diapers so that they are folded below the umbilical cord and do not dampen the cord with urine.

2. Change the diaper frequently to prevent urine from soaking the diaper and cord.

3. Keep the site clean and dry per agency protocol ❶. **Rationale:** *Wetness and moistness promote growth of microorganisms.*

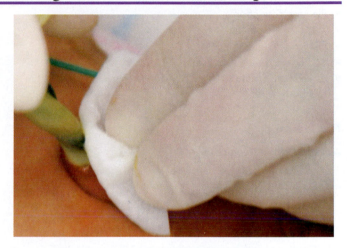

❶ The umbilical cord base is carefully cleaned.

4. Assess the cord for signs and symptoms of infection (foul smell, redness, and greenish-yellow drainage, localized heat and tenderness) or bleeding.

5. Document the condition of the cord in the medical record as part of routine assessment.

Cord Clamp Removal

Cord clamps are removed once the site is dry and before discharge. The cord should look dark and dried up before falling off.

1. Verify that the stump is thoroughly dry.

2. Apply the cord clamp removal device or insert scissors into the loop at the base of the clamp.

3. Cut through the loop, directing the tool away from the cord and baby.

4. Observe for any oozing or bleeding.

5. Instruct parents regarding care of the site. Advise them to contact their primary care provider if bleeding, oozing, or odor is noticed.

6. Document the condition of the cord and teaching in the medical record.

SKILL 16.23 Assisting with Circumcision and Providing Circumcision Care

Equipment

- Infant warmer
- Circ board
- Iodine skin prep
- Circ tray
- Analgesia medications
- Pacifier
- Sucrose solution
- Petroleum gauze or ointment
- Clean diaper
- Gloves

Preparation

- Check physician's orders and confirm that consent has been obtained and documented properly.
- Medicate the infant for pain if ordered.
- Plan for distraction.
- Plan for safe positioning.
- Plan to prevent unnecessary heat loss.
- Obtain necessary supplies.
- Coordinate timing to avoid performing the procedure within 3 to 4 hours after feeding.

Procedure

Assisting with Circumcision

The goal of assisting with circumcision is to provide for the safety of the newborn and to relieve discomfort during the procedure.

1. Check the identity of the newborn, comparing the ID number on the infant's band with the number in the medical record with the circumcision order.
2. Confirm that the newborn has been NPO as ordered.
3. Have equipment and medications available for medicating the newborn for pain as ordered. Perform hand hygiene and provide privacy.
4. Assist the physician during this procedure. Provide comfort and safety for newborn, including securing the infant to the circ board using Velcro straps or other restraint devices; restrain only the legs. Apply warm blankets to the upper body.
5. Provide sucrose as ordered for comfort. Offer a pacifier for nonnutritive sucking. Lightly stroke the infant's head.

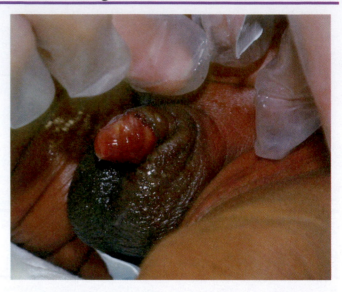

① Following circumcision, petroleum ointment may be applied to the site for the next few diaper changes.

Care Following Circumcision

The goal of care following circumcision is to reduce trauma to the surgical site and to observe for signs of complications **①**.

1. Apply petroleum gauze or ointment to the head of the penis. **Rationale:** *Prevents the diaper from adhering to the surgical site and helps avoid trauma.*
2. Apply a clean diaper. Fasten diaper over penis snugly enough so that it does not move and rub the tender glans.
3. Assess the ability to void. Document urination following the procedure in the medical record. **Rationale:** *Swelling or damage may obstruct the urethral opening.*
4. Return the newborn to his parents. Explain the procedure.
5. Teach parents to apply petroleum gauze to the site and use A&D ointment to prevent adherence of the diaper to the surgical site (unless a Plastibell is in place). Teach them that the glans is sensitive and to avoid placing the newborn on his stomach for the first day after the procedure.
6. Monitor temperature.
7. Check the site hourly till discharge.
8. Document any bleeding, discharge, abnormal temperature, or inability to void in the medical record.

SKILL 16.24 Giving the Initial Newborn Bath

Equipment

- Clean gloves
- Warm water
- Washcloths
- Blankets or towels for drying

Preparation

- The baby should be resting in a radiant warmer or an incubator.
- Prewarm all baby blankets to be used.
- Gather equipment and supplies.

Procedure

1. Perform hand hygiene, following infection control measures, and verify newborn's identity. Provide comfort and safety for newborn.
2. Assess newborn's temperature. Once the newborn has demonstrated the ability to maintain a stable temperature greater than 36.6°C (97.9°F), a first bath can be given. **Rationale:** *Temperature instability introduces a threat to newborn adaptation that can lead to serious complications, including respiratory distress, hypoglycemia, and acidosis. Preventing cold stress is an important goal for newborn care.*

SKILL 16.24   Giving the Initial Newborn Bath (*continued*)

3. Bathe the baby under the radiant warmer. If feasible, position the warmer close to a sink for a source of warm water. Alternatively, fill a basin with warm water. **Rationale:** *The human newborn cannot maintain his or her temperature independently but requires protection against heat loss in the form of warm, dry blankets and hats, or an external heat source such as the warmth of the mother's body or a warmer.*

4. Using a clean, warm, wet washcloth, clean the eyes, washing from the inner to outer canthus of each eye, moving to a clean portion of the washcloth for each eye.

5. Wash the remainder of the face, cleaning the washcloth after each use.

6. A mild soap may be used for the remainder of the bath. Wash the folds of skin in the neck and axilla. Wash between the fingers and toes.

> **CLINICAL ALERT**
> Use only a small amount of soap. Excessive soap and lather can be difficult to rinse off.

7. Wash the belly, extremities, and back. Wash the groin and diaper area. Dry the baby after each area is washed.

8. Complete cord care according to agency policy.

9. The hair and scalp can be washed using a mild shampoo, typically at a sink. To do so, wrap the baby in a warm blanket with arms tucked inside the blanket out of the way. Hold the infant in a football hold with head extended over the sink. Use the free, cupped hand to bring water from the faucet to the infant's head. Wet the scalp, apply a small quantity of shampoo, lather, and rinse, again using a cupped hand to bring water to the newborn's head. Dry the head thoroughly and apply a cap. (*Note:* The head may also be shampooed over a basin.) **Rationale:** *The infant is wrapped for the shampoo to prevent excessive heat loss. Because significant heat loss can occur through the scalp, it is important to work quickly and to dry the head thoroughly. The cap helps retain heat.*

> **CLINICAL ALERT**
> Some nurses prefer to begin the bath with the shampoo.

10. Repeat assessment of temperature. If the temperature is normal and stable, dress the newborn in a shirt, diaper, and cap. Wrap the baby and return to parents in an open crib. If the baby's axillary temperature is below 36.4°C (97.5°F), return the baby to the radiant warmer.

11. Document the bath, any significant findings, and temperature in the medical record.

SKILL 16.25   Providing Phototherapy for an Infant

Equipment

- Bank of phototherapy lights
- Eye patches
- Small scale to weigh diapers

Preparation

- Check physician's order and gather equipment and supplies.
- Explain to the parent(s) the purpose of phototherapy, the procedure itself (including the need to use eye patches), and possible side effects such as dehydration.
- Note evidence of jaundice in the skin, sclera, and mucous membranes (in infants with darkly pigmented skin). Be sure that recent serum bilirubin levels are available. **Rationale:** *The decision to use phototherapy is based on a careful assessment of the newborn's condition over a period of time. The most recent results prior to starting therapy serve as a baseline to evaluate the effectiveness of therapy.*

Procedure

1. Perform hand hygiene and verify newborn's identity. Provide comfort and safety for newborn. Obtain vital signs, including the axillary temperature. **Rationale:** *This provides baseline data.*

2. Remove all of the infant's clothing except the diaper. **Rationale:** *Exposure of the newborn to high-intensity light (a bank of fluorescent light bulbs or bulbs in the blue-white spectrum) decreases serum bilirubin levels in the skin by aiding biliary excretion of unconjugated bilirubin. Because the tissue absorbs the light, best results are obtained when there is maximum skin surface exposure.*

3. Apply eye coverings (eye patches or a bili mask) to the infant according to agency policy. **Rationale:** *Eye coverings are used because it is not known if phototherapy injures delicate eye structures, particularly the retina.*

4. Place the infant in an open crib or isolette (more commonly used in preterm infants and infants who are sicker) about 45 to 50 cm (18 to 20 in.) below the bank of phototherapy lights ❶. Reposition every 2 hours. **Rationale:** *The isolette helps the infant maintain his or her temperature while undressed. Repositioning exposes different areas of skin to the lights, prevents*

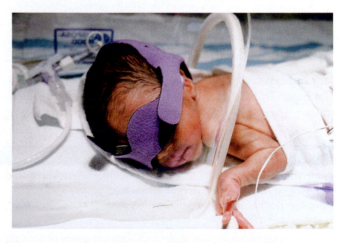

❶ Infant receiving phototherapy. The phototherapy light is positioned over the incubator or crib. Bilateral eye patches are always used during photo light therapy to protect the baby's eyes.
Source: Courtesy of Lisa Smith-Pedersen, RNC, MSN, NNP-BC.

(*continued on next page*)

SKILL 16.25 Providing Phototherapy for an Infant (continued)

the development of pressure areas on the skin, and varies the stimulation the infant receives.

5. Monitor vital signs every 4 hours with axillary temperatures. **Rationale:** *Temperature assessment is indicated to detect hypothermia or hyperthermia. Deviation in pulse and respirations may indicate developing complications.*

6. Check the lights using a bilimeter to ensure safe effective treatment.

7. Cluster care activities. **Rationale:** *Care activities are clustered to help ensure that the newborn has maximum time under the lights.*

8. Discontinue phototherapy and remove eye patches at least once per 8- hour shift. Also discontinue phototherapy and remove patches when feeding the infant and when the parents visit. **Rationale:** *Eye patches are removed to assess for signs of complications such as excessive pressure, discharge, or conjunctivitis. Patches are also removed to provide some social stimulation and to promote parental attachment.*

CLINICAL ALERT

If the area of jaundice about the eyes begins to disappear, it is probable that the eye patches are allowing light to enter and better eye protection is needed.

9. Maintain adequate fluid intake. Evaluate the need for IV fluids.

10. Monitor intake and output carefully. Weigh diapers before discarding. Document quantity and characteristics of each stool. **Rationale:** *Infants undergoing phototherapy treatment have increased water loss and loose stools as a result of bilirubin excretion. This increases their risk of dehydration.*

11. Assess specific gravity with each voiding. Weigh the newborn daily. **Rationale:** *Specific gravity provides one measure of urine concentration. Highly concentrated urine is associated with a dehydrated state. Weight loss is also a sign of developing dehydration in the newborn.*

12. Observe the infant for signs of perianal excoriation, and institute therapy if it develops. **Rationale:** *Perianal excoriation may develop because of the irritating effect of diarrheal stools.*

13. Ensure that serum bilirubin levels are drawn regularly according to orders or agency policy. Turn the phototherapy lights off while the blood is drawn. **Rationale:** *Serum bilirubin levels provide the most accurate indication of the effectiveness of phototherapy. They are generally drawn every 12 hours, but at least once daily. The phototherapy lights are turned off to ensure accurate serum bilirubin levels.*

14. Examine the newborn's skin regularly for signs of developing pressure areas, bronzing, maculopapular rash, and changes in degree of jaundice. Document pertinent information. **Rationale:** *Pressure areas may develop if the infant lies in one position for an extended period. A benign, transient bronze discoloration of the skin may occur with phototherapy when the infant has elevated direct serum bilirubin levels or liver disease. A maculopapular rash is another transient side effect of phototherapy that develops occasionally.*

15. Avoid using lotion or ointment on the exposed skin. **Rationale:** *Lotion and ointments on a newborn receiving phototherapy may cause skin burns.*

16. Provide parents with opportunities to hold the newborn and assist in the infant's care. Answer their questions accurately and keep them informed of developments or changes. **Rationale:** *A sick infant is a source of great anxiety for parents. Information helps them deal with their anxiety. Moreover, they have a right to be kept well informed of their baby's status so that they are able to make informed decisions as needed.*

17. Alternatively, provide phototherapy using lightweight fiberoptic blankets ("bili blankets").

Note: With fiberoptic blankets, the newborn is readily accessible for care, feedings, and diaper changes. The baby does not get overheated, and fluid and weight loss are not complications of this system. The infant is accessible to the parents, and the procedure seems less alarming to parents than standard phototherapy. A combination of a fiberoptic light source in the mattress under the baby and a standard phototherapy light source above is also used by some agencies. In addition, many agencies and pediatricians use fiberoptic blankets for home care.

▶ CRITICAL THINKING OPTIONS FOR UNEXPECTED OUTCOMES

Not all unexpected outcomes require further nursing intervention; however, many times they do. When the client demonstrates a change in signs/symptoms indicating an emerging problem, the nurse should immediately assess and troubleshoot what is happening. The assessment data must be processed quickly to formulate a hypothesis so the nurse can make a clinical judgment. The nurse then decides how best to resolve the problem and improve the client's situation for a better appropriate outcome.

EXPECTED OUTCOME	PROBLEM SOLVING	NURSING ACTIONS
Antepartum Care There are no signs of side effects or allergic responses at the injection site of administered Rh immune globulin.	Client complains about tenderness at the injection site.	■ Monitor for temperature elevation. ■ Apply local warmth to the injection site. ■ Monitor for signs and symptoms of infection of site. ■ Notify physician if needed.
Client experiences no physical problems during pregnancy.	Client complains of constipation in the second trimester.	■ Encourage client to drink adequate fluids. ■ Encourage client to eat fibrous foods. ■ Ask physician about medication interventions like stool softeners, laxatives, or enemas.

EXPECTED OUTCOME	PROBLEM SOLVING	NURSING ACTIONS
Client experiences no physical problems during pregnancy (cont.).	Client has a urinary tract infection.	▪ Take antibiotics and medication for discomfort as ordered by physician. ▪ Encourage client to drink adequate fluids. ▪ Reinforce good perineal hygiene practices, like wearing panty liners. ▪ Perform Kegel exercises. ▪ Maintain bladder emptying pattern.
Intrapartum Care Induction of labor with Pitocin progresses without evidence of fetal distress.	Fetal distress is noted with a client receiving Pitocin during intrapartum care.	▪ Stop the Pitocin infusion. ▪ Stay with the client, and help her reposition to her side. ▪ Administer supplemental oxygen following facility guidelines. ▪ Monitor maternal vital signs and fetal heartbeat. ▪ Monitor contractions. ▪ Notify physician.
Ongoing fetal heartbeat documentation occurs with external electronic fetal monitoring.	The electronic fetal monitoring system stops producing fetal heartbeat strips.	▪ Manually check fetal heartbeat rate. ▪ Check monitoring system for available recording paper, and replace empty roll with new roll if needed. ▪ Check placement of transducer and belt. ▪ Continue monitoring with printed documentation of fetal heartbeat rate and rhythm.
Postpartum Care The client has progressively less lochia every day.	Lochia remains bright red with heavier flow.	▪ Assess vital signs and tenderness. ▪ Assess for recent activity of client (may indicate client has increased activities too much and too soon). ▪ Notify physician if client states there has not been an increase in activity and the flow remains heavy and bright red (may indicate postpartum hemorrhage, which is a medical emergency).
Newborn Care The newborn's cord is kept clean and dry.	The newborn's umbilical cord is moist with a reddened base.	▪ This response is indicative of infection. ▪ Antibiotic ointment may be prescribed. ▪ Clean area periodically and keep it dry. ▪ Monitor for any bleeding or drainage until cord is dried and occluded.

17 Safety

Skills-at-a-Glance

A safe physical environment is one in which people can function without injury and feel a sense of security. The skills in this chapter focus on those measures the nurse can take to reduce the risk of client injury as a result of unsafe movement within and out of a bed or chair. These include measures that are taken in anticipation of and in the event of a seizure during which the client cannot control physical movement and is at risk of sustaining an injury. Attention to the dignity and well-being of clients must be maintained at all times. Many clients will have strong emotional responses around issues of falling, being restrained, and having a seizure. Embarrassment, fear, and a decreased sense of autonomy and control can all compromise a client's healing potential. The holistic nurse will demonstrate therapeutic presence while providing the skills presented in this chapter.

▶ HOME CARE SAFETY

Expected Outcomes

1. Nurse's safety is maintained during home visit.
2. All personal articles and call light are within easy reach of the client.
3. If oxygen is used, appropriate safety measures are in effect.
4. Toxic substances are removed by lavage/not absorbed.
5. Client is safely repositioned or transferred without injury to client or caregiver.
6. Appropriate assistive devices are utilized to transfer client.
7. Caregiver is able to manage turning, repositioning, and assistive devices.
8. Appropriate body mechanics are utilized by caregiver.

SKILL 17.1   Maintaining Nurses' Safety

Procedure

1. Evaluate safety of nurse prior to the visit.
   - Call the client before the visit to determine convenient time.
   - Confirm directions to home.
   - Determine if household pets are present; if so, ask that they be secured during visit.
   - Check neighborhood to determine need for assistance from police to make home visit.
2. Wear identifying name badge. Most agencies request that the nurse wear a lab coat.
3. Wear flat shoes to allow you to walk quickly or to run if necessary.
4. Maintain personal safety while traveling in the car.
   - Keep car in good working order and stocked with necessary equipment.
   - Keep gas tank at least half full at all times.
   - Obtain automobile club membership for emergency use. **Rationale:** *To call for assistance with car problems.*
   - Keep a windshield cover with CALL POLICE sign available. **Rationale:** *To alert neighbors you need immediate assistance.*
   - Have cell phone available and charged at all times.
   - Keep blanket in car. **Rationale:** *To keep warm in the winter if you need to wait for assistance.*
   - Keep thermos of water in car at all times. **Rationale:** *In case you need to wait for assistance in hot weather.*
   - Keep doors locked and windows up at all times.
   - Park in full view of neighbors, preferably directly in front of home.
   - Lock all personal items and valuables in trunk of the car before leaving home or office.
   - Keep all equipment in the trunk of the car. **Rationale:** *To prevent car break-ins and theft.*
   - Restock the nurses' bag before the visits for the day. Keep nurses' bag on front seat.
   - Keep money in car for phone calls if necessary.
5. Maintain personal safety while walking on the street.
   - Keep one arm and hand free when walking from car to house.
   - Walk directly to client's residence.
   - When approaching a group of strangers, cross the street or walkway, if appropriate.
   - When leaving a residence, keep keys in your hand with the pointed end of the key facing outward. **Rationale:** *The keys can act as a weapon if necessary.*
   - Carry a chemical spray and whistle within easy reach. *Note:* Attendance at a class may be necessary in some states before it is legal to carry a chemical spray such as mace.

CLINICAL ALERT

If your safety is in jeopardy, use one of the following defensive strategies: Scream or yell "FIRE" or "STRANGER." Kick the individual in the shin or groin. Bite or scratch the individual. Use chemical spray or blow a whistle. If you feel your personal safety is in question, do not make a visit or stay in the residence.

6. Maintain personal safety when making home visit.
   - Use common walkways or hallways. Do not park behind a building or in a dark area.
   - Knock on the door and wait for permission to enter.
   - Keep a clear pathway to the door if the situation is potentially unsafe.
   - Introduce self and verify client's identity. Perform hand hygiene, following infection control measures. Provide comfort and safety for client and self. Explain what is to be done and why.
   - Observe home environment for safety hazards (i.e., weapons, unsanitary conditions).
   - Make a joint visit with another agency staff member or ask for an escort if there is a potentially unsafe situation.
   - Call for police support if the visit is essential and the situation is unsafe. **Rationale:** *There may be times when a visit is essential, but it is unsafe for one individual to make a visit.*
   - Make visit in the morning when good visual support exists if neighborhood is unsafe.
   - Close the case if the situation is unsafe and there are no alternative actions that can guarantee the nurse's safety.

SKILL 17.2   Evaluating Client's Safety

Procedure

1. Introduce self and identify client. Provide privacy. Provide comfort and safety for client and self. Perform hand hygiene. Explain what is to be done and why. Evaluate client's cognitive abilities: level of consciousness, orientation, ability to make appropriate judgments, ability to follow commands and directions.
   - Knowledge of how to operate appliances (e.g., stoves and heaters)
   - History of alcohol or drug abuse
   - Knowledge of medication times and doses to be taken
   - Knowledge of how to call for help: physician, nurse, fire, police.
2. Evaluate client's sensory and motor function.
   - Hearing and vision acuity
   - Ability to ambulate with assistance
   - Need for assistive devices or support in ambulation.
3. Determine client's ability to manage self-care.
   - Bathing, grooming, and dressing
   - Preparing food and feeding
   - Toileting
   - Housekeeping, shopping, transportation to physician and pharmacy.

4. Assess if client needs alternatives to physical restraints.
   - Determine if environment needs to be modified by removing unsafe objects or barriers.
   - Remove wheels from chairs or bed.
   - Install bed check system or alarm device.
   - Decrease auditory and visual stimuli.
   - Place supplies close to bed or chair (e.g., tissues, water).
   - Develop routine for client.
5. Evaluate most effective type of restraint, if absolutely necessary.
   - Determine that less restrictive methods have been attempted.
   - Assess purpose of restraint to determine most appropriate type.
   - Obtain physician's order for restraint. Order must include reason, type, and time of restraints.
   - Obtain informed consent from client or guardian before applying.
   - Explain purpose of restraints to client and family members.
   - Ensure caregiver is instructed on use of restraints.
   - Evaluate effectiveness and continued need for restraints. The safety issues are the same as for clients in the hospital.
6. Determine client's financial support.
   - Determine healthcare insurance plan, workers' compensation, Medicare, Medicaid, and need for social services.
7. Document findings in client's chart.

SKILL 17.3   Assessing for Abuse

Procedure

1. Introduce self and identify client. Provide privacy. Provide comfort and safety for client and self. Perform hand hygiene. Explain what is to be done and why. Assess client for indications of neglect: failure to have adequate food, clothing, medical assistance, or assistance with ADLs provided. Check body for signs of cleanliness. Determine if emotional abuse is present. Ask about threats, intimidation, or isolation.
2. For an adult client, identify if financial abuse has occurred, such as misuse of finances or property.
3. For all clients, assess for signs of physical abuse: signs of restraining; hitting, biting, burning; black and blue marks on trunk, abdomen, buttocks, upper thighs; scars; and abrasions. Bilateral bruises or parallel injuries may indicate forceful restraining; shaking may cause parallel injuries of upper arms. Sexual abuse may cause edema, bruising, or tearing in the genital or anal area. Accidental injuries affect knees, back of hands, forehead, and elbows.
4. Assess for signs of malnourishment or dehydration.
5. Check skin for pressure ulcers.
6. Assess for signs of sprains, dislocations, or fractures from pulling or pushing the client.

7. Ask about visits to the hospital emergency department (ED). (If the client is a child, ask the parent.) Ask why client sought medical care and how much time elapsed between injury and visit to ED.
8. Assess for signs of emotional abuse. Observe if client is fearful of strangers, becomes quiet when caregiver enters room, refuses to answer if caregiver is present, or craves attention and socialization.
9. Document findings in client's chart.

Questions to Ask If Abuse Is Suspected

- Who cares for you at home?
- Did someone hurt you?
- Are you happy with where you live?
- Tell me about your daily routine.
- Who assists you with everyday activities?
- Do you feel safe living here?
- Adult client: Who manages your money?
- How did the injury (or bruises) occur?
- Did you receive medical attention?
- Has this type of injury happened before?

SKILL 17.4   Assessing Caregiver's Safety

Procedure

1. Introduce self and identify caregiver. Provide privacy. Provide comfort and safety for caregiver and self. Perform hand hygiene. Explain what is to be done and why to the client. Determine caregiver's cognitive function.

   - Ability to understand and carry out interventions
   - Ability to make safe decisions and judgments
   - Willingness to care for client.
2. Determine caregiver's sensory and motor function.
   - Ability to hear client's needs

SKILL 17.4   Assessing Caregiver's Safety *(continued)*

- Visual acuity to read directions, medication labels
- Ability to feel temperature changes (e.g., water for bathing).
3. Determine caregiver's motor function and strength.
   - Ability to assist client in transfer, moving, turning, and ADLs
   - Ability to provide treatments and care for client
   - Ability to prepare food and do housekeeping chores
   - Ability to do shopping and provide transportation for physician visits.
4. Determine need for client care assistance with ADLs.
   - Type of wheelchair, with or without removable arms
   - Shower chairs that fit over toilet or in shower
   - Toilet seat risers.
5. Determine need for type of transfer assist devices for safe client handling.
   - Gait belts: provide secure grip without holding onto client's clothes or limbs. **Rationale:** *Prevents caregiver strain*

because client weight is closer to caregiver and he or she can assume upright position.
   - Small slide/transfer board: used for seated lateral transfers, such as between bed and wheelchair or commode. **Rationale:** *Caregiver does not need to lift client manually.*
   - Turning discs: used to pivot seated clients who can bear weight and stand. The client is guided to a standing position without adjusting their feet. The client must be able to stand or the caregiver will have to exert excessive force in an awkward position.
   - Mechanical lift devices such as the lean–stand assist lift and sling-type full lift are used for clients who cannot support their own weight.
   - Repositioning devices: mechanically pull client up in bed without need for caregiver to assist client.
   - Trapeze lifts: a bar device suspended above the bed that allows clients with upper body strength to reposition.
6. Document findings in client's chart.

▶ ENVIRONMENTAL SAFETY

Expected Outcomes

1. Client is acclimated to home environment and is able to provide safe self-care after a period of support from agency staff.
2. Client is provided appropriate home care modalities.
3. Client's environment is safe from potential mechanical, chemical, fire, and electrical hazards.
4. All electrical equipment is intact and operating safely.
5. Safe environment provides for client safety in home.

SKILL 17.5   Providing Safety for Clients During a Fire

Equipment

- Appropriate extinguisher for fire:
- Water type
- Soda-acid type
- Foam type
- Dry chemical type
- ABC extinguisher

Procedure

1. Introduce self, explain what is to be done and why. Provide safety for client and self. Follow hospital policy and procedure for type of fire safety program and for ringing the fire alarm to summon help.
2. Remove all clients from the immediate area to a safe place. Be familiar with fire exits and agency evacuation plan.
3. To remove a client safely from the fire, use carrying method that is most comfortable for you and safe for client.
   - Place blanket (or bedspread) on floor. Lower client onto blanket. Lift up head end of blanket and drag client out of danger.
   - Use two-person swing method. Place client in sitting position. Form a seat by having two people clasp forearms or shoulders. Lift client into "seat" and carry out of danger.

- Carry client using "back-strap" carry method. Step in front of client. Place client's arms around your neck. Grasp client's wrists and hold tight against your chest. Pull client onto your back and carry to safety.
4. Activate fire alarm.
5. Secure the burning area by closing all doors and windows.
6. Shut off all possible oxygen sources and electrical appliances in the fire area.
7. If possible, employ the appropriate extinguishing method without endangering yourself. Fire extinguishers should not be used directly on an individual.
8. Be familiar with the different types of fire extinguishers and their locations ❶.

Class A
- Water-under-pressure type or soda-acid type.
- Use on cloth, wood, paper, plastic, rubber, or leather.
- Never use on electrical or chemical fires due to danger of shock.

Class B
- Foam, dry chemical type.
- Use on fires such as gasoline, alcohol, acetone, oil, grease, or paint thinner and remover.
- Class A extinguisher is never used on Class B fires.

(continued on next page)

SKILL 17.5   Providing Safety for Clients During a Fire (continued)

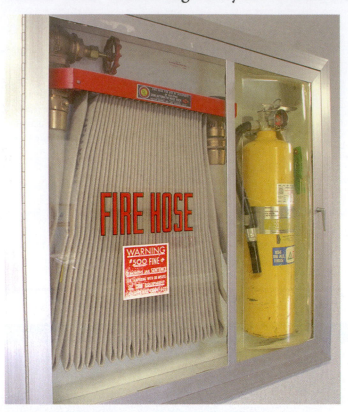

❶ Become familiar with the location and use of fire extinguishers in the hospital.

Class C
- Dry chemical or carbon dioxide types.
- Use on electrical wiring, electrical equipment, or motors.
- Class A or Class B extinguishers are never used on Class C fires.

Class ABC Combination
- Contains graphite.
- Use on any type of fire.
- Most common extinguisher in use.

9. Keep fire exits clear at all times.

RACE: Priorities for Fire Safety

R   Rescue and remove all clients in immediate danger.
A   Activate fire alarm.
C   Confine the fire; close doors, window, turn off oxygen supplies and electrical equipment.
E   Extinguish fire when possible.

SKILL 17.6   Preventing Thermal/Electrical Injuries

Equipment
- Fire extinguishers

Procedure

1. Make sure that all electrical apparatuses are routinely checked and maintained. Look for safety inspection expiration dates on biomedical equipment.
2. Have all electrical appliances brought to the hospital by client (radios, electric razors, hair dryers, etc.) inspected by hospital maintenance staff. It is best to discourage use of nonhospital equipment.
3. Make sure water in the tub or shower is not more than 43°C (110°F) (or 35°C [95°F] for those with circulatory insufficiency).
4. When heating pads, sitz bath, or hot compresses are used, check the client frequently for redness. Maximum temperature should not exceed 41°C (105°F) (or 35°C [95°F] for those with circulatory insufficiency).
5. Hospitals do not allow smoking in the facility. There may be designated smoking areas outside the building. Inform clients and visitors about the hospital's smoking regulations. Do not allow confused, sedated, or severely incapacitated clients to smoke without direct supervision.

CLINICAL ALERT

Older clients and those who are diabetic or comatose are especially vulnerable to thermal injuries.

6. Store all combustible materials securely to prevent spontaneous combustion.
7. Make sure that all staff and employees participate in and understand fire safety measures, such as extinguishing fires, and the plan for evacuating clients.
8. Report and do not use any apparatus that produces a shock, has a broken plug or ground pin, or has a frayed cord.
9. Never apply direct heat (e.g., heating pad) to ischemic tissue—doing so increases the tissues need for oxygen.
10. Turn equipment off before unplugging it. **Rationale:** *This prevents sparks that can cause a fire.*
11. Plug devices that require a high current (i.e., ventilators or radiant warmers) into separate outlets. **Rationale:** *This prevents overloading the circuit that could lead to a fire.*
12. Use only three-pronged grounded plugs.

SKILL 17.7   Evaluating the Home Environment

Equipment

- Home Assessment Checklist
- Outcome and Assessment Information Act (OASIS-B1)

Procedure

1. Introduce self and identify client. Explain what is to be done and why. Identify type of dwelling (i.e., client owned, boarding home, rental, mobile home).
2. Identify water source.
3. Identify sewer source.
4. Identify type of plumbing available.
5. Determine if any pollutants are present in the environment.
6. Assess exterior of the home for:
   - Condition of sidewalks and steps
   - Presence of railings on steps
   - Barriers that prevent easy access to the home
   - Adequacy of lighting
   - Adequacy of roof and windows.
7. Assess interior of the home for:
   - Presence of scatter rugs or worn carpeting
   - Uncluttered pathways throughout the house
   - Adequacy of lighting
   - Doorways wide enough to permit assistive devices
   - Cleanliness of house
   - Presence of insects, rodents, or infective agents
   - Presence of functioning smoke detectors
   - Adequate heating and cooling systems
   - Presence of running water.
8. Determine if hazardous materials are safely stored.
9. Assess for presence of lead-based paint.
10. Determine if medications can be adequately stored out of reach of children and impaired individuals.
11. Assess stairway and halls for:
    - Adequacy of light
    - Handrails that are securely fastened to wall
    - Flooring in good repair
    - Rugs or carpeting in good repair
    - Light switches in easy reach and accessible at both ends of stairs or hallway.
12. Assess kitchen for:
    - Properly functioning stove
    - Adequacy of light surrounding stove and sink
    - Condition of small appliances
    - Accessibility of appliances to clients in wheelchairs
    - Adequacy of sewage disposal.
13. Assess bathroom for:
    - Skidproof strips or mat in tub or shower
    - Handrails around toilet and tub or shower
    - Accessibility of medicine cabinet
    - Adequate space if wheelchairs or walkers are used
    - Temperature of hot water from faucets in sink, tub, or shower.
14. Assess bedroom for:
    - Accessibility of closets and cabinets
    - Ease in getting into and out of bed
    - Adequate space, if commode or wheelchair is required
    - Night light availability
    - Accessibility of medications, water on a nightstand
    - Calling system to alert healthcare provider
    - Flooring in good repair and nonslippery surface.
15. Document findings.

SKILL 17.8   Administering Poison Control Agents

Equipment

- Large (37–40 Fr) soft Ewald tube (Physician may insert; client who is comatose must have endotracheal tube in place.)
- Lukewarm tap water or saline for lavage
- Container for aspirated contents
- Large irrigating syringe with catheter tip
- 50–100 g activated charcoal or prepackaged charcoal/sorbitol product mixed with water to consistency to administer through tube

  or

- Balanced polyethylene glycol–electrolyte solution (e.g., GoLYTELY) for bowel irrigation

Preparation

(See Preparation section for Skill 12.4, Inserting a Nasogastric Tube.)

Procedure

1. Check physician's orders and gather supplies. Introduce self and identify client. Perform hand hygiene and provide privacy. Provide comfort and safety for client and self. Place comatose intubated client in a head-down, left side-lying position or place cooperative alert client on commode.
2. Don clean gloves. Insert large-bore (37–40 Fr) flexible tube nasogastrically or orogastrically.
3. Aspirate gastric contents and save specimen for analysis.
4. Lavage repeatedly with 50–100 mL of fluid until return is clear.
5. Administer activated charcoal slurry and repeat if ordered or, for cooperative client, administer balanced electrolyte solution per nasogastric tube at a rate of 1–2 L/hr until rectal runout is clear.
6. Remove gloves and perform hand hygiene. Document the procedure, significant events during the procedure, and client's response to the procedure.

CLINICAL ALERT

For a known toxin, one should call a regional poison control center by dialing 800-222-1222.

Activated Charcoal for Ingested Poisons

Activated charcoal adsorbs significant amounts of certain poisons, especially when an individual overdoses. The earlier charcoal is given, the more effective it is. The amount given is 5 to 10 times that of the suspected poison or, if the poison is unknown, 50 to 100 g for adults.

▶ IMMOBILIZERS AND RESTRAINTS

Expected Outcomes

1. Client is prevented from injuring self or others.
2. Restraints are applied appropriately.
3. Client does not develop complications due to restraint use (e.g., agitation, pressure ulcers, circulatory disturbance).
4. Child is prevented from reaching an incision site, IVs, or tubes.
5. Client remains in restraints for a limited amount of time.
6. Client does not endure undue psychological stress while being placed in restraints.

SKILL 17.9   Applying a Papoose Board Immobilizer

Equipment

- Immobilization board (papoose) to fit the child's size
- Sheet
- Infection control supplies as needed

Preparation

1. Check physician's order and gather equipment and supplies for the procedure. **Rationale:** *Having supplies prepared reduces the time the child spends in temporary restraint devices and reduces the anxiety felt by the child.*
2. Introduce self to the child and parent. Verify client's identify. Explain the reason for immobilization to the child and parent and how long it will be needed. Tell the child how the restraint will feel. **Rationale:** *Young children will be less anxious if the explanation about what they will feel is placed in nonthreatening, developmentally appropriate terms.*
3. Have an assistant (or the parent) available to help position and hold a body part if needed. **Rationale:** *The papoose is most often used when the nurse does not have an assistant available or a parent willing to restrain the child for a procedure.*

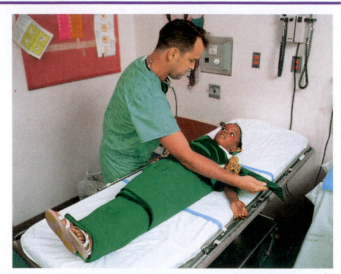

❶ Child on a papoose board.

Procedure

1. Perform hand hygiene and provide privacy. Provide comfort and safety for client. Place a towel or sheet over the board.
2. Have the child lie supine on the board, with the head at the top ❶.
3. Place the fabric wrappings around the child, and secure the Velcro fasteners. To be most effective, the fabric wrappings should be secure over the elbows, hips, and knees to prevent flexion. **Rationale:** *This action prevents the child from pulling apart the wrappings or from kicking.*
4. After the procedure, release the child and allow the parents to provide comfort. Document findings and client response.

SKILL 17.10   Applying a Mummy Immobilizer

Equipment

- Soft blanket or sheet two to three times larger than the child

Preparation

1. Check physician's order and have supplies and materials for the procedure collected and ready for use.
2. Explain the procedure to the child and parent.

Procedure

Infant

1. Introduce self to parent and verify client's identity. Perform hand hygiene and provide privacy. Provide comfort and safety for client. Put the blanket (or sheet) on the bed or examination table. Fold down one corner until it reaches the middle of the blanket.
2. Place the infant in a diagonal position with his or her neck on the folded edge.
3. Bring one side of the blanket over the infant's arm and then under the back. Tuck that edge under and over the other arm and around the back. It may be helpful to roll the infant on the side to smooth the blanket behind the back, and then roll the infant onto the back over the smoothed section of blanket.
4. Bring the other side of the blanket around the body and tuck underneath the body.
5. Bring the bottom corner of the blanket up and over the abdomen.

Toddler and Older Child

1. Put the blanket (or sheet) on the bed or examination table. Fold down one corner until it reaches the middle of the blanket.

SKILL 17.10   Applying a Mummy Immobilizer (*continued*)

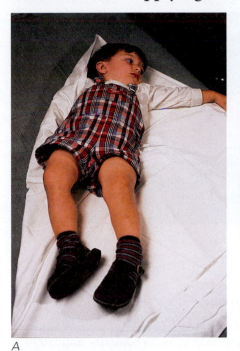

A

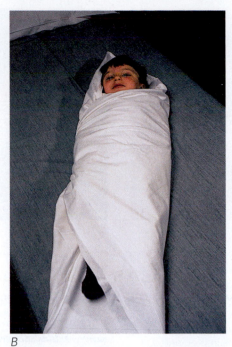

B

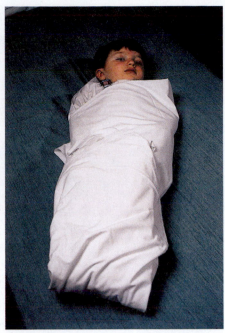

C

1 Steps in applying mummy immobilization.

2. Place the child on the blanket, positioning so that there is sufficient material to wrap the knees and lower legs. If necessary, fold down the top edges of the blanket to the shoulders.

3. Bring one side of the blanket over the arm, body, and legs, and tuck it under the other arm and around the back and legs **1**.

4. Bring the other side of the blanket up and around the body, and tuck underneath the back and legs. **Rationale:** *The child should not be able to flex the knees and kick or it may be impossible to perform the procedure.*

SKILL 17.11   Applying a Wrist or Ankle Restraint

Delegation

The nurse must make the determination that restraints are appropriate in specific situations, select the proper type of restraints, evaluate the effectiveness of the restraints, and assess for potential complications from their use. Application of ordered restraints and their temporary removal for skin monitoring and care may be delegated to UAP who have been trained in their use.

Equipment

■ Appropriate type and size of restraint

Procedure

1. Check physician's order. If no order, call physician or licensed independent practitioner (LIP) for restraint order before applying restraints. If restraints must be placed before the order is obtained, ensure the order is obtained within 1 hour for either a nonbehavioral health client or a behavioral health client. **Rationale:** *Physician's order is required to apply restraints.*

2. Gather equipment and supplies. Prior to performing the procedure, introduce self and verify the client's identity using agency protocol. Explain to the client and family what you are going to do, why it is necessary, and how they can participate. Allow time for the client to express feelings about being restrained. Provide needed emotional reassurance that the restraints will be used only when absolutely necessary and that there will be close contact with the client in case assistance is required.

3. Perform hand hygiene and observe other appropriate infection control procedures.

4. Provide for client privacy if indicated. Provide comfort and safety for client.

5. Apply the selected restraint.

Wrist or Ankle Restraint

■ Pad bony prominences on the wrist or ankle if needed to prevent skin breakdown.

■ Apply the padded portion of the restraint around the ankle or wrist.

■ Pull the tie of the restraint through the slit in the wrist portion or through the buckle and ensure the restraint is not too tight **1**.

■ Using a half-bow knot, attach the other end of the restraint to the movable portion of the bed frame. **Rationale:** *If the ties are attached to the movable portion, the wrist or ankle will not be pulled when the bed position is changed.*

6. Adjust the plan of care as required, for example, to include releasing the restraint, providing skin care and range-of-

(continued on next page)

SKILL 17.11 Applying a Wrist or Ankle Restraint (continued)

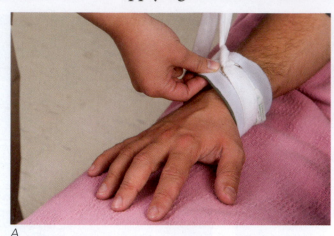

A

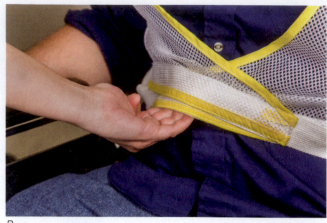

B

❶ Ensure that a finger can be inserted between the restraint and, *A*, the wrist and, *B*, the chest.

motion exercises, and attending to the client's physical needs by providing fluids, nutrition, and toileting.

7. Document on the client's chart the behavior(s) indicating the need for the restraint, all other interventions implemented in an attempt to avoid the use of restraints and their outcomes, and the time the primary care provider was notified of the need for restraint. Also record:

- The type of restraint applied, the time it was applied, and the goal for its application
- The client's response to the restraint, including a rationale for its continued use (Anstine, 2007)
- The times that the restraints were removed and skin care given
- Any other assessments and interventions
- Explanations given the client and significant others.

Sample Documentation

7/10/2015 1200 Confused. Disoriented to time and place. Reoriented frequently. Pulling at central IV line, NG tube, and chest tube. Medicated for pain relief. Lights dimmed. _____ M. Murray, RN

1245 Continues to pull at IV and tubes. Dr. Jones notified. Received an order to apply mitt restraints. Family notified and situation explained. Family member to come and sit with client. Mitt restraints applied, relaxation music initiated. _____ M. Murray, RN

1330 Son arrived and sitting with client. Calm though still disoriented. Mitts removed, skin intact, hands warm with good color and mobility. Vital signs stable. _____ M. Murray, RN

Developmental Considerations

INFANTS

Elbow restraints are used to prevent infants or small children from flexing their elbows to touch or reach their face or head, especially after surgery. Ready-made elbow restraints are available commercially (e.g., No-No's).

A mummy restraint is made by folding a blanket or sheet around the infant, in a certain way to prevent movement during a procedure such as gastric washing, eye irrigation, or collection of a blood specimen.

CHILDREN

- A human restraint (parent or assistant) can be used during intramuscular injections.
- A papoose board immobilizer can be used for toddlers and larger children.
- A crib net is simply a device placed over the top of a crib to prevent active young children from climbing out of the crib. At the same time, it allows them freedom to move about in the crib. The crib net or dome is not attached to the movable parts of the crib so that the caregiver can have access to the child without removing the dome or net.
  - Place the net over the sides and ends of the crib.

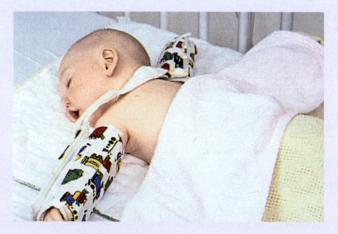

Infant with elbow restraints.

- Secure the ties to the springs or frame of the crib. The crib sides can then be freely lowered without removing the net.
- Test with your hand that the net will stretch if the child stands against it in the crib.

SKILL 17.11   Applying a Wrist or Ankle Restraint (*continued*)

Setting of Care

While other measures should always be tried first, restraints may be necessary for clients in wheelchairs or in the home. Safety guidelines apply in all cases. Assess the knowledge and skill of all caregivers in the use of restraints and educate as indicated.

- Use means other than restraints as much as possible, and stay with the client. Remember that the goal is a restraint-free environment.
- Pad bony prominences, such as wrists and ankles, if needed before applying a restraint over them.

- Tie restraints with half-bow (quick release) knots that will not tighten when pulled, and to parts of the wheelchair that do not move and release quickly in case of emergency. Tie to parts of the wheelchair that do not move.
- Assess restrained limbs for signs of impaired blood circulation.
- Always stay with a client whose restraint is temporarily removed.

Many institutions use a restraint monitoring and intervention flow sheet to ensure careful documentation.

SKILL 17.12   Applying a Torso/Belt Restraint

Equipment

- Safety belt restraint (usually 2-in. soft webbing material) with waist and side belts (for bed)

Procedure

1. Check physician's order and gather belt and supplies. Belts usually have a key-locked buckle ❶. **Rationale:** *To prevent slipping and to provide a snug fit.*
2. Perform hand hygiene and observe other appropriate infection control procedures.
3. Provide for client privacy if indicated.
4. Identify client using two identifiers and explain necessity for safety belt to client and family.
5. Provide for client comfort and safety. Apply torso restraint as follows:
   - Slip waist belt through flat buckle, adjusting to client's size.
   - Snap hinged plate shut by hooking plain end of key over cross bar and lifting upward.
   - Attach side belts to bed frame in similar manner.
   - Release restraint by hooking green end of key over cross bar from below and pulling downward.
6. Document time, rationale, and type of safety belt used in nurses' notes, along with client monitoring, client response, frequency of care measures, and time and rationale for discontinuing restraint. Documentation must be done every 15 minutes.

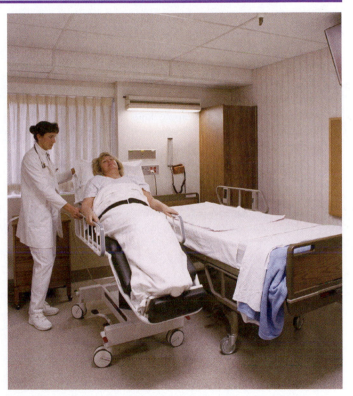

❶ Some belts have a key-locked buckle to prevent slipping and to provide a snug fit.

SKILL 17.13   Managing Clients in Restraints

Equipment

- Appropriate restraint: limb, torso, or vest

Preparation

- Identify and evaluate if less restrictive measures have been explored before the client is placed in restraints.
- Check physician's order. If no order, call physician or licensed independent practitioner (LIP) for restraint order before applying restraints. If restraints must be placed before the order is obtained, ensure the order is obtained within 1 hour

for either a nonbehavioral health client or a behavioral health client. **Rationale:** *Physician's order is required to apply restraints.*

Note: Follow guidelines for obtaining restraint orders and updating orders according to hospital policy.

- Ensure that a face-to-face assessment is completed on the client within 8 hours for a nonbehavioral health client, and 1 hour for a behavioral (psychiatric) health client. **Rationale:** *Frequent assessments prevent complications.*

(continued on next page)

SKILL 17.13   Managing Clients in Restraints (continued)

- Ensure that restraint orders are renewed every 24 hours or sooner according to facility policy for nonbehavioral health clients, or every 2 to 4 hours for behavioral health clients. Children from ages 12 to 17 must have orders renewed every 2 hours, for a maximum of 24 hours. **Rationale:** *Restraints should be discontinued as soon as possible.*
- Establish and implement a plan of care for the client to eliminate the need for restraints.
- Introduce self. Perform hand hygiene. Provide for client privacy as appropriate. Provide for client comfort and safety. Discuss the use of restraints with the client and family members. If possible, elicit the support of the family or use sitters to stay with the client rather than place the client in restraints.

CLINICAL ALERT

Restraints are indicated only if there is no other viable option available to protect the client, and then they are implemented only when the client is assessed and evaluated by an appropriate LIP.

Three types of restraints are used in clinical practice:

1. *Chemical:* Sedating psychotropic drugs to manage or control behavior. Psychoactive medication used in this manner is an inappropriate use of medication.
2. *Physical:* Direct application of physical force to a client, without the client's permission, to restrict his or her freedom of movement.
3. *Seclusion:* Involuntary confinement of a client in a locked room. Physical force may be applied by individuals, mechanical devices, or a combination of any of them.

Procedure

1. Gather appropriate restraint and perform hand hygiene.
2. Identify client using two identifiers and seek the client's cooperation with restraint procedure, if possible.
3. Apply restraint according to manufacturer's specific directions.
4. Monitor and assess the client every 15 minutes, or according to facility policy.

5. Release restraint at least every 2 hours or sooner (per the Joint Commission). **Rationale:** *Releasing restraints allows the client to be provided with the following:*
   - Toileting
   - Fluids and food
   - Hygiene care such as brushing teeth or washing face and hands
   - Circulation checked; skin care provided
   - Body alignment checked
   - Range of motion to all joints, particularly those in restraints.

CLINICAL ALERT

In acute medical and postsurgical care, a restraint may be necessary to ensure that an IV or tube feeding is not removed, or the client cannot be allowed out of bed following surgery. This type of medical restraint may be used temporarily to limit mobility or prevent injury to the client.

Additional types of activities that may constitute a restraint include:

- Tucking a client's sheet so tight that he or she cannot move
- Using a side rail to prevent a client from voluntarily getting out of bed
- Placing the client in a geri-chair with a table
- Placing a wheelchair-bound client so close to the wall that it prevents him or her from moving.

6. Avoid application of force on long bone joints and pad bony prominences beneath restraint. **Rationale:** *Reduces pressure on skin.*
7. Take vital signs every 8 hours unless indicated more frequently.
8. Bathe client every 24 hours or more often as needed.
9. Do not interrupt the client's sleep unless indicated by his or her medical condition.
10. Ensure that a new order and the physician or LIP completes a medical assessment every 24 hours.
11. Obtain a physician's order and discontinue restraints as soon as it is clinically indicated.
12. Document all assessments and findings on appropriate forms.

SKILL 17.14   Using a Bed or Chair Exit Safety Monitoring Device

Delegation

Risk factors for falls may be observed and recorded by persons other than the nurse. The nurse is responsible for assessing the client and confirming that there is a risk of the client falling when getting out of a chair or bed unassisted. The nurse develops a plan of care that includes a variety of interventions that will protect the client. If indicated, use of a safety monitoring device may be delegated to unlicensed assistive personnel (UAP) who have been trained in its application and monitoring.

Equipment

- Alarm and control device
- Sensor
- Connection to nurse call system

Procedure

1. Prior to performing the procedure, introduce self and verify the client's identity using agency protocol. Explain to client

SKILL 17.14   Using a Bed or Chair Exit Safety Monitoring Device (*continued*)

and family the purpose and procedure for using a safety monitoring device. Explain that the device does not limit mobility in any manner; rather, it alerts the staff when the client is about to get out of the bed or a chair. Explain that the nurse must be called when the client needs to get out of the bed or a chair.

2. Perform hand hygiene and observe other appropriate infection control procedures.

3. Provide for client privacy.

4. Test the battery device and alarm sound. **Rationale:** *Testing ensures that the device is functioning properly prior to use.*

5. Apply the leg band or sensor pad.
   - Place the leg band according to the manufacturer's recommendation. Place the client's leg in a straight horizontal position. **Rationale:** *The alarm device is position sensitive; that is, when it approaches a near-vertical position (such as in walking, crawling, or kneeling as the client attempts to get out of bed), the audio alarm will be triggered.*
   - For the bed or chair device, the sensor is usually placed under the buttocks area.
   - For a bed or chair device, set the time delay to 1 to 12 seconds for determining the client's movement patterns.
   - Connect the sensor pad to the control unit and the nurse call system.

6. Instruct the client to call the nurse when the client wants or needs to get up, and assist as required.
   - When assisting the client up, deactivate the alarm.
   - Assist the client back to the bed or chair, and reattach the alarm device.

7. Ensure client safety with additional safety precautions.
   - Place call light within client reach, lift side rails per agency policy, and lower the bed to its lowest position. **Rationale:** *The alarm device is not a substitute for other precautionary measures.*
   - Place fall risk or fall precaution signs on the client's door, chart, and other relevant locations.

8. Document the type of alarm used, where it was placed, and its effectiveness in the client record using forms or checklists supplemented by narrative notes when appropriate. Record all additional safety precautions and interventions discussed and employed.

Sample Documentation

7/2/15 1130 Found out of bed despite frequent verbal reminders to use call light for assistance. Explained about using a magnetic box mobility alarm to ensure own safety from possible fall. Verbalized agreement. Alarm device applied. Reminded again of importance to call the nurse for assistance. Call light placed within client's reach. _____ J. Wallace, RN

Setting of Care

If a monitoring device is used in the home, instruct caregivers to do the following:

- Test the monitoring device every 12 to 24 hours to ensure that it is working.
- Check the volume of the alarm to ascertain they can hear it.
- Although these devices are sensitive and alarms can be triggered by normal movement, instruct family to investigate all alarms, and not to assume a false alarm. They may, however, adjust the alarm controls.

Use of the device does not take the place of proper supervision of clients at risk for falling. Assessment of the reasons for falling, especially among older adults, can lead to effective prevention.

▶ CRITICAL THINKING OPTIONS FOR UNEXPECTED OUTCOMES

Not all unexpected outcomes require further nursing intervention; however, many times they do. When the client demonstrates a change in signs/symptoms indicating an emerging problem, the nurse should immediately assess and troubleshoot what is happening. The assessment data must be processed quickly to formulate a hypothesis so the nurse can make a clinical judgment. The nurse then decides how best to resolve the problem and improve the client's situation for a better appropriate outcome.

EXPECTED OUTCOMES	PROBLEM SOLVING	NURSING ACTIONS
Home Care Safety All personal articles and call light are within easy reach of the client.	Client with history of falling has developed acute cognitive changes.	■ Alert all personnel that client is high risk for fall. ■ Review medication regimen (e.g., Demerol and psychoactive drugs can cause acute confusion). ■ Assess for physiological causes (e.g., hypoxemia, infection, pain) and address alterations. ■ Place bedside commode away from bed and remove all obstacles; provide good lighting as well as night-light.

EXPECTED OUTCOMES	PROBLEM SOLVING	NURSING ACTIONS
		■ Reduce environmental stimuli (e.g., television). ■ Reorient client with each encounter. ■ Move client for better surveillance. ■ Employ monitoring alarm/device or engage family attendance. ■ Request floor mattress or recliner chair.
Toxic substances are removed by lavage/not absorbed.	Client has ingested a large number of tablets that cannot be removed by lavage.	■ Whole-bowel irrigation is more effective for ingestion of enteric-coated or sustained-release tablets. ■ Repeated dose of activated charcoal may be indicated to speed drug elimination. ■ Prepare for possible arrangement for hemodialysis.
Client is safely repositioned or transferred without injury to client or caregiver.	Unable to transfer client from bed to wheelchair due to excess weight.	■ Determine if wheelchair without arms or transfer board can aid in transfer. ■ Contact social services to obtain bariatric assist devices. ■ Determine if other family members can assist with transfer. ■ May need home health aide services to assist with transfer.
Caregiver is able to manage turning, repositioning, and assistive devices.	Injury occurs to client when caregiver attempts transfer to wheelchair.	■ Do not continue to reposition client; place in bed. ■ Conduct a complete sensory, motor, and pain assessment. ■ Notify physician. ■ Document findings.
Environmental Safety Client is acclimated to home environment and is able to provide safe self-care after a period of support from agency staff.	Client is noncompliant with treatments, safety procedures, and taking medications at home.	■ Explain rationale for following home care plan. ■ Discuss reason with client, caregiver, and family members to determine whether change in plan would increase compliance. ■ Remind client that if he or she refuses to follow plan, he or she will be taken off services. ■ Document appropriately on all forms indicating noncompliance issues. ■ Notify physician.
Client's environment is safe from potential mechanical, chemical, fire, and electrical hazards.	The client, nurse, or visitor experiences an accident or injury related to mechanical, chemical, or thermal trauma.	■ Provide immediate first aid or care. ■ Assess vital signs and notify physician. ■ Report the incident according to hospital procedure. Unusual occurrence forms are used to protect the injured individual, the nurse, and the hospital. ■ Review safety procedures to ensure a safe environment. ■ Report all malfunctioning equipment immediately to the proper department.
	Unfamiliarity with hospital fire and disaster protocol results in poor performance.	■ Review protocols frequently to update knowledge base. ■ Participate in fire and disaster drills to become familiar with protocols.
Immobilizers and Restraints Client does not develop complications due to restraint use (e.g., agitation, pressure ulcers, circulatory disturbance).	Skin abrasion, maceration, or rash occurs after application of restraints.	■ Reassess absolute need for restraint. ■ Reassess application method. ■ Increase padding of soft restraints before application. ■ Keep restraints off as much as possible and have staff or family member stay with client.
	Impaired circulation or edema evidenced by change in color, sensation, movement, and blanching of nail beds.	■ On observation of signs of neurovascular changes, immediately release restraints. ■ Massage area gently to increase circulation. ■ If extremity is edematous, elevate extremity above level of heart. Encourage range-of-motion movements. ■ Request order for different type of restraint.

EXPECTED OUTCOMES	PROBLEM SOLVING	NURSING ACTIONS
Restraints are applied appropriately.	Client unties restraints.	■ Camouflage restraint to decrease client's awareness. ■ Reassess need for restraint. ■ Exhaust alternative measures to promote safety. ■ Anticipate and attend to client's needs.
Child is prevented from reaching an incision site, IVs, or tubes.	Child is able to reach incision site even with elbow restraints in place.	■ Make sure the elbow restraints are tight enough and extend over the elbow. ■ Tie the one elbow restraint to the opposite elbow restraint by placing the tie under the child's back and securing the tie with the upper tie on the opposite restraint. ■ Check that the restraint is large enough to completely immobilize the elbow. If not, obtain a larger size or use two restraints and tie them together securely.

RELATED CONCEPTS

The Concept of Tissue Integrity

Exemplar 21.1
Burns

Exemplar 21.2
Contact Dermatitis

Exemplar 21.3
Pressure Ulcers

Exemplar 21.4
Wound Healing

Skills-at-a-Glance

The skin serves a variety of functions, including protecting the individual from injury. Impaired skin integrity is not a frequent problem for most healthy people, but is a threat to older adults and clients with restricted mobility, chronic illness, trauma, and those undergoing invasive procedures. When the skin or underlying tissues are damaged, the inflammatory process of the individual's immune response acts to eliminate any foreign material, if possible, and prepare the injured area for healing. This injured body area is called a **wound**. The nurse plays an important role in assessing client risk for developing wounds, in preventing wounds, and in treating various types of wounds (Table 18–1 ●).

CLINICAL ALERT

For many years, evidence has supported that moist wounds heal faster and with a lower rate of infection than dry wounds. With occlusive dressings, optimal tissue building components found in wound exudate are retained with less scab formation and pain. Cells can continue to function effectively. Wound healing is negatively affected by too much moisture.

TABLE 18–1 Types of Wounds

TYPE	CAUSE	DESCRIPTION & CHARACTERISTICS
Incision	Sharp instrument (e.g., knife or scalpel)	Open wound; deep or shallow
Contusion	Blow from a blunt instrument	Closed wound; skin appears ecchymotic (bruised) because of damaged blood vessels
Abrasion	Surface scrape, either unintentional (e.g., scraped knee from a fall) or intentional (e.g., dermal abrasion to remove pockmarks)	Open wound involving the skin
Puncture	Penetration of the skin and often the underlying tissues by a sharp instrument, either intentional or unintentional	Open wound
Laceration	Tissues torn apart, often from accidents (e.g., with machinery)	Open wound; edges are often jagged
Penetrating wound	Penetration of the skin and the underlying tissues, usually unintentional (e.g., from a bullet or metal fragments)	Open wound

Evidence-Based Nursing Practice

Medieval Remedies: Leeches, Maggots, and Bee Stings

Medieval remedies, like using maggots for bedsores, bee stings for multiple sclerosis, and leeches to improve blood flow after surgery, are enjoying a comeback, but not all are supported by research.

Leeches, used for thousands of years in medical treatments, fell out of use with the introduction of antibiotics. However, in recent years they have shown their value, especially with microvascular surgery. For example, in reattachment surgery it is fairly easy to reconnect large arterial blood vessels but very difficult to reconnect thinner, more delicate venous vessels. Subsequent pooling of blood and swelling can choke off blood flow completely. Leeches relieve this congestion, allowing blood to flow. Their natural anticoagulants prevent clotting and ensure blood flow to the reattached limb until the venous blood vessels can reconnect and survive.

Maggot treatment or conventional treatment for wound debridement was provided to 119 clients (Opletalová, 2012). Each client had a nonhealing, sloughy wound 40 cm² or smaller, less than 2 cm deep, and an ankle brachial index of 0.8 or higher. Results showed a significantly greater rate of cleaning on day 8 in clients being treated with maggots. However, the improvement rate did not continue; by day 15 results were about the same for both groups. This study concluded that maggot debridement has significant benefit in the first week of treatment, but that in the second week another type of dressing should be used.

Bee stings have been used as alternative therapy for treatment of such wide-ranging conditions as multiple sclerosis, debilitation after stroke, and arthritis, and have been used in China for acupuncture (Bee sting therapy, 2013). However, reports of its success have been anecdotal. There have been no controlled studies of bee stings that provide scientific evidence of its value as therapy. Further research may show a role for bee stings (e.g., in the treatment of pain), but the National Multiple Sclerosis Society and the American Cancer Society both specifically caution the public that evidence does not support use of bee stings as treatment for multiple sclerosis or cancer.

Data from Medicinal leeches (2011), Opletalová et al. (2012), and Bee sting therapy (2013).

▶ ASSESSMENT OF TISSUE INTEGRITY

Expected Outcomes

1. Client's wound does not become infected.
2. Client's wound remains intact following staple and/or suture removal.
3. Wound care is provided for contaminated wound and healing occurs.
4. Drainage system functions without obstructions.
5. Wound irrigation is completed using sufficient pressure to cleanse wound bed.
6. Client maintains adequate fluid and nutrition.
7. Client's buttocks and perineal area remain free from urine and stool.
8. Client is periodically repositioned.

SKILL 18.1 Obtaining a Wound Drainage Specimen

Delegation

Obtaining a wound culture is an invasive procedure that requires the application of sterile technique, knowledge of wound healing, and potential problem solving to ensure client safety. Therefore, the nurse needs to perform this skill and does not delegate it to unlicensed assistive personnel (UAP).

Equipment

- Clean gloves
- Protective eyewear, if appropriate
- Sterile gloves
- Moisture-resistant bag
- Sterile dressing set
- Normal saline and irrigating syringe
- Culture tube with swab and culture medium (aerobic and anaerobic tubes are available) or sterile syringe with needle for anaerobic culture.
- Completed labels for each container
- Completed requisition to accompany the specimens to the laboratory

Preparation

- Check the physician's orders to determine if the specimen is to be collected for an **aerobic** (growing only in the presence of oxygen) or **anaerobic** (growing only in the absence of oxygen) culture. Aerobic organisms are generally found on the surface of the wound, whereas anaerobic organisms would be found in deep wounds, tunnels, and cavities.
- Administer an analgesic 30 minutes before the procedure if the client is complaining of pain at the wound site to prevent unnecessary discomfort during the procedure.

Procedure

1. Prior to performing the procedure, introduce self and verify the client's identity using agency protocol. Explain to the client what you are going to do, why it is necessary, and how he or she can participate. Discuss how the results will be used in planning further care or treatments.
2. Perform hand hygiene and observe other appropriate infection control procedures.
3. Provide for client privacy.
4. Remove any moist outer dressings that cover the wound.
   - Apply clean gloves.
   - Remove the outer dressing, and observe any drainage on the dressing. Hold the dressing so that the client does not see the drainage. **Rationale:** *The appearance of the drainage could upset the client.*
   - Determine the amount, color, consistency, and odor of the drainage. For example, "one 4 × 4 gauze saturated with yellow-greenish, thick, malodorous drainage."
   - Discard the dressing in the moisture-resistant bag. Handle it carefully so that the dressing does not touch the outside of the bag. **Rationale:** *Touching the outside of the bag will contaminate it.*
   - Remove and discard gloves. Perform hand hygiene.

5. Open the sterile dressing set using sterile technique.
6. Assess the wound.
   - Apply sterile gloves.
   - Assess the appearance of the tissues in and around the wound and the drainage. Infection can cause reddened tissues with a thick discharge, which may be foul smelling, whitish, or colored.
7. Cleanse the wound.
   - Using gauze swabs or irrigation, cleanse the wound with normal saline until all visible exudates have been removed.
   - After cleansing, apply a sterile gauze pad to the wound. **Rationale:** *This absorbs excess saline.*
   - If a topical antimicrobial ointment or cream is being used to treat the wound, use a swab to remove it. **Rationale:** *Residual antiseptic must be removed prior to culture.*
   - Remove and discard sterile gloves.
8. Obtain the aerobic culture.
   - Apply clean gloves.
   - Open a specimen tube and place the cap upside down on a firm, dry surface so that the inside will not become contaminated, or if the swab is attached to the lid, twist the cap to loosen the swab. Hold the tube in one hand and take out the swab with the other.
   - Rotate the swab back and forth over clean areas of granulation tissue from the sides or base of the wound. **Rationale:** *Microorganisms most likely to be responsible for a wound infection reside in viable tissue.*
   - Do not collect pus or pooled exudates to culture. **Rationale:** *These secretions contain a mixture of contaminants that are not the same as those causing the infection.*
   - Avoid touching the swab to intact skin at the wound edges. **Rationale:** *This prevents the introduction of superficial skin organisms into the culture.*
   - Return the swab to the culture tube, taking care not to touch the top or the outside of the tube ❶. **Rationale:** *The outside of the container must remain free of pathogenic microorganisms to prevent their spread to others.*

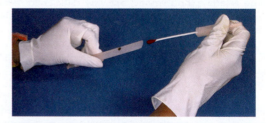

❶ A culturette tube for a wound specimen.

   - Crush the inner ampule containing the medium for organism growth at the bottom of the tube. **Rationale:** *This ensures that the swab with the specimen is surrounded by culture medium.*
   - Twist the cap to secure.
   - If a specimen is required from another site, repeat the steps. Specify the exact site (e.g., inferior drain site or lower aspect of incision) on the label of each container. Be sure to put each swab in the appropriately labeled tube.

SKILL 18.1   Obtaining a Wound Drainage Specimen (*continued*)

9. Dress the wound.
   - Apply any ordered medication to the wound.
   - Cover the wound with a sterile moist transparent wound dressing.
   - Remove and discard gloves. Perform hand hygiene.
10. Arrange for the specimen to be transported to the laboratory immediately. Be sure to include the completed requisition.
11. Document all relevant information.
   - Record on the client's chart the taking of the specimen and source.
   - Include the date and time; the appearance of the wound; the color, consistency, amount, and odor of any drainage; the type of culture collected; and any discomfort experienced by the client.

Sample Documentation

5/27/15 1000 Obtained specimen from (R) hip for anaerobic culture. Pressure ulcer 3 × 3 cm, 6 mm deep, minimal amt. thick, yellow drainage. No odor. Skin around wound reddened. Rates pain at 0 on 0–10 scale.
                                                                  N. Jamaghani, RN

VARIATION: OBTAINING A SPECIMEN FOR ANAEROBIC CULTURE USING A STERILE SYRINGE AND NEEDLE

- Apply clean gloves.
- Insert a sterile 10-mL syringe (without needle) into the wound, and aspirate 1 to 5 mL of drainage into the syringe.
- Attach the needle to the syringe, and expel all air from the syringe and needle.
- Immediately inject the drainage into the anaerobic culture tube.

or

- Use an anaerobic culture swab system in which the swab is immediately placed into a tube filled with an oxygen-free gas or gel environment.
- Label the tube appropriately.
- Remove and discard gloves. Perform hand hygiene.
- Send the tube of drainage to the laboratory immediately. Do not refrigerate the specimen.

▶ DRESSINGS AND BINDERS

Expected Outcomes

1. Client's wound heals without complications.
2. Abdominal binder supports client's abdominal wound.
3. Compression dressing is applied to vascular ulcer site.

SKILL 18.2   Performing a Dry Dressing Change

Delegation

Due to the need for aseptic technique and assessment skills, most dressing changes are not delegated to UAP. In some states, UAP may apply dry dressings to clean, chronic wounds. UAP should observe an exposed wound or dressing during usual care and must report abnormal findings to the nurse. In some agencies, UAP may be permitted to reinforce the dressing (apply additional dry dressings over a saturated bandage), but this must be reported to the nurse as soon as possible. Assessment of the wound and abnormal findings must be validated and interpreted by the nurse.

Equipment

- Clean gloves
- Sterile gloves (optional)
- 4 × 4 gauze
- Hypoallergenic tape, tie tapes, or binder
- Bath blanket (if necessary)
- Moisture-proof bag
- Mask (optional)
- Acetone or another solution (if necessary to loosen adhesive)

- Sterile dressing set; if none is available, gather the following sterile items
  - Drape or towel
  - Gauze squares
  - Container for the cleaning solution
  - Antimicrobial solution
  - Forceps
- Additional supplies required for the particular dressing (e.g., extra gauze dressings and ointment or powder, if ordered)

Preparation

- Check physician's order and gather supplies.
- Acquire assistance for changing a dressing on a restless or confused adult. **Rationale:** *The person might move and contaminate the sterile field or the wound.*
- Make a cuff on the moisture-proof bag for disposal of the soiled dressings, and place the bag within reach. **Rationale:** *Making a cuff keeps the outside of the bag free from contamination by the soiled dressings and prevents subsequent contamination of*

(continued on next page)

SKILL 18.2   Performing a Dry Dressing Change *(continued)*

the nurse's hands or of sterile instrument tips when discarding dressings or sponges. Placement of the bag within reach prevents the nurse from reaching across the sterile field and the wound and potentially contaminating these areas.

Procedure

1. Prior to performing the procedure, introduce self and verify the client's identity using agency protocol. Explain to the client what you are going to do, why it is necessary, and how he or she can participate. Discuss how the results will be used in planning further care or treatments.

2. Perform hand hygiene and observe other appropriate infection control procedures.

3. Provide for client privacy. Assist the client to a comfortable position in which the wound can be readily exposed. Expose only the wound area, using a bath blanket to cover the client, if necessary. **Rationale:** *Undue exposure is physically and psychologically distressing to most people.*

4. Apply a face mask, as indicated. **Rationale:** *A mask may be worn for surgical dressing changes to prevent contamination of the wound by droplet spray from the nurse's respiratory tract.*

5. Remove outer dressings.
   - Apply clean gloves.
   - If adhesive tape was used, remove it by holding down the skin and pulling the tape gently but firmly toward the wound. **Rationale:** *Pressing down on the skin provides countertraction against the pulling motion. Tape is pulled toward the incision to prevent strain on the sutures.*
   - Use a solvent to loosen tape, if required. **Rationale:** *Moistening the tape with acetone or a similar solvent lessens the discomfort of removal, particularly from hairy surfaces.*
   - Lift the dressing so that the underside is away from the client's face. **Rationale:** *The appearance and odor of the drainage may be upsetting to the client.*

6. Dispose of soiled dressings.
   - Place the soiled dressing in the moisture-proof bag without touching the outside of the bag. **Rationale:** *Contamination of the outside of the bag is avoided to prevent the spread of microorganisms to the nurse and subsequently to others.*
   - Remove gloves, dispose of them in the moisture-proof bag, and perform hand hygiene.

7. Remove inner dressings.
   - Open the sterile dressing set, using aseptic technique.
   - Place the sterile drape beside the wound or on the bedside table to form a sterile field. Open individual sterile equipment and place on the field. Apply sterile gloves (optional).
   - Remove the underdressings with forceps or sterile gloves. **Rationale:** *Forceps or gloves are used to prevent contamination of the wound by the nurse's hands and contamination of the nurse's hands by wound drainage.*
   - Assess the location, type (color, consistency), and odor of wound drainage, and the number of gauzes saturated or the diameter of drainage collected on the dressings.
   - Discard the soiled dressings in the moisture-proof bag.
   - After the dressings are removed, discard the forceps, or set them aside from the sterile field. **Rationale:** *These are now contaminated by the wound drainage.*
   - Remove and discard sterile gloves if applied. Perform hand hygiene.

8. Assess the overall appearance of the wound and measure wound size.

9. Clean the wound if indicated.

CLINICAL ALERT

Normal saline and Ringer solution are widely advocated as fluids of choice for cleansing and irrigating wounds. Iodine and chlorhexidine are cytotoxic, particularly to fibroblasts. In severely infected wounds, antimicrobial irrigations may be used.

Povidone-iodine, hydrogen peroxide, Dakin solution, and other agents are not used on acute wounds. They are drying agents and, as such, the wound bed is dried, and the exudates and all its beneficial cells are removed from the area. Wounds maintained in a moist environment have a lower inflection rate than dry wounds.

- Clean the wound, using a new pair of forceps, clean gloves, and moistened swabs.
- Keep the forceps tips lower than the handles at all times. **Rationale:** *This prevents their contamination by fluid traveling up to the handle and nurse's wrist and back to the tips.*
- Clean with strokes from the top to the bottom, starting at the center and continuing to the outside ❶.

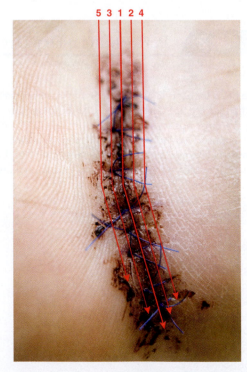

❶ Cleaning a wound from top to bottom. (Samuel Ashfield/Science Source)

SKILL 18.2 Performing a Dry Dressing Change (continued)

or
- Clean outward from the wound ❷. **Rationale:** *The wound is cleaned from the least to the most contaminated area.*

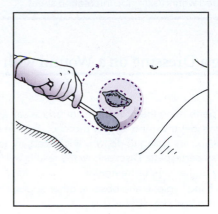

❷ Cleaning a wound from the center outward.

- Use a separate swab for each stroke, and discard each swab after use. **Rationale:** *This prevents the introduction of microorganisms to other wound areas.*
- Repeat the cleaning process until all drainage is removed.
- Remove and discard gloves. Perform hand hygiene.

> **CLINICAL ALERT**
> Gauze dressings do not support healing or prevent entry of exogenous bacteria.

10. Apply sterile dressings.
    - Apply sterile dressings one at a time over the wound, using sterile forceps or sterile gloves. Start at the center of the wound and move progressively outward. The final Surgipad can be picked up by hand, touching only the outside, which is often marked by a blue line down the center.
    - Remove and discard gloves if used. Perform hand hygiene.
11. Secure the dressing with tape, tie tapes, or a binder.
    - Place the tape so that the dressing cannot be folded back to expose the wound. Place strips at the ends of the dressing, and space tapes evenly in the middle ❸.

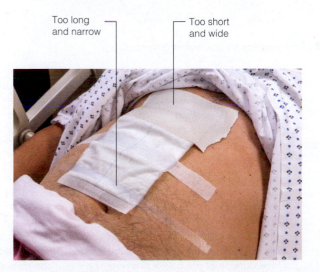

Too long and narrow   Too short and wide

❸ Taping the dressing.

- Ensure that the tape is long and wide enough to adhere to the skin but not so long or wide that it loosens with activity.
- Place the tape in the opposite direction from the body action, for example, across a body joint or crease, not lengthwise ❹.

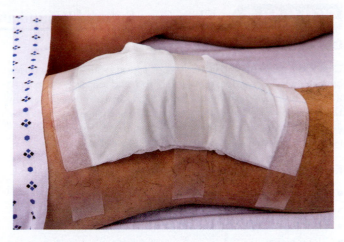

❹ Dressings over moving parts taped at right angle to the joint movement.

- Montgomery straps (tie tapes) are commonly used for wounds requiring frequent dressing changes ❺. **Rationale:** *These straps prevent the skin irritation and discomfort caused by removing the adhesive each time the dressing is changed.*

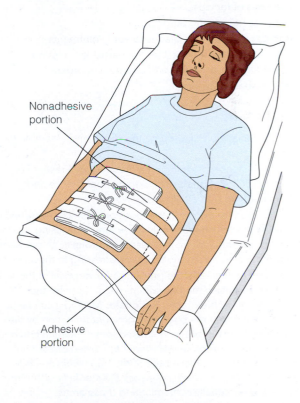

Nonadhesive portion

Adhesive portion

❺ Montgomery straps, or tie tapes, are used to secure large dressings that require frequent changing.

(continued on next page)

SKILL 18.2 Performing a Dry Dressing Change (continued)

- For clients with tape allergies or other conditions in which tape should not be applied directly to the skin, wrap over the dressing and around the body part with rolled gauze, and tape only the gauze.

12. Document the dressing change and the client's response in the client record using forms or checklists supplemented by narrative notes when appropriate. Many agencies use a designated wound/skin documentation sheet.

SKILL 18.3   Cleaning a Sutured Wound and Changing a Dressing on a Wound with a Drain

Delegation

Cleaning a newly sutured wound, especially one with a drain, requires application of knowledge, problem solving, and aseptic technique. As a result, this procedure is not delegated to UAP. The nurse can ask the UAP to report soiled dressings that need to be changed or if a dressing has become loose and needs to be reinforced. The nurse is responsible for the assessment and evaluation of the wound.

Equipment

- Bath blanket (if necessary)
- Moisture-proof biohazard bag
- Mask (optional)
- Clean gloves
- Sterile gloves
- Sterile dressing set; if none is available, gather the following sterile items:
  - Drape or towel
  - Gauze squares
  - Container for the cleaning solution
  - Cleaning solution (e.g., normal saline)
  - Two pairs of forceps
  - Gauze dressings and Surgipad
  - Applicators or tongue blades to apply ointments
- Additional supplies required for the particular dressing (e.g., extra gauze dressings and ointment, if ordered)
- Tape, tie tapes, or binder

Preparation

- Check physician's order, prepare the client, and assemble the equipment.
- Acquire assistance for changing a dressing on a restless or confused adult. **Rationale:** *The person might move and contaminate the sterile field or the wound.*
- Assist the client to a comfortable position in which the wound can be readily exposed. Expose only the wound area, using a bath blanket to cover the client, if necessary. **Rationale:** *Undue exposure is physically and psychologically distressing to most people.*
- Make a cuff on the moisture-proof bag for disposal of the soiled dressings, and place the bag within reach. It can be taped to the bedclothes or bedside table. **Rationale:** *Making a cuff helps keep the outside of the bag free from contamination by the soiled dressings and prevents subsequent contamination of the nurse's hands or of sterile instrument tips when discarding dressing or sponges. Placement of the bag within reach prevents the nurse from reaching across the sterile field and the wound and potentially contaminating these areas.*
- Apply a face mask, if required. **Rationale:** *Some agencies require that a mask be worn for surgical dressing changes to prevent contamination of the wound by droplet spray from the nurse's respiratory tract.*

Procedure

1. Prior to performing the procedure, introduce self and verify the client's identity using agency protocol. Explain to the client what you are going to do, why it is necessary, and how he or she can participate. Discuss how the results will be used in planning further care or treatments.
2. Perform hand hygiene and observe other appropriate infection control procedures.
3. Provide for client privacy.
4. Remove binders and tape.
   - Remove binders, if used, and place them aside. Untie tie tapes, if used. Montgomery straps (tie tapes) are commonly used for wounds requiring frequent dressing changes ❶. **Rationale:** *These straps prevent the skin irritation and discomfort caused by removing the adhesive each time the dressing is changed.*

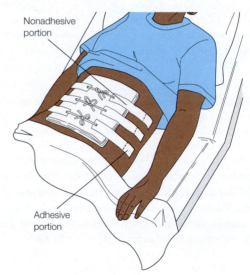
Nonadhesive portion

Adhesive portion

❶ Montgomery straps holding dressing.

   - If adhesive tape was used, remove it by holding down the skin and pulling the tape gently but firmly toward the wound. **Rationale:** *Pressing down on the skin provides countertraction against the pulling motion. Tape is pulled toward the incision to prevent strain on the sutures or wound.*
5. Remove and dispose of soiled dressings appropriately.
   - Apply clean gloves, and remove the outer abdominal dressing or Surgipad.
   - Lift the outer dressing so that the underside is *away* from the client's face. **Rationale:** *The appearance and odor of the drainage may be upsetting to the client.*
   - Place the soiled dressing in the moisture-proof bag without touching the outside of the bag. **Rationale:** *Contamination of the outside of the bag is avoided to prevent the spread of microorganisms to the nurse and subsequently to others.*

SKILL 18.3 Cleaning a Sutured Wound and Changing a Dressing (continued)

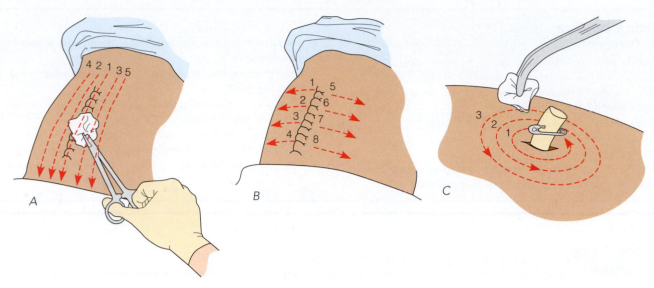

2 Methods of cleaning surgical wounds: *A*, cleaning the wound from top to bottom, starting at the center; *B*, cleaning a wound outward from the incision; *C*, cleaning around a Penrose drain site. For all methods, a clean sterile swab is used for each stroke.

- Remove the underdressings, taking care not to dislodge any drains. If the gauze sticks to the drain, support the drain with one hand and remove the gauze with the other.
- Assess the location, type (color, consistency), and odor of wound drainage, and the number of gauzes saturated or the diameter of drainage collected on the dressings.
- Discard the soiled dressings in the bag as before.
- Remove and discard gloves in the moisture-proof bag. Perform hand hygiene.
6. Set up the sterile supplies.
   - Open the sterile dressing set, using surgical aseptic technique.
   - Place the sterile drape beside the wound.
   - Open the sterile cleaning solution, and pour it over the gauze sponges in the plastic container.
   - Apply sterile gloves.
7. Clean the wound, if indicated.
   - Clean the wound, using your gloved hands or forceps and gauze swabs moistened with cleaning solution.
   - If using forceps, keep the forceps tips lower than the handles at all times. **Rationale:** *This prevents their contamination by fluid traveling up to the handle and nurse's wrist and back to the tips.*
   - Use the cleaning methods illustrated and described **2** or one recommended by agency protocol.
   - Use a separate swab for each stroke, and discard each swab after use. **Rationale:** *This prevents the introduction of microorganisms to other wound areas.*
   - If a drain is present, clean it next, taking care to avoid reaching across the cleaned incision. Clean the skin around the drain site by swabbing in half or full circles from around the drain site outward, using separate swabs for each wipe.
   - Support and hold the drain erect while cleaning around it. Clean as many times as necessary to remove the drainage.
   - Dry the surrounding skin with dry gauze swabs as required. Do not dry the incision or wound itself. **Rationale:** *Moisture facilitates wound healing.*
8. Apply dressings to the drain site and the incision **3**.

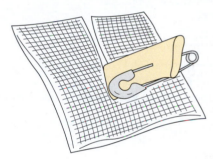

3 Precut gauze in place around a Penrose drain.

- Place a precut 4 × 4 gauze snugly around the drain, or open a 4 × 4 gauze to 4 × 8, fold it lengthwise to 2 × 8, and place the 2 × 8 gauze around the drain so that the ends overlap. **Rationale:** *This dressing absorbs the drainage and helps prevent it from excoriating the skin. Using precut gauze or folding it as described, instead of cutting the gauze, prevents any threads from coming loose and getting into the wound, where they could cause inflammation and provide a site for infection.*
- Apply the sterile dressings one at a time over the drain and the incision. Place the bulk of the dressings over the drain area and below the drain, depending on the client's usual position. **Rationale:** *Layers of dressings are placed for best absorption of drainage, which flows by gravity.*
- Apply the final Surgipad. Remove and discard gloves. Secure the dressing with tape or ties. Perform hard hygiene.
9. Document the procedure and all nursing assessments.

Sample Documentation

3/21/15 1100 Abdominal dressing changed. Small amount of serosanguineous drainage—size of a half dollar—in middle of dressing. Incision approximated with slight redness at edges. Sutures intact. Tolerated well.

————————————————————— S. Jones, RN

(continued on next page)

SKILL 18.3 **Cleaning a Sutured Wound and Changing a Dressing** (*continued*)

Setting of Care

Instruct caregivers to:

- Provide pain medication approximately 30 minutes before the procedure if the wound care causes pain or discomfort.
- Wash hands thoroughly and dry prior to handling wound care supplies and providing wound care.
- Clean and wipe dry a flat surface for the sterile field.
- Keep pets out of the area when setting up for and performing sterile procedures.
- Acquire all needed supplies before starting a sterile procedure.
- Maintain sterile or clean technique as instructed.

- Handle all sterile supplies from the outside of the wrapper or the edges.
- Avoid touching the parts of supplies or equipment that will touch the client.
- Avoid skin injury by using paper tape or Montgomery straps instead of adhesive tape.
- Report any increasing wound drainage, pain, or redness, increasing swelling, or opening or gaping of wound edges.
- Place any soiled dressing materials in a waterproof bag and dispose of it according to public health recommendations.

SKILL 18.4 **Applying Wet-to-Moist Dressings**

Equipment

- Sterile 4 × 8 noncotton gauze dressings
- Semiocclusive dressing, optional
- Sterile gloves
- Clean gloves
- Tape
- Plastic bag or receptacle for contaminated dressings
- Sterile normal saline solution
- Sterile receptacle (round basin or emesis basin) if dressing not in commercial pack
- Montgomery straps, if desired

Preparation

- Check physician's orders and gather supplies.
- Perform hand hygiene and observe other appropriate infection control procedures.
- Identify client by checking the client's identity band and asking client to state name and birth date.
- Explain procedure to client.
- Provide for client privacy.

- Raise bed to HIGH position, and lower side rail nearest you.
- Remove tape by pulling it toward the wound. **Rationale:** *This action prevents injury to newly formed tissue.*
- Don clean gloves.
- Remove wound packing by gently grasping the gauze without touching the wound and tear it away at a right angle from the wound surface. **Rationale:** *Touching only the gauze prevents contamination of the wound.*
- Place soiled dressings in disposable bag.
- Remove gloves, and dispose of them in bag.
- Perform hand hygiene.

Procedure

1. Open packages of dressings making sure sterility is maintained ❶.
2. Pour sterile normal saline solution over dressings ❷.
3. Don sterile gloves.
4. Pick up sterile gauze dressings one at a time.
5. Fluff each dressing, and place over wound ❸. **Rationale:** *If packed tightly, dressing can prevent wound edges from contact with capillaries.*

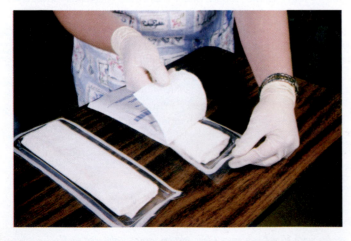

❶ Open sterile packages before beginning dressing change.

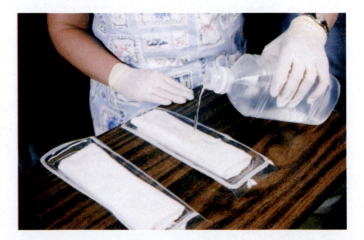

❷ Pour sterile saline solution over dressings to moisten.

SKILL 18.4   Applying Wet-to-Moist Dressings *(continued)*

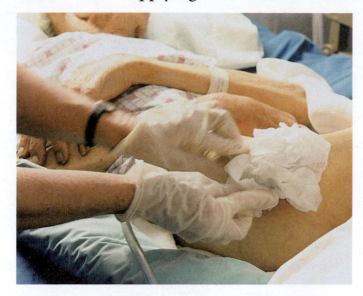

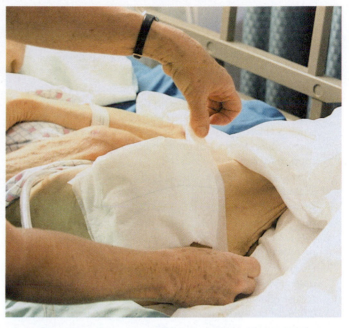

❸ Fluff dressings and apply over wound, covering all exposed surfaces.

❹ Place moist ABD pad over dressings, then cover with dry pad.

6. Place gauze in the wound, covering all exposed surfaces. Press gauze lightly into depressions or cracks. **Rationale:** *Necrotic tissue is more prevalent in these areas.*
7. Unfold a moist, sterile, 4 × 8 (ABD pad) dressing into a single layer and place it on top of wet dressings covering the wound area (not on skin) ❹.
8. Place a dry 4 × 8 pad over the dressing to hold it in place. Some protocols call for semiocclusive dressing in place of pad.
9. Remove gloves, and place in plastic bag.
10. Tape only the edges of the dressing. Montgomery tapes may be used to prevent excessive skin irritation and damage due to frequent dressing changes.

CLINICAL ALERT

Wet-to-dry dressings are used only to debride wounds, because they can cause tissue damage. Maceration of healthy tissue can occur with dressings that are always wet. Dry dressings cause damage to granulating tissue if removed without first soaking the gauze.

Heat lamps should not be used to treat pressure ulcers. Preferred wound care is to promote a clean, moist environment.

11. Position client for comfort. Lower bed, and raise side rail to UP position, if appropriate.
12. Discard soiled material in appropriate container.
13. Perform hand hygiene.
14. Document the procedure in the client's record. Include the date and time; the appearance of the wound; the color, consistency, amount, and odor of any drainage; the type of dressing applied; and how the client responded.
15. Observe wound for excessive drainage or drying out of dressing between dressing changes. Remoisten dressing if dry. **Rationale:** *Unless excessive drainage occurs, or dressing dries out, dressings are usually changed every 8 hours.*
16. Provide client or family teaching regarding wound care, if appropriate.

Note: These dressings function as osmotic dressings. Normal saline is isotonic. As water evaporates from a saline dressing, the dressing becomes hypertonic and fluid from wound tissue is drained into the dressing.

SKILL 18.5   Applying an Abdominal Binder

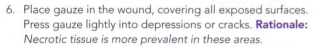

Equipment

- Abdominal binder: woven-cotton, synthetic, or elasticized material (Most facilities use commercial Velcro binders.) Safety pins for binders without Velcro closure

Procedure

1. Check physician's order and gather supplies.
2. Perform hand hygiene and observe other appropriate infection control procedures.

(continued on next page)

SKILL 18.5 Applying an Abdominal Binder (*continued*)

3. Explain use of binder to client.
4. Place client in supine position.
5. Ask client to raise hips, and then slide the binder under client's hips at level of gluteal fold. Place top of binder at client's waist.
6. Bring ends of binder around client, and secure by pressing Velcro surfaces together. If using non-Velcro binder, secure binder with safety pins placed vertically along edges. Start pinning at bottom of binder and pin toward waist. **Rationale:** *Pinning binder from bottom to waist provides uplifting support for abdominal muscles.*
7. Observe for wrinkles in binder. **Rationale:** *Wrinkles can cause pressure areas especially over iliac crest.*
8. Assess client's ability to move freely, breathe deeply, and feel secure pressure over abdominal incision. **Rationale:** *A binder that is too tight may compromise breathing or place pressure on incisional area.*
9. Document the procedure in the client's record. Include the date and time and how the client responded.
10. Assess effectiveness of binder every 4 hours, and rewrap every 8 hours if non-Velcro binder is used. Many clients use this binder only when ambulating ❶.

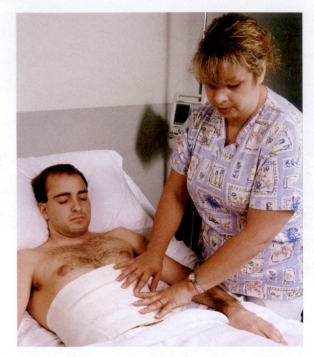

❶ Assess effectiveness of binder every 4 hr.

SKILL 18.6 Applying Bandages and Binders (Elastic Bandages)

Delegation

Application of binders can be delegated to UAP or family members/caregivers after the nurse has performed initial assessment that these persons can perform this skill safely. Application of bandages over wounds may be taught to clients or family members/caregivers for home care purposes.

Equipment

- Clean bandage or binder of the appropriate material and size
- Padding, such as abdominal pads or gauze squares
- Tape, clips, or Velcro

Procedure

1. Check physician's orders and gather supplies.
2. Prior to performing the procedure, introduce self and verify the client's identity using agency protocol. Explain to the client what you are going to do, why it is necessary, and how he or she can participate. Discuss how the results will be used in planning further care or treatments.
3. Perform hand hygiene and observe other appropriate infection control procedures.
4. Provide for client privacy.
5. Position and prepare the client appropriately.
   - Provide the client with support for the area to be bandaged. For example, if a hand needs to be bandaged, ask the client to place the elbow on a table, so that the hand does not have to be held up unsupported. **Rationale:** *Because bandaging takes time, holding up a body part without support can fatigue the client.*
   - Make sure that the area to be bandaged is clean and dry. Wash and dry the area if necessary. Perform wound care as

indicated. **Rationale:** *Washing and drying remove microorganisms, which flourish in dark, warm, moist areas.*
   - Align the part to be bandaged with slight flexion of the joints, unless this is contraindicated. **Rationale:** *Slight flexion places less strain on the ligaments and muscles of the joint.*
6. Apply the bandage. Apply the beginning of the bandage to the most distal part of the body to be bandaged first. **Rationale:** *Wrapping from distal to proximal facilitates venous return and diminishes swelling.*

Circular Turns

- Hold the bandage in your dominant hand, keeping the roll uppermost, and unroll the bandage about 8 cm (3 in.). **Rationale:** *This length of unrolled bandage allows good control for placement and tension.*
- Hold the end down with the thumb of the other hand ❶.

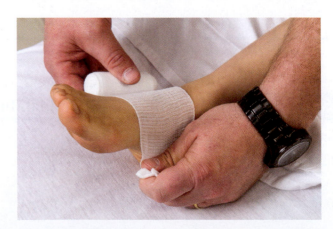

❶ Starting a bandage with circular turns.

SKILL 18.6   Applying Bandages and Binders (Elastic Bandages) *(continued)*

- Encircle the body part a few times or as often as needed, making sure that each layer overlaps one half to two thirds of the previous layer. This provides even support to the area.
- The bandage should be firm, but not too tight. Ask the client if the bandage feels comfortable. A tight bandage can interfere with blood circulation, whereas a loose bandage does not provide adequate protection.
- Secure the end of the bandage with tape or clips if there is no Velcro fastener.

Spiral Turns

- Make two circular turns. **Rationale:** *Two circular turns anchor the bandage.*
- Continue spiral turns at about a 30-degree angle, each turn overlapping the preceding one by two thirds the width of the bandage ❷.
- Terminate the bandage with two circular turns, and secure the end as described for circular turns.

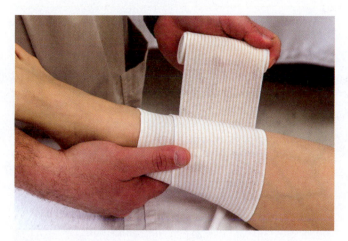

❷ Applying spiral turns.

Spiral Reverse Turns

- Anchor the bandage with two circular turns, and bring the bandage upward at about a 30-degree angle.
- Place the thumb of your free hand on the upper edge of the bandage ❸. **Rationale:** *The thumb will hold the bandage while it is folded on itself.*
- Unroll the bandage about 15 cm (6 in.), and then turn your hand so that the bandage falls over itself.

- Continue the bandage around the limb, overlapping each previous turn by two thirds the width of the bandage. Make each bandage turn at the same position on the limb so that the turns of the bandage will be aligned.
- Terminate the bandage with two circular turns, and secure the end as described for circular turns.

Recurrent Turns

- Anchor the bandage with two circular turns.
- Fold the bandage back on itself, hold it with the thumb of the other hand, and bring it centrally over the distal end to be bandaged ❹.

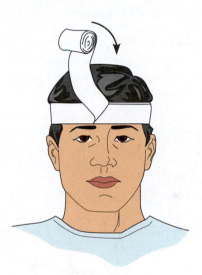

❹ Start a recurrent bandage.

- Bring the bandage back over the end to the right of the center bandage but overlapping it by two thirds the width of the bandage.
- Bring the bandage back on the left side, also overlapping the first turn by two thirds the width of the bandage.
- Continue this pattern of alternating right and left until the area is covered. Overlap the preceding turn by two thirds the bandage width each time.
- Terminate the bandage with two circular turns ❺. Secure the end appropriately.

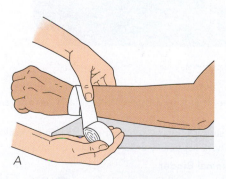

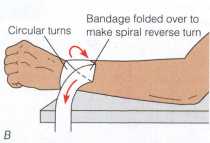

Circular turns

Bandage folded over to make spiral reverse turn

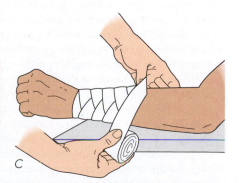

A   *B*   *C*

❸ Applying spiral reverse turns.

(continued on next page)

SKILL 18.6 Applying Bandages and Binders (Elastic Bandages) (*continued*)

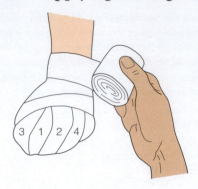

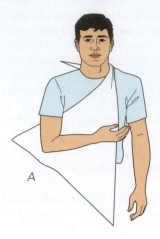

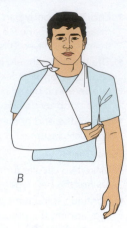

5 Completing a recurrent bandage.

Figure-Eight Turns

- Anchor the bandage with two circular turns.
- Carry the bandage above the joint, around it, and then below it, making a figure eight **6**.

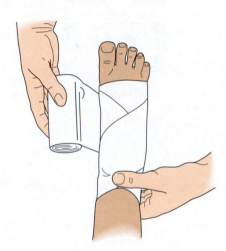

6 Applying a figure-eight bandage.

- Continue above and below the joint, overlapping the previous turn by two thirds the width of the bandage.
- Terminate the bandage above the joint with two circular turns, and then secure the end appropriately.

Arm Sling

- Ask the client to flex the elbow to an 80-degree angle or less, depending on the purpose. The thumb should be facing upward or inward toward the body. **Rationale:** *An 80-degree angle is sufficient to support the forearm, to prevent swelling of the hand, and to relieve pressure on the shoulder joint (e.g., to support the paralyzed arm of a stroke client whose shoulder might otherwise become dislocated). A more acute angle is preferred if there is swelling of the hand (see how to apply a sling for maximum hand elevation, below).*
- If a triangle is used, place one end of the unfolded binder over the shoulder of the uninjured side so that the binder falls down the front of the chest of the client with the point of the triangle (apex) under the elbow of the injured side **7**.
- Take the upper corner, and carry it around the neck until it hangs over the shoulder on the injured side.
- Bring the lower corner of the binder up over the arm to the shoulder of the injured side. Using a square knot, secure

7 A triangle arm sling.

this corner to the upper corner at the side of the neck on the injured side. **Rationale:** *A square knot will not slip. Tying the knot at the side of the neck prevents pressure on the bony prominences of the vertebral column at the back of the neck.*
- Fold the sling neatly at the elbow, and secure it with safety pins or tape. It may be folded and fastened at the front.
- If a commercial sling is used, it may also include a second strap that goes around the back of the client's chest from the finger end of the sling to the elbow **8**. **Rationale:** *This strap holds the arm close to the body at all times, providing shoulder immobilization such as is used following a shoulder dislocation or surgery.*

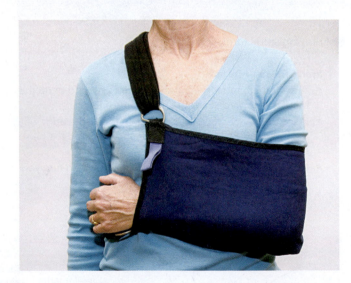

8 A commercial arm sling.

- Make sure the wrist is supported. **Rationale:** *This maintains alignment.*
- Remove the sling periodically to inspect the skin for indications of irritation, especially around the site of the knot.

Straight Abdominal Binder

- Place the binder smoothly around the body **9**. **Rationale:** *A binder placed too high interferes with respiration; one placed too low interferes with elimination and walking.*

SKILL 18.6   Applying Bandages and Binders (Elastic Bandages) (continued)

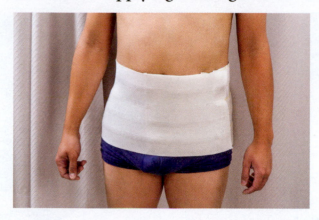

❾ A straight abdominal binder.

- Apply padding over the iliac crests if the client is thin.
- Bring the ends around the client, overlap them, and secure them with clips or Velcro.

7. Document the application of the bandage or binder and the client's response in the client record using forms or checklists supplemented by narrative notes when appropriate.

Sample Documentation

6/3/15 1900 c/o severe sharp and cramping pain in shoulder when moving it. Commercial sling c̄ shoulder immobilizer applied to L arm c̄ elbow flexed 60°. Upper extremity warm, no wounds or lesions, peripheral pulses strong, brisk capillary refill. Able to move fingers and wrist c̄ pain. Client verbalizes understanding of need to request assistance c̄ ADLs.

————————————————————————— L. Morris, RN

Developmental Considerations

CHILDREN

- Allow the child to help with the procedure by holding supplies, opening boxes, counting turns, and so on.
- If a young client is apprehensive, demonstrate the procedure on a doll or stuffed animal.
- Encourage the child to decorate her or his bandage.
- Teach the caregivers to apply bandages and binders safely.

OLDER ADULTS

- Older clients may need extra support during the procedure, especially if arthritis, contractures, or tremors are present.
- Avoid constricting the client's circulation with a tight bandage or binder. Observe skin and bony prominences frequently for signs of impaired circulation. The risk for skin breakdown increases with age.

Setting of Care

- Assess the client's or caregiver's ability and willingness to perform the bandaging procedure.
- Ensure that the client has the proper supplies and knows how to obtain replacement supplies.
- The client should have two binders so that one is available to wear while the other is being washed. Bandages and binders should be washed inside a mesh laundry bag to keep them from becoming twisted and to prevent Velcro or hooks from catching on other laundry.
- Instruct the client's caregiver to:
  a. Cleanse hands thoroughly before handling dressing supplies and applying the bandage.
  b. Report skin breakdown, redness, pain, or pallor of the affected area.
  c. Check for adequate peripheral circulation after applying the bandage.

SKILL 18.7   Changing a Dressing for a Venous Ulcer

Equipment

- Cleansing solution
- Normal saline solution
- Sterile 4 × 4 dressings
- Moisture-retentive dressings (hydrocolloid, transparent film or foam for light-to-moderate drainage)
- Absorbent dressings (foams, alginates, and absorptive dressings) for moderate to heavy exudate
- Compression dressing
- Clean gloves
- Sterile gloves
- Biohazard bag
- Scissors
- Absorbent pad

Preparation

- Check physician's orders and gather supplies ❶.
- Prior to performing the procedure, introduce self and verify the client's identity using agency protocol. Explain to the client what

you are going to do, why it is necessary, and how he or she can participate.

- Perform hand hygiene and observe other appropriate infection control procedures.
- Provide for client privacy.
- Raise bed to HIGH position and lower side rails.
- Open sterile packages, and arrange on overbed table.
- Place absorbent pad under wound.

Procedure

1. Don clean gloves.
2. Remove compression bandage and old dressing, and place in biohazard bag ❷. Compression dressings may be left in place for 3 to 7 days depending on amount of drainage and type of dressing.
3. Assess and measure wound ❸ ❹. **Rationale:** *This determines effectiveness of treatment.*
4. Cleanse off debris by pouring cleansing solution over wound.
5. Rinse wound with sterile normal saline ❺ ❻.

(continued on next page)

SKILL 18.7 **Changing a Dressing for a Venous Ulcer** (*continued*)

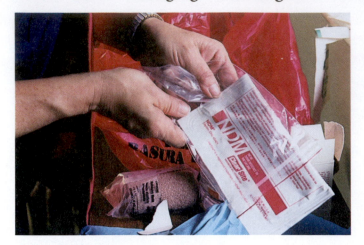

❶ Obtain appropriate wound dressing kit, if available.

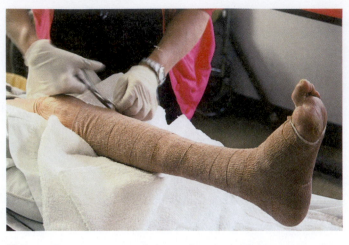

❷ Remove compression dressing, being careful not to cut skin.

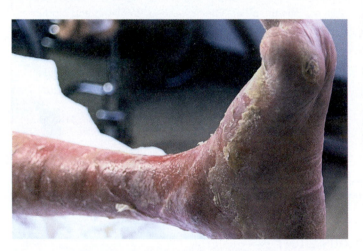

❸ Assess wound healing and evaluate progress (stage II).

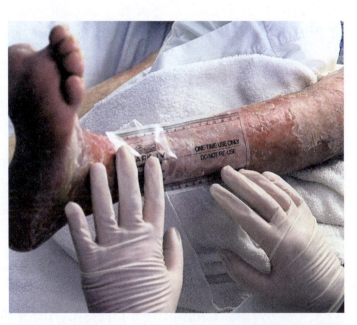

❹ Measure wound to evaluate effectiveness of treatment.

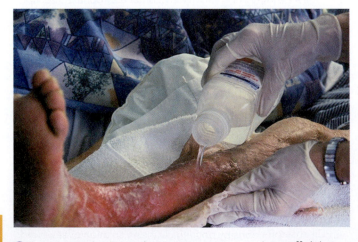

❺ Pour normal saline solution over wound to clean off debris.

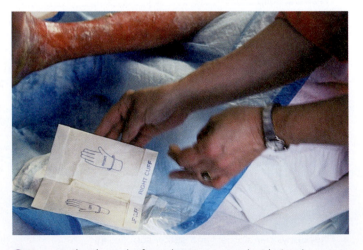

❻ Don sterile gloves before cleaning wound with 4 × 4 gauze pads.

SKILL 18.7 Changing a Dressing for a Venous Ulcer (continued)

CLINICAL ALERT

The wound bed should be kept moist to promote granulation and reepithelialization and to reduce pain. Ointments provide the most occlusive moisturizer because they contain oil and water.

6. Debride wound, if ordered, using one of the following methods:
   - *Autolytic:* Applying occlusive dressings that assist in maintaining a moist wound environment, therefore promoting reepithelialization. **Rationale:** *Autolytic dressings use the body's own enzymes and moisture to rehydrate, moisten, and slough tissue.*
   - *Chemical:* Apply enzyme debriding agents (Accuzyme, collagenase, papain, etc.). *Note:* The major disadvantage of this method is that viable tissue is removed with necrotic tissue.
   - *Mechanical:* Apply wet-to-dry dressings, use hydrotherapy, irrigation.

7. Dry wound using sterile 4 × 4 dressings. Place in biohazard bag **7**.
8. Remove gloves and don sterile gloves.
9. Apply medicated moisturizer over wound, if ordered **8**.
   Rationale: *This keeps wound area moist.*
10. Remove backing on moisture-retentive dressing, and place over open wound site **9**. These dressings prevent entry of bacteria from surface of dressing.
11. Palpate arterial system; dorsalis pedis, posterior, or tibial pulse. If pulses are nonpalpable obtain an ankle–brachial index (ABI) reading.
12. Apply compression dressing if ABI is greater than 0.6 **10** **11**.
    Rationale: *Effective compression bandages generate 40 to 70 mmHg pressure. If arterial insufficiency is present another ulcer can occur.*

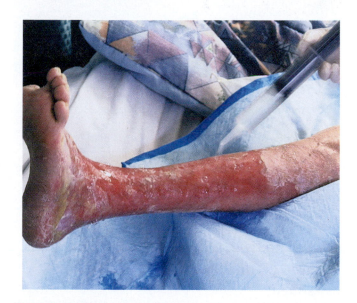

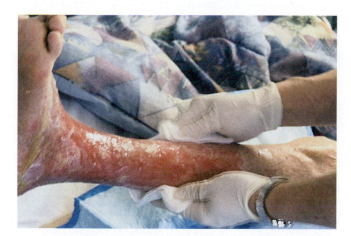

7 Dry with 4 × 4 gauze pad after cleansing.

8 Apply medicated moisturizer over wound, if ordered.

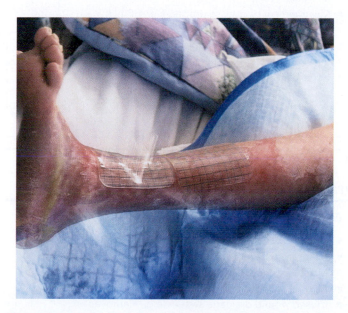

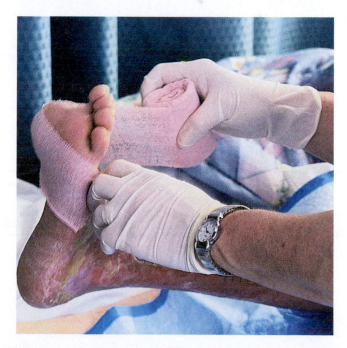

9 Apply moisture-retentive dressing over wound site.

10 Apply compression dressing for venous or lymphatic conditions.

(continued on next page)

SKILL 18.7 Changing a Dressing for a Venous Ulcer (continued)

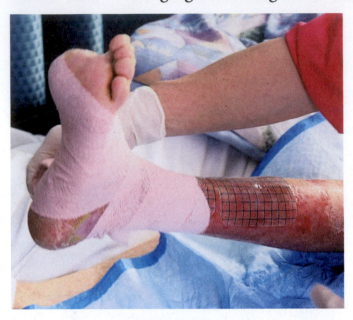

⑪ Cover entire area with compression dressing.

13. Reposition leg in elevated position. Leg should be elevated 18 cm (7 in.) above the heart for 2 to 4 hours during the day and night. **Rationale:** *This prevents edema and venous stasis, and promotes healing.*
14. Remove gloves, and place in biohazard bag. Place all used supplies in bag.
15. Place biohazard bag in appropriate receptacle.

16. Perform hand hygiene.
17. Lower bed and raise side rails.
18. Document the dressing change in the client's record. Include the date and time; appearance of the wound; the color, consistency, amount, and odor of any drainage; the type of dressing applied; and how the client responded.
19. Assess peripheral circulation every 4 hours. **Rationale:** *This ensures compression dressing is not too tight.*

CLINICAL ALERT
Use of semiocclusive dressings reduces the incidence of wound infections by more than 50%. They maintain a moist environment, reduce airborne bacteria, and provide a mechanical barrier for bacterial entry.

COMPRESSION THERAPY
Inelastic System
An Unna boot is frequently used to control edema in lower extremities. An inelastic bandaging system is applied to the lower extremity. As it dries it becomes rigid and when calf muscles press against the rigid bandage it pumps blood more effectively. This system can be used for both mobile and immobile clients. As edema subsides the boot becomes less effective.

Elastic Therapy
Graduated compression and multilayer compression stockings and compression pumps are more effective in increasing venous return. Both mobile and immobile clients can use these stockings, although it is more difficult for the client who is mobile. The stockings are available in different pressures.

Arterial Ulcers

ASSESSMENT
- Assess arterial flow; dorsalis pedis, femoral, popliteal, or posterior tibial.
- Use Doppler to assess pulses if necessary.
- Assess ankle–brachial index; below 0.5 indicates severe arterial insufficiency.
- Assess temperature of skin.
- Observe color of extremities.
- Assess for presence of pain when client resting.

TREATMENT
- Debridement.
- Pain control.

- Occlusive dressings: reduce pain, protect the wound from infection, control exudates, enhance autolytic debridement, maintain moist wound environment.
- Secure dressing with gauze; do not use tape as skin is fragile and tears easily.
- Management of disease process (i.e., BP, eliminate smoking, control blood glucose).
- Surgical intervention to improve circulation.
- Vacuum compression therapy.
- Hyperbaric oxygen therapy.

SKILL 18.8 Maintaining Closed Wound Drainage (Jackson-Pratt Drain)

Delegation
Assessment of the wound, wound drainage, and patency of the wound suction require application of knowledge and problem solving and is the responsibility of the nurse and is not delegated to UAP. The UAP, however, can empty the drainage unit, measure the drainage, and record the amount on the intake and output record. The nurse must ensure that the UAP knows how to empty the unit without contaminating it.

Equipment
- Clean gloves
- Calibrated drainage receptacle
- Moisture-proof pad
- Alcohol sponge
- Closed wound drainage system (e.g., Hemovac or Jackson-Pratt)

SKILL 18.8   Maintaining Closed Wound Drainage (Jackson-Pratt Drain) *(continued)*

Preparation

- Check physician's orders and gather supplies.
- Determine the type and placement of the client's closed wound drainage.

Procedure

1. Prior to performing the procedure, introduce self and verify the client's identity using agency protocol. Explain to the client what you are going to do, why it is necessary, and how he or she can participate. Discuss how the results will be used in planning further care or treatments.
2. Perform hand hygiene and observe other appropriate infection control procedures.
3. Provide for client privacy.
4. Empty the drainage unit.
   - Apply clean gloves.
   - Place the Hemovac or Jackson-Pratt unit on the waterproof pad.
   - Open the plug of the drainage unit.
   - Invert the unit and empty it into the collecting receptacle ❶.

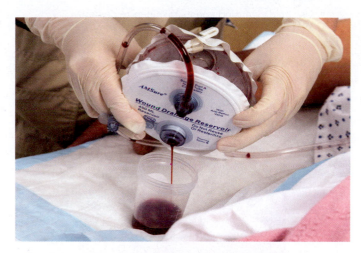

❶ Emptying drainage from Hemovac drainage system.

5. Reestablish suction.

   Hemovac
   - Place the unit on a solid, flat surface with port open.
   - Place palm of hand on unit and press the top and the bottom together.

- While holding the top and bottom together, cleanse the opening and plug with alcohol swab.
- Replace the drainage plug before releasing hand pressure. **Rationale:** *This reestablishes the vacuum necessary for the closed drainage system to work.*

   Jackson-Pratt Drain
   - Compress the bulb with the port open.
   - While maintaining tight compression on the bulb, cleanse the ends of the emptying port.
   - Insert the plug into the emptying port. **Rationale:** *This reestablishes the vacuum necessary for the closed drainage system to work.*

6. Secure the unit to the client's gown or position suction unit on the bed.
   - Ensure that the unit is below the level of the wound ❷. **Rationale:** *This facilitates drainage.*

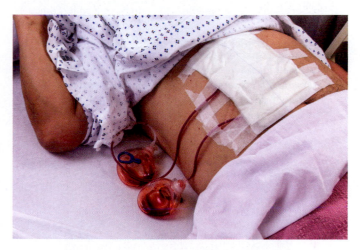

❷ Two Jackson-Pratt devices compressed to facilitate collection of exudates.

7. Remove and discard gloves. Perform hand hygiene.
8. Document all relevant information.
   - Record the emptying of the drainage unit and the nursing assessments.
   - Record the amount and type of drainage on the intake and output record.

Setting of Care

- Schedule regular nursing visits to teach wound care and to observe the drainage site.
- Teach the client or a caregiver to empty, measure, and record the drainage at least once daily.
- Instruct the caregiver to observe the wound daily for signs of infection, such as redness, edema, tenderness, or purulent drainage. The client's temperature should be measured twice daily. **Rationale:** *Elevated temperature can indicate infection.*
- Ensure that the client has the proper supplies and knows how to obtain new items as needed.
- Notify the primary care provider of excess drainage, signs of infection, or occlusion of the tube.
- Determine when the primary care provider plans to remove the drain, and help the client keep the appointment.

► WOUND CARE

Expected Outcomes

1. Stage of pressure ulcer is accurately accessed.
2. Pressure ulcer is treated effectively according to stage of ulcer formation.
3. Pressure ulcer heals within usual time frame.
4. Skin remains free of breakdown in surrounding areas of pressure ulcer.
5. Absence of additional pressure ulcer formation.
6. Granulation tissue is evident using adjunctive therapy.
7. Periwound area remains healthy without evidence of maceration.
8. Moist wound environment is maintained.

9. Wound progresses through usual phases with electrical stimulation.
10. Wound healing occurs faster with radiant heat dressing.
11. Exudate is removed and wound healing occurs using negative pressure wound therapy.
12. Hyperbaric oxygen therapy is effective in treating the leg ulcers of clients with diabetes.
13. Client's stump wound heals without complication.
14. Client's stump maintains functional alignment.
15. Client's stump is prepared for prosthesis use.

SKILL 18.9 Preventing Pressure Ulcers

Procedure

1. Inspect skin at least on admission and once a shift, particularly over bony prominences. Heels and sacrum are most common areas for skin breakdown. Use Braden or Norton scale for assessment ❶–❻. Document assessment findings. **Rationale:** *If skin is red or skin breakdown is evident on admission, Medicare and other payers will reimburse for treatment. If not evident on admission, treatment costs will not be reimbursed.*

2. Individualize client's bathing schedule. Daily baths are not essential. **Rationale:** *Daily cleansing can destroy the skin's natural barrier, making it more susceptible to external irritants.*
   - Avoid hot bath water. **Rationale:** *Tepid water prevents injury to skin.*
   - Use mild cleansing agents to minimize dryness.
   - Cleanse skin immediately if urine, fecal incontinence, or wound drainage seeps onto skin.
   - Provide humidity to prevent drying of skin.
   - Use cream or thin layer of corn starch to protect skin.

❶ Stage I pressure ulcer.

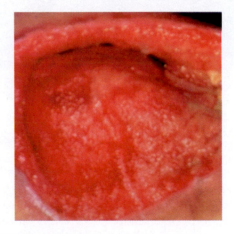

❸ Stage III pressure ulcer.

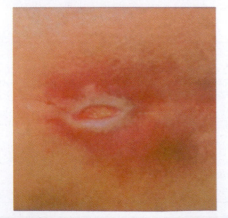

❷ Stage II pressure ulcer.

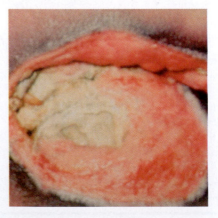

❹ Stage IV pressure ulcer.

SKILL 18.9 Preventing Pressure Ulcers *(continued)*

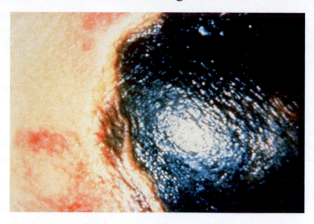

5 Eschar must be removed by debridement before staging is done.

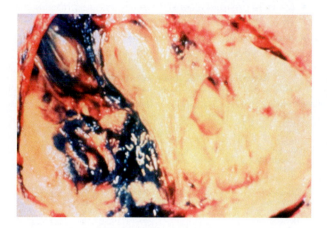

6 Clinical signs of infection.

3. Avoid massaging bony prominences. **Rationale:** *Massaging can lead to deep tissue trauma.*
   - Keep bony prominences from direct contact with one another.
   - Use pillow, foam wedges, or other positioning devices.
   - Use elbow pads and heel elevators.
4. Promote adequate dietary intake of protein, calories, and nutrients. Protein should be approximately 1.2 to 1.5 g/kg body weight daily. **Rationale:** *Adequate protein intake in addition to vitamins and minerals helps prevent pressure ulcer formation.*

CLINICAL ALERT

Be alert to altered skin integrity when pressure is reduced in one anatomical area by turning and repositioning, because the newer location may be placed at risk for pressure ulcer formation.

Air-Fluidized Bed

Air-fluidized beds and low-air-loss beds are recommended to manage pressure ulcers, especially in clients with large or multiple ulcers. Warm, pressurized air circulates through beads in the bed and creates a support surface. A polyester sheet allows for moisture and air to pass through, keeping skin dry. Treatment can take several months. Use of this bed is very expensive.

Low-Air-Loss Bed

Head and foot of bed can be elevated. Bed is a modified standard bed frame, lighter and more portable than an air-fluidized bed. The bed circulates cool air. Urine and feces do not pass through fabric on the bed. Bed is portable and lightweight.

5. Ensure adequate fluid intake. **Rationale:** *Prevent dehydration, which is a risk factor for pressure ulcer formation.*
6. Reposition bedridden client every 1 to 2 hours.
   - Do not position directly on trochanter.
   - Do not turn more than a 30-degree angle.
   - Raise heels off bed by placing pillows under legs; allow heels to hang over edges.
   - Use trapeze or turning sheet to reposition client.
7. Encourage mobility or range-of-motion (ROM) exercises. **Rationale:** *ROM exercises promote activity and reduce effects of pressure on tissue.*
8. Minimize force and friction on skin when turning or moving client. Use turning sheets or Hoyer lift.
9. Maintain head of bed at lowest degree of elevation consistent with medical problem; below 30 degrees if possible.
10. Place at-risk clients on pressure-reducing devices, in both bed and chair, such as foam, static-air, alternating gel, water mattress, or air-fluidized mattress.
11. Place client on specialty bed or mattress if the client already has a pressure ulcer or is at high risk for ulcer formation.
12. Encourage chair-fast clients to shift position every 15 minutes.
13. Document turning and repositioning in the client's record and how the client responded. Document any skin changes in color, texture, or integrity.

Evidence-Based Nursing Practice
Pressure Relief in Surgical Clients

Numerous factors put clients at risk for developing pressure ulcers during surgery. Among these are very low or high body mass index, impaired sensation due to condition or anesthesia, and procedures lasting more than 3 hours. Repositioning—the normal way of relieving pressure on a body part—may be impractical or contraindicated during surgery. Certain types of surgery (cardiac, general, thoracic, orthopedic, and vascular procedures) are associated with increased incidence of pressure ulcer development.

A deliberate strategy is needed to prevent pressure ulcer formation in the surgical suite. The Braden Scale can be used on admission to identify clients who are at increased risk for pressure ulcer

formation. It is recommended that a member of the surgical team take the role of monitoring the client's skin condition before, during, and after surgery, communicating any concerns to the rest of the healthcare team. Support surfaces with pressure redistributing properties should be supplied for any client identified as at risk for pressure ulcers. Thicker pads with variable densities and several layers have been shown to provide greater pressure redistribution than single-layer pads. Use of thick, multilayer pads is more critical for heavier clients than lighter ones. Also, appropriate lifting devices and methods should be used to prevent friction and shearing injuries during transfers.

Data from Minnesota Hospital Association (2013), Baron & MacFarlane (2009), and Tschannen et al. (2012).

(continued on next page)

SKILL 18.9 Preventing Pressure Ulcers (continued)

Pressure Ulcer Formation

There has been no definitive research on whether pressure ulcers begin to form from the skin down or from deep tissue up. However, there is agreement that pressure ulcers form most commonly over bony prominences, often affect deep tissue, and are associated with prolonged immobility and inadequate perfusion of cells. At times skin breakdown may begin superficially, either from friction (as in sliding the client up in bed) or from shearing forces (movement of deep tissue in one direction while skin is pulled in the opposite direction). Most often, sustained pressure that traps deep tissue between bone and a hard surface (e.g., a wheelchair) is implicated in pressure ulcer formation. Moisture of the skin (from sweat, urine, etc.) and poor nutrition (especially lack of protein) are also associated factors.

Pressure ulcers are difficult and costly to treat. The best strategy is to prevent formation of pressure ulcers by moving clients carefully, repositioning regularly, and keeping skin clean and dry.

Data from Wake (2010), Mayo Clinic (2011), and WebMD (2014).

SKILL 18.10   Providing Care for a Client with Pressure Ulcers

Procedure

1. Check physician's orders and gather equipment and supplies.
2. Monitor client's overall condition daily ❶. **Rationale:** *Clients who are dying will have the tendency to develop new skin breakdown (skin failure) as other organs fail. Existing pressure ulcers of lesser staging (I and II) almost always worsen over time and become at least stage III.*
3. Differentiate type of ulcer, pressure versus nonpressure.
4. Determine stage of ulcer.
5. Monitor and assess ulcer characteristics daily.
   - Observe dressing to determine if dry, intact, and not leaking.
   - Observe ulcer bed, if appropriate, and document findings.
6. Assess pain level of client and provide adequate pain relief.
7. Photograph ulcer according to facility policy. **Rationale:** *To determine progress of ulcer healing.*
8. Monitor progress toward healing and for potential complications.
   - Measure pressure ulcer size weekly using a pressure ulcer scale. Usual healing time is 2 to 4 weeks.
   - If healing is not progressing or has not healed in usual time frame, reevaluate treatment plan and client's condition.

SAMPLE PRESSURE ULCER ASSESSMENT GUIDE

Patient Name: _____   Date: _____ Time: _____

Ulcer 1:
Site _____
Stage[a] _____
Size (cm)
  Length _____
  Width _____
  Depth _____

Ulcer 2:
Site _____
Stage[a] _____
Size (cm)
  Length _____
  Width _____
  Depth _____

	Ulcer 1	Ulcer 2
Sinus Tract	☐☐	☐☐
Tunneling	☐☐	☐☐
Undermining	☐☐	☐☐
Necrotic Tissue		
Slough	☐☐	☐☐
Eschar	☐☐	☐☐
Exudate		
Serous	☐☐	☐☐
Serosanguineous	☐☐	☐☐
Purulent	☐☐	☐☐
Granulation	☐☐	☐☐
Epithelialization	☐☐	☐☐
Pain	☐☐	☐☐
Surrounding Skin:		
Erythema	☐☐	☐☐
Maceration	☐☐	☐☐
Induration	☐☐	☐☐

Description of Ulcer(s): _____

Indicate Ulcer Sites:

Anterior   Posterior
(Attach a color photo of the pressure ulcer[s] [Optional])

[a]Classification of pressure ulcers:
Stage I: Nonblanchable erythema of intact skin, the heralding lesion of skin ulceration. In individuals with darker skin, discoloration of the skin, warmth, edema, induration, or hardness may also be indicators.
Stage II: Partial thickness skin loss involving epidermis, dermis, or both.
Stage III: Full thickness skin loss involving damage to or necrosis of subcutaneous tissue that may extend down to, but not through, underlying fascia. The ulcer presents clinically as a deep crater with or without undermining adjacent tissue.
Stage IV: Full thickness skin loss with extensive destruction, tissue necrosis, or damage to muscle, bone, or supporting structures (e.g., tendon or joint capsule).

NUTRITIONAL ASSESSMENT OF CLIENT WITH PRESSURE ULCER(S)

Client Name: _____   Date: _____ Time _____

To be filled out for all clients at risk on initial evaluation and every 12 weeks thereafter, as indicated. Trends will document the efficacy of nutritional support therapy.

Protein Compartments

Somatic:
Current Weight (kg)   _____
Previous Weight (kg)   _____   (_____date)
Percent Change in Weight   _____

Height (cm)   _____
Height/Weight
Current Body Mass Index (BMI) _____   [wt/(ht)²]
Previous BMI   _____   (_____date)
Percent Change in BMI   _____

Visceral:
Serum Albumin   _____
    (Normal ≥ 3.5 mg/dL)
Total Lymphocyte Count (TLC)   _____   (optional)
    (White Blood Cell count x percent Lymphocytes/100)

Guide to TLC:
• Immune competence   ≥ 1,800 mm³
• Immunity partly impaired < 1,800 but ≥ 900 mm³
• Anergy   < 900 mm³

State of Hydration

24-Hour Intake _____ mL   24-Hour Output _____ mL

Note: Thirst, tongue dryness in non-mouth-breathers, and tenting of cervical skin may indicate dehydration. Jugular vein distention may indicate overhydration.

Estimated Nutritional Requirement

Estimated Nonprotein Calories (NPC) _____ /kg   Estimated Protein _____ (g/kg)
Actual NPC   _____ /kg   Actual Protein   _____ (g/kg)

Recommendations/Plan

1.
2.
3.
4.

A   B

❶ A, Pressure ulcer assessment guide; B, nutritional assessment of client with pressure ulcer(s).
Source: Pressure Ulcer Treatment: Quick Reference Guide for Clinicians, No. 15. U.S. Department of Health and Human Services, AHCPR.

SKILL 18.10   Providing Care for a Client with Pressure Ulcers *(continued)*

9. Maintain turning and positioning schedule to promote healing and prevent additional ulcer formation.
10. Complete a nutritional assessment. Positive nitrogen balance and protein intake are necessary for healing.
11. Complete a psychosocial assessment to determine client's adherence to pressure ulcer treatment regimens.
12. Complete dressing change according to facility policy and type of dressing used. Follow manufacturer's guidelines for performing dressing changes. **Rationale:** *Dressing changes are based on a combination of factors, such as manufacturer suggested use, pressure ulcer characteristics, and goals for healing.*
13. Document the procedure, pictures, and assessment data in the client's record. Include the date and time; the appearance of the wound; the color, consistency, amount, and odor of any drainage; the type of dressing applied; and how the client responded.

CLINICAL ALERT

Clients near the end of life have the right to refuse ulcer care. However, do-not-resuscitate orders do not relieve the staff from providing quality pressure ulcer prevention or treatment.

The Centers for Medicare and Medicaid Services has indicated that long-term care facilities must implement evidence-based protocols of prevention and care for pressure ulcers.

SKILL 18.11   Applying a Transparent Film Dressing

Equipment

- Sterile normal saline
- Transparent dressing (e.g., OpSite, Tegaderm, Bioclusive)
- Sterile 4 × 4 gauze pads
- Scissors
- Hypoallergenic tape
- Clean gloves
- Plasticizing agent (e.g., skin prep) (optional)
- Syringe with 26-gauge needle, if needed

Preparation

- Check physician's orders and client care plan.
- Check type of dressing ordered. **Rationale:** *These dressings are very important in preventing pressure ulcers; they prevent friction and shear over bony prominences when moving clients.*
- Gather supplies ❶.
- Obtain appropriately sized transparent dressing ❷. Dressing can be applied to flat surface. (Coccyx area cannot be treated with this type of dressing.)
- Perform hand hygiene and observe other appropriate infection control procedures.
- Identify client by checking the client's identity band and asking client to state name and birth date. Explain procedure to client.
- Provide for client privacy.

Procedure

1. Raise bed to HIGH position, and lower side rail on working side of bed.
2. Don clean gloves.
3. Remove old dressing, "walk off" dressing from one edge to the other, and discard in appropriate receptacle.
4. Wash pressure ulcer with sterile gauze pads moistened with sterile normal saline.
5. Dry thoroughly with sterile gauze pad.
6. Measure wound using pliable device ❸. **Rationale:** *To determine appropriate size dressing and to obtain comparison measurements, which assist in determining effectiveness of treatment.*
7. Apply plasticizing agent (skin prep, skin gel) over surrounding tissue if ordered. **Rationale:** *Do not apply directly on ulcer area because the agent contains alcohol, which burns the*

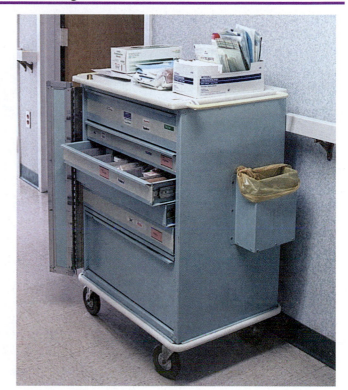

❶ Dressing carts may be used to keep supplies closer to client area.

ulcer area. Alternate treatment: If skin is irritated, apply No Sting barrier film spray to area surrounding tissue. **Rationale:** *To protect/prevent skin breakdown.*

CLINICAL ALERT

Transparent film dressings remain in place for 5 to 7 days. These dressings are adhesive and permeable to moisture, vapor, and atmospheric gases. They are bacteria proof and waterproof. It is imperative to observe the ulcer area daily to determine if a large amount of secretions or serous fluid has accumulated under the dressing. If fluid has increased, aspirate with a 26-gauge needle. These dressings are not used for infected areas.

(continued on next page)

SKILL 18.11 Applying a Transparent Film Dressing (continued)

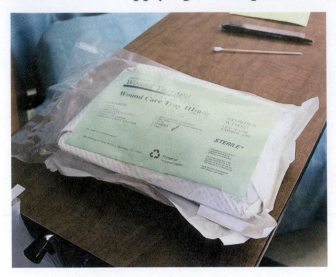

2 Obtain specific dressing tray for ordered treatment.

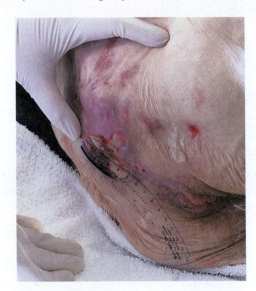

3 Assess size of wound to determine appropriate size of transparent dressing.

8. Loosen transparent dressing from one side of backing paper **4**.

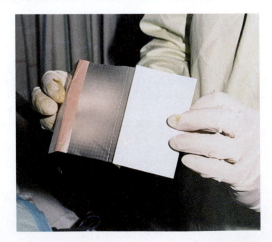

4 Remove backing from OpSite dressing before applying.

9. "Walk on" dressing: Start at one edge of site and gently lay the dressing down, keeping it free of wrinkles. Allow at least a 4-cm (1.5-in.) margin of dressing beyond the ulcer margin **5**. **Rationale:** *This ensures coverage of entire wound area.*

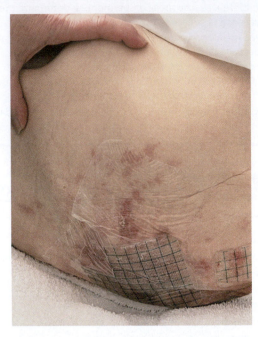

5 Apply transparent adhesive dressing over wound.

10. Cut off tabs if using OpSite after wound is completely covered.
11. Tape edges with hypoallergenic tape. **Rationale:** *This assists in preventing frequent dressing changes due to loose dressings. These dressings can remain in place for 1 week.*
12. Remove gloves, and discard in appropriate receptacle.
13. Position client for comfort.
14. Lower bed, and raise side rails.
15. Remove and discard equipment.
16. Perform hand hygiene.
17. Document the procedure in the client's record. Include the date and time; the appearance of the wound; the color, consistency, amount, and odor of any drainage; the type of dressing applied; and how the client responded.

Hydrogel Dressings

- Hydrogel dressings contain 95% water; they are very absorbent and dehydrate easily when not covered with a secondary dressing.
- Dressings cannot absorb much exudate; they should be used for dry wounds such as skin tears, surgical wounds, and radiation therapy burns.
- Dressings are nonadhesive, can be transparent and conform to wound surfaces.
- Sterile aqueous hydrogen fiber is used to fill cavity with gel; also used to fill dead space in large wounds. Do not overfill wounds to prevent tissue damage.
- Hydrogel sheets are placed in direct contact with wound bed and margins; air bubbles and plastic covering on sheet must be removed. The unique cooling properties soothe painful wounds.

SKILL 18.12 Irrigating a Wound

Delegation

Due to the need for aseptic technique and assessment skills, wound irrigations are not delegated to UAP. However, UAP may observe the wound and dressing during usual care and must report abnormal findings to the nurse. Abnormal findings must be validated and interpreted by the nurse.

Equipment

Although a wound may already be contaminated, sterile equipment is usually used during irrigation to prevent the possibility of adding new nonresident microorganisms to the site. In settings outside of hospitals, some reusable supplies such as irrigating syringes or basins may be cleaned and used again for a specific wound.

- Sterile dressing equipment and dressing materials
- Sterile irrigation set or individual supplies, including:
  - Sterile syringe (e.g., a 30- to 60-mL syringe) with a catheter of an appropriate size (e.g., #18 or #19) or an irrigating tip syringe
  - Splash shield for syringe (optional)
  - Sterile graduated container for irrigating solution
  - Basin for collecting the used irrigating solution
  - Moisture-proof sterile drape
  - Moisture-proof bag
  - Irrigating solution, usually 200 mL (6.5 oz) of solution warmed to body temperature, according to the agency's or primary care provider's choice
  - Goggles, gown, and mask
  - Clean gloves
  - Sterile gloves (optional)

Preparation

- Check physician's orders and gather equipment and supplies.
- Check that the irrigating fluid is at the proper temperature.

Procedure

1. Prior to performing the procedure, introduce self and verify the client's identity using agency protocol. Explain to the client what you are going to do, why it is necessary, and how he or she can participate. Discuss how the results will be used in planning further care or treatments.
2. Perform hand hygiene and observe other appropriate infection control procedures.
3. Provide for client privacy.
4. Prepare the client.
   - Assist the client to a position in which the irrigating solution will flow by gravity from the upper end of the wound to the lower end and then into the basin.
   - Place the waterproof drape under the wounds and over the bed.
   - Apply clean gloves and remove and discard the old dressing.
5. Measure and assess the wound and drainage.
   - If indicated, clean the wound.
   - Remove and discard gloves. Perform hand hygiene.

6. Prepare the equipment.
   - Open the sterile dressing set and supplies.
   - Pour the ordered solution into the solution container.
   - Position the basin below the wound to receive the irrigating fluid.
7. Irrigate the wound.
   - Apply clean gloves.
   - Instill a steady stream of irrigating solution into the wound. Make sure all areas of the wound are irrigated.
   - Use either a syringe with a catheter attached or with an irrigating tip to flush the wound ❶.

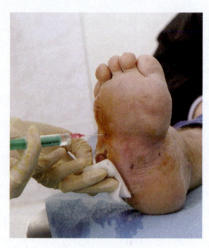

❶ Irrigating an open wound. (BSIP/Photoshot)

   - If you are using a catheter to reach tracts or crevices, insert the catheter into the wound until resistance is met. Do not force the catheter. **Rationale:** *Forcing the catheter can cause tissue damage.*
   - Continue irrigating until the solution becomes clear (no exudate is present).
   - Dry the area around the wound. **Rationale:** *Moisture left on the skin promotes the growth of microorganisms and can cause skin irritation and breakdown.*
   - Remove and discard gloves. Perform hand hygiene.
8. Assess and dress the wound.
   - Assess the appearance of the wound again, noting in particular the type and amount of exudate still present and the presence and extent of granulation tissue.
   - Using sterile technique, don gloves and apply a sterile dressing to the wound based on the amount of drainage expected.
   - Remove and discard sterile gloves. Perform hand hygiene.
9. Document the irrigation and the client's response in the client record using forms or checklists supplemented by narrative notes when appropriate. Many agencies use a designated wound/skin documentation sheet.

Sample Documentation

5/31/15 1000 Wound on (R) hip 3 × 3 cm, 6 mm deep, draining minimal amt. thick yellow. No odor. Skin around wound erythematous. Pain 0 on 0–10 scale. Irrigated c̄ NS until clear. Redressed c̄ sterile technique.
                                                                    N. Jamaghani, RN

SKILL 18.13   Using Alginates on Wounds

Delegation

Due to the need for aseptic technique and assessment skills, alginate dressing changes are not delegated to UAP. However, UAP may observe the dressing during usual care and must report abnormal findings to the nurse. Abnormal findings must be validated and interpreted by the nurse.

Equipment

- Alginate dressing
- Sterile dressing equipment and secondary dressing materials
- Solution for irrigation (e.g., sterile saline or water)
- Irrigating syringe
- Bowl
- Basin to collect irrigation
- Forceps or cotton-tipped applicators (optional)
- Moisture-proof bag
- Clean gloves
- Sterile gloves (optional)

Procedure

1. Check physician's orders and gather equipment and supplies.
2. Prior to performing the procedure, introduce self and verify the client's identity using agency protocol. Explain to the client what you are going to do, why it is necessary, and how he or she can participate. Discuss how the results will be used in planning further care or treatments.
3. Perform hand hygiene and observe other appropriate infection control procedures.
4. Prepare the client. Assist the client to a comfortable position in which the wound can be readily exposed.
5. Provide for client privacy. Expose only the wound area, using a bath blanket to cover the client, if necessary. **Rationale:** *Undue exposure is physically and psychologically distressing to most people.*
6. Prepare the supplies.
   - Open the sterile dressing set and supplies.
   - Pour the ordered solution into the solution container.
   - Position the basin below the wound to receive the irrigating fluid.
7. Remove the existing dressing and alginate.
   - Apply clean gloves, remove and discard the outer secondary dressing in the moisture-proof bag.
   - Irrigate the wound with the prescribed solution until all of the alginate dressing has been removed.
   - If the alginate dressing does not remove easily with irrigation, either the secondary dressing is not maintaining a moist environment or the wound is no longer producing enough exudate to warrant alginate dressing.
8. Assess the wound.
9. Clean the wound if indicated
   - Remove and discard gloves. Perform hand hygiene.
10. Pack the wound with the alginate.
    - Apply sterile gloves.
    - Pack the alginate into all depressions and grooves of the wound. Cover all exposed surfaces.
11. Dress the wound.
    - Cover the alginate with petrolatum gauze, foam, or other secondary dressing that will keep the alginate in place and provide a moist wound environment.
    - Remove and discard gloves. Perform hand hygiene.
12. Document the dressing change and the client's response in the client record using forms or checklists supplemented by narrative notes when appropriate. Many agencies use a designated wound/skin documentation sheet.

Client Teaching

Perform appropriate client teaching for promoting wound healing and maintenance of healthy skin.

Maintaining Intact Skin

- Discuss relationship between adequate nutrition (especially fluids, protein, vitamins B and C, iron, and calories) and healthy skin.
- Demonstrate appropriate positions for pressure relief.
- Establish a turning or repositioning schedule.
- Demonstrate application of appropriate skin protection agents and devices.
- Instruct to report persistent reddened areas.
- Identify potential sources of skin trauma and means of avoidance.

Wound Care

- Instruct family about hygiene and medical asepsis, hand cleansing before and after dressing changes, and using a clean area for storage of dressing supplies.
- Instruct the client and family on where to obtain needed supplies. Be sensitive to the cost of dressings (e.g., transparent barriers are costly) and suggest less expensive alternatives if necessary. Be creative in the use of household items for padding pressure areas.
- Instruct the client and family in proper disposal of contaminated dressings. All contaminated items should be double bagged in moisture-proof bags.

Developmental Considerations

INFANTS

- The skin of infants is more fragile than that of older children and adults, and more susceptible to infection, shearing from friction, and burns. Keep skin hydrated by applying lotion daily.

CHILDREN

- *Staphylococcus* and fungus are two major infectious agents affecting the skin of children. Abrasions or small lacerations, commonly experienced by children, provide an entry in

SKILL 18.13   Using Alginates on Wounds (continued)

the skin for these organisms. Minor wounds should be cleansed with warm, soapy water, and covered with a sterile bandage.

- With more serious skin lesions, remind the child not to touch the wound, drains, or dressing. Cover with an appropriate bandage that will remain intact during the child's usual activities. Cover a transparent dressing with opaque material if viewing the site is distressing to the child. Restrain only when all alternatives have been tried and when absolutely necessary.

- For younger children, demonstrate wound care on a doll. Reassure that the wound will not be permanent and that nothing will fall out of the body.

OLDER ADULTS

- Hold wrinkled skin taut during application of a transparent dressing. Obtain assistance if needed.

- Skin of older adults is more fragile and can easily tear with removal of tape (especially adhesive tape). Use paper tape and tape remover as indicated, keeping tape use to the minimum required. Use extreme caution during tape removal. If possible, use conforming gauze bandage (e.g., Elastomull, Flexicon, Kerlix Lite, or Kling) to hold dressing in place.

- Older adults who are in long-term care facilities often have the following factors: immobility, malnutrition, and incontinence, all of which increase the risk for development of skin breakdown.

- Skin breakdown can occur as quickly as within 2 hours, so assessments should be done with each repositioning of the client.

- A thorough assessment of a client's heels should be done every shift. The skin can break down quickly from friction of movement in bed. Whenever possible, heels should be suspended off the mattress using pillows or other mechanisms.

Setting of Care

- Discuss importance of adequate nutrition (especially fluids, protein, vitamins B and C, iron, and calories).

- Instruct in wound assessment and provide mechanism for documenting.

- Emphasize principles of asepsis, especially hand cleansing and proper methods of handling used dressings.

- Provide information about signs of wound infection and other complications to report.

- Reinforce appropriate aspects of pressure ulcer prevention.

- Demonstrate wound care techniques such as wound cleansing, dressing change.

- Discuss pain control measures, if needed.

- Verify how the client may bathe with the wound (i.e., does the wound need to be covered with a waterproof barrier or should it be cleansed in the shower?).

- Tap water may be used to cleanse wounds instead of normal saline (Fernandez & Griffiths, 2008).

SKILL 18.14   Using a Hydrocolloid Dressing

Equipment

- Sterile normal saline
- Hydrocolloid dressing (e.g., DuoDERM, Restore, Ultec, Comfeel Plus) ❶

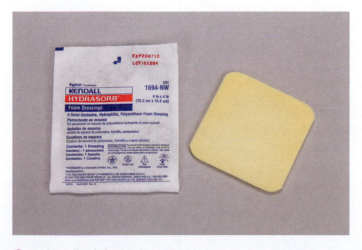

❶ Hydrocolloid dressing.

- Hydrogel (ClearSite, Aquasorb), if needed
- Sterile 4 × 4 gauze pads
- Hypoallergenic tape
- Clean gloves
- Skin prep, optional

Note: These dressings are a combination of adhesive and gelling polymers that are impermeable to oxygen, water, and water vapor (**Table 18–2** ● and **18–3** ●). They promote a moist wound environment, aid in autolytic debridement, and have no toxic components. They are waterproof and bacteria proof. These dressings are best used in clients who have partial- to full-thickness wounds with minimal to moderate exudates such as pressure ulcers, skin tears, surgical wounds, and burns.

Procedure

1. Check physician's orders and gather supplies.
2. Select dressing size to ensure coverage 3 cm (1 1/4-inch) beyond ulcer margin. (Dressing available in 4 × 4 to 8 × 8 sizes.) **Rationale:** *This ensures complete covering of wound. Use for small ulcers and in stage II and III.*

(continued on next page)

SKILL 18.14 Using a Hydrocolloid Dressing (*continued*)

Note: These dressings can be used for dry wounds because they contain 95% water. They are occlusive and do not allow water or bacteria into the wound. Hydrocolloid causes the pH of the wound surface to drop, and this acidic environment can inhibit bacterial growth.

3. Perform hand hygiene and don clean gloves.
4. Cleanse skin with gauze pad moistened with sterile normal saline and pat dry with gauze pad.
5. Measure wound using pliable device.

6. Apply skin prep to surrounding skin to protect, if ordered.
7. Fill ulcer area with Hydrogel if ordered (usually used with stage III or IV pressure ulcer of the hip when exudate is present). Do not overfill with gel. **Rationale:** *Facilitates autolytic debridement of devitalized tissue.*
8. Warm dressing by holding in hands. **Rationale:** *To increase activity of adhesive and make the dressing more pliable.*

TABLE 18–2 Additional Moist Wound Dressings

TYPE OF ALTERNATIVE	USE	OUTCOME OF TREATMENT	CONSIDERATIONS
Hydrogel sheet	■ Interacts with aqueous solutions. ■ Used with minor wounds with light to moderate drainage. ■ Absorbs minimal to heavy exudates. ■ Is nonadherent.	Softens necrotic tissue. Creates moist environment.	Use outer dressing to prevent wounds from drying out. Change dressing every 1–2 days.
Impregnated gauze dressing	■ Absorbs minimal to moderate exudates. ■ Is nonadherent.	Conforms to irregular surfaces. Eliminates dead space. Creates moist environment.	Requires outer dressing. Change daily. Is nonabsorptive.
Alginates*	■ Absorbs heavy exudates. ■ Converts to gel when comes in contact with wound drainage. ■ Is easily removed from wound. ■ Is nonadherent. ■ Absorbs up to 20 times its weight in fluid. ■ Can be used in infected and uninfected wounds.	Maintains moist environment. Promotes fast healing of wound.	Not to be used on dry wounds. It dehydrates wound, delays healing eschar-covered wounds, third-degree burns or surgical wounds.
Foams	■ Absorbs minimal to heavy exudates. ■ Is highly absorbent. ■ Used for deep cavity wounds.	Maintains moist environment. Decreases tissue trauma when removed. Increases time between dressing changes (3–4 days).	Requires external dressing. Can cause drying effect on wound.
Hydrophilic	■ Is a type of foam dressing. ■ Is nonadherent. ■ Is very absorbent.	Cushions wound. Traps exudate.	Used in wounds with moderate to heavy drainage.
Hydrophobic	■ Is a nonadherent flexible dressing. ■ Used with minimal or no necrotic tissue. ■ Used with lightly to moderately exudating wounds.	Resists fluid penetration into wound. Is used on lightly draining wounds. Provides cushion to irritated skin.	
Medical hydrolysate of collagen	■ Soluble and degrades in wound site. ■ Absorbs wound exudates. ■ Is interactive with wound site to provide mechanical protection against physical and bacterial insult.	Absorbs up to 30 times own weight. Used in stage I through IV pressure ulcers. Accelerates tissue remodeling and reduces scarring.	Cover with nonstick dressing. Soak dressing in warm water before removing.
Anticoat 7 silver-coated contact dressing	■ Used for wounds with moderate to heavy exudates. ■ Has antimicrobial barrier to protect against bacterial contamination and infection. ■ Calcium in the dressing provides antimicrobial to protect against bacterial contamination and infection. ■ Kills bacteria faster than any other forms of silver dressing.	Use for leg, pressure, and diabetic foot ulcers and for burns.	Stays in place for up to 3 days to provide moist environment.

*Alginates are made from acids that are obtained from brown seaweed. The calcium salts of alginic, mannuronic, and guluronic acids are processed into nonwoven, biodegradable fibers. When the fibers come into contact with fluids, sodium, and calcium ions, a soluble sodium gel forms.

SKILL 18.14 Using a Hydrocolloid Dressing (continued)

TABLE 18–3 Comparisons of Moisture-Retentive Dressings

	TRANSPARENT	HYDROCOLLOID
Common brands	Tegaderm OpSite Bioclusive	Tegasorb DuoDERM Comfeel Plus Restore
Characteristics	Provides a sterile, semipermeable membrane with hypoallergenic adhesive. Is permeable to oxygen and moisture vapor. Allows oxygen exchange. Is impermeable to bacteria and prevents contamination.	Is impermeable to oxygen. Dressing gel maintains moist environment that promotes autolysis. Is impermeable to external bacteria and contamination. Is minimally to moderately absorptive.
Function	Provides moist environment. Promotes autolysis and protects newly formed tissue. Assists with debridement.	Dressing contains hydroactive particles that absorb exudates to form a hydrated gel over wound. When dressing removed, gel separates from dressing, which protects newly formed tissue.
Use	Easy assessment of wound; dressing is transparent. Is nonabsorbable. Used for nondraining or minimally draining wounds only; pressure ulcers, stage I and some stage II; and minor burns and lacerations.	Absorbs exudates while preserving moist environment needed for autolysis of slough. Irrigate gel with saline to allow for assessing wound. Used for pressure ulcers, some stage III and some clean stage IV; wounds with mild or moderate exudates; wounds with necrosis or slough.
Contraindications	Infected wounds Wounds with fragile surrounding skin	Wounds that need frequent assessment, not transparent Wounds with heavy exudate

9. Remove silicone release paper backing from dressing. Minimize finger contact with adhesive surface. **Rationale:** *Dressing is sterile and contamination should be avoided.*

10. Center dressing over affected area and extend at least 2.5 cm (1 in.) onto periwound skin. Gently roll dressing over pressure ulcer—do not stretch dressing. **Rationale:** *Stretching the dressing may cause wrinkling of dressing, which allows air to enter wound.*

11. Placing dressing one third above wound and two thirds below wound maximizes time between dressing changes. **Rationale:** *Increases absorption capacity of dressing.*

12. Mold the dressing gently to skin, and hold down with hand for approximately 1 minute.

13. Apply skin prep to area that is to be covered by tape if ordered. Allow to dry. Do not apply skin prep under hydrocolloid dressing. **Rationale:** *Hydrocolloid dressings are placed over broken skin; skin prep may cause damage to skin.*

14. Use silk or hypoallergenic tape to "window frame" the sides of the hydrocolloid dressing.

15. Check dressing each shift for impaired integrity.

16. Change dressing at first sign of impaired integrity. Dressings should not be left on longer than 7 days; they are usually left in place for 3 to 4 days.

Note: DuoDERM is removed when exudate seeps from edges of dressing or white blister appears under dressing. Comfeel Plus is changed when dressing becomes transparent or there is leakage.

17. Remove dressing by pressing hand down on adjacent skin surface while carefully lifting edge of dressing from skin. Continue lifting dressing around periphery until all edges are released, then lift dressing carefully away from wound.

18. Remove gloves and perform hand hygiene.

19. Record stage, size, and appearance of ulcer; date; and reason for removal of hydrocolloid dressing.

Note: Although frequently listed as wound care alternatives, topical disinfectant agents such as iodine and silver sulfadiazine are very controversial in wound care. Iodine is cytotoxic to fibroblasts and can impair wound healing. Silver solutions are sometimes used to prevent bacterial colonization in infection-prone areas. They do not eliminate existing infections.

SKILL 18.15 Using Electrical Stimulation

Equipment

- Normal saline solution
- Bag for soiled dressings
- Gauze pads
- Two sterile basins
- Hydrogel sheets
- Electrode
- Bandage tape
- Alligator clip
- Stimulator
- Two pair clean gloves
- Sterile gloves

Preparation

- Check physician's order. Determine if client is candidate for electrical stimulation.
- Determine phase of wound healing. **Rationale:** *This determines the correct treatment protocol.*
- Set the stimulator settings according to manufacturer's directions, based on client's phase in wound healing. The settings include polarity, pulse rate, intensity, duration, and frequency.
- Explain procedure to client.
- Gather equipment.

(continued on next page)

SKILL 18.15   Using Electrical Stimulation (*continued*)

- Perform hand hygiene and observe other appropriate infection control procedures.
- Provide for client privacy.

Procedure

1. Raise bed to high position, lower side rails as needed.
2. Place client in position to enable staff to work with wound area and equipment. (Placement depends on wound site.)
3. Place supplies on overbed table, near working area.
4. Open all supply packages, maintaining sterility.
5. Pour sterile normal saline into one basin.
6. Don clean gloves.
7. Place disposal bag near wound. **Rationale:** *For ease in disposing of soiled dressings.*
8. Remove dressing carefully to avoid interfering with granulation tissue.
9. Remove clean gloves; place in disposal bag. Don sterile gloves.
10. Place sterile basin next to wound to catch irrigation solution as wound is cleansed.
11. Pour sterile normal saline into wound to cleanse wound. **Rationale:** *To remove exudates, slough, and petrolatum products. Current will not be conducted into wound tissue if petrolatum products remain in the wound.*
12. Remove excess irrigation solution using sterile gauze pads.
13. Place fluffed gauze pads into normal saline solution, squeeze out excess liquid.
14. Fill wound cavity with gauze including any undermined/tunneled spaces. Pack gently.
15. Place surface (active) electrode in wound bed, over gauze packing. **Rationale:** *This transfers electrical energy into wound bed, producing positive effects on necessary components for wound healing (i.e., blood flow, oxygen uptake, DNA, and protein synthesis).*
16. Cover with dry gauze pad.
17. Tape dry pad securely.
18. Connect alligator clip to foil.
19. Connect to stimulator lead.
20. Place a wet washcloth over area where dispersive electrode will be placed.
21. Select a dispersive pad that is larger than the sum of areas of active electrodes and wound packing.
22. Place dispersive electrode proximal to wound, over soft tissue, avoiding bony prominences.

Note: The greater the separation between two electrodes, the deeper the current path. Larger separation space is used to treat deep and undermined wounds. Closer separation space is used for shallow or partial-thickness wounds. Ensure electrodes do not touch.

23. Ensure all edges of electrode are in good contact with skin. Hold electrode in place with nylon elasticized strap.
24. Place client in position of comfort. Electrical stimulation treatments usually last 60 minutes.
25. Remove gloves and discard.
26. Perform hand hygiene.
27. Don clean gloves.
28. Remove electrode from wound following treatment.
29. Remove saline-soaked gauze and cover wound with occlusive dressing.
30. Document care and client response.

Note: Hydrogel sheets or amorphous hydrogel-impregnated gauze can be used to conduct current. If hydrogel gauze is the conductor, it is changed BID.

Candidates for Electrical Stimulation

- Pressure ulcers, stage I–IV.
- Diabetic ulcers
- Venous ulcers, ischemic ulcer
- Traumatic wounds
- Surgical wounds
- Wound flap
- Donor site, burn wound

SKILL 18.16   Using Noncontact Normothermic Wound Therapy

Equipment

- Warm-up therapy system components:
  - Warming cover (latex free)
  - Warming card
  - Temperature control unit (TCU)
  - AC adapter
- Wound measuring guide
- Sterile normal saline solution
- Skin scalant
- Carrying pouch
- Sterile normal saline
- Skin sealant
- Gauze pads
- Moisture-proof pad
- Sterile basin and irrigating syringe
- Sterile gloves
- Clean gloves
- Disposable bag

Preparation

- Check physician's orders and client care plan.
- Gather equipment. Select appropriately sized wound cover and warming card after measuring wound.
- Check that temperature control unit's battery is charged; if not, recharge with battery pack or wall outlet power source.
- Explain procedure to client.
- Provide for client privacy.
- Perform hand hygiene and observe other appropriate infection control procedures.

Procedure

1. Place equipment on overbed table.
2. Open sterile normal saline bottle, gauze pads, and basin with irrigating syringe.
3. Place disposable bag near wound site.
4. Position client for easy access to wound.
5. Remove compression stockings, if used.

SKILL 18.16   Using Noncontact Normothermic Wound Therapy *(continued)*

6. Don clean gloves.
7. Remove old dressing and place in disposal bag.
8. Remove gloves and discard in disposal bag. Don sterile gloves.
9. Fill irrigating syringe with normal saline. **Rationale:** *Using the syringe will increase pressure in wound to assist with removing debris and slough.*
10. Place moisture-proof pad or sterile basin under wound site.
11. Irrigate wound using the prescribed amount of irrigating solution.
12. Cleanse the surrounding skin with normal saline.
13. Dry periwound skin area.
14. Apply scalant to periwound area. **Rationale:** *This protects periwound area from exudates.*
15. Select appropriately sized wound cover based on wound size. **Rationale:** *To ensure that there is adequate healthy periwound skin between edge of foam and wound.*
16. Hold wound cover near edges only. Pull away one half of wound cover liner.
17. Place wound cover over wound, so wound can be seen through window. Do not stretch wound cover over skin while applying. **Rationale:** *Damage can occur to skin.*
18. Check for holes in wound cover, wrinkling, and folding of its edges. **Rationale:** *Wound cover will not be a barrier if this occurs.*
19. Press adhesive portion of cover to skin.
20. Pull away other half of wound cover liner and press adhesive portion to skin.
21. Gently smooth adhesive portion of wound cover with your fingertips to ensure adhesive sticks to skin.
22. Instruct the client that wound cover is worn 24 hours per day and requires no additional dressing.
23. Attach wound cover to Warm-Up® therapy system.
24. Remove and discard gloves. Perform hand hygiene. Document application of wound cover.

To Use Warm-Up® Therapy System ❶

1. Select appropriately sized warming card based on size of wound cover.
2. Plug warming card into gray socket on temperature control unit (TCU).

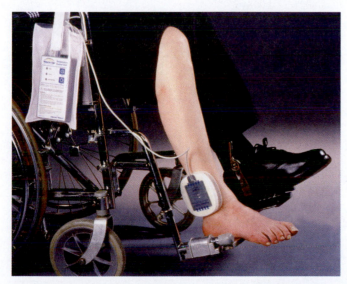

❶ Warm-Up® therapy unit. *(Courtesy of Augustine Medical, Inc., Eden Prairie, MN)*

CLINICAL ALERT

This warming treatment is done three times a day for 1 hour each treatment. Ensure that there is at least 1 hour between treatments. You can expect a significant increase in exudate for at least 7 to 10 days. This is considered a normal consequence of the wound healing process.

The wound cover is sterile and protects wound from contamination and trauma. The cover maintains a moist and warm wound, which creates a healing environment. The cover is a thin shell with a window and a foam frame. The shell has an adhesive border, is water resistant, and can be cleaned. It is flexible and moves with the client. The foam cover absorbs excess exudates to protect the periwound area from maceration. The foam frame keeps the pocket above the wound surface, so the warming card does not come in contact with the wound. The window is in the center of the cover and contains a pocket for the warming card.

Do not use compression therapy while warming card and TCU are in place. Client injury could occur.

3. Insert warming card into wound cover pocket. The warming card is used throughout warming therapy and is only for one client; it can be cleaned with damp cloth and clean water, if needed. Do not apply the warming card directly to the periwound area. Always cover the card with the wound cover. **Rationale:** *To prevent thermal injury.*
4. Turn off TCU.
5. Select mode of power (can use battery or AC adapter wall outlet).
6. Check that battery has sufficient charge for therapy session, usually 1 hour.
   - If battery needs charging, plug AC adapter into TCU, then plug the AC adapter into wall outlet.
   - Charge TCU until amber light on AC adapter flashes rapidly. It takes up to 2 hours to fully charge battery.
7. Plug AC adapter into black socket on the TCU, if using the TCU with the AC adapter. Plug AC adapter into wall outlet.
8. Position TCU and warming card cable to allow client some movement. Instruct client not to lie on any electronic components, cables, cords, or the wound cover.
9. Press the ON button to begin therapy. Follow physician orders for length of time for therapy. The unit will automatically turn off after 2 hours of continuous use.
10. Shut off TCU and remove warming card by grasping edge of card and sliding it out of wound cover pocket. Place card in plastic pouch for storage between treatments. DO NOT REMOVE WOUND COVER. **Rationale:** *Wound cover is only replaced if drainage occurs, the cover comes loose, the periwound area becomes macerated, or it has been in place 72 hours.*
11. Replace compression therapy if ordered.
12. Document procedure and assessment.

To Change Wound Cover

1. Check wound cover to ensure it needs to be changed.
2. Gather equipment for new wound cover.

(continued on next page)

SKILL 18.16   Using Noncontact Normothermic Wound Therapy *(continued)*

3. Explain procedure to client.
4. Perform hand hygiene and observe other appropriate infection control procedures.
5. Follow Preparation steps at the beginning of this skill.
6. Don clean gloves.
7. Place disposal bag near wound.
8. Gently press down on skin along one edge of wound cover.
9. Carefully lift edge of wound cover.
10. Slowly peel away wound cover until all edges are loose.
11. Discard wound cover in disposal bag.
12. Remove and discard gloves. Perform hand hygiene.
13. Reapply new wound cover.
14. Document the procedure and length of time for therapy in the client's record. Include the date and time; the appearance of the wound; the color, consistency, amount, and odor of any drainage; and how the client responded.

LEGAL ALERT

Wound care practitioners are at risk for litigation. Clients who experience wounds frequently believe it is because of neglect by healthcare workers. Wound care practitioners may face liability for:

- Negligence
- Violations of Medicare and Medicaid fraud and abuse prohibitions
- Abandonment for terminating services to clients.

PROVING NEGLIGENCE

To prove negligence, a client must show that the provider owed the client a duty, breached the duty owed the client, and the breach of duty must result in injury or damage to the client. Owing a duty of reasonable care to a client incorporates the standards of wound care. Breaching a duty occurs when the healthcare practitioner does something that should not have been done. To be charged with causing injury, the client would need to prove that injuries occurred as a result of practitioner error.

SKILL 18.17   Using Negative Pressure Wound Therapy (Wound VAC)

Evidence-Based Nursing Practice

Vacuum-Assisted Closure (V.A.C.®) for Sternal Wounds: A First-Line Therapeutic Management Approach.

A retrospective review of 103 clients was completed at one institution. The clients underwent vacuum-assisted closure therapy after median sternotomy between June 1999 and March 2004. The clients' wounds were classified as sterile wounds, superficial sternal infections, and mediastinitis. The wound closure device was applied sterilely to all wounds over a layer of Acticoat. The results indicated that vacuum-assisted closure was utilized in the treatment of 103 clients with sternal wounds (67 males and 36 females). The median age was 52 years (3 months to 91 years). Client comorbidities included diabetes, chronic obstructive pulmonary disease, end-stage renal disease, immunosuppression, and other conditions. The therapy was utilized for 11 days per client. Sixty-eight of the clients had definitive chest closure with open reduction internal fixation and/or flap closure. The remaining 32% of the clients had no definitive closure method. The overall mortality rate was 28%, although none of the four deaths was directly related to the use of the therapy. The conclusion indicated that vacuum-assisted closure therapy has been shown to decrease wound edema, decrease time to definitive closure, and reduce wound bacterial colony counts.

Source: Agarwal et al. (2005).

Equipment

- Foam, black or white V.A.C.® kit ❶
- Gauze pads
- Sterile normal saline
- Irrigating syringe
- Moisture-proof pad or sterile basin
- Skin prep agent (optional)
- Razor (optional)
- Clean gloves
- Sterile gloves
- Disposal bag
- Sterile scissor

Preparation

- Check physician's orders.
- Evaluate if client is candidate for V.A.C. therapy: nutritionally stable, able to use device 22 hours each day, and can use a pressure support surface if wound is over bony prominence.

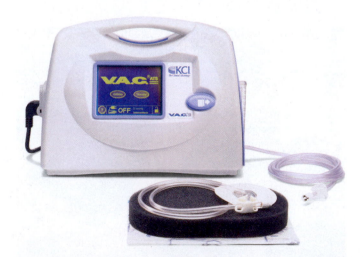

❶ V.A.C. unit.

SKILL 18.17   Using Negative Pressure Wound Therapy (Wound VAC) *(continued)*

Rationale: *If therapy is turned off longer than 2 hours, the dressing must be removed and replaced with a traditional dressing.*

- Assess wound to determine if therapy can be implemented.
  a. Wound surrounded by at least 2 cm (0.8 in.) of intact peri-wound tissue to maintain airtight seal.
  b. Wound open enough to insert foam dressing that touches all edges.
  c. Wound debrided.
  d. Sufficient circulation to assist in healing process.
- Select correct foam dressing according to size and type of wound. Black foam has larger pores and is used to stimulate granulation tissue and wound contraction. White (soft) foam is used when granulation tissue needs to be restricted or client cannot tolerate pain associated with black foam. White foam is used with superficial wounds, shallow chronic ulcers, and tunneling or undermining wounds.
- Gather equipment and supplies.
- Provide for client privacy.
- Explain procedure to client and determine client's willingness to use this therapy.
- Perform hand hygiene and observe other appropriate infection control procedures.

Procedure

1. Place disposal bag near wound.
2. Open supplies and place on overbed table. Open kit while maintaining sterility.
3. Draw up normal saline irrigating solution in syringe.
4. Don clean gloves.
5. Place moisture-proof pad or sterile basin under wound. **Rationale:** *Protects skin and bed during irrigation.*
6. Clean wound using aggressive irrigation. If debridement is to be done, only a trained professional can perform the skill. Notify the appropriate person. **Rationale:** *Devitalized tissue should be removed as areas of soft or stringy slough delays the healing process.*
7. Remove and discard gloves. Perform hand hygiene.
8. Don sterile gloves.
9. Dry wound and prepare periwound tissue with skin preparation agent if necessary. **Rationale:** *To promote an airtight seal.*
10. Cut the V.A.C. foam to fit the shape and entire wound cavity, including tunneling or undermined areas. White foam is used for tunneled wounds ❷.
11. Size and trim drape to cover foam dressing, leaving a 3.5-cm (1.5 in.) border per wound area.
12. Gently place the foam into wound, ensuring entire wound is covered.

CLINICAL ALERT

Do not pack foam into any areas of the wound. Forcing foam dressings in a compressed manner into any wound may lead to risk of adverse health issues.

For deep wound, reposition tubing to minimize pressure on wound edges every 2 hours. Excess foam can be used to cushion skin under tubing.

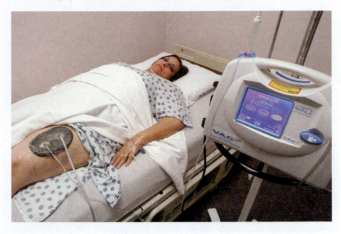

❷ V.A.C. foam cut to fit shape and wound cavity, with tubing attached to vacuum pump.

13. Apply tubing to foam. Tubing can be laid on top of foam or placed inside foam dressing. Keep tubing away from bony prominences.
14. Cover foam and 3.5 cm (1.5 in.) per wound area with drape. Do not stretch drape or compress foam with drape. **Rationale:** *This ensures a tight seal without causing tension or a shearing force on periwound tissue.*
15. Lift tubing and place on drape that has been bunched up to protect skin from pressure of tube.
16. Secure tubing with additional piece of drape or tape several centimeters away from dressing. **Rationale:** *This prevents pulling on the dressing, leading to a leak.*
17. Remove gloves and discard.
18. Remove canister from sterile package and push it into the V.A.C. unit until you hear it click in place. Alarm will sound if canister is not properly inserted into unit.
19. Connect dressing tubing to canister tubing.
20. Open both clamps, one on the dressing tubing and the other on the canister tubing.
21. Place V.A.C. unit on level surface or hang from footboard.
22. Press power button ON.
23. Adjust V.A.C. unit settings according to physician's orders or Guidelines for Treating Wound Types in the reference manual that comes with the unit. Target pressure should be set for 5 minutes on and 2 minutes off (intermittent therapies on machine). Intensity of setting sets the negative pressure.
24. Assess dressing in 1 minute. **Rationale:** *The dressing should collapse unless air leak is present.*
25. Dressing changes must be completed every 48 hours unless wound is infected, then change every 12 to 24 hours.
26. Document relevant information.

Procedure for Removing Dressing

1. Perform hand hygiene.
2. Don clean gloves.
3. Raise tube connector above level of pump unit.
4. Tighten clamp on dressing tube.
5. Separate canister tube and dressing tubes by disconnecting the connector.
6. Allow pump unit to pull exudates in canister tube into canister; then tighten clamps on canister tube.
7. Press Therapy ON/OFF to deactivate pump.

(continued on next page)

SKILL 18.17   Using Negative Pressure Wound Therapy (Wound VAC) *(continued)*

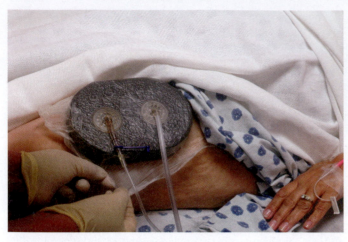

③ Remove adhesive drape by gently pulling away from skin.

8. Stretch drape horizontally and slowly pull up from skin. Gently remove it from skin. Do not peel it off skin **③**.
9. Discard disposable equipment including gloves in appropriate bag or container.
10. Perform hand hygiene.
    Note: Dressing changes are completed every 48 hours; if infected, every 12 hours.
11. Document the procedure in the client's record. Include the appearance of the wound; the color, consistency, amount, and odor of any drainage; and how the client responded.

Procedure for Disconnecting V.A.C. Unit

1. Turn the unit to OFF.
2. Clamp both clamps on tubing.
3. Press quick-release connector to separate dressing tubing from canister tubing.

4. Cover ends of tubing with gauze and secure.
5. Document cessation of therapy and assessments.

Procedure for Reconnecting V.A.C. Unit

1. Remove gauze from ends of tubing.
2. Connect tubing.
3. Unclamp clamps.
4. Press V.A.C. green power button to ON.
5. Select NO at new client prompt. Unit will resume previous settings.
6. Press therapy to ON. Document reinitiation of therapy.

Procedure for Changing Canister

1. Don clean gloves.
2. Assess that canister unit is full. Unit will alarm when full.
3. Tighten clamps on canister tubing from dressing tubing.
4. Pull back on release knob on V.A.C. unit at same time as you pull canister from slot.
5. Put canister in biohazard disposable bag and place in designated area for disposal.
6. Remove and discard gloves. Perform hand hygiene. Document canister change.
   Note: Average length of treatment is 4 to 6 weeks. Home systems are available as well.

V.A.C. GranuFoam® Silver

- Provides continuous delivery of silver directly to wound bed.
- Provides a protective barrier to reduce aerobic, gram-negative, and gram-positive bacteria, yeast, and fungi, and it may reduce infections in wounds.
- Indicated for client with chronic, acute, traumatic, and dehisced wounds, partial-thickness burns, and pressure ulcers.

SKILL 18.18   Applying a Transparent Wound Barrier

Delegation

Due to the need for aseptic technique and assessment skills, most dressing changes are not delegated to UAP. In some states, UAP may apply dry dressings to clean, chronic wounds. UAP should observe an exposed wound or dressing during usual care and must report abnormal findings to the nurse. In some agencies, UAP may be permitted to reinforce the dressing (apply additional dry dressings over a saturated bandage), but this must be reported to the nurse as soon as possible. Assessment of the wound and abnormal findings must be validated and interpreted by the nurse.

Equipment

- Clean gloves
- Sterile gloves (optional)
- Hair scissors or clippers
- Alcohol or acetone
- Moisture-proof bag
- Sterile gauze and the wound-cleaning agents specified by the primary care provider or agency (e.g., sterile saline)
- Wound barrier dressing
- Scissors
- Paper tape

Preparation

- Review the physician's orders regarding frequency and type of dressing change, and determine agency protocol about solutions used to clean the wound and whether clean or sterile technique is to be used. Many agencies recommend clean rather than sterile technique for chronic wounds such as a pressure ulcer. If possible, schedule the dressing change at a time convenient for the client. Some dressing changes require only a few minutes and others can take much longer.

Procedure

1. Prior to performing the procedure, introduce self and verify the client's identity using agency protocol. Explain to the client what you are going to do, why it is necessary, and how he or she can participate. Discuss how the results will be used in planning further care or treatments.
2. Perform hand hygiene and observe other appropriate infection control procedures.
3. Provide for client privacy. Assist the client to a comfortable position in which the wound can be readily exposed. Expose only the wound area, using a bath blanket to cover the client, if necessary. **Rationale:** *Undue exposure is physically and psychologically distressing to most people.*

SKILL 18.18   Applying a Transparent Wound Barrier (*continued*)

4. Remove the existing dressing.
5. Assess the wound.
6. Thoroughly clean the skin area around the wound.
   - Apply clean gloves.
   - Clean the skin well with normal saline or a mild cleansing agent. Always rinse the adjacent skin well before applying a dressing.
   - Clip the hair about 5 cm (2 in.) around the wound area if indicated. Do not use a standard bladed razor because they can cause small nicks in the skin and create or spread infection (Woo et al., 2009).
   - Remove gloves and dispose of them in the moisture-proof bag. Perform hand hygiene.
7. Clean the wound if indicated.
   - Apply clean or sterile gloves in accordance with agency protocol.
   - Clean the wound with the prescribed solution.
   - Dry the surrounding skin with dry gauze.
8. Apply the wound barrier.
   - Review the instructions on the barrier package. Remove part of the paper backing on the dressing ❶.
   - Apply the dressing at one edge of the wound site, allowing at least 2.5-cm (1-in.) coverage of the skin surrounding the wound.
   - Gently lay or press the barrier over the wound. Keep it free of wrinkles, but avoid stretching it too tightly. **Rationale:** *A stretched dressing restricts mobility and can pull loose easily.*
   - Remove and discard gloves. Perform hand hygiene.
9. Reinforce the dressing only if absolutely needed. **Rationale:** *Additional dressing over the transparent barrier will constrict the flow of gases.*
   - Apply paper or other porous tape to "window frame" the edges of the dressing.

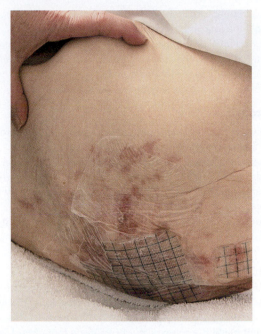

❶ Transparent wound dressing.

10. Assess the wound at least daily.
    - Determine the extent of serous fluid accumulation under the dressing, wound healing, and the need to repair the dressing.
    - If excessive serum has accumulated, consider replacing the transparent wound barrier with a more absorbent type of dressing, such as hydrocolloid.
    - If the dressing is leaking, remove it and apply another dressing.
11. Document the dressing change and the client's response in the client record using forms or checklists supplemented by narrative notes when appropriate. Many agencies use a designated wound/skin documentation sheet.

SKILL 18.19   Positioning and Exercising a Client's Stump

Equipment

- Pillows

Preparation

- Check physician's orders.
- Identify client by checking the client's identity band and asking client to state name and birth date. Explain purpose of positioning and exercising.
- Perform hand hygiene and observe other appropriate infection control procedures.
- Provide for client privacy.

Procedure

For Preoperative Care

1. Evaluate nutritional status and request nutritional consult if indicated. **Rationale:** *Adequate protein is necessary to promote wound healing.*
2. Recruit assistance of OT, PT, and social worker for early multidisciplinary care planning. A prosthetist explains future prosthetic care to the client and possibly organizes amputee peer visit, because this helps lessen anxiety about living with an amputation.
3. Explain importance of exercises to client. Tell client that because flexor muscles are stronger than extensors, stump will be permanently flexed and abducted unless the client practices extension and adduction exercises. **Rationale:** *Exercises increase muscle strength and improve mobility of amputated extremity. Both are necessary for optimal ambulation with a prosthesis.*
4. Teach client quadriceps-setting exercises with a below-the-knee amputation.
   - Extend leg and try to push back of knee into bed; try to move patella proximally.
   - Contract quadriceps and hold contraction for 10 seconds.
   - Repeat this procedure four or five times.
   - Repeat the exercise at least four times a day.
5. Teach use of ambulatory aids. **Rationale:** *Prepares client for postsurgery mobility.*

(continued on next page)

SKILL 18.19   Positioning and Exercising a Client's Stump *(continued)*

6. Explain phantom limb sensation; the client may continue to "feel" the lost limb postsurgery.
7. Counsel families, for they also mourn the loss of a visible body part. **Rationale:** *They too need psychological support and education about rehabilitation and necessary skills for self-care.*
8. Document care, teaching, and client response.

For Postoperative Care

1. Monitor for complications: hemorrhage, infection, unrelieved pain, wound that will not heal.
2. Assess for excessive wound drainage. Keep tourniquet at bedside. **Rationale:** *If excessive bleeding occurs, tourniquet must be applied, because hemorrhage is a potentially life-threatening complication.*
3. Administer ordered pain medication and continually assess to determine if pain is controlled.

> **CLINICAL ALERT**
> Adequate pain management in the preoperative period can reduce the occurrence of phantom limb pain postoperatively.

4. Do not place stump on pillow, but elevate foot of bed for first 24 hours ONLY to reduce stump edema and pain. **Rationale:** *Elevation on a pillow can promote flexion contracture of stump.*
5. Turn client to prone or supine position for at least 1 hour every 4 hours. **Rationale:** *This promotes hip extension and helps counteract possible flexion contracture formation.*
6. Avoid dependent positioning of stump. **Rationale:** *To prevent edema and discomfort. Edema may be present for up to 4 months after amputation.*
7. While washing the stump, tap and massage the stump skin toward the incision line. **Rationale:** *To prevent development of painful adhesions.*
8. Teach stump extension exercises.
   - Lie in a prone position with foot hanging over the end of the bed.

- Keep stump next to intact leg to extend stump and to contract gluteal muscles.
- Hold the contraction for 10 seconds.
- Repeat this exercise at least four times a day.
9. Teach adduction exercise.
   - Place a pillow between the client's thighs.
   - Squeeze the pillow for 10 seconds and then relax for 10 seconds.
   - Repeat this exercise at least four times a day.
10. Have the client keep track of time spent with the stump flexed and then spend an equal amount of time with the stump extended.
11. Encourage appropriate use of trapeze: Use both hands to pull up with trapeze; place foot flat on mattress to lift body. Do not use heel to push in the mattress. **Rationale:** *Pushing with the heel can lead to pressure ulcers.*
12. After stump incision heals, have client begin to bear weight on stump, initially pressing into padded surface (pillow on chair seat). **Rationale:** *To reduce pain and help prepare the stump for prosthesis.*

> **CLINICAL ALERT**
> Keep a tourniquet nearby in the event of excessive stump incision bleeding.

Amputees use more energy in ambulation than nonamputees. Older adults with an AKA must put forth an effort 100% above normal to walk at a slow rate. The longer the residual limb, the less energy the client must expend for ambulation.

13. Document exercising, care, and teaching in the client's record. Document any stump changes, incision site appearance, and how the client responded.

SKILL 18.20   Shrinking/Molding a Client's Stump

Equipment

- Two elastic bandages: 10 cm (4 in.) for below-the-knee amputation (BKA), 15 cm (6 in.) for above-the-knee amputation (AKA)
- Tape or safety pins
- Commercial stump shrinker (sheath)

Preparation

- Review client's record to check physician's orders and to determine date and type of amputation.
- Gather equipment.
- Identify client by checking the client's identity band and asking client to state name and birth date. Explain rationale for procedure.
- Perform hand hygiene and observe other appropriate infection control procedures.
- Provide for client privacy.

Procedure

1. Wash stump with soap and water and allow to dry for at least 10 minutes before bandaging. Do not use lotions, powders, or alcohol.
2. Inspect and encourage client to assess stump for circulatory status, pressure areas, wound healing, and edema.
3. Explain that purpose of wrap is to form a conical AKA stump to prepare for prosthesis use ❶.
4. Explain that wrap is to be worn at all times except during bathing or when wearing a prosthesis.
5. Start by placing bandage end outer surface on distal stump. **Rationale:** *The pressure gradient of the bandage should be greatest at the distal stump.*
6. Wrap bandage medially and diagonally around stump. Have client assist by holding turns. Stretch bandages to two thirds of the limit of the elastic.
7. Continue to wrap smoothly up the stump with medially directed spirals or figure eight turns (not circular). Progress up

SKILL 18.20 Shrinking/Molding a Client's Stump *(continued)*

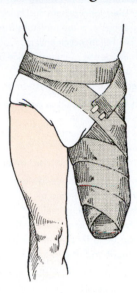

❶ Compression bandage may be used following amputation to mold and shrink stump in preparation for prosthesis.

the stump and well into groin area. **Rationale:** *Circular turns constrict circulation. Medial turns help correct stump tendency toward abduction.*

8. Finish bandaging with a "spica" turn over and around the client's pelvis, then back down to stump. **Rationale:** *Large "spica" turn prevents bandage from slipping.*

9. Secure the bandage with tape or (cautiously) with safety pins. Do not use bandage clips. **Rationale:** *Clips can pierce the skin, or easily come loose.*

10. Reapply elastic bandage every 4 to 6 hours, or when loose. **Rationale:** *It must never be in place for more than 12 hours without being rewrapped.*

11. If client has a stump "shrinker sheath," roll down and stretch the sheath using plastic ring. Fit onto stump end and apply, making sure there are no wrinkles ❷.

12. Teach client home care of residual limb and prosthesis (washing; assessing for redness, pressure points, irritation, swelling skin breakdown; socket, stump, socks, liners, mechanical parts, etc.).

13. Document the procedure in the client's record. Include the date and time; actions performed; type of dressing applied; and how the client responded.

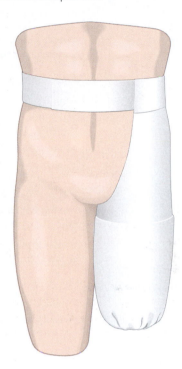

❷ "Commercial shrinkers" may be used for AKA amputations.

▶ CRITICAL THINKING OPTIONS FOR UNEXPECTED OUTCOMES

Not all unexpected outcomes require further nursing intervention; however, many times they do. When the client demonstrates a change in signs/symptoms indicating an emerging problem, the nurse should immediately assess and troubleshoot what is happening. The assessment data must be processed quickly to formulate a hypothesis so the nurse can make a clinical judgment. The nurse then decides how best to resolve the problem and improve the client's situation for a better appropriate outcome.

EXPECTED OUTCOME	PROBLEM SOLVING	NURSING ACTIONS
Assessment of Wound Integrity Client's wounds do not become infected.	Wound drainage increases.	▪ Decrease time between dressing changes. Change every 4 hours. ▪ Obtain order for culture and sensitivity to determine whether different microorganisms are present or antibiotic medication is not sensitive to microorganism.
Moist wound environment is maintained.	Dressings dry between dressing changes.	▪ Moisten dressing with sterile normal saline before removing to prevent debridement of granulation tissue. ▪ Ensure that dressing is moist when applied to wound and cover with moist dressing. ▪ Moisten and change dressing more frequently. ▪ Semiocclusive dressing should be considered.
Client maintains adequate fluid and nutrition.	Nutritional or hydration deficit occurs.	▪ Monitor nutritional and fluid intake accurately. ▪ Obtain order for vitamin supplements if client is not already on vitamins. ▪ Increase protein intake by supplementing with high-protein drinks.

EXPECTED OUTCOME	PROBLEM SOLVING	NURSING ACTIONS
Client's buttocks and perineal area remain free from urine and stool.	Skin is exposed to moisture.	■ Establish bowel or bladder program and select absorbent products for wound area that wick the moisture from skin. ■ Cleanse skin with pH-balanced cleansers, avoiding friction and dry skin after each incidence of incontinence and dry thoroughly. ■ Apply skin barrier product. ■ Consider use of fecal management system or urinary catheter.
Client is periodically repositioned.	Shearing and friction occur secondarily related to immobility or reduced activity.	■ Keep head of bed at lowest position possible to prevent client from sliding down in bed. ■ Use lifting devices to move client up in bed or out of bed to prevent friction on skin. ■ Instruct client on use of trapeze to assist in repositioning.
Dressings and Binders Wound heals without complications.	Client's wound does not heal with traditional types of treatments.	In client care conference discuss the following: ■ Is everyone following same treatment? ■ Are causative agents preventing healing? ■ Should treatment be adjusted or changed? ■ Would use of a support surface be effective? ■ Is surgical debridement and grafting necessary for healing?
	Fault light is flashing and an alarm is sounding on TCU.	■ Reconnect warming card; it may be disconnected. ■ Warming card or cable could be bent or damaged. Replace warming card. ■ TCU is broken. Turn TCU on and off. If light continues and alarm continues, turn off TCU and obtain new unit.
	Foam is not collapsed in wound bed.	■ Ensure therapy is on. Ensure clamps are open and tubing is not kinked. ■ Check for leaks and patch.
Wound Care Exudate is removed and wound healing occurs with negative wound therapy.	Wound is too large for V.A.C. kit.	■ Use more than one foam piece. ■ Place pieces so they touch each other. ■ Use only one tubing piece to one of the foam pieces.
Periwound area remains healthy without evidence of maceration.	Periwound skin is fragile.	■ Use skin prep prior to applying drape. ■ Frame wound with skin barrier or DuoDERM. ■ Cut drape large enough to enclose foam dressing and skin barrier layer.
Moist wound environment is maintained.	Dressing adheres to wound with negative pressure system.	■ Instill sterile water or normal saline into dressing, let sit for 15–20 minutes, then gently remove dressing from wound.
Hyperbaric oxygen therapy is effective in treating diabetic leg ulcers.	Client exhibits signs of anxiety when providing education regarding use of hyperbaric chamber.	■ Place client in multichamber where nurse is present to assess client with anxiety-reducing interventions.
Client is periodically repositioned.	Client sits in chair most of day and keeps stump elevated on a pillow while in bed.	■ Discuss hip and knee contracture complications that occur with prolonged flexion positioning of the stump. ■ Review and reinforce exercises that promote stump adduction and extension to prevent contractures and facilitate prosthesis use.
Client's wounds do not become infected.	Stump edema occurs in spite of compression bandage application.	■ Evaluate wrapping procedure. ■ Ensure that wraps are applied with pressure greater at distal stump and reapplied several times a day. Instruct client to avoid prolonged dependent positioning of stump. ■ Consult prosthetist for possible rigid shrinker use. ■ Apply shrinker before client gets out of bed.
Wound care is provided for contaminated wound and healing occurs.	Client expresses fear of losing other leg.	■ Teach client to care for the remaining extremity. ■ Inspect for lesions; wash and dry daily; use lotion for dry skin (not between toes); keep nails trimmed straight across; avoid mechanical, chemical, or thermal injury; wear shoes that are wide and deep enough for toes. ■ Exercise daily and avoid smoking. ■ Consult podiatrist for individual foot care or shoe orthotic adaptations, especially if client has diabetes. ■ Consult physician for management of diabetes or atherosclerosis.

REFERENCES

CHAPTER 1

Adiyaman, A., Tosun, N., Elving, L. D., Deinum, J., Lenders, J. W. M., & Thien, T. (2007). The effect of crossing legs on blood pressure. *Blood Pressure Monitoring, 12,*189–193.

American Academy of Ophthalmology (2012) *Pediatric eye evaluations: Preferred practice pattern.* Retrieved from http://one.aao.org/CE/PracticeGuidelines/PPP_Content.aspx?cid=2e30f625-1b04-45b9-9b7c-c06770d02fe5

Barness, L. A., Gilbert-Barness, E., & Fauber, D. (2009). *Handbook of pediatric physical and clinical diagnosis* (8th ed., p. 20). New York, NY: Oxford Press.

D'Amico, D., & Barbarito, C. (2011). *Health and physical assessment in nursing* (2nd ed.). Upper Saddle River, NJ: Prentice Hall Health.

Daniel, E. (2007) Noise and hearing loss: A review. *Journal of School Health, 77,* 225–231. doi:10.1111/j.1746-1561.2007.00197.x

Dossey, B. M., & Keegan, L. (2008). *Holistic nursing: A handbook for practice* (5th ed.). Sudbury, MA: Jones & Bartlett.

El-Radhi, A. S., & Barry, W. (2006). Thermometry in paediatric practice. *Archives of Disease in Childhood, 91*(4), 351–356. Retrieved from http://www.ncbi.nlm.nih.gov/pmc/articles/PMC2065972

Hausfater, P., Zhao, Y., Defrenne, S., Bonnet, P., & Riou, B. (2008). *Emerging Infectious Diseases, 14*(8), 1255–1258. Retrieved from http://www.ncbi.nlm.nih.gov/pubmed/18680649

Howlin, F. (2010). Cardiovascular assessment in children: Assessing pulse and blood pressure. *Paediatric Nursing, 22*(1), 25–35.

Kavey, R. W., Daniels, S. R., & Flynn, J. T. (2010). Management of high blood pressure in children and adolescents. *Cardiology Clinics, 28,* 597–607.

Knecht, K. R., Seller, J. D., & Alpert, B. S. (2009). Korotkoff sounds in neonates, infants, and toddlers. *American Journal of Cardiology, 103,* 1165–1167. doi:10.1016/j.amjcard.2008.12.038

Ogedegbe, G., & Pickering, T. (2010). Principles and techniques of blood pressure measurement. *Cardiology Clinics, 28*(4), 571–586.

Pinar, R., Ataalkin, S., & Watson, R. (2010). The effect of crossing legs on blood pressure in hypertensive patients. *Journal of Clinical Nursing, 19,* 1284–1288. doi:10.1111/j.1365-2702.2009.03148.x

Qaseem, A., Snow, V., Barry, P., Hornbake, E. R., Rodnick, J. E., Tobolic, T., . . . Joint

American Academy of Family Physicians/American College of Physicians Panel on Deep Venous Thrombosis/Pulmonary Embolism. (2007). Current diagnosis of venous thromboembolism in primary care: A clinical practice guideline from the American Academy of Family Physicians and the American College of Physicians. *Annals of Internal Medicine, 146,* 454–458.

Schell, K., Bradley, E., Bucher, L., Seckel, M., Lyons, D., Wakai, S., . . . Simpson, K. (2005). Clinical comparison of automatic, noninvasive blood pressure in the forearm and upper arm. *American Journal of Critical Care, 14*(3), 232–241.

Valdez-Lowe, C., Ghareeb, S. A., & Artinian, N. T. (2009). Pulse oximetry in adults. *American Journal of Nursing, 109*(6), 52–59. doi:10.1097/01.NAJ.0000352474.55746.81

Whittington, A., Whitlow, G., Hewson, D., Thomas, C., & Brett, S. J. (2009). Bacterial contamination of stethoscopes on the intensive care unit. *Anesthesia, 64*(6), 620–624.

CHAPTER 2

American Dental Association. (n.d.). *Cleaning your teeth and gums.* Retrieved from http://www.ada.org/2624.aspx

American Society for Parenteral and Enteral Nutrition. (2009). A.S.P.E.N. enteral nutrition practice recommendations. *Journal of Parenteral and Enteral Nutrition, 33,* 122–167. doi:10.1177/0148607108330314

Andrews, M. M., & Boyle, J. S. (2008). *Transcultural concepts in nursing care* (5th ed.). Philadelphia, PA: Lippincott Williams & Wilkins.

Bower, L. M. (2005). Is your patient's metered-dose inhaler technique up to snuff? *Nursing, 35*(8), 50–51.

Cohen, H. (2008). Let's work together to improve medication safety. *Nursing, 38*(4), 6.

Downey, L., & Lloyd, H. (2008). Bed bathing patients in hospital. *Nursing Standard, 22*(34), 35–40.

Fayaz, M., Sultana, A., & Rai, M. E. (2009). Comparison between efficacy of MDI+spacer and nebuliser in the management of acute asthma in children. *Journal of Ayub Medical College, Abbottabad, 21*(1), 32–34.

Immunization Action Coalition. (2009). *Administering vaccines: Dose, route, site, and needle size* (Technical content reviewed by the Centers for Disease Control and Prevention, February 2009). Retrieved from http://www.vdh.virginia.gov/Epidemiology/immunization/VFC/documents/forms/VVFCToolkit/Fulltoolkit.pdf

Institute for Safe Medication Practices. (2010). *Oral dosage forms that should not be crushed.* Retrieved from http://www.ismp.org/Tools/DoNotCrush.pdf

Jacobs, C. (2008). Ear irrigation. *Primary Health Care, 18*(7), 36–39.

Joint Commission. (2011). *Official "do not use" list.* Used with permission. Retrieved from http://www.jointcommission.org/topics/patient_safety.aspx

Joint Commission. (2014a). *National patient safety goals.* Retrieved from http://www.jointcommission.org/assets/1/6/2014_HAP_NPSG_E.pdf

Joint Commission. (2014b). *National patient safety goals slide presentation.* Retrieved from http://www.jointcommission.org/2014_national_patient_safety_goals_slide_presentation

Kraszewski, S. (2008). Safe and effective ear irrigation. *Nursing Standard, 22*(43), 45–48.

Minnesota Department of Health. (2013). *Nervanas Caring Hands Inc. neglect causes death of resident* (Case No. HL26052001). Retrieved from http://www.health.state.mn.us/divs/fpc/directory/surveyapp/ohfc-findings/hl26052001.pdf

National Academy of Sciences, Institute of Medicine. (2006). *Preventing medication errors: Quality chasm series.* Retrieved from http://iom.edu/Reports/2006/Preventing-Medication-Errors-Quality-Chasm-Series.aspx

National Library of Medicine, National Institutes of Health. (2014). *Nitroglycerin.* Retrieved from http://www.nlm.nih.gov/medlineplus/druginfo/meds/a601086.html#how

Nursing World. (2008). 2008 Study of nurses' views on workplace safety and needlestick injuries. Retrieved from http://www.nursingworld.org/MainMenuCategories/WorkplaceSafety/Healthy-Work-Environment/SafeNeedles/2008-Study/2008InviroStudy.pdf 2008

Penzer, R. (2008). Providing patients with information on caring for skin. *Nursing Standard, 23*(9), 49–55.

Phillips, L. D. (2010). *Manual of I.V. therapeutics: Evidence based practice for infusion therapy* (5th ed.). Philadelphia, PA: F. A. Davis.

Pump up the volume—Tips for increasing error reporting. (2009). *Nurse Advise-ERR, 7*(7), 1–3.

Rubin, B., & Durotoye, L. (2004). How do patients determine that their metered-dose inhaler is empty? *Chest, 126,* 1134–1137.

Sucre, M. J., & De Nicola, A. (2009). Economic comparison of the traditional bathing method with the basinless bathing method in coma patients. *Critical Care 2009, 13*(Suppl. 1): 459.

U.S. Food and Drug Administration. (2010). *A guide to bed safety: Bed rails in hospitals, nursing homes and home health care: The facts.* Retrieved from http://www.fda.gov/downloads/MedicalDevices/ProductsandMedicalProcedures/GeneralHospitalDevicesandSupplies/HospitalBeds/ucm125857.pdf

CHAPTER 3

Phillips, L. D. (2010). *Manual of I.V. therapeutics: Evidence-based practice for infusion therapy* (5th ed.). Philadelphia, PA: F. A. Davis.

CHAPTER 4

Andrews, M. M., & Boyle, J. S. (2012). *Transcultural concepts in nursing care* (6th ed.). Philadelphia, PA: Lippincott Williams & Wilkins.

Ball, J., & Bindler, R. (2012). *Principles of pediatric nursing: Caring for children* (5th ed.). Upper Saddle River, NJ: Prentice Hall.

D'Arcy, Y. M. (2009). The effect of culture on pain. *Nursing, 17*(3), 5–7.

Davidson, J. E. (2009). Family-centered care: Meeting the needs of patients' families and helping families adapt to critical illness. *Critical Care Nurse, 29*(3), 28–34. Retrieved from http://www.aacn.org/WD/CETESTS/media/C093.pdf?origin=publication_detail

Field, M. J., & Behrman, R. E. (Eds.). (2003). *When children die: Improving palliative and end-of-life care for children and their families.* Washington, DC: National Academies Press. Retrieved from http://www.nap.edu/catalog/10390.html

Harvard Mental Health Letter. (2011). Understanding the stress response. Retrieved from http://www.health.harvard.edu/newsletters/Harvard_Mental_Health_Letter/2011/March/understanding-the-stress-response

Kagawa-Singer, M., & Blackhall, L. J. (2001). Negotiating cross-cultural issues at the end of life. *Journal of the American Medical Association, 286*(23), 2992–3001.

Lawrence, J., Alcock, D., McGrath, P., Kay, J., MacMurray, S. B., & Dulberg, C. (1993). The development of a tool to assess neonatal pain. *Neonatal Network, 12*(6), 59–66.

Merkel, S. I., Voepel-Lewis, T., Shayevitz, J. R., & Malviya, S. (1997). The FLACC: A behavioral scale for scoring postoperative pain in young children. *Pediatric Nursing, 23*(3), 293–297.

Midori, A. Y., & Hemmen, T. M. (2010). Therapeutic hypothermia for brain ischemia: Where have we come and where do we go? *Stroke, 41,* S72–S74. Retrieved from http://stroke.ahajournals.org/content/41/10_suppl_1/S72.long

Morrow, C. (2010). Reducing neonatal pain during routine heel lance procedures. *American Journal of Maternal Child Nursing, 35*(6), 346–354.

National Hospice and Palliative Care Organization (2012). *Facts and figures: Hospice care in America 2012.* Alexandria, VA: Author.

Searight, H. R., & Gafford, J. (2005). Cultural diversity at the end of life: Issues and guidelines for family physicians. *American Family Physician, 71*(3), 515–522. Retrieved from http://www.aafp.org/afp/2005/0201/p515.html

Spector, R. (2012). *Cultural diversity in health and illness* (8th ed.). Upper Saddle River, NJ: Prentice Hall Health.

Truog, R. D., Cist, A. F., Brackett, S. E., Burns, J. P., Curley, M. A., Danis, M., . . . Hurford, W. E. (2001). Recommendations for end-of-life care in the intensive care unit: The Ethics Committee of the Society of Critical Care Medicine. *Critical Care Medical, 29*(12), 2332–2348.

Waterman, B., Walker, J. J., Swaims, C., Shortt, M., Todd, M. S., Machen, S. M., & Owens, B. D. (2012). The efficacy of combined cryotherapy and compression compared with cryotherapy alone following anterior cruciate ligament reconstruction. *Journal of Knee Surgery, 25*(2), 155–160.

CHAPTER 5

Grant, R., Biglin, A., Zeuschner, C., Guy, T., Pearce, R., Hokin, B., & Ashton, J. (2008). The relative impact of a vegetable-rich diet on key markers of health in a cohort of Australian adolescents. *Asia Pacific Journal of Clinical Nutrition, 17*(1), 107–115.

Siegel, J. D., Rhinehart, E., Jackson, M., Chiarello, L., & Healthcare Infection Control Practices Advisory Committee. (2007). *2007 Guideline for isolation precautions: Preventing transmission of infectious agents in healthcare settings.* Retrieved from http://www.cdc.gov/ncidod/dhqp/pdf/isolation2007.pdf

CHAPTER 6

Centers for Disease Control and Prevention. (2009). *Guideline for prevention of catheter-associated urinary tract infections, 2009.* Retrieved from http://www.cdc.gov/hicpac/cauti/02_cauti2009_abbrev.html

Chung, H. F., Spigt, M. G., Knottnerus, J. A., & vanMastrigt, R. (2008). Comparative analysis of the reproducibility and applicability of the condom catheter method for noninvasive urodynamics in two Dutch centers. *Urologia Internationalis, 81,* 139–148. doi:10.1159/000144051

Dumont, C., & Wakeman, J. (2010). Preventing catheter associated UTIs: Survey report. *Nursing, 40*(12), 24–30.

Fallis, Wendy. (2005). Indwelling Foley catheters: Is the current design a source of erroneous measurement of urine output? *Critical Care Nurse, 25*(2), 44–46, 48–51.

Gray, M. (2008). Securing the indwelling catheter. *American Journal of Nursing, 108*(12), 44–51.

Kim, B. R., Park, J. H., Shin, H. S., Jung, Y. S., & Rim, H. (2012). Survival by time of day of hemodialysis in Korean patients: A single center study. *British Journal of Medicine and Medical Research, 3*(1), 108–115. Retrieved from http://www.sciencedomain.org/abstract.php?iid=163&id=12&aid=759#.UtgEtWeA1jp

Lo, E. (2008). Strategies to prevent catheter-associated urinary tract infections in acute care hospitals. *Infection Control and Hospital Epidemiology, 29*(1), S41–S50.

Martelly-Kebreau, Y., & Farren, M. (2009). Research on prevention of urinary incontinence and catheter management. *Home Healthcare Nurse, 27,* 468–474. doi:10.1097/01.NHH.0000360920.11109.7f

Mayo Clinic. (2013a). *Chronic constipation in older patients.* Retrieved from http://www.mayoclinic.org/medical-professionals/clinical-updates/digestive-diseases/chronic-constipation-older-patients-educational-approach

Mayo Clinic. (2013b). *Cranberry (Vaccinium macrocarpon).* Retrieved from http://www.mayoclinic.org/drugs-supplements/cranberry/background/hrb-20059059

Newman, D. (2007). The indwelling urinary catheter: Principles for best practice. *Journal of Wound, Ostomy and Continence Nursing, 34,* 655–663. doi:10.1097/01.WON.0000299816.82983.4a

Perakis, K. E., Stylianou, K. G., Kyriazis, J. P., Mavroeidi, V. N., Katsipi, I. G., Vardaki, E. A., . . . Daphnis, E. K. (2009). Long-term complication rates and survival of peritoneal dialysis catheters: The role of percutaneous versus surgical placement. *Seminars in Dialysis, 22,* 569–575. doi:10.1111/j.1525-139X.2009.00621.x

Registered Nurses Association of Ontario. (2005, March). *Prevention of constipation in the older adult population* (revised). Toronto, Canada: Author.

Saint, S., Kaufman, S. R., Thompson, M., Rogers, M. A., & Chenoweth, C. E. (2005). A reminder reduces urinary catheterization in hospitalized patients. *Journal on Quality and Patient Safety, 31*(8), 455–462.

Villanueva, C., & Hemstreet, G. P. (2008). Difficult male urethral catheterization: A review of different approaches. *International Brazilian Journal of Urology, 34,* 401–412.

Willson, M., Wilde, M., Webb, M., Thompson, D., Parker, D., Harwood, J., . . . Gray, M. (2009). Nursing interventions to reduce the risk of catheter-associated urinary tract infection. *Journal of Wound, Ostomy and Continence Nursing, 36*(2), 137–154.

CHAPTER 7

Bertolino, G., Pitassi, A., Tinelli, C., Staniscia, A., Guglielmana, B., Scudeller, L., & Luigi Balduini, C. (2012). Peripheral intravenous catheters in a medical department: a pragmatic cluster-randomized controlled study. *Worldviews on Evidence-Based Nursing, 9*(4), 221–226.

Centers for Disease Control and Prevention. (2011). *2011 Guidelines for the prevention of intravascular catheter-related infections.* Retrieved from http://www.cdc.gov/hicpac/bsi/03-bsi-summary-of-recommendations-2011.html

Hadaway, L. (2005). Caring for a nontunneled CVC site. *Nursing, 35*(12), 54–56.

Hadaway, L. (2007). Infiltration and extravasation. *American Journal of Nursing, 107*(8), 64–72.

Hadaway, L. C. (2008). Targeting therapy with central venous access devices. *Nursing, 38*(6), 34–40.

Hadaway, L. (2009). Protect patients from I.V. infiltration. *American Nurse Today, 4*(7), 10–11.

Infusion Nurses Society (INS). (2006). Infusion nursing standards of practice. *Journal of Infusion Nursing, 29*(1), S1–S92.

Institute for Healthcare Improvement. (2012). *How-to guide: Prevent central line-associated bloodstream infections (CLABSI).* Cambridge, MA: Author. Available at www.ihi.org

Joint Commission. (2013). *2013 National patient safety goals, hospital.* Retrieved from http://www.jointcommission.org/assets/1/6/HAP_NPSG_Chapter_2014.pdf

Maki, D. G., Genihner, D., Hua, S., Chiacchierini, R. P., et al. (2000). *An evaluation of Biopatch Antimicrobial Dressing compared to routine standard of care in the prevention of catheter-related bloodstream infection.* Johnson & Johnson Medical Division of ETHICON, Inc., www.ethicon.com.

Moureau, N. L., & Dawson, R. B. (2010). Keeping needleless connectors clean, part 2. *Nursing, 40*(6), 61–63.

Movahedi, A. F., Rostami, S., Salsali, M., Keikhaee, B., & Moradi, A. (2007). Effect of local refrigeration prior to venipuncture on pain related responses in school age children. *Australian Journal of Advanced Nursing, 24*(2), 51–55.

Phillips, L. D. (2010). *Manual of I.V. therapeutics. Evidence based practice for infusion therapy* (5th ed.). Philadelphia, PA: F. A. Davis.

Rodriguez, W. (n.d.). To heparinize or not to heparinize? *Children's Hospital of Orange County.* Retrieved from http://www.choc.org/userfiles/file/RodriguezW0209.pdf

Timsit, J. F. (2009). Chlorhexidine gluconate-impregnated sponges reduced rate of catheter-related infections in ICU. *Journal of the American Medical Association, 301,* 1231–1241.

U.S. Food and Drug Administration. (2005, September). *FDA issues bar code regulation, 2004.* Retrieved from http://www.fda.gov/oc/initiatives/barcode

CHAPTER 8

Arias, K. M. (2010). *Contamination and cross contamination on hospital surfaces and medical equipment.* Retrieved from http://www.initiatives-patientsafety.org/Initiatives4.pdf

Arrowsmith, V. A., & Taylor, R. (2012). *Removal of nail polish and finger rings to prevent surgical infection.* Retrieved from http://www.ncbi.nlm.nih.gov/pubmed/22592690

Centers for Disease Control and Prevention. (2013). *Handwashing: Clean hands save lives.* Retrieved from http://www.cdc.gov/handwashing

Dossey, B. M., & Keegan, L. (2008). *Holistic nursing: A handbook for clinical practice* (5th ed.). Sudbury, MA: Jones & Bartlett.

U.S. Department of Health and Human Services, Agency for Healthcare Research and Quality. (2013). *Electronic hand hygiene monitoring system significantly reduces health care–associated infections.* Retrieved from http://www.innovations.ahrq.gov/content.aspx?id=3348

World Health Organization (WHO). (2009a). *Summary of the indications for gloving and for glove removal (Use information leaflet).* Geneva, Switzerland: Author. Retrieved from http://www.who.int/gpsc/5may/Glove_Use_Information_Leaflet.pdf

World Health Organization (WHO). (2009b). *WHO guidelines on hand hygiene in health care* (p. 133). Geneva, Switzerland: Author. Retrieved from http://whqlibdoc.who.int/publications/2009/9789241597906_eng.pdf

CHAPTER 9

Abo, A., Chen, L., Johnston, P., & Santucci, K. (2010). Positioning for lumbar puncture in children evaluated by bedside ultrasound. *Pediatrics, 125*(5), e1149–e1153. doi:10.1542/peds.2009-0646

Comprehensive Advanced Life Support (CALS). (2011). *Acute care 30: Glasgow Coma Scale—Adult, pediatric, infant.* Retrieved from http://calsprogram.org/manual/volume1/section1/neurology/acute_care_30.html

Hockenberry, M., & Wilson, D. (2012). *Wong's nursing care of infants and children* (9th ed.). St. Louis, MO: Mosby/Elsevier.

Rainbow Rehabilitation Centers. (2009). *The Glasgow Coma Scales.* Retrieved from http://www.rainbowrehab.com/RainbowVisions/article_downloads/articles/Art-TECH-GComaScale.pdf

Rangel-Castillo, L., Gopinath, S., & Robertson, C. S. (2008). Management of intracranial hypertension. *Neurology Clinics, 26,* 521–541.

CHAPTER 10

Alsulami, Z., Conroy, S., & Choonara, I. (2012). Double checking the administration of medicines: What is the evidence? A systematic review. *Archives of Disease in Childhood, 97,* 833–837.

Intermountain University. (n.d.). *Medication high-alert double check.* Retrieved from http://www.ppag.org/attachments/courses/medcheck/medcheck.swf

CHAPTER 11

Bakody, E. (2009). Orthopaedic plaster casting: Nurse and patient education. *Nursing Standard, 23*(51), 49–56.

Carlson, M. E., Suetta, C., Conboy, M. J., Aagaard, P., Mackey, A., Khaer, M., & Conboy, I. (2009). Molecular aging and rejuvenation of human muscle stem cells. *EMBO Molecular Medicine, 1,* 381–391. doi:10.1002/emmm.200900045

Filek, S., Leach-Macleod, K., Brims, M., Binsted, G., & Jakobi, J. (2010). *Changing the sheets. The slider sheet system—Phase two: Incorporating lessons learned from phase one; Final report: WorkSafeBC* (Innovation at Work Grant RS2008–IG12). Retrieved from http://www.wcb.ns.ca/app/DocRepository/5/Prevention/Education/McGovern_Slider_Sheet_Phase_2.pdf

Handoll, H. H., Queally, J. M., & Parker, M. J. (2011, December). Pre-operative traction for hip fractures in adults. *Cochrane Database of Systematic Reviews,* Issue 7. Art. No.: CD000168. Retrieved from http://www.ncbi.nlm.nih.gov/pubmed/22161361

Hoch, D. B., & Zieve, D. (2008). *Radial nerve dysfunction.* Retrieved from http://www.clarian.org/ADAM/doc/OrthopedicsCenter/1/000790.htm

Hockenberry, M., & Wilson, D. (2012). *Wong's nursing care of infants and children* (9th ed.). St. Louis, MO: Mosby/Elsevier.

Kunkler, C. E. (2007). Therapeutic modalities. In *Core curriculum for orthopaedic nursing* (6th ed., pp. 227–257). Boston, MA: Pearson Custom Publishing.

Kutash, M., Short, M., Shea, J., & Martinez, M. (2009). The lift team's importance to a successful safe patient handling program. *Journal of Nursing Administration, 39,* 170–175. doi:10.1097/NNA.0b013e31819c9cfd

Lethaby, A., Temple, J., & Santy, J. (2008). Pin site care for preventing infections associated with external bone fixators and pins. *Cochrane Database of Systemic Reviews,* Issue 4. Art. No.: CD004551. doi:10.1002/14651858.CD004551.pub2

National Institute for Occupational Safety and Health. (2013). *Workplace safety & health topics: Safe patient handling.* Retrieved from http://www.cdc.gov/niosh/topics/safepatient

Occupational Safety and Health Administration. (2011). *Safe patient handling programs: Effectiveness and cost savings.* Retrieved from https://www.osha.gov/dsg/hospitals/documents/3.5_SPH_effectiveness_508.pdf

Patterson, M., Mechan, P., Hughes, N., & Nelson, A. (2009). Safe vertical transfer of patient with extremity cast or splint. *Orthopaedic Nursing, 28*(2), S18–S23. doi:10.1097/NOR.0b013e318199d1bb

Waters, T. R. (2007). When is it safe to manually lift a patient? *American Journal of Nursing, 107*(8), 53.

Waters, T. R., Nelson, A., Hughes, N., & Menzel, N. (2009). *Safe patient handling training for schools of nursing curricular materials.* National Institute for Occupational Safety and Health. Retrieved from http://www.cdc.gov/niosh/docs/2009-127/pdfs/2009-127.pdf

CHAPTER 12

Centers for Disease Control and Prevention. (2011). *Botulism.* Retrieved from http://www.cdc.gov/nczved/divisions/dfbmd/diseases/botulism

de Aguilar-Nascimento, J., & Kudsk, K. (2007). Use of small-bore feeding tubes: Successes and failures. *Current Opinion in Clinical Nutrition & Metabolic Care, 10,* 291–296. doi:10.1097/MCO.0b013c3280d64a1d

DiMaria-Ghalili, R. A., & Guenter, P. A. (2008). How to try this: The Mini-Nutritional Assessment. *American Journal of Nursing, 108*(2), 50–59.

Durai, R., Venkatraman, R., & Ng, P. (2009). Nasogastric tubes. 1: Insertion technique and confirming the correct position. *Nursing Times, 105*(16), 12–13.

Gaskin, D. J., & Ilich, J. Z. (2009). Lactose maldigestion revisited: Diagnosis, prevalence in ethnic minorities, and dietary

recommendations to overcome it. *American Journal of Lifestyle Medicine, 3,* 212–218. doi:10.1177/1559827609331555

Grant, R., Biglin, A., Zeuschner, C., Guy, T., Pearce, R., Hodkin, B., & Ashton, L. (2008). The relative impact of a vegetable-rich diet on key markers of health in a cohort of Australian adolescents. *Asia Pacific Journal of Clinical Nutrition, 17*(1), 107–115.

Madsen, D., Sebolt, T., Cullen, L., Folkedahl, B., Mueller, T., Richardson, T., & Titler, M. (2005). Listening to bowel sounds: An evidence-based practice project. The *American Journal of Nursing, 105*(12), 40–49.

Ogden, C. L., Carroll, M. D., & Flegal, K. M. (2008). High body mass index for age among US children and adolescents, 2003–2006. *Journal of the American Medical Association, 299,* 2401–2405. doi:10.1001/jama.299.20.2401

Rauen, C. A., Chulay, M., Bridges, E., Vollman, K. M., & Arbour, R. (2008). Seven evidence-based practice habits: Putting some sacred cows out to pasture. *Critical Care Nurse, 28*(2), 98–123.

Rolfes, S. R., Pinna, K., & Whitney, E. (2009). *Understanding normal and clinical nutrition* (8th ed.). Belmont, CA: Wadsworth, Cengage Learning.

Stock, A., Gilbertson, H., & Babl, F. (2008). Confirming nasogastric tube position in the emergency department: pH testing is reliable. *Pediatric Emergency Care, 24,* 805–809. doi:10.1097/PEC.0b013e31818eb2d1

CHAPTER 13

Barnett, M. (2007). Prescribing oxygen therapy. *Nurse Prescribing, 5*(8), 345–351.

Benson, H. (1996). *Timeless healing: The power and biology of belief.* New York, NY: Scribner.

Berg, R. A., Hemphill, R., Abella, B. S., Aufderheide, T. P., Cave, D. M., Hazinski, M. F., . . . Swor, R. A. (2010). Part 5: Adult basic life support: 2010 American Heart Association guidelines for cardiopulmonary resuscitation and emergency cardiovascular care. *Circulation, 122*(Suppl. 3), S685–S705. doi:10.1161/CIRCULATIONAHA.110.970939

Bindler, R. C., Ball, J. W., London, M. L., & Ladewig, P. W. (2014). *Clinical skills manual for maternal & child nursing care* (4th ed.). Upper Saddle River, NJ: Prentice Hall Health.

Bridget, P. (2009). Pulse points. *Nursing 2009, 39*(2), 8.

Briggs, D. (2010). Nursing care and management of patients with intrapleural drains. *Nursing Standard, 24*(21), 47–56.

Centers for Disease Control and Prevention. (2012). *Ventilator-associated pneumonia*

(VAP). Retrieved from http://www.cdc.gov/hai/vap/vap.html

Feider, L., Mitchell, P., & Bridges, E. (2010). Oral care practices for orally intubated critically ill adults. *American Journal of Critical Care, 19,* 175–183. doi:10.4037/ajcc2010816

Halm, M. A. (2007). To strip or not to strip? Physiological effects of chest tube manipulation. *American Journal of Critical Care,* 16, 609–612.

Hazinski, M. F. (Ed.). (2010). *Highlights of the 2010 American Heart Association Guidelines for CPR and ECC.* Dallas, TX: American Heart Association.

Howlett, M., Alexander, G., & Tsuchiya, B. (2010). Health care providers' attitudes regarding family presence during resuscitation of adults: An integrated review of the literature. *Clinical Nurse Specialist, 24,* 161–174. doi:10.1097/NUR.0b013e3181dc548a

Hunter, J. (2008). Chest drain removal. *Nursing Standard, 22*(45), 35–38.

Ireton, J. (2007). Tracheostomy suction: A protocol for practice. *Paediatric Nursing, 19*(10), 14–18.

Jerath, R., & Barnes, V. A. (2009). Augmentation of mind–body therapy and role of deep slow breathing. *Journal of Complementary & Integrative Medicine, 6*(1), 1–7. doi:10.2202/1553-3840.1299

Joint Commission. (2011). *National patient safety goals.* Retrieved from http://www.jointcommission.org

Jones, C. U., Sangthong, B., & Pachirat, O. (2010). An inspiratory load enhances the antihypertensive effects of home-based training with slow deep breathing: A randomized trial. *Journal of Physiotherapy, 56,* 179–186.

Kleinman, M. E., de Caen, A. R., Chameides, L., Atkins, D. L., Berg, R. A., Berg, M. D., . . . Pediatric Basic and Advanced Life Support Chapter Collaborators. (2010). Part 10: Pediatric basic and advanced life support: 2010 international consensus on cardiopulmonary resuscitation and emergency cardiovascular care science with treatment recommendations. *Circulation, 122,* S466–S515. doi:10.1161/CIRCULATIONAHA.110.971093

Lemone, P., & Burke, K. (2012). *Medical-surgical nursing* (4th ed.). Upper Saddle River, NJ: Prentice Hall Health.

Mutchner, L. (2007). The ABCs of CPR—Again. A review of the latest changes to the American Heart Association's cardiopulmonary resuscitation and emergency cardiovascular care guidelines. *American Journal of Nursing, 107*(1), 60–69.

National Heart Lung and Blood Institute. (2007). *National asthma education and prevention program expert report 3: Guidelines* for the diagnosis and management of asthma (NIH Publication No. 08-5846). Washington, DC: U.S. Department of Health and Human Services. Retrieved from http://www.nhlbi.nih.gov/guidelines/asthma/asthgdln.pdf

Shalli, S., Saeed, D., Fukamachi, K., Gillinov, A. M., Coh, W. E., Perrault, L. P., & Boyle, E. (2009). Chest tube selection in cardiac and thoracic surgery: A survey of chest tube related complications and their management. *Journal of Cardiac Surgery, 24,* 503–509. doi:10.1111/J.1540–8191.2009.00905.X

SOS-KANTO Study Group. (2007). Cardiopulmonary resuscitation by bystanders with chest compression only (SOS-KANTO): An observational study. *The Lancet, 369*(9565), 920–926.

CHAPTER 14

Christakou, A., & Zakynthinos, S. (2014). The effectiveness of early mobilization in hospitalized patients with deep venous thrombosis. *Hospital Chronicles 2014, 9*(1), 11–16. Retrieved from http://www.hospitalchronicles.gr/index.php/hchr/article/view/553

Johns Hopkins Medical Letter: Health After 50. (2013a). Compression stockings: One size definitely does not fit all: Lower extremity review. Retrieved from http://lowerextremityreview.com/special-section/diabetic-foot-care/compression-stockings-one-size-definitely-does-not-fit-all

Johns Hopkins Medical Letter: Health After 50. (2013b). Pulmonary embolism/DVT. Retrieved from http://www.healthcommunities.com/pulmonary-embolism-dvt/compression-stockings.shtml

Pal, S. (2011). Compression stockings: One size definitely does not fit all. *Lower Extremity Review.* Retrieved from http://lowerextremityreview.com/special-section/diabetic-foot-care/compression-stockings-one-size-definitely-does-not-fit-all

Rauen, C. A, Chulay, M., Bridges, E., Vollman, K. M., & Arbour, R. (2008). Seven evidence-based practice habits: Putting some sacred cows out to pasture. *Critical Care Nurse, 28*(2), 98–123.

CHAPTER 15

American Academy of Orthopaedic Surgeons. (2014). *Joint Commission guidelines: Guidelines for implementation of the universal protocol for the prevention of wrong site, wrong procedure and wrong person surgery.* Retrieved from http://www3.aaos.org/member/safety/guidelines.cfm

Association of periOperative Nurses (AORN). (2007). Statement on the role of the scrub person. In *AORN standards, recommended practices, and nursing guidelines.* Denver, CO: Author.

Broex, E. C., van Asselt, A. D., Bruggeman, C. A., & van Tiel, F. H. (2009). Surgical site infections: How high are the costs? *Journal of Hospital Infection, 72*(3), 193–201. Retrieved from http://www.ncbi.nlm.nih.gov/pubmed/19482375

Centers for Disease Control and Prevention. (2011). *Guideline for prevention of surgical site infection, 1999.* Retrieved from http://www.cdc.gov/hicpac/SSI/004_SSI.html

Joint Commission. (2010). *Universal protocol for preventing wrong site, wrong procedure, wrong person surgery.* Retrieved from http://www.jcaho.org/accredited+organizations/patient+safety/universal+protocol/faq_uphtm.

Joint Commission. (2014). *Facts about the Universal Protocol.* Retrieved from http://www3.aaos.org/member/safety/guidelines.cfm

Knight, N., & Aucar, J. (2010). Use of an anatomic marking form as an alternative to the universal protocol for preventing wrong site, wrong procedure and wrong person surgery. *American Journal of Surgery, 200*(6), 803–809. Retrieved from http://www.americanjournalofsurgery.com/article/S0002-9610(10)00537-4/abstract

Neily, J., Mills, P. D., Eldridge, N., Dunn, E. J., Samples, C., Turner, J. R., . . . Bagian, J. P. (2009). Incorrect surgical procedures within and outside of the operating room. *Archives of Surgery, 144,* 1028–1034. Retrieved from http://www.psnet.ahrq.gov/resource.aspx?resourceID=17108

Reichman, D. E., & Greenberg, J. A. (2009). Reducing surgical site infections: A review. *Reviews in Obstetrics and Gynecology, 2*(4), 212–221. Retrieved from http://www.ncbi.nlm.nih.gov/pmc/articles/PMC2812878

Stahel, P. F., Sabel, A. L., Victoroff, M. S., Varnell, J., Lembitz, A., Boyle, D. J., . . . Mehler, P. S. (2010). Wrong-site and wrong-patient procedures in the universal protocol era: analysis of a prospective database of physician self-reported occurrences. *Archives of Surgery, 145*(10), 978–84. Retrieved from http://www.ncbi.nlm.nih.gov/pubmed/20956767

CHAPTER 16

American Congress of Obstetricians and Gynecologists. (2013). *Study finds adverse effects of Pitocin in newborns.* Retrieved from https://www.acog.org/About_ACOG/News_Room/News_Releases/2013/Study_Finds_Adverse_Effects_of_Pitocin_in_Newborns

Davidson, M., London, M., & Ladewig, P. (2012). *Olds' maternal-newborn nursing &* *women's health across the lifespan* (9th ed.). Upper Saddle River, NJ: Pearson/Prentice Hall.

Haws, R. A., Yakoob, M. Y., Soomro, T., Menezes, E. V., Darmstadt, G. L., & Bhutta, Z. A. (2009). Reducing stillbirths: Screening and monitoring during pregnancy and labour. *BMC Pregnancy Childbirth, 9*(Suppl. 1), S5. doi:10.1186/1471-2393-9-S1-S5

Lalor, J. G., Fawole, B., Alfirevic, Z., & Devane, D. (2008). Biophysical profile for fetal assessment in high risk pregnancies. *Cochrane Database of Systematic Reviews,* Issue 1. Art. No.: CD000038. Retrieved from http://www.ncbi.nlm.nih.gov/pubmed/18253968

Mayo Clinic. (2011, July 23). *Inducing labor: When to wait, when to induce. Considering inducing labor? Understand who makes a good candidate for inducing labor and why the intervention isn't for everyone.* Retrieved from http://www.mayoclinic.org/inducing-labor/art-20047557

Myles, M. F. (1975). *Textbook for midwives* (p. 246). Edinburgh, Scotland: Churchill-Livingstone.

O'Neill, E., & Thorp, J. (2012). Antepartum evaluation of the fetus and fetal well being. *Clinical Obstetrics and Gynecology, 55*(3), 722–730. Retrieved from http://www.ncbi.nlm.nih.gov/pmc/articles/PMC3684248

Siddique, A. (2013, May 7). *Pitocin may have adverse effects on newborn babies.* Retrieved from http://www.medicaldaily.com/pitocin-may-have-adverse-effects-newborn-babies-245641

U.S. Food and Drug Administration. (2013). *IDI-Strep B assay—K022504.* Retrieved from http://www.fda.gov/MedicalDevices/ProductsandMedicalProcedures/DeviceApprovalsandClearances/Recently-ApprovedDevices/ucm083015.htm

CHAPTER 17

Anstine, J. P. (2007). Understanding the new standards for patient restraint and seclusion. *American Nurse Today, 2*(6), 15–17.

CHAPTER 18

Agarwal, J. P., Ogilvie, M., Wu, L. C., Lohman, R. F., Gottlieb, L. J., Franczyk, M., & Song, D. H. (2005). Vacuum-assisted closure for sternal wounds: A first-line therapeutic management approach. *Plastic Reconstructive Surgery, 116*(4), 1035–1040.

Baron, S., & MacFarlane, G. (2009, May 20). *White paper: Reducing pressure ulcer risk in the operating room (D-770444-A1).* Acton, MA: Allen Medical Company. Retrieved from http://www.allenmedical.com/uploads/files/pdf/AllenWhitePaper_D770444-A1.pdf

Bee sting therapy treats illnesses from arthritis to cancer in China, but U.S. health experts call it "quackery." (2013, August 19). Retrieved from http://www.nydailynews.com/life-style/health/bee-sting-therapy-causing-buzz-china-article-1.1430797#ixzz2sNVfEQws

Fernandez, R., & Griffiths, R. (2008). Water for wound cleansing. *Cochrane Database of Systematic Reviews,* Issue 1. Art. No.: CD003861. doi:10.1002/14651858.CD003861.pub2

Joint Commission. (2013). *National patient safety goals effective January 1, 2014, hospital accreditation program.* Retrieved from http://www.jointcommission.org/standards_information/npsgs.aspx

Mayo Clinic. (2011). *Bedsores (pressure sores).* Retrieved from http://www.mayoclinic.org/diseases-conditions/bedsores/basics/causes/con-20030848

Medicinal leeches: Nature's finest surgical tool from the swamps. (2011, August 8). *Yale Journal of Medicine and Law.* Retrieved from http://www.yalemedlaw.com/2011/08/medicinal-leeches-natures-finest-surgical-tool-from-the-swamps

Minnesota Hospital Association. (2013). *Pressure ulcer prevention in the O.R.: Recommendations and guidance.* Retrieved from http://www.mnhospitals.org/Portals/0/Documents/ptsafety/skin/OR-pressure-ulcer-recommendations.pdf

Opletalová, K., Blaizot, X., Mourgeon, B., Chêne, Y., Creveuil, C., Combemale, P., . . . Dompmartin, A. (2012). Maggot therapy for wound debridement: A randomized multicenter trial. *Archives of Dermatology, 148*(4), 432–438. Retrieved from http://archderm.jamanetwork.com/article.aspx?articleid=1150957

Tschannen, D., Bates, O., Talsma, A., & Guo, Y. (2012). Patient-specific and surgical characteristics in the development of pressure ulcers. *American Journal of Critical Care, 21*(2), 116–124. Retrieved from http://www.aacn.org/wd/Cetests/media/A1221021.pdf

Wake, W. T. (2010). Pressure ulcers: What clinicians need to know. *Permanente Journal, 14*(2), 56–60. Retrieved from http://www.ncbi.nlm.nih.gov/pmc/articles/PMC2912087

WebMD. (2014). *Pressure sores—Topic overview.* Retrieved from http://www.webmd.com/skin-problems-and-treatments/tc/pressure-sores-topic-overview

Woo, K. Y., Sibbald, R. G., Ayello, E., Coutts, P. M., & Garde, D. (2009). Peristomal skin complications and management. *Advances in Skin & Wound Care, 22,* 522–532. doi:10.1097/01.ASW.0000305497.15768.cb

CREDITS

Note: Listings are by page number and source in consecutive order.

5, Audrey Berman & Shirlee J. Snyder, SKILLS IN CLINICAL NURSING, 7e, © 2012. Printed and Electronically reproduced by permission of Pearson Education, Inc., Upper Saddle River, New Jersey; 8, Daniel Dempster/Alamy; 9 (left), 377, 439 (bottom), 440 (top left), 447, 448, 449, 548, George Dodson/Pearson Education, Inc.; 11 (right), 12 (bottom left), 12 (top right), 16, 17 (bottom), 18, 19 (bottom right), 22 (bottom right), 23, 67, 76, 89 (bottom), 194, 195, 300 (right), 355 (top left), 360, 363, 364 (middle), 365, 366, 370, 372 (bottom right), 372 (top right), 373, 383, 422, 428 (bottom left), 430, 432, 442, 444, 445 (left), 454 (right), 459 (right), 473, 474 (top), 480 (left), 495, 496, 560, 571 (bottom left), 571 (top right), 577 (top left), 579, 583 (left), Rick Brady/Pearson Education, Inc.; 12 (bottom right), Courtesy of Illinois State Library digital archives; 25 (bottom), St-fotograf/Fotolia; 26, Thinkstock/Getty Images; 27, Andy Crawford/Dorling Kindersley Ltd.; 30 (A), Michael P. Gadomski/Science Source; 30 (B), Hercules Robinson/Alamy; 30 (C), Olavs silis/Alamy; 30 (D), DermPics/Science Source; 30 (E), Harout Tanielian/Science Source; 30 (F), Scott Camazine/Science Source; 30 (G), Mediscan/Medical-on-Line/Alamy; 30 (H), Ted Kinsman/Science Source; 37, 41 (top), 42, 43, 44, 48 (top), 52 (top), 53, 56, 73 (bottom), 73 (top left), 329, 345 (top right), 346 (bottom right), 346 (middle left), 347 (top left), 348, 349 (bottom right), 349 (middle left), 350 (top left), 350 (top right), 353 (middle right), 526, Pat Watson/Pearson Education, Inc.; 40, 47, 48 (bottom), 58, 61, 62, 64 (top), 77 (top), 78 (bottom), 79, Richard Tauber/Pearson Education, Inc.; 50, courtesy of the National Society to Prevent Blindness; 52 (bottom), CNRI/Science Source; 73 (top right), Southern Illinois University/Science Source; 77 (bottom), 78 (top), Ollyy/Shutterstock; 89 (top), Fotolia XXII/Fotolia; 125 (top), Milena Boniek/PhotoAlto/Alamy; 127, 399 (left), 405 (bottom), 412, Patrick Watson/Pearson Education, Inc.; 149 (bottom left), 149 (bottom right), SPL/Custom Medical Stock Photo; 161, 421 (right), Science Photo Library/Alamy; 168, Pain Management Flow Sheet from Sunrise Hospital and Medical Center and Sunrise Children's Hospital. Published by Sunrise Hospital and Medical Center and Sunrise Children's Hospital; 169, The FACES Rating Scale from The Wong-Baker FACES™ Foundation. Used by permission of by The Wong-Baker FACES™ Foundation; 219, James E. Knopf/Shutterstock; 221 (right), 273 (top right), 274, 275, 281, 427, 428 (top), 431 (left), 435 (left), 435 (bottom right), 436 (left), 439 (top), 454 (left), 455 (top left), 458 (bottom), 497, 578 (bottom right), George Draper/Pearson Education, Inc.; 248 (left), Pavel Marjanovic/Shutterstock; 273, Slaven MD/Custom Medical Stock Publishers; 277, Villareal/Science Source; 279, David L. Moore—Healthcare/Alamy; 328 (bottom), Karen M. Burke, Elaine L. Mohn-Brown, Linda Eby, MEDICAL-SURGICAL NURSING CARE, 3e © 2012. Printed and Electronically reproduced by permission of Pearson Education, Inc., Upper Saddle River, New Jersey; 332, Audrey Berman, Shirlee J. Snyder, SKILLS IN CLINICAL NURSING, 7e © 2012. Printed and Electronically reproduced by permission of Pearson Education, Inc., Upper Saddle River, New Jersey; 333, Audrey Berman; Shirlee J. Snyder, SKILLS IN CLINICAL NURSING, 7e © 2012. Printed and Electronically reproduced by permission of Pearson Education, Inc., Upper Saddle River, New Jersey; 335 (left bottom), 335 (right), John Thys/Reporters/Science Source; 335 (left top), Life in View/Science Source; 336, Sandra F. Smith, Donna J. Duell, Barbara C. Martin, CLINICAL NURSING SKILLS: BASIC TO ADVANCED SKILLS, EIGHTH EDITION © 2012, 2008 and 2004. Printed and Electronically reproduced by permission of Pearson Education, Inc., Upper Saddle River, New Jersey; 364 (bottom), B. Slavin/Custom Medical Stock Photo; 396 (left), Monkey Business Images/Shutterstock; 400 (right), Bodenham, LTH NHS Trust/Science Source; 421 (left), MediaforMedical/Emmanuel Rogue/Alamy; 428 (middle), 428 (right), Shirlee Snyder; 429 (bottom right), 72/Fotolia; 429, Rick Brady/Pearson Education, Inc.; 431 (bottom), B. Kramer/Custom Medical Stock Photo; 433, ZUMA Press/Alamy; 445 (right), 3660 Group/Custom Medical Stock Photo; 455 (bottom), 457, Roman Milert/Alamy; 455 (top right), Ian Miles-Flashpoint Pictures/Alamy; 456 (left), Burger/Phanie/Science Source; 456 (right), Martin/Custom Medical Stock Photo; 458 (left), Dr. P. Marazzi/Science Source; 458 (top right), wunkley/Alamy; 459 (left), Audrey Berman; 460, Lee F. Snyder/Science Source; 462, Daviles/Fotolia; 463 (top), Roman Milert/123RF; 463 (bottom), Jules Selmes/Getty Images; 498, BSIP SA/Alamy; 526, 527, Alexander Raths/Fotolia; 538, Roy Ramsey/Pearson Education, Inc.; 543 (bottom), 544, 545, Courtesy of Brigitte Hall; 546, Tom McCarthy/Photoedit; 547, George Dodson/Pearson Education, Inc.; 549, Smith-Pedersen, Lisa; 570, Samuel Ashfield/Science Source; 583 (right), Rick Brady/Pearson Owned; 589, BSIP/Photoshot; 595, Eden Prairie/Pearson Education, Inc.

INDEX

Tympanogram, 55*f*
Tympanometry, 55, 55*f*

PEARSON SOURCES

The following authors from Pearson generously allowed us to repurpose their work for this project:

- Audrey Berman, Shirlee J. Snyder, *Skills in Clinical Nursing*, Seventh Edition
- Audrey Berman, Shirlee J. Snyder, Barbara Kozier, and Glenora Erb, *Kozier & Erb's Fundamentals of Nursing: Concepts, Process, and Practice*, Ninth Edition

- Ruth C. McGillis Bindler, Jane W. Ball, Marcia L. London, Michele R. Davidson, *Clinical Skills Manual for Maternal & Child Nursing Care*, Fourth Edition
- Karen M. Burke, Elaine L. Mohn-Brown, Linda Eby, *Medical-Surgical Nursing Care*, Third Edition
- Sandra F. Smith, Donna J. Duell, Barbara C. Martin, *Clinical Nursing Skills: Basic to Advanced Skills*, Eighth Edition

Skills List by Key Word

Skills List by Key Word

(continued on next page)

translations of the work of al-Khwārizmī and other Islamic authors. There was also some awareness that much of plane and spherical trigonometry could be attributed to Islamic authors. Thus, although the first pure trigonometrical work in Europe, *On Triangles* by Regiomontanus, written around 1463, did not cite Islamic sources, Gerolamo Cardano noted a century later that much of the material there on spherical trigonometry was taken from the twelfth-century work of the Spanish Islamic scholar Jābir ibn Aflaḥ.

By the seventeenth century, European mathematics had in many areas reached, and in some areas surpassed, the level of its Greek and Arabic sources. Nevertheless, given the continuous contact of Europe with Islamic countries, a steady stream of Arabic manuscripts, including mathematical ones, began to arrive in Europe. Leading universities appointed professors of Arabic, and among the sources they read were mathematical works. For example, the work of Ṣadr al-Ṭūsī (the son of Naṣīr al-Dīn al-Ṭūsī) on the parallel postulate, written originally in 1298, was published in Rome in 1594 with a Latin title page. This work was studied by John Wallis in England, who then wrote about its ideas as he developed his own thoughts on the postulate. Still later, Newton's friend, Edmond Halley, translated into Latin Apollonius's *Cutting-off of a Ratio*, a work that had been lost in Greek but had been preserved via an Arabic translation.

Yet in the seventeenth and eighteenth centuries, when Islamic contributions to mathematics may well have helped Europeans develop their own mathematics, most Arabic manuscripts lay unread in libraries around the world. It was not until the mid-nineteenth century that European scholars began an extensive program of translating these mathematical manuscripts. Among those who produced a large number of translations, the names of Heinrich Suter in Switzerland and Franz Woepcke in France stand out. (Their works have recently been collected and republished by the Institut für Geschichte der arabisch-islamischen Wissenschaften.) In the twentieth century, Soviet historians of mathematics began a major program of translations from the Arabic as well. Until the middle of the twentieth century, however, no one in the West had pulled together these translations to try to give a fuller picture of Islamic mathematics. Probably the first serious history of Islamic mathematics was a section of the general history of medieval mathematics written in 1961 by A. P. Yushkevich, already mentioned earlier. This section was translated into French in 1976 and published as a separate work, *Les mathématiques arabes* (*VIIIᵉ–XVᵉ siècles*). Meanwhile, the translation program continues, and many new works are translated each year from the Arabic, mostly into English or French.

By the end of the twentieth century, all of these scholarly studies and translations of the mathematics of these various civilizations had an impact on the general history of mathematics. Virtually all recent general history textbooks contain significant sections on the mathematics of these five civilizations. As this sourcebook demonstrates, there are many ideas that were developed in these five civilizations that later reappeared elsewhere. The question that then arises is how much effect the mathematics of these civilizations had on what is now world mathematics of the twenty first-century. The answer to this question is very much under debate. We know of many confirmed instances of transmission of mathematical ideas from one of these cultures to Europe or from one of these cultures to another, but there are numerous instances where, although there is circumstantial evidence of transmission, there is no definitive documentary evidence. Whether such will be found as more translations are made and more documents are uncovered in libraries and other institutions around the world is a question for the future to answer.

Skills List by Key Word

(continued on inside back cover)